Emergency Management of Infectious Diseases

Second Edition

Emergency Management of Infectious Diseases

Second Edition

Edited by

Rachel L. Chin
Professor of Emergency Medicine
Department of Emergency Medicine
University of California, San Francisco School of Medicine
Zuckerberg San Francisco General Hospital and Trauma Center
San Francisco, CA

Bradley W. Frazee
Department of Emergency Medicine
Alameda Health System – Highland Hospital
Oakland, CA
Clinical Professor of Emergency Medicine
University of California, San Francisco School of Medicine
San Francisco, CA

Associate Editor
Zlatan Coralic
Assistant Clinical Professor of Emergency Medicine
Emergency Medicine Clinical Pharmacist
University of California, San Francisco
San Francisco, CA

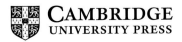

CAMBRIDGE
UNIVERSITY PRESS

CAMBRIDGE
UNIVERSITY PRESS

University Printing House, Cambridge CB2 8BS, United Kingdom

One Liberty Plaza, 20th Floor, New York, NY 10006, USA

477 Williamstown Road, Port Melbourne, VIC 3207, Australia

314–321, 3rd Floor, Plot 3, Splendor Forum, Jasola District Centre, New Delhi – 110025, India

79 Anson Road, #06-04/06, Singapore 079906

Cambridge University Press is part of the University of Cambridge.

It furthers the University's mission by disseminating knowledge in the pursuit of education, learning and research at the highest international levels of excellence.

www.cambridge.org
Information on this title: www.cambridge.org/9781107153158
DOI: 10.1017/9781316597095

© Cambridge University Press (2008) 2018

First published: 2008
Second edition: 2018

Printed and bound in Great Britain by Clays Ltd, Elcograf S.p.A.

A catalogue record for this publication is available from the British Library

ISBN 978-1-107-15315-8 Hardback

....

Contents

Preface

The diagnosis and treatment of infectious disease represents a large and very important part of emergency medicine practice. Challenges faced by acute care practitioners on a daily basis range from the definitive treatment and discharge of a patient with a simple abscess, to recognition of a rare infection in a traveler, to resuscitation and stabilization of a patient with septic shock.

In this second edition of *Emergency Management of Infectious Diseases*, we have endeavored to produce a practical, clinically oriented, systems-based overview of the most important infectious diseases encountered in emergency practice. Our textbook covers the gamut of common viral, bacterial, fungal, and parasitic infections. For each disease, we briefly discuss microbiology, pathophysiology, and epidemiology, but the emphasis is on emergent diagnosis and treatment. The narrative is supplemented with photographs and tables highlighting key diagnostic findings and current antimicrobial recommendations, including dosing.

Acute care practitioners also act as sentinels for outbreaks of communicable and emerging infections, and are likely to be the first to encounter victims of biological weapons. In this edition, we include chapters on recent emerging infections such as Ebola and Zika, as well as rare but deadly infectious agents that can be weaponized, such as anthrax and smallpox.

We hope that our textbook can be of use to every type of practitioner that cares for patients with infectious diseases, including emergency physicians, primary care physicians and specialists, nurse practitioners, physician assistants, residents, and medical students.

We thank the many nationally and internationally respected clinicians, educators, and researchers who contributed, and hope that this second edition of *Emergency Management of Infectious Diseases* will prove an invaluable reference for practitioners confronting the spectrum of infectious disease.

Bradley W. Frazee, MD
Rachel L. Chin, MD
Zlatan Coralic

Contributors

Nicole Abolins, PharmD, BCPS
Medical Outcomes Specialist, Director
Pfizer, Inc.
Greensboro, NC

Fredrick M. Abrahamian, DO, FACEP, FIDSA
Health Sciences Clinical Professor of Emergency Medicine
David Geffen School of Medicine at UCLA
Los Angeles, CA

Nisa S. Atigapramoj, MD
Assistant Clinical Professor
Department of Emergency Medicine and Pediatrics
UCSF Benioff Children's Hospital
Zuckerberg San Francisco General Hospital and
Trauma Center
University of California, San Francisco School of Medicine
San Francisco, CA

Camille Beauduy, PharmD
Infectious Diseases Clinical Pharmacist
Department of Pharmacy Services
Zuckerberg San Francisco General Hospital
San Francisco, CA

Greg Bever, MD
Department of Ophthalmology
University of California, San Francisco School of
Medicine
San Francisco, CA

Nisha Bhatia, MD
Neurology Attending Physician
The Permanente Medical Group
Vallejo, CA
Steven Bin, MD
Associate Clinical Professor
Departments of Emergency Medicine and Pediatrics
UCSF Benioff Children's Hospital
Zuckerberg San Francisco General Hospital and
Trauma Center
University of California, San Francisco School of Medicine
San Francisco, CA

William D. Binder, MD
Associate Professor of Emergency Medicine
Alpert School of Medicine, Brown University
Providence, RI

Robert Blount, MD
Pulmonary and Critical Care Medicine
University of Iowa
Iowa City, IA

Katherine C. Bonsell, DO
Neurological Care
Evergreen Health Neuroscience Institute
Kirkland, WA

Justin Bosley, MD, CAQSM
Emergency Medicine Attending Physician
The Permanente Medical Group
Oakland, CA

Robert Brown, MD
Department of Emergency Medicine
University of Maryland School of Medicine
Baltimore, MD

Amy Bryant, MD, MSCR
Assistant Professor of Obstetrics and Gynecology
Department of Obstetrics and Gynecology
University of North Carolina at Chapel Hill
Chapel Hill, NC

Jeffrey Bullard-Berent, MD, FAAP, FACEP
Professor Emergency Medicine and Pediatrics
Vice Chair Emergency Medicine
Medical Director, Child Ready
Virtual Pediatric Emergency Department
University of New Mexico School of Medicine
Albuquerque, NM

Cordelia W. Carter, MD
Assistant Professor of Orthopaedic Surgery
Yale Department of Orthopaedics and Rehabilitation
Yale University School of Medicine
New Haven, CT

Adithya Cattamanchi, MD
Associate Professor of Medicine
Zuckerberg San Francisco General Hospital and
Trauma Center
University of California, San Francisco School of Medicine
San Francisco, CA

Rachel L. Chin, MD
Professor of Emergency Medicine
Department of Emergency Medicine
University of California, San Francisco School of Medicine
Zuckerberg San Francisco General Hospital and Trauma Center
San Francisco, CA

Deborah Cohan, MD, MPH
Professor of Obstetrics, Gynecology, and
Reproductive Sciences
University of California, San Francisco School of Medicine
Medical Director, HIVE
Zuckerberg San Francisco General Hospital and Trauma Center
San Francisco, CA

Zlatan Coralic, PharmD
Assistant Clinical Professor of Emergency Medicine
Emergency Medicine Clinical Pharmacist
University of California, San Francisco
San Francisco, CA

Bryan Darger, MD
Emergency Medicine Physician
Department of Emergency Medicine
University of California, San Francisco School of Medicine
Zuckerberg San Francisco General Hospital and Trauma
Center
San Francisco, CA

Michael S. Diamond, MD, PhD
The Herbert S. Gasser Professor
Departments of Medicine, Molecular Microbiology,
Pathology, and Immunology
Associate Director, The Andrew M. and Jane M. Bursky
Center for Human Immunology and Immunotherapy
Programs
Washington University School of Medicine
St. Louis, MO

Edwin Dietrich, MD
Emergency Medicine Attending Physician
The Permanente Medical Group
Oakland, CA

Erik R. Dubberke, MD
Assistant Professor of Medicine
Clinical Director, Transplant Infectious Diseases
Washington University School of Medicine
St. Louis, MO

Christopher J. Edwards, PharmD, BCPS
Clinical Associate Professor – Department of Pharmacy
Practice
University of Arizona College of Pharmacy
Marana, AZ

Joseph Engelman, MD, MPH
Clinical Professor of Medicine
San Francisco Department of Public Health Physician
Specialist
University of California, San Francisco School of Medicine
San Francisco, CA

Christopher Fee, MD
Professor of Clinical Emergency Medicine
Associate Chair for Education
Emergency Medicine Residency Program Director
University of California, San Francisco School of Medicine
San Francisco, CA

Jorge Fernandez, MD
Assistant Clinical Professor of Emergency Medicine
Associate Residency Program Director
University of California, San Diego School of Medicine
San Diego, CA

Alexander C. Flint, MD, PhD
Department of Neuroscience
Division of Research
The Permanente Medical Group
Redwood City, CA

Bradley W. Frazee, MD
Department of Emergency Medicine
Alameda Health System – Highland Hospital
Oakland, CA
Clinical Professor of Emergency Medicine
University of California, San Francisco School of Medicine
San Francisco, CA

Gus M. Garmel, MD
Clinical Professor (Affiliate) of Emergency Medicine
Stanford University School of Medicine
Stanford, CA
Senior Staff Emergency Physician, The Permanente
Medical Group
Santa Clara, CA
Senior Editor, The Permanente Journal
Portland, OR

Elisabeth Giblin, MD
Attending Physician
Department of Emergency Medicine
Northwest Community Hospital
Arlington Heights, IL

Robert Goodnough, MD
Emergency Medicine Physician
Department of Emergency Medicine
University of California, San Francisco School of Medicine
Zuckerberg San Francisco General Hospital and Trauma
Center
San Francisco, CA

Christopher Hahn, MD
Assistant Professor of Emergency Medicine
Icahn School of Medicine at Mount Sinai
Assistant Program Director
Department of Emergency Medicine
Mount Sinai St. Lukes-Roosevelt
New York, NY

Charles Hartis, PharmD, BCPS
Clinical Pharmacy Specialist
Forsyth Medical Center
Davie Medical Center – Wake Forest Baptist Health
Advance, NC

Laurence Huang, MD, FCCP, ATSF
Professor of Medicine
Chief, HIV/AIDS Chest Clinic
Positive Health Program at San Francisco General
Zuckerberg San Francisco General Hospital and
Trauma Center
University of California, San Francisco School of Medicine
San Francisco, CA

Paul Ishimine, MD
Clinical Professor of Emergency Medicine and Pediatrics
Program Director, Pediatric Emergency Medicine Fellowship
Division of Pediatric Emergency Medicine
Rady Children's Hospital, San Diego
Department of Emergency Medicine
University of California, San Diego School of Medicine
San Diego, CA

Asim A. Jani, MD, MPH, FACP
Hospital Epidemiologist
Orlando Health
Orlando, FL

Cheryl A. Jay, MD
Clinical Professor of Neurology
University of California, San Francisco School of Medicine
Zuckerberg San Francisco General Hospital and Trauma
Center
San Francisco, CA

Tamara John, MD
Yale Department of Orthopaedics and Rehabilitation
Yale University School of Medicine
New Haven, CT

Jaime Jordan, MD
Assistant Clinical Professor of Emergency Medicine
Vice Chair, Acute Care College
David Geffen School of Medicine at UCLA
Associate Director, Residency Training Program
Department of Emergency Medicine
Harbor-UCLA Medical Center
Torrance, CA

Shruti Kant, MD
Associate Clinical Professor
Departments of Emergency Medicine and Pediatrics
UCSF Benioff Children's Hospital
Zuckerberg San Francisco General Hospital and
Trauma Center
University of California, San Francisco School of Medicine
San Francisco, CA

Janel Kittredge-Sterling, DO
St. Vincent Mercy Medical Center
Perrysburg, OH

Michael A. Kohn, MD, MPP
Professor of Epidemiology and Biostatistics
University of California, San Francisco School of Medicine
San Francisco, CA
Attending Emergency Physician
Mills-Peninsula Medical Center
Burlingame, CA

Aaron Kornblith, MD
Assistant Clinical Professor
Departments of Emergency Medicine and Pediatrics
UCSF Benioff Children's Hospital
Zuckerberg San Francisco General Hospital and
Trauma Center
University of California, San Francisco School of Medicine
San Francisco, CA

Anita A. Koshy, MD
Associate Professor of Neurology
Department of Neurology, Department of Immunobiology,
BIO5 Institute
University of Arizona, College of Medicine
Tucson, AZ

Leah T. Le, MPH
Research Coordinator
Department of Neurology
Yale University School of Medicine
New Haven, CT

Suzanne Lippert, MD, MS
Emergency Medicine Attending Physician
The Permanente Medical Group
Oakland, CA

Jill Logan, PharmD, BCPS
Emergency Medicine Clinical Pharmacist
Silver Spring, MD

Conan MacDougall, PharmD, MAS, BCPS-AQ ID
Professor of Clinical Pharmacy
University of California, San Francisco School of Pharmacy
San Francisco, CA

Debbie Yi Madhok, MD
Assistant Clinical Professor
Department of Emergency Medicine
Director, Emergency Stroke Program
Zuckerberg San Francisco General Hospital and
Trauma Center
University of California, San Francisco School of Medicine
San Francisco, CA

William Mallon, MD, DTMH, FACEP, FAAEM
Professor of Clinical Emergency Medicine
Director: Division of International Emergency Medicine
Department of Emergency Medicine
Stony Brook University (SUNY)
Stony Brook, NY

Catherine A. Marco, MD
Professor of Emergency Medicine
Wright State University Boonshoft School of Medicine
Dayton, OH

Maureen McCollough, MD, MPH, FACEP, FAAEM
Assistant Professor of Emergency Medicine and
Pediatrics
Director, Pediatric Emergency Department
Department of Pediatrics
Medical Director, Department of Emergency Medicine
Los Angeles County+USC Medical Center
Keck School of Medicine
University of Southern California
Los Angeles, CA

Mary P. Mercer, MD, MPH, FAEMS
Associate Clinical Professor
Department of Emergency Medicine
University of California, San Francisco
Associate Director, EMS/Disaster Medicine Fellowship
Zuckerberg San Francisco General Hospital and Trauma Center
San Francisco, CA

Roland C. Merchant, MD, MPH
Associate Professor
Emergency Medicine and Epidemiology
Rhode Island Hospital
Alpert Medical School
Brown University
Providence, RI

Siamak Moayedi, MD
Assistant Professor
Department of Emergency Medicine
University of Maryland School of Medicine
Baltimore, MD

Kareem Moussa, MD
Department of Ophthalmology
University of California, San Francisco School of
Medicine
San Francisco, CA

Megan Musselman, PharmD, MS, BCPS, BCCCP
Emergency Medicine Clinical Pharmacy Specialist
PGY1 Pharmacy Residency Coordinator
North Kansas City Hospital
North Kansas City, MO

Payam Nahid, MD
Professor of Medicine
University of California, San Francisco School of
Medicine
Zuckerberg San Francisco General Hospital and
Trauma Center
San Francisco, CA

Rachel Najafi, MD
Hospitalist, Medical Service
Veteran's Hospital, Palo Alto
Clinical Instructor (Affiliated)
Stanford University School of Medicine
Palo Alto, CA

Allison Nazinitsky, MD
Infectious Disease Physician
Oklahoma City VA Health Care System
Oklahoma City, OK

Anh T. Nguyen, MD, MS
Department of Neurosurgery
Houston Methodist Neurocritical Care
Houston, TX

Tu Carol Nguyen, MD
Clinical Instructor
Department of Emergency Medicine
University of Maryland School of Medicine
Baltimore, MD

Jessica L. Osterman, MD
Assistant Professor of Clinical Emergency Medicine
Assistant Program Director
Los Angeles County+USC Medical Center
Keck School of Medicine
University of Southern California
Los Angeles, CA

Michelle Y. Peng, MD
Department of Ophthalmology
University of California, San Francisco School of Medicine
San Francisco, CA

Nicholas Pokrajac, MD
Attending Physician
Department of Emergency Medicine
University of California San Diego Health System
San Diego, CA

Kavita Radhakrishnan, MD
Department of Medicine, Division of Gastroenterology
University of California, San Francisco School of
Medicine
San Francisco, CA

Lisa Rahangdale, MD
Associate Professor of Obstetrics and Gynecology
Department of Obstetrics and Gynecology
University of North Carolina School of Medicine
Chapel Hill, NC

Saras Ramanathan, MD
Associate Professor of Ophthalmology
Department of Ophthalmology
University of California, San Francisco School of
Medicine
San Francisco, CA

Michael J. A. Reid, MD, MA, MPH
Assistant Professor of Medicine
Division of HIV, Infectious Diseases, and Global
Medicine
Zuckerberg San Francisco General Hospital
University of California, San Francisco
San Francisco, CA

Ashley Rider, MD
Emergency Medicine Physician
Department of Emergency Medicine
Alameda Health System – Highland Hospital
Oakland, CA

Jada L. Roe, MD
Emergency Medicine Physician
Department of Emergency Medicine
David Geffen School of Medicine at UCLA
Los Angeles, CA

R. James Salway, MD
Clinical Assistant Professor of Emergency Medicine
Department of Emergency Medicine
SUNY Downstate Medical Center / Kings County Hospital
Center
Brooklyn, NY

Kimberly A. Schertzer, MD, FACEP
Associate Director of Simulation
Simulation Fellowship Director
Department of Emergency Medicine
Stanford University School of Medicine
Stanford, CA

Jonathan Schimmel, MD
Attending Physician
Department of Emergency Medicine
University of Colorado School of Medicine
Aurora, CO

Daniel Schnorr, MD
Attending Physician
Department of Emergency Medicine
Harbor-UCLA Medical Center
Torrance, CA

Dominika Seidman, MD, MAS
Assistant Professor of Obstetrics, Gynecology and
Reproductive Sciences
Department of Obstetrics, Gynecology and
Reproductive Sciences
University of California, San Francisco School of Medicine
Zuckerberg San Francisco General Hospital and
Trauma Center
San Francisco, CA

Ghazala Sharieff, MD, MBA
Clinical Professor
University of California, San Diego School of Medicine
Corporate Vice President, Chief Experience Officer,
Scripps Health
San Diego, CA

Melinda Sharkey, MD
Associate Professor of Orthopaedic Surgery
Yale Department of Orthopaedics and Rehabilitation
Yale University School of Medicine
New Haven, CT

Scott C. Sherman, MD
Associate Professor of Emergency Medicine
Department of Emergency Medicine
Cook County (Stroger) Hospital
Rush Medical College
Chicago, IL

Jan M. Shoenberger, MD
Associate Professor of Clinical Emergency Medicine
Residency Program Director
Los Angeles County+USC Medical Center
Keck School of Medicine
University of Southern California
Los Angeles, CA

Colgan Sloan, PharmD, BCPS
Clinical Pharmacy Specialist - Emergency Medicine
Department of Pharmacy Services
University of Utah Health
Salt Lake City, UT

Eric Snoey, MD
Vice Chair
Department of Emergency Medicine
Alameda Health System – Highland Hospital
Oakland, California
Clinical Professor of Emergency Medicine
University of California, San Francisco School of Medicine
San Francisco, CA

Aparajita Sohoni, MD
Attending Emergency Physician
California Pacific Medical Center
San Francisco, CA

Serena S. Spudich, MD
Professor of Neurology
Division Chief, Neurological Infections and Global Neurology
Department of Neurology
Yale University School of Medicine
New Haven, CT

David M. Stier, MD
Director, Communicable Disease Prevention Unit
Medical Director, AITC Immunization and Travel Clinic
Medical Epidemiologist, Communicable Disease Control Unit
Population Health Division, San Francisco Department of Public Health
San Francisco, CA

Elena Strunk, MD
Research Instructor
Department of Emergency Medicine
George Washington University Hospital
Washington, DC

Sukhjit S. Takhar, MD
Attending Physician
Mills-Peninsula Emergency Medical Associates
Burlingame, CA

Michele M. Tana, MD, MHS
Assistant Professor of Medicine
Department of Medicine, Division of Gastroenterology
University of California, San Francisco School of Medicine
Zuckerberg San Francisco General Hospital and Trauma Center
San Francisco, CA

David Thompson, MD
Clinical Associate Professor of Emergency Medicine
Department of Emergency Medicine
University of California, San Francisco School of Medicine
Zuckerberg San Francisco General Hospital and Trauma Center
San Francisco, CA

Phyllis C. Tien, MD, MPH
Professor of Medicine
University of California, San Francisco School of Medicine
UCSF Positive Health Program
Zuckerberg San Francisco General Hospital and Trauma Center
San Francisco, CA

Mercedes Torres, MD
Clinical Assistant Professor
Department of Emergency Medicine
University of Maryland School of Medicine
Baltimore, MD

Tracy Trang, PharmD, BCPS
Emergency Medicine and Infectious Disease Pharmacist
Downey, CA

Timothy M. Uyeki, MD, MPH, MPP
Chief Medical Officer, Influenza Division
Centers for Disease Control and Prevention,
Atlanta, GA
Clinical Associate Professor
Department of Pediatrics
University of California, San Francisco School of Medicine
San Francisco, CA

Hugh West, MD, FACEP, FAAEM
Associate Clinical Professor of Emergency Medicine
University of California, San Francisco School of Medicine
San Francisco, CA

Chapter 1

Infective Endocarditis

Jorge Fernandez and Jessica L. Osterman

Introduction

Infectious endocarditis (IE) is a difficult diagnosis to make in the emergency setting. Early diagnosis and management requires an understanding of endocarditis risk factors, typical and atypical clinical presentations, and current diagnostic and empiric treatment strategies.

Epidemiology and Microbiology

In developed countries, the incidence of IE is roughly 5 cases per 100,000 persons per year. It more commonly affects males (2:1). Well-recognized risk factors for IE include presence of a prosthetic heart valve (which carry an annual incidence of approximately 1%), congenital heart disease, endocardiac devices, injection drug use (see Chapter 61), and a prior history of endocarditis. Rheumatic heart disease is now an uncommon predisposing risk factor in the United States. However, in modern series, there is no easily identifiable risk factor for underlying valve damage in approximately 50% of endocarditis cases. Such cases are believed to be due to age-related degenerative valve disease and subtle immunosuppresion from diabetic endocarditis and other factors. Health-care associated cases, often in the elderly, account for a growing proportion of endocarditis in the United States.

Infective endocarditis occurs when circulating pathogens adhere to damaged endothelium and form a vegetation, usually on or around a cardiac valve. Abnormal turbulent flow and damaged endothelium lead to fibrin and platelete deposition which presents a nidus for bacterial infection during bacteremia. In the setting of frequent bacteremia, such as intravenous drug use and dental infection, IE may occur even without an identifiable pathologic valvular lesion. Growth of the infected vegetation eventually leads to valve destruction and impaired function, typically regurgitation, and eventually heart failure. Invasion of the myocardium can lead to paravalvular abscess and heart block. Large, mobile vegetations are associated with embolization and metastatic infection (see below).

The list of pathogens that have been reported to cause IE is enormous and includes fungi and protozoa. The most common etiolgies, however, are gram-positive cocci, including *Staphylococcus* species, both *S. aureus* and coagulase negative *Staphylococcus*, and Streptococcal species, particularly viridans Streptococci and group D *Streptococcus*. *S. aureus* is both the most common etiology and the pathogen most often associated with metastatic complications. *Enterococcus* is common in the elderly. The clinical setting may suggest the pathogen involved: *S. aureus* is the most common in injection drug users, viridans Streptococci in patients with recent dental procedures, and gram-negative bacilli in patients that have undergone invasive genitourinary procedures.

Pathogens that are less commonly implicated in IE include the "HACEK" (*Haemophilus aphrophilus*, *Haemophilus paraphrophilus*, *Haemophilus parainfluenzae*, *Actinobacillus actinomycetemcomitans*, *Cardiobacterium hominis*, *Eikenella corrodens*, *and Kingella kingae*) group of fastidious bacteria, *Bartonella*, chlamydia, *Legionella*, and fungi. Infections with these organisms may be difficult to detect because they do not always grow in routine blood cultures.

Clinical Features

The presentation of IE (see Table 1.1 and Figure 1.1) ranges from the well-appearing patient with non-specific symptoms to the toxic patient in severe septic shock with multi-organ failure. Symptoms are often frustratingly non-specific, and may include low-grade fever, malaise, myalgias, headache, and anorexia. Patients with mild symptoms are often misdiagnosed as having a viral syndrome. Approximately 80% of patients with IE will have a fever during their initial emergency department stay. The presence of a new murmur may be helpful;

Table 1.1 Clinical Features: Infective Endocarditis

Pathogens	*Staphylococcus aureus* *Staphylococcus epidermidis* Viridans *Streptococcus bovis* *Enterococcus* spp. HACEK Immuno-compromised: fungal, rickettsial, protozoan
Signs and symptoms	Fever, malaise, weight loss, night sweats, myalgias, headache, chest/neck/back pain, cough, dyspnea, hepatosplenomegaly, hematuria, arthritis, edema, neurologic symptoms, jaundice, rash.
Laboratory and radiologic findings	**Duke Clinical Criteria:** 2 Major *or* 1 Major + 3 Minor *or* 5 Minor **Major (microbiology):** Typical organisms × 2 blood cultures (*S. viridans*, *S. bovis*, HACEK, *S. aureus*, or *Enterococcus*) Persistent bacteremia (≥ 12 hours) 3/3 or 3/4 positive blood cultures **Major (valve):** Positive echocardiogram New valve regurgitation **Minor:** Predisposing heart condition or IDU Fever ≥ 38 °C (100.4 °F) Vascular phenomenon (arterial embolism, mycotic aneurysm, intracerebral bleed, conjunctival hemorrhage, Janeway lesions) Immune phenomenon (glomerulonephritis, Osler node, Roth spot, rheumatoid factor) Positive blood culture not meeting above criteria Echocardiogram – abnormal but not diagnostic

IDU – intravenous drug use.

however, the high prevalence of a baseline murmur in older adults makes this finding non-specific.

Patients with a more indolent or subacute presentation may display physical findings that result from the deposition of immune complexes in end-vessels throughout the body. These findings include the classic stigmata of IE: *Roth spots* (exudative lesions on the retina), *Janeway lesions* (painless erythematous lesions on the palms and soles), and *Osler nodes* (painful violet lesions on the fingers or toes), as well as hematuria (due to glomerulonephritis), subungual splinter hemorrhages, or petechiae of the palate and conjunctiva. These subtle signs of IE should be sought on examination; however, they are actually quite uncommon and their absence does not rule out IE.

In left-sided endocarditis, arterial embolization may occur in any organ system. The central nervous system is the most common location. Infections that initially appear to be focal or localized, particularly when due to *S. aureus*, may actually be the result of septic emboli from IE. Examples include stroke and spinal cord syndromes, mycotic aneurysms, osteomyelitis, epidural abscesses, septic arthropathies, necrotic skin lesions, and cold, pulseless extremities. Mycotic aneurysms may cause meningitis, headaches, or focal neurological deficits. Destruction of the mitral or aortic valve can cause acute respiratory failure and cardiogenic shock. Right-sided endocarditis may present with septic pulmonary emboli, which cause respiratory symptoms that may be mistaken for pneumonia or pulmonary embolism. Mechanical failure of the pulmonic or tricuspid valves can cause signs and symptoms of acute right-sided heart failure.

Other serious sequelae of endocarditis include intravascular hemolysis, and disseminated intravascular coagulation. Abscesses around the annulae of the cardiac valves may result in conduction blocks and bradydysrhythmias. Ventricular wall rupture may lead to cardiac tamponade or hemorrhagic shock, and extension into the coronary arteries may cause acute coronary syndrome.

Differential Diagnosis

The differential diagnosis of IE includes both acute and chronic infections, malignancies, and a wide spectrum of inflammatory and autoimmune disorders. However, IE should be suspected in any febrile patient with the following risk factors:

- injection drug use
- rheumatic heart disease
- valvular insufficiency
- indwelling catheter
- pacemaker

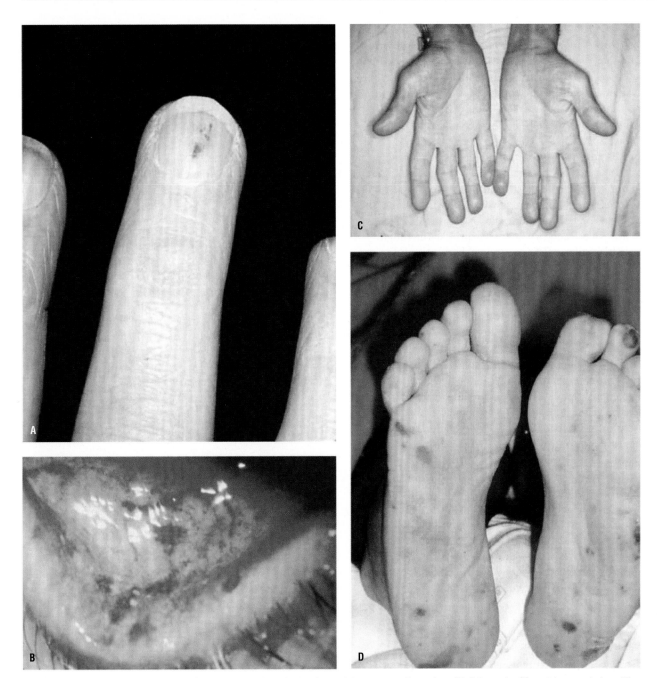

Figure 1.1 Classic physical examination findings in IE. Splinter hemorrhages (A); conjunctival petechiae (B); Osler nodes (C); and Janeway lesions (D).

- prosthetic heart valve
- congenital heart disease
- prior endocarditis

In more severe cases, the differential diagnosis will depend on the presenting signs and symptoms:

- severe sepsis with end-organ dysfunction: pneumonia, urinary tract infection, peritonitis, soft-tissue infections, and meningitis
- left- or right-sided heart failure: myocardial infarction, acute myocarditis, decompensated valvular disease, pulmonary embolism, or aortic dissection
- systemic embolization: carotid stenosis, vascular dissection, or cardiac dysrhythmias
- altered mental status with fever: meningitis, encephalitis, brain abscess

Laboratory and Radiographic Findings

Blood cultures are a crucial basis for the definitive diagnosis of IE. Thus, it is important for emergency providers to obtain blood cultures prior to giving antibiotics whenever IE is suspected. At least two and preferably three sets of blood cultures should be drawn with aseptic technique, be of sufficient volume (10 mL), and be drawn at multiple sites. The sensitivity of three sets of blood cultures approaches 90% in patients who have not received antibiotics. Serologies for Bartonella, Brucella, and Coxiella Burnetii (Q fever) may be indicated if standard cultures are negative. Other routine blood tests such as inflammatory markers (complete blood count [CBC], erythrocyte sedimentation rate [ESR], C-reactive protein [CRP]) lack specificity.

Endocarditis produces abnormal findings on standard diagnostic tests that can lead the clinician to an incorrect initial diagnosis. For example, an abnormal urinalysis may lead to a diagnosis of cystitis or glomerulonephritis, infiltrates on a chest X-ray may be interpreted as pneumonia, or abnormalities on a lumbar puncture may lead to a diagnosis of primary meningitis.

Electrocardiography (ECG) is seldom helpful in establishing the diagnosis of IE. The most common ECG abnormality in IE is sinus tachycardia. A valve ring abscess can produce heart block, particularly an elongating PR interval. Cardiac ischemia may result if IE extends into a coronary artery lumen.

Like blood cultures, echocardiography is an essential test in establishing the definitive diagnosis of IE. However, its main utility in the emergency setting is in the detection of life-threatening complications such as pericardial effusion, cardiac tamponade, and valvular rupture. Transthoracic echocardiography is useful if positive for a clear-cut vegetation; however, transesophageal echocardiography has higher sensitivity and is generally required in suspected IE if the transthoracic echocardiogram is negative.

The Duke Criteria (see Table 1.1) are a widely accepted, structured diagnostic tool for assisting in the often challenging diagnosis of IE. However, these criteria have limited utility in the emergency setting. Emergency providers must maintain constant vigilance for IE, have a low threshold for obtaining blood cultures and echocardiography in suspicious cases, and must exercise judgment in when to admit patients for empiric therapy.

Treatment and Prophylaxis

Empiric therapy targeting common IE bacterial pathogens is indicated when the diagnosis is strongly suspected. The empiric regimen should be tailored to whether or not there is a prosthetic valve, and, when possible, to the current hospital antibiogram (see Table 1.2). The duration of therapy is typically 4 to 6 weeks. It may be appropriate to withhold antibiotics pending culture results in patients with chronic, intermittent fevers who otherwise appear well, provided that close follow-up is available.

Antibiotic prophylaxis was previously recommended to all patients at risk from IE prior to certain invasive dental, gastrointestinal, and genitourinary procedures; however, this practice has now become controversial, with conflicting guidelines in the United States and Europe. While most procedures routinely performed in the emergency department do not require prophylaxis, prophylaxis should be strongly considered for dental or skin abscess incision and drainage (see Table 1.3) or

Table 1.2 Empiric Treatment for Infective Endocarditis

Patient Category	Empiric Therapy Recommendation*
Adults	**Native valve:** Vancomycin 15–20 mg/kg/dose IV every 8–12 hours *and* Ceftriaxone 2 g IV every 24 hours (alternate: ciprofloxacin 400 mg IV every 12 hours) **Prosthetic valve:** Vancomycin 15–20 mg/kg/dose IV every 8–12 hours *and* Gentamicin 1 mg/kg IV every 8 hours *and* Rifampin 300 mg PO/IV every 8 hours
Children	Vancomycin 15–20 mg/kg/dose IV every 6 hours *and* Gentamicin 1.5–2.5 mg/kg IV every 8 hours
Pregnant women	Vancomycin 15–20 mg/kg/dose IV every 8–12 hours *and* Ceftriaxone 2 g IV every 24 hours *and* Rifampin 300 mg PO/IV every 8 hours (if prosthetic heart valve)
Immunocompromised	As above, depending on age and pregnancy status

* Vancomycin and gentamicin dosing may need to be adjusted based on renal function and ideal body weight. Trough monitoring with both agents is strongly recommended. Rifampin has many clinically important drug–drug interactions and may require other drug-level monitoring.

IV – intravenous.

skin infections (with vancomycin 20mg/kg IV × 1) in very high risk patients: those with a prior history of IE; prosthetic valve; heart transplant with abnormal valve function; repaired congenital heart disease.

Complications and Admission Criteria

The treatment of septic and mechanical complications of endocarditis can be challenging. In cases of suspected acute valvular dysfunction with pump failure, emergent echocardiography and consultation with a cardiothoracic surgeon and cardiologist are indicated. Anticoagulation with heparin is not recommended for septic emboli because it does not reduce further embolization and the risk of hemorrhagic transformation is very high. Limb-threatening emboli (e.g. a cold, pulseless extremity) may require revascularization with interventional or surgical techniques, such as the administration of local fibrinolytics.

Patients for whom the diagnosis of IE is suspected should generally be admitted for further work-up and empiric intravenous antibiotics. In selected cases, it may be appropriate to discharge febrile but otherwise well-appearing patients home with blood cultures pending, provided that reliable, urgent

Table 1.3 Antibiotic Prophylaxis for Invasive Procedures in Highest Risk Patients

Patient Category	Recommended Antibiotic for ED Dental Procedures
Adults	Amoxicillin 2 g PO × 1
	if PCN allergy
	Clindamycin 600 mg PO × 1
	Unable to take oral medications:
	Ceftriaxone 1 g IV/IM × 1
	if PCN allergy
	Clindamycin 600 mg IV/IM × 1
Children	Amoxicillin 50 mg/kg PO × 1 (max. 2 g/dose)
	if PCN allergy
	Clindamycin 20 mg/kg PO × 1 (max. 600 mg/dose)
	Unable to take oral medications:
	Ceftriaxone 50 mg/kg IV/IM × 1 (max. 1 g/dose)
	if PCN allergy
	Clindamycin 20 mg/kg IV/IM × 1 (max. 600 mg/dose)
Pregnant women	As above
Immunocompromised	As above

IM – intramuscular; IV – intravenous; PCN – penicillin; PO – by mouth.

follow-up is available. Patients with septic or mechanical complications of IE should be managed in a closely monitored setting, preferably one in which cardiothoracic surgical intervention is readily available.

Pearls and Pitfalls

1. Endocarditis is important to consider in any febrile patient with a predisposing valve disease or other risk factors.
2. Emergency providers can play an essential role in IE diagnosis by obtaining blood cultures prior to empiric antibiotics.
3. Mechanical complications of IE may require emergent cardiovascular surgery.
4. Do not heparinize patients with septic emboli and endocarditis.

References

Alexiou, C., Langley, S. M., Stafford, H., *et al.*, Surgery for active culture-positive endocarditis: determinants of early and late outcome. *Ann. Thorac. Surg.* 2000; 69(5): 1448–54.

Cabell, C. H., Jollis, J. G., Peterson, G. E., *et al.*, Changing patient characteristics and the effect on mortality in endocarditis. *Arch. Intern. Med.* 2002; 162(1): 90–4.

Calder, K. K. and Severyn, F.A., Surgical emergencies in the intravenous drug user. *Emerg. Med. Clin. North. Am.* 2003; 21(4): 1089–116.

Cresti, A., Chiavarelli, M., Scalese, M., *et al.*, Epidemiology and mortality trends in infective endocarditis, a 17-year population-based prospective study. *Cardiovasc. Diagn. Ther.* 2017; 7(1): 27–35.

Habib, G., Hoen, B., Tornos, P., *et al.*, Guidelines on the prevention, diagnosis, and treatment of infective endocarditis (new version 2009): the Task Force on the Prevention, Diagnosis, and Treatment of Infective Endocarditis of the European Society of Cardiology (ESC). *Eur. Heart J.* 2009; 30(19): 2369–2413.

Li, J. S., Sexton, D. J., Mick, N., *et al.*, Proposed modifications to the Duke Criteria for the diagnosis of infective endocarditis. *Clin. Infect. Dis.* 2000; 30(4): 633–8.

Mitchell, R. S., Kumar, V., Robbins, S. L., Abbas, A. K., and Fausto, N. *Robbins Basic Pathology*, 8th edn. (Philadelphia, PA: Saunders/Elsevier, 2007), pp. 406–8.

Olaison L. and Pettersson G., Current best practices and guidelines indications for surgical intervention in infective endocarditis. *Infect. Dis. Clin. North Am.* 2002; 16(2): 453–75.

Pawsat, D. E. and Lee, J. Y., Inflammatory disorders for the heart. Pericarditis, myocarditis, and endocarditis. *Emerg. Med. Clin. North Am.* 1998; 16(3): 665–81.

Samet, J. H., Shevitz, A., and Fowle J., Hospitalization decision in febrile intravenous drug users. *Am. J. Med.* 1990; 89(1): 53–7.

Sandre, R. M. and Shafran, S. D., Infective endocarditis: review of 135 cases over 9 years. *Clin. Infect. Dis.* 1996; 22(2): 276–86.

Sexton, D. J. and Spelman, D., Current best practices and guidelines. Assessment and management of complications in infective endocarditis. *Infect. Dis. Clin. North Am.* 2002; 16(2): 507–21.

Thornhill, M. H., Dayer, M. J., Forde, J. M., *et al.*, Impact of the NICE guideline recommending cessation of antibiotic prophylaxis for prevention of infective endocarditis: before and after study. *BMJ* 2011; 342: d2392.

Towns, M. L. and Reller, L. B., Diagnostic methods current best practices and guidelines for isolation of bacteria and fungi in infective endocarditis. *Infect. Dis. Clin. North Am.* 2002; 16(2): 363–76.

Wilson, L. E., Thomas, D. L., Astemborski, J., *et al.*, Prospective study of infective endocarditis among injection drug users. *J. Infect. Dis.* 2002; 185(12): 1761–6.

Wilson, W., Taubert, K. A., Gewitz, M., *et al.*, Prevention of infective endocarditis: guidelines from the American Heart Association: a guideline from the American Heart Association Rheumatic Fever, Endocarditis, and Kawasaki Disease Committee, Council on Cardiovascular Disease in the Young, and the Council on Clinical Cardiology, Council on Cardiovascular Surgery and Anesthesia, and the Quality of Care and Outcomes Research Interdisciplinary Working Group. *Circulation* 2007; 116(15): 1736–54.

Young, G. P., Hedges, J. R., Dixon, L., *et al.*, Inability to validate a predictive score for infective endocarditis in intravenous drug users. *J. Emerg. Med.* 1993; 11(1): 1–7.

Additional Readings

Baddour, L. M., Wilson, W. R., Bayer, A. S., *et al.*, Infective endocarditi in adults: diagnosis, antimicrobial therapy, and management of complications. A scientific statement for healthcare professionals from the American Heart Association. *Circulation* 2015; 132(15): 1435–86.

Hoen, B. and Duval, X., Infective endocarditis. *N. Engl. J. Med.* 2013; 368(15): 1425–33.

Chapter

2

Pericarditis and Myocarditis

Jessica L. Osterman and Jorge Fernandez

Introduction

Cardiac infections are classified by the affected site: pericardium, myocardium, or endocardium. Since pericarditis and myocarditis often coexist, and the infectious etiologies are very similar, these will be discussed together here. Endocarditis is a fundamentally different type of infection that is covered in Chapter 1. Pericarditis is a common cause of chest pain that has the potential to result in significant morbidity and mortality. Acute care providers should be well versed in the identification, risk stratification, and evidence-based management of this common condition.

Pericarditis

The pericardium is composed of two layers of fibrous tissue, the visceral and parietal, which envelop and protect the heart. The visceral layer is firmly attached to the epicardium, whereas the parietal layer moves freely within the mediastinum. Approximately 15 to 50 mL of fluid is normally present within the pericardial sac.

Pericarditis is defined as inflammation of the pericardium. It frequently causes a small pathologic pericardial effusion and may be associated with adjacent myocardial inflammation or infection, termed myopericarditis. Large pericardial fluid accumulations may occur in pericarditis, which can result in cardiac tamponade, if they develop rapidly.

The majority of infectious pericarditis and myocarditis are due to direct viral infection or less commonly bacterial seeding of the pericardium. Contiguous spread to the pericardium from pleural, pulmonary, or mediastinal infections, or from endocarditis, can also occur. There are also numerous non-infectious causes of both pericarditis and myocarditis.

Epidemiology and Microbiology

While the epidemiology of pericarditis is not well described, it is clearly a common condition, estimated to account for 5% of non-ischemic chest pain cases seen in emergency departments (EDs). Pericarditis commonly affects young men, for reasons that are not well understood.

Acute pericarditis is often idiopathic, in that routine evaluation reveals no definite cause; the majority of such cases are presumed to be viral. When a pathogen is identified, viruses predominate, including coxsackieviruses, echoviruses, influenza, EBV, VZV, mumps, and hepatitis. Human immunodeficiency virus (HIV) can cause pericarditis and myocarditis and remains a common cause of pericardial disease in developing countries where HIV is prevalent.

Bacterial pericarditis, termed purulent pericarditis, is fortunately rare. It can result from hematogenous seeding or direct spread, usually from pneumonia. Myriad bacteria have been reported to cause pericarditis, with the most common pathogens being *Staphyloccus aureus* and *Streptococcus pneumoniae*. Pneumococcal pneumonia and empyema and *S. aureus* endocarditis (via endomyocardial abscess) are the infections that classically spread directly to the pericardium. Mediastinitis, penetrating trauma, and thoracic surgery can also lead to purulent pericarditis. *S. aureus* is the predominant pathogen in hematogenous cases.

Mycobacterium tuberculosis is considered to be the most uncommon etiology of infectious endocarditis in developing countries. Fungi are a relatively uncommon cause of

Table 2.1 Important Causes of Pericarditis and Myocarditis

Idiopathic	**Fungal infections**	**Malignancy**
Viral infections	*Histoplasma capsulatum*	**Medications**
Coxsackievirus A and B	*Aspergillus* species	Penicillin
Echoviruses	**Mycobacterial infections**	Sulfa drugs
Adenoviruses	*M. tuberculosis*	Procainamide
HIV	**Parasitic infections**	Hydralazine
Bacterial infections	Chagas disease	Isoniazid
Gram-positive species	Trichinosis	Phenytoin
Gram-negative species	Toxoplasmosis	Chemotherapeutic agents
Anaerobes	**Autoimmune-mediated**	**Metabolic disorders**
Mycoplasma	Acute rheumatic fever	Hypothyroidism
Rickettsial infections	Dressler's syndrome	Uremia (dialysis-related)
RMSF	Systemic lupus erythematosus	**Radiation exposure**
Q fever	Rheumatoid arthritis	**toxins/environmental**
Scrub typhus	Vasculitis (e.g. Kawasaki)	Cocaine
Spirochetes	Sarcoidosis	Amphetamines
Lyme disease	Postvaccination	Carbon monoxide
Syphilis	Postpericardiotomy syndrome	Lead
		Stings/bites
		Trauma or surgery

Adapted from A. M. Ross and S. E. Grauer, Acute pericarditis. Evaluation and treatment of infectious and other causes. *Postgrad Med.* 2004 March; 115(3): 67–75.
RMSF – Rocky Mountain spotted fever.

pericarditis. Histoplasomosi pericarditis is seen in endemic regions of the United States and *Candida* species are a common etiology in nosocomial cases.

The list of non-infectious causes of acute pericarditis is very long (see Table 2.1). These include uremia, trauma, malignancy (lymphoma, cancers of the breast, lung, and kidney), radiation, chemotherapy, drug reactions (penicillin, minoxidil), post-cardiotomy or thoracic surgery, and autoimmune disorders (systemic lupus erythematosus [SLE], rheumatoid arthritis [RA], Dressler's syndrome after myocardial infarction postpericardiotomy syndrome).

Clinical Features

The clinical presentation of infectious pericarditis varies depending on the pathogen and the the host immune response (see Table 2.2). Most patients with acute viral (or ideopathic) pericarditis have mild symptoms, which include low-grade fever, malaise, and substernal chest pain. There may be a history of a preceeding viral respiratory or gastrointestinal illness. The pain is typically described as sharp or stabbing, but may be squeezing. It usually has a pleuritic quality – worsened by inspiration and cough. The pain is commonly postural: lying supine exacerbates the pain, whereas sitting upright or leaning slightly forward relieves it. The phrenic nerve traverses the pericardium, so the pain of pericarditis is often described as radiating to the trapezial ridges. Patients with pericarditis may also complain of cough, odynophagia, or dysphagia, presumably secondary to the spread of the inflammatory process to adjacent structures.

Patients with slowly accumulating effusions, such as in uremic or autoimmune pericarditis, may have no chest pain and limited hemodynamics signs. Those with rapidly accumulating effusions may present with tamponade and shock. This classically occurs from malignancy, in patients on anticoagulants and in purulent pericarditis. Associated myocarditis can lead to rapid heart failure, cardiogenic shock, and arrythmias.

Patients with purulent pericarditis usually appear toxic with an acute febrile illness and may have evidence of pneumonia, empyema, endocarditis, or mediastinal infection. Tuberculous pericarditis generally presents as an indolent illness with nonspecific symptoms such as fever, night sweats, weight loss, and fatigue.

The classic physical finding in acute pericarditis is a pericardial friction rub, which is typically a three-phase "scratchy" heart sound that comes and goes, best heard while the patient leans forward. Signs of pericardial tamponade are discussed under "Complications and Admission Criteria."

Differential Diagnosis

The differential diagnosis of a patient complaining of chest pain or dyspnea in an emergent or urgent setting includes the following:

- aortic dissection
- pulmonary embolism
- pneumothorax and tension pneumothorax
- acute coronary syndrome
- esophageal perforation
- myopericarditis
- mediastinitis
- pneumonia
- pleurisy

Table 2.2 Clinical Features: Pericarditis and Myocarditis

	Pericarditis	Myocarditis
Signs and symptoms: adults	• Fever, malaise, night sweats • Chest pain (typically sharp, pleuritic) • Pericardial friction rub • Tamponade: tachycardia, Beck's triad, pulsus paradoxus	• Fever, malaise, night sweats • Chest pain uncommon unless associated pericarditis • Dyspnea, orthopnea • Left and right-sided heart failure signs: lung crackles, hypoxemia, hypotension, JVD, HSM, peripheral edema • Dysrhythmia or conduction disturbance
Signs and symptoms: infants	• As above • Non-specific – lethargy, poor feeding, cyanosis	• As above • Non-specific – lethargy, poor feeding, cyanosis
Laboratory and ECG findings	• Elevated WBC, CRP, ESR • ECG findings include: • Sinus tachycardia and non-specific ST-T changes • Diffuse ST-segment elevation • PR depression • T wave inversion without Q wave formation • Ultrasound – pericardial effusion, possible signs of tamponade	• Elevated WBC, CRP, ESR, and cardiac biomarkers • ECG findings non-specific: • Sinus tachycardia and non-specific ST-T changes • ST-segment elevation or depression • Decreased QRS amplitude and Q waves • Atrial or ventricular ectopy • Bundle branch blocks • Ultrasound – decreased left ventricular function

CRP – C-reactive protein; DOE – dyspnea on exertion; ECG – electrocardiography; ESR – erythrocyte sedimentation rate; JVD – jugular venous distention; HSM – hepatosplenomegaly; TB – tuberculosis; WBC – white blood (cell) count.

- gastroesophageal reflux disease
- costochondritis
- panic attack
- herpes zoster
- cholecystitis

The diagnosis of pericarditis and/or myocarditis should be considered when chest pain, dyspnea, dysrhythmias, heart failure, or cardiac tamponade accompanies a recent viral-seeming upper respiratory or gastrointestinal illness, or in the setting of an underlying autoimmune disorder, malignancy, renal failure, recent cardiac surgery, or exposure to tuberculosis.

Acute pericarditis can be mistaken for ST-segment elevation myocardial infarction resulting in inappropriate treatment with fibrinolytic agents and/or anticoagulants. Electrocardiographic findings should distinguish these disorders: ST elevations of pericarditis generally occur diffusely, whereas acute coronary syndrome (ACS) involves a specific coronary artery territory. Likewise, pericarditis can be difficult to distinguish from other pain syndromes associated with underlying immunologic disease, or from pulmonary embolism in a patient with underlying cancer.

Laboratory and Radiographic Findings

In the acute care setting, routine studies in patients presenting with chest pain or dyspnea include pulse oximetry, chest X-ray, and electrocardiography. Echocardiography is recommended in all cases of suspected pericardial disease.

While blood tests may not always be necessary in an otherwise healthy patient presenting with typical findings of acute pericarditis and normal vital signs, most patients require further risk stratification. Laboratory findings in pericarditis may include leukocytosis, elevated CRP, and increased ESR. Negative inflammatory markers argue against pericarditis.

A single set of biomarkers is recommended; elevated cardiac biomarkers suggest associated myocarditis (myopericarditis). Blood culture should be drawn in patients with a high fever or signs of toxicity. Skin testing and sputum testing for acid-fast bacilli should be considered in the appropriate setting.

Chest X-ray is useful in excluding pneumonia and pneumothorax, and it may reveal a pleural effusion, lung mass, or infiltrate suggestive of active tuberculosis, which can focus the differential diagnosis. A large pericardial effusion or severe myocarditis with heart failure will cause cardiomegaly (see Figure 2.1).

Electrocardiography is a cornerstone of pericarditis diagnosis. Typical findings are shown in Figure 2.2. Acute pericarditis causes a characteristic progression of ECG findings through four distinct phases. Stage one lasts for days and is characterized by diffuse ST elevation in all leads except avR and V1 and PR segment depression. Stage two is normalization of the ST and PR segments. Stage 3 is characterized by diffuse T wave inversion without Q wave formation, and stage 4 is ECG normalization. In the case of a large effusion, these signs are usually not seen; rather, there may be tachycardia, loss of QRS voltage, and electrical alternans.

Echocardiography is recommended for risk stratification in suspected pericarditis (See Figure 2.4). In typical acute idiopathic pericarditis, a small effusion may or may not be seen. An effusion greater than 20 mm is considered high risk, generally necessitating admission. Echocardiographic evidence of tamponade (discussed below under "Complications and Admission Criteria") or decreased ventricular function, suggesting associated myocarditis, also necessitate admission.

Diagnostic pericardiocentesis should be considered in patients with a significant effusion and fever, to rule out purulent pericarditis, in those with tamponade or impending tamponade, and to work up suspected malignant pericardial effusion.

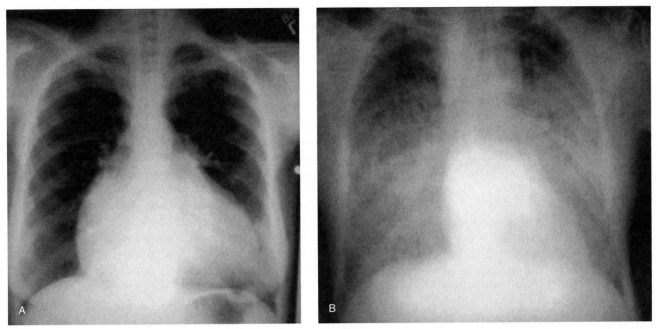

Figure 2.1 Chest X-ray findings in pericarditis and myocarditis. (A) Cardiomegaly from pericardial effusion. (B) Acute pulmonary edema in myocarditis.

Reprinted with permission from W. J. Brady, J. D. Ferguson, E. A. Ullman, and A. D. Perron, Myocarditis: emergency department recognition and management. *Emerg. Med. Clin. North Am.* 2004; 22(4): 865–85.

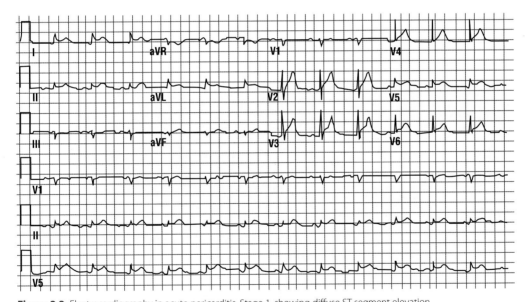

Figure 2.2 Electrocardiography in acute pericarditis. Stage 1, showing diffuse ST segment elevation.

Reprinted with permission from A. M. Ross and S. E. Grauer, Acute pericarditis. Evaluation and treatment of infectious and other causes. *Porstgrad. Med.* 2004; 115(3): 67–75.

Treatment and Prophylaxis

Symptomatic treatment of pericarditis should be undertaken after ruling out other life-threatening causes of chest pain and life-threatening complications of pericarditis (see Table 2.3). Treatment of pain and inflammation with aspirin or non-steroidal agents like ibuprofen is the mainstay of pericarditis treatment. Based on trial data showing a reduction in recurrence, routine addition of colchicine is now recommended for acute uncomplicated pericarditis. No definitive treatment benefit of corticosteroids has been documented, except when there is an underlying collagen vascular disease such as SLE or RA. Additionally, the use of steroids in acute pericarditis appears to increase the risk of recurrent or chronic pericarditis. Exercise restriction until symptom resolution and normalization of inflammatory markers is recommended in young patients with idiopathic or viral pericarditis.

Complications and Admission Criteria

Important complications of pericarditis include myocarditis, tamponade, and recurrence (see Table 2.4). Patients with purulent or tuberculous pericarditis are at risk from progression of the infection itself. Signs of myocarditis should always be sought.

Evaluation of a patient with suspected pericarditis should routinely include assessment for signs of hemodynamic compromise and pericardial tamponade. These signs include pulsus paradoxus, tachycardia, and Beck's triad of hypotension, JVD, and muffled heart sounds. Electrical alternans, characterized by alternating voltage of the P wave, QRS segment, and T wave, is pathognomonic of a large, hemodynamically significant pericardial effusion. Echocardiography is the gold standard test for diagnosis. Diagnostic findings include pericardial effusion, inferior vena cava dilation, diastolic collapse of the right atrial or ventricular, and leftward bowing of the septum with inspiration (see Figure 2.3). Cardiac tamponade requires aggressive fluid resuscitation followed by emergent pericardiocentesis if a patient does not immediately improve with IV fluids.

Recurrence occurs in up to 38% of patients with idiopathic pericarditis who are not treated with colchicine and 17% of those who are. Recurrecnt of pericarditis is thought to be autoimmune and can prove difficult to manage.

In the setting of a normal echocardiogram, patients with acute pericarditis who are well appearing may be safely discharged. Small or moderate effusions can be followed with serial echocardiograms; large effusions may require pericardiocentesis or placement of a pericardial window.

Table 2.3 Initial Treatment for Pericarditis

Patient Category	Therapy Recommendation
Adults	**Non-steroidal anti-inflammatories (avoid if isolated myocarditis):** Aspirin 650–1000 mg PO TID *or* Ibuprofen 600–800 mg PO TID *or* Indomethacin 50 mg PO TID *plus* Colchicine 0.6 mg PO BID
Children	**Non-steroidal anti-inflammatories (avoid if isolated myocarditis):** Ibuprofen 5–10 mg/kg PO QID *or* Naproxen 5–10 mg/kg PO BID *plus* Colchicine 0.3–0.6 mg PO daily
Pregnant women	Acetaminophen 500 mg PO every 6 hours
Immunocompromised	As above, depending on age and pregnancy status
PO – by mouth.	

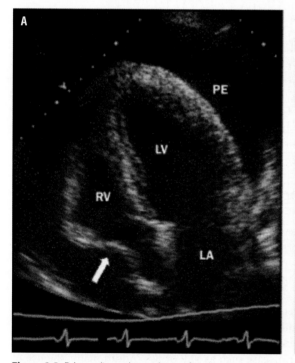
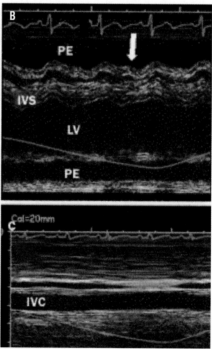

Figure 2.3 Echocardiographic evidence of cardiac tamponade. Echocardiographic images of large pericardial effusion with features of tamponade. (A) Apical four-chamber view of LV, LA, and RV that shows large PE with diastolic right-atrial collapse (arrow). (B) M-mode image with cursor placed through RV, IVS, and LV in parasternal long axis. The view shows circumferential PE with diastolic collapse of RV free wall (arrow) during expiration. (C) M-mode image from subcostal window in same patient that shows IVC plethora without inspiratory collapse. Reprinted with permission from Elsevier (*The Lancet,* 2004, vol. 363, pp. 717–27).

Photo and text from R. W. Troughton, C. R. Asher, and A. L. Klein, Pericarditis. Lancet 2004; 363(9410): 717–27.

IVC – inferior vena cava; IVS – interventricular septum; LA – left atrium; LV – left ventricle; PE – pericardial effusion; RV – right ventricle.

Guidelines recommend hospitalization for pericarditis patients with any of the following high risk features:

- temperature >38 °C
- subacute onset
- pericardial effusion >20 mm
- cardiac tamponade
- lack of response to anti-inflammatory treatment after 1 week
- evidence of myopericarditis
- immunosuppression
- trauma
- oral anticoagulant therapy

Myocarditis

Myocarditis, inflammation of the myocardium, can occur on its own or be associated with concurrent pericarditis. Though most cases are infectious, there are many non-infectious forms of myocarditis too. Generally speaking, idiopathic, viral, and lymphocytic myocarditis are synonymous. Manifestations range from mild dyspnea and chest pain in the setting of a viral illness to sudden, progressive heart failure and cardiogenic shock.

Epidemiology and Microbiology

The epidemiology of myocarditis is difficult to gauge, since the majority of cases are mild, self limited, and often associated with generalized viral syndrome. Studies of coxsackievirus outbreaks suggest myocarditis may occur in up to 5% of patients. Evidence of myocarditis is found in 5–10% of young athletes with sudden death and approximately 10% of cases of unexplained dilated cardiomyopathy in children and adults. Myocarditis is obviously a much more common cause of cardiomyopathy in children than adults.

Etiologies of mycarditis mirror those of endocarditis or pericarditis (see Table 2.1). Infectious causes include viruses, bacteria, fungi, rickettsia, spirochetes, and parasites. In all types of infection, myocardial damage may result from direct effects of the invasive pathogen, or from immune-mediated lysis of infected cells. In developed nations, viruses represent the most common infectious cause. In North America, the most common viral pathogens are coxsackievirus, adenovirus, and parvovirus B 19. Other viral etiolgies include influenza virus, echovirus, herpes simplex virus (HSV), varicella-zoster virus (VZV), Epstein-Barr virus (EBV), cytomegalovirus (CMV), and the hepatitis viruses. Human immunodeficiency virus (HIV) infection may also cause myocarditis, either directly from HIV-induced cytotoxicity during any phase of the infection, or indirectly as a result of other opportunistic infections. Most cases of viral myocarditis are preceded by an upper respiratory infection or gastrointestinal illness by 1 to 2 weeks.

Bacterial myocarditis is unusual and most often caused by direct extension from infected endocardial or pericardial tissue. Certain exotoxin-mediated bacterial illnesses, such as diphtheria, may also cause myocarditis.

Tick-borne illnesses caused by rickettsia (Rocky Mountain spotted fever, Q fever, and scrub typhus) and spirochetes (Lyme disease) have all been associated with myocarditis. Lyme myocarditis should be suspected in patients from endemic areas presenting with atrioventricular block. Similarly, in patients from rural South and Central America presenting with heart block or regional wall motion abnormalities or ventricular aneurisms, Chagas cardiomyopathy, caused by the parasite *Trypanosoma cruzi*, should be suspected. Immunocompromised patients may develop myocarditis secondary to toxoplasmosis.

There are a variety of non-infectious causes of myocarditis, including autoimmune disorders, medications, and environmental toxins. Autoimmune causes include systemic lupus erythematosus (SLE), rheumatoid arthritis (RA), sarcoidosis, and various vasculitides (Kawasaki disease and giant cell arteritis). A variety of drugs and chemotherapeutics can directly induce myocardial inflammation, including cocaine, amphetamines, lithium, phenothiazines, zidovudine (AZT), chloroquine, and doxorubicin. Hypersensitivity reactions to penicillin and sulfonamides may trigger inflammatory changes in the myocardium, resulting in myocarditis. Environmental toxins such as carbon monoxide, lead, and arsenic, as well as stings from spiders, scorpions, and wasps, can also result in myocardial inflammation.

Clinical Features

Like pericarditis, the virulence of the pathogen and the host immune response dictate the clinical course in myocarditis, resulting in a wide spectrum of severity. Typically, myocarditis presents with symptoms such as fatigue, dyspnea on exertion, palpitations, syncope, and occasionally chest pain. There will often be a history of a viral syndrome that may include fever, upper respiratory symptoms, gastrointestinal symptoms, or myalgias. Chest pain, particulary if pleuritic, suggests concurrent pericarditis, but coronary-artery spasm can also occur. Dyspnea on exertion is common; dyspnea at rest and orthopnea suggest severe disease. Palpitations, light-headedness, or syncope suggest associated dysrhythmia. Neonates and infants frequently present with non-specific symptoms, such as fever, respiratory distress, cyanosis, or poor feeding.

Physical exam findings in myocarditis may include signs of left-sided heart failure such as tachypnea, hypoxemia, and pulmonary rales. Right-sided heart failure presents with JVD, hepatosplenomegaly, and peripheral edema. Some patients, including children, present with fulminant cardiomyopathy characterized by pulmonary edema and/or cardiogenic shock. Tachyarrhythmias, bradyarrhythmias, and heart block can occur. Myocarditis can be the cause of sudden cardiac death.

Differential Diagnosis

In the case of myopericarditis with chest pain, the differential diagnosis includes the diseases listed in the pericarditis section. In the case of new onset heart failure in an adult, the main considerations are ischemic cardiomyopathy and hypertensive cardiomyopathy. Lack of risk factors or pre-existing hypertension, and a preceeding viral illness, favor myocarditis. A history of immunologic disease, prior chemotherapy or radiation

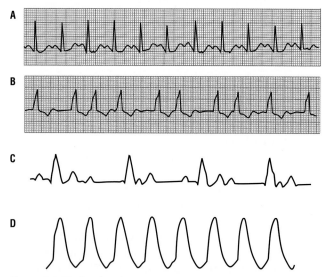

Figure 2.4 Rhythm disturbances in acute myocarditis. (A) Sinus tachycardia. (B) Atrial fibrillation with bundle-branch block morphology. (C) Third-degree (complete) atrioventricular block with wide QRS complex escape. (D) Wide QRS complex tachycardia.

Reprinted with permission from W. J. Brady, J. D. Ferguson, E. A. Ullman, and A. D. Perron, Myocarditis: emergency department recognition and management. *Emerg. Med. Clin. North Am.* 2004; 22(4): 865–85.

therapy, or heavy alcohol, cocaine, or amphetamine use should be sought. A careful medication history is crucial, looking for potentially cardiotoxic agents.

Laboratory and Radiographic Findings

Myocarditis will present with the diagnostic test findings of heart failure. The chest X-ray will demonstrate cardiomegaly and signs of pulmonary congestions (see Figure 2.1). Brain natiuretic peptide (BNP) may be elevated. Cardiac biomarkers are often elevated reflecting myocardial necrosis. While these findings confirm the diagnosis of heart failure, they are obviously not specific for infectious myocarditis.

ECG findings are likewise non-specific. Sinus tachycardia, ectopic beats, and non-specific ST-T changes are the rule (see Figure 2.4). Lyme carditis classically presents with heart block. ST segment elevation, when present, can be diffuse if there is associated pericarditis, or regional.

Echocardiography is a crucial diagnostic test in cases of suspected myocarditis, since it is the gold standard for ventricular dysfunction. Wall motion abormalities are typically global, but can be regional. Echocardiography may demonstrate concomitant pericardial involvement.

Myocarditis, as the cause of ventricular dysfunction, particularly in adults, is a diagnosis of exclusion. In adults, normal coronary angiography is generally required prior to diagnosis of myocarditis. While endomyocardial biopsy is considered the gold standard test to establish the diagnosis of myocarditis, and to help determine the underlying etiology, many patients with presumed myocarditis never undergo this invasive test. A diagnostic biopsy will show mononuclear inflammatory infiltrate and necrosis of the myocardium. The added diagnostic value of viral genome PCR is uncertain. Cardiac

magnetic resonance imaging (MRI) has emerged as an alternative to endomyocardial biopsy. MRI is increasingly being used to detect occult myocarditis in younger patients who present with idiopathic dysrhythmias and have normal electrophysiology testing.

Treatment and Prophylaxis

The treatment of myocarditis is primarily supportive, with cardiac monitoring, cardiovascular support, and diuresis as indicated. Congestive heart failure with acute pulmonary edema may require aggressive treatment with vasodilators such as nitrates and angiotensin-converting enzyme inhibitors. Beta-blockers should be avoided, as they are not only contraindicated in acute congestive heart failure, but have also been shown to worsen cardiac inflammation in animal models. While non-steroidal agents are a mainstay of treatment for cases of pericarditis, some studies suggest that these drugs are potentially harmful in cases of isolated myocarditis. As with pericarditis, no definitive benefit of corticosteroids or intravenous gamma globulin has been documented in myocarditis, except when caused by a specific collagen vascular disease such as SLE or Kawasaki's disease. Other specific immunomodulator and antiviral drugs have yet to be proven beneficial. Antitrypanosomal therapy is not recommended in established Chagas cardiomyopathy. Patients with suspected or diagnosed myocarditis should limit activity for 6 months.

Complications and Admission Criteria

All cases of suspected myocarditis should be admitted, preferably to a telemetry or intensive care unit setting for cardiac monitoring.

In the emergent setting, the main complications of myocarditis are dysrhythmias, pulmonary edema, respiratory failure, cardiogenic shock, and tamponade due to concomitant pericarditis (see Table 2.4). For the emergency management of bradycardia or tachydysrhythmias, standard advanced cardiovascular life support (ACLS) protocols should be followed. Because conduction disturbances are generally transient, insertion of a transvenous pacemaker is usually not necessary in cases of myocarditis-induced bradycardia.

Hemodynamic support with vasopressors and/or inotropes may be needed. Intubation is frequently needed in patients with fulminant myocarditis. Emergent placement of an intra-aortic balloon pump or left-ventricular assist device in adults may serve as a bridge to transplantation. Extracorporial membrane oxygenation is used frequently in children as a bridge to recovery or transplantation. Cardiac transplantation may be life saving in cases of fulminant myocarditis; however, these patients are at high risk of recurrent myocarditis or rejection.

Most cases of viral myocarditis, particularly those with clinical myopericarditis, have a benign course and resolve spontaneously without sequelae. Cases with severe and biopsy-proven cardiomyopathy, however, have an approximately 20% 1 year mortality. Unfortunately, a subset of both children and adults

Table 2.4 Complications of Pericarditis and Myocarditis and Recommended Treatment

Complication	Recommended Therapy
Congestive heart failure	Nitroglycerin 5–300 mcg/min IV drip titrated to effect, and Captopril 25 mg SL/PO × 1, and Furosemide 0.5–1 mg/kg IV × 1, and BiPAP Note: Beta-blockers are contraindicated.
Cardiac tamponade	Aggressive fluid resuscitation Pericardiocentesis
Heart block and tachydysrhythmias	As per ACLS or APLS protocols
Cardiogenic dhock	Dobutamine 1–20 mcg/kg/min IV drip titrated to effect (may need additional pressor support) Intra-aortic balloon pump Extracorporeal membrane oxygenation Cardiac transplantation

APLS – advanced pulmonary life support; BiPAP – bilevel positive airway pressure; IV – intravenous; PO – by mouth.

with infectious cardiomyopathy will go on to develop chronic dilated cardiomyopathy and/require transplantation.

Pearls and Pitfalls

1. Most cases of myocarditis and pericarditis are viral and have a benign course; consider alternative causes in toxic appearing patients.
2. Serious complications of myocarditis include congestive heart failure, conduction disturbances, and tachydysrhythmias.
3. Echocardiography is recommended for all patients with newly diagnosed pericarditis or myocarditis prior to discharge.
4. Hospital admission is indicated for all cases of myocarditis, as well as pericarditis when associated with fever, trauma, oral anticoagulants, immunosuppression, or pericardial effusion >20 mm.

References

Acker, M. A. Mechanical circulatory support for patients with acute-fulminant myocarditis. *Ann. Thorac. Surg.* 2001; 71(3 Suppl.): S73–6.

Adler, Y., Charron, P. Imazio, M., *et al.*, 2015 ESC Guidelines for the diagnosis and management of pericardial diseases: The Task Force for the Diagnosis and Management of Pericardial Diseases of the European Society of Cardiology (ESC). Endorsed by: The European Association for Cardio-Thoracic Surgery (EACTS). *Eur. Heart J.* 2015; 36: 2921–64.

Barbaro, G., Fisher, S. D., Gaincaspro, G., and Lipshultz, S. E. HIV-associated cardiovascular complications: a new challenge for emergency physicians. *Am. J. Emerg. Med.* 2001; 19(7): 566–74.

Caforio, A. L. P., Pankuweit, S., Arbustini, E., *et al.* Curent state of knowledge on aetiology, diagnosis, management, and therapy of myocarditis: a position statement of the European Society of Cardiology Working Group on Myocardial and Pericardial Diseases. *Eur. Heart J.* 2013; 34: 2636–48.

Carapetis, J. R., McDonald, M., and Wilson, N. J. Acute rheumatic fever. *Lancet* 2005; 366(9480): 155–68.

Cilliers, A. M., Manyemba, J., and Saloojee, H. Anti-inflammatory treatment for carditis in acute rheumatic fever. *Cochrane Database Syst. Rev.* 2003; (2): CD003176.

Imazio, M., Spodick, D. H., Brucato, A., and Trinchero, R. Controversial issues in the management of pericardial diseases. *Circulation* 2010; 121(7): 916–28.

Imazio, M. and Trinchero, R. Myopericarditis: etiology, management and prognosis. *Int. J. Cardiol.* 2008; 127(1): 17–26.

Klein, A. L., Abbara, S., Agler, D. A., *et al.* American Society of Echocardiography clinical recommendations for multimodality cardiovascular imaging of patients with pericardial disease. *J. Am. Soc. Echocardiogr.* 2013; 26(9): 965–1012.

Meune, C., Spaulding, C., Lebon, P., and Bergman, J. F. Risks versus benefits of NSAIDs including aspirin in myocarditis: a review of the evidence from animal studies. *Drug Saf.* 2003; 26(13): 975–81.

Pawsat, D. E. and Lee, J. Y. Inflammatory disorders for the heart. Pericarditis, myocarditis, and endocarditis. *Emerg. Med. Clin. North Am.* 1998; 16(3): 665–81.

Ross, A. M. and Grauer, S. E. Acute pericarditis. Evaluation and treatment of infectious and other causes. *Postgrad. Med.* 2004; 115(3): 67–75.

Stollerman, G. H. Rheumatic fever in the 21st century. *Clin. Infect. Dis.* 2001; 33(6): 806–14.

Trautner, B. W. and Darouiche, R. O. Tuberculous pericarditis: optimal diagnosis and management. *Clin. Infect. Dis.* 2001; 33(7): 954–61.

Additional Readings

Brady, W. J., Ferguson, J. D., Ullman, E. A., and Perron, A. D. Myocarditis: emergency department recognition and management. *Emerg. Med. Clin. North Am.* 2004; 22(4): 865–85.

Chan, T. C., Brady, W. J., and Pollack, M. Electrocardiographic manifestations: acute myopericarditis. *J. Emerg. Med.* 1999; 17(5); 865–72.

Cooper, L. T. Myocarditis. *N. Eng. J. Med.* 2009; 360: 1526–38.

LeWinter, M. M. Acute pericarditis. *N. Eng. J. Med.* 2014; 371: 2410–16.

Cardiac Implantable Electronic Device Infections

Jorge Fernandez and Nicholas Pokrajac

Introduction

Cardiac implantable electronic devices (CIEDs) include permanent pacemakers (PPMs), automatic implantable cardioverter defibrillators (AICDs), and long-term ventricular assist devices (VADs), including left-ventricular assist devices (LVADs), right-ventricular assist devices (RVADs), and biventricular assist devices (BiVADs). These devices are increasingly prevalent because of the improved quality of life and survival they afford to patients with cardiac disease. As a result, infectious complications arising from these devices are increasingly encountered in emergency department (ED) settings. This chapter summarizes the clinical presentation and ED management of CIED infections.

Epidemiology and Microbiology

The rate of CIED implantation in the United States continues to grow. One study demonstrated a 19% and 60% increase in implantation rate of PPMs and AICDs, respectively, from 1997 to 2004. LVAD implantations increased from 107 in 2004 to 612 in 2011 among Medicare beneficiaries.

Despite less invasive techniques and increasing surgical expertise, multiple studies identify a rise in CIED-related infections. For every 1,000 Medicare beneficiaries, the rate of CIED infections increased from 0.94 to 2.11 between 1990 and 1999. and hospitalizations for cardiac device infections increased by a factor of 3.1 between 1996 and 2003, with AICD-related infections predominating. Ventricular assist devices have a high rate of infection, with one study showing a rate of 72%. Increases in CIED use and associated infections requires that ED providers be familiar with presentation and management.

The majority of PPM- and AICD-related infections are caused by *Staphylococcus*, with a recent clinical update identifying *S. aureus* and *coagulase negative Staphylococcus* in 60 to 80% of cases (see Table 3.1). Methicillin resistance is common and should be assumed until susceptibility results return. Gram-negative bacilli, such as *Escherichia coli*, are the second most common infectious etiology, while polymicrobial and fungal device infections have also been described. A recent retrospective case review of VAD-related infections found that *Staphylococcus* species were responsible for the majority, though gram-negative (including nosocomial pathogens such as *Pseudomonas*), anaerobic, and mixed etiologies also occured. One 2001 study found a high rate of *Candida* in LVAD recipients with bloodstream infections, though this was not borne out in more recent studies.

Pathogenesis

CIED infection may occur by several mechanisms. Initial implantation carries risk of direct contamination of the device, such as the pulse generator or intravascular leads, or surrounding tissue. Subcutaneous infection in the pulse generator pocket is common. Erosion of the generator body or wires through the skin, or an overlying soft tissue infection, can lead to local spread of infection to the device. Exiting drivelines from the skin required by VADs represent a constant potential source of inoculation. Hematogenous seeding of device can occur from urinary tract infections or other sources of bacteremia. Vegetations can form on the intravascular portion of the leads in the right side of the heart, with or without associated valvular endocarditis. Various device factors influence bacterial adherence to the device itself, including its material composition and shape.

Bacterial biofilms play an important role in CIED infections and their resistance to antimicrobial therapy. Biofilm formation allows bacteria to stick together on a surface through the production of an extracellular matrix. Biofilms prevent antibiotic penetration and create islands of developing antibiotic resistance. The clinical implication is that all confirmed CIED

Table 3.1 Causative Pathogens of CIED Infections*

Organism	PPM/AICD	VAD
Staphylococcus sp. and other gram positives	Most frequent 60–80%	Most frequent 50%
Gram negatives (*Escherichia coli, Pseudomonas aeruginosa, Proteus, Serratia*)	10%	25–30%
Polymicrobial	10%	15–20%
Fungal	Rare	5–7%
Mycobacterial	Rare	Rare

* Approximate values.

Box 3.1 Risk Factors for CIED Infection

Device type: VAD > AICD > PPM
Pulse generator location: intra-abdominal > pectoral
Prior device implantation
Recent (< 3 months) device implantation, revision, or generator change
Pre-procedural transvenous pacing
Congestive heart failure
Diabetes mellitus
Chronic renal disease
Use of immunosuppressive agents
Obesity

---

infections require device removal, in addition to a course of antibiotic therapy, for definitive cure. When removal is not possible, long-term antibiotic suppression therapy is generally required.

Patient Risk Factors

Comorbidities such as congestive heart failure, kidney disease, diabetes mellitus, and other forms of immunosuppression are associated with an increased risk of CIED infections (see Box 3.1). The presence of a fever 24 hours prior to implantation and pre-procedural temporary transvenous pacing also increases the risk. Replacement or revision of devices carry increased incidence of infection. AICDs carry a greater risk of infection than PPMs. For all devices, the risk of acute or subacute device infection persists for 3 months.

Certain factors appear to be protective, such as the pre-procedural use of antibiotic prophylaxis. In addition, device implantation by pectoral approach carries less risk of infection than intra-abdominal approach or by thoracotomy.

Clinical Features and Presentation

Symptoms of an underlying cardiac device infection are variable. In general, systemic complaints are present in approximately 80% of patients with a CIED infection. Vague complaints such as fatigue, decreased appetite, or a general sense of unwellness should prompt clinical concern. Infectious symptoms such as fevers and chills may be present, but often are not. Cardiopulmonary manifestations such as chest pain, shortness of breath, and decreased exercise

tolerance are also possible. In local infections there may be a history of increased pain and drainage from either generator site or exiting drivelines in the case of VADs. Physical examination may reveal erythema, tenderness, fluctuance, or purulent drainage near the pulse generator, or evidence of erosion of the generator or wires. Manifestations of endocarditis such as a new cardiac murmur or splinter hemorrhages may also occur. Device infections may present with overt sepsis or septic shock.

CIED infections may also, though less commonly, present initially with downstream, extra-cardiac symptoms. Persistent cough or hemoptysis may signify septic pulmonary emboli and abscess. CIED infection may rarely present as osteomyelitis, septic phlebitis, or septic emboli to other solid organs.

Differential Diagnosis

Since CIED infections often manifest with vague complaints, a broad differential diagnosis is required. Patients requiring CIED implantation frequently have multiple comorbidities, such as heart failure and chronic obstructive pulmonary disease (COPD), that may cloud the diagnostic picture. Many patients with CIEDs, and all those with VADs, are anticoagulated and at high risk of gastrointestinal bleeding and anemia. The bleeding risk may be increased if patients are given antibiotics that interfere with anticoagulant metabolism. Infectious symptoms, which should prompt concern for a CIED infection, may derive from an alternative source such as pneumonia or a urinary tract infection (UTI). Associated metabolic derangements from acute or chronic kidney disease, as well as hepatic dysfunction, may also occur.

Laboratory and Radiographic Findings

Any significant clinical suspicion of a CIED infection by history and physical exam should prompt consultation of the relevant specialist and a low threshold for admission. In general, any visit to the ED by a VAD patient warrants a discussion with their specialist. Laboratory and radiographic modalities provide useful adjuncts to aid in diagnosis.

Laboratory Findings

Non-specific inflammatory markers such as C-reactive protein are elevated in CIED infections up to 96% of the time. Leukocytosis may be present, though one review of LVAD-associated infections found leukocytosis in only 50% of cases. Non-specific findings like anemia, renal insufficiency, and hypoalbuminemia are all associated with infections, but can also be due to comorbidities and so have limited diagnostic utility. Although it does not affect ED decision making, the most important diagnostic test is blood cultures. Two sets should be obtained in all patients with suspected device infection prior to antibiotic administration. Bacteremia even without localized signs can signify device involvement; however, when CIED patients are referred to the ED for positive blood cultures but no evidence of local infection, other sources of bacteremia should be investigated.

Radiographic Findings

Chest X-ray has limited utility, but may reveal an alternative diagnosis such as pneumonia, or may suggest septic pulmonary emboli or abscess. Most PPM and AICD infections are due to *Staphylococcus* species, which are also prone to causing endocarditis. Transthoracic echocardiography (TTE) has limited sensitivity, but may reveal a valve vegetation or a mass adherent to pacing wires. The fact that thrombus adherent to pacing wires may not be infected complicates the diagnosis. If TTE is not definitive, it is recommended that all patients with suspected CIED infection should undergo non-emergent transesophageal echocardiography (TEE) for further evaluation.

Treatment

A true cardiac device infection ultimately requires complete removal for definitive care. However, depending on the indication for the device, particularly in the case of ventricular assist devices, immediate removal is often not possible. Chronic antibiotic suppression therapy is indicated when devices cannot be removed. Suspected infections in the ED necessitate broad-spectrum empiric treatment after obtaining cultures, unless a recent culture is available for targeted therapy. Initial therapy for suspected PPM and AICD infections should include coverage for Methicillin-resistant *Staphylococcus* spp., usually with vancomycin. For patients with sepsis syndrome and VAD patients, anti-psuedomonal coverage is indicated.

A dilemma for the ED provider is whether localized signs of infection over a pulse generator site are due to a superficial or incision infection, or a true device infection, as the treatments are vastly different. While device infections necessitate removal of hardware or long-term suppression therapy, a superficial infection may be treated with 7 to 10 days of oral antibiotics and follow-up. Superficial or incisional infections overlying a generator pocket site presenting with a fluctuant, erythematous mass should generally not be incised or aspirated for cultures in the ED for concern of seeding and causing a device infection. Localized erythema and drainage may surround exiting VAD drivelines from local trauma alone, though this frequently does progress to true infection.

Complications and Admission Criteria

Numerous local complications may arise from an infected CIED. Cardiac or chest wall abscesses have been reported. Local extension into the mediastinum may provoke an infectious mediastinitis. Similarly, spread into surrounding bony structures may result in clavicular or thoracic osteomyelitis. Venous thrombosis or septic thrombophlebitis, particularly of the internal jugular, with associated bacteremia, can occur. Specific to VADs, infection surrounding the pump-pocket or exiting drivelines is common. Valvular endocarditis or endocarditis arising from pacer leads accounts for roughly 10% of CIED infections.

Virtually any distal site of infection may arise from an infected CIED due to septic emboli. Infected right-sided leads can cause septic pulmonary emboli and multifocal pneumonia or a pulmonary abscess. Mycotic or bacterial pulmonary arterial aneurysms have been described. Skeletal infections include osteomyelitis, spinal diskitis, spinal epidural abscess, and septic arthritis. Deep soft tissue or muscle abscesses may occur. Similarly, renal emboli, infarction, abscess, and perinephric abscess can occur. Septic cranial emboli result in brain abscess or meningitis. Bacteremia may be associated with severe sepsis and septic shock.

The high mortality associated with CIED infections is due to the associated complications and the patients' dependence on their device. One study of confirmed PPM and AICD infections demonstrated a 6-month mortality rate of 18%, though the rate varies significantly across available evidence. LVAD infections carry a 5.5% 30-day mortality and 40% 2-year mortality. Long-term survival is especially dismal in VAD fungal infections.

Because of the need for empiric intravenous antibiotics and high associated complication and mortality rate, suspected cardiac device infections require inpatient admission until infection is either confirmed or sufficiently ruled out. It may be appropriate to trial outpatient management, in consultation with the cardiologist, in cases of apparent superficial infection.

Pearls and Pitfalls

1. Vague presenting complaints in a patient with a CIED should raise suspicion of an underlying infection.
2. In suspected cases, always obtain blood cultures prior to initiation of broad spectrum antibiotics.
3. The initial antibiotic in the ED should cover MRSA (usually vancomycin). In unstable or septic patients, additional broad-spectrum antibiotics with *Pseudomonas* coverage should be provided.
4. Patients on chronic antibiotic suppression therapy may still develop CIED-associated complications due to resistance mechanisms.
5. Outpatient oral antibiotics are reasonable only when a superficial infection is present.
6. Avoid incision or aspiration of apparently superficial infections overlying the pulse generator.
7. Whenever possible, manage these cases in consultation with a cardiologist who is responsible for the device.

Table 3.2 Infectious Complications

Local	Systemic	VAD-Specific
Superficial wound infection	Septic emboli	Driveline infection
Generator-pocket infection	Left-sided endocarditis	Pump-pocket infection
Right-sided endocarditis	Osteomyelitis	
Chest wall abscess	Spinal epidural abscess	
Septic thrombophlebitis	Septic arthritis	
Mediastinitis	Muscle abscess	
	Sepsis	

References

Athan, E., Chu, V. H., Tattevin, P., *et al.* Clinical characteristics and outcome of infective endocarditis involving implantable cardiac devices. *JAMA* 2012; 307(16): 1727–35.

Baman, T. S., Gupta, S. K., Valle, J. A., and Yamada, E. Risk factors for mortality in patients with cardiac device-related infection. *Circ. Arrhythm. Electrophysiol.* 2009; 2(2): 129–34.

Baddour, L. M., Epstein, A. E., Erickson, C. C., *et al.* Update on cardiovascular implantable device infections and their management: a scientific statement from the American Heart Association. *Circulation* 2010; 121(3); 458–77.

Cabell, C. H., Heidenreich, P. A., Chu, V. H., *et al.* Increasing rates of cardiac device infections among Medicare beneficiaries: 1990–1999. *Am. Heart J.* 2004; 147(4): 582–6.

Darouiche, R. O. Device-associated infections: a macroproblem that starts with microadherence. *Clin. Infect. Dis.* 2001; 33(9): 1567–72.

Gordon, S. M., Schmitt, S. K., Jacobs, M., *et al.* Nosocomial bloodstream infections in patients with implantable left ventricular assist devices. *Ann. Thorac. Surg.* 2001; 72(3): 725–30.

Klug, D., Balde, M., Pavin, D., *et al.* Risk factors related to infections of implanted pacemakers and cardioverter-defibrillators: results of a large prospective study. *Circulation.* 2007; 116(12): 1349–55.

Kojic, E. M. and Darouiche, R. O. *Candida* infections of medical devices. *Clin. Microbiol. Rev.* 2004; 17(2): 255–67.

Lampropulos, J. F., Kim, N., Wang, Y., *et al.* Trends in left ventricular assist device use and outcomes among Medicare beneficiaries, 2004–2011. *Open Heart* 2014; 1: doi:10.1136/openhrt-2014-000109.

Le, K. Y., Sohail, M. R., Friedman, P. A., *et al.* Impact of timing of device removal on mortality in patients with cardiovascular implantable electronic device infections. *Heart Rhythm* 2011; 8(11): 1678–85.

Maniar, S., Kondareddy, S., and Topkara, V. Left ventricular assist device-related infections: past, present and future. *Expert Rev. Med. Devices* 2011; 8(5): 627–34.

Mela, T., McGovern, B. A., Garan, H., *et al.* Long-term infection rates associated with pectoral versus abdominal approach to cardioverter-defibrillator implants. *Am. J. Cardiol.* 2001; 88(7): 750–3.

Monkowski, D. H., Axelrod, P., Fekete, T., *et al.* Infections associated with ventricular assist devices: epidemiology and effect on prognosis after implantation. *Transpl. Infect. Dis.* 2007; 9(2): 114–20.

Nienaber, J. J., Kusne, S., Riaz, T., *et al.* Clinical manifestations and management of left ventricular assist device-associated infections. *Clin. Infect. Dis.* 2013; 57(10): 1438–48.

Sandoe, J. A., Barlow, G., Chambers, J. B., *et al.* Guidelines for the diagnosis, prevention and management of implantable cardiac electronic device infection. Report of a joint Working Party project on behalf of the British Society for Antimicrobial Chemotherapy, British Heart Rhythm Society, British Cardiovascular society, British Heart Valve Society and British Society for Echocardiography. *J. Antimicrob. Chemother.* 2015; 70(2): 325–59.

Sohail, M. R., Uslan, D. Z., Khan, A. H., *et al.* Management and outcome of permanent and implantable cardioverter-defibrillator infections. *J. Am. Coll. Cardiol.* 2007; 49(18): 1851–9.

Sohail, M. R., Uslan, D. Z., Khan, A. H., *et al.* Infective endocarditis complicating permanent pacemaker and implantable cardioverter-defibrillator infection. *Mayo Clin. Proc.* 2008; 83(1): 46–53.

Voigt, A., Shalaby, A., and Saba, S. Rising rates of cardiac rhythm management device infections in the United States: 1996 through 2003. *J. Am. Coll. Cardiol.* 2006; 48(3): 590–1.

Zhan, C., Baine, W. B., Sedrakyan, A., and Steiner, C. Cardiac device implantation in the United States from 1997 through 2004: a population-based analysis. *J. Gen. Intern. Med.* 2007; 23(Suppl. 1): 13–19.

Altered Mental Status in HIV-Infected Patients

Nisha Bhatia and Cheryl A. Jay

Introduction

Patients who test positive for human immunodeficiency virus (HIV) are vulnerable to developing altered mental status (AMS). The increased risk is related to HIV itself, the accompanying immune dysfunction, major systemic illness, comorbid psychiatric disorders, and complicated medication regimens. Combination antiretroviral therapy (ART) has decreased the incidence of central nervous system (CNS) opportunistic infections (OIs) and HIV-associated dementia, but the beneficial effects are not absolute. Moreover, patients with undiagnosed or untreated HIV infection may present with AMS. In addition to CNS OIs and complications of complex multisystem disease, immune reconstitution events developing in the early weeks and months after initiating ART may affect the brain and cause AMS.

Epidemiology

Before ART became the standard of HIV care in resource-rich countries, approximately half of HIV-infected patients developed symptomatic central or peripheral nervous system disease, with neuropathology observed in nearly all individuals dying with HIV/acquired immunodeficiency syndrome (AIDS). Since the advent of ART, the incidence of dementia, the major cerebral OIs (cryptococcal meningitis, toxoplasmosis, progressive multifocal leukoencephalopathy), and primary CNS lymphoma has fallen. HIV-associated dementia is also less common among patients on ART and milder and more indolent than before. In the United States, fewer patients now develop the mutism, quadriparesis, and incontinence that were typically seen in the early years of the AIDS epidemic.

Clinical Features

As with any patient with AMS presenting to the emergency department (ED) for evaluation, important elements of the history include the temporal progression of symptoms, drug use (prescription, over-the-counter, illicit), trauma, and in particular focal symptoms (aphasia, neglect, hemianopsia, hemiparesis, hemisensory loss), seizures, or symptoms suggesting increased intracranial pressure (ICP), such as progressive or morning headache.

Additional important details in the HIV-infected patient include recent and nadir CD4 counts, viral load, and, for patients on ART, the specific agents that comprise the patient's regimen and the duration of therapy. Regardless of treatment history, patients with CD4 counts below 200/mm³ are at highest risk for cerebral OIs, primary CNS lymphoma, and HIV-associated dementia. Patients with prior cerebral toxoplasmosis or cryptococcal meningitis require secondary prophylaxis unless ART increases CD4 counts to greater than 200/mm³ for 3 months; consequently, a patient with a history of either of these cerebral OIs, low CD4 count, and poor medication adherence presenting with AMS may be experiencing a relapse.

For patients recently begun on ART, additional diagnostic considerations include medication side effects (e.g. efavirenz) or immune reconstitution inflammatory syndrome (IRIS). Patients with CD4 counts above 200/mm³ may be at risk for major HIV-related brain disorders if treatment was begun within the past 6 months or if there is evidence of treatment failure, such as falling CD4 count, rising viral load, or both.

An important concept in evaluating HIV-infected patients with AMS, particularly at lower CD4 counts, is that the immune dysfunction that predisposes to cerebral infections also masks

Table 4.1 Key Points in Recognizing Subtle CNS Infections in Advanced HIV Disease

- Absence of fever or headache does not exclude cerebral infections.
- Absence of meningismus does not exclude meningitis.
- Neurological exam should focus on identifying increased ICP and focal cerebral dysfunction.

Table 4.2 Differential Diagnosis of AMS in the High-Risk HIV Population

IDU	• Drug intoxication or withdrawal • Endocarditis with septic encephalopathy • Ischemic (septic embolism) or hemorrhagic (mycotic aneurysm rupture) stroke • Brain abscess or meningitis
Cocaine and methamphetamine	• Seizures • Ischemic or hemorrhagic strokes
Medications	Prescription: • Efavirenz • Psychotropic drugs • Opiates and other analgesics Non-prescription: • Antihistamines • Ethanol (intoxication or withdrawal) Illicit: • Heroin • Stimulants • Other drugs of abuse
Multisystem disease	• Uremic encephalopathy • Hepatic encephalopathy • Electrolyte abnormalities
Focal cerebral dysfunction	See Table 4.2
Diffuse cerebral dysfunction	See Table 4.3
IDU – injection drug user.	

the symptoms and signs associated with similar disorders in immunocompetent individuals.

In particular, the absence of fever or headache should not be used to exclude CNS infection, nor should the absence of meningismus be used to exclude meningitis on clinical grounds (see Table 4.1). Neurologic examination should focus on identifying evidence of increased ICP (anisocoria, papilledema) or focal cerebral dysfunction, such as visual field deficit, lateralized motor (pronator drift, hemiparesis, reflex asymmetry, unilateral Babinski sign) or sensory deficit, and, in patients alert enough to walk, gait disorder.

The history and physical exam should also be aimed at categorizing the AMS as a manifestation of focal cerebral dysfunction or diffuse cerebral dysfunction, because this approach will help narrow the long list of HIV-specific conditions (see Tables 4.3 and 4.4).

Differential Diagnosis

HIV-positive patients are often at high risk for non-infectious causes of altered mental status. Acute care providers need to maintain a broad differential diagnosis for the cause of acute altered mental status in the high-risk HIV population. A careful history and physical exam may reveal one or more of the etiologies listed in Table 4.2. Whether the patient's AMS appears to be a manifestation of focal or diffuse cerebral dysfunction helps focus the long list of diagnostic considerations.

Focal Cerebral Dysfunction

Patients with signs or symptoms suggesting lateralized brain disturbance may have AMS by several mechanisms, which can coexist in a given patient (see Table 4.3). Brainstem or cerebellar lesions may impair level of alertness early. Patients with solitary hemispheric lesions are awake unless there is significant mass effect or concomitant meningitis or toxic-metabolic encephalopathy. Dominant hemisphere lesions cause aphasia (often with associated right homonymous hemianopsia, hemiparesis, or hemisensory loss) and non-dominant hemisphere processes cause neglect or inattention with left-sided visual, motor, or sensory dysfunction. Patients with old focal brain lesions, such as prior trauma, stroke, tumor, or infection, may experience a worsening of stable focal deficits with drug intoxication, metabolic derangement, meningitis, or after a seizure. In general, CNS OIs and primary CNS lymphoma are more common in patients with CD4 below $200/mm^3$, whereas cerebrovascular disease (which may complicate CNS infection, particularly tuberculosis [TB] or syphilitic meningitis) is more common in HIV-positive patients with focal cerebral deficit at higher CD4 counts.

Diffuse Cerebral Dysfunction

Patients with depressed level of alertness or milder cognitive or behavioral disturbances without aphasia, neglect, or lateralizing motor, reflex, or sensory findings may have multiple brain lesions, meningitis, delirium, psychiatric decompensation, or had an unwitnessed seizure (see Table 4.4). Dementia is a risk factor for delirium, but dementia alone does not cause depressed level of alertness (lethargy, obtundation, or stupor) except in its very advanced stages.

Other Causes of Altered Mental Status

In up to 40% of patients, the first weeks and months after initiation of ART may be complicated by the immune reconstitution inflammatory syndrome (IRIS), with paradoxical

Table 4.3 Clinical Features: Focal Cerebral Dysfunction in HIV/AIDS

Common Etiologies of Focal Dysfunction (usually CD4 <200/mm³)	
Cerebral toxoplasmosis	• Altered mental status, focal cerebral symptoms, or seizure usually evolving over days to weeks, often with fever and headache
	• Reactivation of previously acquired, often asymptomatic, infection with the parasite *Toxoplasma gondii*
	• Unusual in patients on trimethoprim-sulfamethoxazole for *Pneumocystis* prophylaxis, because the drug also provides primary prophylaxis against toxoplasmosis
Progressive multifocal leukoencephalopathy (PML)	• Focal deficit, often homonymous hemianopsia or hemiparesis, steadily progressive over months without headache or fever
	• Reactivation of previously acquired, often asymptomatic, infection with the JC virus
Primary CNS lymphoma	• Gradually progressive focal deficit or cognitive dysfunction, sometimes with headache, evolving over months
	• Almost always associated with EBV in tumor cells in HIV-positive patients
Less Common Infectious Causes	
CMV ventriculoencephalitis	• CD4 <100
	• Cognitive impairment with brainstem findings (cranial neuropathies, ataxia)
	• Sometimes associated with polyradiculitis (cauda equina syndrome with paraparesis, incontinence, and hyporeflexia) evolving over days to weeks
	• CSF profile may resemble bacterial meningitis with elevated protein, polymorphonuclear pleocytosis, and low or normal glucose
Brain abscess (bacterial or fungal)	• Progressive focal cerebral deficit, with or without headache
	• Consider in patients with proven or suspected bacteremia (injection drug use, indwelling line, chronic skin infection, prosthetic heart valve) or craniofacial infection
	• Consider angioinvasive fungi (*Mucor* or *Aspergillus*, discussed below) in patients with CD4 <50 and associated sinus infection
Tuberculoma	• Presentation similar to brain abscess
	• Rare, but may develop as immune reconstitution inflammatory syndrome in patients on antituberculous therapy for systemic TB (or tuberculous meningitis) in the first weeks to months of ART
Stroke	
Meningovascular syphilis	• Occurs with or after secondary syphilis as ischemic stroke(s) with or without clinically apparent meningitis
Angioinvasive fungi (*Aspergillus*, *Mucor*)	• CD4 <50, associated sinus infection or palatal lesion or brain abscess, in addition to hemorrhagic or ischemic stroke(s)
VZV vasculopathy	• Multiple small-vessel strokes with recent or remote history of shingles
Bacterial endocarditis	• Septic embolism (infarction, abscess, or both), mycotic aneurysm rupture, bacterial meningitis

CMV – cytomegalovirus; CSF – cerebrospinal fluid; EBV – Epstein-Barr virus; JC virus – John Cunningham virus; VZV – varicella-zoster virus.

worsening of previously diagnosed or subclinical OIs or development of autoimmune disorders. IRIS affects most organ systems, including the brain. Patients with tuberculosis may be at particular risk of IRIS, and tuberculous meningitis or tuberculoma are among the reported manifestations. In the setting of immune reconstitution, clinical exacerbation of cryptococcal meningitis, worsening PML, and rapidly progressive dementia have been described. IRIS should be considered when patients develop AMS in the first several months after starting ART.

Patients with HIV are at increased risk for substance abuse, affective disorders, and psychosis. Injection drug users with HIV remain at risk for the neurologic sequelae of endocarditis, including ischemic stroke from septic embolism, hemorrhagic stroke from mycotic aneurysm rupture, brain abscess, and meningitis. Additionally, HIV patients who use cocaine or methamphetamine are at risk for seizures and ischemic and hemorrhagic stroke.

Medications used to treat HIV disease or associated conditions may also contribute to AMS. Antiretroviral agents, particularly the non-nucleoside reverse transcriptase inhibitor efavirenz, can cause cerebral side effects, including psychiatric syndromes, as can the myriad other drugs used to treat HIV/AIDS and comorbid medical conditions.

Finally, as a multisystem illness, HIV infection can cause AMS even without primary neurologic, psychiatric, or iatrogenic illness. For example, patients with HIV-associated nephropathy are subject to the neurologic complications of uremia, including encephalopathy. Patients coinfected with hepatitis C are at risk for hepatic encephalopathy with advanced liver disease or cognitive dysfunction even in the absence of cirrhosis and portal hypertension.

Laboratory and Radiographic Findings

Initial evaluation proceeds as for any patient with AMS, with particular attention to evidence of increased ICP, first-time seizure, trauma, or focal cerebral deficit (see Table 4.5).

Appropriate laboratory studies include electrolytes, blood urea nitrogen (BUN) and creatinine, liver function tests, complete blood count (CBC), prothrombin time, and toxicology screen.

Table 4.4 Clinical Features: Diffuse Cerebral Dysfunction in HIV/AIDS

Common Etiologies of Diffuse Dysfunction (usually CD4 <200/mm³)	
HIV-associated dementia	• Cognitive, behavioral, and motor slowing over months with hyperreflexia and, in more advanced disease, gait disturbance • More common in patients with untreated HIV disease • Alertness is typically preserved except in end-stage dementia or if there is a coexisting cause for altered mental status
Cryptococcal meningitis	• Most common complaint is mild to moderate headache • Some patients present with symptomatic increased intracranial pressure, including coma • Severe headache with prominent meningismus is unusual, except as a manifestation of immune reconstitution inflammatory syndrome
Less Common Types of Meningitis	
Tuberculous meningitis	• Usually presents as chronic meningitis with typical symptoms (headache, meningismus, altered mental status, cranial neuropathies), sometimes with small-vessel ischemic stroke • Risk of extrapulmonary disease, including meningitis or tuberculoma, is increased in HIV-positive patients • May present as immune reconstitution event in patients with systemic TB or as exacerbation of TB meningitis (in the first weeks to months of ART)
Syphilitic meningitis	• Occurs weeks to years after primary infection, usually as an aseptic or chronic meningitis with or without cranial neuropathies • May be complicated by ischemic stroke (meningovascular syphilis), seizures, or hydrocephalus
Lymphomatous meningitis	• Presents as headache, altered mental status, cranial neuropathies, or cauda equina syndrome, individually or in combination • Usually with history of systemic lymphoma, though may occasionally be presenting feature
Bacterial meningitis	• Consider *Listeria monocytogenes*, in addition to pneumococcus and meningococcus.
Other Etiologies of Diffuse Dysfunction	
Multifocal brain disease	• Toxoplasmosis and Primary CNS Lymphoma may occasionally present as diffuse brain dysfunction
Drug ingestion	• Prescription: efavirenz, psychotropic drugs, opiates and other analgesics, among many others • Non-prescription: antihistamines, ethanol • Illicit: heroin, stimulants, and other drugs of abuse
Metabolic encephalopathies	• Renal or hepatic failure, electrolyte abnormalities (in particular sodium, calcium), hypo- or hyperglycemia, hypothyroidism, B12 deficiency

Although magnetic resonance imaging (MRI) is more sensitive for many HIV-related cerebral disorders, multidetector computed tomographic (CT) scanners are preferable for agitated and otherwise unstable patients.

Studies of the yield of non-contrast CT in HIV-infected patients presenting to the ED with neurologic dysfunction indicate that AMS was significantly associated with abnormal findings on CT.

For patients with CD4 count less than 200/mm³, who are at highest risk for HIV-related cerebral complications, CT with and without contrast can sometimes obviate the need for lumbar puncture (LP) if the findings suggest toxoplasmosis (see Figure 4.1), primary CNS lymphoma (see Figure 4.2), or PML (see Figure 4.3).

Whereas neuroradiologic findings in PML are relatively distinct, toxoplasmosis and primary CNS lymphoma can be difficult to distinguish definitively, even by MRI. In patients with meningitis, CT may reveal complications such as edema, infarction, or obstructive or communicating hydrocephalus.

If there are contraindications to iodinated contrast, non-contrast CT can identify hydrocephalus, hemorrhage, or large mass lesions that would contraindicate lumbar puncture.

Patients with mass lesions should have serum *Toxoplasma* IgG antibodies sent, because a negative serology significantly decreases the likelihood that mass lesions are due to *T. gondii*.

If laboratory studies have not revealed the cause of the patient's AMS and CT reveals no contraindication to LP, cerebrospinal fluid (CSF) examination should be performed. In addition to opening pressure, CSF should be sent for protein, glucose, cell count, cryptococcal antigen, and venereal disease research laboratory (VDRL) serology, as well as for bacterial, fungal, and acid-fast bacillus (AFB) smears and cultures. If possible, additional CSF should be obtained and held in the laboratory for possible polymerase chain reaction (PCR) testing for JC virus (PML), EBV, primary CNS lymphoma, or herpes viruses (cytomegalovirus [CMV], varicella-zoster virus [VZV], herpes simplex virus).

The CSF opening pressure is critical for the management of cryptococcal meningitis, because increased ICP (>200 mm H_2O) contributes to the morbidity and mortality associated with the infection. Markedly elevated ICP may require serial LPs, lumbar drainage, or ventriculoperitoneal shunting; measurement of initial opening pressure at the time of admission is very helpful in guiding subsequent management. Acetazolamide and steroids do not have a role in ICP management in HIV-associated cryptococcal meningitis.

Table 4.5 Selected HIV-Related Brain Disorders: Neuroimaging, CSF

Cerebral toxoplasmosis	• Toxoplasma IgG positive: serologic screening is part of routine HIV care, so results may be available in patients with established HIV diagnosis
	• CT/MRI (see Figure 4.1): ring-enhancing lesions with marked surrounding edema in basal ganglia or cortical/subcortical junction
	• Enhancing lesions with negative *Toxoplasma* serology are more likely to be other infectious cause or primary CNS lymphoma
	• LP may be contraindicated, depending on imaging results: elevated protein, normal glucose, lymphocytic/monocytic pleocytosis; *Toxoplasma* serologies usually not done routinely
Primary CNS lymphoma	• CT/MRI (see Figure 4.2): homogeneously enhancing lesion or lesions in periventricular regions or corpus callosum, with mild to moderate surrounding edema
	• LP may be contraindicated, depending on imaging results: elevated protein, normal glucose (unless associated lymphomatous meningitis, in which case glucose may be low), lymphocytic pleocytosis, sometimes with positive EBV PCR or more rarely cytology
PML	• CT/MRI (see Figure 4.3): non-enhancing, asymmetric white matter lesion or lesions, often in parietal or occipital white matter, without surrounding edema in most patients. May be confused with ischemic stroke – sparing of cortical ribbon in PML is a helpful clue
	• Patients who have just started ART and have IRIS may have atypical imaging findings of enhancement and mass effect
	• LP: elevated protein, normal glucose, mild lymphocytic pleocytosis, positive JC virus PCR
Cryptococcal meningitis	• CT/MRI: normal (or generalized atrophy) or may show hydrocephalus or cerebral edema
	• LP: elevated opening pressure, normal or elevated protein, normal or low glucose, lymphocytic pleocytosis, positive cryptococcal antigen
HIV-associated dementia	• CT/MRI: generalized atrophy with mild, symmetric periventricular white matter abnormalities especially bifrontally
	• LP: normal opening pressure, normal or elevated protein (<100 mg/dL), normal glucose, mild lymphocytic pleocytosis
Tuberculous meningitis	• CT/MRI: normal or basilar enhancement, hydrocephalus or small-vessel infarctions
	• LP: elevated opening pressure, elevated protein, low glucose, lymphocytic pleocytosis; negative AFB smear does not exclude diagnosis and cultures are not always positive
Syphilitic meningitis	• CT/MRI: normal or basilar enhancement, sometimes with infarction (meningovascular syphilis)
	• LP: normal or elevated opening pressure, elevated protein, normal or low glucose, lymphocytic pleocytosis; CSF VDRL is ≤70% sensitive, so diagnosis may depend on positive serum serology with compatible CSF profile and overall clinical picture
CMV ventriculoencephalitis	• CT/MRI: normal or periventricular enhancement, with or without hydrocephalus
	• LP: may resemble bacterial meningitis with elevated protein, polymorphonuclear pleocytosis, and low or normal glucose, positive CMV PCR

Patients whose altered mental status remains unexplained after blood work, CT, and CSF examination may require electroencephalogram (EEG) to exclude non-convulsive status epilepticus.

CSF cryptococcal antigen is very informative because the sensitivity exceeds 95%. India ink smear is specific, but not sensitive, and cultures may take weeks or months to grow the organism. Similar considerations apply in tuberculous meningitis; hence a negative CSF AFB smear or prior negative CSF culture does not exclude the diagnosis. Typical CSF findings of chronic meningitis (markedly elevated protein, normal or low glucose, and lymphocytic pleocytosis) are not always seen in cryptococcal meningitis in the setting of HIV disease. Routine CSF studies (protein, glucose, cell count) may occasionally be entirely normal in cryptococcal meningitis, highlighting the importance of the cryptococcal antigen as a diagnostic test. In patients who refuse LP or have other contraindications to the procedure, serum cryptococcal antigen can be useful because it is only rarely negative in cryptococcal meningitis.

One challenge in interpreting CSF results from patients with HIV infection is the high prevalence of mild protein elevation (<100 mg/dL) and lymphocytic pleocytosis (<50/mm³), particularly in patients with CD4 counts above 50/mm³ or who are not on ART. More marked abnormalities in CSF protein or cell count, low glucose, or polymorphonuclear pleocytosis at any CD4 count warrants investigation for causes other than HIV, as does pleocytosis in patients with CD4 count below 50/mm³ or whose HIV disease is well controlled on ART. If the CSF profile resembles bacterial meningitis, with elevated protein, polymorphonuclear pleocytosis, and low or normal glucose, an additional diagnostic consideration, particularly in patients with CD4 counts less than 50/mm³, is CMV ventriculoencephalitis. In such patients, CT may be normal or reveal mild hydrocephalus, periventricular enhancement, or both. CSF polymerase chain reaction for CMV nucleic acids can establish the diagnosis.

Complications and Admission Criteria

Except for patients with a secure diagnosis of a rapidly reversible and definitively treatable toxic-metabolic encephalopathy, such as hypoglycemia or opiate overdose, or seizure with full recovery (and negative work-up), most patients with AMS and HIV disease require admission for further evaluation and management. Patients with focal CNS infection, meningitis, or primary CNS lymphoma are at risk for seizures and

Left **Center** **Right**

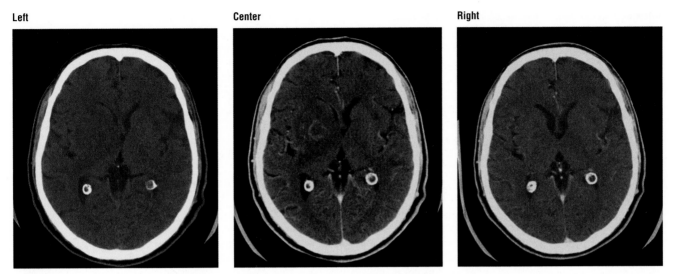

Figure 4.1 Cerebral toxoplasmosis. Head CT pre- (left) and post- (center) from a patient who presented with headache, speech difficulty, and left arm weakness demonstrated a ring-enhancing lesion with surrounding edema in the right globus pallidus (and a smaller lesion in the left temporal lobe not seen on this image). HIV serology came back positive, with positive *Toxoplasma* IgG. The patient's headache and focal deficits resolved with empiric therapy for toxoplasmosis. Repeat post-contrast head CT 2 months later (right) showed decreased edema and resolution of abnormal enhancement.

Left **Right**

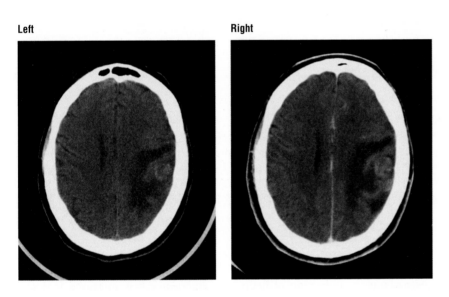

Figure 4.2 Primary CNS lymphoma. Head CT pre- (left) and post- (right) contrast from an untreated AIDS patient who presented with a generalized seizure after a week of dysarthria and right-sided weakness and numbness demonstrated an intrinsically hyperdense left frontoparietal lesion with mass effect and slight homogeneous enhancement. *Toxoplasma* serology was negative, and brain biopsy revealed primary CNS lymphoma.

Left **Right**

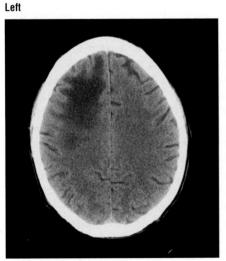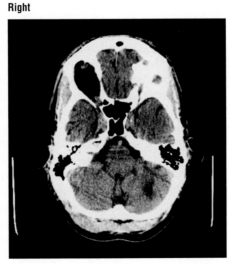

Figure 4.3 Progressive multifocal leukoencephalopathy. Non-contrast head CT from an AIDS patient with left-sided weakness showed a right frontal white matter lesion without mass effect (left) and a clinically silent lesion in the left cerebellar white matter (right). The lesions were not enhanced on gadolinium MRI (not shown). Brain biopsy confirmed the presumptive diagnosis of PML.

Table 4.6 Initial Treatment of Selected CNS Infections in HIV/AIDS

Cerebral toxoplasmosis	Pyrimethamine 200 mg PO × 1, followed by 50 mg PO daily (≤ 60 kg), or 75 mg PO daily (≥ 60 kg) *plus* Sulfadiazine 1 g PO QID (≤ 60 kg) or 1.5 g PO QID (≥ 60 kg) *plus* Leucovorin 10–25 mg PO daily (pyrimethamine hematologic toxicity prophylaxis) *For patients with a sulfonamide allergy, substitute sulfadiazine with:* Clindamycin 600 mg PO/IV QID • Consult infectious diseases specialist for patients with antibiotic allergies or who cannot take oral medications • Anticonvulsants should be administered only to patients with a history of toxoplasmosis and seizures, not recommended as prophylaxis
Cryptococcal meningitis	Liposomal amphotericin B 3–4 mg/kg/dose IV daily *plus* Flucytosine 25 mg/kg/dose PO QID (caution if significant marrow failure) for at least 2 weeks, followed by fluconazole 400 mg PO daily for a minimum of 8 weeks • Consult infectious disease specialist for patients with renal insufficiency and starting antiretroviral treatment • Consider high-dose oral fluconazole >800 mg (1200 mg preferred) PO daily, with flucytosine 25 mg/kg/dose PO QID (caution if significant marrow failure) for patients without intravenous access or who decline admission • Start ART 14 days after induction therapy
PML	• None (ART in treatment-naive patients)
Tuberculous meningitis	• Four-drug therapy; consult infectious disease specialist due to complex drug–drug interactions between many antituberculous drugs, particularly rifampin, and many ART regimens • Start adjunctive intravenous dexamethasone 0.3–0.4 mg/kg/day tapered over 6–8 weeks or prednisone 1 mg/kg/day for 2 weeks tapered over 6–8 weeks as soon as possible.
Neurosyphilis	• Penicillin G 3–4 million units IV every 4 hours × 10–14 days *or* • Procaine penicillin G 2.4 million units IM once daily *plus* • Probenecid 500 mg PO QID × 10–14 days
VZV encephalitis	• Acyclovir 10–15 mg/kg/dose IV every 8 hours
CMV encephalitis	• Ganciclovir with or without foscarnet or cidofovir; consult infectious disease specialist
Bacterial meningitis	• Consider adjunctive dexamethasone, with first or prior to initial dose of antibiotics, 0.15 mg/kg/dose IV every 6 hours for proven or suspected pneumococcal meningitis • Cover for *Listeria monocytogenes* (ampicillin), in addition to meningococcus and pneumococcus (ceftriaxone and vancomycin) • See Chapter 78 for detailed antibiotic recommendations for empiric bacterial meningitis treatment in immunosuppressed patients

IM – intramuscular; IV – intravenous; PO – by mouth.

increased ICP. Antiepileptic drugs (AEDs) are not given as routine prophylaxis without a documented seizure. Elevated ICP may develop as a consequence of focal or generalized cerebral edema, hydrocephalus, or both. Patients with meningitis may develop cranial neuropathies, and ischemic stroke may complicate syphilitic, tuberculous, or acute bacterial meningitis. Additional considerations in patients with CNS infection or lymphoma who decompensate in the ED during evaluation or while awaiting hospitalization include medication effects, unwitnessed seizure, or intercurrent electrolyte disorder, particularly hyponatremia from the syndrome of inappropriate antidiuretic hormone secretion or cerebral salt wasting, or hypernatremia from diabetes insipidus.

Treatment and Prophylaxis

Therapy will depend on the cause of altered mental status, and may not always be started in the ED for HIV-related cerebral OIs if there is significant diagnostic uncertainty and no indication of neurologic emergency (e.g. increased ICP, seizure, bacterial meningitis, or acute stroke) (see Table 4.6).

Increased ICP is managed in the usual fashion, as is status epilepticus. The recurrence risk for seizures in patients with HIV disease appears to be higher than in seronegative patients; hence it is reasonable to consider AED therapy for a single seizure, in the absence of an obvious toxic-metabolic precipitant such as ethanol or other sedative-hypnotic withdrawal, cocaine or methamphetamine use, hypoglycemia, hyponatremia, hypocalcemia, and so forth. That decision is particularly complicated in patients on ART, because first-line AEDs such as phenytoin and carbamazepine, as hepatic enzyme inducers, have adverse drug–drug interactions with most ART regimens. Failure of antiretroviral therapy has been reported in this context, highlighting the importance of prescribing very carefully in patients on ART. Newer AEDs such as lamotrigine, levetiracetam, and lacosamide may be used, but with careful consideration of potential interactions with the current antiretroviral treatment regimen, generally in consultation with an HIV specialist.

In tuberculous meningitis, treatment with intravenous steroids should be started as early as possible with change to oral therapy according to clinical improvement. The use of steroids in bacterial meningitis remains controversial; however, patients with pneumococcal and *Hemophilus influenzae* meningitis may benefit from adjuvant steroid therapy.

Infection Control

Other than usual universal precautions and consideration of respiratory isolation in patients with proven or suspected TB, no additional infection control measures are required in HIV-positive patients with AMS.

Pearls and Pitfalls

1. Key elements of the history in HIV-infected patients with AMS are recent and nadir CD4 count, recent viral load, prior neurologic or psychiatric disorders, and detailed medication history, including antibiotic use and allergies, illicit and other non-prescribed drugs, and duration of ART.

2. AMS in the first weeks to months of ART should prompt consideration of a medication-related effect if efavirenz is one of the prescribed drugs or an immune reconstitution event occurs such as tuberculous or cryptococcal meningitis or PML.

3. For patients experiencing AMS from efavirenz, modifications to ART should be discussed with the patient's HIV provider or an infectious disease consultant.

4. The risk of major cerebral opportunistic infections and malignancies is highest for patients with CD4 $<200/mm^3$. The absence of headache, fever, or meningismus should not be used to exclude these diagnoses on clinical grounds.

5. Non-contrast head CT is indicated in the evaluation of AMS in HIV-positive patients; contrast-enhanced CT should be considered in patients with CD4 $<200/mm^3$ or symptoms or signs of focal cerebral dysfunction.

6. Cerebral toxoplasmosis is a common cause of fever and focal cerebral dysfunction in patients with AIDS and ring-enhancing lesions on neuroimaging studies; *Toxoplasma* IgG serology is usually positive.

7. AIDS patients with headache with or without altered mental status, non-focal examination, and absence of focal abnormalities on neuroimaging may have cryptococcal meningitis.

8. Serum cryptococcal antigen can help suggest or exclude the diagnosis in patients who refuse or have other contraindications to lumbar puncture.

9. Medications should be prescribed carefully for patients on ART, because of numerous complex drug–drug interactions, particularly for hepatic enzyme-inducing agents such as older antiepileptic drugs and rifampin.

References

Birbeck, G. L., French, J. A., Perucca, E., *et al.* Antiepileptic drug selection for people with HIV/AIDS: evidence-based guidelines from the ILAE and AAN. *Epilepsia* 2012; 53(1): 207–14.

Chang, C. C., Sheikh, V., Sereti, I., and French, M. A. Immune reconstitution disorders in patients with HIV infection: from pathogenesis to prevention and treatment. *Curr. HIV/AIDS Rep.* 2014; 11(3): 223–32.

Kirmani, B. F. and Mungall-Robinson, D. Role of anticonvulsants in the management of AIDS related seizures. *Front. Neurol.* 2014; 5: 10.

Kranick, S. M. and Nath, A. Neurologic complications of HIV-1 infection and its treatment in the era of antiretroviral therapy. *Continuum (Minneapolis, MN)* 2012; 18(6 Infectious Disease): 1319–37.

McArthur, J. and Smith, B. Neurologic complications and considerations in HIV-infected persons. *Curr. Infect. Dis. Rep.* 2013; 15(1): 61–6.

McNicholl, I. R. and Peiperl, L. (eds.). HIV InSite Database of Antiretroviral Drug Interactions, http://hivinsite.ucsf.edu/arvdb?page=ar-0002 (accessed December 3, 2014).

Panel on Opportunistic Infections in HIV-Infected Adults and Adolescents. Guidelines for the prevention and treatment of opportunistic infections in HIV-infected adults and adolescents: recommendations from the Centers for Disease Control and Prevention, the National Institutes of Health, and the HIV Medicine Association of the Infectious Diseases Society of America, https://aidsinfo.nih.gov/contentfiles/lvguidelines/adult_oi.pdf (accessed March 8, 2018).

Perfect, J. R., Dismukes, W. E., Dromer, F., *et al.* Clinical practice guidelines for the management of cryptococcal disease: 2010 update by the Infectious Diseases Society of America. *Clin. Inf. Dis.* 2010; 50(3): 291–322.

Price, R. W., Spudich, S. S., Peterson, J., *et al.* Evolving character of chronic central nervous system HIV infection. *Semin. Neurol.* 2014; 34(1): 7–13.

Quagliarello, V. Adjunctive steroids for tuberculous meningitis – more evidence, more questions. *New Engl. J. Med.* 2004; 351(17): 1792–4.

Rothman, R. E., Keyl, P. M., McArthur, J. C., *et al.* A decision guideline for emergency department utilization of noncontrast head computerized tomography in HIV-infected patients. *Acad. Emerg. Med.* 1999; 6(10): 1010–19.

Snider, W. D., Simpson, D. M., Nielsen, S., *et al.* Neurological complications of acquired immune deficiency syndrome: analysis of 50 patients. *Ann. Neurol.* 1983; 14(4): 403–18.

Spudich, S. S., Nilsson, A. C., Lollo, N. D., *et al.* Cerebrospinal fluid HIV infection and pleocytosis: relation to systemic infection and antiretroviral treatment. *BMC Infect. Dis.* 2005; 5: 98.

Tate, D. F., Khedraki, R., McCaffrey, D., *et al.* The role of medical imaging in defining CNS abnormalities associated with HIV-infection and opportunistic infections. *Neurotherapeutics* 2011; 8(1): 103–16.

Treisman, G. J. and Kaplin, A. I. Neurologic and psychiatric complications of antiretroviral agents. *AIDS* 2002; 16(9): 1201–15.

Tso, E. L., Todd, W. C., Groleau, G. A., and Hooper, F. J. Cranial computed tomography in the emergency department evaluation of HIV-infected patients with neurologic complaints. *Ann. Emerg. Med.* 1993; 27: 70–7.

Tunkel, A. R., Hartman, B. J., Kaplan, S. L., *et al.* Practice guidelines for the management of bacterial meningitis. *Clin. Infect. Dis.* 2004; 39(9): 1267–84.

Botulism

David M. Stier and Mary P. Mercer

Introduction and Microbiology

Botulism is a disease caused by exposure to botulinum toxin produced from *Clostridium* species, mainly *Clostridium botulinum*. Clinical forms of the disease include foodborne, inhalational, wound, infant, adult intestinal toxemia, and iatrogenic. *C. botulinum* is a gram-positive, strictly anaerobic, spore-forming bacillus naturally found in soil and aquatic sediments. There are seven types of the toxin based on antigenic differences, labeled A through G. Types A, B, and E (and rarely, F) are pathogenic in humans. Types C, D, and E cause illness in other mammals, birds, and fish. Botulinum toxin lacks color, odor, and taste and is the most lethal toxin known. Death is caused by doses of less than 1 µg. Antibiotics have no activity against the toxin itself.

In response to unfavorable environmental conditions (changes in pH, temperature, and water or nutrient availability), *C. botulinum* bacteria "sporulate." *C. botulinum* spores are hardy, resistant to desiccation, heat, ultraviolet (UV) light, and alcohols, and can survive boiling for up to 4 hours; however, they are readily killed by chlorine-based disinfectants. Once spores encounter more favorable conditions, such as are found in contact with human tissues, they "germinate," thereby producing growing cells that are capable of reproducing and elaborating toxin.

The five predominant forms of botulism are:

- foodborne, in which pre-formed toxin is ingested most frequently occurring from home-canned foods
- infant botulism, the most common form, in which spores are ingested and bacteria then growing in the intestine produce the toxin
- adult intestinal toxemia, an extremely rare adult equivalent of infant botulism

- wound botulism, in which toxin is elaborated from an infected wound (also discussed in Chapter 61, Infectious Complications of Injection Drug Use and
- iatrogenic botulism, resulting from accidental overdose of injected medical botulinum toxin, most commonly used for cosmetic purposes

The Working Group for Civilian Biodefense considers botulism to be a dangerous potential biological weapon because of the pathogen's "extreme potency and lethality; its ease of production, transport, and misuse; and the need for prolonged intensive care among affected persons." Use of botulism as a biological weapon is expected to produce severe medical and public health outcomes.

Epidemiology
Naturally Occurring Botulism

Reservoirs

The sporulated form of the bacterium is commonly found in soils and aquatic sediments. Cistern water, dust, and foods, including honey, can become contaminated from contact with the soil.

Mode of Transmission

Botulism is caused by exposure to botulinum toxin. Humans can become infected in a number of ways:

- inhalation of toxin (inhalational)
- consumption of toxin (foodborne)
- consumption of *C. botulinum* spores (infant; adult intestinal toxemia)

- contamination of a tissue with *C. botulinum* spores (wound) and
- contamination of a tissue with toxin (iatrogenic)

Worldwide Occurrence

In the late 1700s, botulism emerged as a disease because of changes in sausage production in Europe. In fact, *botulus* means sausage. Soon thereafter in the early 1800s, botulism associated with consumption of fermented fish was recognized in Russia. Wound and infant botulism were discovered much later in the mid- to late 1900s. From 1999 to 2000, more than 2,500 cases of foodborne botulism were reported in Europe. The highest incidence is found in countries of the former Soviet Union and in Asia and is related to improper food handling. Type B is more common in Europe, whereas type E is more common in Scandinavia and Canada and is frequently linked to improper storage of fish and marine mammals.

Occurrence in the United States

In the United States, naturally occurring botulism is a rare disease with an annual incidence of under 200 cases. In the most recent year of Centers for Disease Control and Prevention (CDC) reporting for 2014, there were 163 reported cases (infant, 128; wound, 27; foodborne, 20; and unknown etiology, 2). More than half of foodborne cases occur in the western states of California, Oregon, Washington, Alaska, and Colorado. Type E is more common among Alaskan natives because of their diet of fermented meat from aquatic mammals and fish. Type A is found mainly in western states and type B is more common in the east. Most cases of wound botulism result from injection drug use with black tar heroin, which is more common in the western states. No case of iatrogenic botulism has been documented in the United States since 2004.

Botulinum Toxin as a Biological Weapon

State-sponsored military programs have researched and weaponized botulinum toxin dating back to the 1930s. Botulism has also been used as a weapon by a terrorist group. Unfortunately, botulism is ubiquitous in nature and therefore access to it cannot be easily controlled.

Likely modes of dissemination for toxin used as a weapon include:

- **Contamination of food or beverages.** Possible food or beverage vehicles for botulism toxin are those that are not heated at 85°C (185°F) for 5 minutes before consumption or those that are contaminated after appropriate heating. Typical pasteurization does not remove all toxin.
- **Dispersion of aerosolized toxin.** Animal studies and rare cases of laboratory accidents have confirmed the pathogenicity of aerosolized toxin. One study estimates that aerosolizing 1 g of botulinum toxin could kill up to 1.5 million people; another estimates that a point source exposure could kill 10% of the population 500 meters downwind. Technical factors make such dissemination difficult.

- **Contamination of a water supply.** This is a possibility, but not likely because of the quantity of toxin needed to effectively contaminate a water supply. Additionally, standard drinking water treatment inactivates the toxin quickly and, in fresh water, it is inactivated through natural decay (temperature extremes, humidity, and ultraviolet light irradiation) in 3 to 6 days.

An intentional release of botulinum toxin would have the following characteristics:

- Clustering in time: multiple similarly presenting cases of rapidly progressing acute flaccid symmetric paralysis with prominent bulbar palsies, generally 12 to 36 hours after release.
- Atypical host characteristics: cases of unusual botulinum toxin type (C, D, F, G, and possibly E) *or* cases without typical gastrointestinal symptoms of nausea, vomiting, and diarrhea.
- Unusual geographic clustering: cases in geographic proximity during the week before symptom onset, but lack common food exposure (aerosol exposure) *or* toxin type outside of typical geographic range.
- Absence of risk factors: multiple outbreaks without an association with a common food source.

Clinical Features

The disease generally begins with absorption of toxin by mucosal surfaces in the gastrointestinal system, the eye, or non-intact skin. Regardless of the route of exposure, the same clinical neurologic syndrome develops (see Table 5.1). Botulism is an afebrile descending symmetric paralytic illness. After absorption of the toxin, cranial nerve dysfunction ensues within hours to days, followed by muscle weakness beginning with the proximal muscle groups. Severity of disease is variable, ranging from mild cranial nerve dysfunction to flaccid paralysis (see Figure 5.1). Both the severity of disease and the rapidity of onset correlate with the amount of toxin absorbed into the circulation.

Botulinum toxin blocks acetylcholine release at the neuromuscular junction of skeletal muscle neurons and peripheral muscarinic cholinergic autonomic synapses. It binds irreversibly to presynaptic receptors to inhibit the release of acetylcholine and cause neuromuscular weakness and autonomic dysfunction. The effect lasts weeks to months, until the synapses and axonal branches regenerate. Death from botulism results acutely from airway obstruction or paralysis of respiratory muscles.

The case fatality rate was close to 60% prior to the advent of critical care. Even today, the mortality rate is high if treatment is not immediate and proper. In an outbreak setting, the mortality rate for the first case is 25% and for all other cases is less than 4%. A shorter incubation period has been linked to higher mortality, possibly reflecting a dose-dependent response. Fatality doubles in persons above the age of 60.

Foodborne botulism occurs from the consumption of preformed botulinum toxin in food. Waterborne botulism has not been seen. Toxin types A, B, and E account for most cases

27

Table 5.1 Clinical Features: Botulism

Incubation period	• 2 hours to 8 days
Transmission	• Inhalation of toxin • Consumption of toxin or *C. botulinum* spores • Contamination of a tissue with toxin or *C. botulinum* spores
Signs and symptoms	**Cardinal signs:** • Afebrile • Symmetrical neurological manifestations • Normal mental status, though may appear lethargic and have difficulty with communication • Normal to slow heart rate without the presence of hypotension • Normal sensory nerve function, other than vision **Early presentation – cranial nerve abnormalities:** • Fatigue and vertigo • Double and blurred vision, intermittent ptosis and disconjugate gaze • Difficulty swallowing food **Later presentation – descending paralysis:** • Difficulty moving eyes and mild pupillary dilation and nystagmus • Tongue weakness, decreased gag reflex, indistinct speech, dysphagia, dysphonia • Symmetrical, descending progressive muscular weakness, especially arms and legs • Unsteady gait • Extreme weakness, including postural neck muscles and occasional mouth breathing • Autonomic nerve dysfunction; may include urinary retention, orthostasis • Constipation **Ingestional:** • Dry mouth and dysarthria • Nausea and vomiting, except when exposure is purified toxin **Inhalational:** • Mucus in throat • Serous nasal discharge, salivation **Infant:** • Inability to suck and swallow • Constipation • Weakened voice • Floppy neck
Progression and complications	• Respiratory failure and possible aspiration pneumonia • Residual fatigue, dry mouth or eyes, dyspnea on exertion several years later
Laboratory and radiographic findings	• Normal CSF values • Normal CBC • Normal imaging of brain and spine (CT scan or MRI) Characteristic EMG findings include: • Decremented response to repetitive nerve stimulation at low frequency (3 Hz) • Facilitated response to repetitive nerve stimulation at high frequencies (10–50 Hz) • Low compound muscle action potential

CBC – complete blood count; CSF – cerebrospinal fluid; CT – computed tomographic; EMG – electromyogram; MRI – magnetic resonance imaging.

of foodborne botulism. Minute amounts of toxin can cause disease. A case in which a contaminated potato was spat out before being swallowed resulted in 6 months of hospitalization.

In order for foodborne botulism to occur, the following conditions must exist:

• *C. botulinum* spores must contaminate the food
• anaerobic, non-acidic, low sugar and salt, and warm conditions must be met during the food preservation so that the spores can survive, germinate, and produce toxin
• the food must not be reheated sufficiently to inactivate the heat-labile toxin before the food is consumed (≥85°C for 5 minutes)

Inhalational botulism does not occur in nature; however, three human cases occurred in 1962 in lab technicians working with aerosolized botulinum toxin. It has also been produced experimentally in laboratory animals.

Wound botulism is caused by toxin absorbed into the circulation through a wound. Most cases are related to injection drug use, especially in association with use of black tar heroin being injected into soft tissue ("skin popping"). This topic is covered in detail in Chapter 61, Infectious Complications of Injection Drug Use.

Infant botulism occurs from the consumption of *C. botulinum* spores. The spores invade the gastrointestinal tract,

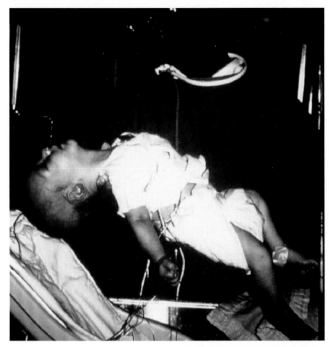

Figure 5.1 Infant with botulism. From the US Centers for Disease Control and Prevention, Public Health Image Library at http://phil.cdc.gov/phil/home.asp.

replicate, and release toxin, which is absorbed into the circulation. The source of spores typically is unknown, though ingestion of corn syrup or raw honey accounts for some cases.

Adult intestinal toxemia (or undefined) botulism occurs from the consumption of *C. botulinum* spores. Characteristics include unknown source of toxin, presence of toxin in stool, and abnormal gastrointestinal pathology (e.g. Billroth surgery, Crohn's disease, and peptic ulcer disease) or antimicrobial drug use.

Iatrogenic botulism has been noted very rarely after medical use or misuse of the botulinum toxin. Purified, highly diluted, injectable botulinum toxin is used to treat a range of spastic or autonomic muscular disorders. Toxin type A (Botox) is used in extremely minute doses for the treatment of facial wrinkles and blepharospasm, cervical dystonia strabismus, glabellar lines, and primary axillary hyperhidrosis. Toxin type B (Myobloc, Neurobloc) is used to treat cervical dystonia. Dysphagia, limited paresis, and other neuromuscular impairment of the toxin are symptoms that have been seen.

Differential Diagnosis

Diagnosis of botulism during the initial stages requires a high index of suspicion because of the lack of readily available rapid confirmatory tests.

Important questions to ask include:

- recent history of eating: home-canned or home-prepared vegetable, fruit, including foil-wrapped baked potato, lightly preserved or fermented meat and fish products, including seafood products from Alaska, Canada, or the Great Lakes;

- other known individuals with similar symptoms;
- injection drug use, particularly with black tar heroin

Other conditions to consider are:

- Guillain-Barré syndrome (especially Miller–Fisher syndrome);
- myasthenia gravis;
- stroke or CNS tumor;
- CNS infections (particularly of brainstem);
- Lambert–Eaton syndrome;
- tick paralysis;
- sudden infant death syndrome;
- hyperemesis gravidarum;
- saxitoxin (paralytic shellfish poisoning);
- tetrodotoxin (puffer fish poisoning);
- laryngeal trauma;
- diabetic neuropathy;
- poliomyelitis/West Nile acute flaccid paralysis;
- psychiatric illness (i.e. conversion paralysis);
- inflammatory myopathy;
- streptococcal pharyngitis;
- viral syndrome;
- hypothyroidism;
- over-exertion;
- diphtheria;
- Wernicke's encephalopathy;
- intoxication with CNS depressants (atropine, aminoglycoside, magnesium, ethanol, organophosphates, nerve gas, carbon monoxide)

Key features that distinguish botulism are the constellation of:

- afebrile illness;
- normal mental status;
- cranial nerves prominently involved;
- descending paralysis;
- symmetric bilateral impairment;
- absence of paresthesias;
- normal cerebrospinal fluid (CSF) studies;
- characteristic electromyogram (EMG) findings

Laboratory and Radiographic Findings

Routine laboratory and radiographic findings for specific clinical presentations of botulism are listed in Table 5.1.

Although laboratory confirmation should be initiated as soon as possible if testing facilities are available, the clinical presentation should guide clinical management and public health interventions. Laboratory confirmation is challenging, but can be achieved in most cases by detection of botulinum toxin in serum, respiratory secretions, and stool via mouse bioassay, in which mice are injected with the patient sample and observed for the development of characteristic symptoms. Serum specimens must be taken *before* antitoxin treatment to demonstrate the presence of botulinum toxin. The test requires 1 to 4 days to complete and is performed only at reference laboratories. Electromyography provides diagnostic information more rapidly. Repetitive nerve stimulation at 20 to 50 Hz differentiates between various etiologies of acute flaccid paralysis. Electromyography is not recommended for infants.

Because the laboratory diagnosis of botulism may take several days to complete, health department officials can authorize the release of antitoxin prior to laboratory confirmation on the basis of clinical findings and may be able to provide other rapid detection tests that are currently investigational (e.g. time-resolved fluorescence assay, toxin micronanosensor, ganglioside-liposome immunoassay, enzyme-linked immunosorbent assay [ELISA]).

Treatment and Prophylaxis

Treatment

Outcome is based on early diagnosis and treatment. Supportive care (including airway protection, mechanical ventilation, and feeding by central tube or parenteral nutrition) and timely administration of equine botulinum antitoxin are keys to the successful management of botulism. Establish a means of communication early, because sometimes conditions such as debilitating headaches are not communicated after the onset of paralysis.

Antitoxin

Following the clinical diagnosis, immediate administration of botulism antitoxin is the key to reducing morbidity and mortality. Antitoxin administration should not be delayed for laboratory confirmation, because antitoxin does not reverse disease or existing paralysis, but only stops progression of disease. Administration in less than 12 hours from the time of diagnosis is associated with a significant reduction in respiratory failure, length of intubation, and overall hospital stay. A study showed that patients given antitoxin within the first 24 hours after symptom onset had shorter hospital stays, shorter duration of ventilatory support, and a lower fatality rate (10%) than those given antitoxin more than 24 hours after onset (15%) or those who did not receive antitoxin at all (46%).

In the United States, antitoxin is obtained from state health departments and the CDC (the CDC hotline number is 770-488-7100). The CDC authorizes release of antitoxin from designated storage facilities; emergency departments and hospital pharmacies should have a policy for emergency delivery of antitoxin.

In 2010, the FDA approved the first heptavalent equine botulism antitoxin (H-BAT), which neutralizes toxin subtypes A to G. H-BAT contains less than 2% intact equine-derived immunoglobulin G, and in a clinical trial with 228 subjects, none experienced anaphylaxis, and less than 1% experienced severe adverse reactions. Pre-treatment skin testing is therefore no longer recommended. The usual dose is a single vial, usually containing 10 to 20 mL of antitoxin solution. Consult public health authorities regarding dosage, because recommendations change. The patient should be monitored for signs of allergy, with diphenhydramine and epinephrine at the bedside.

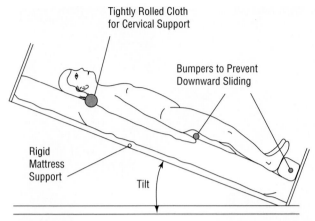

Figure 5.2 Bed position that is best for botulism patients with respiratory muscle weakness.

A. Arnon, R. Schecter, T. V. Inglesby, et al., Botulinum toxin as a biological weapon: medical and public health management. JAMA 2001; 285: 1059–70.

Supportive Care

Ventilatory support may be required for several weeks or more. One study found the mean time on a ventilator for botulism cases was 58 days.

With modern intensive care methods, case-fatality rates for botulism in the United States have dropped to less than 10%. In a mass casualty setting, measurement and management of ventilatory function may pose challenges because of limited ventilator capacities. Local health departments can request supplemental laryngoscopes, endotracheal tubes, and Ambu bags from the CDC. If personnel are limited, consider recruiting healthy civilians for bag ventilation.

A reverse Trendelenburg positioning with cervical vertebral support has been beneficial in terms of respiratory mechanics and airway protection in non-ventilated infants with botulism, but has not been tested in adults (see Figure 5.2). In adults, especially those with obesity, a 20- to 25-degree angle may be beneficial.

Utilize physical therapy and physical turning to minimize intensive care complications.

Secondary Infections

Antibiotics may be used for treatment of secondary infections; however, aminoglycosides and clindamycin are contraindicated because they may exacerbate the neuromuscular blockade.

Post-Exposure Prophylaxis

There is currently no available post-exposure prophylaxis for asymptomatic exposed persons. Such persons should be educated regarding the signs and symptoms of clinical botulism and instructed to seek medical care immediately if symptoms occur. Not all exposed persons will develop clinical symptoms. Exposed persons and their families may experience anxiety and/or somatic symptoms that may include neurologic symptoms. These patients should be carefully assessed. Antitoxin supplies are limited, and therapy will be reserved for patients with compatible neurological findings.

Vaccine

Pre-exposure immunization with botulinum toxoid is restricted to certain laboratory and military personnel. Supplies are extremely limited and would not be available for the public.

Complications and Admission Criteria

In patients with botulism, cranial nerve dysfunction progresses inexorably to a symmetric, descending muscle weakness or paralysis. Respiratory failure occurs in 40 to 70% of botulism patients because of declining upper airway and ventilatory muscle strength. Additional complications of botulism include secondary infection of the respiratory system and sequelae related to intubation and mechanical ventilation, prolonged immobilization, and autonomic dysfunction. Diminished respiratory muscle function and easy fatigability were described by botulism patients 2 years after recovery.

Hospital admission is required for protection of the airway, mechanical ventilatory support, and fluid and nutritional management until normal muscular function returns.

Infection Control and Decontamination

Clinicians should notify local public health authorities and their laboratory of any suspected botulism case. Health authorities may conduct epidemiologic investigations and implement disease control interventions to protect the public. Both HICPAC (Hospital Infection Control Practices Advisory Committee) of the CDC and the Working Group for Civilian Biodefense recommend standard precautions for botulism patients in a hospital setting without the need for isolation. Person-to-person transmission does not occur.

After exposure to toxin, wash clothes and skin with soap and water. Inactivation of the toxin in the environment can take 2 days; however, changes in temperature and humidity can affect the rate of decomposition. Contaminated surfaces and spills of cultures or toxin can be disinfected with sodium hypochlorite (0.1% which is a 1:50 dilution of household bleach) or sodium hydroxide (0.1 N), which inactivates the toxin. Moist heat at 120°C for at least 15 minutes destroys spores.

Pearls and Pitfalls

1. Botulism is often misdiagnosed as a polyradiculopathy (Guillain–Barré syndrome or Miller-Fisher syndrome), myasthenia gravis, or other diseases of the central nervous system. Botulism is distinguished from other flaccid paralyses by its initial presentation with prominent cranial neuropathy, its subsequent descending, symmetrical paralysis, and its absence of sensory nerve deficits.

2. In the United States, botulism is more likely than Guillain–Barré syndrome, chemical poisoning, or poliomyelitis to cause a cluster of cases of acute flaccid paralysis.

3. Botulism antitoxin neutralizes freely circulating toxin, but does not dislodge toxin already bound to presynaptic receptors. Early administration of antitoxin can help to inhibit further paralysis, but does not reverse paralysis that has already occurred.

4. Botulism antitoxin is limited in quantity and is available only through public health authorities. Because the laboratory diagnosis of botulism requires an in vivo assay and may take several days to complete, health department officials often authorize the release of antitoxin prior to laboratory confirmation, on the basis of clinical findings.

References

Black, R. E. and Gunn, R. A. Hypersensitivity reactions associated with botulinum antitoxin. *Am. J. Med.* 1980: 69(4): 567–70.

Centers for Disease Control (CDC). Botulism, www.cdc.gov/botulism (accessed March 19, 2018).

CDC. Drug service: general information, www.cdc.gov/laboratory/drugservice/formulary.html#tbat (accessed March 19, 2018).

CDC. National Enteric Disease Surveillance: Botulism Surveillance Overview, www.cdc.gov/laboratory/drugservice/formulary.html#tbat (accessed March 19, 2018).

Chertow, D. S., Tan, E. T., Maslanka, S. E., *et al*. Botulism in 4 adults following cosmetic injections with an unlicensed, highly concentrated botulinum preparation. *JAMA* 2006; 296(20): 2476–9.

Chin, J. *Control of Communicable Diseases Manual*, 17th edn. (Washington, DC: American Public Health Association, 2000).

Franz, D. R., Jahrling, P. B., Friedlander, A. M., *et al*. Clinical recognition and management of patients exposed to biological warfare agents. *JAMA* 1997; 278(5): 399–411.

Hodowanec, A. and Bleck, T. P. *Clostridium botulinum* in J. E. Bennett, R. Dolin, and M. J. Blaser (eds.), *Mandell, Douglas, and Bennett's Principles and Practice of Infectious Diseases*, 8th edn. (Philadelphia, PA: Elsevier/Saunders, 2015).

Horowitz, B. Z. Botulinum toxin. *Crit. Care Clin.* 2005; 21(4): 825–39.

Kongsaengdao, S., Samintarapanya, K., Rusmeechan, S., *et al*. An outbreak of botulism in Thailand: clinical manifestations and management of severe respiratory failure. *Clin. Infect. Dis.* 2006; 43(10): 1247–56.

Middlebrook, J. L. and Franz, D. R. Botulinum toxins in F. R. Sidell, E. T. Takafuji, and D. R. Franz (eds.), *Medical Aspects of Chemical and Biological Warfare* (Textbook of Military Medicine, pt. I, vol. 3) (Washington, DC: Office of the Surgeon General, 1997), pp. 643–54.

Nishiura, H. Incubation period as a clinical predictor of botulism: analysis of precious izushi-borne outbreaks in Hokkaido, Japan, from 1951 to 1965. *Epidemiol. Infect.* 2006; 135(1): 126–30.

Peck, M. W. *Clostridium botulinum* and the safety of minimally heated, chilled foods: an emerging issue? *J. Appl. Microbiol.* 2006; 101(3): 556–70.

Shapiro, R. L., Hatheway, C., Becher, J., *et al*. Botulism surveillance and emergency response: a public health strategy for a global challenge. *JAMA* 1997; 278(5): 433–5.

Sobel, J. Botulism. *Clin. Infect. Dis.* 2005; 41(8): 1167–73.

Sobel, J., Tucker, N., McLaughlin, J., *et al*. Foodborne botulism in the United States, 1990–2000. *Emerg. Infect. Dis.* 2004; 10(9): 1606–11.

Additional Readings

Arnon, S. A., Schechter, R., Inglesby, T. V., *et al.* Botulinum toxin as a biological weapon: medical and public health management. Working Group on Civilian Biodefense. *JAMA* 2001; 285(8): 1059–70.

Center for Infectious Disease Research and Policy (CIDRAP). Botulism: current, comprehensive information on pathogenesis, microbiology, epidemiology, diagnosis, and treatment, retrieved March 5, 2007, www.cidrap.umn.edu/infectious-disease-topics/botulism (accessed March 19, 2018).

Fever and Focal Cerebral Dysfunction

Serena S. Spudich and Leah T. Le

Introduction

A focal cerebral neurological finding in the presence of fever suggests infection or inflammation of the brain or surrounding tissues, or a cerebral complication of systemic infection. Typical findings of focal cerebral infection are asymmetrical motor or sensory deficits, such as one-sided weakness or numbness, or language dysfunction. However, subtle presentations include perceptual deficits such as deficits in reading comprehension, visual field cuts, apraxias, ataxia, confusion, or personality changes. Cerebral infections may be accompanied by headache and focal or generalized seizures. Fever may be absent or intermittent in infectious cerebral disease, so making the correct diagnosis on clinical grounds can be challenging. Focal neurological findings in the setting of suspected or known infection constitute an emergency.

This chapter focuses on focal cerebral infections in immunocompetent hosts. The most common serious causes of fever and focal neurological deficit are intracranial abscess, arising from either a local or hematogenous source, and focal encephalitis, which is most commonly due to herpes simplex virus. Other diagnoses to consider are shown in Table 6.1. For a discussion of causes of meningitis and encephalitis: fever and headache, see Chapter 8. Altered mental status in HIV-infected patients is discussed in Chapter 4.

Intracranial Abscess

Intracranial abscesses may be categorized as an intraparenchymal brain abscess, subdural empyema, or intracranial epidural abscess, also termed extradural abscess. Intraparenchymal brain abscesses are the most common. These focal infections within the cranial vault are due to introduction of infection via one of three routes:

- local spread from adjacent infected site, such as the mastoid bone, frontal sinuses, or middle ear
- bloodborne infection from intravascular source (endocarditis) or other remote site (dental abscess, lung infection, osteomyelitis)
- seeding through penetrating brain injury from trauma or a neurosurgical procedure

Intracranial abscesses due to contiguous otitis are most common in children, whereas those secondary to sinusitis are found most often in young adults. Elderly and mildly

Table 6.1 Other Diagnoses to Consider with Fever and Focal Deficit

• Exacerbation of chronic deficit in setting of systemic infection	• Acute thiamine deficiency
• Bacterial or aseptic meningitis	• Paraneoplastic encephalitis
• Lyme disease or neuroborreliosis	• Cerebral septic thrombophlebitis
• West Nile virus encephalomyelitis	• Mitochondrial myopathy, encephalopathy, lactic acidosis, and stroke-like episodes (MELAS)
• Poliomyelitis enterovirus meningoencephalitis	
• Enterovirus 71	
• CNS Whipple disease	• Vasculitis of the nervous system
• Listeria monocytogenes brainstem encephalitis	• Hemorrhagic leukoencephalitis
• Inflammatory myopathy	• Neuro-Behçet's disease
• Acute intermittent porphyria	
• Subarachnoid hemorrhage	
• Oto-rhinocerebral infection	
• Neoplasm	

CNS – central nervous system.

Table 6.2 Intraparenchymal Brain Abscess: Etiologic Organisms Based on Predisposing Condition

Sinusitis	*Streptococcus, Bacteroides, Fusobacterium, Haemophilus*
Dental abscess	*Streptococcus, Bacteroides, Fusobacterium*
Ear infection	*Enterobacteriaceae, Streptococcus, Staphyloccus, Pseudomonas, Bacteroides*
Lung infection	*Streptococcus, Fusobacterium, Actinomyces, Nocardia*
Endocarditis	*Streptococcus viridans, Staphylococcus aureus*
Congenital cardiac disease	*Streptococcus, Haemophilus*
Penetrating head trauma or post-neurosurgery	*Staphylococcus aureus, Enterobacter, Clostridium, Streptococcus, Pseudomonas*

immunocompromised patients (e.g. those with diabetes or chronic alcoholism) are at increased risk of hematogenous infection, often originating from the lungs. Also at risk of hematogenous infection are those with congenital heart disease with right-to-left shunting and pulmonary arteriovenous fistula. Brain abscess occurs in approximately 7% of cases of infective endocarditis.

Epidemiology and Microbiology

Though recent incidence data is lacking, an estimated 10,000 cases of brain abscess are reported in the United States each year. This condition has a mortality rate between 10 and 20% even in the current era of antibiotics and a high neurological morbidity rate in survivors of up to 70%. Because the risk of neurological sequelae and death is directly correlated with time to diagnosis and treatment, early identification and management of this condition are essential.

Streptococci (both aerobic and anaerobic), *Staphylococcus aureus*, and *Bacteroides* are the most common organisms isolated in brain abscesses. Aerobic organisms are found in 33%, anaerobic organisms are found in 17%, and multiple organisms are found in 4% of brain abscesses. In intraparenchymal abscess, the specific typical causative organisms vary depending on the route and source of infection, as presented in Table 6.2.

Clinical Features

Intraparenchymal Brain Abscess

The most common means of infection is from extension of infection from adjoining tissues. Contiguous infections tend to lead to single abscesses located in the cortex in locations related to the initial site of infection: otitis leads to temporal or cerebellar lesions, sinusitis usually to frontal or deep temporal lobe abscesses. In hematogenous infections, there are often multiple abscesses that form at the gray–white junction. The middle cerebral artery territory is the most common location.

Risk factors for intracranial abscess include:

- recent dental work
- recent ear infection, mastoiditis, sinusitis, tooth abscess, or pneumonia
- recent head trauma or neurological surgery
- history of valvular disease, congenital heart disease, or endocarditis
- history of chronic infection, such as osteomyelitis
- injection drug use

The classic presentation of a brain abscess includes rapid development over days of headache, focal neurological dysfunction, and fever (see Table 6.3). However, the complete triad is rare, especially in the earliest stages of disease. Notably, a temperature greater than 38.5°C is present in only 53% of cases. Approximately 47% of patients with brain abscess exhibit signs of increased intracranial pressure, such as nausea and vomiting. Furthermore, signs and symptoms may be indolent, progressing over weeks. Often, an indolent, largely asymptomatic course is punctuated by the sudden onset of generalized or focal seizures (25%), leading to hospital presentation and diagnostic work-up.

Though the earliest stages of cerebritis and abscess capsule formation may be relatively asymptomatic, a mature abscess can cause symptoms by direct tissue compression or from the surrounding inflammatory reaction. As a result, the clinical presentation can be identical to that of malignant or inflammatory CNS lesions.

Epidural Brain Abscess and Subdural Empyema

Subdural empyema is an infectious collection occurring between the dura and the arachnoid, which most commonly occurs in the setting of infection in adjoining otic structures or sinuses (70 to 90% of cases), or along tracts created by trauma or surgery. Subdural empyema typically presents with fulminant headache, fever, and signs of increased intracranial pressure. The condition may progress rapidly over days and can be fatal if not promptly drained. The main means of differentiating between intraparenchymal brain abscess and epidural brain abscess or subdural empyema is via neuroimaging.

Rarely, abscesses external to the brain but within the intracranial layers of the meninges can lead to focal neurological deficits. Intracranial epidural abscesses, by definition occurring in the space between the dura and the skull, are far less common than parenchymal abscesses, subdural empyema, or spinal epidural infections. They occur almost exclusively in the setting of underlying local infection such as mastoiditis, sinusitis, or otitis and often develop adjacent to a parenchymal or subdural pus collection, or in conjunction with septic venous thrombophlebitis. Their clinical presentation is characterized predominantly by headache. Focal neurological deficits are usually related to cortical structures located near the lesion and include disruptions of language, primary motor functions, or sensation.

Differential Diagnosis

Because classic signs and symptoms of infection, such as fever, are often absent, a high index of suspicion is necessary to

Table 6.3 Clinical Features: Intraparenchymal Brain Abscess

Abscess development	• 1–3 days: focal cerebritis after local seeding • 4–9 days: necrosis of capsule core, angiogenesis around abscess • >10 days: collagen capsule formation around abscess, inflammation and edema
Signs and symptoms	**Initial phase:** • May be neurologically asymptomatic or have progressive headache • If abscess due to dental, ear, sinus, or pulmonary infection, may have associated symptoms **Subacute phase:** • Progressively worsening headache (69%) • Focal neurological deficit (48%) • Symptoms of increased intracranial pressure (47%) • May or may not have signs of systemic infection (~50% in most series) • May progress to seizures (25%), sudden loss of consciousness with high fever if abscess ruptures into ventricle, or brain herniation and death
Laboratory and radiologic findings	• Peripheral white blood count is mildly elevated in two-thirds of patients • ESR is elevated in 72% of patients • CSF cultures are rarely diagnostic, LP often contraindicated • Blood cultures positive in 28% of patients, most informative in those with systemic signs of infection • CT with contrast may demonstrate a hazy hypointense (dark) lesion that becomes surrounded by a bright ring of enhancement on the administration of contrast • MRI shows a distinctly hypointense lesion on T1 sequences, encircled by a ring of contrast after IV injection of gadolinium; extensive edema around the lesion is seen on T2 sequences; pyogenic abscesses appear bright on DWI sequences (see Figure 6.1)

CSF – cerebrospinal fluid; CT – computed tomography; DWI – diffusion-weighted imaging; ESR – erythrocyte sedimentation rate; IV – Intravenous; LP – lumbar puncture; MRI – magnetic resonance imaging.

differentiate brain abscesses from other causes of focal neurological symptoms. An indolent brain abscess most often mimics the weeks- to months-long course of a primary or metastatic tumor, though occasionally the natural history is punctuated by sudden clinical worsening due to rupture into a ventricle or rapid expansion of the mass.

Other conditions to consider include:

- primary brain tumor
- epidural hematoma
- metastatic brain tumor
- ischemic or hemorrhagic stroke
- inflammatory or granulomatous disease (e.g. sarcoidosis)
- demyelinating disease
- subdural hematoma

Key features that distinguish intracranial abscess from other conditions are:

- presence of infection at other sites, including intravascular or local contiguous source
- focal neurological symptom and predominant headache in the setting of signs or symptoms of systemic infection

Laboratory and Radiographic Findings

The diagnosis of brain abscess is made by neuroimaging. While evaluation usually begins with CT scan with IV contrast, MRI is more sensitive. In early cerebritis, CT scan may appear normal or show a hazy hypointense (dark) region that does not enhance following IV injection with contrast. The most typical CT findings of an established abscess are a hypointense lesion surrounded by a bright enhancing ring with the administration

of contrast. An abscess or a malignant lesion may be surrounded by a large hypointense area of edema, which may be accompanied by mass effect and displacement of brain structures.

MRI can be more helpful in differentiating an infectious abscess from a neoplastic lesion. In T1-weighted MRI scan, abscesses demonstrate a hypointense core surrounded by a smooth ring of contrast when gadolinium is administered (see Figure 6.1). T2-weighted MRI scans show a hyperintense lesion, a slightly hypointense surrounding rim, and extensive hyperintense surrounding signal representing edema. A diffusion-weighted imaging (DWI) sequence can be crucial in differentiating a non-infectious or inflammatory lesion from a pyogenic brain abscess as bacterial brain abscess restricts diffusion of water and results in a homogenously and intensely bright signal on DWI.

The gold standard for diagnosis of brain abscess is direct examination and culture of tissue obtained through a stereotactic biopsy or excision of the lesion.

Lumbar puncture is almost always contraindicated in the evaluation of a patient with suspected or confirmed brain abscess, because of the frequently associated mass effect and elevated intracranial pressure (ICP) that increase the risk of cerebral herniation. A meta-analysis found that 7% of patients who underwent LP in the setting of brain abscess or subdural empyema experienced clinical deterioration, including death. In the same meta-analysis, 24% of cerebrospinal fluid (CSF) cultures obtained from these patients yielded an etiological organism found in the abscess cavity, whereas 28% of blood cultures were diagnostic. Based on the high risk of severe morbidity and the lack of information provided by CSF sampling,

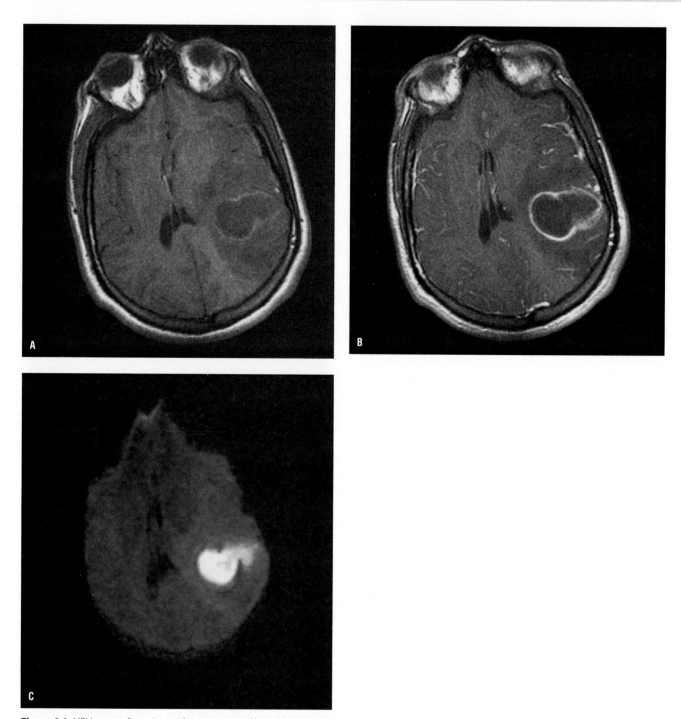

Figure 6.1 MRI images of a patient with a streptococcal brain abscess in the setting of congenital heart disease. T1-weighted images without contrast (A) show a bi-lobed lesion with a hypointense (dark) core, surrounded by a brighter capsule, causing significant local edema and mass effect upon the ventricles. After administration of contrast, a typical outline of the lesion with contrast appears (B). The core of the lesion appears dramatically bright on diffusion-weighted imaging, typical of a pyogenic abscess (C).

CSF analysis is not indicated in the evaluation of suspected brain abscess or subdural empyema.

Treatment and Prophylaxis

Management of brain abscess involves prompt hospitalization, close clinical monitoring, IV antibiotic therapy, and a plan for definitive diagnosis. Initial antibiotic therapy should be chosen based on the suspected route (hematogenous, local, or direct trauma or instrumentation) and source of infection (see Table 6.4). Dexamethasone 10 to 25 mg IV (loading dose) followed by 4 to 10 mg IV every 6 hours can be given as an adjunct to antibiotic therapy in patients with life-threatening edema and mass effect. However, corticosteroids may decrease penetration of antibiotics, interfere with formation of an abscess

Table 6.4 Intracranial Abscess: Initial Empiric IV Antibiotic Therapy Based on Predisposing Route of Infection

Presumed Route of Infection	Therapy Recommendation (Same Doses for Each Drug for Each Indication)
Sinusitis, dental abscess, ear infection	Metronidazole 15 mg/kg/dose IV × 1 as a loading dose, followed by 7.5 mg/kg/dose IV every 8 hours *plus* Penicillin G (24 million units per day IV in six equally divided doses) *or* Ceftriaxone 2 g IV every 12 hours *or* Cefotaxime 2 g IV every 4 hours
Lung infection or congenital cardiac disease	Vancomycin 15–20 mg/kg/dose IV every 8–12 hours (target trough 15–20 mg/L) *plus* Ceftriaxone 2 g IV every 12 hours *plus* Metronidazole 15 mg/kg/dose IV × 1 as a loading dose, followed by 7.5 mg/kg/dose IV every 8 hours Sulfadiazine (PO) and pyramethamine (PO) should be added if *Nocardia* or *Toxoplasma* is in consideration as etiological agent in pulmonary infection
Endocarditis	Vancomycin 15–20 mg/kg/dose IV every 8–12 hours (target trough 15–20 mg/L) *plus* Ceftriaxone 2 g IV every 12 hours
Penetrating Head Trauma or Post Neurosurgery	Vancomycin 15–20 mg/kg/dose IV every 8–12 hours (target trough 15–20 mg/L) *plus* Cefepime 2 g IV every 8 hours *or* Ceftazidime 2 g IV every 8 hours

PO – by mouth.

capsule, and have long-term immunosuppressive effects; therefore, corticosteroids should be discontinued promptly once the mass effect is surgically or medically reduced.

In most cases, surgical intervention is required for effective treatment of brain abscesses, and it is the only means of definitive diagnosis. Although a causative pathogen is not always isolated, the majority of samples obtained via surgical drainage or excision yield at least one organism. Although antibiotic therapy prior to sampling may reduce the yield of culture, a Gram stain may still be revealing in this setting.

Duration of treatment with antibiotics is usually 6 to 8 weeks, though the clinical course and the appearance of lesions on neuroimaging should inform duration of therapy. Usually, neurological deficits improve promptly with reduction of mass effect by surgical intervention or antibiotic treatment, and signs of generalized infection, such as fever, improve in response to antibiotic treatment. Appearance of edema on neuroimaging resolves within weeks of therapy, though residual enhancement around the abscess cavity can persist even in the setting of successful treatment.

For suspected or confirmed brain abscess, prophylactic antiepileptic therapy is often given because of the relatively high incidence (25%) of seizures in the course of the disease. Neurologists often recommend prophylactic IV loading doses of phenytoin or fosphenytoin as soon as an infectious brain lesion is suspected. Seizure therapy may eventually be discontinued in patients who have significant resolution with appropriate surgical or medical therapy, usually after several months and after further evaluation with electroencephalography.

Complications and Admission Criteria

All patients with suspected or confirmed brain abscess should be admitted for diagnosis, monitoring, and treatment. Potential complications include progressive loss of consciousness from increasing intracranial pressure, development of generalized seizures or status epilepticus, and sudden loss of consciousness and high fever in the setting of abscess rupture into the ventricles. These infections may be associated with septic venous thrombophlebitis, leading to cerebral infarction and metastatic infections.

Herpes Simplex Virus Encephalitis

Focal encephalitis is most commonly due to infection with the herpes simplex virus type 1 (HSV-1) and can rapidly lead to severe neurological dysfunction, coma, and death. HSV-1 tends to cause temporal lobe necrosis. Despite the availability of pathogen-specific antiviral treatment and supportive care, mortality from HSV-1 encephalitis remains at 30%. Early treatment decreases both morbidity and mortality, making early detection and antiviral intervention critical.

Epidemiology

Approximately 650 to 1,300 cases of HSV-1 encephalitis are identified in the United States each year. These infections occur in all age groups with a bimodal distribution: a third of

Table 6.5 Clinical Features: Herpes Simplex Encephalitis

Symptoms at onset (typically days 1 through 3)	• Reduced level of consciousness or confusion (97%) • Fever (90%) • Headache (80%) • Behavior change (70%) • Seizure (67%)
Symptoms at presentation	• Fever (90%) • Behavior change (85%) • Aphasia (75%) • Hemiparesis (40%) • Continued seizures, may develop focal or generalized status epilepticus • Progressive confusion, somnolence, may progress to coma
Laboratory findings	• CSF typically shows lymphocytic pleocytosis 10–500 cells/mm^3 • CSF may have xanthochromia or elevated red blood cells from hemorrhagic necrosis in cerebral lesions • Approximately 5% of patients may have normal CSF cell count • CSF protein is elevated in 80% of cases • CSF glucose may be normal or mildly reduced • Blood serologies and cultures are uninformative • CSF PCR for HSV-1 DNA is both >90% sensitive and specific before antibiotic therapy; sensitivity declines to 80% after one or more weeks

PCR – polymerase chain reaction.

infections affect children and young adults, but the peak incidence of disease is in the seventh decade. Although infants younger than 1 year old may be affected, the majority of cases of encephalitis are due to reactivation of prior infection rather than primary infection. HSV-1 exhibits no seasonal or geographic predilection.

Clinical Features

Typically, HSV-1 encephalitis presents with a rapid clinical course over days, characterized by somnolence or disorientation, personality change, fever, headache, and focal or generalized seizures (see Table 6.5). The classic focal findings of aphasia and hemiparesis indicate involvement of the temporal and frontal lobes and may be evident early in the course of disease or develop only after an initial period of seemingly diffuse encephalopathy. A clue suggesting HSV-1 is a history of vesicle or rash on the lips or face. Any change in mentation in the setting of fever or other signs of infection should raise the possibility of HSV-1 encephalitis, even in the absence of more focal features, which may manifest later.

Differential Diagnosis

Although these patients occasionally present with focal seizures or language dysfunction that immediately suggests a focal encephalitis, they most commonly present with a non-specific clinical picture that requires a high index of suspicion for encephalitis.

Although temporal or frontal lobe focal involvement is thought to be a hallmark of HSV-1 encephalitis, other viruses (cytomegalovirus, Epstein-Barr virus, and varicella-zoster virus, as well as West Nile virus and a variety of enteroviruses) can cause focal signs and symptoms, though none of these has a particular predilection for the temporal lobes. Involvement of the temporal lobes is also typical in encephalitis due to HHV-6,

and in the paraneoplastic limbic encephalitis classically associated with small-cell lung cancer.

Other conditions to consider are:

- subarachnoid hemorrhage
- middle cerebral artery territory ischemic stroke
- aseptic or bacterial meningitis
- early stage brain abscess
- non-herpes viral encephalitides (West Nile, Enterovirus 71, St. Louis, alphavirus, enterovirus)
- varicella-zoster virus encephalitis
- human immunodeficiency virus (HIV)-1 encephalitis
- hemorrhagic leukoencephalitis
- acute disseminated encephalomyelitis (ADEM)
- paraneoplastic encephalitis
- human herpes virus-6 (HHV-6) encephalitis
- non-infectious encephalopathy

Key features that distinguish HSV-1 encephalitis from other conditions are:

- aphasia or hemiparesis, indicating focal involvement of the temporal and frontal lobes
- neuroimaging or electroencephalographic (EEG) findings that localize focal lesions to the temporal or frontal lobes
- hemorrhagic lesions on imaging or evidence of blood in CSF, suggestive of typical necrotic lesions of HSV
- changes in personality, behavior, and level of consciousness reflect involvement of the cerebral parenchyma rather than inflammation of the meninges that characterizes isolated meningitis

Laboratory and Radiographic Findings

The gold standard for diagnosis of HSV-1 encephalitis is brain biopsy, though a highly sensitive and specific PCR assay for

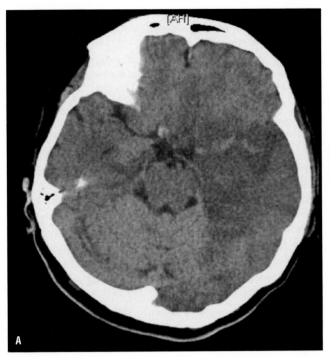
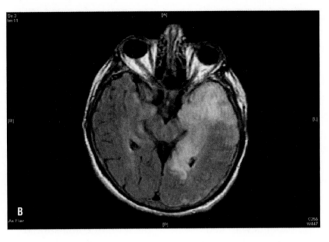

Figure 6.2 Brain images of a patient with HSV-1 encephalitis. CT scan (A) shows an area of hypodensity (darkness) in the temporal lobe on the right side of the image, suggesting edema and necrosis. Fluid attenuated inversion recovery (FLAIR) MRI image (B) better demonstrates extensive bright signal in the cortex of the temporal lobe on the same side, typical in location and appearance of HSV-1 encephalitis.
Images courtesy of Dr. Steven Feske.

HSV-1 DNA from CSF has obviated the need for biopsy in most cases.

If a patient has seizures, focal neurological signs or symptoms, or an altered level of consciousness, neuroimaging should precede LP to exclude a mass lesion that would place the patient at risk for herniation. CT without contrast is usually the initial imaging study before LP and will be negative in most patients early in the course of HSV-1 encephalitis, though it may show hypointense lesions in the temporal lobes, indicating edema or necrosis. MRI is far more sensitive for the early abnormalities of HSV-1 encephalitis, but may also be normal in up to 10% of patients with evidence of disease by PCR. Typical findings on MRI are hypointense areas in the temporal and frontal lobes on T1 sequences that may hazily enhance with administration of gadolinium (see Figure 6.2). Edema is especially evident on T2 sequences, and gradient echo sequences may show evidence of petechial hemorrhage in the most necrotic areas of the lesions.

Once a mass lesion and severe cerebral edema are excluded, CSF should be obtained and sent for cell count, protein and glucose, Gram stain, culture, and HSV-1/HSV-2 polymerase chain reaction (PCR). CSF HSV-1 PCR has diminishing sensitivity over the course of treatment, but also may be negative very early in the course. Herpes simplex rarely grows in culture from CSF, but if the diagnosis of HSV-1 encephalitis is incorrect, culture may yield the true etiologic pathogen.

CSF analysis for detection of viral DNA or paraneoplastic antibodies should be considered on a case-by-case basis in conjunction with PCR testing for HSV-1. Similarly, special CSF studies (e.g. tests for Lysteria monocytogenes, fungal or mycobacterial cultures and stains, cryptococcal antigen) may be indicated, depending on the clinical suspicion for alternate entities.

Treatment and Prophylaxis

As soon as HSV-1 encephalitis is suspected, patients should be hospitalized for intensive supportive care and treated with IV acyclovir 10 mg/kg every 8 hours for 14 to 21 days. Prompt initiation of antiviral therapy improves survival and clinical outcome. Although the yield of CSF HSV-1 PCR declines through the course of therapy, the effect has been noted over the first weeks of therapy rather than the first hours. Thus, treatment with IV acyclovir should be initiated in the emergency department when a diagnosis of HSV-1 encephalitis is being considered and may be started prior to neuroimaging and CSF collection if these tests are delayed.

Except when clearly contraindicated, such as in the setting of unstable heart failure, all patients should receive IV hydration during IV acyclovir therapy, to prevent crystalluria and acquired renal disease. There is no systematic evidence to support the use of oral antiviral agents or adjunctive corticosteroids in the treatment of HSV-1 encephalitis, though this may be beneficial in certain settings and this is an area of current research. Additionally, a large recent study showed that there was no outcome benefit from prolonged oral acyclovir in patients with HSV-1 encephalitis.

When there is high clinical suspicion for HSV-1 encephalitis, antimicrobial therapy should continue even with negative HSV-1 PCR results, pending definitive brain biopsy.

Like brain abscess, many patients develop seizures during the natural history of treated HSV-1 encephalitis. Therefore, antiepileptic medications are recommended.

Complications and Admission Criteria

All patients with suspected encephalitis need to be admitted to the hospital for neurological monitoring and treatment. Progressive involvement of temporal and orbitofrontal lobes may result in focal language difficulties, memory loss, agitation, hallucinations, and autonomic dysfunction that may evolve over days even after initiation of acyclovir. Patients who develop drowsiness and pupillary asymmetry should be transferred to an intensive care setting for monitoring of intracranial pressure. Patients who deteriorate to the level of coma should be evaluated emergently by a neurosurgeon for potential craniectomy and brain decompression. Typical complications related to treatment include renal impairment from acyclovir therapy and electrolyte disturbances from fluid and acyclovir administration.

Infection Control

Person-to-person transmission of HSV-1 encephalitis has not been documented. Therefore, standard precautions are considered adequate for patients with HSV-1 encephalitis. No isolation is required.

Pearls and Pitfalls

1. In brain abscess, lumbar puncture is almost always contraindicated and CSF analysis is often uninformative.
2. Typical signs of systemic infection (fever, elevated erythrocyte sedimentation rate [ESR] or markedly elevated peripheral white blood cell count [WBC]) are absent in up to 80% of patients with brain abscess.
3. Diffusion-weighted imaging on MRI is sensitive and specific in differentiating brain tumors from pyogenic abscesses in the brain, subdural, and epidural space.
4. HSV-1 encephalitis should be considered in all patients who present with symptoms and signs of encephalitis.
5. Patients presenting with any focal signs or lesions on examination, neuroimaging, or electroencephalogram without another etiologic explanation should be presumed to have HSV-1 encephalitis and empirically treated with acyclovir while a work-up is initiated.
6. CSF cell count may be normal in a small minority (5%) of patients with HSV-1 encephalitis.

References

Brock, D. G. and Bleck, T. P. Extra-axial suppurations of the central nervous system. *Semin. Neurol.* 1992; 12: 263–72.

Brouwer, M. C., Coutinho, J. M., and van de Beek, D. Clinical characteristics and outcome of brain abscess: systematic review and meta-analysis. *Neurology* 2014; 82(9): 806–13.

Brouwer, M. C., Tunkel, A. R., McKhann, G. M., and van de Beek, D. Brain abscess. *N. Engl. J. Med.* 2014; 371(5): 447–56.

Butler, J. M., Rapp, S. R., and Shaw, E. G. Managing the cognitive effects of brain tumor radiation therapy. *Curr. Treat. Options Oncol.* 2006; 7(6): 517–23.

Carpenter, J., Stapleton, S., and Holliman, R. Retrospective analysis of 29 cases of brain abscess and review of the literature. *Eur. J. Clin. Microbiol. Infect. Dis.* 2007; 26(1): 1–11.

Chun, C. H., Johnson, J. D., Hofstetter, M., and Raff, M. J. Brain abscess. A study of 45 consecutive cases. *Medicine (Baltimore)* 1986; 65(6): 415–31.

Fitch, M. T. and van de Beek, D. Drug insight: steroids in CNS infectious diseases – new indications for an old therapy. *Nat. Clin. Pract. Neurol.* 2008; 4(2): 97–104.

Gnann, J. W., Sköldenberg, B., Hart, J., *et al.* Herpes simplex encephalitis: lack of clinical benefit of long-term valacyclovir therapy. *Clin. Infect. Dis.* 2015; 61(5): 683–91.

Kao, P. T., Tseng, H. K., Liu, C. P., *et al.* Brain abscess: clinical analysis of 53 cases. *J. Microbiol. Immunol. Infect.* 2003; 36(2): 129–36.

Kastrup, O., Wanke, I., and Maschke, M. Neuroimaging of infections. *NeuroRx* 2005; 2(2): 324–32.

Kennedy, P. G. Viral encephalitis: causes, differential diagnosis, and management. *J. Neurol. Neurosurg. Psychiatry* 2004; 75(1): i10–15.

McGrath, N., Anderson, N. E., Croxson, M. C., and Powell, K. F. Herpes simplex encephalitis treated with acyclovir: diagnosis and long term outcome. *J. Neurol. Neurosurg. Psychiatry* 1997; 63(3): 321–6.

Menon, S., Bharadwaj, R., Chowdhary, A., *et al.* Current epidemiology of intracranial abscesses: a prospective 5 year study. *J. Med. Microbiol.* 2008; 57(10): 1259–68.

Sonneville, R., Mirabel, M., Hajage, D., *et al.* Neurologic complications and outcomes of infective endocarditis in critically ill patients: the ENDOcardite en REAnimation prospective multicenter study. *Crit. Care Med.* 2011; 39(6): 1474–81.

Schmutzhard, E. Viral infections of the CNS with special emphasis on herpes simplex infections. *J. Neurol.* 2001; 248(6): 469–77.

Steiner, I. Herpes simplex virus encephalitis: new infection or reactivation? *Curr. Opin. Neurol.* 2011; 24(3): 268–74.

Tseng, J. H. and Tseng, M. Y. Brain abscess in 142 patients: factors influencing outcome and mortality. *Surg. Neurol.* 2006; 65(6): 557–62.

Tunkel, A. R., Glaser, C. A., Bloch, K. C., *et al.* The management of encephalitis: clinical practice guidelines by the Infectious Diseases Society of America. *Clin. Infect. Dis.* 2008; 47(3): 303–27.

Tyler, K. L. Herpes simplex virus infections of the central nervous system: encephalitis and meningitis, including Mollaret's. *HERPES* 2004; 11(2): 57A–64A.

Whitley, R. J. Herpes simplex encephalitis: adolescents and adults. *Antiviral Res.* 2006; 71(2): 141–8.

Whitley, R. J., Kimberlin, D. W., and Roizman, B. Herpes simplex viruses. *Clin. Infect. Dis.* 1998; 26(3): 541–53.

Whitley, R. J., Soong, S. J., Linnemann, C., *et al.* Herpes simplex encephalitis: clinical assessment. *JAMA* 1982; 247(3): 317–20.

Additional Readings

Carpenter, J., Stapleton, S., and Holliman, R. Retrospective analysis of 29 cases of brain abscess and review of the literature. *Eur. J. Clin. Microbiol. Infect. Dis.* 2007; 26(1): 1–11.

Domingues, R. B., Tsanaclis, A. M., Pannuti, C. S., *et al.* Evaluation of range of clinical presentations of herpes simplex encephalitis by using polymerase chain reaction assay of cerebrospinal fluid samples. *Clin. Infect. Dis.* 1997; 25(1): 86–91.

Mathisen, G. E. and Johnson, J. P. Brain abscess. *Clin. Infect. Dis.* 1997; 25(4): 763–79.

Ramos-Estebanez, C., Lizarraga, K. J., and Merenda, A. A systematic review on the role of adjunctive corticosteroids in herpes simplex virus encephalitis: is timing critical for safety and efficacy? *Antivir. Ther.* 2014; 19(2): 133–9.

Tselis, A. C. and Booss, J. Neuroimaging of viral infections of the central nervous system in M. J. Aminoff, F. Boller, and D. F. Swaab (eds.), *Neurovirology: Handbook of Clinical Neurology Series* (Amsterdam: Elsevier, 2014), vol. 123, p. 149.

Whitley, R. J., Kimberlin, D. W., and Roizman, B. Herpes simplex viruses. *Clin. Infect. Dis.* 1998; 26(3): 541–53.

Infections Affecting the Spinal Cord

Anh T. Nguyen and Debbie Yi Madhok

Introduction

Among infections affecting the spinal cord, spinal epidural abscess is the most critical. Rapid diagnosis and prompt initiation of treatment in the case of spinal epidural abscess can avert irreversible neurologic damage. Therefore, acute care physicians need to be well versed on the presentation and diagnostic appoach to this uncommon infection. Spinal epidural abscess is the main topic covered in this chapter and is also discussed in Chapter 61, Infectious Complications of Injection Drug Users.

Although the combination of an acute febrile illness and focal weakness should always raise the possibility of spinal epidural abscess, there are other critical diagnoses that may present similarly. These are covered in the Differential Diagnosis section, below. The physical exam can often help localize a lesion to the brain, spinal cord, nerve root(s), peripheral nerve(s), neuromuscular junction, or muscles.

Epidemiology and Microbiology

Spinal epidural abscess is a rare disorder, accounting for 0.2 to 20 per 10,000 hospital admissions. Reported risk factors include diabetes mellitus, immunocompromised individuals, intravenous (IV) drug use, prior spine surgery, trauma, and alcohol abuse. Spinal epidural abscess has been documented as a potential complication of epidural catheter placement and epidural injection of steroids or local anesthetics. As many as 5% of patients with epidural abscess may have a recent history of epidural anesthesia. More unusual risk factors include duodenolumbar fistula, bacterial endocarditis, and a recent history of tattooing.

Staphylococcus aureus is the most common causative organism in epidural spinal abscesses, reported in 65 to 73% of patients. Depending on the institution, methicillin-resistant *S. aureus* (MRSA) accounts for 15 to 40% of all staphylococcal epidural spinal abscesses. Other important agents include *Streptococcus* species and *Escherichia coli*. Cases have been reported with a wide range of other bacterial species, and more unusual causes include *Nocardia*, *Brucella*, *Cryptococcus*, and *Aspergillus*. Specific agents may be associated with particular clinical settings. For example, in the postpartum setting, group B *Streptococcus* can cause an epidural abscess, and in the setting of endocarditis, an epidural abscess can develop from direct hematogenous spread.

Clinical Features

In a patient presenting with weakness and suspected infection, a careful neurological exam can often localize the lesion. Table 7.1 presents a schematic approach to localizing the lesion within the nervous system.

The classic symptoms of an epidural abscess with spinal cord compression include neck or back pain, fever, leukocytosis, and focal motor deficit, though the entire constellation is present only in a minority of cases. Back or neck pain is present in 72 to 97% in various case series, while fever is reported in only 33%, leukocytosis in 60 to 78%, and some neurologic deficit in 41% including senory loss, weakness, and urinary incontinence. Symptoms of nerve root irritation, such as radicular pain or a positive straight leg raise test are reported in only 19 to 47% of cases.

Epidural abscesses are more likely to occur around the spine than around the brain, likely because the cranial epidural space is a potential space and the spinal epidural space is a true space filled with fat and venous structures. Anatomically, spinal epidural abscesses are most often thoracic (35%) or lumbosacral (30%), and can be either anterior or posterior predominant. There can be isolated involvement of the epidural space, or additional involvement of neighboring vertebrae (osteomyelitis) and intervertebral disks ("diskitis"). Involvement of adjacent structures occurs in both bacterial and tuberculous epidural abscesses, but is more frequent in tuberculous disease (Pott's disease).

Table 7.1 "First-Pass Neurological Localization" Relevant to the Weak, Febrile Patient

Anatomical Location	Classic Signs and Symptoms
Brain	Cortical signs (aphasia, neglect, higher cognitive dysfunction) Hemiparesis (face, arm, and leg all contralateral to lesion, but usually *not* equally affected) Hemisensory loss (face, arm, and leg all contralateral to lesion, but usually *not* equally affected)
Brainstem	Cranial nerve symptoms (e.g. diplopia, dysarthria, dysphagia) Cranial nerve signs (e.g. abnormal eye movements, decreased hemifacial sensation, facial droop, tongue deviation, or impaired pupillary, corneal, or gag reflexes) Neurological deficit involving a hemifacial distribution and a contralateral extremity or extremities (e.g. lower motor neuron left facial paresis with right hemiparesis of the arm and leg)
Spinal cord	Weakness of both legs, or both legs and both arms Sensory loss in a bilateral distribution, with a sensory level that approximates the level of the lesion Hemicord "Brown-Sequard" pattern of symptoms (weakness and loss of position or vibration sense in one arm and leg, loss of pain or temperature sense in the other arm and leg) Bladder and/or bowel symptoms Hyperactive reflexes (variable, dependent on acuity) Increased muscle tone (variable, dependent on acuity)
Conus medullaris of spinal cord	Little or no weakness Sensory loss in "saddle" area or perineum Bladder and/or bowel symptoms Will have pain if roots involved by lesion as well
Nerve roots (general)	Pain Weakness (distribution variable) Sensory loss (distribution variable) Hypoactive or absent reflexes Decreased tone
Nerve roots (cauda equina)	Pain Weakness in bilateral legs Sensory loss including legs and "saddle" area and perineum Hypoactive or absent reflexes Decreased muscle tone Bladder and/or bowel symptoms
Peripheral nerves	Weakness and sensory loss involving a distal > proximal distribution Hypoactive or absent reflexes Decreased muscle tone
Neuromuscular junction	Time-dependent weakness (worse or better over course of day or with repeated activity) No sensory involvement
Muscle	Proximal > distal weakness, often symmetric in the arms and legs No sensory involvement Muscle tenderness to palpation

Lesions causing extrinsic compression of the spinal cord produce dysfunction of the long tracts that control motor, sensory, bowel, and bladder function. Because extrinsic compressive lesions usually exert a mass effect on both sides of the cord, either anteriorly or posteriorly, they often produce bilateral symptoms. Sensory symptoms will usually, but not always, occur at the level of the lesion and below. In contrast, a lesion at any level of the cord can produce bowel or bladder dysfunction. This dysfunction may present as new or worsening nocturia, well before frank urinary incontinence develops. Because frank stool incontinence is a relatively late finding, the anal sphincter tone and anal wink reflexes are essential parts of the spinal cord neurological exam.

Lesions of the conus medullaris, the lowest portion of the spinal cord, have several distinguishing features. If the conus is impinged out of proportion to the roots of the cauda equina, the patient may have a selective "saddle anesthesia" without motor or sensory dysfunction in the legs. Because the conus contains the lower motor neurons controlling bowel, bladder, and sexual function, these functions may be profoundly affected. In isolated lesions of the conus medullaris, radicular pain may be absent.

Lesions of the cauda equina, instead, produce radicular pain as a rule and lead to motor and sensory dysfunction of many or all of the lumbar and sacral roots. Classically, there is motor dysfunction in both legs and a pattern of sensory loss in the legs and saddle area, with prominent bowel, bladder, and sexual dysfunction.

It is important to note the distinction between the spinal cord level and vertebral body level, especially in the lower aspects of the spinal column. For example, an epidural abscess at the level of the T12 to L2 vertebral bodies would likely compress the conus, the cauda equina, or both, because the spinal cord ends at approximately the L1 vertebral body level. If a spinal sensory level is obtained on exam at approximately L1, this might correspond to a vertebral body level of T11. This anatomical distinction is of practical importance because focused MRI studies must usually be ordered as either thoracic or lumbosacral studies.

In addition, because the axons of the upper motor neurons controlling leg motor function and bladder control course from the medial surface of the cortex, a midline frontal lesion can cause bilateral leg weakness and bladder dysfunction, mimicking a spinal cord lesion. Such lesions may also cause signs and symptoms of higher cortical dysfunction such as cognitive dysfunction, perseveration, or abulia (loss or impairment of the ability to make decisions or act independently).

Because morbidity and mortality are increased by a delay in surgical decompression and antibiotic therapy, early diagnosis is critical. Unfortunately, a delay in diagnosis is common. In one series, 30% of patients were initially misdiagnosed and discharged from an emergency department (ED) or clinic setting. The two most common misdiagnoses are meningitis and vertebral disc prolapse. The variety and subtlety of presentations, the relative rarity of the diagnosis, and the serious consequences of missing it make a high degree of suspicion crucial.

Differential Diagnosis

Pott's disease, or spinal tuberculosis, unlike bacterial epidural abscess, usually involves multiple tissue compartments (see Table 7.2). These include the vertebral bodies, intervening disk spaces, the epidural space, and the paravertebral soft tissues. The course of the disease is generally subacute to chronic, in contrast to bacterial epidural abscess. Because most patients presenting with Pott's disease do not have active pulmonary tuberculosis (TB), clinicians should consider TB as a cause of compressive myelopathy in all patients who have risk factors, come from endemic areas, or exhibit a more insidious course than would be expected for a bacterial epidural abscess.

Intrinsic lesions of the cord producing fever and weakness include viral myelitis, which can affect any area of the cord, and poliomyelitis, which is a selective infection of the anterior gray matter of the cord (the lower motor neurons). Paralytic poliomyelitis caused by poliovirus presents with fever, back pain, and rapidly progressive lower motor neuron weakness, with decreased muscle tone and eventual atrophy and fasciculations. Although poliomyelitis has not caused an outbreak of paralytic disease in the United States in many years as a result of widespread vaccination, a series of non-paralytic cases in a Amish community in Minnesota in 2005 makes it clear that this disease could become more common in the absence of vaccination. Poliomyelitis is now regularly reported as a result of infection with West Nile virus, either as an isolated syndrome or together with encephalitis. Fungal and parasitic causes of myelitis are very rare, but should be considered in immunocompromised patients or in travelers to or residents of endemic areas. Intramedullary bacterial abscess is very rare

and is clinically indistinguishable from epidural spinal abscess, but can be identified by magnetic resonance imaging (MRI).

Botulism presents as a descending weakness starting with cranial nerve signs and symptoms, progressing to respiratory weakness requiring mechanical ventilation. There is usually a documented exposure (home canning or injection drug use) to a potential source of *Clostridium botulinum*. Fever in botulism is variable. Tetanus is similarly easy to distinguish from spinal causes of fever and focal weakness, by the uniform presence of spasms induced by the toxins elaborated by *Clostridium tetani*. Tetanus can occur in local, cephalic, or generalized forms, but in all cases there is both tonic muscle contraction (rigidity) and superimposed painful muscle contractions, both stimulus-evoked and spontaneous.

Pyomyositis is a localized infection and abscess formation in proximal muscles and usually presents with fever and weakness. Pyomyositis, like spinal epidural abscess, is usually caused by *Staphylococcus aureus* and often requires surgical drainage in addition to antibiotic therapy. Clinically, pyomyositis should be easily distinguishable from spinal causes of fever and weakness by the presence of proximal muscle weakness with warm, erythematous, swollen, and tender muscles. Contrast computed tomography (CT), ultrasound, or MRI of the affected muscles confirms the diagnosis.

Syphilis, though often considered in neurological differential diagnoses as the "great mimicker," is a rare cause of progressive myelopathy in the modern era. Several features distinguish syphilitic myelopathy, due to either tabes dorsalis or gummatous myelopathy, from more acute causes of myelopathy with fever. Regardless of the subtype of syphilis, the course is indolent, and fever and signs of active systemic infection are almost always absent at the tertiary stage.

Lyme radiculoneuropathy is a slowly progressive infectious or parainfectious process that diffusely involves the spinal roots and peripheral nerves and can involve the cervical cord as well (Lyme myeloradiculoneuropathy). Although Lyme disease is often entertained in a wide variety of neurological presentations, this condition is usually not acute enough to mimic epidural abscess.

A brain abscess can present with a focal weakness in the setting of similar risk factors to spinal epidura abscess, but clinical features such as cortical dysfunction with hemiparesis or hemisensory loss distinguish this from a spinal process.

Human immunodeficiency virus (HIV) myelopathy is a common process in acquired immunodeficiency syndrome (AIDS) patients, but is also slowly progressive and usually manifests as posterior column sensory deficits without fever, unless another opportunistic process is present. Cytomegalovirus (CMV) radiculitis presents almost exclusively in AIDS patients with very low CD4 counts as a rapidly progressive painful polyradiculopathy with ascending weakness in the legs.

Vasculitic neuropathy can be accompanied by fever and presents as a "mononeuritis multiplex" (focal and patchy involvement of multiple distinct peripheral nerves) or as a polyneuropathy (more diffuse, often symmetric and distal neuropathic picture). The neuropathy can be painful, but the neuropathic quality of the pain and lack of back pain should

Table 7.2 Distinguishing Features among Infections Presenting with Focal Weakness

Differential Diagnosis	Distinguishing Features	Specific Testing
Spinal epidural abscess	• Fever and acute to subacute spinal syndrome • Elevated ESR	MRI WBC, ESR, CRP BCx
Pott's disease (spinal TB)	• Fever and subacute to chronic spinal syndrome • History of TB or exposure • Immunocompromised host	Plain films MRI WBC, ESR, CRP BCx, AFB PPD
Intramedullary spinal abscess	• Fever and acute to subacute spinal syndrome • Elevated ESR	Distinguished from epidural abscess by MRI
Viral myelitis	• Acute to subacute spinal syndrome • Can be in setting of viral syndrome	MRI LP, including viral studies
Poliomyelitis	• Fever • Back pain • Rapidly progressive lower motor neuron syndrome	LP EMG/NC
Fungal or parasitic myelitis	• Acute to subacute spinal syndrome, compromised host or exposure to endemic area	MRI LP, including fungal studies, O&P, wet prep
CMV radiculitis	• Almost always in setting of AIDS, painful progressive polyradiculopathy	EMG/NC LP
Vasculitic neuropathy	• Mononeuritis multiplex	EMG/NC LP
Botulism	• Descending weakness, cranial neuropathies, exposure to source	EMG/NC LP Bedside respiratory testing
Tetanus	• Painful spasms (evoked and spontaneous), trismus, rigidity	EMG/NC Bedside respiratory testing
Myasthenic crisis	• Descending weakness and cranial neuropathies, worse during day and with repetition	EMG/NC Edrophonium test (MG diagnosis) Bedside respiratory testing
Pyomyositis	• Proximal muscle weakness, swollen, warm, erythematous muscles	CT, MRI, or US of muscle
Brain abscess	• Fever, acute to subacute cortical or subcortical syndrome, elevated ESR	MRI
Guillain-Barré syndrome	• Febrile illness, then delayed onset of ascending weakness, areflexia	LP (elevated CSF protein) EMG/NC
Post-infectious transverse myelitis	• Febrile illness, then delayed acute to subacute spinal syndrome	MRI LP
ADEM	• Febrile illness or vaccine, then delayed acute to subacute cortical or subcortical with or without spinal syndrome	MRI brain and spine LP
Lyme radiculoneuropathy	• Subacute to chronic nerve root and peripheral nerve syndrome, rarely cord involvement	LP Lyme titers from blood and CSF MRI
Syphilis	• Chronic, slowly progressive spinal syndrome; usually history of primary or secondary syphilis	RPR LP with CSF VDRL MRI
HIV myelopathy	• Slowly progressive posterior column syndrome	MRI EMG/NC
Leptomeningeal carcinomatosis	• Slowly progressive radiculopathy or spinal syndrome	MRI with enhancement of leptomeninges LP for cytology

AFB – acid-fast bacilli preparation; BCx – blood cultures; CRP – cross-reactive protein; CSF – cerebrospinal fluid; EMG/NC – electromyography and nerve conduction studies; ESR – erythrocyte sedimentation rate; LP – lumbar puncture; MG – myasthenia gravis; O&P – ova & parasites; PPD – purified protein derivative; VDRL – venereal disease research laboratory; WBC – white blood (cell) count.

aid in distinguishing this entity from spinal causes of fever and weakness. The overall course is typically subacute and can be chronic, but the onset of each peripheral neuropathy in a mononeuritis multiplex is usually acute.

A myasthenic crisis is an acute exacerbation of myasthenia gravis, an autoimmune disorder that causes destruction and dysfunction of postsynaptic nicotinic acetylcholine receptors at the neuromuscular junction. A myasthenic crisis is commonly provoked by a febrile illness, so it is possible to see a febrile and acutely weak patient in the ED with the diagnosis of a myasthenic crisis. Although there is usually a history of myasthenia, an acute crisis in the setting of a febrile illness is not an uncommon first presentation of the disease. The diagnosis of this entity at first presentation relies on historic elements and physical findings of time- and use-dependent weakness, in addition to an edrophonium test, which can be performed in the ED with sufficient monitoring and rescue atropine at the bedside. The key in the management of patients with a suspected myasthenic crisis is to consider endotracheal intubation earlier than for other causes of respiratory deterioration. Non-invasive positive pressure ventilation has been shown to be helpful in patients without hypercapnea. If the patient with myasthenia develops significant oxygen desaturation, he or she should have been intubated earlier. Other useful tests that can be easily done in the ED to assess the degree of neuromuscular respiratory weakness include measurement of vital capacity and peak inspiratory pressure, and the bedside "counting on one breath" test. Vital capacity of less than 20 mL/kg or a peak inspiratory pressure of less than 30 cm H_2O is generally accepted as a criterion for intubation. Having the patient take a deep breath and attempt to count as high as possible on breath is a crude but often useful tool to assess neuromuscular respiratory strength – the inability to count higher than 20 on a single breath is a cause for alarm and should at least indicate the need for urgent vital capacity and peak inspiratory pressure measurement.

Guillain–Barré syndrome is a subacute ascending weakness with areflexia caused by an autoimmune reaction against motor, more than sensory, peripheral nerves and roots. Signs and symptoms often develop 2 to 3 weeks following a febrile illness or, very rarely, following vaccinations. It is unusual for a patient with Guillain–Barré to still have signs of systemic illness by the time weakness develops. Post-infectious transverse myelitis and acute disseminated encephalomyelitis (ADEM) can both cause a fulminant myelopathy that may or may not be associated with a history of fever or infectious illness.

Leptomeningeal carcinomatosis (also known as carcinomatous meningitis) is metastatic cancer of the spinal subarachnoid space and is usually slowly progressive and without accompanying fever. In rare cases, fever is present and the disease can progress more rapidly. MRI should accurately distinguish between carcinomatosis and epidural abscess.

Laboratory and Radiographic Findings

There are no signs, symptoms, or laboratory tests that reliably exclude a spinal epidural abscess. When a patient presents with concerning risk factors and objective findings, an emergent MRI with contrast is indicated, as early detection correlates with improved morbidity and mortality (see Figure 7.1). It is prudent to image the entire spine as multiple skip lesions may be present. MRI findings of central spinal canal narrowing by more than half, contrast enhancement of the abscess, and abnormal spinal cord signal are all associated with long-term weakness. Serial MRI scans may be useful to follow the clinical response to therapy.

Patients with viral myelitis may have a normal MRI acutely or may show a diffuse or patchy T2-prolongation of intrinsic cord signal, easily distinguished from extrinsic compressive infectious processes or even other intramedullary infectious processes. If imaging demonstrates the extensive bony and disk involvement typical of TB vertebral osteomyelitis, or an intramedullary lesion, a TB test and infectious disease consult are indicated.

When MRI is not available or is contraindicated, CT myelography is a useful alternate study. A CT myelogram is usually positive when a high degree of clinical suspicion is present. However, CT myelography is invasive and its sensitivity and specificity for epidural abscess have not been systematically compared to MRI, so results should be interpreted in light of the clinical scenario.

The erythrocyte sedimentation rate (ESR) is very commonly elevated upon presentation in cases of spinal epidural abscess and has been reported as greater than 20 mm/hr in 94 to 100% of patients, depending on the series. In a large meta-analysis, the average reported ESR in patients with confirmed epidural abscess was 77 mm/hr (range 2–150). By comparison, the average WBC count was only 15,700 leukocytes/μL (range 1,500–42,000).

Blood cultures should be obtained prior to initiating antibiotic treatment. These are positive in more than half of patients with spinal epidural abscess and may be more likely to be positive if the causative organism is *Staphylococcus aureus*. Although the CSF is usually abnormal, with a pattern typically suggestive of bacterial infection, the CSF Gram stain and culture are rarely positive. Care should be taken with lumbar puncture to avoid seeding the subarachnoid space with a spinal needle that has traversed the abscess.

Treatment and Prophylaxis

Once the diagnosis of spinal epidural abscess is made, prompt neurosurgical decompression and antibiotic therapy remain the mainstay of therapy for an epidural spinal abscess causing a myelopathy. Although successful non-surgical antibiotic therapy for epidural abscess without significant myelopathy has been reported, the success rate of this approach is unclear from published series. Percutaneous CT-guided drainage in selected patients with little or no myelopathy has been reported, both by direct needle aspiration and by catheter placement. A minimally invasive surgical technique involving limited laminectomies and drainage catheter placement has also been reported.

Empiric antibiotics should be begun as soon as possible in the ED after two sterile sets of blood cultures are obtained

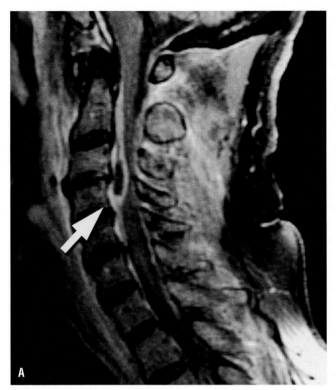
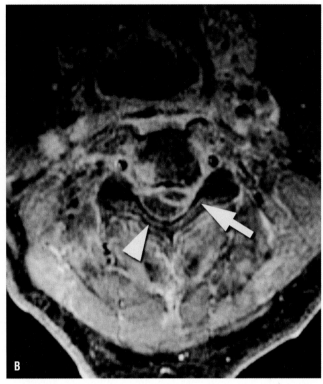

Figure 7.1 MRI of a spinal epidural abscess. (A) Sagittal T1-weighted MRI after administration of gadolinium contrast shows abnormal enhancement anterior to the cervical spinal cord and posterior to the cervical vertebral bodies. In this case, there is a cystic, non-enhancing component with the abscess visible adjacent to the C3 and C4 vertebral bodies (arrow). (B) Axial view of the same abscess, showing the anterior and lateral position of the abscess (arrow) relative to the spinal cord (arrowhead), which is deviated laterally and posteriorly, with mass effect on the cord and effacement of the normal CSF space surrounding the cord.

(see Table 7.3). It is unlikely that a single dose of parenteral antibiotics will sterilize the surgical specimen culture. Empiric antibiotics should be active against staphylococci, Streptococci, and gram-negative bacilli. The optimal antibiotic choice depends on the local prevalence of methicillin-resistant *Staphylococcus aureus* (MRSA), the patient's general immune status, and the likely cause of the infection (i.e. related to prior surgery or instrumentation). Although vancomycin is often a reasonable choice to cover MRSA when the suspected organism is *S. aureus*, vancomycin alone may be insufficient therapy for serious MRSA infections. It is therefore appropriate to cover with both vancomycin and a third- or fourth-generation cephalosporin until isolates and sensitivities are obtained. The addition of a third- or fourth-generation cephalosporin will also cover *Enterobacteriaceae* and gram-negative bacteria. An empiric antibiotic regimen should be utilized unless there is a known pathogen from culture or aspirate.

Complications and Admission Criteria

All patients diagnosed with epidural abscess should be admitted for parenteral antibiotics, monitoring, and immediate neurosurgical consultation. Those with myelopathic signs and symptoms require urgent neurosurgical decompression. The main complication of spinal epidural abscess is irreversible spinal cord damage and paraplegia, which occurs in 4 to 22% of patients. It is worth emphasizing that the risk of irreversible neurologic damage is directly correlated with delay to diagnosis and definitive care.

Table 7.3 Initial Antibiotic Therapy for Spinal Epidural Abscess

Patient Category	Therapy Recommendation
Adults	Vancomycin 15–20 mg/kg/dose IV every 8–12 hours *plus* Ceftriaxone 2 g IV every 12 hours *or* Cefepime 2 g IV every 8 hours
Children	Consider infectious disease consultation – unusual in this group

Many other antibiotics and antibiotic combinations have been reported for empiric therapy of patients with a spinal epidural abscess. Therapy should be based on local resistance patterns and the most likely source for the abscess.

Infection Control

Universal precautions should be observed. No isolation is required, except in cases of suspected concomitant pulmonary TB.

Pearls and Pitfalls

1. Because extrinsic compression lesions such as epidural abscesses usually exert a mass effect on both sides of the cord, there are often bilateral symptoms.
2. A lesion at any level of the cord can produce bowel or bladder dysfunction.

3. New or worsening nocturia may be the first sign of cord pathology, well before frank urinary incontinence develops.

4. A midline frontal lesion can cause bilateral leg weakness and bladder dysfunction, mimicking a spinal cord lesion.

5. Consider TB when the MRI shows involvement of multiple tissue compartments.

6. When neuromuscular disorders are in the differential, always assess respiratory function and consider early intubation.

References

Bouchez, B., Arnott, G., and Delfosse, J. M. Acute spinal epidural abscess. *J. Neurol.* 1985; 231(6): 343–4.

Brazis, P. W., Masdeu, J. C., and Biller, J. *Localization in Clinical Neurology* (New York: Lippincott Williams & Wilkins, 2001).

Bremer, A. A. and Darouiche, R. O. Spinal epidural abscess presenting as intra-abdominal pathology: a case report and literature review. *J. Emerg. Med.* 2004; 26(1): 51–6.

Brust, J. C. M. *The Practice of Neural Science: From Synapses to Symptoms* (New York: McGraw-Hill, 2000).

Centers for Disease Control and Prevention (CDC). Poliovirus infections in four unvaccinated children – Minnesota, August–October 2005. *MMWR Morb. Mortal. Wkly. Rep.* 2005; 54(Dispatch): 1–3.

Chowfin, A., Potti, A., Paul, A., and Carson, P. Spinal epidural abscess after tattooing. *Clin. Infect. Dis.* 1999; 29(1): 225–6.

Clark, R., Carlisle, J. T., and Valainis, G. T. *Streptococcus pneumoniae* endocarditis presenting as an epidural abscess. *Rev. Infect. Dis.* 1989; 11(2): 338–40.

Cwikiel, W. Percutaneous drainage of abscess in psoas compartment and epidural space. Case report and review of the literature. *Acta Radiol.* 1991; 32(2): 159–61.

Danner, R. L. and Hartman, B. J. Update on spinal epidural abscess: 35 cases and review of the literature. *Rev. Infect. Dis.* 1987; 9(2): 265–74.

Darouiche, R. O. Spinal epidural abscess. *N. Engl. J. Med.* 2006; 355(19): 2012–20.

Darouiche, R. O., Hamill, R. J., Greenberg, S. B., *et al.* Bacterial spinal epidural abscess. Review of 43 cases and literature survey. *Medicine (Baltimore)* 1992; 71(6): 369–85.

Flikweert, E. R., Postema, R. R., Briel, J. W., *et al.* Spinal epidural abscess presenting with abdominal pain. *Eur. J. Pediatr. Surg.* 2002; 12(2): 141–3.

Fukui, T., Ichikawa, H., Kawate, N., *et al.* Acute spinal epidural abscess and spinal leptomeningitis: report of 2 cases with comparative neuroradiological and autopsy study. *Eur. Neurol.* 1992; 32(6): 328–33.

Grewal, S., Hocking, G., and Wildsmith, J. A. Epidural abscesses. *Br. J. Anaesth.* 2006; 96(3): 292–302.

Gupta, R. K., Agarwal, P., Rastogi, H., *et al.* Problems in distinguishing spinal tuberculosis from neoplasia on MRI. *Neuroradiology* 1996; 38(Suppl. 1): S97–104.

Gupta, R. K., Gupta, S., Kumar, S., *et al.* MRI in intraspinal tuberculosis. *Neuroradiology* 1994; 36(1): 39–43.

Hanigan, W. C., Asner, N. G., and Elwood, P. W. Magnetic resonance imaging and the nonoperative treatment of spinal epidural abscess. *Surg. Neurol.* 1990; 34(6): 408–13.

Harston, P. K. Spinal epidural abscess as a complication of duodenolumbar fistula. A Case Report. *Spine* 1992; 17(5): 593–6.

Hendrix, W. C., Arruda, L. K., Platts-Mills, T. A., *et al. Aspergillus* epidural abscess and cord compression in a patient with aspergilloma and empyema. Survival and response to high dose systemic amphotericin therapy. *Am. Rev. Respir. Dis.* 1992; 145(6): 1483–6.

Hlavin, M. L., Kaminski, H. J., Ross, J. S., and Ganz E. Spinal epidural abscess: a ten-year perspective. *Neurosurgery* 1990; 27(2): 177–84.

Huang, R. C., Shapiro, G. S., Lim, M., *et al.* Cervical epidural abscess after epidural steroid injection. *Spine* 2004; 29(1): E7–9.

Jenkin, G., Woolley, I. J., Brown, G. V., and Richards, M. J. Postpartum epidural abscess due to group B *Streptococcus. Clin. Infect. Dis.* 1997; 25(5): 1249.

Jinkins, J. R., Gupta, R., Chang, K. H., and Rodriguez-Carbajal, J. MR imaging of central nervous system tuberculosis. *Radiol. Clin. North Am.* 1995; 33(4): 771–86.

Joshi, S. M., Hatfield, R. H., Martin, J., Taylor, W. Spinal epidural abscess: a diagnostic challenge. *Br. J. Neurosurg.* 2003; 17(2): 160–3.

Khatib, R., Riederer, K. M., Held, M., Aljundi, H. Protracted and recurrent methicillin-resistant *Staphylococcus aureus* bacteremia despite defervescence with vancomycin therapy. *Scand. J. Infect. Dis.* 1995; 27(5): 529–32.

Knight, J. W., Cordingley, J. J., and Palazzo, M. G. Epidural abscess following epidural steroid and local anaesthetic injection. *Anaesthesia* 1997; 52(6): 576–8.

Koppel, B. S., Tuchman, A. J., Mangiardi, J. R., *et al.* Epidural spinal infection in intravenous drug abusers. *Arch. Neurol.* 1988; 45(12): 1331–7.

Latronico, N., Tansini, A., Gualandi, G. F., *et al.* Successful nonoperative treatment of tuberculous spinal epidural abscess with cord compression: the role of magnetic resonance imaging. *Eur. Neurol.* 1993; 33(2): 177–80.

Lawn, N. D., Fletcher, D. D., Henderson, R. D., *et al.* Anticipating mechanical ventilation in Guillain-Barré syndrome. *Arch. Neurol.* 2001; 58(6): 893–8.

Leys, D., Lesoin, F., Viaud, C., *et al.* Decreased morbidity from acute bacterial spinal epidural abscesses using computed tomography and nonsurgical treatment in selected patients. *Ann. Neurol.* 1985; 17(4): 350–5.

Li, J., Loeb, J. A., Shy, M. E., *et al.* Asymmetric flaccid paralysis: a neuromuscular presentation of West Nile virus infection. *Ann. Neurol.* 2003; 53(6): 703–10.

Lyu, R. K., Chen, C. J., Tang, L. M., and Chen, S. T. Spinal epidural abscess successfully treated with percutaneous, computed tomography-guided, needle aspiration and parenteral antibiotic therapy: case report and review of the literature. *Neurosurgery* 2002; 51(2): 509–12; discussion 512.

Mampalam, T. J., Rosegay, H., Andrews, B. T., *et al.* Nonoperative treatment of spinal epidural infections. *J. Neurosurg.* 1989; 71(2): 208–10.

Maslen, D. R., Jones, S. R., Crislip, M. A., *et al.* Spinal epidural abscess. Optimizing patient care. *Arch. Intern. Med.* 1933; 153(14): 1713–21.

Messer, H. D., Lenchner, G. S., Brust, J. C., and Resor, S. Lumbar spinal abscess managed conservatively. Case report. *J. Neurosurg.* 1977; 46(6): 825–9.

Numaguchi, Y., Rigamonti, D., Rothman, M. I., *et al.* Spinal epidural abscess: evaluation with gadolinium-enhanced MR imaging. *Radiographics* 1993; 13(3): 545–59; discussion 559–60.

Nussbaum, E. S., Rigamonti, D., Standiford, H., *et al.* Spinal epidural abscess: a report of 40 cases and review. *Surg. Neurol.* 1992; 38(3): 225–31.

Panagiotopoulos, V., Konstantinou, D., Solomou, E., *et al.* Extended cervicolumbar spinal epidural abscess associated with paraparesis successfully decompressed using a minimally invasive technique. *Spine* 2004; 29(14): E300–3.

Patten, J. *Neurological Differential Diagnosis* (London: Springer-Verlag, 1996).

Pirofski, L. and Casadevall, A. Mixed staphylococcal and cryptococcal epidural abscess in a patient with AIDS. *Rev. Infect. Dis.* 1990; 12(5): 964–5.

Reihsaus, E., Waldbaur, H., and Seeling W. Spinal epidural abscess: a meta-analysis of 915 patients. *Neurosurg. Rev.* 2000; 23(4): 175–204; discussion 205.

Rigamonti, D., Liem, L., Sampath, P., *et al.* Spinal epidural abscess: contemporary trends in etiology, evaluation, and management. *Surg. Neurol.* 1999; 52(2): 189–96; discussion 197.

Sadato, N., Numaguchi, Y., Rigamonti, D., *et al.* Spinal epidural abscess with gadolinium-enhanced MRI: serial follow-up studies and clinical correlations. *Neuroradiology* 1994; 36(1): 44–8.

Sarubbi, F. A. and Vasquez, J. E. Spinal epidural abscess associated with the use of temporary epidural catheters: report of two cases and review. *Clin. Infect. Dis.* 1997; 25(5): 1155–8.

Shintani, S., Tanaka, H., Irifune, A., *et al.* Iatrogenic acute spinal epidural abscess with septic meningitis: MR findings. *Clin. Neurol. Neurosurg.* 1992; 94: 253–5.

Siao, P., McCabe, P., and Yagnik, P. Nocardial spinal epidural abscess. *Neurology* 1989; 39(7): 996.

Sillevis Smitt, P., Tsafka, A., van den Bent, M., *et al.* Spinal epidural abscess complicating chronic epidural analgesia in 11 cancer patients: clinical findings and magnetic resonance imaging. *J. Neurol.* 1999; 246(9): 815–20.

Soehle, M. and Wallenfang, T. Spinal epidural abscesses: clinical manifestations, prognostic factors, and outcomes. *Neurosurgery* 2002; 51(1): 79–85; discussion 86–7.

Solera, J., Lozano, E., Martinez-Alfaro, E., *et al.* Brucellar spondylitis: review of 35 cases and literature survey. *Clin. Infect. Dis.* 1999; 29(6): 1440–9.

Tabo, E., Ohkuma, Y., Kimura, S., *et al.* Successful percutaneous drainage of epidural abscess with epidural needle and catheter. *Anesthesiology* 1994; 80(6): 1393–5.

Tessman, P. A., Preston, D. C., and Shapiro, B. E. Spinal epidural abscess in an afebrile patient. *Arch. Neurol.* 2004; 61(4): 590–1.

Tung, G. A., Yim, J. W., Mermel, L. A., *et al.* Spinal epidural abscess: correlation between MRI findings and outcome. *Neuroradiology* 1999; 41(12): 904–9.

Walter, R. S., King, J. C. Jr., Manley, J., and Rigamonti, D. Spinal epidural abscess in infancy: successful percutaneous drainage in a nine-month-old and review of the literature. *Pediatr. Infect. Dis. J.* 1991; 10(11): 860–4.

Wheeler, D., Keiser, P., Rigamonti, D., and Keay, S. Medical management of spinal epidural abscesses: case report and review. *Clin. Infect. Dis.* 1992; 15(1): 22–7.

Wu, L. L., Chen, S. T., and Tang, L. M. Nonsurgical treatment of spinal epidural abscess: report of a case. *J. Formos. Med. Assoc.* 1994; 93(3): 253–5.

Meningitis

Katherine C. Bonsell and Anita A. Koshy

Introduction

Although there is a broad differential in a patient presenting with fever and headache, a few infectious diagnoses need to be ruled in or out immediately. Acute bacterial meningitis is a critical diagnosis because delay of appropriate antimicrobial therapy increases morbidity and mortality. Distinguishing between bacterial, viral, and more chronic meningitides requires careful interpretation of multiple clinical and laboratory findings. The microbiology of meningitis is discussed below.

Epidemiology

The most recent US data studying hospitalizations for meningitis estimates that more than 800,000 people were hospitalized for meningitis from 1988 to 1999. The majority of these hospitalizations were for viral (50%) and bacterial meningitis (23%). Fungal meningitis accounted for 9% of the hospitalizations and unspecified for 18%. As these numbers describe only hospitalized patients, they underrepresent the actual incidence, especially of viral meningitis. Although recent data on meningitis as a whole is lacking, the incidence of acute bacterial meningitis fell 31% between 1998 and 2011, primarily because of increased vaccination in the United States during these years. However, there are still estimated to be over 4,000 reported cases of bacterial meningitis annually in the United States. The case-fatality rate has remained relatively stable over 1998 to 2007, though limited data

suggests that widespread use of adjuvant corticosteroid therapy may be reducing the mortality rate of pneumococcal meningitis.

Microbiology

Acute Bacterial Meningitis

Causes of acute bacterial meningitis vary by age. Neonates acquire organisms such as group B *Streptococcus*, *Escherichia coli*, or less commonly, *Listeria monocytogenes*, from passage through the mother's birth canal. Beyond the first month of life, the most common organisms are *Neisseria meningitidis* (meningococcus) and *Streptococcus pneumoniae*, with age-dependent differences in incidence (see Table 8.1). Previously, infants and children made up the majority of acute bacterial meningitis cases, but with the development of multiple vaccines for routine childhood vaccination, adults (greater than age 18) now account for the majority of these cases in developed countries.

Streptococcus Pneumoniae

Since the advent of the Hib vaccine, *S. pneumoniae* has emerged as the most common cause of bacterial meningitis in patients older than 1 month. This is related to a "replacement phenomenon," rather than an absolute increase in the incidence. Additionally, since the introduction of the heptavalent vaccine in 2000, the overall incidence of *S. pneumonia* meningitis has also declined by ~25%, with children between 2 and 23 months of age showing

Table 8.1 Acute Bacterial Meningitis Pathogens

Organism	Gram Stain	Associated Risks
Streptococcus pneumoniae	• Gram-positive coccus that forms diplococci or very short chains	• Most common cause of bacterial meningitis in patients older than 1 month • Declining overall incidence since advent of vaccine, with an increase in cases caused by strains not targeted by the vaccine
Neisseria meningitidis	• Gram-negative coffee-bean diplococcus • Can be intracellular or extracellular	• Second most common cause of bacterial meningitis, declining in incidence • Bimodal age distribution: <1 year of age and young adults in close proximity (college, military) • Most common cause of petechial rash associated with meningitis
Haemophilus influenza B (Hib)	• Gram-negative coccobacillus	• Generally affects children <6 years old • Declining incidence since advent of vaccine
Listeria monocytogenes	• Gram-positive rod	• Age >50, on steroids or other immunosuppressant drugs, history of alcohol abuse or cancer • Outbreaks have been associated with contaminated coleslaw, raw vegetables, unpasteurized milk or cheese, cantaloupe, caramel apples
Rickettsia rickettsii	Intracellular pathogen that requires special staining Small gram-negative rod (when cultured)	• Acquired by a tick bite • Uniformly fatal if not treated • Most commonly found in the South Atlantic United States, but has been reported in majority of United States • Presents late spring to early fall • Generally affects children <16 years old • Rash beginning on wrist, ankles around 3–5 days, often involves palms and soles

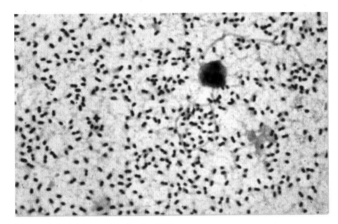

Figure 8.1 *S. pneumoniae* in the CSF.
Courtesy of Dr. Ellen Jo Baron, Stanford University.

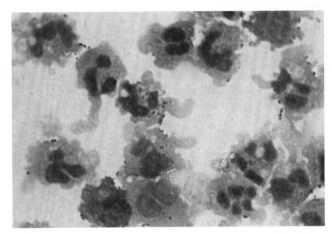

Figure 8.2 Intracellular gram-negative diplococci of *N. meningitides*, from a cytospin.
Courtesy of Dr. Ellen Jo Baron, Stanford University.

the steepest decline in incidence (~60%). *S. pneumoniae* is a gram-positive bacterium that forms diplococci or very short chains (see Figure 8.1). It is ubiquitous and can cause severe disease in any patient. The mortality of pneumococcal meningitis is approximately 20 to 30%, even with appropriate antibiotic treatment. Relatively recent studies using adjuvant steroid therapy have shown a decrease in mortality from *S. pneumoniae*, but only in developed countries and in HIV-negative persons (see Treatment section below). One study suggests that *S. pneumoniae* mortality has declined since 2004, when the Infectious Diseases Society of America (IDSA) guidelines recommended the use of adjuvant steroid therapy for this disease. This finding is consistent with a study in the Netherlands that showed a 10% decline in pneumococcal meningitis mortality after the widespread use of adjuvant steroids.

Neisseria Meningitidis

N. meningitidis is a gram-negative diplococcus that can be observed intracellularly or extracellularly (see Figure 8.2).

It is the second most common cause of acute bacterial meningitis and usually causes disease in a bimodal age distribution: in infants younger than 12 months of age, and then again in young adults. Similar to pneumococcal meningitis, meningococcal meningitis rates have been falling, though this decline appears to pre-date the widespread use of the tetravalent vaccine. From 1997 to 2010, there was an 86% decrease in the incidence of meningococcal meningitis in all age groups. Of note, the tetravalent vaccine introduced in 2005 does not contain serogroup B, which is responsible for 50% of meningococcal infections in the United States and >90% in many European countries as of 2010. This risk is highlighted by the recent college campus outbreaks of serogroup B meningococcal disease (MenB). In October 2014, the FDA approved the first MenB specific vaccine in the United States, with a second vaccine approved in January 2015. Clinically, meningococcal

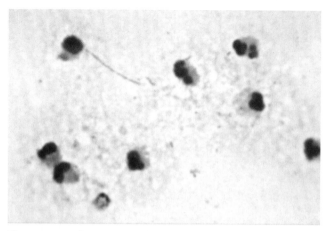

Figure 8.3 *H. influenzae* B in CSF.
Courtesy of Dr. Ellen Jo Baron, Stanford University.

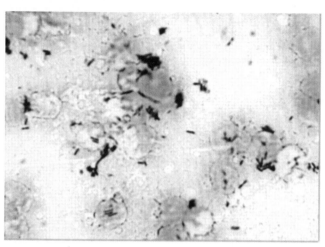

Figure 8.4 *L. monocytogenes* in blood.
Courtesy of Dr. Ellen Jo Baron, Stanford University.

disease frequently (50%) presents with a petechial rash, and the mortality rate of meningococcal meningitis without associated sepsis is approximately 7%. Close contacts should receive chemoprophylaxis (see below).

Haemophilus Influenzae

Haemophilus influenzae is a gram-negative coccobacillus that, prior to the availability of a vaccine, accounted for 45 to 58% of acute bacterial meningitis cases in the United States, with serotype B causing ~90% of this disease (see Figure 8.3). With the widespread introduction of the Hib vaccine in the late 1980s, *H. influenza* meningitis now only accounts for ~7% of cases, with most cases being caused by non-type b serotypes. Unfortunately, akin to measles and mumps, outbreaks of invasive Hib have been seen in various states, in part secondary to hesitations about vaccination, as well as vaccine shortages. Chemoprophylaxis for contacts of a patient with *H. influenza* meningitis is described in the Infection Control section below.

Listeria Monocytogenes

L. monocytogenes is a gram-positive rod commonly found in soil, dust, water, and sewage (see Figure 8.4). It is responsible for approximately 8% of bacterial meningitis cases. It occurs more commonly in neonates, older adults, and patients with a history of immunosuppressive therapy, alcohol abuse, or cancer. While pregnant women are at high risk for listerial bacteremia, for reasons that are unclear, unless they have other risk factors, they do not commonly develop listerial meningitis. However, newborns whose mothers have listerial bacteremia are at high risk for contracting listeria and developing meningits. With exception of this vertical transmission, person-to-person spread is not seen in *Listeria*. Outbreaks of listeriosis have been traced to contaminated coleslaw, raw vegetables, unpasteurized milk products, cantaloupe, and caramel apples. The incidence of listerial meningitis is also decreasing, potentially secondary to decreases in contamination of ready-to-eat foods, or because of high-risk groups avoiding potentially contaminated food, or both. Listerial meningitis is thought to

commonly involve the brainstem and present with altered mental status and seizures, though in a recent prospective study of listerial meningitis cases, the patients presented with signs and symptoms typical of acute bacterial meningitis (fever, headache, neck stiffness > altered sensorium). In patients at risk for listerial meningitis, ampicillin should be included in the empiric antibiotic regimen.

Key features that distinguish acute bacterial from viral or chronic meningitis include:

- sepsis
- altered mental status (can be seen late in the course of chronic meningitis)
- petechial rash

Aseptic Meningitis and Viral Meningitis

Aseptic meningitis refers to patients who have signs and symptoms of meningitis without evidence of purulent bacterial infection. Thus, aseptic meningitis encompasses viral meningitis, atypical bacterial meningitis, chemical meningitis, carcinomatosis meningitides, granulomatous disease (such as sarcoidosis), and fungal meningitis (discussed below). The majority of these entities will present with an indolent course.

The etiology of viral meningitis is identified in 55 to 70% of cases. The herpes viruses, enteroviruses, flaviviruses, and retroviruses have all been implicated (see Table 8.2). The occurrence of symptomatic meningitis from these agents is estimated at 1 in 3,000 cases. Excluding the neonatal period, the morbidity and mortality from viral meningitis is low. The treatment of viral meningitis is generally supportive.

Viral *encephalitis*, however, may present with fever, headache, and focal features, such as seizures, hallucinations, aphasia, and hemiparesis. Herpes simplex virus is the most common cause of fatal infectious encephalitis in the United States. As acyclovir has been shown to significantly decrease the morbidity and mortality of herpes simplex encephalitis, a suspected diagnosis of encephalitis requires emergent antiviral therapy to limit morbidity and mortality. Other herpes viruses (varicella (VZV), Epstein–Barr, cytomegalovirus, and

Table 8.2 Viral Meningitis Pathogens

Organism	Signs and Symptoms	Associated Risks
Non-polio enteroviruses	• Prodrome of flu-like illness and sore throat • Nausea, vomiting, fever, meningismus, and possible viral exanthem	• Causes up to 90% of viral meningitis when etiology identified • Found worldwide • Presents in summer and fall in temperate climates, and year-round in tropical and subtropical climates • Children infected most often **Treatment:** Supportive
Polio	• Symptoms same as above • Can affect motor and ANS neurons leading to permanent paralysis	• Rare cause of meningitis in vaccinated countries • Important cause of aseptic meningitis in endemic areas: Afghanistan, Pakistan, and Nigeria • Anticipated eradication if immunization universal **Treatment:** Supportive
Flavivirus – includes Japanese encephalitis complex, St. Louis encephalitis (SLE) virus, tick-borne encephalitis virus, and West Nile virus (WNV)	• CNS involvement depends on the virus • Most infections asymptomatic or mild febrile illnesses without CNS involvement	• Each complex has a general geographic distribution and seasonality • SLE is seen in the south and southeastern states • WNV follows bird migrations and is now found throughout the United States • Older (age >50) and immunocompromised patients generally have the most severe disease • Vector-borne (mosquito or tick) **Treatment:** Supportive
HIV	• Acute HIV infection is often associated with fever, pharyngitis, lymphadenopathy, and rarely a rash	• Risk factors would be unprotected sex and sharing of contaminated needles **Treatment:** supportive, but close follow-up necessary to determine appropriate time to start HAART
Herpes viruses – includes HSV-1 and 2, VZV, CMV, EBV, and HHV-6	• Fever, headache, neck stiffness • Altered mental status, seizures, focal neurologic findings define meningoencephalitis	• In immunocompetent patients, HSV-2 is the most common cause • Usually associated with a primary genital outbreak • In immunocompromised patients, any of these viruses can be seen **Treatment:** • Immunocompetent patients – no treatment guidelines for meningitis • Immunocompromised patients or any patient with meningoencephalitis: HSV and VZV, acyclovir 10 mg/kg/dose IV every 8 hours, and for CMV, EBV, or HHV-6 ganciclovir 5 mg/kg/dose IV every 12 hours or foscarnet
Lymphocytic choriomeningitis (LCMV)	• Asymptomatic	• Can cause congenital hydrocephalus, micro- or macrocephaly, chorioretinitis, intracranial calcifications, and nonimmune hydrops • Risk factors: exposure to rodents such as lab workers, pet owners, and those living in non-hygienic conditions, and transplant recipients on immunosuppression **Treatment:** Supportive
Mumps	• Fever, headache, neck stiffness • Can be associated with parotitis, precede parotitis, or be the only manifestation of an infection	• Present in winter and spring, usually infects unimmunized and partially immunized children, college students • Affects males more often than females **Treatment:** Supportive

ANS – autonomic nervous system.

human herpes virus-6 [HHV-6]) have also been associated with encephalitis. These are more commonly present in immunocompromised patients, though VZV can be seen in the immunocompetent. Suspicion for these viruses depends on the clinical scenario and may require institution of intravenous ganciclovir instead of acyclovir (CMV, HHV-6, EBV). For most other causes of viral encephalitis, the treatment is supportive. See Chapter 6 for a discussion of Fever and Focal Cerebral Dysfunction.

Enteroviruses

The most common causes of viral meningitis are the non-polio enteroviruses, which account for up to 90% of viral meningitis in which an etiology is identified. These viruses are found worldwide and cause disease in summer and fall months in temperate climates, and year-round in tropical and subtropical climates. They most often affect children, but epidemics in adults and adolescents have been reported. A prodrome of a flu-like illness and sore throat is not unusual, and is often followed by nausea, vomiting, fever, headache, meningismus, and occasionally a viral exanthem. In immunocompetent patients, the morbidity and mortality of enteroviral meningitis is very low. In patients with agammaglobulinemia, enteroviruses can cause a severe, chronic meningoencephalitis. In neonates, especially those less than 2 weeks old, enteroviral meningitis or encephalitis can present with severe sepsis.

Polio Virus

Polio is an enterovirus, but is a very rare cause of viral meningitis in the developed world where vaccinations are routinely given. The oral live attenuated form of the polio vaccine can rarely cause an aseptic meningitis, but currently in the United States, only the injected form is used. In the unimmunized who live in, or have recently traveled to, endemic countries (Afghanistan, Nigeria, and Pakistan), polio is still an important, though infrequent, cause of aseptic meningitis.

Flaviviruses

This family includes Japanese encephalitis complex, St. Louis encephalitis (SLE) virus, tick-borne encephalitis virus, and West Nile virus (WNV). Most often, infection with these viruses is asymptomatic or causes a mild febrile illness without central nervous system (CNS) involvement. In the United States, SLE is seen in the southern and southeastern states, though a small outbreak of non-neuroinvasive disease was seen in Arizona in 2015. West Nile virus is present throughout the continental United States, though most prevalent in the southwest and central regions. The likelihood of CNS involvement depends on the viral strain, and the immune status of the host. Older adults (age >50) or those who are immunocompromised are at increased risk for severe infection.

Human Immunodeficiency Virus

In the acute phase of infection, human immunodeficiency virus (HIV) can invade the CNS and cause aseptic meningitis. Usually, this meningitis is accompanied by an acute retroviral (ARS) syndrome that includes fever, pharyngitis, lymphadenopathy, and sometimes a rash. In a patient with risk factors, serum HIV screening should be considered.

Herpes Viruses

Herpes simplex virus (HSV) 1 and 2, varicella-zoster virus (VZV), cytomegalovirus (CMV), and Epstein–Barr virus (EBV) have all been associated with aseptic meningitis. In an immunocompetent host, the most likely to cause aseptic meningitis is HSV-2, usually in association with a primary genital outbreak. Herpes zoster (VZV) has also been associated with aseptic meningitis, while *zoster sine herpete* is a VZV reactivation causing viral meningitis without the cutaneous lesions. CMV, EBV, and now human herpes virus-6 (HHV-6) are much better known for causing encephalitis in the immunocompromised, but have been reported to cause meningitis as well.

Although it is clear that in HSV encephalitis, treatment with acyclovir decreases the morbidity and mortality, treatment with antivirals for immunocompetent patients with herpes virus meningitis remains unclear. One retrospective review of 42 patients found no difference in neurologic outcome for immunocompetent patients with HSV meningitis who were treated with acyclovir compared to those who were not. On the other hand, this same study found that immunocompromised patients were at increased risk of neurologic sequelae if not treated with antivirals. Therefore, in the immunocompromised, or in those with evidence of encephalitis, it is recommended to treat HSV and VZV with acyclovir, and CMV, EBV, and HHV-6 with ganciclovir or foscarnet. Prophylactic treatment can be considered in patients diagnosed with Mollaret's meningitis, a recurrent aseptic meningitis associated with HSV-2 outbreaks, though a recent double-blinded, placebo -controlled trial from Sweden found that patients in the treatment prophylaxis group (valacyclovir 500 mg BID) were not protected from recurrent meningitis compared to the placebo group, and had an increased incidence of meningitis after they discontinued the treatment.

Lymphocytic Choriomeningitis Virus (LCMV)

This arenavirus is a rare cause of aseptic meningitis in individuals with exposure to rodents: lab workers, pet owners, and those living in unhygienic conditions. It most commonly presents in the fall. Although the affected patient rarely suffers sequelae, a devastating congenital infection can occur. Lethal infections have been described in organ transplant recipients that are treated with potently immunosuppressive drugs.

Mumps

Prior to the introduction of widespread vaccination, mumps was a relatively common cause of aseptic meningitis. It occurs most often in winter and spring, and usually infects children. However, there have been recent US outbreaks, even among vaccinated and partially vaccinated adolescents and young adults, particularly on college campuses. The meningitis can be associated with parotitis, precede parotitis, or be the only manifestation of an infection. The disease is generally benign in terms of neurologic outcomes. The vaccine has rarely (1–10/10,000 vaccinations) been associated with aseptic meningitis.

Key features that may help to distinguish viral from bacterial or chronic meningitis are:

- patients are generally not obtunded or truly altered
- not septic
- acute onset

Clinical Features

Meningitis is classically characterized as a triad of fever, neck stiffness, and altered mental status, though it may be more appropriate to consider the triad of fever, headache, and meningismus (see Table 8.3). Fewer than half of the patients with acute bacterial meningitis will present with the complete "classic" triad, though most present with headache. In retrospective studies, fever is the most common symptom, though many of these did not evaluate for headache as a clinical feature of meningitis. In the only prospective study of adults with bacterial meningitis, headache was the most common complaint (87%), then neck stiffness (83%), fever (77%), and altered mental status (69%). Of the patients studied, 95% had at least two of these four symptoms, and 99% had at least one. A petechial rash is present in more than 50% of cases of meningitis caused by *Neisseria meningitides*, but can be seen with any organism that causes meningitis; in particular, *Streptococcus pneumoniae*, *Staphylococcus aureus*, group B *Streptococcus*, and *Rickettsia rickettsii* meningitis can present with a rash.

In infants and children, the presentation of acute bacterial meningitis is often less specific than in adults, though fever does tend to be a cardinal symptom. Neonates can appear septic and may present with hypotension and apnea. Young children may present with fever and irritability or lethargy. About one-third of children with *S. pneumoniae* or *Haemophilus influenza* B (Hib) meningitis will present with seizures. Clinicians should have a high index of suspicion for meningitis in febrile children, even in the absence of localizing complaints. See also Chapter 50 on Fever in the Newborn and Chapter 51 on The Febrile Child.

Both viral meningitis and chronic meningitis (etiologies discussed below) also present with fever and headache. Viral meningitis is usually relatively abrupt in onset, but the patients are less symptomatic than those with bacterial meningitis and should not have an alteration in mentation. Chronic meningitis is characterized by more gradual onset of symptoms and an indolent course. Any meningitis can present with cranial neuropathies, though these neuropathies are more commonly described with basilar meningitides, such as tuberculous, Lyme, fungal, or sarcoid meningitis.

Differential Diagnosis

It is important to distinguish infectious meningitis from its mimics (see Table 8.4). When CSF evaluation reveals an apparent aseptic meningitis, the many causes of chronic meningitis (discussed below) are also on the differential diagnosis.

Laboratory and Radiographic Findings

A lumbar puncture (LP) should be done in all patients with suspected meningitis, but imaging studies are not necessary in all patients prior to LP. These studies have been shown to delay antibiotic treatment which increases morbidity and mortality. Conversely, the theoretical risk of cerebral herniation secondary to LP is poorly studied, but likely small. The IDSA guidelines do recommend imaging prior to LP in patients who are immunocompromised, who present with focal neurologic deficits or recent seizures, who present with moderate-to-severe impairment of consciousness, and, according to some sources, patients aged 60 years or older, and patients who have a history of CNS lesion(s) (see Table 8.5). However, in 2009, the Swedish guidelines removed impaired consciousness as an indication for imaging. Following these changes, a study compared time to antibiotics, and morbidity and mortality from 2005–2009 to 2010–2016 (adjuvant steroid use was the same in both groups). Patients in the 2010–2016 era received antibiotics in < 2 hours more frequently than in the 2005–2009 era, and had a decreased mortality and morbidity. Importantly, in patients with GCS <11 or GCS<8 (impaired consciousness), LP without imaging was not associated with an increase in mortality or morbidity. These data suggest that alterations in consciousness do not increase the risk of post-LP herniation, but the associated delay

Table 8.3 Clinical Features of Acute Meningitis

Children: signs and symptoms	• Fever • Neonates can appear septic • Irritability or lethargy • Seizures (one-third of children with *S. pneumoniae* or *Haemophilus influenza* B (Hib) meningitis) • Petechial rash (favors *N. meningitidis*, but can be present with any organism that causes meningitis)
Adults: signs and symptoms	• Fever, headache, neck stiffness, altered mental status • Seizures are very rare • Petechial rash (favors *N. meningitidis*, but can be present with any organism that causes meningitis)

Table 8.4 Differential Diagnosis of Acute Bacterial Meningitis

Etiology	Key Features
Meningitis	• Fever, headache, meningismus • May have history of otitis media or sinusitis • See the rest of chapter to distinguish acute bacterial, viral, and chronic
Sinusitis	• Sinus headache, facial pain, nasal congestion, • Purulent nasal drainage • Subacute symptoms
Bacterial brain abscess	• Progressive headache • History of pulmonary hereditary hemorrhagic telangiectasia • History of recent dental abscess or procedure • Subacute symptoms • May have focal neurologic findings and fever • Poor dentition when oropharynx is examined
Encephalitis	• Headache, altered mental status, seizures • Fever
Subarachnoid hemorrhage	• Acute onset headache, often severe • No fever or meningismus early on (later can develop central fever and will develop meningismus) • Can have focal neurologic findings, especially cranial neuropathies

Table 8.5 IDSA Guidelines for Imaging Prior to Lumbar Puncture for Adults with Suspected Bacterial Meningitis

Head imaging prior to LP	• Age ≥60 • History of CNS disease (mass lesion, stroke, focal infection) • Immunocompromised • History of seizure ≤1 week before presentation • Abnormal neurologic exam*
Immunocompetent	• Non-contrast image sufficient
Immunocompromised	• Image with and without contrast to evaluate for parenchymal enhancing lesions

* Abnormal level of consciousness, inability to answer two consecutive questions or follow two consecutive commands, gaze palsy, abnormal visual fields, facial palsy, arm and/or leg drift, abnormal language.

Table 8.6 Suggested CSF Studies

Routine studies on all CSF	Cell count, glucose, protein, routine bacterial culture
Acute aseptic meningitis	Consider enterovirus PCR, WNV IgM/IgG
Immunocompromised	Same list as above, and VZV, CMV, EBV, HHV-6 PCR
Chronic aseptic meningitis, immunocompetent	VDRL, coccidioidomycosis serology and complement fixation, cryptococcal antigen, MTB (minimum 10 mL), cytology (minimum 10–20 mL)
Immunocompromised	Same list as above, and consider infectious disease and/or neurology consult
Eosinophilic meningitis*	Consider cysticercosis serology, coccidioidomycosis serology and CF titer, MTB in appropriate patient

* Defined as >10 eosinophils and/or >10% eosinophils on cell count.

CF – complement fixation; MTB – *Mycobacterium tuberculosis*; RT-PCR – reverse transcriptase polymerase chain reaction; VDRL – venereal disease research laboratory.

in administration of antibiotics does negatively impact the outcomes of patients with acute bacterial meningitis (ABM). This consideration is particularly important as mounting evidence continues to suggest that imaging is over-used and delays appropriate antibiotic +/– steroid treatment.

CSF Studies

Ideally, the LP should be performed with the patient in a lateral decubitus position, so that an accurate opening pressure can be measured. After measuring and recording the opening pressure, we recommend collection of 2 mL of fluid in tubes 1 and 2, 6 mL in tube 3, and 10 mL in tube 4. Tube 1 is typically sent for cell count, tube 2 for protein and glucose, and tube 3 for microbiologic studies (see Table 8.6). Tube 4 can be used for a second cell count to assess whether the tap was traumatic, for cytology, or for extra cultures, serologies, or PCR studies.

Interpreting the CSF

Generally, in ABM, the white blood cell (WBC) count is elevated, often above 1,000, with a neutrophilic predominance (see Tables 8.7 and 8.8). Mildly elevated WBC counts (>5) can be seen in healthy premature infants and neonates, and chronic HIV infection can cause a mild, clinically asymptomatic CSF pleocytosis. Lymphocytic predominance can be seen in *Listeria* meningitis, neonatal gram-negative rod meningitis, and in both partially and fully treated bacterial meningitis. In ABM, the protein is usually greater than 100 mg/dL, and the glucose is usually less than 40 mg/dL. When the patient has a very elevated serum blood glucose, as in diabetes, estimating the CSF:serum glucose ratio can be helpful. Generally, ratios below 0.31 are more likely to indicate bacterial meningitis.

In viral meningitis, a milder lymphocytic pleocytosis (often 10 to 1,000), with no or only mildly elevated opening pressure, is the rule. The protein is also mildly elevated, usually ranging between 50 and 80, whereas glucose is generally normal, above 40, and the CSF:serum ratio generally is greater than 0.31.

Treatment

The rapid administration of appropriate antibiotics is the most important step in the treatment of ABM (see Table 8.9). If brain imaging is required prior to LP (see Table 8.5), empiric antibiotics (+/– steroids, see below) should be given immediately after drawing blood cultures, but prior to imaging and LP. The CSF pleocytosis will persist, though the likelihood of isolating a bacterial pathogen from the CSF culture decreases with time from antibiotic administration.

Steroids

In 2002, a prospective, double-blinded, randomized study of adults with bacterial meningitis showed an overall benefit from treatment with four days of dexamethasone initiated with or before the first dose of antibiotics, with all of the benefit being secondary to effects in patients with pneumococcal meningitis. Although this study has been criticized and debated for years, recent studies from the Netherlands suggest that widespread use of adjuvant steroids has led to a decline in both pneumococcal and non-pneumococcal meningitis mortality. Similarly, a US study also suggested that the use of adjuvant steroids led to a decreased mortality in US *S. pneumoniae* patients. Despite these findings, a more recent study that looked at several Connecticut community hospitals found that less than 8% of

Table 8.7 General Guidelines for CSF Parameters in Different Diagnoses

Etiology	OP (mm H$_2$O)	Cell Count	Differential	Protein (mg/dL)	Glucose (mg/dL)	Other
Normal:						
Term*		0–22	61% PMN	20–170	34–119	
Child*	80–110	0–7	5% PMN	5–40	40–80	
Adult	<200	0–5	0%–rare	<45	>55	
Acute bacterial meningitis	Elevated	>1,000†	PMNs predominate	Elevated	Low (CSF:serum ratio often <0.31)	Gram stain +
Viral meningitis	Normal to mildly elevated	<1,000	Monocytic‡	Normal to mild elevation	Normal to mildly low	Patient not septic or obtunded
Fungal or MTB	Often elevated	<500	Monocytic	Mild to highly elevated	Low	High volume for culture

* Adapted from J. Robertson, Blood chemistry and body fluids in J. Robertson and N. Shilkofski (eds.), *Harriet Lane Handbook: A Manual for Pediatric Housestaff*, 17th edn. (Philadelphia, PA: Elsevier Mosby; 2005), Table 25–3.

† Can be low to absent in the immunocompromised.

‡ Refers to all cells that are not polymorphonuclear.

MTB – *Mycobacterium tuberculosis*; OP – opening pressure; PM –, polymorphonuclear neutrophil leukocyte.

Table 8.8 Differential Diagnoses of CSF Findings

Cell	Differential	Protein	Glucose	Differential Diagnosis
>1,000	PMNs mostly	Elevated	Low	Bacterial meningitis, very early viral (generally <1,000 cells)
<1,000	Monocytic*	Normal or mildly elevated	Normal or mildly low	Viral, partially treated bacterial, parameningeal focus (usually <100 cells), TB meningitis (though usually protein very elevated, glucose low), syphilis, carcinomatous meningitides (atypical cells in cell count or cytology)
<1,000	>10 absolute, and/or >10% eosinophils	Normal to elevated	Low	*A. cantonensis*, *C. immitis*, neurocysticercosis, sarcoidosis, MTB

* Refers to all cells that are not polymorphonuclear.

MTB – *Mycobacterium tuberculosis*; PMN – polymorphonuclear neutrophil leukocyte.

patients were given IDSA-recommended adjuvent steroids (or appropriate antibiotics).

IDSA guidelines recommend, in adults, giving dexamethasone 0.15 mg/kg intravenously (IV) with or before the first dose of antibiotics and every 6 hours thereafter to patients with suspected or proven bacterial meningitis, except for those who are in septic shock. There is no clear consensus on whether or not to continue the steroids in patients who are found not to have pneumococcal meningitis, though many experts recommend discontinuing steroids if *S. pneumoniae* is not identified. Based on the results of several other studies, at this time, empiric adjuvant steroids are not recommended in patients with HIV or in developing countries. Based on animal models, there had been concern that dexamethasone decreases vancomycin penetration into the CNS. This issue was partially addressed by a prospective 2007 study that showed that patients with resistant pneumococcal meningitis, and placed on both steroids and empirical antibiotics, had adequate CSF vancomycins levels, and none of the patients had positive cultures on repeat LP. The caveat to this study is that a continuous vancomycin infusion was used.

In the pediatric population, dexamethasone given before or with the first dose of antibiotics decreased the incidence of hearing loss and other neurologic complications, especially in children with Hib meningitis. Thus, in children with Hib, the recommendation is to give 0.15 mg/kg every 6 hours for 2 to 4 days. The evidence is less clear for pneumococcal meningitis, and the current recommendation is to consider dexamethasone in children with pneumococcal disease. For infants less than 6 weeks old, there are not enough data to make a recommendation for or against adjuvant dexamethasone.

Chronic Meningitis, Fungal Meningitis, and Unusual Pathogens

Chronic meningitis can present with fever, headache, and mild meningismus, but as the name implies, it is chronic or subacute in nature. In general, chronic meningitis CSF studies demonstrate a monocytic pleocytosis, a normal or mildly elevated protein, and a normal or low glucose. The infectious etiologies below generally present as chronic meningitis with some exceptions (e.g. *Naegleria fowleri*) which are noted on a case-by-case basis.

Fungal Meningitis

Although fungal meningitis occurs most commonly in the immunocompromised or in patients with a prolonged hospital

Table 8.9 Treatment of Bacterial Meningitis

Patient Category	Organisms	Empiric Treatment*
Neonates (<1 month)	• Group B *Streptococcus* • *E. coli, K. pneumoniae* • *L. monocytogenes*	Ampicillin: 0–7 days old: 200 mg/kg/day IV (divided every 8 hours) 8–28 days: 300 mg/kg/day IV (divided every 6 hours) *plus* Cefotaxime: 0–7 days: 100–150 mg/kg/day IV (divided every 8–12 hours) 8–28 days: 150–200 mg/kg/day IV (divided every 6–8 hours) *or* Gentamicin: 0–7 days: 5 mg/kg/day IV (divided every 12 hours) 8–28 days: 7.5 mg/kg/day IV (divided every 8 hours)
1 month–5 years	• *N. meningitidis* • *S. pneumoniae* • *H. influenza*	Vancomycin 20 mg/kg/dose IV every 6 hours *plus* Ceftriaxone 50 mg/kg/dose IV every 12 hours *or* Cefotaxime 225–300 mg/kg/day IV (divided every 6–8 hours)
6–50 years	• *N. meningitidis* • *S. pneumoniae*	Vancomycin Pediatric: see previous box Adult: 15–20 mg/kg/dose IV every 8–12 hours *plus* Ceftriaxone Pediatric: see previous box Adult: 2 g IV every 12 hours *or* Cefotaxime Pediatric: see previous box Adult: 2 g IV every 4 hours
>50 years	• *S. pneumoniae* • *N. meningitidis* • *L. monocytogenes*	Vancomycin (dose as above) *plus* Ceftriaxone or cefotaxime (dose as above) *plus* Ampicillin 2 g IV every 4 hours

* Refer to institutional guidelines regarding dosing adjustments for gestational age and renal impairment.

stay, there are several fungi which can also infect immuno-competent hosts (see Table 8.10). In general, fungal meningitis presents with a mild CSF pleocytosis and an abnormally low CSF glucose level. The clinical presentation is often a basilar meningitis, which can affect cranial nerves or cause hydrocephalus.

Cryptococcus neoformans is distributed worldwide and can infect immunocompetent patients, but more commonly infects patients with acquired immunodeficiency syndrome (AIDS) or a history of prolonged, high-dose steroid use. In the immunosuppressed patient, the inflammatory response can be blunted, though fever is usually evident of the presentation. Immunocompromised patients may lack a pleocytosis, which is a negative prognostic indicator. Increased intracranial pressure is a common feature and associated with death in those with cryptococcal meningitis. When suspicion for *Cryptococcus* is high if the opening pressure on LP is greater than 250 mm H$_2$O, and symptoms of increased intracranial pressure are present, enough CSF should be drained to decrease the opening pressure by 50% if extremely high, or to below 200 mm H$_2$O. Lowering the intracranial pressure will reduce complications such as cranial neuropathies, herniation, and death. CSF cryptococcal

antigen testing is highly sensitive and specific for this disease and can be analyzed within 24 hours at most institutions.

Coccidioides immitis, a dimorphic fungus endemic to the southwestern United States, Mexico, and Central and South America, usually causes an asymptomatic or mildly symptomatic pulmonary infection, but can disseminate and cause meningitis in immunocompetent patients. Certain ethnic groups, Filipinos, African Americans, and Latinos, are much more likely to have disseminated coccidioidomycosis. Testing for coccidioidomycosis requires serum and CSF serology, which, if positive, should be confirmed with complement fixation titers. The complement fixation titers help determine the likelihood of disseminated disease and can be followed for treatment effectiveness. CSF eosinophilia is common. Direct testing for coccidioides antigens is expected to be available soon.

Meningitis caused by *Candida* species is seen most often in those who are at risk for invasive candidiasis: neonates, prematurely born infants, neutropenic patients, and those exposed to long courses of broad-spectrum antibiotics. Neonates with candidemia appear to have a much higher risk of meningeal involvement than adults with candidemia. Patients with

Table 8.10 Fungal Meningitis

Fungus*	Associated Risks
Cryptococcus neoformans	• Found worldwide and can infect immunocompetent patients • Most commonly found in patients with AIDS or prolonged high-dose steroid use • Subacute symptoms common in all immunocompromised hosts: headache with or without fever and no nuchal rigidity • CSF can lack a pleocytosis, which is a bad prognostic sign • If the opening pressure is >250 mm H_2O, CSF should be drained to <200 mm H_2O or half of opening pressure • Diagnosis is made with the CSF cryptococcal antigen test, which is highly sensitive
Coccidioides immitis (Coccidioidomycosis)	• Most often seen in immunocompetent patients of certain ethnic groups (Filipinos, African Americans, and Latinos) • Endemic to the southwestern United States, Mexico, Central and South America • CSF eosinophilia is a hallmark, though it does not have to be present • Diagnosis requires serum and CSF serology, which, if positive, should be confirmed with complement fixation titers • Direct testing for coccidioides antigens is expected to be available soon.
Candida spp.	• Seen in neonates, premature infants, neutropenic patients, those exposed to long courses of broad-spectrum antibiotics, and those with ventricular shunts • Neonates with candidemia have a higher risk of meningeal involvement compared to adults • Patients with CNS prosthetics, such as shunts, are predisposed to candidal meningitis without candidemia
Rare fungal infections in severely immunocompromised hosts	• *Aspergillus* spp., *Histoplasmosis capsulatum*, *Pseudallescheria boydii*, and *Penicillium marneffei* • Zygomycetes (*Rhizopus* spp.) in diabetics after a bout of DKA

* Fungal infections of the CNS often present with basilar meningitis, which can affect cranial nerves or cause hydrocephalus, leading to decreased levels of consciousness.

ventricular shunts are predisposed to candidal meningitis without concomitant candidemia.

In the severely immunocompromised host, such as the immunosuppressed transplant patient or AIDS patient, meningitis can be caused by relatively unusual fungi, including, *Histoplasma capsulatum*, *Pseudallescheria boydii*, and *Penicillium marneffei* (usually in AIDS patients from Southeast Asia). Zygomycete meningitis, such as *Rhizopus* species, can be seen secondary to invasion from the sinuses in poorly controlled diabetics, classically after an episode of diabetic ketoacidosis (DKA). *Aspergillus* meningitis is rare, and though invasive *Aspergillus* CNS disease is usually seen in severely immunocompromised patients, a recent study suggests pure *Aspergillus* meningitis more commonly occurs in the immunocompetent. Finally, in 2012, a multi-state outbreak of *Exserohilum rostratum* meningitis occurred in association with epidural injection of contaminated methylprednisolone acetate. At this time, the outbreak is considered over and no further cases are anticipated.

Tuberculous Meningitis

Tuberculosis (TB) is the most common cause of chronic bacterial meningitis worldwide. Risk factors include immigration from a country endemic for TB, homelessness, history of TB exposure, history of incarceration, and risk factors for immunosuppression (HIV, alcohol abuse, diabetes mellitus, elderly age, and immunosuppressive drugs, especially anti-TNF-alpha antibodies). Of the immunosuppressive risk factors, untreated HIV/AIDS is associated with the highest likelihood of developing active TB (reactivation or new infection), including extra-pulmonary disease. In areas of the world endemic for TB, children 0 to 4 years old are the most likely to develop TB meningitis.

The CSF in tuberculous meningitis is characterized by a monocytic pleocytosis, occasionally a mild eosinophilia, low glucose, and moderately elevated protein. Definitive diagnosis is made by positive CSF PCR for TB DNA or culture for acid-fast bacilli, which requires high volumes of CSF and can take 4 to 8 weeks for results to return. A newer real-time PCR assay (Xpert MTB/RIF) holds promise for a more rapid and sensitive test for TB meningitis, but a number of issues have limited its in the developing world, where the need is highest. Both adult and pediatric patients with TB meningitis will generally present with greater than 5 to 6 days of symptoms and commonly have fever. Meningismus is often lacking early on, but will develop as the disease progresses. Adults more commonly present with headache, while children present with vomiting and malaise/anorexia. Multiple neurologic complications can result from TB meningitis and can often be the presenting complaint. Of these, altered mentation, hydrocephalus, cranial neuropathies, and seizures are relatively common, with hydrocephalus and seizures being more common in children, and alterations in mentation being seen more commonly in adults. If clinical suspicion is high enough, and the CSF compatible with a diagnosis of tuberculous meningitis, initiating empiric four-drug therapy in consultation with an infectious disease specialist is appropriate. If the patient is HIV-negative, in both children and adults, adjuvant treatment with glucocorticoids is also warranted, as it has been demonstrated to decrease mortality, though some debate about this adjuvant therapy still exists.

Syphilis

Syphilis is caused by the spirochete bacterium *Treponema pallidum*, and is usually acquired through sexual contact. The incidence of syphilis in the United States declined most dramatically after the introduction of penicillin, and then again from 1990 to 2001. However, rates have increased annually from 2001. While the increase in syphilis was originally driven by men who have sexual intercourse with men, from 2013 to 2015, the rates increased in both men and women, which, not surprisingly, has led to an increase in cases of congenital syphilis. Men who have sexual intercourse with men and men aged 20 to 29 continue to have the highest rate of syphilis (both primary and secondary). HIV-positive patients have a high incidence of neurosyphilis and treatment failures.

Neurologic complications of syphilis can occur in all stages of syphilis (primary, secondary, and tertiary), though the meningeal forms of syphilis generally occur within the first several years of infection, and can either present acutely or chronically. Early complications of neurosyphilis include asymptomatic and symptomatic meningitis, both of which can often be found in association with other manifestations of secondary syphilis, particularly the characteristic rash on the palms and soles. Symptomatic meningitis presents with headache, photophobia, nausea, vomiting, meningismus, and cranial nerve deficits. Cranial nerves VII and VIII are most commonly affected. With asymptomatic meningitis, patients have CSF findings consistent with inflammation, but not clinical signs of CNS disease. However, if these patients remain untreated, they are at increased risk of developing other manifestations of neurosyphilis.

CSF studies in syphilitic meningitis are non-specific, showing a mononuclear predominant pleocytosis, elevated protein, and decreased glucose. Given the difficulty in culturing *T. pallidium*, serologic tests are routinely used to aid in the diagnosis of neurosyphilis. The gold standard is a positive CSF VDRL assay, but given its sensitivity of <30%, a negative CSF VDRL cannot exclude syphilitic meningitis. CSF fluorescent treponemal antibody absorption testing has a lower specificity, but higher sensitivity, and is often used to exclude the diagnosis. Serum studies for VDRL and RPR assays should also be done if syphilis is suspected. Ultimately, the diagnosis of syphilitic meningitis (except in those with florid secondary syphilis) is complicated and requires the integration of CSF abnormalities, clinical findings, and risk factors. Given this complexity, the diagnosis of syphilitic meningitis should be done in coordination with neurologic and infectious disease consultation. Penicillin is the treatment of choice, but dose and route of administration depend upon the stage of disease.

Other rare causes of chronic meningitis include *Borrelia burgdorferi*, *Leptospirosis* spp., *Brucella* spp., *Francisella tularensis*, and rickettsial diseases (other than Rocky Mountain spotted fever, which presents acutely).

Parasitic Meningitis

Taenia solium is the etiologic agent of cysticercosis, and thus neurocysticercosis, which is the most common cause of seizures worldwide. Although neurocysticercosis usually presents as a new seizure secondary to active or degenerating cysts in the brain parenchyma, cysts can develop in the ventricular system and produce subacute meningitis. If the cyst ruptures in the ventricle, a more acute decline can ensue. Neurocysticercosis meningitis is often accompanied by typical parenchymal lesions (see Table 8.11). Treatment recommendations should be made in consultation with a neurologist.

Angiostrongylus cantonensis is found in Southeast Asia and the Pacific basin, which includes Hawaii. It generally presents as acute meningitis, often accompanied by cranial neuropathies and paresthesias in the limbs, trunk, or face. Treatment is supportive, but the symptoms can linger for weeks.

Both of the above entities often produce CSF eosinophilia.

Naegleria fowleri is a free-living ameba found in warm fresh water, such as lakes, rivers, hot springs, and wells. It can cause primary amebic meningoencephalitis, which is usually fatal. *Naegleria* reaches the brain via the olfactory nerve, and should be suspected in patients presenting with a clinical picture consistent with ABM and who have a recent history of swimming or diving in fresh water. It cannot be contracted by drinking untreated water, but has been contracted by bathing in contaminated well water. If *Naegleria* is suspected, given the high rate of mortality (approaches 100%), infectious disease consultation should be urgently initiated to define the appropriate multidrug regimen, including miltefosine, which is now available in the United States.

There are a variety of non-infectious causes of chronic meningitis (see Table 8.12). These causes often present with the same subacute complaints as infectious chronic meningitis, except most lack fever as one of the presenting signs. Table 8.4 includes non-infectious mimics of acute meningitis.

Key features that may help to distinguish chronic meningitis from viral or bacterial meningitis are:

- time course (subacute in chronic meningitis, acute in bacterial or viral meningitis)

Table 8.11 Parasitic Meningitis

Etiology	Associated Risks
Taenia solium	• Found in various areas of the world, but not common in the United States • Etiologic agent of cysticercosis and neurocysticercosis • Cysts can develop in the ventricular system and produce subacute meningitis
Angiostrongylus cantonensis	• Found in Southeast Asia and the Pacific basin, including Hawaii • Generally presents as an acute meningitis • Often causes cranial neuropathies and paresthesias in the limbs, trunk, or face
Naegleria fowleri	• Warm fresh water, associated with water sports, has been associated with bathing in contaminated well water • Presents like ABM, often spring or summer

Table 8.12 Chronic Non-Infectious Meningitis

Non-Infectious* Causes of Meningitis	Etiology
Chemical	• NSAIDs • Antibiotics (trimethoprim, amoxicillin, cephalosporins) • Immunosuppressants (azathioprine, cytarabine, OKT3 antibody)
Rheumatologic	• SLE • Sarcoidosis (often as basilar meningitis) • Wegener's granulomatosis • Behçet's • Vogt–Koyanagi–Harada syndrome (bilateral ocular disease and chronic meningitis)
Tumor	• Carcinomatous meningitides – often the glucose is very low and cytology shows atypical cells • Send large volume (some recommend approximately 20 mL) for cytology, which should be done on same day as LP
Intrathecal	• Contrast • Chemotherapy

* Except for vasculitis and lymphoma, these non-infectious etiologies will generally not present with fever.

NSAID – non-steroidal anti-inflammatory drug.

- mild meningismus
- immunocompromised patients may be afebrile

Special Considerations

In 2017, IDSA released the first ever guidelines for health-care-associated ventriculitis and meningitis. The guidelines do provide some guidance for patients who have external or internal shunts, basilar skull fractures, and/or history of neurosurgical procedures. As there are few randomized controlled trials in this area, expert opinion is often utilized. Overall, the guidelines recommend that if these patients present with symptoms of meningitis or ventriculitis, health-care-associated ventriculitis or meningitis should be considered. Evaluation of these patients will generally require imaging (ideally an MRI with/without contrast), CSF studies, and consultation with infectious disease specialists and neurosurgery.

Shunt Infections

Generally, the diagnosis of CSF infections secondary to internalized or externalized shunts, such as ventriculoperitoneal or ventriculoatrial shunts, will require tapping of the shunt or obtaining CSF from the external shunt. Patients often present with shunt malfunction and signs of increased intracranial pressure such as headache, nausea, and decreased level of consciousness or lethargy. They may or may not have fever. Infecting organisms are often coagulase-negative *Staphylococcus*, *Staphylococcus aureus*, *P. acnes*, *E. coli*, *Klebsiella*, *Proteus*, or *Pseudomonas aeruginosa*. Additionally, they can be predisposed to candidal meningitis without concomitant candidemia. Given this range of organisms, the recommendation is to start vancomycin, and a cephalosporin (e.g. ceftazidime or cefepime), or carbapenem (e.g. meropenem) with anti-pseudomonal activity. Most often, infected shunts must be removed. Of note, while the IDSA guidelines recommend peri-procedural antibiotics for neurosurgical procedures (including placement of external ventricular devices (EVDs)), they recommend against prolonged prophylactic antibiotics for the duration of EVD use.

Skull Fractures, Penetrating Trauma, or History of Neurosurgical Procedure

There are no data to support prophylactic antibiotics to prevent meningitis in patients with basilar skull fractures. If a patient with a known history of skull fracture or CSF leak presents with symptoms consistent with meningitis, then empiric antibiotics should again include vancomycin and a cephalosporin, or carbapenem with anti-pseudomonal activity.

Immunocompromised Patients

Immunocompromised patients include those with HIV and CD4 count below 500 or AIDS, those with a history of transplant who are on immunosuppressive therapy, and those taking chronic steroids above 20 mg daily. Immunocompromised patients have a blunted inflammatory response and may lack meningismus or fever in the setting of meningitis. All immunocompromised patients should have neuroimaging with contrast prior to lumbar puncture. Additionally, because immunocompromised patients may have meningitis without an associated pleocytosis, the general guidelines for evaluating CSF may not apply. Finally, viral meningitis in the immunocompromised can be life-threatening. Consultation with an infectious disease specialist is recommended for the immunocompromised patient that is suspected of having meningitis.

Complications and Admission Criteria

Any patient with proven or highly suspected bacterial meningitis should be admitted. Patients with viral meningitis may require admission if they are unable to keep down food and liquids, or require IV medications for pain control. A patient with suspected viral meningitis may be discharged when there is a friend or family member available to monitor the patient for signs or symptoms requiring return to the emergency department: not improving in 24 to 48 hours, unable to keep down food or liquids, increasing lethargy, or altered mental status. Patients with chronic meningitis, who do not appear to have hydrocephalus or other concerns for increased intracranial pressure, can also be discharged from the ED if they have reliable follow-up.

Increased intracranial pressure (ICP) can be a complication of any form of meningitis, though it is generally not seen in viral meningitis. Uncontrolled increased ICP can lead to permanent neurologic sequelae or death. Several mechanisms can lead to elevated ICP, including diffuse inflammation associated with bacterial meningitis, or hydrocephalus associated with arachnoiditis in subacute meningitis. Symptoms of elevated ICP include headache, lethargy, nausea, and vomiting, all of which are progressive. Measures used to control ICP include hyperventilation, IV mannitol, hypertonic saline, or removal of CSF by repeat lumbar punctures or external ventricular drainage.

Infection Control

In general, most etiologies of meningitis do not require contact isolation. The exceptions are *N. meningitides* and tuberculous meningitis. Patients with meningococcal disease will need to have droplet precautions for the first 24 hours after appropriate antibiotics are started. Patients with proven or suspected tuberculous meningitis should be placed in respiratory isolation until an active respiratory infection can be ruled out. Depending on state-specific guidelines, these cases may require reporting to the department of public health, who may initiate contact screening.

Table 8.13 outlines the use of chemoprophylaxis in meningitis. Provision of chemoprophylaxis to household contacts and staff with exposure to respiratory droplets from a case of meningococcal meningitis often falls to the acute care provider. In the case of meningococcal outbreak secondary to serotype b, MenB, vaccination efforts with either of the two FDA-approved MenB vaccines are recommended. Patients with Hib meningitis do not need isolation precautions, but chemoprophylaxis for household, school, or daycare contacts may be necessary.

In general, patients with viral meningitis do not need to be isolated, though contact precautions should be considered in cases associated with severe enterovirus diarrhea.

Pearls and Pitfalls

1. Never delay appropriate antibiotic therapy for neuroimaging.
2. In neonates and infants, meningitis can present with fever and non-specific signs.
3. Viral meningitis does not cause obtundation or sepsis (except rarely in neonates and the immunocompromised).
4. Immunocompromised patients with meningitis can present with relatively mild symptoms, and they may have a very mild or no CSF pleocytosis.
5. If a lumbar puncture is considered, it should probably be done.
6. Give steroids prior to or with antibiotics.

References

Antinori, S., Corbellino, M., Meroni, L., *et al.* *Aspergillus* meningitis: a rare clinical manifestation of central nervous system aspergillosis. Case report and review of 92 cases. *J. Infection* 2013; 66(3): 218–38.

Aurelius, E., Franzen-Rohl, E., Glimaker, M., *et al.* Long-term valacyclovir suppressive treatment after herpes simplex virus type 2 meningitis: a double-blind, randomized controlled trial. *Clin. Infect. Dis.* 2012; 54(9): 1304–13.

Table 8.13 Chemoprophylaxis

Organism	Contact	Antibiotic Regimen
N. meningitidis	• All household contacts • Child-care or school contacts • Contacts with exposure to secretions of index case (including health-care workers) • Contact in above categories occurring ≤7 days prior to onset of illness in index case	Rifampin*: Neonate: 5 mg/kg PO/IV BID × 2 days ≥1 mo: 10 mg/kg PO BID × 2 days Adults: 600 mg PO BID × 2 days Ceftriaxone: <15 years 125 mg IM once ≥15 years 250 mg IM once Ciprofloxacin: ≥18 years: 500 mg PO once
H. influenzae B	• All household contacts, if household includes any susceptible child† • Nursery or child-care contacts if contain susceptible children *and* if there have been ≥2 cases at the nursery or child-care facility within 60 days • Index case if ≤2 years old or has a susceptible household member *and* index case treated with antibiotics other than ceftriaxone or cefotaxime	Rifampin*: Neonates: 10 mg/kg PO daily × 4 days ≥1 month old: 20 mg/kg PO daily × 4 days

* rifampin is not recommended in pregnant women due to teratogenicity.

† Unimmunized or partially immunized children <4 years old or immunocompromised children regardless of age and immunization status.

IM – intramuscular; PO – by mouth.

Adapted from American Academy of Pediatrics, Haemophilus influenzae infections in L. K. Pickering, C. J. Baker, S. S. Long, and J. A. McMillan (eds.), *Red Book: 2006 Report of the Committee on Infectious Disease*, 27th edn. (Elk Grove Village, IL; American Academy of Pediatrics, 2006), pp. 310–18.

Bennett, J. E. Chronic meningitis in J. E. Bennett, R. Dolin, and M. J. Blaser (eds.), *Mandell, Douglas, and Bennett's Principles and Practice of Infectious Diseases*, 8th edn. (Philadelphia, PA: Elsevier/Saunders, 2015), pp. 1138–43.

Bijlsma, M. W., Brouwer, M. C., Kasanmoentalib, E. S., *et al.* Community-acquired bacterial meningitis in adults in the Netherlands, 2006–14: a prospective cohort study. *Lancet Infect. Dis.* 2016; 16(3): 339–47.

Castellblanco, R. L., Lee, M. J., and Hasbun, R. Epidemiology of bacterial meningitis in the USA from 1997 to 2010: a population-based observational study. *Lancet Infect. Dis.* 2014; 14(9): 813–19.

Chia, D., Yavari, Y., Kirsanov, E., *et al.* Adherence to standard of care in the diagnosis and treatment of suspected bacterial meningitis. *Am. J. Medical Quality* 2015; 30(6): 539–42.

Cho, T. Clinical approach to the syndromes of viral encephalitis, myelitis, and meningitis in A. Tselis and J. Booss (eds.), *Handbook of Clinical Neurology* (Amsterdam: Elsevier, 2014), vol. 123, pp. 89–121.

Clauss, H. E. and Lorber, B. Central nervous system infection with Listeria monocytogenes. *Curr. Infect. Dis. Rep.* 2008; 10(4): 300–6.

Centers for Disease Control and Prevention (CDC). Listeria outbreaks, www.cdc.gov/listeria/outbreaks/ (accessed: March 16, 2017).

CDC. Meningococcal disease, https://www.cdc.gov/meningococcal/outbreaks/index.html (accessed November 9, 2015).

CDC. Mumps: mumps cases and outbreaks, www.cdc.gov/mumps/outbreaks.html (accessed March 16, 2017).

CDC. Naegleria fowleri – primary amebic meningoencephalitis (PAM) – amebic encephalitis, www.cdc.gov/parasites/naegleria/treatment.html (accessed March 16, 2017).

CDC. Rocky Mountain spotted fever, www.cdc.gov/ncidod/dvrd/rmsf/index.htm (accessed January 3, 2015).

CDC. West Nile virus, www.cdc.gov/westnile/ (accessed March 16, 2017).

CDC. Syphilis, www.cdc.gov/std/syphilis/ (accessed February 24, 2017).

Fishman, R. A. *Cerebrospinal Fluid in Diseases of the Nervous System*, 2nd edn. (Philadelphia, PA: Saunders, 1992).

Garcia-Monco, J. C. Tuberculosis in A. Tselis and J. Booss (eds.), *Handbook of Clinical Neurology* (Amsterdam: Elsevier, 2014), vol. 121, pp. 1485–99.

Glimaker, M., Johansson, B., Grindborg, O., *et al.* Acute bacterial meningitis: earlier treatment and improved outcome following guideline revision prompting prompt lumbar puncture. *Clin. Infect. Dis.* 2015; 60(8): 1162–9.

Granoff, D. M. Review of meningococcal group B vaccines. *Clin. Infect. Dis.* 2010; 50(2): S54–65.

Lawrence, D., Cresswell, F., Whetham, J., *et al.* Syphilis treatment in the presence of HIV: the debate goes on. *Curr. Opin. Infect. Dis.* 2015; 28(1): 44–52.

Noska, A., Kyrillos, R., Hansen, G., *et al.* The role of antiviral therapy in immunocompromised patients with herpes simplex virus meningitis. *Clin. Infect. Dis.* 2015; 60(2): 237–42.

Pappas, P. G. Lessons learned in the multistate fungal infection outbreak in the United States. *Curr. Opin. Infect. Dis.* 2013; 26(6): 545–50.

Prasad, K. and Singh, M. B. Corticosteroids for managing tuberculous meningitis. *Cochrane Database Syst. Rev.* 2008: CD002244.

Sejvar, J. Neuroepidemiology and the epidemiology of viral infections of the nervous system in A. Tselis and J. Booss (eds.), *Handbook of Clinical Neurology* (Amsterdam: Elsevier, 2014), vol. 123, pp. 67–87.

Thigpen, M. C., Whitney, C. G., Messonnier, M. E., *et al.* Bacterial meningitis in the United States, 1998–2007. *N. Eng. J. Med.* 2011; 364(21): 2016–25.

Thwaites, G. E., van Toorn, R., and Schoeman, J. Tuberculous meningitis: more questions, still too few answers. *Lancet Neurol.* 2013; 12(10): 999–1010.

Tunkel, A. R., Hartman, B. J., Kaplan, S. L., *et al.* Practice guidelines for the management of bacterial meningitis. *Clin. Infect. Dis.* 2004; 39(9): 1267–84.

Tunkel, A. R. Acute meningitis in J. E. Bennett, R. Dolin, and M. J. Blaser (eds.), *Mandell, Douglas, and Bennett's Principles and Practice of Infectious Diseases*, 8th edn. (Philadelphia, PA: Elsevier/Saunders, 2015), pp. 1097–137.

Tunkel, A. R., Hasbun, R., Bhimraj, A., *et al.* Clinical practice guidelines for healthcare-associated ventriculitis and meningitis. *Clin. Infect. Dis.* 2017; doi 10.1093/cid/ciw861.

Zunt, J. and Baldwin, K. J. Subacute and chronic meningitis. *Continuum* 2012; 18(6 Infectious Disease): 1290–318.

Additional Readings

Brower, M. C., Tunkel, A. R., and van de Beek, D. Epidemiology, diagnosis, and antimicrobial treatment of acute bacterial meningitis. *Clin. Microbiol. Rev.* 2010; 23(3): 467–92.

DeBiasi, R. L. and Tyler, K. L. Viral meningitis and encephalitis. *Continuum* 2006; 12(2): 58–94.

Ricard, J.D., Wolff, M., Lacherade, J. C., *et al.* Levels of vancomycin in cerebrospinal fluid of adult patients receiving adjunctive corticosteroids to treat pneumococcal meningitis: a prospective multicenter observational study. *Clin. Infect. Dis.* 2007; 44(2): 250–5.

Perfect, J. R., Dismukes, W. E., Dromer, F., *et al.* Clinical practice guidelines for the management of cryptococcal disease: 2010 updates by the Infectious Disease Society of America. *Clin. Infect. Dis.* 2010; 50(3): 291–322.

van de Beek, D., de Gans, J., Spanjaard, L., *et al.* Clinical features and prognostic factors in adults with bacterial meningitis. *N. Engl. J. Med.* 2004; 351(18): 1849–59.

Chapter

9

Rabies

Fredrick M. Abrahamian and Jada L. Roe

Introduction and Microbiology

Rabies is a highly fatal yet preventable disease through proper wound care and timely administration of rabies post-exposure prophylaxis. Rabies virus is a single-stranded negative-polarity RNA virus belonging to the genus *Lyssavirus* of the Rhabdoviridae family. Once the virus gains entry into its host, it begins to replicate within the cells of striated muscle. It then travels within the peripheral nervous system to the dorsal root ganglia at a rate of 5 to 10 centimeters per day, but then progresses rapidly up the spinal cord and to the brain. The virus then disseminates to peripheral organs such as the salivary glands, heart, lungs, liver, kidneys, and skeletal muscle via the autonomic nervous system.

Rabies is primarily a disease of wildlife and rarely occurs in humans in the United States. The predominant wildlife reservoir species include bats, foxes, raccoons, and skunks. The majority of human cases of rabies acquired in the United States are often associated with a bat rabies virus variant. The decline of human rabies cases in the United States and other developed countries is attributed to control of the disease in domestic animals, as well as effective pre- and post-exposure vaccination programs. Since there are no proven treatment modalities for rabies and mortality approaches 100% in patients with symptoms of infection, attention is directed at prevention of exposures and proper pre- and post-exposure rabies prophylaxis.

Epidemiology

The epidemiology of human rabies for a specific geographic region is related to the prevalence of rabies in animals, and the extent of human contact with them. In the United States, rabies is most commonly reported in animals such as raccoons, skunks, bats, and foxes. Other animals that can potentially transmit the disease include bobcats, coyotes, and mongooses.

Smaller mammals such as squirrels, rabbits, mice, and rats are considered to be at a lower risk for transmitting the disease. If infected, these animals often succumb quickly to the disease, and therefore have a very limited chance of spreading the disease. Non-mammalian bites (e.g. birds and reptiles) pose no risk of rabies transmission.

In the United States, dogs, cats, ferrets, and livestock are considered to be at a lower risk of being infected with rabies virus because of effective vaccination practices. However, in comparison to other parts of the United States, dogs along the border of the United States and Mexico (e.g. Texas–Mexico) and cats that roam freely in endemic areas with rabid terrestrial animals (e.g. raccoons in the northeastern United States) should be considered at higher risk.

Exposure to rabies most commonly occurs from the bite of an infected animal, which has the greatest potential for disease transmission. Bites from bats may go unnoticed because their small, thin, and sharp teeth bites are not felt. Transmission requires infected neural tissue or saliva to come into contact with broken skin (e.g. through a scratch) or mucous membranes. Handling, petting, or contact with low-risk bodily fluids (e.g. blood, urine, and stool) from terrestrial animals carries a low risk of disease transmission. Human-to-human rabies transmission has been reported in the setting of organ transplantation.

Clinical Features

The clinical manifestation of rabies can be categorized into three distinct phases: the prodromal phase, acute neurologic phase (encephalitic), and coma (see Table 9.1). The incubation period is variable and can range from 7 days to more than a year. In the majority of cases, the incubation period is 1 to 3 months. In comparison to bites of the extremities, bites to the head have shorter incubation periods.

Table 9.1 Clinical Features of Rabies

Incubation period	Typically 1–3 months
Organisms	Rabies virus, a single-stranded RNA virus belonging to the genus *Lyssavirus*
Signs and symptoms	**Prodromal phase:** non-specific symptoms (e.g. fever, headache, myalgia, malaise, fatigue, anorexia, nausea, vomiting, sore throat, non-productive cough, irritability, agitation, and anxiety) **Acute neurologic phase (encephalitic):** Confusion, delirium, hallucinations, incoordination, excessive salivation, hydrophobia, dysphasia, aerophobia, aphasia, seizures, hyperthermia, postural hypotension, and nuchal rigidity. In the paralytic form, paralysis is the predominant clinical feature either localized to the bitten extremity or diffuse. An ascending paralysis similar to Guillain-Barré syndrome may also occur. **Coma and death**
Laboratory findings	There are no specific laboratory findings that can reliably make the diagnosis of rabies in the emergency department
Treatment	Management is directed at supportive measures and the prevention of complications

The prodromal phase typically has a duration of 2 to 10 days, with non-specific symptoms that include fever, headache, myalgia, malaise, fatigue, anorexia, nausea, vomiting, sore throat, non-productive cough, irritability, agitation, or anxiety. Prodromal symptoms that are suggestive of rabies (occurring in 50 to 80% of patients) are paresthesia and fasciculation at or near the site of the bite.

The acute neurological (encephalitic) phase commonly lasts less than 1 week. This phase is diagnosed when there are objective signs of central nervous system disease (e.g. confusion, delirium, hallucinations, incoordination, aphasia, dysphasia, and seizures). This phase is often described in two forms: furious rabies (80%) and paralytic rabies (20%). Patients with furious rabies exhibit disorientation, hallucinations, and bizarre behavior. Early within this period, lucid and calm periods may intersperse with abnormal behavior. Patients also exhibit hydrophobia and aerophobia to a variable degree. The act of swallowing liquids or inspiring deeply results in violent contractions of the pharyngeal muscles, diaphragm, and the accessory muscles of inspiration. This is due to exaggerated respiratory tract protective reflexes and is an indication of central nervous system dysfunction. The presence of these symptoms should raise a high suspicion for rabies. Other symptoms can include autonomic dysfunction (e.g. excessive salivation, hyperthermia, and postural hypotension), nuchal rigidity, and convulsions. In the paralytic form of rabies, paralysis is the predominant clinical feature, which can either be localized (to the extremity that was bitten) or diffuse. The paralysis may also occur in an ascending pattern similar to Guillain–Barré syndrome.

In the final stages, the disease progresses to coma and eventually death. Death usually occurs from complications of the disease such as respiratory failure and cardiac dysfunction.

Differential Diagnosis

Other conditions to consider include:

- encephalitis from other pathogens (e.g. herpes viruses)
- meningitis
- poliomyelitis
- Guillain-Barré syndrome
- transverse myelitis
- intracranial mass lesions (e.g. brain abscess)
- cerebrovascular accident
- tetanus
- severe alcohol withdrawal
- adrenergic or cholinergic poisoning

Key features that may help to distinguish rabies are:

- A prodromal symptom suggestive of and often reported in patients with rabies, including paresthesia and fasciculation at or near the site of the bite.
- The majority of patients with rabies exhibit hydrophobia and aerophobia, symptoms that should raise a high suspicion for rabies.
- In comparison to rabies, patients with tetanus most often have normal mental status and normal cerebrospinal fluid.

Laboratory Diagnosis

There are no specific laboratory findings that can reliably make the diagnosis of rabies. Similar to other viral infections, the cerebrospinal fluid may demonstrate mild pleocytosis with lymphocytosis, mildly elevated protein, and a normal glucose. The ultimate antemortem diagnosis of rabies rests on the isolation of the organism from bodily fluids (e.g. saliva, cerebrospinal fluid) or an infected tissue sample (e.g. nape of the neck). Other diagnostic tools include the demonstration of the viral antigen or nucleic acid in the patient's saliva or tissue sample. Additionally, the discovery of a specific antibody in the serum of a previously unvaccinated person or presence of the antibody in the cerebrospinal fluid may be helpful.

Treatment

Once a patient develops signs and symptoms consistent with clinical rabies, there is no specific therapy. Interventions are directed at supportive measures and the prevention of complications.

Complications

Death from rabies occurs from complications of the disease such as respiratory failure (e.g. adult respiratory distress syndrome, hypoxia) and cardiac dysfunction (e.g. dysrhythmias).

Post-Exposure Prophylaxis

When evaluating a patient who has potentially been exposed to rabies virus, it is imperative to gather the following information: type of animal exposure, whether the animal is available for quarantine and brain testing, vaccination history (both for the patient and the animal), when and where the exposure occurred, and whether the attack was provoked or unprovoked (see Figure 9.1).

Rabies post-exposure prophylaxis includes administration of rabies vaccine and, depending on the patient's immunization history, human rabies immune globulin (HRIG). Rabies vaccine provides active immunity, whereas HRIG provides passive immunity. If indicated, pregnant women may receive rabies post-exposure prophylaxis.

HRIG is only administered to patients who have never been vaccinated against rabies. It is administered only once on the initial visit (day 0) at a dose of 20 international units/kg. Adherence to the dosing regimen is important, as administration of higher doses of HRIG may have interference with active production of rabies virus antibody. If possible, the full dose should be infiltrated intramuscularly around the bite wounds. The remaining dose should be infiltrated intramuscularly at a site distant from where the first vaccine dose was administered. If not given during the initial visit, it can be given once within 7 days of the rabies vaccine administration. The same syringe should not be used for administration of HRIG and rabies vaccine.

Immunocompetent individuals who have not been previously immunized should receive rabies vaccine on days 0, 3, 7, and 14. The four-dose rabies vaccination regimen replaced the historically recommended five-dose regimen based on data indicating no increase in favorable outcomes with the addition of a fifth dose of rabies vaccine. Immunocompromised patients should still receive a fifth dose on day 28. Previously vaccinated patients should receive the vaccine only on days 0 and 3. In adults and older children, rabies vaccine should be administered intramuscularly in the deltoid area. In young children, the preferred injection site is the outer aspect of the upper thigh. The vaccine should not be administered in the gluteal area as administration of vaccine in this region results in lower neutralizing antibody titers.

Local wound care should include cleansing the wound with a solution of soap and water. If possible, irrigate wounds with copious amounts of iodine-based virucidal cleansing solution (e.g. diluted povidone-iodine solution). Necrotic and devitalized tissues should be debrided. As indicated, tetanus prophylaxis and administration of antibiotics should be initiated.

Infection Control

Standard precautions aimed at preventing contact with potentially infectious bodily fluids such as saliva, cerebrospinal fluid, and tears are adequate for the care of patients with rabies. Blood, urine, and feces are not considered infectious. These patients do not require respiratory isolation. To reduce the potential for precipitating agitation, it is best to place patients in rooms that are quiet, limit procedures, and minimize patient manipulation and stimulation.

Pearls and Pitfalls

1. In the United States, animal rabies is most commonly reported in raccoons, skunks, bats, and foxes.
2. Dogs along the border of the United States and Mexico and cats that roam freely in endemic areas with rabid terrestrial animals should be considered at higher risk of being infected with rabies virus.
3. A prodromal symptom suggestive of rabies includes paresthesia and fasciculation at or near the site of the bite.
4. Hydrophobia and aerophobia should raise a high suspicion for rabies.
5. Consider rabies in the differential diagnosis of ascending paralysis.
6. Previously rabies vaccinated patients should not receive HRIG.

References

Centers for Disease Control and Prevention (CDC), Rupprecht, C. E., Briggs, D., *et al.* Use of a reduced (4-dose) vaccine schedule for postexposure prophylaxis to prevent human rabies: recommendation of the advisory committee on immunization practices. *MMWR Morb. Mortal. Wkly. Rep.* 2010; 59(RR-2): 1–9.

CDC. Human rabies prevention – United States, 2008: recommendations of the Advisory Committee on Immunization Practices. *MMWR Morb. Mortal. Wkly. Rep.* 2008; 57(RR-3): 1–28.

CDC. Human rabies, Mississippi, 2005. *MMWR Morb. Mortal. Wkly. Rep.* 2006; 55(8): 207–8.

CDC. Human rabies prevention – United States, 1999. *MMWR Morb. Mortal. Wkly. Rep.* 1999; 48(RR-1): 1–21.

Coleman, P. G., Fevre, E. M., and Cleaveland, S. Estimating the public health impact of rabies. *Emerg. Infect. Dis.* 2004; 10(1): 140–2.

Dyer, J. L., Wallace, R., Orciari, L., *et al.* Rabies surveillance in the United States during 2012. *J. Am. Vet. Med. Assoc.* 2013; 243(6): 805–15.

Dyer, J. L., Yager, P., Orciari, L., *et al.* Rabies surveillance in the United States during 2013. *J. Am. Vet. Med. Assoc.* 2014; 245(10): 1111–23.

Krebs, J. W., Long-Marin, S. C., and Childs, J. E. Causes, costs and estimates of rabies postexposure prophylaxis treatments in the United States. *J. Public Health Manage. Pract.* 1998; 4(5): 56–62.

Krebs, J. W., Mandel, E. J., Swerdlow, D. L., *et al.* Rabies surveillance in the United States during 2004. *J. Am. Vet. Med. Assoc.* 2005; 227(12): 1912–25.

McQuiston, J., Yager, P. A., Smith, J. S., *et al.* Epidemiologic characteristics of rabies virus variants in dogs and cats in the United States, 1999. *J. Am. Vet. Med. Assoc.* 2001; 218(12): 1939–42.

Noah, D. L., Drenzek, C. L., Smith, J. S., *et al.* Epidemiology of human rabies in the United States, 1980–1996. *Ann. Intern. Med.* 1998; 128(11): 922–30.

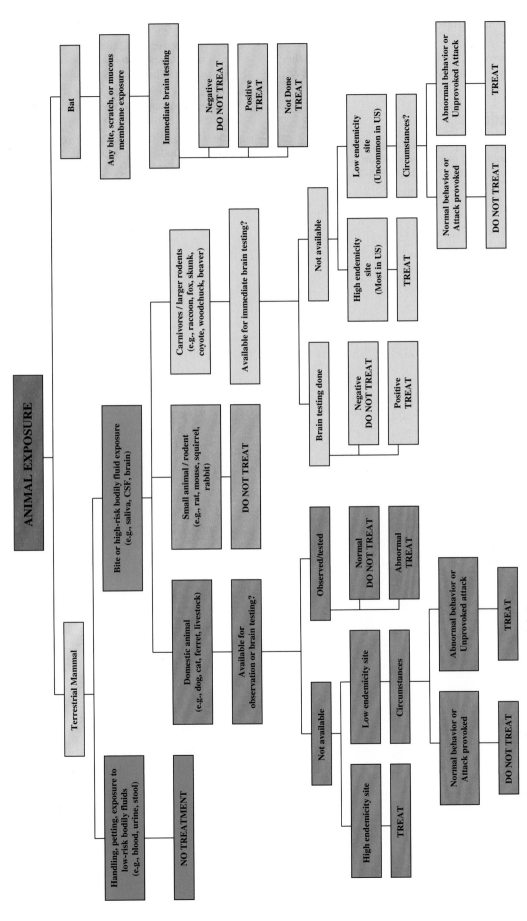

Figure 9.1 Algorithm for initiating rabies post-exposure prophylaxis.

Weiss, H. B., Friedman, D. I., Coben, J. H. Incidence of dog bite injuries treated in emergency departments. *JAMA* 1998; 279(1): 51–3.

Willoughby, R. E., Tieves, K., Hoffman, G. M., *et al.* Survival after treatment of rabies with induction of coma. *N. Engl. J. Med.* 2005; 352(24): 2508–14.

Additional Readings

Chutivongse, S., Wilde, H., Benjavongkulchai, M., *et al.* Postexposure rabies vaccination during pregnancy: effect on 202 women and their infants. *Clin. Infect. Dis.* 1995; 20(4): 818–20.

Dreesen, D. W. A global review of rabies vaccines for human use. *Vaccine* 1997; 15(Suppl.): S2–6.

Feder, H. M. Jr., Petersen, B. W., Robertson, K. L., *et al.* Rabies: still a uniformly fatal diseases? Historical occurrence, epidemiological trends, and paradigm shifts. *Curr. Infect. Dis. Rep.* 2012; 14(4): 408–22.

Moran, G. J., Talan, D. A., Mower, W., *et al.* Appropriateness of rabies postexposure prophylaxis treatment for animal exposures. *JAMA* 2000; 284(8): 1001–7.

Rupprecht, C. E. and Gibbons, R. V. Prophylaxis against rabies. *N. Engl. J. Med.* 2004; 351(25): 2626–35.

Warrell, M. J. and Warrell, D. A. Rabies and other lyssavirus diseases. *Lancet* 2004; 363(9413): 959–69.

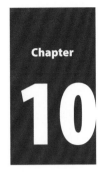

Chapter

10

Tetanus

Fredrick M. Abrahamian and Jada L. Roe

Introduction and Microbiology

Clostridium tetani is an obligatory anaerobic spore-forming microorganism. Spore germination and proliferation occurs in environments with low oxygen tension (e.g. necrotic tissue, frostbite, crush injuries). The two main toxins released by *C. tetani* are tetanospasmin and tetanolysin.

Tetanolysin damages cell membranes and lowers the oxygen content of tissue, providing a favorable environment for proliferation of the organism. Tetanospasmin, also known as tetanus toxin, is a neurotoxin that is responsible for the clinical manifestations of tetanus. It enters the nervous system through the neuromuscular junctions of alpha motor neurons. Tetanospasmin travels to the motor neuron body by retrograde axonal transport and then spreads transsynaptically to other neurons preventing the release of inhibitory neurotransmitters such as glycine and gamma-aminobutyric acid (GABA). Uninhibited motor neuron excitation results in muscle spasms, rigidity, contractions, and a hypersympathetic state.

Although now uncommon in developed countries, tetanus can occur in unvaccinated individuals. Recognition of the clinical presentation and basic management remains essential. Moreover, acute care providers play an important role in tetanus prevention.

Epidemiology

Tetanus is rare in the developed world, but remains widespread in developing countries, with an estimated 1 million cases worldwide per year. Large-scale immunization protocols, especially for infants and school-aged children, have significantly reduced the number of cases worldwide. Other factors such as availability of tetanus immunoglobulin, improved wound care management and childbirth practices, and advances in supportive care and airway management have also resulted in a decline in tetanus-associated morbidity and mortality.

In the United States, tetanus occurs primarily in adults, with most of the cases reported in older adults and injection drug users (IDUs). Other at-risk populations include immigrants from outside North America and Western Europe and persons lacking a formal education past grade school.

Clinical Features

Clinically, tetanus is classified into generalized, local, cephalic, and neonatal tetanus. Generalized tetanus, the most common form of the disease, results from the hematogenous spread of the toxin to myoneural junctions throughout the body (see Table 10.1). The incubation period can vary from 2 days to greater than 4 weeks, with the majority of cases occurring within 14 days. The incubation period is defined as the time from initial injury to the first symptom (e.g. trismus). A common symptom at presentation is trismus or "lockjaw," which is due to masseter muscle contraction and rigidity. Isolated trismus is the most common subtle finding at the time of presentation and the diagnosis can easily be missed at this stage. Other initial symptoms can include dysphagia and neck, back, and shoulder pain and stiffness.

As the disease progresses, patients develop generalized muscle rigidity and spasms, which may occur spontaneously or be precipitated by an external stimulus such as touch, light, or noise. A sardonic smile (risus sardonicus) occurs from sustained contraction and rigidity of facial muscles. Opisthotonos is another classical finding, where the head and feet are drawn backward and the spine arches forward. Elevated levels of catecholamines lead to a hypersympathetic state and autonomic dysfunction. This typically occurs around the second week of the disease, with clinical manifestations including fever, blood pressure extremes, and cardiac arrhythmias.

Table 10.1 Clinical Features: Generalized Tetanus

Incubation period	Variable (3–21 days); majority of cases occur within 14 days
Organisms	*Clostridium tetani*
Signs and symptoms	Trismus, dysphagia, neck, back, and shoulder pain and stiffness, risus sardonicus, opisthotonos
Laboratory findings	There are no specific laboratory findings that can reliably make the diagnosis of tetanus
Treatment	• Stabilization of the airway • Aggressive control and management of muscle spasms and rigidity with benzodiazepines or possibly paralytics • Passive immunization with human tetanus immune globulin • Active immunization with age-specific tetanus toxoid-containing vaccine • Antibiotics (e.g. metronidazole) • Control of autonomic instability • General wound care (e.g. debridement, incision and drainage of abscesses) and supportive measures
IM – intramuscular; IV – intravenous.	

Local tetanus manifests with rigidity and muscular spasms around the inciting wound and has the potential of becoming generalized. Affected muscles are painful at rest and during contractions, and deep tendon reflexes are more pronounced. These symptoms may persist for weeks to months. Local tetanus has a better prognosis than other forms of tetanus.

Cephalic tetanus is a specific type of local tetanus that affects the cranial nerves. It is usually associated with ear infections or wounds to the head following trauma. The initial presentation typically includes trismus and cranial nerve palsy. Most commonly the organism affects the facial nerve. Cephalic tetanus is considered a severe form of tetanus because of its potential for rapid progression to the generalized form.

Neonatal tetanus occurs in newborns of mothers who are unvaccinated or inadequately vaccinated for tetanus. The most common source of infection is the umbilical stump, through either contamination from a non-sterile delivery or improper umbilical cord care practices. Clinical manifestations occur within 10 days of birth and include generalized weakness, inability to suck, and irritability. The mortality rate is high, and survivors are often afflicted with mental and growth retardation.

Differential Diagnosis

Other conditions to consider include:

• generalized convulsive seizures
• extrapyramidal reaction
• malignant neuroleptic syndrome
• hypocalcemic tetany
• hyperventilation syndrome
• black widow spider bite
• strychnine poisoning
• drug withdrawal
• peritonitis
• temporomandibular joint dislocation
• rabies
• progressive fluctuating muscular rigidity (stiff-man syndrome)
• conversion reaction

Key features that may help to distinguish tetanus are:

• generalized muscle rigidity and spasms precipitated by an external stimulus such as touch, light, or noise; development of trismus, risus sardonicus, or opisthotonos
• history of a tetanus-prone injury
• lack of fever, muscle weakness, sensory symptoms, or mental status changes distinguish tetanus from most of the alternate diagnoses

Laboratory Diagnosis

There are no specific laboratory findings that can reliably make the diagnosis of tetanus. *C. tetani* is rarely isolated from wounds, and as a result, the diagnosis does not depend on bacterial confirmation. Even with isolation of the organism, routine bacteriologic studies cannot determine whether that strain possesses the plasmid required for tetanospasmin production.

The tetanus toxoid antibody titer is potentially helpful in assessing the susceptibility of a patient, but is not diagnostic. There have been case reports of tetanus occurring in individuals with high serum tetanus antibody titers that are assumed to be in the "protective" range.

Electromyographic studies may be helpful in documenting denervation and lack of intraspinal inhibition, and for tracking the progress of reinnervation in individual patients.

Treatment and Prophylaxis

All patients with tetanus should initially be managed in a closely monitored area, preferably the intensive care unit. Stabilization and control of the airway should be a priority, and the patient should be intubated at the first sign of airway compromise since pharyngeal and chest wall muscle spasms can result in aspiration or apnea. Environmental triggers should be minimized by creating a dark, quiet room, and limiting procedures and patient manipulation.

Muscle spasms and rigidity are controlled with benzodiazepines. In addition, benzodiazepines provide sedative, amnestic, and anxiolytic effects. Patients typically require large doses of intravenous (IV) benzodiazepines to achieve control of the muscle spasms. At these high doses, there have been reports of patients developing metabolic acidosis secondary to the accumulation of propylene glycol, a solvent vehicle for certain benzodiazepines. To avoid this complication, a constant infusion of midazolam (a water-soluble agent that does not contain propylene glycol) is recommended. Other drugs, such as propofol, intrathecal baclofen, dantrolene, magnesium sulfate, chlorpromazine, and barbiturates have also been used to treat tetanus-induced muscle spasms.

When muscle spasms are refractory to the above-mentioned medications, prolonged neuromuscular blockade is recommended to prevent rhabdomyolysis. Non-depolarizing neuromuscular blocking agents (e.g. vecuronium or rocuronium) are preferred because of their minimal cardiovascular effects. Benzodiazepines should be continued alongside neuromuscular blockade to ensure adequate sedation.

Human tetanus immune globulin (HTIG) passively immunizes patients by neutralizing unbound circulating tetanospasmin. In adults, HTIG should be administered intramuscularly (IM) into the deltoid muscle, and in infants and children into the anterolateral aspect of the upper thigh muscles. The efficacy of injecting a portion of the HTIG dose locally around the wound has not been established. HTIG should be given on the side opposite to where the tetanus toxoid was administered. Muscle spasms should be controlled prior to the administration of HTIG, because IM injections may precipitate additional spasms.

The recommended dosage of HTIG for the *treatment of active tetanus* ranges from 500 to 6,000 units with no definitive consensus on an optimal dose. HTIG does not cross the blood–brain barrier and has no effect on intraneural bound toxin. Because of its long half-life (~23 days), there is no need for repeated injections. Weight-adjusting the dose is also not necessary, as the amount of toxin produced in the body is independent of the patient's body mass. Dosage adjustments are not necessary in patients with renal failure. HTIG may be administered to pregnant patients when indicated.

Active immunization with tetanus toxoid-containing vaccine is also necessary because the disease does not confer immunity. The first two doses are given 4 to 6 weeks apart, and the third dose is given 6 to 12 months after the second dose. Tetanus toxoid should not be administered in the same syringe or at the same site as HTIG.

Local wound care (e.g. debridement, incision and drainage of abscesses, removal of foreign bodies) and antibiotics are routinely given in an attempt to eliminate the source of toxin production. It is essential that HTIG be given prior to any wound manipulation and antibiotic administration because both interventions have the potential to release additional free toxin into the bloodstream. Recommended antibiotics include metronidazole (500 mg IV every 6 to 8 hours), penicillin G (24 million units per day in divided doses), or doxycycline (100 mg IV every 12 hours) for 7 to 10 days. Some authorities recommend against penicillin, however, because of its centrally acting GABA antagonist activity and the potential to amplify the effects of tetanospasmin.

Autonomic instability may result in hemodynamic failure and unexpected cardiac arrest. There is no consensus as to a drug of choice for the sympathetic overactivity associated with tetanus. Bradydysrhythmias are less common and may require cardiac pacing.

Post-Exposure Prophylaxis

Post-exposure prophylaxis is based on the wound type and the patient's vaccination history (see Table 10.2). Wounds are classified as either low- or high-risk for tetanus. Clean, superficial (≤1 cm in depth), minor, acute (≤6 hours) wounds are considered to be at low risk for harboring *C. tetani*. High-risk wounds for tetanus include deep wounds (>1 cm in depth); puncture wounds; wounds contaminated with dirt, feces, soil, and saliva; and wounds associated with missiles, avulsions, crush injuries, devitalized or necrotic tissue, burns, and frostbite.

There are two important points to consider in the patient's vaccination history. First is whether or not the patient has received a primary immunization series, which consists of at least three doses of tetanus toxoid-containing vaccine. The second is the time elapsed from the last tetanus booster to possible exposure. Many people do not recall whether they have completed a primary series of tetanus immunization. All individuals who have served in the military or who went to elementary school in North America or Western Europe after 1950 likely have received their primary immunization series. Conversely, immigrants from outside North America or Western Europe and persons uneducated beyond grade school are more likely to lack the tetanus primary immunization series.

Primary immunization should begin in infancy with IM injections of diphtheria–tetanus–acellular pertussis vaccine adsorbed (DTaP) at 2, 4, and 6 months of age. The first and second boosters with DTaP should occur at 15 to 18 months and 4 to 6 years of age, respectively. The next tetanus booster is recommended at age 11 to 12 years with tetanus toxoid, reduced diphtheria toxoid, and acellular pertussis (Tdap) vaccine. Subsequent routine vaccinations are recommended with adult tetanus and diphtheria toxoids (Td) vaccine adsorbed every 10 years. For adults who require tetanus toxoid-containing vaccine, a single dose of Tdap is preferred to Td if they have not previously received Tdap.

Currently, Boostrix and Adacel are the two formulations of Tdap available in the United States. Boostrix is Food and Drug Administration (FDA)-approved for ages 10 years and older, while Adacel is approved for ages 11 to 64 years. However, if Boostrix is not available, Adacel can be administered to a patient over the age of 64 years. The most current recommended immunization schedule can be obtained through the Centers for Disease Control and Prevention National Immunization Program.

An additional historical question with regard to the patient's vaccination history is the time elapsed from the last tetanus booster to possible exposure. For low-risk tetanus wounds, it is recommended that a patient receive tetanus prophylaxis if it has been 10 or more years since the last tetanus toxoid-containing vaccine dose. This time span decreases to 5 years in the case of a high-risk tetanus wound.

Post-exposure prophylaxis with HTIG is recommended for patients with high-risk wounds who never received their primary immunization series (i.e. history of fewer than three

Table 10.2 Current Summary Guide to Tetanus Prophylaxis in Routine Wound Management

History of Adsorbed Tetanus Toxoid (Doses)	Clean, Minor Wounds		All Other Wounds*	
	Tdap or Td† (0.5 mL IM)	TIG (250 units IM)	Tdap or Td† (0.5 mL IM)	TIG (250 units IM)
Unknown or < three	Yes	No	Yes	Yes
Three or more	No‡	No	No§	No

* Such as, but not limited to, wounds contaminated with dirt, feces, soil, or saliva; puncture wounds; avulsions; and wounds resulting from missiles, crush injuries, burns, or frostbite.

† Tdap is preferred to Td for adolescents aged 11–18 years and adults who have never received Tdap. The preferred tetanus toxoid-containing vaccine for children aged <7 years is the pediatric diphtheria and tetanus toxoid and acellular pertussis vaccine (DTaP). Minimum age for DTaP administration is 6 weeks and maximum age is 6 years.

‡ Yes, if ≥10 years have elapsed since the last tetanus toxoid-containing vaccine dose.

§ Yes, if ≥5 years have elapsed since the last tetanus toxoid-containing vaccine dose.

Tdap – tetanus–diphtheria–acellular pertussis vaccine adsorbed formulated for use in adolescents and adults (Boostrix approved for use in persons 10 years of age or older; Adacel approved for use in persons aged 11–64 years); Td – adult diphtheria–tetanus vaccine adsorbed (minimum age: 7 years); TIG – tetanus immunoglobulin.

doses of adsorbed tetanus toxoid-containing vaccine) or for patients who are unaware of their vaccination history. The dose for post-exposure prophylaxis is 250 units IM into the deltoid muscle or anterolateral aspect of the upper thigh muscles (preferred site for infants and small children). HTIG will provide adequate antitoxin levels from 2 days to 4 weeks following administration.

Immunosuppressed individuals may receive tetanus toxoid, though there is some question as to whether these patients mount an adequate immunologic response to the vaccine.

Current recommendations are for all women to receive Tdap during every pregnancy. Optimal timing is between 27 and 36 weeks gestation. Both Td and Tdap are acceptable for administration during breastfeeding.

Complications

A shorter incubation period (<7 days) between injury and clinical tetanus, treatment delay greater than 24 hours, and early signs suggestive of autonomic dysfunction are factors commonly associated with poor prognosis. Tetanus associated with wound types such as burns, surgical procedures, umbilical stump infections, and septic abortions also carries a poor prognosis.

Hemodynamic failure may result from poorly controlled autonomic instability and nosocomial infections. Currently, these are the leading causes of mortality associated with tetanus. Respiratory failure used to be the leading cause of death before the ability to paralyze and mechanically ventilate patients, but is now less common. However, several respiratory complications still contribute to the morbidity and mortality of the disease (e.g. aspiration, pneumonia, acute respiratory distress syndrome). Prolonged muscle spasms may lead to rhabdomyolysis and subsequent hyperkalemia and renal failure.

Infection Control

Tetanus is not contagious. Standard contact precautions are adequate for the care of patients with tetanus. These patients do not require isolation.

Pearls and Pitfalls

1. Isolated trismus is the most common initial symptom of tetanus.
2. Populations at higher risk for developing tetanus in the United States include the elderly, IDUs, individuals with an incomplete or unknown vaccination history, immigrants from developing countries, and persons who have not completed elementary school.
3. A patient's tetanus vaccination history should include whether or not the patient has received a primary immunization series and the time elapsed from the last tetanus booster to possible exposure.
4. Post-exposure prophylaxis is based on the wound type and the patient's vaccination history; patients with tetanus-prone wounds who have gone more than 5 years since last vaccination should receive tetanus toxoid.
5. For adults, a single dose of Tdap is preferred to Td if they have not previously received Tdap.

References

Abrahamian, F. M. Management of tetanus: a review. *Curr. Treat. Options Infect. Dis.* 2001; 3: 209–16.

Abrahamian, F. M., Pollack, C. V., Lovecchio, F., *et al.* Fatal tetanus in a drug abuser with "protective" antitetanus antibodies. *J. Emerg. Med.* 2000; 18(2): 189–93.

Afshar, M., Raju, M., Ansell, D., *et al.* Narrative review: tetanus – a health threat after natural disasters in developing countries. *Ann. Intern. Med.* 2011; 154: 329–35.

Centers for Disease Control and Prevention (CDC). Advisory Committee on Immunization Practices recommended immunization schedules for persons aged 0 through 18 Years – United States, 2016. *MMWR Morb. Mortal. Wkly. Rep.* 2016; 65(4): 86–7.

CDC. Advisory Committee on Immunization Practices recommended immunization schedule for adults aged 19 years or older – United States, 2016. *MMWR Morb. Mortal. Wkly. Rep.* 2016; 65(4): 88–90.

CDC. Diphtheria, tetanus, and pertussis: recommendations for vaccine use and other preventive measures. *MMWR Morb. Mortal. Wkly. Rep.* 1991; 40(RR-10): 1–28.

CDC. Update: vaccine side effects, adverse reactions, contraindications, and precautions. *MMWR Morb. Mortal. Wkly. Rep.* 1996; 45(RR-12): 1–35.

Cook, T. M., Protheroe, R. T., and Handel, J. M. Tetanus: a review of the literature. *Br. J. Anaesth.* 2001; 87(3): 477–87.

Ergonul, O., Erbay, A., Eren, S., *et al.* Analysis of the case fatality rate of tetanus among adults in a tertiary hospital in Turkey. *Eur. J. Clin. Microbiol. Infect. Dis.* 2003; 22(3): 188–90.

Ernst, M. E., Klepser, M. E., Fouts, M., *et al.* Tetanus: pathophysiology and management. *Ann. Pharmacother.* 1997; 31(12): 1507–13.

Gergen, P. J., McQuillan, G. M., Kiely, M., *et al.* A population-based serologic survey of immunity to tetanus in the United States. *N. Engl. J. Med.* 1995; 332(12): 761–6.

Hsu, S. S. and Groleau, G. Tetanus in the emergency department: a current review. *J. Emerg. Med.* 2001; 20(4): 357–65.

Saltoglu, N., Tasova, Y., Midikli, D., *et al.* Prognostic factors affecting deaths from adult tetanus. *Clin. Microbiol. Infect.* 2004; 10(3): 229–33.

Santos, M. L., Mota-Miranda, A., Alves-Pereira, A., *et al.* Intrathecal baclofen for the treatment of tetanus. *Clin. Infect. Dis.* 2004; 38(3): 321–8.

Trujillo, M. H., Castillo, A., Espana, J., *et al.* Impact of intensive care management on the prognosis of tetanus. *Chest* 1987; 92(1): 63–5.

Additional Readings

Abrahamian, F. M. Tetanus: an update on an ancient disease. *Infect. Dis. Clin. Pract.* 2000; 9(6): 228–35.

Attygalle, D. and Rodrigo, N. New trends in the management of tetanus. *Expert Rev. Anti-Infect. Ther.* 2004; 2(1): 73–84.

Centers for Disease Control and Prevention (CDC). Updated recommendations for the use of tetanus toxoid, reduced diphtheria toxoid and acellular pertussis vaccine (Tdap) in pregnant women – Advisory Committee on Immunization Practices (ACIP). *MMWR Morb. Mortal. Wkly. Rep.* 2013; 62(7): 131–5.

CDC. Updated recommendations for use of tetanus toxoid, reduced diphtheria toxoid, and acellular pertussis (Tdap) vaccine in adults aged 65 years and older – Advisory Committee on Immunization Practices (ACIP). *MMWR Morb. Mortal. Wkly. Rep.* 2012; 61(25): 468–70.

Talan, D. A., Abrahamian, F. M., Moran, G. J., *et al.* Tetanus immunity and physician compliance with tetanus prophylaxis practices among emergency department patients presenting with wounds. *Ann. Emerg. Med.* 2004; 43(3): 305–14.

West Nile Encephalitis Virus

Michael S. Diamond

Introduction and Microbiology

West Nile encephalitis virus (WNV) is a small, enveloped, mosquito-transmitted, positive-polarity RNA virus of the *Flaviviridae* family. This virus is closely related to other arthropod-borne viruses that cause human disease, including Dengue, Zika, yellow fever, and Japanese encephalitis viruses. WNV normally cycles in nature between mosquitoes and birds, but during epidemics will infect and cause disease in humans, horses, and other vertebrate animals. WNV is still considered the most important cause of arbovirus disease in the United States, though epidemics of the related Zika virus may change this soon. Manifestations of WNV infection range from asymptomatic infection to severe neurological disease, which usually occurs within 1 to 2 weeks after mosquito inoculation and is more frequent in elderly and immunocompromised individuals. Acute care providers should be well versed in the early recognition and initial management of WNV infection.

Epidemiology

WNV historically caused sporadic outbreaks of a mild febrile illness in regions of Africa, the Middle East, Asia, and Australia. However, in the 1990s, the epidemiology of infection changed. New outbreaks in parts of Eastern Europe were associated with higher rates of severe neurological disease. In 1999, WNV entered North America, and caused seven human fatalities in the New York area, as well the deaths of a large number of birds and horses. Since then, WNV has spread to all 48 of the lower United States, as well as to parts of Canada, Mexico, and the Caribbean. Because of the increased range, the number of human cases has continued to rise: in the United States between 1999 and 2017, more than 48,000 clinical cases were diagnosed and associated with 2,128 deaths.

Approximately 85% of human infections in the United States occur in the late summer with a peak number of cases in August and September. This pattern reflects the seasonal activity of the *Culex* mosquito vectors and a requirement for virus amplification in the late spring and early summer in one of several different bird hosts, including blue jays, sparrows, and grackles. In warmer parts of the country, however, virtually year-round transmission has been documented. WNV infection tends to be fatal in some birds such as crows. The number of dying birds in a community in the early summer often predicts the number of human cases weeks later.

The vast majority of human cases of WNV are acquired after mosquito inoculation. Seroprevalence studies suggest that most (approximately 80%) cases are subclinical or undiagnosed. About 1 in 150 WNV infections result in the most severe and potentially lethal neuroinvasive form of the disease. During an epidemic, on a human population scale, the seroconversion rate ranges from 3 to 20% and the attack rate for severe disease is about 7 per 100,000. The risk of severe WNV infection is greatest in the elderly, with an estimated 20-fold increased risk of neuroinvasive disease and death in those over 50 years of age. Comorbidities such as immunosuppression, diabetes mellitus, and alcohol abuse are also associated with increased risk and poor outcome.

Although most human WNV infections occur after the bite of an infected mosquito, human-to-human transmission has been documented via transfusion, organ transplantation, transplacental transmission, and breastfeeding.

Clinical Features

The clinical spectrum of WNV infection is broad and includes apparently asymptomatic cases, to a mild flu-like illness, to a more severe febrile illness that can progress to polio-like

Table 11.1 West Nile Virus Infection: Clinical Features

Organism	West Nile virus
Incubation period	2–14 days
Transmission	Mosquito bite Blood transfusion Organ recipient Intrauterine transmission
West Nile fever	Fever, headache, flu-like illness, myalgia, arthralgia, GI complaints, macular rash, fatigue, difficulty concentrating
West Nile meningitis	Fever, headache, myalgia, arthralgia, vomiting, back pain, macular rash, fatigue, difficulty concentrating
West Nile encephalitis	Fever, headache, myalgia, arthralgia, vomiting, back pain, macular rash, fatigue, memory problems, dysarthria, dysphagia, focal motor exam, paralysis
West Nile acute flaccid paralysis	Fever, flaccid paralysis
Post-WNV infection syndrome	Fatigue, weakness, difficulty concentrating, muscle weakness
Laboratory and radiologic findings	Serum: leukopenia, lymphopenia, thrombocytopenia CSF: lymphocytic pleocytosis (early neutrophilia or no WBC) MRI: signal abnormalities in basal ganglia, thalamus, and brain stem
Laboratory diagnosis	Serum for anti-WNV IgM Paired acute and convalescent serum for anti-WNV IgG (fourfold rise in titer) Serum for WNV RT-PCR or nucleic acid amplification test (NAAT) (within first 8 days of symptoms) CSF for anti-WNV IgM
Therapy	Investigational clinical trials – none at present

paralysis, meningitis, and encephalitis (see Table 11.1). These syndromes present within 1 to 2 weeks after a mosquito bite or exposure. Most individuals who come to clinical attention have a self-limited West Nile fever (WNF), which is characterized by fever and some or all of the following signs and symptoms: headache, neck pain, poor concentration, myalgia, arthralgia, weakness, gastrointestinal complaints, and/or macular rash. This non-neuroinvasive form nonetheless can be severe as 38% of patients with WNF were hospitalized with a mean length stay of 5 days.

Less common non-neurological clinical manifestations include hepatitis, pancreatitis, myocarditis, rhabdomyolysis, cardiac arrhythmias, orchitis, and ocular findings. Several studies also suggest that WNV can cause ocular disease, including chorioretinitis, vitritis, intraretinal hemorrhages, iritis, optic neuritis, and retinal artery occlusions.

WNV neuroinvasive disease occurs in less than 1% of infected individuals and manifests as meningitis, encephalitis, or paralysis. The clinical presentation of meningitis and encephalitis appears to differ slightly as patients with meningitis were more likely to have nausea, vomiting, myalgia, rash, back pain, and arthralgia, whereas those with encephalitis typically had memory problems, dysarthria, dysphagia, and focal motor abnormalities. Notably, no differences in the frequency of seizure, limb weakness, or tremor were observed in the meningitis and encephalitis patient groups. The acute paralysis that occurs with WNV infection is generally flaccid in nature and is due to infection and injury of anterior horn lower motor neurons. Because of the location and severity of neuron injury, it is referred to as a poliomyelitis-like syndrome. More rarely, inflammatory changes associated with central nervous system infection can result in additional neuromuscular manifestations, including Guillain–Barré syndrome and demyelinating neuropathies.

Laboratory and Radiographic Findings

Routine clinical laboratory studies (complete blood count, serum chemistries, hepatic panels, coagulation tests) do not distinguish WNV from other viral infections. Nonspecific laboratory findings include mild leukopenia, mild to severe lymphopenia, and thrombocytopenia. Patients with neuroinvasive disease (meningitis or encephalitis) generally have a lymphocytic pleocytosis in their cerebrospinal fluid (CSF), though neutrophils or even an absence of cells may occur early in the course of infection. Notably, transplant recipients that naturally acquire WNV infection may have atypical lymphocytes in their CSF. In cases of WNV encephalitis, computer tomography (CT) of the head rarely shows abnormalities; however, magnetic resonance imaging (MRI) can show signal abnormalities in the basal ganglia, thalamus, and brain stem.

Although clinical criteria for assessment of patients with suspected WNV infection have been defined, definitive diagnosis depends on the detection of antibodies, viral nucleic acid, or infectious virus in the blood or cerebrospinal fluid (see Table 11.2). Few clinical laboratories have the ability to isolate virus directly from infected clinical samples. Because viremia is relatively transient and often precedes the severe neurological manifestations of the WNV infection, nucleic acid testing, though quite specific, can have relatively low sensitivity, especially with delayed clinical presentation.

At present, the most common method for diagnostic confirmation is detection of WNV IgM in the serum and/or CSF by antibody capture ELISA. The tests, which are performed by both state and commercial laboratories, are reasonably

Table 11.2 Interpretation of West Nile Virus Antibody Test Results

Tests	Results	Interpretation
IgM IgG	Negative Negative	Antibody not detected (no infection, unless sample taken early in course prior to seroconversion)
IgM IgG	Negative Positive	Infection with a flavivirus at undetermined time
IgM IgG	Positive Negative	Possible evidence of recent or current infection; further confirmatory testing necessary*
IgM IgG	Positive Positive	Evidence of recent or current infection
IgM IgG	Indeterminate Negative	Inconclusive † request convalescent serum

Owing to heterotypic antibody responses and/or cross-reactions, serologic results should be interpreted on the basis of clinical and epidemiological information.

* False positive IgM results may occur.
† Paired acute and convalescent serum samples may demonstrate seroconversion.

sensitive (60 to 90%) when carried out by day 8 of illness. Antibody testing within the first 72 hours of clinical presentation may yield false negative results because of the kinetics of the anti-WNV IgM response. False positive results are also possible, because the ELISA test also detects antibodies against related flaviviruses (e.g. St. Louis and Japanese encephalitis virus and possibly Dengue or Zika viruses). Thus, it is important to obtain a history of recent vaccination (e.g. yellow fever virus) or foreign travel and at present definitive serological diagnosis of WNV infection requires a comparison of antigen or neutralization activity among related flavivirus family members. Newly developed assays that utilize purified WNV structural and non-structural proteins appear more specific, and may allow distinction between natural infection, vaccination, and immunity. One cautionary note is that WNV IgM can persist in serum of some individuals for up to 500 days after onset of infection; this could confound interpretation of serologic results in patients presenting subsequently with clinical syndromes that resemble WNV infection.

Differential Diagnosis

WNV infection should be considered in the differential diagnosis for any ill, febrile patient when indicators of WNV activity are present in the community and especially in patients who have had intensive mosquito exposure. Updated maps of active mosquito, animal, and human WNV transmission can be found on the Center for Disease Control and Prevention (CDC) website (www.cdc.gov/ncidod/dvbid/westnile/). WNV infection should be considered especially for elderly or immunocompromised patients in endemic areas who present with non-specific febrile illnesses, and who lack leukocytosis or neutrophilia or obvious signs of bacterial infection. These patients may present in the early stages of WNV infection, which can subsequently progress to severe, life-threatening CNS disease.

The differential diagnosis of West Nile encephalitis includes both infectious and non-infectious causes. Among the infectious causes, several viruses can cause initial similar presentations with acute encephalopathy and fever:

- herpes simplex virus
- St. Louis encephalitis virus (which is closely related to WNV and will cross-react by serology but not by nucleic acid testing: this is now rare except in regions of Texas and Arkansas)
- (Eastern, Western, and Venezuelan equine encephalitis viruses
- California and La Crosse encephalitis viruses
- enterovirus
- cytomegalovirus
- rabies virus
- varicella-zoster virus
- Epstein–Barr virus

In addition to the typical bacterial causes of community–acquired meningitis, which in the early stages may be difficult to distinguish from encephalitis, *Listeria*, *Legionella*, and *Mycoplasma* can cause encephalitis, especially in pregnant women and the immunocompromised.

Non-infectious causes of acute encephalopathy include toxic ingestions or exposures, metabolic causes (e.g. hyponatremia), hepatic failure, systemic lupus erythematosis, granulomatouis angiitis, CNS metastatic disease, cerebrovascular accidents, and CNS hemorrhage.

Treatment

At present, no specific therapy has been approved for use in humans with WNV infection, and thus current treatment is supportive. Among the challenges will be to develop therapeutics that efficiently cross the blood–brain barrier into the central nervous system, clear virus from infected neurons, and have a beneficial effect on patient outcome. Investigational studies have begun to evaluate candidate therapies. The most up-to-date information on WNV therapeutic trials is located on the CDC website (www.cdc.gov/ncidod/dvbid/westnile/clinicalTrials.htm).

Ribavirin

Ribavirin is a broad-spectrum antiviral agent and has been used clinically to treat respiratory syncytial, hepatitis C, Lassa, Hantaan, and La Crosse viruses. Ribavirin has inhibitory activity against WNV infection in cell culture. Limited in vivo pre-clinical studies have been performed with WNV and the results have not been promising. However, no clinical benefit of ribavirin was observed in mouse, hamster, or monkey models of flavivirus infection. In a human trial during a WNV outbreak in Israel in 2000, a high mortality rate (41%) was observed in patients who received ribavirin. Thus, ribavirin is *not* recommended as therapy for WNV.

Interferon (IFN)-α

IFNs comprise an important immune system control against viral infections. IFNs induce an antiviral state within cells through the upregulation and activation of antiviral proteins and by modulating adaptive immune responses. Pre-treatment of cells in vitro with IFN potently inhibits WNV infection. However, the inhibitory effect of IFN is markedly attenuated after viral replication has begun as WNV proteins specifically inhibit IFN signaling and gene transcription. Treatment with IFN-α has been used in an uncontrolled manner to treat small numbers of human cases of WNV encephalitis. It is not clear that it provides any benefit.

Immune Antibody

In animals, passive administration of anti-WNV antibodies is both protective and therapeutic. Passive administration of immune serum, purified immune human γ-globulin, or monoclonal antibodies prior to WNV infection protected rodents from infection. Passive transfer of immune antibody also improved outcome in animals even after WNV had disseminated into the CNS. Small numbers of human patients have received monoclonal and polyclonal neutralizing antibody preparations as therapy against WNV infection. Individual case reports suggested clinical improvement. Clinical trials with antibodies were largely equivocal, possibly due to a failure to enroll enough subjects to show efficacy. Immune γ-globulin or anti-WNV monoclonal antibodies currently are not available.

Vaccines

Progress has been made toward the development of a WNV vaccine. Attenuated, DNA plasmid, and heat-killed vaccines have been developed and deployed for immunization of exotic birds, horses, and other veterinary animals with varying degrees of efficacy. Similar strategies are being used to develop vaccine candidates for pre-clinical and clinical assessment in humans, though none has been approved for clinical use.

Complications and Admission Criteria

Most immunocompetent patients that present to the ED with WNV fever or mild meningitis will not require hospital admission. However, in specific high-risk populations (elderly, immunocompromised, pregnant women, or infants) severe, potentially life-threatening complications can occur and a low threshold for hospitalization should be maintained. When such patients present with severe illness or any neurological symptoms, they should be monitored in a hospital setting for the development of neuroinvasive disease. Patients with encephalitis, moderate to severe meningitis, or exacerbation of underlying chronic conditions should be admitted.

Severe complications of WNV infection include aspiration pneumonia (secondary to altered mental status), respiratory failure, encephalopathy, encephalitis, seizures, paralysis, and a sepsis-like syndrome. Neurological complications of WNV are common in hospitalized cases and are more common in the elderly. Fulminant encephalitis can occur rapidly in at-risk populations and result in severe long-term disability (cognitive, motor, and sensory) and death.

Infection Control

WNV is primarily transmitted by mosquito bite, though other routes of transmission such as blood transfusion are possible. There are no data to support non-blood-borne person-to-person transmission of WNV infection. Thus, standard precautions are adequate for patients with WNV infection, and isolation is not necessary. Articles contaminated with infected or bloody material should be bagged, labeled, and sent for decontamination by autoclave. Contaminated surfaces should be cleaned with a hospital-approved disinfectant or a 10% bleach solution.

Pearls and Pitfalls

- In endemic regions with active WNV infection, consider the diagnosis in febrile patients that present with some of the typical signs and symptoms: headache, fatigue, weakness, cognitive defects, rash, and focal weakness. Check the CDC website for current WNV activity in your area: www.cdc.gov/ncidod/dvbid/westnile/.
- CSF usually has lymphocytic pleocytosis, but can have neutrophil predominance or no cells early in the course of disease.
- Head CT is usually negative; MRI may have signal abnormalities in several regions of the brain.
- Laboratory diagnosis is by detection of viral RNA in serum or WNV antibodies (IgM or IgG) in serum or CSF.

References

Bakri, S. J. and Kaiser, P. K. Ocular manifestations of West Nile virus. *Curr. Opin. Ophthalmol.* 2004; 15(6): 537–40.

Bode, A. V., Sejvar, J. J., Pape, W. J., *et al.* West Nile virus disease: a descriptive study of 228 patients hospitalized in a 4-county region of Colorado in 2003. *Clin. Infect. Dis.* 2006; 42(9): 1234–40.

Cunha, B. A. Differential diagnosis of West Nile encephalitis. *Curr. Opin. Infect. Dis.* 2004; 17(5): 413–20.

DeSalvo, D., Roy-Chaudhury, P., Peddi, R., *et al.* West Nile virus encephalitis in organ transplant recipients: another high-risk group for meningoencephalitis and death. *Transplantation* 2004; 77: 466–9.

Diamond, M. S. Progress on the development of therapeutics against West Nile virus. *Antiviral Res.* 2009; 83(3): 214–27.

Granwehr, B. P., Lillibridge, K. M., Higgs, S., *et al.* West Nile virus: where are we now? *Lancet Infect. Dis.* 2004; 4(9): 547–56.

Hall, R. A. and Khromykh, A. A. West Nile virus vaccines. *Expert Opin. Biol. Ther.* 2004; 4(8): 1295–305.

Hayes, E. B., Sejvar, J. J., Zaki, S. R., *et al.* Virology, pathology, and clinical manifestations of West Nile virus disease. *Emerg. Infect. Dis.* 2005; 11(8): 1174–9.

Kleinschmidt-DeMasters, B. K., Marder, B. A., Levi, M. E., *et al.* Naturally acquired West Nile virus encephalomyelitis in transplant recipients: clinical, laboratory, diagnostic, and neuropathological features. *Arch. Neurol.* 2004; 61(8): 1210–20.

Leis, A. A. and Stokic, D. S. Neuromuscular manifestations of human West Nile virus infection. *Curr. Treat. Options Neurol.* 2005; 7(1): 15–22.

Monath, T. P., Liu, J., Kanesa-Thasan, N., *et al.* A live, attenuated recombinant West Nile virus vaccine. *Proc. Natl. Acad. Sci. USA* 2006; 103(17): 6694–9.

Mostashari, F., Bunning, M. L., Kitsutani, P. T., *et al.* Epidemic West Nile encephalitis, New York, 1999: results of a household-based seroepidemiological survey. *Lancet* 2001; 358(9278): 261–4.

Nash, D., Mostashari, F., Fine, A., *et al.* The outbreak of West Nile virus infection in the New York City area in 1999. *N. Engl. J. Med.* 2001; 344(24): 1807–14.

Pealer, L. N., Marfin, A. A., Petersen, L. R., *et al.* Transmission of West Nile virus through blood transfusion in the United States in 2002. *N. Engl. J. Med.* 2003; 349(13): 1236–45.

Rossi, S. L., Ross, T. M., and Evans, J. D. West Nile virus. *Clin. Lab. Med.* 2010; 30(1): 47–65.

Sejvar, J. J., Haddad, M. B., Tierney, B. C., *et al.* Neurologic manifestations and outcome of West Nile virus infection. *JAMA* 2003; 290(4): 511–15.

Suthar, M. S., Diamond, M. S., and Gale, M. Jr. West Nile virus infection and immunity. *Nat. Rev. Microbiol.* 2013; 11(2): 115–28.

Watson, J. T., Pertel, P. E., Jones, R. C., *et al.* 2004. Clinical characteristics and functional outcomes of West Nile Fever. *Ann. Intern. Med.* 141(5): 360–5.

Bacterial Skin and Soft-Tissue Infections

Bradley W. Frazee

Outline

Introduction

Skin and soft-tissue infections, comprising abscess, cellulitis, and necrotizing soft-tissue infection (NSTI), account for 1.8 million annual emergency department (ED) visits in the United States alone. Terminology and definitions of the main types of skin and soft-tissue infections are presented in Table 12.1. Starting in the late 1990s, a shift occurred in the bacteriology of these infections, with a dramatic rise in the prevalence of community-acquired methicillin-resistant *Staphylococcus aureus* (CA-MRSA), which required change in empiric antibiotic strategies. Emergency physicians are often the first to diagnose and begin treatment of skin and soft-tissue infections. In the case of potentially lethal NSTI rapid diagnosis can reduce morbidity and mortality and requires familiarity with diverse presentations and the limitations of diagnostic tests.

Abscess

Epidemiology and Microbiology

Risk factors for abscess formation include injection drug use (IDU), shaving, and known colonization or infection with CA-MRSA. *Staphylococcus aureus* is the primary pathogen, found in about 75% of routine abscess and purulent cellulitis cases, with 40 to 84% of isolates being MRSA, depending on geographic location. The emergence of CA-MRSA as an endemic pathogen in the United States has manifested largely as a rise

in spontaneous skin abscesses (furuncles). Nearly all *S. aureus* strains secrete exotoxins (including hemolysins, nucleases, proteases, lipases, hyaluronidase, and collagenase) that convert host tissues into nutrients required for bacterial growth. Additionally, some methicillin-sensitive *S. aureus* (MSSA) and the majority of CA-MRSA strains carry genes for Panton–Valentine leukocidin (PVL), a cytotoxin causing leukocyte destruction, tissue necrosis, and enhanced abscess formation.

Abscesses may also contain a mix of anaerobes and aerobes. Oral flora (including *Streptococcus milleri*, *Eikenella*, and *Peptostreptococcus*) are commonly found in abscesses associated with injection drug use (IDU). Gut flora such as *E. coli* and *Bacteroides fragilis* may be found in abscesses occurring around the groin and anal area.

Clinical Features

The initial diagnostic approach (see Figure 12.1) to acute cutaneous erythema, warmth, and tenderness should be to look for evidence of a purulent fluid collection, as indicated by fluctuance on exam or a hypoechoic fluid pocket on bedside ultrasound (see Figure 12.2). Blind needle aspiration in the absence of these findings is generally not recommended. The presence of pus usually mandates immediate drainage and often obviates the need for antibiotics. In the absence of pus, diagnostic possibilities include both simple cellulitis and NSTI.

Abscess usually presents as a localized, circular area of erythema, warmth, and tenderness (see Figure 12.3). Palpable

Table 12.1 Skin and Soft-Tissue Infections: Definitions

Abscess	Subcutaneous collection of pus
Furuncle ("boil")	An infection originating in a hair follicle that produces a localized subcutaneous abscess
Carbuncle	Coalescence of multiple furuncles, typically involving the deep subcutaneous tissues of the neck and upper back
Cellulitis	Acute spreading infection of the dermis and subcutaneous tissue
NSTI (includes necrotizing fasciitis and myonecrosis)	Characterized by necrosis of deep structures such as fascia and muscle Fulminant course with eventual development of systemic manifestations

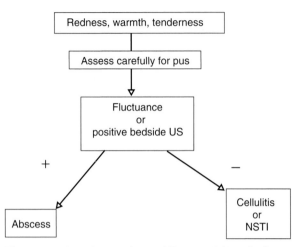

Figure 12.1 General approach to undifferentiated skin and soft-tissue infections.

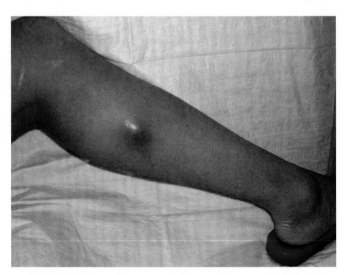

Figure 12.3 Cutaneous furuncle (superficial skin abscess).

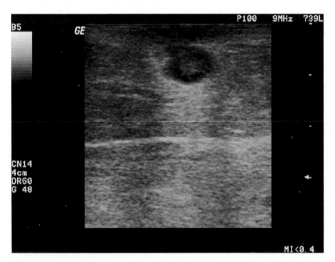

Figure 12.2 An abscess visualized by ultrasound demonstrating a hypoechoic fluid pocket with farfield enhancement.

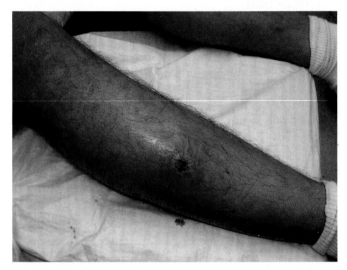

Figure 12.4 Ruptured and healing furuncle with shallow ulcer and eschar and mild surrounding purulent cellulitis.

fluctuance is a critical sign that can be subtle, and a deep abscess can easily be missed. After spontaneous drainage, an ulcer and eschar may form (see Figure 12.4). Abscesses may be accompanied by a significant surrounding so-called purulent cellulitis. However, a uniform rim of reactive erythema and dense induration is often present around an uncomplicated abscess, and does not necessarily signify an infectious cellulitis (see Figure 12.5). Overlying necrosis and drainage may be present in a mature abscess. Fever can occur, and large abscesses accompanied by fever are associated with up to a 20%

incidence of bacteremia. In contrast, bacteremia appears to be uncommon in afebrile patients with abscesses, either before or immediately after drainage.

Hidradenitis suppurativa is a disease defined by multiple and recurrent abscesses involving the apocrine glands of the axilla and inguinal region. There is usually a personal and/or family history of multiple abscesses. Although incision and drainage of individual abscesses is frequently necessary,

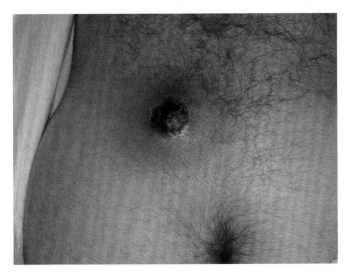

Figure 12.5 Purulent cellulitis centered around an abscess.

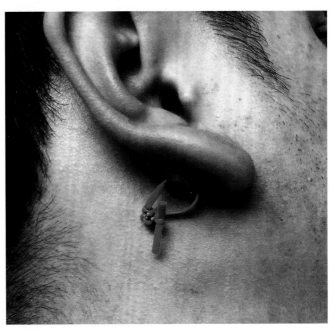

Figure 12.6 Loop drain that has just been placed in a small abscess on the auricle.

it is rarely sufficient for cure. More aggressive treatments include extensive debridement of the affected areas with skin grafts. Topical clindamycin and long-term (3 months) tetracycline therapy are considered effective, though data are limited. Inhibitors of tumor necrosis factor have shown promise for moderate to severe disease.

Differential Diagnosis

As emphasized above, when faced with skin tenderness, erythema, and edema concerning for bacterial infection, the crucial initial distinction is between abscess, cellulitis, and NSTI (see Table 12.1).

Laboratory and Radiologic Findings

Bedside ultrasound has emerged as a useful adjunct to the physical exam for the diagnosis of cutaneous abscesses when fluctuance is not obvious. Abscess cavities usually appear as hypo- or anechoic on ultrasound, and acoustic enhancement may be seen farfield of the collection (see Figure 12.2). Computed tomographic (CT) scan likely represents the gold standard for diagnosis of deep subcutaneous or intramuscular abscesses, though it is rarely indicated. Traditionally, culturing of abscesses has not been recommended; however, culture results may be informative if the community prevalence of CA-MRSA is unclear, if the abscess is health-care associated or if one of the risk factors enumerated in Table 12.2 is present.

Treatment

In most cases of abscess, the host defense has successfully walled off infection and simple drainage is curative. Abscesses should undergo immediate drainage in almost all cases, as antibiotics alone are unlikely to result in cure. Aspiration with a large-bore needle may be sufficient for small superficial abscess, though in most cases, scalpel incision and blunt dissection of loculations is required. Use of wall suction is advised for evacuating pus from large abscesses and irrigation is generally necessary. Studies have shown that gauze packing is not required

after drainage of small abscesses. If used, packing should be removed at 12 to 48 hours and the wound inspected by medical personnel. An alternative to packing is loop drainage, where a rubber drain is looped through the abscess cavity, out through adjacent intact skin and tied loosely over the skin (see Figure 12.6). Post-drainage care by the patient must include twice-daily removal of dressings and packing followed by vigorous cleaning or soaks in soapy water. A major advantage of rubber loops is that they are left in place during cleaning.

Local anesthesia provides sufficient analgesia for incision and drainage in many cases. Other options include peripheral nerve block, regional anesthesia, and procedural sedation.

Pre-drainage parenteral antibiotics should be considered in patients at high risk for infectious endocarditis, including those with congenital heart disease, major valvular abnormalities, or a history of endocarditis. Routine use of adjunctive (post-drainage) antibiotics is controversial. Meta analyses of multiple small trials conducted since the emergence of CA-MRSA found that for uncomplicated abscesses, adjunctive antibiotics offer no benefit compared to incision and drainage alone. This is reflected in current practice guidelines that recommend witholding antibiotics after drainage of mild purulent infections. However, two recent, large, high-quality trial demonstrated a 7–14% improvement in the cure rate of uncomplicated abscesses with adjunctive trimethoprim-sulfamethoxazole or clindamycin versus placebo. Adjunctive antibiotics are strongly recommended for immunosuppressed patients or those at extremes of age, and for abscesses accompanied by fever or significant surrounding purulent cellulitis (see Table 12.3). Empiric antibiotics need only cover *S. aureus*, including MRSA. Trimethoprim-sulfamethoxazole is the first-line oral agent because it has a narrow spectrum, has retained excellent activity against CA-MRSA strains, is inexpensive, and is taken twice per day.

Complications and Admission Criteria

When incision and drainage of abscess is successful, the need for admission is rare. Exceptions include:

- abscesses requiring drainage in the operating room
- significant surrounding cellulitis requiring parenteral antibiotics
- evidence of severe sepsis suggesting bacteremia
- immunocompromised patients (diabetes, HIV, end-stage renal disease [ESRD])

Cellulitis

Epidemiology and Microbiology

Risk factors for cellulitis include processes that disrupt the skin barrier, such as wounds, bites, surgical procedures, inject-ion drug use, body piercing, and dermatophytoses, as well as conditions that render local immune defenses less effective, such as morbid obesity and peripheral edema. Rarely, cel-lulitis can be due to a subjacent primary infection such as osteomyelitis, or due to hematogenous spread in the setting of bacteremia. Most cases of non-purulent cellulitis are caused by β-hemolytic streptococcal species; in addition to Group A *Streptococcus*, Group B and G species are increasingly rec-ognized as causes of cellulitis. *Staphylococcus aureus* seems to be a less common cause of non-purulent cellulitis, unless there is associated abscess or penetrating trauma. Purulent cellulitis associated with an abscess, on the other hand, is almost always due to *S. aureus*. There are a few notable risk factors for cellu-litis associated with other organisms (see Table 12.2).

Clinical Features

Even when non-purulent cellulitis seems likely on initial exam, consideration should be given to the approach outlined in Figure 12.1, because purulent cellulitis, that is associated with an unsuspected abscess, is very common. Non-purulent cel-lulitis presents with erythema, warmth, and tenderness, but unlike the circular erythema around an abscess, when present on an extremity, non-purulent cellulitis is usually circumfer-ential (see Figure 12.7). There may be an irregular margin or blotchy appearance. While fluid-filled blisters occasionally occur, non-purulent cellulitis by definition lacks an associated

pus pocket and it is not walled off, but rather spreads laterally. Unlike most abscesses, cellulitis is often associated with some degree of systemic toxicity such as a low-grade fever. Areas of superficial hemorrhagic transformation can be seen in severe cellulitis, but such findings should always raise concern for a necrotizing infection requiring urgent surgical intervention. Lymphangitis and fever may be present and are considered markers of severity (see Figure 12.8). A portal of entry, such as a recent site of drug injection or fungal infection of the feet, may or may not be evident.

Erysipelas is a specific form of cellulitis caused by group A *Streptococcus* and isolated to the superficial dermis (see Figure 12.9). It is characterized by bright erythema with a sharp, raised margin and peau d'orange appearance caused by subcutaneous edema around hair follicles. It typically occurs on the face or on the lower extremities in the setting of pre-existing edema.

Differential Diagnosis

As emphasized above, when faced with skin tenderness, erythema, and edema concerning for bacterial infection, the crucial initial distinction is between abscess, cellulitis, and NSTI. Other superficial skin infections with a distinc-tive appearance, such as impetigo and fungal infections, are easily diagnosed in most cases. Impetigo is a staphylococcal or streptococcal infection common in young children and characterized by discrete pustules or bullae on the face and extremities that rupture and give rise to a lacquer-like crust.

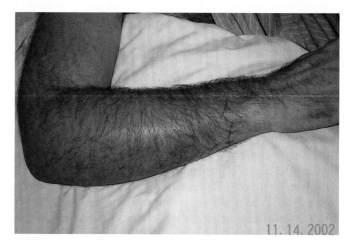

Figure 12.7 Upper extremity non-purulent cellulitis.

Table 12.2 Risk Factors and Pathogens Associated with Severe or Unusual Forms of Cellulitis

Clinical Presentation	Likely Organisms
Diabetic foot ulcer	Gram-positive cocci, gram-negative rods (including *Pseudomonas*), and anaerobes (including *Bacteroides*)
Cat bite	*Pasteurella multocida*
Human bite	*Eikenella corrodens*, anaerobes
Fresh water exposure	*Aeromonas hydrophila*
Salt water exposure	*Vibrio vulnificus*
Fish tank owner or fish handler	*Erysipelothrix rhusiopathiae*

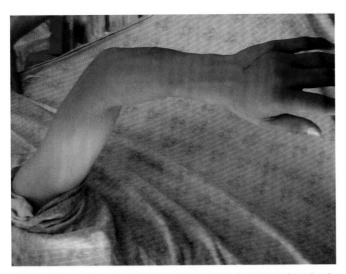

Figure 12.8 Lymphangitis. (This example happens to be due to a large local allergic reaction to a bee sting on the hand.)

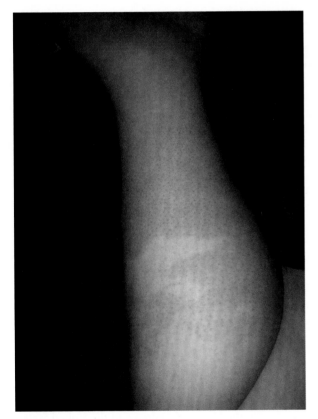

Figure 12.9 Erysipelas on the lower extremity.

Fungal infections typically produce round, plaque-like lesions with discrete borders.

Other conditions that are sometimes difficult to differentiate from cellulitis include viral exanthems, autoimmune rashes, dermatitis, allergic reactions to insect bites and stings, gout, deep venous thrombosis (DVT), and chronic changes associated with edema and venous stasis. Dermatitis and autoimmune rashes typically produce lesions with a distinctive appearance, or pattern, such as target lesions, serum-filled bullae, scales, and

plaques. Of note, dermatitis and infection often coexist, as many chronic inflammatory skin conditions are prone to bacterial superinfection. Large local reactions to insect envenomation, particularly bee stings, can develop an area of erythema, warmth, a peau d'orange appearance and even lymphangitis that closely mimics non-purulent cellulitis; the difference is that tenderness is minimal and pruritis is intense and large local reactions, while categorized as delayed allergic reactions, usually begin within several hours of envenomation, earlier than would be expected with superinfection (see Figure 12.8).

Laboratory and Radiologic Findings

The Infectious Diseases Society of America recommends that all patients with soft-tissue infection accompanied by signs and symptoms of systemic toxicity (including fever or hypothermia, heart rate greater than 100 beats/min, or systolic blood pressure less than 90 mm Hg or 20 mm Hg below baseline) have blood drawn for studies, including culture, complete blood count (CBC) with differential, serum chemistries, creatine phosphokinase (CPK), and C-reactive protein (CRP) (though routine use of CRP has yet to be integrated into US emergency practice). A lactate level should be obtained in all cases when signs of sepsis are present.

Studies of the etiology of cellulitis have relied on needle aspiration of the infected area, punch biopsies, and acute and convalescent serologies, though there is no role for these tests in routine care. Blood cultures prior to admission for cellulitis are no longer recommended in most immunocompetent patients, as the yield is around 5% and even positive cultures rarely change management. Cultures are indicated in patients with lymphangitis, rigors, or high fever suggesting bacteremia; in immunosuppressed patients, including those with human immunodeficiency virus (HIV), severe renal disease, diabetes mellitus (DM), or neutropenia; and in all cases of cellulitis associated with animal bites, or with salt or fresh water immersion.

The main role of imaging in suspected cellulitis is to rule out an occult abscess, a necrotizing infection, or a foreign body.

Treatment

Cellulitis can be treated with oral therapy if close follow-up is available. The first step in selecting antibiotic therapy is to distinguish non-purulent from purulent cellulitis. Treatment of purulent cellulitis is discussed above under Abscess. For uncomplicated non-purulent cellulitis, empirical therapy must cover *Streptococcus* species (see Table 12.3). Staphylococcal coverage is not needed; however, most recommended agents do cover methicillin susceptible *Staphylococcus*, though not MRSA. Antistaphylococcal penicillins or first-generation cephalosporins are first-line agents. Macrolides are no longer recommended for penicillin-allergic patients because of rising resistance in group A *Streptococcus* isolates. Clindamycin is a second-line agent that is also active against MRSA. In patients who fail to respond within 48 hours of starting antibiotics, MRSA coverage should be added. Adjunctive therapies include elevation of the infected area and treatment of any underlying predisposing condition, particularly fungal dermatitis and eczema.

Table 12.3 Initial Treatment for Abscess and Cellulitis*

Incision and drainage required for abscess (often sufficient for cure without antibiotics)

Antibiotics	
Purulent cellulitis (associated with abscess or wound infection)	Oral antibiotics (for 7–10 days): TMP/SMX DS 1–2 tab PO BID *or* Clindamycin 300–450 mg PO TID *or* Doxycycline 100 mg PO BID IV antibiotics: Vancomycin 15–20 mg/kg/dose IV every 8–12 hours
Non-purulent cellulitis	Oral antibiotics: PenicillinVK 500 mg PO QID *or* Cephalexin 500 mg PO QID *or* Dicloxacillin 500 mg PO QID *or* Clindamycin 300–450 mg PO TID IV antibiotics: Cefazolin 1 g IV every 8 hours *or* Vancomycin 15–20 mg/kg/dose IV every 8–12 hours

* Always consider local and institutional susceptibility patterns.

IV – intravenous; PO – by mouth; TMP/SMX DS – trimethoprim/sulfamethoxazole double-strength tablet (160/800 mg).

Complications and Admission Criteria

The Infectious Diseases Society of America recommends admission for all patients with skin and soft-tissue infections accompanied by hypotension, elevated creatinine, low serum bicarbonate, creatine phosphokinase at two to three times the upper limit of normal, marked left shift, or a CRP level above 13 mg/L. Additionally, a lactate level above 4 mmol/L mandates admission. Immunosuppressed states such as diabetes or social factors such as homelessness, which might prevent elevation of an infected limb, should lower the threshold for hospitalization.

Patients with cellulitis should be admitted in the following cases:

- failure of outpatient therapy
- fever or extreme leukocytosis
- cellulitis of the hand after a bite
- cellulitis in the setting of fresh or salt water exposure
- concern for compliance with outpatient therapy
- immunocompromised states (e.g. diabetes, HIV, ESRD)

Necrotizing Soft-Tissue Infection (NSTI)

Epidemiology and Microbiology

Although NSTI can develop after minor wounds or trauma, most cases are associated with at least one of the following risk factors: IDU, diabetic foot ulcers, surgery, trauma, peripheral vascular disease, malnutrition, or alcoholism (see Table 12.4). IDU is by far the most common risk factor for community-acquired NSTI in the United States. Emersion in brackish water is a risk factor for *Vibrio vulnificus* NSTI.

Depending on the study, approximately one-third to two-thirds of NSTIs are polymicrobial. Staphylococcal species (*aureus* and *epidermidis*) are the most common isolates, and CA-MRSA NSTI has been reported. Oral and bowel flora such as non-group-A streptococcal species, gram-negative rods, and non-clostridial anaerobes are common in polymicrobial infections. Clostridial species (*perfringens*, *sordellii*) are a major cause of severe NSTIs in IDUs and *C. perfringens* is the main pathogen implicated in myonecrosis and gas gangrene. Group A *Streptococcus* causes a distinct monomicrobial form of NSTI that is often associated with only trivial or occult prior injury. The pathophysiology of these often fulminant infections involves bacterial exotoxins, like those produced by *C. perfringens* and group A *Streptococcus*, and release of cytokines such as tumor necrosis factor.

Clinical Features

Recognition of NSTI can be difficult because the initial clinical features are non-specific. On average, the diagnosis of NSTI is made 3 to 4 days from onset of symptoms. Pain out of proportion to skin signs, though considered a classic finding that may indicate underlying myonecrosis, is actually uncommon. Induration and erythema are the most common findings, and a characteristic woody edema extending beyond the border of erythema may be apparent. Classic findings that are frequently absent include bullae, crepitus, skin sloughing, hemorrhage, necrosis, and cutaneous sensory deficit (see Figure 12.10). These findings usually appear late in the course of necrotizing infections, if at all. Fever is present in 40% of cases of NSTI, leukocytosis in about 85%, and hypotension occurs in 9 to 50%.

A number of community-acquired NSTI deserve special mention. NSTI due to group A *Streptococcus* infection and accompanied by *Streptococcus* toxic shock syndrome classically follows varicella infection in children; however, it is actually more common in adults, who often lack risk factors or an obvious portal of entry. Clustered outbreaks in both children and adults have been described. IDU-related NSTI is common in the western United States, usually related to intramuscular injection, "skin popping," of black tar heroin. Outbreaks have been described in the United Kingdom and the United States, implicating contaminated batches of drugs or paraphernalia. IDU-associated NSTI may present with massive swelling of the extremity near the site of injection, often with spread to the trunk. Case mortality exceeds 25%. Other classic presentations of NSTI include:

- diabetic foot ulcer with associated extremity swelling or signs of systemic inflammation
- infection of the scrotum and perineum, particularly in men (Fournier's gangrene)
- odontogenic infection in which swelling extends into the floor of the mouth or the neck (Ludwig's angina)

Table 12.4 Necrotizing Soft-Tissue Infections

Polymicrobial (Type I)	Associated with devitalized tissue: • post-op. setting • battlefield injuries • injection drug use • decubitus or diabetic foot ulcer
	Polymicrobial synergistic infection often involving anaerobes such as clostridial species
	Includes gas gangrene, Fournier's gangrene, Ludwig's angina
Monomicrobial (Type II)	Typified by group A *Streptococcus*, *V. vulinificus* • Trivial or occult injury in many cases • Produces streptococcal toxic shock syndrome

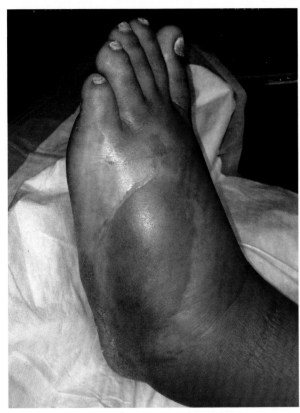

Figure 12.10 Hemorrhagic bullus due to a necrotizing skin and soft-tissue infection of the foot.

Given the non-specific and varied presenting signs and symptoms, and the limitations of imaging (see below), maintaining a high index of suspicion for NSTI is imperative. A systematic review of 1,463 NSTI cases reported a 71% initial misdiagnosis rate. In a series of 15 cases of group A streptococcal necrotizing fasciitis that were missed on initial outpatient presentation, the leading incorrect diagnoses were musculoskeletal pain, influenza, gastroenteritis, and first-degree burn.

Laboratory and Radiographic Findings

All patients suspected of having NSTI should have a CBC, metabolic panel, CPK, lactate, and blood cultures sent. Unfortunately, there is no sensitive laboratory or imaging finding that can be used to rule out NSTI. Leukocytosis is neither sensitive nor specific for the diagnosis, but a markedly elevated white blood cell count (WBC) (>20) is frequently seen and should raise concern for NSTI. There are some data suggesting that NSTI is distinguished by the combination of leukocytosis and hyponatremia. An elevated anion gap or lactate may be present. Azotemia and other signs of organ dysfunction usually are not evident on initial presentation.

Plain soft-tissue X-rays reveal subcutaneous gas in 25% of cases, typically in a stippled pattern that follows tissue planes. CT and MRI can delineate the extent of inflammation and identify small gas pockets and fluid along the fascial planes. CT has emerged as the imaging modality of choice, whereas MRI is time-consuming, costly, and dangerous for unstable patients. Use of bedside ultrasound to diagnose necrotizing fasciitis has been described by one group. A significant fluid stripe adjacent to the deep fascia was reported to be diagnostic, though these findings have yet to be validated. No patient with a suspected diagnosis of NSTI should have definitive surgical evaluation and treatment delayed for an imaging study, as these infections progress on the order of minutes to hours.

Ultimately, the rapid diagnosis of NSTI requires a high index of suspicion on the part of the emergency physician, immediate surgical consultation, and a low threshold for surgical exploration in the operating room. Surgical findings, which remain the diagnostic gold standard, include grayish, non-bleeding subcutaneous tissue, tissue planes that separate easily with blunt dissection, swollen fascia and "dishwater pus." Surgical cultures should be obtained with careful attention to proper anaerobic collection and transport, though the yield remains frustratingly low. Gram stain of surgical specimens can guide antibiotic treatment.

Treatment

Any suspicion of NSTI should prompt immediate surgical consultation without delay for laboratory or imaging results. The surgical approach to diagnosis has been likened to the traditional approach to appendicitis, where more patients should be taken to surgery and explored than actually have the disease. Underscoring the importance of early surgical intervention, numerous studies have found that delay to surgery is the major determinant of mortality. Delay of greater than 12 to 24 hours

Table 12.5 Initial IV Therapy for Necrotizing Fasciitis

Prompt surgical debridement

Aggressive fluid resuscitation

Vancomycin 15–20 mg/kg/dose IV every 8–12 hours

plus

Piperacillin-tazobactam 4.5 g IV every 6 hours

plus

Clindamycin 900 mg IV every 8 hours

(Alternative for penicillin-allergic patients: aztreonam 2 g IV every 8 hours)

quadruples mortality rates. Diagnostic delay has been correlated with admission to a medical service and "negative" blind needle aspiration.

Surgical intervention with wide debridement of the affected area is the major therapeutic modality. Initial empiric antibiotic therapy should be extremely broad-spectrum (see Table 12.5) and must cover *Staphylococcus aureus*, including MRSA, and group A *Streptococcus*, as well as gram negatives and anaerobes. Vancomycin is recommended for its MRSA activity, whereas high-dose clindamycin is recommended both for its activity against Streptococcal species and anaerobes and because it suppresses toxin production. An advanced penicillin plus beta-lactamase inhibitor, such as piperacillin-tazobactam, is generally recommended as these offer gram-negative, gram-positive, and anaerobic activity. Additional measures include aggressive fluid resuscitation, hemodynamic monitoring, vasopressors as needed, and ample analgesia.

Complications and Admission Criteria

All patients suspected to have NSTI should be treated empirically, taken emergently for surgical exploration, and subsequently admitted to a monitored setting.

Infection Control

Other than universal precautions, no additional infection control measures are required.

Pearls and Pitfalls

1. In an undifferentiated skin and soft-tissue infection, a pus pocket is present more often than not, and, when present, must be drained.

2. Bedside ultrasound can reveal and localize an unsuspected abscess.

3. With the emergence of CA-MRSA, trimethoprim-sulfamethoxetal is now the main oral antimicrobial for purulent infections.

4. In the evaluation of cellulitis, always consider risk factors (such as animal bites or water exposure) that are associated with esoteric pathogens and severe cellulitis, as well as the possibility of a necrotizing infection.

5. In NSTI, time to surgical debridement significantly affects morbidity and mortality. Request an immediate surgical consult as soon as the diagnosis is suspected. Do not delay for laboratory or imaging studies.

6. NSTIs are usually accompanied by signs of sepsis at the time of presentation. Aggressive IV fluid resuscitation is required.

References

Chen, J. L., Fullerton, K. E., and Flynn, N. M. Necrotizing fasciitis associated with injection drug use. *Clin. Infect. Dis.* 2001; 33(1): 6–15.

Daum, R. S., Miller, L. G., Immergluck, L., *et al.*, Placebo-controlled trial of antibiotics for smaller skin abscesses. *N. Engl. J. Med.* 2017; 376(26): 2545–55.

Goh, T., Goh, L. G., Ang, C. H., and Wong, C. H. Early diagnosis of necrotizing fasciitis. *Br. J. Surg.* 2014; 101(1): e119–25.

Jeng, A., Beheshti, M., Li, J., and Nathan, R. The role of beta-hemolytic streptococci in causing diffuse, nonculturable cellulitis: a prospective investigation. *Medicine (Baltimore)* 2010; 89(4): 217–26.

Kaul, R., McGeer, A., Low, D. E., *et al.* Population-based surveillance for group A streptococcal necrotizing fasciitis: clinical features, prognostic indicators, and microbiologic analysis of seventy-seven cases. Ontario Group A Streptococcal Study. *Am. J. Med.* 1997; 103(1): 18–24.

Ladde, J. G., Baker, S., Rodgers, C. N., and Papa, L. The LOOP technique: a novel incision and drainage technique in the treatment of skin abscesses in a pediatric ED. *Am. J. Emerg. Med.* 2015; 33(2): 271–6.

Leinwand, M., Downing, M., Slater, D., *et al.* Incision and drainage of subcutaneous abscesses without the use of packing. *J. Ped. Surg.* 2013; 48(9): 1962–5.

Moran, G. J., Krishnadasan, A., Gorwitz, R. J., *et al.* Methicillin-resistant *S. aureus* infections among patients in the emergency department. *N. Engl. J. Med.* 2006; 355(7): 666–74.

Moran, G. J., Krishnadasan, A., Mower, W. R., et al., Effect of cephalexin plus trimethoprim-sulfamethoxazole vs cephalexin alone on clinical cure of uncomplicated cellulitis: a randomized clinical trial. *JAMA.* 2017; 317(20): 2088–96.

Squire, B. T., Fox, J. C., and Anderson, C. ABSCESS: applied bedside sonography for convenient evaluation of superficial soft tissue infections. *Acad. Emerg. Med.* 2005; 12(7): 601–6.

Talan, D. A., Krishnadasan, A., Gorwitz, R. J., *et al.* Comparison of Staphylococcus aureus from skin and soft-tissue infections in US emergency department patients, 2004 and 2008. *Clin. Infect. Dis.* 2011; 53(2): 144–9.

Talan, D. A., Mower, W. R., Krishnadasan, A., *et al.* Trimethoprim-sulfamethoxazole versus placebo for uncomplicated skin abscess. *N. Engl. J. Med.* 2016; 374(9): 823–32.

Additional Reading

Stevens, D. L., Bisno, A. L., Chambers H. F., *et al.* Practice guidelines for the diagnosis and management of skin and soft tissue infections: 2014 update by the Infectious Diseases Society of America. *Clin. Infect. Dis.* 2014; 59(2): e10–52.

Stevens, D. L. and Bryant, A. E. Necrotizing soft-tissue infections. *N. Engl. J. Med.* 2017; 377(23): 2253–65.

Chapter 13

Ectoparasites

Jan Shoenberger, William Mallon, and R. James Salway

Outline

Introduction

Ectoparasitosis includes all infestations where parasites live in or on human skin. Most human ectoparasites are arthropods, primarily insects, arachnids, and ticks. Many ectoparasite infestations result in significant morbidity and yet go unrecognized in the acute care setting. Failure to treat affected patients leads to spread of ectoparasites through vulnerable populations both inside and outside the hospital. Recognition and treatment of ectoparasitosis (including resistant strains of pediculosis and scabies) is particularly important because these infestations are increasing geographically and within traditionally less vulnerable populations.

General Ectoparasite Epidemiology and Microbiology

Ectoparasitoses are most prevalent in resource-poor populations, including the homeless, immigrants, refugees, the incarcerated, the malnourished, and those who are underinsured and uninsured. The worldwide prevalence of scabies has been estimated at 300 million cases and growing. Crusted (or Norwegian) scabies is now an important nosocomial disease resulting in a large number of bed closures in intensive care units (ICUs) and wards across the United States. Head lice

result in the loss of 12 to 24 million school days for children annually in the United States. Emerging resistance makes control more difficult, and incidence is also increasing due to the expanded use of steroids for asthma, arthritis, lupus, and other inflammatory diseases. Table 13.1 lists the major ectoparasites encountered worldwide.

Scabies
Clinical Features

Scabies is a common ectoparasitic infestation caused by the mite *Sarcoptes scabiei*. They are also known as "human itch mites." In general, the infestation causes an intensely pruritic rash as the pregnant female mite burrows into the skin and deposits eggs in a burrow. Larvae hatch in 3 to 10 days and migrate to the skin surface while maturing into adults. The pruritic rash of scabies is a result of both the infestation itself and the host's hypersensitivity reaction to the mite and its feces. Superinfections with *Staphylococcus aureus* and *Streptococcus pyogenes* are common. Complications such as poststreptococcal glomerulonephritis, rheumatic fever, and sepsis, though rare, have been reported.

For a primary infestation, the incubation period before symptoms is usually between 3 and 6 weeks (see Table 13.2).

Table 13.1 Major Ectoparasites of the World

Category of Ectoparasite	Scientific/Common Name	Comments
Scabies	*Sarcoptes scabiei*, classic scabies, crusted (Norwegian) scabies	Crusted scabies seen in bed-ridden, malnourished, immunosuppressed
Mites	Bedbugs, dust mites, chiggers	More than 30,000 species
Ticks	Ixodidae (hard ticks), Argasidae (soft ticks)	Important vectors for many viral and bacterial diseases
Tungiasis	*Tunga penetrans*	Sand flea disease. Presents as a slow-growing, sometimes painful nodule from which the parasite must be extracted. Endemic to the West Indies, Africa, India, Latin America. In the United States, a rare disease seen in returning travelers or immigrants from endemic regions.
Bedbugs	*Cimex lectularius* (common bedbug)	Worldwide. Nearly eradicated in the United States 50 years ago, but outbreaks reported in all 50 US states in recent years. Not considered a major vector of disease, but bites can be numerous and can become secondarily infected.
Human louse (pediculosis)	Head louse, body louse, pubic louse	Worldwide. Head lice have greatest impact on children.
Cutaneous larva migrans	Hookworm larvae, "clam-digger's itch"	Disease of travelers who stepped on feces of dogs/cat. Most common travel-associated skin disease.
Myiasis	Flies and maggots (larval stages)	Most are not invasive in the United States

Table 13.2 Clinical Features: Scabies

Incubation period	3–6 weeks for primary infestation 1–3 days for reinfestation
Transmission	Direct (person to person) *or* Indirect (through infested bedding or clothing)
Signs and Symptoms	Pruritis typically worse at night Rash commonly found on the hands, flexor surface of wrists, elbows, knees, genitalia, and breasts Rash usually spares the face, scalp, and head in adults, but can affect those areas in infants
Crusted or Norwegian scabies	Psoriatic hyperkeratotic dermatitis of the hands and feet (with nail involvement) Erythematous, scaly rash on face, neck, scalp, and trunk Highly contagious because of the large number of mites involved Common among immunocompromised patients
Diagnosis	Clinical diagnosis *or* Direct visualization under a light microscope Skin biopsy

Transmission can be direct (person to person) or indirect (through infested bedding or clothing, which can remain infectious for up to several days). Transmission between members of the same household and among institutionalized people is common.

The itching caused by scabies is typically worse at night. The rash is most commonly found on the hands (particularly the webbing between the fingers) and the flexor surfaces of the wrists, elbows, and knees, as well as on the genitalia and breasts of women. The rash usually spares the face, scalp, and head in adults, but can affect those areas in infants. Itching may be reported in areas of the body where no mites are detectable. It is very common to see secondary excoriations, eczematous skin changes, and superinfection (impetigo). In patients who have had a prior scabies infestation, a papular "scabies rash" can be seen on the buttocks, scapular region, and abdomen and is thought to be caused by a delayed hypersensitivity reaction.

There are also "atypical" forms of scabies, such as crusted (or Norwegian) scabies, which cause a psoriatic hyperkeratotic dermatitis of the hands and feet (with nail involvement) and an erythematous, scaly eruption on the face, neck, scalp, and trunk. These lesions are highly contagious because of a high concentration of mites and usually affect immunocompromised and bed-bound patients.

Differential Diagnosis

The differential diagnosis of pruritic rashes is vast and includes infestation by fleas, bedbugs, lice, and other mites. Flea and bedbug bites tend to be punctate. Flea bites tend to be on the extremities, whereas bedbug bites tend to be on areas of exposed skin such as the neck and face. Repeated failed treatment of scabies suggests infestation by free-living arthropods, such as bedbugs and fleas.

Laboratory and Radiographic Findings

The diagnosis of scabies is primarily a clinical one because definitive diagnosis requires microscopic visualization of the mite, eggs, or feces of the mite in skin scrapings from areas with burrows. Samples can be obtained by scraping laterally across the skin with a scalpel blade. Alternatively, strong adhesive tape can be applied over the burrow areas, peeled off, and viewed under the microscope. Under low power, the mites will appear translucent with brown legs and are 0.2 to 0.5 mm long. One challenge to diagnosis is that in classic scabies (the most common form), the mite burden is low and the detection by microscopy is tissue sample and operator dependent. Failure to find mites is common and does not rule out the diagnosis. According to one study at a university hospital, the diagnosis was missed 65% of the time. Diagnosis can sometimes be made by skin biopsy. There have been discussions and research into an improved diagnostic test using mite-expressed sequence tags that remains in development.

In areas of high prevalence, the presence of diffuse itching and visible lesions associated with either at least two typical locations of scabies or a household member with itching can have nearly 100% sensitivity and specificity for the diagnosis.

Treatment and Prophylaxis

Index patients and all close contacts need to be treated to achieve eradication. First-line treatment is 5% permethrin cream given as a single overnight application, with multiple studies showing >90% 14- or 28-day cure rate. These rates improved when a second treatment was given after 1 week. Lindane is no longer a first-line therapy because of reports of neurotoxicity and seizures in children. Though effective, topical therapy has some disadvantages. It is messy, difficult to apply for some, and can burn or sting on excoriated areas. An alternative therapy is oral ivermectin, an arthropod neurotoxin. The only major adverse event reported from ivermectin is a transient, mild increase in itching that occurs after drug ingestion and is thought to be a result of an enhanced hypersensitivity reaction to dead mites. The dose is 200 µg/kg, and the cost is generally higher than for topical agents. Oral ivermectin can also be given as a single dose, but has increased efficacy rivaling permethrin when a second dose is given 14 days later. A combination of topical and oral therapy is recommended for crusted scabies. Table 13.3 summarizes treatment options for scabies.

In addition to pharmacologic treatment, environmental control measures are crucial. All bedding, clothes, and towels used by the patient in the 48 hours prior to treatment should be washed in hot water (125 °F) and dried in a hot drier.

Other Mites

Besides scabies, there are many other mites that result in ectoparasitosis and other medical conditions in humans. Mites have complex symbiotic associations with larger organisms, both plant and animal. The vast majority are very small (fractions of a millimeter) and are visible only under magnification.

Clinical Features

Medical conditions associated with mites include allergic rhinitis, asthma, childhood eczema, dermatitis, and superinfection of lesions due to excoriation (see Table 13.4).

- **Dust and bed mite:** *Dermatophagoides* species survive best in warm, humid locations, particularly in high-traffic areas, upholstered furniture, and especially beds, where they feed on skin flakes, mold, fungus, and household detritus. Both dust and bed mites can become airborne with bed making, cleaning, and vacuuming, causing allergic and dermatologic problems. These mites do not bite, sting, or transmit any disease-causing pathogens.
- **Harvest mite:** *Trombicula autumnalis* will move from plants to people, dogs, cats, and reptiles in the six-legged larval stage, during which they feed on digested keratinized skin. They tend to attach where clothing fits tightly (waistline, socks and armpits) and do not suck blood but inject saliva, which digests skin, particularly near hair follicles. Severely pruritic welts develop 3 to 6 hours after exposure and persist up to 2 weeks. Firm red nodules may result from the host immune response. The mites drop off after feeding for 3 to 4 days.

Table 13.3 Treatment of Scabies

Drug name	Dose	Side Effects	Comments
Permethrin (Elimite)	5% cream applied to entire body and rinsed off in 8–14 hours	May burn or sting	First-line topical therapy. Should reapply 1 week after initial application
Benzyl benzoate	25% (adults) or 10% (children) cream applied to entire body, rinsed off after 24 hours	Skin irritation	Second-line topical therapy in Africa and the United Kingdom, not available in the United States
Lindane (Kwell)	1% lotion or 30 g cream applied to entire body and rinsed off after 8–10 hours	Seizures, muscle spasm, aplastic anemia. Not to be used in infants or lactating mothers	Second-line topical therapy in some countries, though rarely used in the United States
Crotamiton (Eurax)	10% cream applied for 24 hours, rinsed and reapplied for 24 hours	Seizures (rare)	Second- or third-line topical therapy
Ivermectin (Mectizan, Stromectol)	200 µg/kg/dose PO × 1, and second dose 14 days later recommended	Increased itching initially	Literature to support this drug is emerging, especially in crusted scabies; may be more expensive than topical agents

Table 13.4 Clinical Features and Treatment: Mites

Transmission	Direct (person to person)
	or
	Indirect (through infested bedding or clothing)
Dust and bed mite	Survive best in warm humid locations
	Feed on skin flakes, mold, fungus, and detritus
	Allergic and dermatologic problems when they become airborne from cleaning and vacuuming
	Do not bite or sting, nor do they transmit any disease-causing pathogens
Harvest mite	Feed on digested keratinized skin during the larval stage only
	Attach where clothing fits tightly (waistline, socks, and armpits)
	Inject saliva that digests skin, particularly near hair follicles, which causes pruritic welts to develop after 3–6 hours
Bird mite	Often called "bird lice"
	Cannot infest humans, but will bite when no birds are available
	Rash, irritation, pruritis, and secondary bacterial infection are common for up to 2 weeks after being bitten
Chiggers	Feed on keratinized skin during the larval stage only
	Bites around tight-fitting clothes with similar host response to harvest mites
Diagnosis	Clinical diagnosis
	or
	Direct visualization under a microscope of skin scraping or biopsy
Treatment	Antibiotics for superinfected skin excoriations
	Thorough cleaning and vacuuming with a HEPA filter
	Wash clothes and linens at 125 °F
	Symptomatic treatment of pruritis with steroids and antihistamines as needed

Dog, cat, rabbit, fowl, rat, clover and bat mites, straw itch mites, and grain mites can all cause similar medical problems to the species above.
HEPA filter – high-efficiency particulate air filter.

- **Bird mite:** *Ornithonyssus* species, often called "bird lice," populate bird nests and are parasites of common birds. When birds leave the nest, these hematophagous mites are dispersed and may enter human dwellings and bite humans. They cannot infest humans, but will bite when no birds are available. Rash, irritation, pruritis, and secondary bacterial infection are common for up to 2 weeks after bites. Control is best achieved by bird nest control.
- **Chiggers:** *Eutrombicula alfreddugesi* and other species, like the harvest mite, feed only in the larval stage. Common throughout the southeastern United States, they bite around tight-fitting clothes and cause a rash similar to that caused by harvest mites.
- **Dog, cat, rabbit, fowl, rat, clover and bat mites, straw itch mites, and grain mites:** All can cause similar medical problems to the species above. *Cheyletiella* species (including dog, cat, and rabbit mite) infestations tend to appear in very specific patterns on human skin. For example, the pruritis can appear on the arms and across the chest after holding a pet animal. This is the most common diagnostic clue.

Differential Diagnosis

The differential diagnosis would include:

- drug eruptions
- furunculosis
- folliculitis
- other contact dermatitis
- other pruritic papular or nodular processes

Laboratory Findings

Mites are usually diagnosed clinically, but occasionally require skin scrapings or skin biopsy examined with magnification. Sometimes the larvae can be felt crawling on the skin and can be seen with direct inspection. No laboratory tests exist except allergen testing.

Treatment and Prophylaxis

When superinfected excoriations are found, antimicrobial therapy directed toward *Streptococcus* and *Staphylococcus* (including methicillin-resistant *Staphylococcus aureus* [MRSA]) infection may be warranted. Most ectoparasitic infestations due to mites are self-limited and source control should be the primary target. For bed and dust mites, thorough cleaning and vacuuming with a high-efficiency particulate air (HEPA) filter can provide relief. All bed linens and clothing should be washed at 125 °F (52 °C), which kills mites. Raising the bed off the floor and air conditioner filter changes may decrease exposures. Allergy treatment with immunotherapy mite extract injections may help decrease allergic symptoms. Pesticide "bombing" will often be ineffective if the sources (bird nests, rodents, domestic animals) are not removed. Household pets can be treated topically (e.g. pyrethrin, lime sulfur) or with ivermectin as advised by a veterinarian.

Treatment of clothing with permethrin and skin with *N*,*N*-diethyl-*m*-toluamide (DEET)-containing pesticides may provide protection during specific exposures (e.g. field work). Pruritis can be treated with topical or oral steroids and antihistamines.

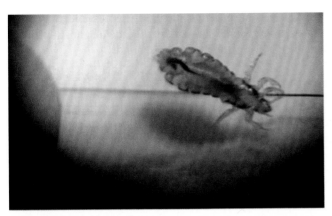

Figure 13.1 *Pediculus corporis* (10).
Photograph courtesy of Dr. Matthew Lewin.

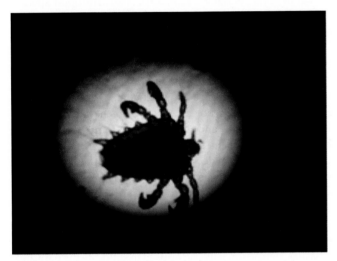

Figure 13.2 *Phthirus pubis* (10).
Photograph courtesy of Dr. Toby Salz.

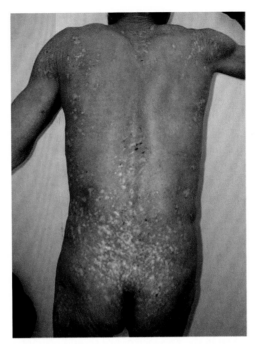

Figure 13.3 Typical distribution of body lice infestation.
Courtesy of Dr. Bradley W. Frazee, MD.

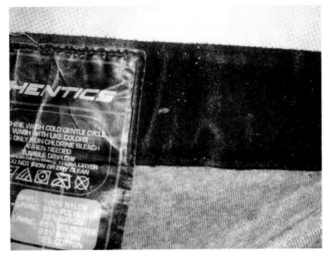

Figure 13.4 Body lice discovered in a clothing seam.

Lice

Three types of infestation with lice are seen in humans – head lice (*Pediculus humanus capitis*), body lice (*Pediculus humanus corporis*; see Figure 13.3), and pubic lice (*Phthirus pubis*; see Figures 13.2 and 13.4). The head louse infests only the human head, but the pubic louse may be found on any short hair (pubic hair, areolar hair, beard, eyebrow or lash, axillary hairs). The Centers for Disease Control and Prevention (CDC) considers infestation with pubic lice a sexually transmitted disease (STD), and co-infection with other STDs is common. Body lice (*Pediculus corporis*; Figure 13.1) is also a major public health concern due to its role in spreading trench fever (*Bartonella quintana*), epidemic typhus (via *Rickettsia prowazekii*), and relapsing fever (via *Borrelia recurrentis*).

Life Cycle and Transmission

Head lice feed on blood and reside close to the scalp. The adult female head louse lays 1 to 6 eggs per day for up to 30 days after mating. The eggs are translucent and are attached to a hair shaft close to the scalp. They hatch in 7 days and the 1-mm-long empty egg casings (nits) then become white and are visible. After 9 to 12 days, the grayish-colored louse becomes an adult about the size of a sesame seed (3–4 mm). Nits (empty egg casings) stay on the hair shaft, and they move away from the scalp as the hair grows. Head lice are usually transmitted through head-to-head contact, but can also be transmitted by fomites (hats, scarves, brushes, etc.). Lice cannot jump or fly.

Pubic lice are spread through sexual activity. If pubic lice are discovered in children, sexual abuse should be suspected. Lice or nits found on an eyelash are almost invariably pubic lice, not head lice.

Body lice are associated with poverty, homelessness, poor levels of personal hygiene, and inability to wash clothes. They live and lay eggs exclusively on clothing, typically within the seams, crawling to the skin to feed multiple times per day. Body lice are often accompanied by simultaneous head lice.

Clinical Features

The most common symptom of infestation is pruritis (Table 13.5). It is possible, however, to have an infestation of head lice without itching. A tickling sensation of something moving in the hair may be noticed. Head lice and their nits are most commonly found behind the ears and on the hairs of the neck and occiput. The excoriated rash from body lice is typically distributed at the nape of the neck and around the waist, corresponding to clothing seams, where they live (see Figure 13.3). Body lice are found by removing clothing, turning it inside out, and examining the seams closely (see Figure 13.4). Pubic lice will be found attached to the base of the pubic hair and the infestation generally results in severe itching. Oftentimes patients susceptible to lice will have delusional parasitosis. However, they may also have lice or both disorders. Patients with psychiatric disorders are particularly prone to the diagnosis of one or the other, if not both. The presence of delusional parasitosis even in the presence of lice should prompt a psychiatric or toxicological evaluation followed by appropriate counseling.

Laboratory Findings

Infestation with head lice is best diagnosed by isolating parasites with a fine-tooth comb. This is more efficient than direct visualization on the hairs and scalp. The comb should be placed in the hair right at the scalp and then drawn down firmly. The entire head of hair should be combed twice and the comb examined after each stroke. It often takes at least a full minute of combing to find the first louse. Finding nits does not necessarily mean active infestation because nits can persist after treatment. Some sources say that the diagnosis can only be made if a living, moving louse is found.

Treatment and Prophylaxis

Treatment of head lice is somewhat controversial and varies from region to region. Some of these differences lie in different resistance patterns. In the United States, chemical pediculicides are the mainstay of therapy. Treatment should be repeated 10 days after initial application because eggs are less effectively killed than adults and it takes 5 to 11 days for eggs to hatch. All close contacts should be treated. Permethrin 5% cream or lotion is first-line therapy (see Table 13.6). Malathion is also recommended as second-line therapy, though it has a strong odor and cannot be used in young children or in people with asthma or severe eczema. Permethrin is an arthropod-specific neurotoxin, but malathion is an acetylcholinesterase inhibitor and can cause severe autonomic dysfunction in humans. Using a nit comb as an adjunct to chemical treatments decreases reinfection rates.

For children younger than 2 years of age, or in cases where parents do not want to use an insecticide, wet combing alone is an alternative. It is not as effective as chemical methods. Brushes, combs, hats, and other possible fomites such as bed sheets and other linens should be cleaned in hot water, but further environmental decontamination is not necessary. Oral ivermectin may also be used and is the preferred treatment in patients unable to comply with topical therapy or who may also have co-infestations (such as scabies). In resistant cases, ivermectin or a combination of topical therapy and oral tri-methoprim–sulfamethoxazole may be used. If lice infest the eyelashes, petroleum jelly can be used to suffocate the parasites.

Table 13.5 Clinical Features: Lice

Incubation period	3–7 days
Head lice (*Pediculus humanus capitis*) Body lice (*Pediculus humanus corporis*) Pubic lice (*Phthirus pubis*)	Infests only human head Rare in African Americans Commonly found behind ears, neck, and occiput hair Lives in clothing seams Does not affect hair Infects any short hair (pubic, areolar, beard, axillary, and eyebrows or lashes) Lice or nits found on an eyelash are always pubic lice and not head lice Should suspect sexual abuse if discovered in children
Transmission	Direct (person to person) *or* Indirect (through infested bedding or clothing) Lice cannot jump or fly
Signs and symptoms	Pruritis Visible insects, eggs, feeling of movement on hair or skin
Diagnosis	Clinical diagnosis *or* Direct visualization under a light microscope Skin biopsy

Table 13.6 Treatment of Head, Body, and Pubic Lice

Topical therapy:

Permethrin (5% Elimite for skin) or (1% Nix for hair) lotion:
- Apply to damp hair and leave on for 10 minutes and rinse
- May itch, burn, or sting
- Comb out lice/nits after treatment
- First-line treatment

Benzyl alcohol 5% lotion
- Apply to dry hair and leave on for 10 minutes
- Usually requires two treatments (7 days apart)
- Comb out lice/nits after treatment
- More expensive
- Approved for children >6 months and pregnant women

Pyrethrin–piperonyl butoxide (RID, A-200):
- Available over-the-counter
- Apply to dry hair for 10 minutes
- Usually requires two treatments
- Less effective than permethrin
- Second- or third-line therapy

Malathion (Ovide) – 0.5% aqueous-based lotions:
- Apply to dry hair and leave on 8–12 hours and rinse
- Flammable, avoid contact with eyes, mucous membranes
- Strong odor
- Not recommended for children <6 years old
- Second- or third-line therapy

Oral therapy:

Ivermectin (Mectizan, Stromectol):
- 200 µg/kg/dose PO × 1, and second dose 10 days later
- Increased itching initially
- Not FDA-approved for treatment of pediculosis
- Usually used in resistant cases

Body lice:

Typically eradicated by improving hygiene alone (clean clothing, wash bedding)

If treatment is desired, a pediculicide may be used

Body lice do not require chemical therapy because they live in the clothing, not on the skin (unless severely infested). In most cases, hot-water laundering of all clothing and bedding is sufficient.

Ticks

Epidemiology and Microbiology of Tickborne Illnesses

In North America, ticks are widely dispersed in rural and suburban areas. Ticks are arachnids closely related to mites and are hematophagous, taking blood meals from humans and animals. Adult ticks are larger than mites and are visible without magnification. However, smaller, immature forms are also hematophagous and may be overlooked. Both immature and adult forms can be disease vectors. Tick-borne diseases have a wide variety of infectious agents, including viruses, spirochetes, and intracellular bacterial pathogens (*Rickettsia* and Ehrlichiae), gram-negative bacteria (*Francisella tularensis*), and protozoa (*Babesia microti*).

Table 13.7 summarizes the major tick-borne illnesses, the vectors, and their geographic distribution. Wherever humans come into contact with ticks, bites and diseases follow. Children are more commonly exposed to ticks, for example, and the peak incidence for Rocky Mountain spotted fever (RMSF) is between ages 5 and 9. Approximately half of patients diagnosed with tick-borne illnesses will recall having had a tick bite. Lyme disease is now the most common tick-borne disease in the United States and is a reportable disease. In 2013, approximately 27,000 cases of Lyme were reported to the CDC (by all states except Arkansas, Colorado, Hawaii, Louisiana, Mississippi, Missouri, New Mexico, and Oklahoma) and the national incidence in 2013 was 8.6 cases per 100,000 population. RMSF is found in all states except Maine, Hawaii, and Alaska and is much more common along the eastern seaboard than the Rocky Mountains, with a peak incidence in 2008 of 8.4 cases per 1 million. In some cases, a single bite may transmit multiple diseases (e.g. human granulocytic ehrlichiosis and Lyme disease). If a high proportion of ticks in a given area are infected, a "treat all" prophylactic strategy is warranted for a potentially disabling disease such as Lyme disease. However, this strategy is not appropriate in most cases, and many people receive unnecessary antibiotics and testing. See also Chapter 14, Fever and Rash in Adults.

Tick Removal

Removal of the tick will cure toxin-mediated ascending tick paralysis and may prevent transmission of Lyme disease, which requires that a tick be attached to its host long enough for the infecting pathogen to move from the gut to the salivary tract of the tick – a process that may take hours to days. Thus, the duration of tick attachment is important for disease transmission. Additionally, the longer the ticks are attached, the more difficult they are to remove.

Traction on the tick using a forceps will allow complete removal of some recently attached ticks (see Figure 13.5). Later on, the biting apparatus of the tick is cemented in place by its secretions. Pulling on the body will often snap it off, leaving the head behind. A scalpel can be used to core out the head to prevent a foreign-body reaction or superinfection.

Myiasis

Myiasis is the infestation of skin (and subcutaneous tissues) with fly larvae and is divided into three subtypes: facultative, obligatory, and accidental (see Table 13.8). Facultative myiasis is commonly referred to as maggots. The usual precondition for facultative myiasis is the exposure of a wound to the ubiquitous house fly. Once a fly deposits eggs within a wound, maggots develop and clean the wound. For physicians, the main elements of the epidemiology are homelessness and substance use, which produces an altered sensorium during which flies can access the wound to lay eggs. Obligatory infestations include *Dermatobia hominis* (botfly), *Cordylobia anthropophaga* (tumbu fly), and screw worm infestations. These organisms have larval stages that require the living tissue of an animal host and may cause significant tissue destruction. Accidental myiasis occurs when egg-stage flies are ingested on contaminated food or come into contact with the genitourinary tract.

Table 13.7 Common Tick-Transmitted Diseases

Disease	Causative Agent	Vector	Geography	Signs and Symptoms	Diagnosis and Findings	Selected Treatments	Comments
Lyme disease	*Borrelia burgdorferi*	Deer tick (black legged) – main reservoir is white-footed mouse	Most in NE or Great Lakes.	Erythema migrans, lymphadenopathy, fever, arthritis, CNS late (three stages)	Clinical. Joint fluid PCR, serology	Doxycycline 100 mg PO BID × 2–3 weeks *or* Amoxicillin 500 mg PO TID × 2–3 weeks Doxycycline prophylaxis: 200 mg PO × 1	"Bell's palsy" should provoke tick bite questions. New vaccine "LymeRix"
Rocky Mountain spotted fever (RMSF)	*Rickettsia rickettsii*	Wood tick, dog tick	All states except CT, KS, MA, NV, SD, VT, and WV	Fever, headache, rash involving palms and soles	Thrombocytopenia, hyponatremia, rash biopsy, immunofluorescence	Doxycycline 100 mg PO BID × 7 days	Not in the Rockies primarily and may not be "spotted"
Ehrlichiosis (HME)	*Ehrlichia chaffeensis*	Lone star tick (south central United States), dog tick (SE United States)	See vector box	Flulike syndrome and a rash	Leukopenia, thrombocytopenia, transaminitis, serology	Doxycycline 100 mg PO BID × 7 days	Treat while diagnostics are pending (RMSF mimic)
Ehrlichiosis (HGE)	*Anaplasma phagocytophilum*	Deer tick	Midwest and NE United States	Flu-like syndrome and a rash	Leukopenia, thrombocytopenia, transaminitis, serology	Doxycycline 100 mg PO BID × 7 days	Treat while diagnostics are pending (RMSF mimic)
Tularemia	*Francisella tularensis*	Lone star tick, wood tick, dog tick – also deer and horse flies	All states except Hawaii	Fever, headache, sore throat, cough, ARDS, chest pain (pericarditis)	Serology, rabbit exposure, CXR (triad of effusion, adenopathy, ovoid opacities)	Gentamicin 5 mg/kg/dose IV every 24 hours × 7–14 days *plus* chloramphenicol for meningitis	"Rabbit fever," possible bioweapon
Babesiosis	*Babesia microti, Babesia divergens*	Deer tick (black legged)	NE United States	Flu-like syndrome, jaundice, renal failure	Hemolytic anemia, "Maltese cross" (on smear), serology, PCR	Clindamycin 600 mg PO/IV every 8 hours *plus* Quinine 650 mg PO TID × 7 days each	Malaria-like
Colorado tick fever	RNA orbivirus	Wood tick	Rocky Mountains	Flu-like syndrome, "saddleback fever"	Serology, immunofluorescence	Supportive care	Treat while diagnostics are pending
Tick paralysis	Non-infectious (neurotoxin)	*Dermacentor andersoni, D. variabilis*, and others	Rocky Mountains – NW United States/Canada	Ascending paralysis	Find feeding tick (usually on a child)	Remove tick	Look for a tick in the scalp region
Relapsing fever	Borrelial spirochete	*Ornithodoros* genus (main reservoir rabbits and rodents)	West of the Mississippi	Flu-like syndrome, epistaxis, myocarditis, iridocyclitis	Splenomegaly, bone marrow aspiration, leukocytosis	Doxycycline 100 mg PO BID until 48 hours no symptoms	Jarisch–Herxheimer reaction
North Asian tick typhus and African tick typhus	*Rickettsia sibirica* and *Rickettsia conorii*	*Ixodes* ticks of Northeast and Central Asia (*R. sibirica*) and subequatorial Africa (*R. conorii*)	Northeast and Central Asia (*R. sibirica*) and subequatorial Africa (*R. conorii*)	Cardinal symptoms of rickettsiosis, but not usually fatal or with high morbidity as with RMSF	Fever, headache, rash, eschar, lymphadenopathy are typical	Doxycycline 100 mg PO BID for 7 to 10 days	

ARDS – acute respiratory distress syndrome; CNS – central nervous system; CXR – chest X-ray; IV – intravenous; PCR – polymerase chain reaction; PO – by mouth.

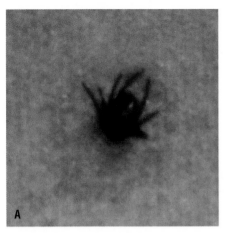
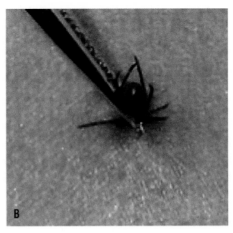
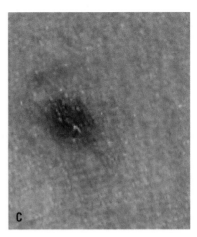

Figure 13.5 Removal of ticks. (A) Deeply embedded *Ixodes pacificus*. (B) Forceps removal with forceps as close to the head as possible and slow, but firm traction. (C) Successful removal of the tick and its head. The patient had been camping in a Lyme-endemic county and was treated with doxycycline for prophylaxis. Photograph courtesy of Dr. Matthew R. Lewin.

Table 13.8 Subtypes of Myiasis Infestation

Facultative (semi-specific) agents	Wounds and ulcers become colonized by maggots, but there is limited live tissue damage. *Fannia canicularis* (lesser house fly) and *Musca domestica* (house fly) are commonly involved. Other species such as the green blowfly and humpback flies can also result in facultative myiasis.
Obligatory (or specific) agents	Have a larval stage that can grow only in the living tissue of an animal host. Tissue destruction and, more rarely, superinfection, follow. *Dermatobia hominis* (botfly) and *Cordylobia anthropophaga* (tumbu fly) are the most common agents. Old and New World screw worms are very invasive obligatory agents that can be quite disfiguring and can even invade bone.
Accidental (non-specific) agents	Egg-stage flies are ingested on contaminated food or come into contact with the genitourinary tract.

Clinical Features

Because larvae are visible to the naked eye, the diagnosis of wound-related myiasis is made by careful examination. The most common presentation is a patient with a chronic wound that has obvious maggot infestation when the wound is undressed (see Table 13.9).

Furuncular cutaneous myiasis presents as a pruritic papule 2 to 3 mm across that gradually increases in size with a diameter of 1 to 3 cm. The respiratory sinuses of the maggot may be seen at the center of this furuncle, and it is through this punctuate opening that the larva breathes. The oft-quoted cure, using a strip of bacon, works because the grease occludes the opening and suffocates the larvae. Because botfly larvae develop for a long period (5 to 12 weeks) in their host tissues, a chronic furunculosis with persistent pruritic papules not responsive to antibiotics is a common historical feature. In the United States, botfly (*D. hominis*) is more commonly found in a traveler who has returned from Central or South America or in military personnel returning overseas from central Asian republics such as Afghanistan. Infestation often does not become apparent until long after the return from the trip, and patients may not associate the travel history with the lesion.

Differential Diagnosis

Important questions to ask include:

- Any travel history within the last 6 weeks?
- History of exposure to biting flies?
- History of furuncular disease?

Key features that distinguish myiasis from infestation by smaller arthropods such as mites, lice, bedbugs, and fleas (see Table 13.10) are:

- the size of lesions and degree of inflammation
- the relatively small number of furuncles in the typical traveler (though massive infestations can occur in the intoxicated who fail to notice the biting)
- there is commonly a readily identifiable punctate opening at the crown of the pruritic papule and a magnifying glass will allow visualization of the breathing apparatus

Other conditions to consider:

- bedbug infestation
- excoriated allergic dermatitis
- primary soft-tissue infection
- skin picking or delusional parasitosis

Laboratory and Radiographic Findings

Exact diagnosis is made by allowing the larvae removed from a patient to pupate and complete its growth to the adult fly, which can then be speciated, though many entomologists can identify species from the larval stages. This is rarely done in practice, however, and diagnosis is often made based on the history and examination.

Table 13.9 Clinical Features: Myiasis

Course	Symptoms develop over weeks to months
Transmission	Fly deposits eggs within a wound
Facultative (semi-specific) agents	Wounds and ulcers become colonized by maggots Limited tissue damage *Fannia canicularis* (lesser house fly), *Musca domestica* (house fly) are commonly involved Green blowfly and humpback flies are also facultative agents
Obligatory (i.e. requires host to complete life cycle)	Furuncular myiasis occurs because the larval stage can only grow in living tissue of host Tissue destruction and rarely superinfection occurs *Dermatobia hominis* (botfly) and *Cordylobia anthropophaga* (tumbu fly) are most common Old and New World screw worms are very invasive agents that can be disfiguring and invade bone
Accidental (non-specific) agents	Occurs when egg-stage flies are ingested on contaminated food leading to infestation of the GI or GU tract and deposition of larvae into feces; may or may not be symptomatic
Signs and symptoms	Obvious visualization of larvae (maggots) Pruritic papules ~2–3 mm in furuncular cutaneous myiasis
Diagnosis	Direct visualization
Treatment	Good wound care Furuncular myiasis – surgical or suffocation removal methods

GI – gastrointestinal; GU – genitourinary.

Table 13.10 Differential Diagnosis of the Persistent Pruritic Papule

Infestation	Physical Characteristics	Location and Historical Features
Scabies	Excoriated papules with burrows	Intertriginous areas with moist, warm skin
Leishmaniasis	Indurated, ulcerated papules and plaques with rolled or raised borders ("cheese pizza lesion")	Travel to an area with sandflies (e.g. military returning from Iraq)
Cutaneous myiasis	Tender, ulcerated papules with central punctum. Nodules may move!	Travel to area with botfly or tumbu fly
Furunculosis	Erythematous perifollicular nodules	Current MRSA epidemic in the United States

Ultrasound may aid in diagnosis and surgical debridement of myiasis. Using a 10-MHz ultrasound probe, a mobile element of a furuncle confirms the presence of the larvae below the skin and may guide surgical removal.

Treatment and Prophylaxis

Myiasis associated with wounds is usually a self-limited problem easily managed by good wound care. The maggots seen in the wound can usually be irrigated away (along with any other eggs). Good wound care and dressings will prevent reinfestation. The psychological aspects of myiasis may be more difficult to manage and may require referral.

Furuncular myiasis due to obligatory agents is more difficult to manage. Surgical incision and extraction of larvae should be performed under local anesthesia. Injecting the area beneath the larvae with lidocaine may force them to surface and allow tweezer extraction. Suffocation techniques with bacon, petroleum jelly, mineral oil (or other substances) may also allow removal. These approaches are particularly useful in endemic areas with few resources. Care must be taken to avoid partial removal. Retention of dead larvae can result in local infection and granuloma formation.

Complications and Admission Criteria

It would be unusual to have to admit a patient for primary arthropod infestations such as lice and scabies. However, these patients frequently have concomitant psychiatric or immune-compromised states that place them at risk for complications from compromised dermis. Infections resulting from bites or the transmission of bacterial and/or viral pathogens by arthropods may cause debilitating or life-threatening disease. Some diseases transmitted by ticks such as *Rickettsia sibirica* can present as fever and fixed lymphadenopathy months after exposure and be mistaken for lymphoma with constitutional symptoms. Others, such as RMSF, can be fatal and require a high degree of clinical suspicion and rapid treatment in order to avert disaster. All patients strongly suspected to have RMSF should be admitted.

Infection Control and Prevention of Infestation

Prevention is the cornerstone of infestation and infection control. Attention to risk factors for exposure and contact identification can prevent major outbreaks of infestation and disease. For common urban infestations such as lice, personal and public hygiene are paramount. Hospitals, psychiatric facilities, jails, and emergency departments are particularly susceptible to minor or major outbreaks of scabies and lice if infested individuals are not treated appropriately, including skin, hair, clothes, and bed sheets. Health-care workers treating patients suspected to have scabies should use universal precautions.

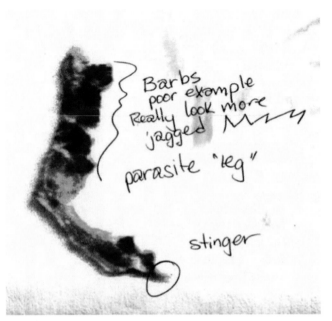

Figure 13.6 Delusional parasitosis. The patient presented with bags and labeled photos of scabs as evidence of infestation. The patient refused to give a urine sample.

Photograph and copy courtesy of Dr. Matthew Lewin.

Diseases such as RMSF and Lyme disease are not transmitted by human-to-human contact.

Pearls and Pitfalls

1. Treatment failures with scabies and lice are becoming more common because of resistance, especially in cases of crusted scabies. Ivermectin has emerged as a simple, effective, albeit more expensive oral treatment option.
2. Mites are ubiquitous ectoparasites that affect humans via their feeding or via their allergenicity, potentially causing asthma, eczema, and dermatitis.
3. Most mites feed in the larval stage, typically resulting in a very pruritic papular or nodular lesion.
4. Ticks are major vectors for a wide array of diseases, and Lyme disease is the most common tick-borne disease in the United States.
5. Most myiasis in the United States is due to facultative organisms that usually cause little or no live tissue damage – these maggots generally debride the wounds they infest.
6. In the United States, obligatory or specific myiasis is primarily a disease of travelers.

7. Delusional parasitosis (see Figure 13.6) is common in psychiatric disorders and, in particular, in abusers of sympathomimetic drugs, such as methamphetamine. Patients may present with samples of lint, scabs, or labeled photographs as "evidence."

References

Boutellis, A., Abi-Rached, L., and Raoult, D. The origin and distribution of human lice in the world. *Infect. Genet. Evol.* 2014; 23: 209–17.

Bratton, R. L. and Corey, R. Tick-borne disease. *Am. Fam. Physician* 2005; 71(12): 2323–30.

Caumes, E. Skin diseases in J. S. Keystone, D. O. Freedman, P. E. Kozarsky, B. A. Connor, and H. D. Nothdurft (eds.), *Travel Medicine*, 3rd edn (New York: Elsevier, 2013).

Centers for Disease Control and Prevention (CDC). Lyme disease data, August 27, 2014, www.cdc.gov/lyme/stats/index.html (accessed November 10, 2017).

CDC. Rocky Mountain spotted fever statistics and epidemiology, September 5, 2013, www.cdc.gov/rmsf/stats/ (accessed November 10, 2017).

Currie, B. J. and McCarthy, J. S. Permethrin and ivermectin for scabies. *N. Engl. J. Med.* 2010; 362(8): 717–25.

Edlow, J. A. Lyme disease and related tick-borne illnesses. *Ann. Emerg. Med.* 1999; 33(6): 680–93.

Fischer, K., Holt, D., Currie, B., *et al.* Scabies: important clinical consequences explained by new molecular studies. *Adv. Parasitol.* 2012; 79: 339–73.

Fuller, L. C. Epidemiology of scabies. *Curr. Opin. Infect. Dis.* 2013; 26(2): 123–6.

Gunning, K., Pippitt, K., Kiraly, B., *et al.* Pediculosis and scabies: treatment update. *Am. Fam. Physician* 2012; 86(6): 535–41.

Heller, M. M., Wong, J. W., Lee, E. S., *et al.* Delusional infestations: clinical presentation, diagnosis and treatment. *Int. J. Dermatol.* 2013; 52(7): 775–83.

Hong, M. Y., Lee, C. C., Chuang, M. C., *et al.* Factors related to missed diagnosis of incidental scabies infestations in patients admitted through the emergency department to inpatient services. *Acad. Emerg. Med.* 2010; 17(9): 958–64.

Mounsey, K. E. and McCarthy, J. S. Treatment and control of scabies. *Curr. Opin. Infect. Dis.* 2013; 26(2): 133–9.

Roberts, R. J. Clinical practice. Head lice. *N. Engl. J. Med.* 2002; 346(21): 1645–50.

Additional Reading

Heukelbach, J. and Feldmeier, H. Ectoparasites – the underestimated realm. *Lancet* 2004; 363(9412): 889–91.

Fever and Rash in Adults

Catherine Marco, Janel Kittredge-Sterling, and Rachel L. Chin

Outline

Introduction

The clinical picture of fever and rash can be caused by a multitude of pathogens, including bacteria, viruses, fungi, protozoa, and helminths. Non-infectious causes include autoimmune diseases and severe drug reactions. This chapter will cover the general approach to fever and rash and focus on several of the most common and serious infectious causes. For the acute care provider, familiarity with the epidemiology, clinical presentations, and initial management of these infections is absolutely essential. Pediatric fever and rash is covered in Chapter 52.

History and Physical Examination

A detailed history and physical are essential in establishing the etiology of fever and rash (see Box 14.1). Attention to general appearance and vital signs is critical since numerous rapidly life-threatening infections can present with fever and rash. The skin should be examined thoroughly, under adequate lighting. Information regarding the lesions should be documented.

Differential Diagnosis

Table 14.1 lists and categorizes causes of fever and rash. The most important distinction for the acute care provider is between diseases with an explosive onset, usually accompanied with high fever or hypothermia, including meningococcemia, Rocky Mountain spotted fever, and toxic shock syndrome – which are rapidly life-threatening – from those with a subacute onset, often presenting primarily as a rash present for days, such as secondary syphilis and Lyme disease. Most viral exanthems lie

somewhere between these two extremes. Several non-infectious causes of fever and rash can also be life-threatening. These include severe drug reactions and toxic epidermal necrolysis.

Clinical Features

Meningococcemia

Meningococcal disease, caused by *Neisseria meningitidis*, a gram-negative diplococcus, presents with a spectrum of disease (see Chapter 8, Meningitis). Most cases in the United States are caused by serogroups B, C, and Y. Approximately 1,400 to 2,800 cases occur annually in the United States. More than 98% of cases are sporadic, though some localized outbreaks occur. Approximately 10 to 14% of cases are fatal. The highest incidence occurs in children 3 months to 3 years, though there has been an increasing incidence in 12 to 29 year olds. The risk of meningococcal disease is increased among infants, asplenic patients, alcoholics, and patients with a terminal (C6–C9) complement deficiency. Meningococcal disease has a peak incidence in midwinter and early spring, and the disease is transmitted by direct respiratory secretion contact (see Table 14.2).

Clinical syndromes associated with meningococcus include respiratory tract infection, meningitis, meningococcal bacteremia, and meningococcemia. Meningococcal bacteremia and meningococcemia are associated with high morbidity and mortality and are often accompanied by characteristic hemorrhagic cutaneous findings. Meningitis and meningococcemia may or may not occur together. Acute fulminant meningococcemia occurs in 10% of cases, presenting

Box 14.1 Focused History and Examination for Fever and Rash

History

- duration of symptoms
- associated symptoms (e.g. fever, headache, gastrointestinal symptoms, pruritus)
- evolution of lesions
- distribution
- history of animal or arthropod bites
- exacerbating and relieving factors (e.g. environmental exposures, foods, medications)
- medical, occupational, and sexual history, medications, illicit drug history, travel, and allergies

Examination

Type of lesions, size, color, secondary findings (e.g. scale, excoriations), and distribution.

Primary lesions may include the following:

- *Macules* are flat lesions defined by an area of changed color (e.g. blanchable erythema).
- *Papules* are raised, solid lesions <5 mm in diameter.
- *Plaques* are lesions >5 mm in diameter with a flat, plateau-like surface.
- *Nodules* are lesions >5 mm in diameter with a more rounded configuration.
- *Wheals* (urticaria, hives) are papules or plaques that are pale pink and may appear annular (ring-like) as they enlarge; classic (non-vasculitic) wheals are transient, lasting only 24 to 48 hours in any defined area.
- *Vesicles* (<5 mm) and *bullae* (>5 mm) are circumscribed, elevated lesions containing fluid.
- *Pustules* are raised lesions containing purulent exudates. Vesicular processes such as varicella or herpes simplex may evolve to pustules.
- *Non-palpable purpura* is a flat lesion that is due to bleeding into the skin. If <3 mm in diameter, the purpuric lesions are termed *petechiae*. If >3 mm, they are termed *ecchymoses*. *Palpable purpura* is a raised lesion that is due to inflammation of the vessel wall (vasculitis) with subsequent hemorrhage.
- An *ulcer* is a defect in the skin extending at least into the upper layer of the dermis.
- *Eschar* is a necrotic lesion covered with a black crust.

Secondary lesions may include:

- scale
- crust
- fissure
- erosions
- ulcer
- scar
- excoriation
- infection
- pigment changes
- lichenification

Color may be:

- normal
- erythematous
- violaceous
- hyperpigmented
- hypopigmented

Patterns of lesions should be established as:

- single
- grouped
- scattered
- linear
- annular
- symmetric
- dermatomal
- central or peripheral
- along Blaschko's lines (specific linear skin patterns thought to be of embryonic origin, usually forming a "V" shape over the spine and "S" shapes over the chest, stomach, and sides)

with shock, hypotension, intracutaneous hemorrhage, and multi-organ failure. Typically, patients present initially with a systemic illness including fever, malaise, coryza, pharyngitis, headache, vomiting, myalgias, and/or arthralgias. Leg pain is a classic presenting symptom.

Cutaneous lesions may be varied in appearance. They include petechiae (50% of patients), papules, purpura, mottling, or morbilliform lesions. The eruption often begins on extremities and becomes generalized. Early lesions may appear as non-specific pink macules and papules. Later lesions may display the classic intracutaneous hemorrhage of petechiae and purpura (see Figure 14.1).

Rocky Mountain Spotted Fever

Rocky Mountain spotted fever is caused by *Rickettsia rickettsii*. It is the most common rickettsial infection in the United States. The organism is transmitted by ticks, especially wood and dog ticks. Annually, there are 500 to 1,000 cases in the United States. The name is actually a misnomer, as less than 5% of cases occur in Rocky Mountain states, whereas more than 50% of cases occur in the south Atlantic states. RMSF is more common in the summer months, and children between the ages of 5 and 9 are commonly affected. Most patients (70%) have a history of tick bite or exposure. The incubation period is 2 to 14 days. If untreated, the disease may be fatal in 25% of cases.

The initial clinical presentation is typically one of systemic illness and may include fever, headache, muscle tenderness (especially the gastrocnemius), photophobia, conjunctival injection, pulmonary symptoms, and gastrointestinal symptoms, including nausea, vomiting, abdominal pain, and splenomegaly (see Table 14.3). Skin lesions occur in 85 to 95% of patients and appear at days 2 to 6. Lesions are typically macular rose-colored blanching lesions, petechiae, or ecchymoses on the extremities with centripetal spread (see Figure 14.2). The lesions are not pathognomonic and the diagnosis should be made clinically based on the constellation of symptoms.

Etiologic tests include fluorescent antibody testing on biopsy and serologic tests. Note that a presumptive diagnosis based on clinical suspicion mandates immediate treatment, long before test results return.

Table 14.1 Selected Causes of Fever and Rash

Etiologies and Categories	Key Features
Bacteria	
Meningococcemia	High fever, altered mental status, shock
Rocky Mountain spotted fever	Tick-borne Rickettsia, centripital rash
Toxic shock syndrome	*S. aureus*, *S. pyogenese*, toxin induced, confluent rash, shock
Secondary syphilis	Sexually transmitted spirochete, subacute
Lyme disease	Tick-borne spirochete, subacute
Viruses	
Measles	Rare in the United States, but occurs in unvaccinated individuals
Rubella	Declared eliminated in the United States
Childhood viral exanthems: roseola, erythema infectiosum, varicella	See Chapter 52
Acute HIV infection	Sexually transmitted, lymphadenopathy, oral lesions, fourth-generation HIV tests usually positive
Mononucleosus (EBV)	Pharyngitis, rash follows aminopenicillin exposure
Connective tissue diseases	
Systemic lupus erythemetosis	Dermatologic findings are typically erythematous macular lesions in light-exposed facial areas
Vasculitis	
Kawasaki disease	Most common childhood vasculitis
Polyarteritis nodosa	Purpura and nodules, multisystem involvement
Severe drug reactions	
Stevens-Johnson syndrome, toxic epidermal necrolysis	Blisters, mucous membrane involvement
Drug rash with eosinophilia and systemic symptoms (DRESS)	Exanthematous rash, fever, organ involvement
Acute generalized exanthematous pustulosis (AGEP)	Rare, acute pustular rash, fever
Other	
Thrombotic thrombocytopenic purpura (TTP)	Microangiopathy, purpuric rash, fever in 20%
Purpura fulminans	Rare, DIC in setting of protein C deficiency
DIC – disseminated intravascular coagulation; EBV – Epstein–Barr virus; HIV – human immunodeficiency virus.	

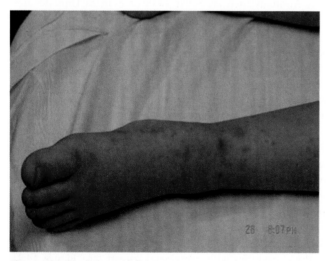

Figure 14.1 Meningococcal disease.
Photograph courtesy of David C. Brancati, DO.

Antimicrobial therapy for RMSF should include doxycycline or tetracycline, for 5 to 7 days. Chloramphenicol may be used as alternative therapy. Aggressive supportive care including mechanical ventilation and dialysis is required in severe cases.

Toxic Shock Syndrome

Toxic shock syndrome is a clinical syndrome associated with *Staphylococcus aureus* infection. Historically, the disease was commonly associated with high-absorbency tampon use, but it may also be seen in association with intravaginal contraceptive devices, nasal packing, post-operative wound infections, and other foreign bodies. More than 5,000 cases have been reported since 1979, though its annual incidence has declined following tampon redesign and public education.

Patients with toxic shock syndrome present with a constellation of symptoms (see Table 14.4). Typically, patients have high fever and an erythematous macular rash, often with extensive desquamation (see Figure 14.3). Hypotension and tachycardia may be seen. Other potential diagnoses must be ruled out, including sepsis, Rocky Mountain spotted fever (RMSF), leptospirosis, measles, hepatitis, mononucleosis, and syphilis.

A minimum of three organ systems must be involved, including gastrointestinal (nausea, vomiting, diarrhea), muscular, renal, hepatic, hematologic, CNS, or mucosal. Abnormal laboratory values that indicate multisystem involvement include elevated creatinine kinase, blood urea nitrogen (BUN)/

Table 14.2 Meningococcemia

Organism	*Neisseria meningitidis*
Signs and symptoms	• Headache, meningismus, cranial nerve palsies or other focal neurologic findings, headache, seizures, myalgia • Rash: petechiae (50% of patients), papules, purpura, mottling, or morbilliform lesions
Laboratory findings	• CSF: typical results OP >30 cm, WBC >500/mL with >80% neutrophils, glucose <40 mg/dL (or <2/3 plasma), and protein >200 mg/dL • Gram-negative, diplococcus, from CSF, blood cultures, or skin lesions
Treatment	Ceftriaxone 2 g IV every 12 hours × 7 days *or* Cefotaxime 2 g IV every 4 hours × 7 days **Alternatives:** Aztreonam 2 g IV every 8 hours × 7 days **Prophylaxis:** household or intimate contact, medical personnel in contact with oral secretions: Rifampin 600 mg PO BID × 2 days *or* Ciprofloxacin 500 mg PO × 1 *or* Ceftriaxone 250 mg IM × 1

CSF – cerebrospinal fluid; IM – intramuscular; IV – intravenous; PO – by mouth; WBC – white blood (cell) count.

Table 14.3 Rocky Mountain Spotted Fever

Organism	*Rickettsia rickettsii*
Signs and symptoms	General: fever, myalgia, sepsis syndrome Skin: petechial rash, begins on extremities, moves toward trunk (centripetal); endothelial cell dysfunction leads to edema of hands and feet; 50% of rashes begin after 3 days of fever Neurological: vasculitis; headache, focal neurological deficits, deafness, meningismus (sometimes with CSF mononuclear/polynuclear pleocytosis), delirium Renal: acute renal failure–ATN and/or intravascular volume depletion; may require hemodialysis Pulmonary: pneumonia (alveolar infiltrates); non-cardiogenic pulmonary edema; ARDS
Laboratory findings	Normal to low WBC; thrombocytopenia characteristic; occasionally mild anemia; coagulopathy (DIC); hyponatremia in 50%; high CK, LDH with tissue injury in severe cases Diagnosis is made by: skin biopsy, direct fluorescent antibody; or serum IFA to detect antibodies to spotted fever group *Rickettsia*
Treatment	Doxycycline (drug of choice in children,* adults, and select pregnant women†): Adults and children ≥8 years old and weighing >45 kg: Doxycycline 100 mg PO/IV BID × 5–7 days or continued treatment for 3 days after defervescence Children <8 years old: Doxycycline 2.2 mg/kg PO/IV BID × 5–7 days Alternative: Adults and children: Chloramphenicol 12.5 mg/kg PO/IV QID × 7 days or 3 days after defervescence Adjunctive steroids not recommended

* Doxycycline or tetracycline recommended for children for two reasons: RMSF can be life-threatening, and a brief course of one of these drugs is unlikely to lead to tooth problems or staining.

† Tetracyclines are generally contraindicated in pregnant women and chloramphenicol is the drug of choice. However, tetracyclines may be preferred in pregnancy during the third trimester, severe disease, and when chloramphenicol is unavailable.

ARDS – acute respiratory distress syndrome; ATN – acute tubular necrosis; CK – creatine kinase; CSF – cerebrospinal fluid; DIC – disseminated intravascular coagulation; IFA – indirect fluorescence assay; LDH – lactate dehydrogenase.

creatinine, bilirubin, aspartate transaminase (AST), alanine aminotransferase (ALT), platelets, and sterile pyuria. Chest radiographic findings may be consistent with acute respiratory distress syndrome secondary to sepsis.

Management is primarily supportive, though removing any possible toxin source, including tampons, wound or nasal packing, contraceptive devices, indwelling lines, or any other foreign body, is crucial to initial management. *S. aureus* produces the enterotoxins toxic shock syndrome toxin-1 (TSST-1), Staphylococcal enterotoxins B (SEB), and Staphylococcal enterotoxins C (SEC). Therapy is aimed at halting toxin production and killing bacteria. Clindamycin inhibits toxin synthesis and is the drug of choice. Antibiotics include clindamycin plus oxacillin or nafcillin for methicillin-sensitive *S. aureus* and clindamycin plus vancomycin for methicillin-resistant *S. aureus*. Supportive care may require aggressive volume

Table 14.4 Toxic Shock Syndrome

Organism	*S. aureus* enterotoxins, TSST-1, SEB, and SEC
Signs and symptoms and laboratory findings	Fever: >38.9°C
	Hypotension and tachycardia
	Rash: diffuse erythematous macular rash and desquamation of palms and soles
	Multisystem involvement (three or more of the following):
	(a) GI: vomiting, diarrhea at onset
	(b) musculoskeletal: CPK >2 × normal or severe myalgia
	(c) renal: BUN/creatinine >2 × normal or sterile pyuria
	(d) hepatic: bilirubin, AST, or ALT >2 × normal
	(e) Hematologic: platelets <100,000/mm³
	(f) CNS: altered mental status without focal neurologic signs
Treatment	Supportive with ICU monitoring
	Clindamycin 900 mg IV every 8 hours + oxacillin or nafcillin 2 g IV every 4 hours for methicillin-sensitive *S. aureus*
	or
	Clindamycin 900 mg IV every 8 hours plus vancomycin 15–20 mg/kg/dose IV every 8–12 hours for methicillin-resistant *S. aureus*
	Some may favor linezolid instead of vancomycin if MRSA concerns, mainly because of protein synthesis inhibition
	Consider IVIG: 2 g/kg IV × 1, repeat in 48 hours if patient remains unstable

CPK – creatine phosphokinase; GI – gastrointestinal; MRSA – methicillin-resistant *Staphylococcus aureus*.

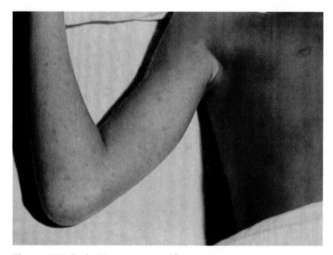

Figure 14.2 Rocky Mountain spotted fever.

Photograph source: Centers for Disease Control Public Health Image Library, http://phil.cdc.gov/Phil/publicdomain.asp.

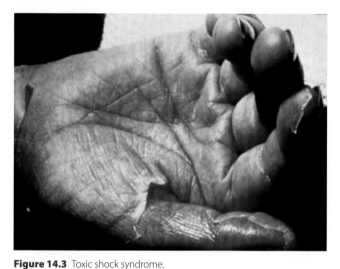

Figure 14.3 Toxic shock syndrome.

Photograph source: Centers for Disease Control Public Health Image Library, http://phil.cdc.gov/Phil/publicdomain.asp.

replacement for severe third spacing, vasopressors, mechanical ventilation, and fresh frozen plasma for coagulopathy. Most patients with *S. aureus* toxic shock syndrome have been shown to lack antibodies to the toxin; though there are no trial data to support its use, experts recommend intravenous immune globulin (IVIG) in severe cases, to boost antibody levels to this common antigen.

Secondary Syphilis

Syphilis is caused by the spirochete *Treponema pallidum*, which typically enters the body through mucous membranes or non-intact skin (see Table 14.5). Syphilis is the third most common reportable sexually transmitted disease in the United States (after chlamydia and gonorrhea) and is spread almost exclusively through sexual contact, with some rare cases of trans-placental transmission. The prevalence of syphilis has risen

since 2005. Syphilis occurs in men more than women and is considered an epidemic among men who have sex with men (MSM). Co-infection with HIV is common. In the United States, syphilis disproportionately affects African Americans and Hispanics. The incubation period is 10 to 90 days after exposure.

Primary syphilis presents as a painless genital chancre (see Chapter 31, Ulcerative Sexual Transmitted Diseases). Often medical care is not sought because the lesion is painless and usually resolves spontaneously, though latent disease persists. Up to 50% of patients with syphilis do not recall any genital lesions.

Secondary syphilis, a systemic infection, occurs 5 to 12 weeks after the chancre appears. Symptoms may include headache, sore throat, adenopathy splenomegaly, and weight loss. Fever may occur, though it is not a prominent feature of

Table 14.5 Syphilis

Organism	*Treponema pallidum*
Incubation period	• Primary (chancre) lesion appears 10–90 days after contact • Secondary (rash) occurs within 6 months of primary lesion
Signs and symptoms	• Mucocutaneous: usually one lesion, may be more, untreated lasts several weeks • Secondary: within 6 months of exposure; palmar-plantar copper coin rash classic; many other rash forms, condyloma latum; other secondary symptoms include alopecia areata, fever • CNS: meningitis (1–2 years after infection), meningovascular (5–7 years), general paresis and tabes dorsalis (10–20 years), gummatous neurosyphilis • Ocular: uveitis, iridocyclitis, Argyll Robertson pupils • Cardiovascular system: ascending aortitis • Bone: arthritis, osteitis, periostitis • Liver: hepatitis
Laboratory findings	Diagnosis is made by dark-field microscopy, non-treponemal serology, or treponemal antibody tests. Non-treponemal serologic tests, including RPR and VDRL, typically correlate with disease progress and become positive 14 days after a chancre appears. Titers are expected to decline or disappear after treatment, though they may remain positive in some patients indefinitely. Treponemal antibody tests, such as FTA-ABS, do not correlate with disease activity, and many patients will remain positive indefinitely. **Primary syphilis:** • May be dark-field positive, but serologically negative; TP-specific test (FTA) may be positive before RPR **Secondary syphilis:** • RPR positive in 99%

CNS – central nervous system; FTA-ABS – fluorescent treponemal antibody absorbed; RPR – rapid plasma reagin; TP – *Treponema pallidum*; VDRL – venereal disease research laboratory.

syphilis. Most patients (75 to 100%) will have skin findings, which may include localized or generalized macules, papules, follicular lesions, nodules, pustules, and annular or serpiginous lesions. Inflammatory lesions of oral and genital mucosa may occur. The trunk, extremities, and genitalia may be affected and lesions usually occur symmetrically (see Figures 14.4 to 14.7). Alopecia and nail changes may also be seen. Secondary syphilis should be considered in the differential diagnosis of any maculopapular lesion involving the trunk, palms, or soles. Condyloma lata is the term for soft, flat-topped, red to pale papules, nodules, or plaques seen in intertriginous or mucous membranes, such as the anogenital region, mouth, interdigital spaces, or axillae. Neurosyphilis may occur during any phase of syphilis. If untreated, secondary syphilis may progress to tertiary syphilis, with meningitis, dementia, neuropathy, or thoracic aneurysm.

Treatment of secondary syphilis may be undertaken prior to establishment of the definitive diagnosis (see Table 14.5). The treatment of choice is benzathine penicillin G (Bicillin-LA, BPG), 2.4 million units intramuscular. It is important to note that the similar combination benzathine–procaine penicillin G (Bicillin-CR) is not appropriate therapy for secondary syphilis. Alternative regimens include doxycycline or ceftriaxone (see Table 14.6).

Lyme Disease

In the United States, Lyme disease is caused by the spirochete *Borrelia burgdorferi* and is transmitted by the deer tick bite (see Chapter 13, Ectoparasites). Most cases occur in the spring and early summer. Endemic areas include the Northeast, Midwest, West, and scattered other areas. Although 36 to 48

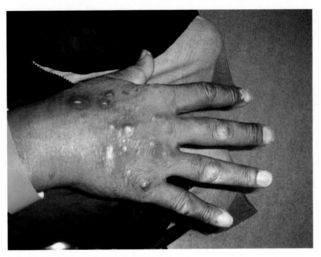

Figure 14.4 Secondary syphilis on hand.

hours of tick attachment is necessary to transmit disease, less than 33% of patients recall a tick bite. The incubation period is 3 to 30 days.

Clinical presentations include three disease stages (see Table 14.7). Stage I occurs early and is manifested by malaise, headache, fever, lymphadenopathy, and arthralgias. Stage I typically resolves in 4 weeks. Erythema migrans occurs in 60 to 80% of cases and manifests as erythematous annular, non-scaling lesion with central clearing (see Figure 14.8). Stage II presents with secondary annular lesions, fever, lymphadenopathy, neurologic manifestations, and/or AV block and may last weeks to months. Stage III manifests as chronic arthritis, CNS disease, and dermatitis.

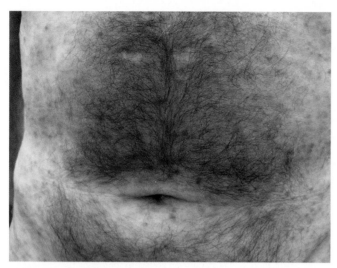

Figure 14.5 Secondary syphilis on trunk.
Photograph courtesy of Joseph Engleman, MD.

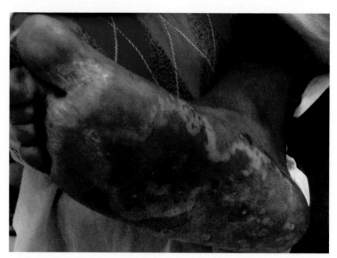

Figure 14.7 Secondary syphilis on the plantar surface of the foot in the setting of AIDS; note atypical hyperpigmentation, hypopigmentation and scaly quality.
Photograph courtesy of Dr. Bradley W. Frazee, MD.

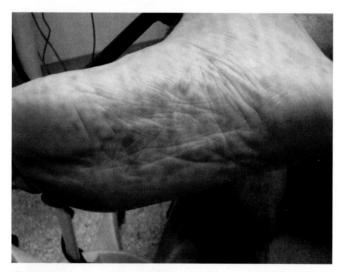

Figure 14.6 Typical secondary syphilis on the plantar surface of the foot.
Photograph courtesy of Joseph Engleman, MD.

Diagnostic tests may include a non-specific elevated erythrocyte sedimentation rate and serologic tests, which are helpful in establishing the definitive diagnosis, but are not available acutely.

Management should include appropriate antibiotic administration (see Table 14.8). The antibiotic regimen may include doxycycline for 10 to 21 days, or as alternates, cefuroxime, ceftriaxone, or penicillin G. Amoxicillin may be used in pediatric and pregnant patients. Antimicrobial prophylaxis after a tick bite with a single dose of doxycycline should be considered in areas with high prevalence of Lyme if the tick was attached for 36 hours or more and if treatment is given within 72 hours of tick removal.

Disseminated Gonococcal Infection

Gonococcal infections are caused by the gram-negative diplococcus species *Neisseria gonorrhoeae*. Approximately 700,000

cases occur annually in the United States. Disseminated gonococcal infection occurs in 1 to 3% of patients with gonococcal infection and occurs disproportionately in women (see Chapter 33, Adult Septic Arthritis).

Systemic symptoms may include mono- or polyarthralgias, tenosynovitis, endocarditis, and meningitis (see Table 14.9). Fever is uncommon. Skin lesions may appear as tender erythematous or hemorrhagic papules or petechiae that may evolve into pustules and vesicles, with predilection for periarticular regions of distal extremities (see Figure 14.9).

Diagnostic tests may include cervical or urethral cultures (80 to 90% sensitive), cultures of joint or skin lesions (20 to 50% sensitive), immunofluorescent staining of pustule contents, and blood cultures.

Treatment should include hospital admission, with supportive care, such as intravenous hydration and antipyretics, as well as antibiotic therapy, such as ceftriaxone 1 g IV QD for 7 to 10 days. Alternative regimens include cefotaxime or ceftizoxime. Quinolone-resistant *Neisseria gonorrhea* (QRNG) continues to be an emerging treatment problem in the United States, and quinolones are no longer recommended. The rate of co-infection with chlamydia is high, and all patients should also be treated with azithromycin or doxycycline.

Viral Infections

Systemic viral infections may cause fever and rash. Common organisms include enterovirus, adenovirus, rotavirus, coxsackievirus, roseola, and numerous others. In many cases, the viral infection is brief and self-limited. Specific viruses of clinical importance, including measles and rubella, are discussed here.

Measles

Measles, or rubeola, caused by a single-stranded RNA paramyxovirus, occurs commonly in the winter months. Overall, the number of reported cases of measles has dropped

Table 14.6 Treatment for Syphilis

Primary and secondary syphilis	PCN G benzathine 2.4 million units IM × 1
	PCN allergy (non-pregnant, preferred):
	Doxycycline 100 mg PO BID × 14 days
	or
	Tetracycline 500 mg PO QID × 14 days
	or
	Ceftriaxone 1 g IM or IV daily × 8–10 days
	All treatments require well-documented close follow-up.
Latent syphilis	Early latent (<1 year duration) (normal CSF exam, if done): PCN G benzathine 2.4 million units IM × 1
	Late latent or latent of unknown duration (normal CSF exam, if done): PCN G benzathine 2.4 million units IM weekly × 3 weeks
	If any PCN dose >2 days late, must recommence the regimen
	PCN allergy recommended: (1) Doxycycline 100 mg PO BID × 4 weeks or (2) Tetracycline 500 mg PO QID × 4 weeks
Neurosyphilis	Only PCN is currently recommended; allergic persons should be desensitized and treated with penicillin
	Recommended: aqueous PCN G 18–24 million units IV per day, administer as 3–4 million units IV every 4 hours × 10–14 days
	Alternative: PCN G procaine 2.4 million units IM daily, plus probenecid 500 mg PO QID × 10–14 days
	PCN is the preferred regimen for all stages of syphilis in HIV-infected persons
Syphilis in HIV-infected individuals	Primary, secondary, and early latent syphilis: use IM PCN G benzathine as for immunocompetent persons; some experts recommend three weekly doses (i.e. as for late latent syphilis)
	PCN-allergic HIV-positive, primary, secondary, or early latent syphilis: can be treated as allergic HIV-negative person
	Late latent syphilis or syphilis of unknown duration requires LP to rule out neurosyphilis; all require PCN-based treatment; desensitization required with allergies
Syphilis in pregnancy	Only PCN is currently recommended; treatment during pregnancy should be the penicillin regimen appropriate to the stage of syphilis diagnosis; desensitization required for PCN-allergic pregnant patients
	Some experts recommend a second dose of PCN G benzathine 2.4 million units IM 1 week after the initial dose for primary, secondary, early latent syphilis in pregnancy

BPG – benzathine PCN G; CSF – cerebrospinal fluid; HIV – human immunodeficiency virus; IM – intramuscular; IV – intravenous; LP – lumbar puncture; PCN – penicillin; PO – by mouth.

Table 14.7 Clinical Features: Lyme Disease

Organism	*Borrelia burgdorferi*
Signs and symptoms	• Stage I occurs early (3–30 days after tick bite): erythema migrans, malaise, headache, fever, and arthralgias
	• Stage II has secondary annular lesions, fever, neurologic manifestations (weakness, lethargy), and cardiac manifestations (AV block).
	• Stage III has chronic arthritis, neurologic manifestations (cranial nerve palsy including Bell's palsy, lymphocytic meningitis, or radiculopathy with pain, paresis, or paresthesias), encephalopathy, and dermatitis
Laboratory findings	Laboratory conformation not typically necessary.
	Elevated ESR, elevated transaminases; EIA or IFA and Western blot – takes 4–6 weeks for seroconversion

AV – atrioventricular; EIA – enzyme immunoassay.

dramatically in the United States since the advent of the measles vaccine. However, a recent outbreak in 2014 was seen in the United States, with over 500 cases, most cases associated with international importation. In recent years, typically <100 cases are seen annually in the United States, compared to the 4 to 5 million cases per year prior to immunization. Measles is most likely to infect unvaccinated individuals, often including preschoolers in low-income homes or in heavily populated areas. Worldwide, approximately 20 million measles cases occur annually and this is the primary cause of death that is preventable by vaccination. Patients are considered to be contagious from 5 days prior to onset of symptoms until 5 to 6 days after the onset of dermatologic involvement.

Symptoms may include fever, cough, coryza, or conjunctivitis preceding the dermatologic findings (see Table 14.10).

Gastrointestinal symptoms of nausea, vomiting, diarrhea, headache, and malaise may also occur. Lymphadenopathy and splenomegaly may occur. Skin lesions are erythematous macules and papules, often beginning on the scalp and head and spreading caudally to neck, trunk, and extremities (see Figure 14.10). Purpura may occur in association with thrombocytopenia. Koplik's spots, small white or blue lesions on an erythematous base, are found opposite the second molars on the buccal mucosa (see Figure 14.11).

The diagnosis is usually made clinically. Complete blood count will often reveal leukopenia with lymphocytopenia. Complement fixing detection of antibodies can be performed to ascertain the diagnosis.

Complications may include pneumonia, otitis media, diarrhea, hepatitis, thrombocytopenia, and encephalitis. Children

Table 14.8 Treatment of Lyme Disease

Tick exposure	Prompt tick removal
	Doxycycline 200 mg PO × 1 if <72 hours in epidemic area
Erythema migrans	Doxycycline 100 mg PO BID × 10–21 days
	Alternatives:
	Amoxicillin 500 mg PO TID × 14–21 days
	or
	Cefuroxime axetil 500 mg PO BID × 14–21 days
Bell's palsy/CNS	Doxycycline 100 mg PO BID × 14–28 days
	or
	Amoxicillin 500 mg PO TID × 21–28 days
	or
	Ceftriaxone 2 g IV daily × 10–28 days
	or
	Cefotaxime 2 g IV every 8 hours × 10–28 days
	or
	PCN G 4 million units IV every 4 hours × 10–28 days
Cardiac first-degree block	Doxycycline 100 mg PO BID × 14–21 days
	or
	Amoxicillin 500 mg PO TID × 14–21 days
	or
	Cefuroxime axetil 500 mg PO BID × 14–21 days
Cardiac second- or third-degree block	Ceftriaxone 2 g IV daily × 21–28 days
	or
	Cefotaxime 2 g IV every 8 hours × 21–28 days
	or
	PCN G 4 million units IV every 4 hours × 21–28 days
	Doxycycline 100 mg PO BID × 28 days
	or
Arthritis	Amoxicillin 500 mg PO TID × 28 days
	or
	Cefuroxime axetil 500 mg PO BID × 28 days

IV – intravenous; PO – by mouth.

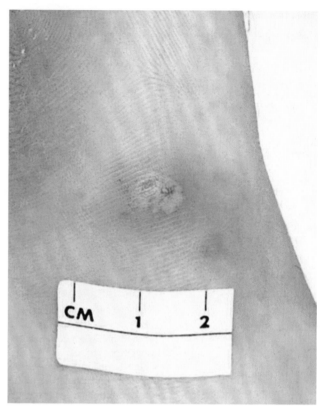

Figure 14.8 Erythema migrans associated with Lyme disease. Photograph courtesy of David C. Brancati, DO.

younger than age 5, immunocompromised individuals, and pregnant women are at highest risk for complications. Pneumonia is the most common cause of death in children with measles.

Supportive therapy, including rest, hydration, and antipyretics, is usually sufficient. Some patients may require intravenous hydration. Immune globulin may shorten the course if given within 6 days of exposure. Prevention of measles by immunization is the primary measure of disease control.

Rubella

Rubella, or German measles, caused by a single-stranded RNA togavirus, occurs commonly in the spring months. Rubella was responsible for major morbidity and mortality in the United States prior to widespread vaccination in the 1960s, but has now been declared eliminated in the United States. However, in some developing countries, rubella remains an important infection.

Rubella typically presents with fever, conjunctivitis, and lymphadenopathy, followed by a rash that appears 1 to 7 days after onset of symptoms (see Table 14.11). Tender suboccipital, posterior cervical, and postauricular adenopathy are common.

The rash typically persists for 2 to 3 days (hence the term "3-day measles"). Lesions appear as erythematous macules with confluence, often beginning in the head and neck and spreading to the trunk and extremities (see Figure 14.12). Forchheimer's sign, seen in 20% of rubella cases, is the eruption of petechiae over the soft palate. Pruritus is common with the rash, and mild desquamation often occurs.

Although the clinical diagnosis is sufficient in most cases, the rubella hemagglutination inhibiting antibody test may be performed at the time of appearance of the rash and repeated 2 weeks later for comparison.

Rarely, complications may include encephalitis, arthritis, thrombocytopenic purpura, and peripheral neuritis. Complications are more prevalent in adolescents and adults. Congenital rubella is a serious condition occurring in utero and is manifest by multiple congenital defects, including deafness, heart disease, and cataracts.

Management includes supportive care, hydration, and antipyretics. Immunization is important to prevent disease.

HIV Infection

Several common cutaneous manifestations of HIV infection and acquired immunodeficiency syndrome (AIDS) are likely to be seen in the acute care setting. Among the most important of these, and most challenging to diagnose, is acute HIV infection (acute retroviral syndrome). In a patient with known HIV infection, the occurrence of fever and rash may signify a systemic bacterial or viral infection, including rising HIV

Table 14.9 Disseminated Gonococcal Infection

Signs and symptoms	• Fever, mono- or polyarthralgias, tenosynovitis, endocarditis, and meningitis • Skin lesions may appear as tender erythematous or hemorrhagic papules that evolve into pustules and vesicles, with predilection for periarticular regions of distal extremities
Laboratory findings	Gram stains: urethral and accessory gland secretions (95% sensitive); female cervical secretions (50%) immunofluorescent staining of pustule contents, blood cultures
Treatment	Recommended: Ceftriaxone 1 g IM or IV every 24 hours Alternative regimens: Cefotaxime 1 g IV every 8 hours *or* Ceftizoxime 1 g IV every 8 hours

Fluoroquinolones (FQs) are no longer recommended due to high rates of developing resistance.

IM – intramuscular; IV – intravenous.

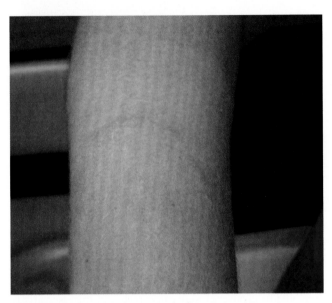

Figure 14.9 Disseminated gonococcal infection.
Photograph courtesy of Centers for Disease Control Public Health Image Library, Dr. S. E. Thompson, http://phil.cdc.gov/Phil/publicdomain.asp.

antigenemia, or autoimmune disorder, or drug reaction. In addition, pre-existing dermatologic conditions may be exacerbated by HIV infection. Common infections and dermatologic conditions may present in an atypical manner. Selected examples of conditions causing fever and rash in the HIV-infected patient are discussed in this section.

Acute HIV infection (acute retroviral syndrome) commonly occurs 2 to 6 weeks after primary exposure and is the clinical manifestation of HIV seroconversion. This syndrome is often undiagnosed or misdiagnosed because of non-specific symptoms. Symptoms may include fever, adenopathy, fatigue, pharyngitis, diarrhea, weight loss, and rash. Myopathy, peripheral neuropathy, or other neurologic or immunologic manifestations may also be seen. Symptoms may persist for 1 to 3 weeks.

Soft-tissue infections occur commonly in the HIV-infected population. These include abscesses, cellulitis, impetigo, ecthyma, folliculitis, and ulcerations. Methicillin-resistant

S. aureus colonization and infection are prevalent in the HIV-infected population and are often associated with low CD4+ cell counts, MSM, anal intercourse, previous MRSA infections, and illicit drug use. Treatment for skin and soft-tissue infections should be initiated with standard antibiotic therapy to treat MRSA and other bacterial infections. Inpatient admission should be considered for patients with fever and significant systemic disease.

Sexually transmitted diseases may occur with increased frequency in HIV-infected patients. In addition to testing for common STDs such as gonorrhea, chlamydia, and herpes infections, serologic testing for syphilis should be performed for all patients with possible sexually transmitted disease. The prevalence of syphilis in the United States has recently increased, and syphilis has been associated with increased susceptibility to HIV infection. Syphilis in the setting of HIV may have an aggressive and atypical course. Because a normal antibody response may be absent in HIV-infected individuals, specific attention must be paid to identify potential cases of syphilis, even with negative serologies. Treatment regimens for syphilis in the setting of HIV are covered in Table 14.6.

Varicella-zoster infection often presents atypically in HIV-infected patients. Eruptions involving several dermatomes are commonly seen in patients with AIDS. Although varicella seropositivity is common among adults (90%), reactivation causing clinical disease is more common in the HIV-infected population, who are seventeen times more likely than the general population to develop dermatomal zoster reactivation. Multidermatomal involvement occurs with increased frequency, and multiple recurrences are common. In the HIV-infected patient with routine dermatomal zoster infection, outpatient management should be initiated with oral famciclovir (5 mg, PO, BID or TID, for 7 days), acyclovir (800 mg, five times daily), or valacyclovir (1000 mg, BID, for 7 days). Admission is indicated if there is evidence of systemic involvement, ophthalmic zoster, or severe multidermatomal zoster. IV acyclovir may be administered at a dosage of 10 mg/kg every 8 hours. Varicella immune globulin may be administered to patients with primary infection and visceral involvement. Postherpetic neuralgia may be

Table 14.10 Measles

Organism	Morbillivirus, RNA virus of paramyxoviridae group
Signs and symptoms	• Fever, cough, coryza, conjunctivitis preceding the dermatologic findings • Skin lesions: erythematous macules and papules, often beginning on the scalp and head and spreading caudally to neck, trunk, and extremities • Koplik's spots are pathognomonic
Laboratory findings	• Laboratory conformation not typically necessary • If necessary, measles EIA IgM helpful for acute infection • IgG to screen immune status • Tissue/secretions may be cultured for virus and/or identified by IFA • Nasopharyngeal aspirate IFA offers rapid diagnosis
Treatment	• Supportive care; disease tends to be more severe in pediatric populations

EIA – enzyme immunoassay; IFA – immunofluorescent antibodies.

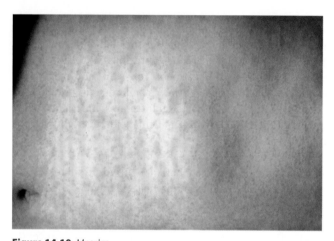

Figure 14.10 Measles.
Photograph courtesy of Centers for Disease Control Public Health Image Library, Dr. Heinz F. Eichenwald, http://phil.cdc.gov/Phil/publicdomain.asp.

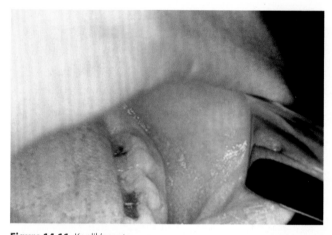

Figure 14.11 Koplik's spots.
Photograph source: Centers for Disease Control Public Health Image Library, http://phil.cdc.gov/Phil/publicdomain.asp.

treated with topical agents, such as capsaicin or lidocaine, or systemic agents, including gabapentin, pregabalin, tricyclic antidepressants, or opiates. The varicella-zoster virus (VZV) vaccine has demonstrated efficacy among geriatric patients in leading to reduced incidence of herpes zoster infections and reduction of incidence of postherpetic neuralgia. The safety and efficacy of its use among HIV-infected patients has not been established.

Adverse drug reactions are common among HIV-infected patients. Several factors account for this increased susceptibility: first, these patients are commonly treated with a variety of drugs known to produce adverse effects, such as antiretroviral agents; and, second, for unclear reasons, HIV-infected individuals may have more frequent or more severe reactions to commonly used medications. Dermatologic reactions are particularly prevalent, and fever may also be seen. Antimicrobial drugs are most commonly implicated. Potential drug interactions should always be considered when prescribing new medications. Common reactions include drug hypersensitivity, Stevens–Johnson syndrome, and toxic epidermal necrolysis. Among antiretroviral agents, the nucleoside reverse transcriptase inhibitors (e.g. NRTIs; zidovudine, lamivudine) cause hypersensitivity reactions in 5 to 10% of patients. The non-nucleoside reverse transcriptase inhibitors

(e.g. NNRTIs; efavirenz) may cause rash and hypersensitivity reactions in up to 17% of patients. Protease inhibitors (e.g. indinavir, saquinavir) cause skin reactions less commonly compared to the NRTIs and NNRTIs.

Systemic Lupus Erythematosus

Systemic lupus erythematosus (SLE) is a multisystem autoimmune disease. It is more common in females (10:1) and most common in the Native American and African American population.

A multitude of clinical signs and symptoms may be seen, including fever, fatigue, weight loss, malaise, arthritis, renal involvement, hemolytic anemia, pericarditis, thrombocytopenia, arthritis, pneumonitis, pleuritis, neurologic disorders, hepatomegaly, splenomegaly, and lymphadenopathy (see Table 14.12). Dermatologic findings are seen in 75% of patients and are typically erythematous macular lesions in light-exposed facial areas, or scattered papules on forearms and hands (see Figure 14.13). The characteristic "butterfly rash" presents with erythema and macular or papular edema over the malar eminences and nose. Patients may also present with alopecia, photosensitivity, discoid lesions, or vasculitis.

Table 14.11 Rubella

Organism	RNA togavirus, genus Rubivirus
Incubation period	12–23 days, and 20–50% of cases may be subclinical
Signs and symptoms	• Erythematous macules, confluence, caudal spread • Soft palate petechiae
Laboratory findings	• Laboratory conformation not typically necessary • Virus can be cultured from respiratory tract or CSF • False-positive IgM has occurred with parvovirus, EBV infections, or patients positive for rheumatoid factor • Positive hemagglutination inhibiting antibody test
Treatment	• Supportive care • Often mild illness, necessitates no therapy • Fever, arthritic complaints may be treated with acetaminophen or other NSAIDs

CSF – cerebrospinal fluid; EBV – Epstein–Barr virus; NSAID – non-steroidal anti-inflammatory drug.

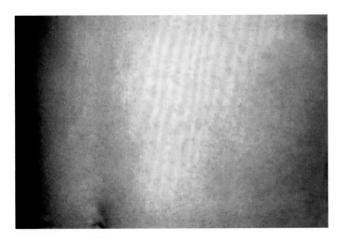

Figure 14.12 Rubella.

Photograph source: Centers for Disease Control Public Health Image Library, http://phil.cdc.gov/Phil/publicdomain.asp.

The diagnosis is made by skin biopsy, antinuclear antibody (ANA) titers, or lupus anticoagulant (which may lead to false positive serology for syphilis).

Management includes supportive therapy, topical steroids, sunblock, systemic steroids, or antimalarial agents and should be undertaken in consultation with a dermatologist or rheumatologist.

Severe Drug Reactions

Adverse drug reactions commonly cause dermatologic symptoms and signs. Patterns include a maculopapular or morbilliform rash difficult to distinguish from a viral exanthem, urticaria, target lesions, and photosensitivity. The most commonly implicated medications are beta-lactam antibiotics, sulfonamides, allopurinol, and antiepileptic medications, particularly carbamazepime, phenytoin, and lamotragine. Fever signifies a more severe type of reaction, as does mucosal involvement. Immunosuppressed patients are at high risk for adverse drug reactions, including HIV-infected patients, patients with SLE, and malignancy. Important, well-characterized forms of severe drug reaction include: Stevens–Johnson and toxic epidermal necrolysis syndrome, drug rash with eosinophilia and systemic symptoms (DRESS), and acute generalized exanthematous pustulosis (AGEP).

Stevens–Johnson Syndrome and Toxic Epidermal Necrolysis

Stevens–Johnson Syndrome (SJS) and toxic epidermal necrolysis (TEN) are acute life-threatening mucocutaneous eruptions caused primarily by drugs, such as phenytoin, sulfa, penicillins, NSAIDs, and transfusions. Other etiologies may include infection and malignancy. Females are affected more than males, and patients with HIV are at high risk.

In SJS, full thickness epidermal detachment involves less than 10% of body surface area (BSA) and in TEN involves 30% or more of BSA. This can lead to a very high mortality rate of up to 40%.

These syndromes usually begin with a prodrome that includes high fever, malaise, and myalgias (see Table 14.13). Dermatologic findings include erythema, warmth, bullae, and extensive full thickness desquamation, and a positive Nikolsky's sign. Mucous membranes are almost always involved and this is considered an important early and characteristic finding.

The diagnosis is based on history and physical examination and may be confirmed by skin biopsy.

Treatment includes supportive care, preferably in a burn unit, removal of the offending agent, and the use of steroids (controversial). Serum plasmapheresis may also be considered.

Dermatologic Conditions Associated with Systemic Infection

Erythema Nodosum

Erythema nodosum is a type of hypersensitivity vasculitis commonly associated with underlying infection, including streptococcal infections, coccidiomycosis, and tuberculosis. Erythema nodosum is also associated with inflammatory bowel disease, drugs (e.g. sulfa, penicillins, oral contraceptives), and sarcoidosis, and is idiopathic in 20 to 50% of cases. It is more common in women, in the third and fourth decades of life.

Lesions are painful, erythematous, or violaceous firm nodules that result from subcutaneous panniculitis (see Table 14.14). Lesions typically are found on extensor surfaces

Table 14.12 Clinical Features: Systemic Lupus Erythematosus

Signs and symptoms	• Fever, fatigue, weight loss, malaise, arthritis, renal involvement, hemolytic anemia, pericarditis, thrombocytopenia, arthritis, pneumonitis, pleuritis, neurologic disorders, hepatomegaly, splenomegaly, and lymphadenopathy • Dermatologic findings are seen in 75% of patients and are typically erythematous macular lesions in light-exposed facial areas, or scattered papules on forearms and hands • Patients may also present with alopecia, photosensitivity, discoid lesions, or vasculitis
Laboratory findings	Skin biopsy, ANA titers, or lupus anticoagulant (which may lead to false positive serology for syphilis)
Treatment	Supportive therapy, topical steroids, sunblock, systemic steroids, or antimalarial agents

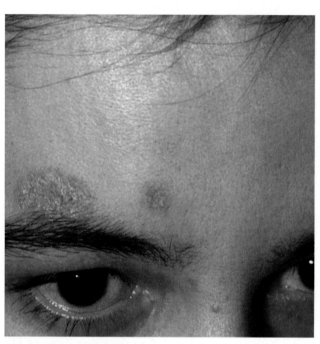

Figure 14.13 Systemic lupus erythematosus.
Photograph source: www.derm101.com, with permission.

of extremities such as the pretibial areas and forearms (see Figure 14.14).

Most cases are self limited, requiring treatment of the underlying disease and symptomatic relief with NSAIDs, bed rest, leg elevation, and treatment with potassium iodide. Corticosteroids can be considered, but are not typically required.

Erythema Multiforme

Erythema multiforme (EM) is a systemic hypersensitivity reaction associated with a variety of infectious and non-infectious diseases. It is characterized by so-called target skin lesions; when there is mucosal involvement, it is referred to as EM major. By far the most common associated underlying infection is herpes simplex virus (see Figure 14.15). Others include *Mycoplasma pneumonia* and other viruses. Leading associated medications are NSAIDs and sulfa antibiotics.

Systemic symptoms may include fever, arthralgias, headache, diffuse burning, and diffuse pruritus (see Table 14.15). Skin lesions are classically described as "target lesions" and may be macular, papular, or bullous with a central area that is typically dusky in appearance, but may be hemorrhagic, or necrotic (see Figures 14.15 and 14.16). Oral mucosa lesions include focal erythema, erosions, or bullae.

Diagnosis is usually made by history and physical examination, but may be confirmed by skin biopsy.

Management of EM includes discontinuing the causal drug, if present, and treating the underlying condition. Empiric treatment with antiviral agents, such as acyclovir and valacyclovir, has demonstrated benefits in small studies, but their efficacy has not yet been definitively established. Systemic steroids may have some benefit. If more than 10% of the body surface area (BSA) is involved, admission for aggressive skin care and hydration management may be beneficial.

Laboratory Diagnosis

Many laboratory tests are discussed above with specific diagnoses. In general, patients with fever and rash should be evaluated with complete physical examination. In selected cases, complete blood count, platelet count, serologic tests, skin biopsy, or cultures of blood or skin lesions are indicated. Any patient with fever and rash who appears acutely ill or has unstable vital signs should immediately have blood cultures, a complete blood count (to assess platelet count) and coagulation studies drawn.

Complications and Admission Criteria

Many patients with fever and rash can be safely discharged home, following appropriate physical and laboratory evaluation, if the patient is clinically stable, with normal vital signs, if the diagnosis is considered relatively benign and no specific inpatient therapy is indicated, and if there is adequate home care and follow-up arrangements have been made.

Certain patients should often be managed as inpatients, including patients with immunosuppression, systemic bacterial infections, sepsis, or unstable vital signs, or those lacking appropriate home resources or medical follow-up.

Infection Control

Patients with fever and rash often do not have a definitive diagnosis made while in the acute care setting. Thus, patients presenting with fever and rash should be considered contagious. Standard precautions should be used when treating patients with fever and rash.

Table 14.13 Stevens–Johnson Syndrome and Toxic Epidermal Necrolysis

Signs and symptoms	Fever, malaise, and myalgias Skin erythema, warmth, bullae, and extensive desquamation Mucous membranes involvement involved; Nikolsky's sign
Laboratory findings	Clinical diagnosis, but may be confirmed by skin biopsy
Treatment	Supportive treatment Management includes discontinuing the causal drug and treating underlying disease Treatment in burn unit is recommended

Table 14.14 Erythema Nodosum

Signs and symptoms	Painful, erythematous or violaceous firm nodules Lesions typically are found on the pretibial areas and forearms
Treatment	Management includes treatment of the underlying disease, NSAIDs, systemic steroids, bed rest, leg elevation, and treatment with potassium iodide, 300–500 mg PO TID

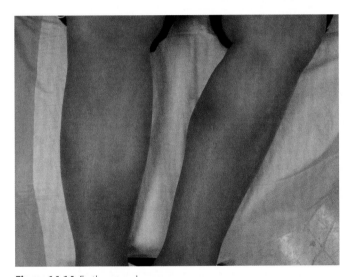

Figure 14.14 Erythema nodosum.
Photograph courtesy of Dr. Bradley W. Frazee, MD.

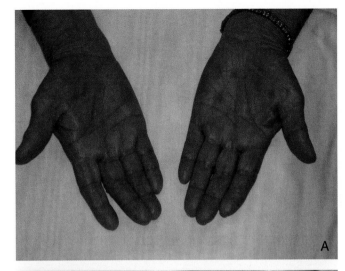
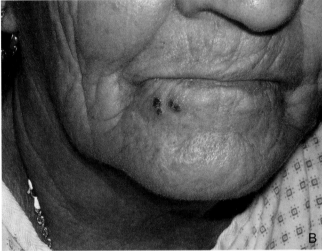

Figure 14.15 Erythema multiforme of the hands with subtle target-like appearance and dusky center (A); associated with simultaneous active herpes simplex labialis (B).

Photograph courtesy of Dr. Bradley W. Frazee, MD.

Appropriate management of sexually transmitted diseases includes treatment of the primary patient, as well as notification of and treatment of sexual contacts. Barrier contraceptive methods are important in reducing the spread of sexually transmitted diseases. Disease reporting is an important component of public health. Gonorrhea and syphilis are reportable diseases in all American states. Chlamydia is a reportable disease in most states.

Close contacts of possible cases of meningococcal disease (including household contacts, child-care contacts, and health-care providers) should undergo prophylactic treatment with rifampin (600 mg PO BID for four doses), ceftriaxone (250 mg IM), or ciprofloxacin (500 mg PO).

Pearls and Pitfalls

1. Evaluation of rash and fever should always begin with consideration of life-threatening infection.
2. Presence of high fever, unstable vital signs, and purpura generally mandates immediate blood cultures and empiric antibiotic treatment.
3. Consider syphilis in any sexually active person with a generalized rash or painless genital ulcer.
4. In suspected toxic shock syndrome, immediately search for and remove or drain any possible toxin source.
5. A drug reaction accompanied by fever or oral mucosal involvement generally requires admission for supportive care, as well as withdrawal of the culprit drug.

References

American College of Physicians. Guidelines for laboratory evaluation in the diagnosis of Lyme disease. *Ann. Intern. Med.* 1997; 127(12): 1106.

Table 14.15 Erythema Multiforme

Signs and symptoms	Skin target lesions, oral mucosal lesions Fever, arthralgias, headache, diffuse burning, and diffuse pruritus Signs of oral or genital HSV recurrence
Laboratory findings	Laboratory conformation not typically necessary May be confirmed by skin biopsy
Treatment	Supportive treatment Management includes discontinuing the causal drug and treating underlying disease or infection For recurrent EM, consider HSV prophylaxis

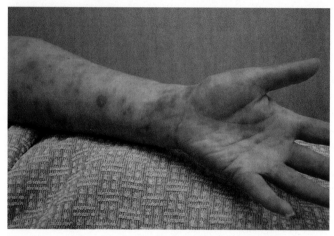

Figure 14.16 Erythema multiforme. Note target-like appearance. Photograph courtesy of Dr. Bradley W. Frazee, MD.

Banatvala, J. E. and Brown, D. W. Rubella. *Lancet* 2004; 363(9415): 1127–37.

Brady, W. J., DeBehnke, D., and Crosby, D. L. Dermatological emergencies. *Am. J. Emerg. Med.* 1994; 12(2): 217–37.

Centers for Disease Control and Prevention (CDC). Reported cases of Lyme disease by year, United States, 1995–2014. Atlanta, GA: US Department of Health and Human Services, CDC, www.cdc.gov/lyme/stats/graphs.html (accessed August 19, 2016).

CDC. Prevention and control of meningococcal disease. *MMWR Morb. Mortal. Wkly. Rep.* 2013; 62(2): 1–28, available at www.cdc.gov/mmwr/PDF/rr/rr6202.pdf (accessed August 19, 2016).

CDC. Sexually transmitted diseases treatment guidelines 2015. *MMWR Morb. Mortal. Wkly. Rep.* 2015; 64 (RR-3): 1–137, available at www.cdc.gov/std/tg2015/ (accessed August 19, 2016).

CDC. Meningococcal disease: technical and clinical information, www.cdc.gov/meningococcal/clinical-info.html (accessed August 19, 2016).

CDC. Tickborne diseases of the United States: a reference manual for health care providers, 3rd edn. (2015), available at www.cdc.gov/lyme/resources/TickborneDiseases.pdf (accessed August 19, 2016).

Cenizal, M. J., Hardy, R. D., Anderson, M., *et al.* Prevalence of and risk factors for methicillin-resistant staphylococcus aureus (MRSA) nasal colonization in HIV-infected ambulatory patients. *J. Acquir. Immune Defic. Syndr.* 2008; 48(5): 567–71.

Clemmons, N. S., Gastañaduy, P. A., Fiebelkorn, A. P., *et al.* Measles – United States, January 4–April 2, 2015. *MMWR Morb. Mortal. Wkly. Rep.* 2015; 64(14): 373–6.

Cunha, B. A. Rocky Mountain spotted fever revisited. *Arch. Intern. Med.* 2004; 164: 221–3.

Dourmishev, L. A. and Dourmishev, A. L. Syphilis: uncommon presentations in adults. *Clin. Dermatol.* 2005; 23(6): 555–64.

Duke, T. and Mgone, C. S. Measles: not just another viral exanthem. *Lancet* 2003; 36(9359): 763–73.

Fleischer, A. B., Feldman, S. R., McConnell, C. F., *et al. Emergency Dermatology: A Rapid Treatment Guide* (New York: McGraw-Hill, 2002).

Gardner, P. Clinical practice: prevention of meningococcal disease. *N. Engl. J. Med.* 2006; 355(14): 1466–73.

Gastañaduy, P. A., Redd, S. B., Fiebelkorn, A. P., *et al.* Measles – United States, January 1–May 23, 2014. *MMWR Morb. Mortal. Wkly. Rep.* 2014; 63(22): 496–9.

Habif, T. P. Hypersensitivity syndromes and vasculitis in T. P. Habif, *Clinical Dermatology: A Color Guide to Diagnosis and Therapy*, 6th edn (St. Louis, MO: Elsevier, 2016), pp. 717–22.

Hajjeh, R. A., Reingold, A., Weil, A., *et al.* Toxic shock syndrome in the United States: surveillance update, 1979–1996. *Emerg. Infect. Dis. J.* 1999; 5(6): 807–10.

Hazelzet, J. A. Diagnosing meningococcemia as a cause of sepsis. *Pediatr. Crit. Care Med.* 2005; 6(3 Suppl.): S50–4.

Hernandez-Salazar, A., Rosales, S. P., Rangel-Frausto, S., *et al.* Epidemiology of adverse cutaneous drug reactions. A prospective study in hospitalized patients. *Arch. Med. Res.* 2006; 37(7): 899–902.

Horio, T., Imamura, S., Danno, K., *et al.* PotassiumIodide in the treatment of EN and Nodular Vasculitis. *Arch. Derm.* 1981; 117(1): 29–31.

Johnson, R. W. and Rice, A. S. D. Postherpetic neuralgia. *N. Engl. J. Med.* 2014; 371(16): 1526–33.

Lamoreux, M. R., Sternbach, M. R., and Hsu, W. T. Erythema multiforme. *Am. Fam. Physician* 2006; 74(11): 1883–8.

Masters, E. J., Olson, G. S., Weiner, S. J., *et al.* Rocky Mountain spotted fever: a clinician's dilemma. *Arch. Intern. Med.* 2003; 163(7): 769–74.

McCann, D. J., Nadel, E. S., and Brown, D. F. Rash and fever. *J. Emerg. Med.* 2006; 31(3): 293–7.

Oster, A. M., Sternberg, M., Nebenzahl, S., *et al.* Prevalence of HIV, sexually transmitted infections, and viral hepatitis by urbanicity, among men who have sex with men, injection drug users, and heterosexuals in the United States. *Sex. Transm. Dis.* 2014; 41(4): 272–9.

Patton, M. E., Su, J. R., Nelson, R., and Weinstock, H. Primary and secondary syphilis – United States, 2005–2013. *MMWR Morb. Mortal. Wkly. Rep.* 2015; 63(18): 402–6.

Pitambe, H. V. and Schulz, E. J. Life-threatening dermatoses due to metabolic and endocrine disorders. *Clin. Dermatol.* 2005; 23(3): 258–66.

Quagliarello, V. and Scheld, M. Treatment of bacterial meningitis. *N. Engl. J. Med.* 1997; 336(10): 708.

Reidner, G., Rusizoka, M., Todd, J., *et al.* Single-dose azithromycin versus penicillin G benzathine for the treatment of early syphilis. *N. Engl. J. Med.* 2005; 353(12): 1236–44.

Robson, K. J. and Piette, W. W. Cutaneous manifestations of systemic disease. *Med. Clin. North Am.* 1998; 82(6): 1359–79.

Rodgers, S. and Leslie, K. S. Skin infections in HIV-infected individuals in the era of HAART. *Curr. Opin. Infect. Dis.* 2011; 24(2): 124–9.

Rosenstein, N. E., Perkins, B. A., Stephens, D. S., *et al.* Meningococcal disease. *N. Engl. J. Med.* 2001; 344(18): 1378–88.

Singh-Behl, D., La Rosa, S. P, and Tomecki, K. J. Tick-borne infections. *Dermatol. Clin.* 2003; 21(2): 237–44.

Socor, M., Pandit, A., and Brady, W. J. Generalized skin disorders in J. E. Tintinalli, J. S. Stapdzynski, A. J. Ma, *et al.* (eds.), *Tintinalli's Emergency Medicine: A Comprehensive Study Guide*, 8th edn (New York: McGraw-Hill Medical Publishing Division, 2016).

Steere, A. Lyme disease. *N. Engl. J. Med.* 2001; 345(2): 115–25.

Young, N. and Brown, K. Mechanisms of disease: parvovirus B19. *N. Engl. J. Med.* 2004; 350(6): 586–97.

Chapter

15

Otitis Externa

Jeffrey Bullard-Berent

Introduction and Microbiology

Acute otitis externa (AOE) or "swimmer's ear" is a cellulitis of the external auditory canal with acute inflammation and edema. In North America, bacteria cause 98% of AOE. *Pseudomonas aeruginosa* (20 to 60%) and *Staphylococcus aureus* (10 to 70%) are by far the most common pathogens. Other gram-negative organisms account for the remainder of the bacterial infections, many of which are polymicrobial. Fungi are an infrequent cause, usually seen in chronic otitis externa or after prolonged antibiotic treatment of AOE. *Aspergillus* species and *Candida albicans* account for the majority of these fungal infections. Less commonly, varicella, herpes, or measles virus may cause AOE. If vesicular eruptions are present, a thorough physical exam is needed to evaluate for the herpes zoster virus-associated Ramsay Hunt syndrome.

Epidemiology

AOE occurs in both children and adults, affecting 1 in 123 people in the United States. Nearly half of all cases of AOE are found in children 5 to 14 years of age. AOE is most common in tropical climates, where heat, humidity, and increased swimming all contribute to an altered ear canal environment, which increases the risk of infection. Persistent water exposure, aggressive cleaning, and over zealous manipulation with cotton tipped applicators or other mechanical devices may remove too much cerumen which protects the ear canal by maintaining a slightly acidic pH. Patients with a history of eczema, atopic dermatitis, and seborrhea may be at higher risk for AOE as they are predisposed to disruption of the auditory canal epidermis.

A history of trauma, laceration, or a recent intra-aural foreign body may be an inciting event. Cotton tipped applicators, pins, paper clips, legs of eyeglasses, and other objects are frequently used in attempt to relieve the discomfort of water in the ear canal or the subsequent inflammation. A vicious cycle of inflammation, itching, and scratching can ensue. A careful history must be elicited in recurrent cases, as patients may stop using cotton tipped applicators as instructed only to be found using other objects to help alleviate their itch.

Clinical Features

AOE presents with pruritis of the ear canal, otalgia, fullness, and hearing loss. Palpation of the tragus and pinna often causes pain disproportionate to what the clinician anticipates from visual inspection. Edema and a foul-smelling whitish discharge from the external auditory canal may be present and make the examination of the proximal canal and tympanic membrane difficult (see Table 15.1).

Vesicles within the external auditory canal or pinna suggest herpes zoster oticus, commonly termed Ramsey Hunt syndrome. In this form of zoster, the crania nerve (CN) VII dermatome is affected, causing the typical rash and pain, as well as unilateral facial paresis, loss of taste to the anterior two-thirds of the tongue, and decreased lacrimation. Any eye involvement should prompt ophthalmologic consultation. Auditory nerve (CN VIII) involvement may result in sensorineural hearing loss and/or vertigo.

Malignant otitis externa (MOE) is a severe form of AOE found primarily but not exclusively in elderly and diabetic patients. It is usually caused by *P. aeruginosa*. Fungal MOE has been reported in patients with AIDS. The hallmark of this infection is underlying osteomyelitis in addition to the classic AOE findings. These patients require admission, intravenous antibiotics, otolaryngology consultation, and may require surgical debridement.

Differential Diagnosis

The differential diagnosis of AOE includes all causes of otalgia and otorrhea. AOE often causes erythema of the canal and may cause erythema of the tympanic membrane. It may be difficult to distinguish AOE from acute otitis media (AOM)

Table 15.1 Clinical Features: Otitis Externa

Organisms	*Pseudomonas aeruginosa* *Staphylococcus aureus* Gram-negative species *Aspergillus* sp. *Candida albicans* Herpes virus Varicella Measles
Signs and symptoms	• Otalgia (ear pain) • Pruritis (ear itching) • Otorrhea (ear drainage), usually foul smelling • Aural fullness • Conductive hearing loss • Vesicles may suggest a herpetic etiology • Hyphae may suggest a fungal etiology
Laboratory and radiographic findings	• Usually not indicated • Refractory AOE may require culture-directed therapy • Imaging may be indicated if progression to malignant OE is suspected
Treatment	• Aural hygiene • Dry ear precautions • Otic antibiotic drops: Acetic acid 2.0% solution Ciprofloxacin 0.2%, hydrocortisone 1.0% suspension Ciprofloxacin 0.3%, dexamethasone 0.1% suspension Neomycin, polymyxin B, hydrocortisone suspension Ofloxacin 0.3% solution Tip: Equivalent concentration ophthalmic drops may be substituted for otic preparations (e.g. ofloxacin); however, never vice versa. See also Box 15.1, Instructions for Patients

and pneumatic otoscopy is recommended to distinguish the red but mobile tympanic membrane of AOE from the red but immobile tympanic membrane of AOM. Even with pneumatic otoscopy the canal may be so inflamed that the patient does not tolerate insertion of the speculum enough to obtain a seal. Cholesteotomas may also be mistaken for AOE and when suspected require otolaryngologist evaluation.

Dermatoses of the ear canal can also mimic AOE. Eczema, atopic dermatitis, and seborrheic dermatitis may all cause white scaly debris in the ear canal, inflammation, and pain. Contact dermatitis (most commonly nickel) and allergic dermatitis (otic drops) can also be confused for AOM. Neomycin, a component of some otic drops, is associated with an allergic reaction in up to 10% of patients.

Otalgia without findings of ear erythema, edema, and discharge suggest that the pain is coming from elsewhere. Temporomandibular joint syndrome, dental caries, infections or fractures, pharyngitis, tonsillitis, peritonsillar abscess, retropharyngeal abscess, carotidynia, styloid process elongation, angina, intrathoracic aneurysms, glossopharyngeal neuralgia, and geniculate neuralgia may all cause otalgia.

Laboratory and Radiographic Findings

Diagnosis is made on clinical examination. Rarely, a diagnostic culture is needed to direct therapy in refractory cases. If Ramsey Hunt is suspected, a Tzank smear or other viral testing may be indicated. Imaging studies are indicated for patients with suspected malignant otitis externa, such as elderly, immunosuppressed, or diabetic patients with severe AOE. CT scan and MRI are considered the initial imaging studies of choice to reveal the subtle osteomyelitis involving the base of the skull that is the hallmark of malignant otitis externa.

Treatment and Prophylaxis

The mainstays of treatment are aural hygiene, topical drops, and pain control. Aural hygiene is performed with gentle cleaning under direct visualization. If the edema of the external auditory canal is so severe that the space is obliterated, a small wick or sponge can be placed in the canal to deliver medicated drops effectively.

A variety of topical ear drops are effective in the treatment of AOE. Antibiotic drops with or without steroids and disinfectant (acetic acid) have similar outcomes in the treatment of AOE. Aminoglycosides, quinolones, and polymixin B antibiotics have efficacy in treating AOE. Drops with potential ototoxicity should be avoided if tympanic membrane perforation is suspected. Aminoglycoside and neomycin-containing drops are implicated in ototoxicity. Quinolone drops are the only FDA-approved antibiotic drops for middle ear use, and are thus recommended if TM perforation is noted. Low pH antiseptic drops (acetic acid) demonstrate similar efficacy in AOE, and are an alternative to antibiotic drops. Duration of treatment with all topical medication is 7 days.

Systemic antibiotics should not be started routinely in AOE. Systemic antibiotics do not improve symptoms and may potentially select for resistant bacteria. Additionally, topical antibiotics allow a much higher concentration of medication at the directed site than the oral alternatives. Systemic antibiotics are reserved for AOE patients with extension of infection beyond the ear or those who are immunosuppressed.

The American Academy of Otolaryngology and Head and Neck Surgery Guidelines stresses the importance of informing the patient on methods to enhance eardrop delivery (see Box 15.1). These include asking for assistance in placing the drops, filling the ear canal with drops, and placing the drops with the affected ear up and maintaining that position for 3 to 5 minutes. In addition, patients should avoid self-instrumentation, refrain from water sports for 7 days, and attempt to keep the ear canal dry during showering by using earplugs or petroleum-jelly-coated cotton.

Pain is often a significant problem in AOE treatment and should be addressed at the first visit. Acetaminophen or NSAIDs are efficacious, but some patients may require a brief course of opioids. Patients who require cleaning, suctioning, or wick placement may require analgesia prior to the procedure, and occasionally patients may require procedural sedation.

Box 15.1 Instructions for Patients

1. If possible, get someone to put the drops in the ear canal for you.

2. Lie down with the affected ear up. Put enough drops in the ear canal to fill it up.

3. Once the drops are in place, stay in this position for 3 to 5 minutes. Use a timer to help measure the time.

4. It is important to allow adequate time for the drops to penetrate into the ear canal.

5. A gentle to-and-fro movement of the ear will sometimes help in getting the drops to their intended destination. An alternate method is to press with an in/out movement on the small piece of cartilage (tragus) in front of the ear.

6. You may then get up and resume your normal activities. Wipe off any excess drops. Keeping the ear dry is generally a good idea while using ear drops.

7. Try not to clean the ear yourself as the ear is very tender and you could possibly damage the ear canal or even the eardrum.

8. If the drops do not easily run into the ear canal, you may need to have the ear canal cleaned by your clinician or have a wick placed in the ear canal to help in getting the drops into the ear canal.

9. If you do have a wick placed, it may fall out on its own. This is a good sign as it means the inflammation is clearing and the infection subsiding. Do not remove the wick yourself unless instructed to do so.

American Academy of Otolaryngolgy and Head and Neck Surgery

Topical pain medications may be used, but require close follow-up, as progressing symptoms may be masked.

Complications and Admission Criteria

AOE typically responds well to treatment, but may cause additional complications. Direct spread of the cellulitis of AOE to the ear canal may cause AOM with perforation (just as the drainage from perforated suppurative otitis media may lead to AOE). Progression of the infection may rarely lead to cellulitis outside of the ear as well as chondritis. Auricular deformity from cartlilage necrosis may result from chondritis, and the treatment requires long-term antibiotics.

Patients with recurrent and chronic OE infections may develop granulation tissue in the external auditory canal, fibrosis, or stenosis. Stenosis of the ear canal may lead to a conductive hearing loss and require surgical intervention.

Careful evaluation is required in the poorly controlled diabetic or immunocompromised patient because there is a risk of progression to malignant otitis externa. Clinical findings include granulation tissue at the floor of the ear canal, paresis or paralysis of cranial nerves, and central neurologic findings. Treatment includes hospital admission, intravenous antibiotics, and imaging such as CT or MRI to evaluate for skull base involvement.

Pearls and Pitfalls

1. Aural hygiene and topical medication is the mainstay of AOE treatment.

2. AOE may be treated with topical antibiotics, antibiotics + corticosteroids, or antiseptic drops. Wick placement may be required for adequate delivery of topical medication.

3. Systemic antibiotics are rarely indicated in AOE.

4. Treat the pain of AOE.

5. Good patient instructions are essential to ensure correct administration of topical drops.

6. If the tympanic membrane is perforated, avoid ototoxic drops.

7. Consider malignant otitis externa in patients who are elderly, diabetic, immunosuppressed, or fail to respond to standard treatment.

References

de Ru, J. A. and van Benthem, P. P. Combination therapy is preferable for patients with Ramsay Hunt syndrome. *Otol. Neurotol.* 2011; 32(5): 852–5.

Kaushik, V., Malik, T., and Saeed, S. R. Interventions for acute otitis externa. *Cochrane Database Syst. Rev.* 2010: CD004740.

Mahdyoun, P., Pulcini, C., Gahide, I., *et al.* Necrotizing otitis externa: a systematic review. *Otol. Neurotol.* 2013; 34(4): 620–9.

Roland, P. S., Belcher, B. P., Bettis, R., *et al.* A single topical agent is clinically equivalent to the combination of topical and oral antibiotic treatment for otitis externa. *Am. J. Otolaryngol.* 2008; 29(4): 255–61.

Rosenfeld, R. M., Schwartz, S. R., Cannon, C. R., *et al.* Clinical practice guideline: acute otitis externa. *Otolaryngol. Head Neck Surg.* 2014; 150(1 Suppl.): S1–24.

Rubin Grandis, J., Branstetter, B. F., 4th, and Yu, V. L. The changing face of malignant (necrotising) external otitis: clinical, radiological, and anatomic correlations. *Lancet Infect. Dis.* 2004; 4(1): 34–9.

Wipperman, J. Otitis externa. *Prim. Care* 2014; 41(1): 1–9.

Otitis Media

Jeffrey Bullard-Berent

Introduction and Microbiology

Historically acute otitis media (AOM) was considered a bacterial infection, but as the reliability of testing for viruses has improved, it is now recognized that AOM pathogens include bacteria, viruses, and mixed infections. Often a predisposing viral upper respiratory infection causes Eustachian tube inflammation and dysfunction, allowing viruses and bacteria normally residing in the nasopharynx to invade the middle ear, causing AOM. The majority of AOM remains bacterial followed by mixed bacterial and viral, and then viral- only infections. Respiratory syncytial virus (RSV), influenza, rhinovirus, and parainfluenza are the most common viral pathogens, whereas *Streptococcus pneumonia*, *Haemophilus influenza*, *Moraxella catarrhalis*, and *Streptococus pyogenes* are the predominant bacterial causes.

Epidemiology

Otitis media remains the most common bacterial infection and the most common reason for antibiotic prescriptions in children. By 36 months, 83% of children have had at least one epidsode of AOM. The peak incidence is between 6 and 15 months. Children with mid-face defects, such as Trisomy 21 or cleft palate, are at higher risk of persistent and recurrent AOM. AOM does occur in adults, but is much less common than in children. Adults predisposed to AOM include those with HIV, other causes of immunosuppression, and recipients of head or neck radiation. Otherwise healthy adults with persistent or recurrent unilateral AOM warrant additional workup for underlying malignancy.

Clinical Features

Acute otitis media is most common in children under 2 years of age, making many symptoms subtle in these mostly nonverbal patients. Generalized irritability, crying, poor feeding, and fever are often seen in AOM, but these are the presenting symptoms of many other pediatric illnesses. Otalgia may manifest in the young child with ear tugging or rubbing. In adults, the symptoms of AOM are rarely subtle, with patients complaining of unilateral otalgia, which is frequently acute in onset, decreased hearing, and occasionally ear drainage.

Current guidelines from the United States, Japan, and multiple European countries emphasize pneumatic otoscopy as crucial to the diagnosis. The tympanic membrane should be evaluated for color (red, yellow, amber, white), contour (bulging, retracted, normal), translucency (translucent, opaque), and mobility (normal, decreased, absent). Obtaining an adequate exam is essential and challenging in an ill child, and requires the proper equipment and positioning. Middle ear effusion (MEE) must be present to make the diagnosis of AOM. Both pneumatic otoscopy and tympanometry may be used to demonstrate MEE. Bulging, movement-impaired, erythematous tympanic membranes suggest AOM (see Table 16.1). Pain must be assessed and treated.

Differential Diagnosis

As fever, irritability, and poor feeding are seen in many pediatric infections, a scrupulous exam is required to narrow the differential diagnosis. Upper respiratory infection, urinary tract infection, herpangina, herpetic stomatitis, cervical adenitis, and a multitude of other childhood illnesses may present with these symptoms, but usually these can be differentiated from AOM with a careful exam.

Acute OM must be distinguished from otitis media with effusion (OME) formerly termed serous otitis media. The definition of AOM is an acute illness with at least one bulging, immobile, erythematous, or purulent-appearing tympanic membrane, with or without otorrhea not caused by otitis externa, observed in the setting of irritability, fever, and otalgia. Otitis media with effusion presents as a non-acute, often incidental finding or upon re-evaluation of an acute episode. It

Table 16.1 American Academy of Pediatrics Diagnostic Criteria for AOM

1	Clinicians should diagnose AOM in children who present with moderate to severe bulging of the TM or new onset of otorrhea not due to acute otitis externa.
2	Clinicians should diagnose AOM in children who present with mild bulging of the TM and recent (less than 48 hours) onset of ear pain (holding, tugging, rubbing of the ear in a non-verbal child), or intense erythema of the TM.
3	Clinicians should not diagnose AOM in children who do not have MEE (based on pneumatic otoscopy and/or tympanometry).

Table 16.2 AAP/AAFP 2013 Guidelines for AOM Treatment

Age	Otorrhea with AOM	Unilateral or Bilateral AOM with Severe Symptoms	Bilateral AOM without Otorrhea	Unilateral AOM without Otorrhea
6 months–2 years	Antibiotic therapy	Antibiotic therapy	Antibiotic therapy	Antibiotic therapy or additional observation
≥2 years	Antibiotic therapy	Antibiotic therapy	Antibiotic therapy or additional observation	Antibiotic therapy or additional observation

may predispose to or persist after AOM, and can be considered in the continuum of AOM.

Multiple prior infections may cause myringosclerosis of the tympanic membrane making it appear dull on visualization; however, pneumotoscopy should reveal a mobile, albeit stiff, tympanic membrane. Cholesteatoma, abnormal deposition of squamous epithelium in the middle ear, may also present as a dull immobile tympanic membrane with foul discharge.

Laboratory and Radiographic Findings

The diagnosis of AOM is made on clinical exam alone. Middle ear culture may be obtained via tympanocentesis or myringotomy, but is not indicated in routine cases. Recurrent or refractory AOM may, however, benefit from tympanocentesis so that therapy can be tailored to the susceptibility of the causative organism. Culture of the fluid obtained from the ear canal after perforation from AOM is often contaminated with skin flora and rarely helpful in selecting treatment. Complete blood count is not recommended unless the patient is very young and febrile (less than 2 months) or appears toxic. CT and MRI will both demonstrate MEE, but are not recommended for the routine diagnosis of AOM.

Treatment and Prophylaxis

Until recently, antibiotic choice was considered the most critical decision in the treatment of AOM. However, with the recognition that AOM is most often a self-limited illness, the question of whether to treat should in most cases replace the question of which antibiotic to choose. Current AOM treatment guidelines in the United States, the United Kingdom, Sweden, Scotland, Israel, and Holland all emphasize the option of watchful waiting, in select patient populations, prior to starting antibiotics. The AAP/AAFP guidelines recommend addressing pain first. Acetaminophen and ibuprofen in adequate doses work well for mild to moderate pain. Opioid medications are rarely required. Opioids can provide additional relief for moderate to severe pain, but with the risk of respiratory

depression, altered mental status, GI upset, and constipation. Topical anesthetics such as lidocaine and benzocaine may offer short-lived pain relief; however, combination benzocaine, antipyrine, and glycerine has been removed from the market in the United States. Home remedies (warm oil to the ear canal, hot or cold to the ear, distraction) and naturopathic remedies have no controlled studies to demonstrate benefit. Decongestants and other over-the-counter cold and cough medicines are not recommended in children.

For those patients with AOM being treated with antibiotics (see Table 16.2), amoxicillin remains the antibiotic of choice. Alternatively, amoxicillin-clavulanate may be started as initial treatment or in situations where amoxicillin was used in the previous 30 days. Recommendations for penicillin-allergic patients (non-type I hypersensitivity reactions) include cefdinir, cefuroxime, cefpodoxime, or ceftriaxone. The structure of these second- and third-generation cephlosporins is unlikely to cause cross reactivity. In patients who do not improve within 48 to 72 hours on amoxicillin, amoxicillin-clavulanate, ceftriaxone, or clindamycin are recommended (see Table 16.3).

Complications and Admission Criteria

The most common complication of AOM is a perforated tympanic membrane that will typically heal on its own. Following perforation, it is important for the patient to keep the ear dry until it has healed. Large perforations that do not close on their own may require subsequent tympanoplasty, a microsurgical closure of the eardrum perforation using graft material.

Acute mastoiditis is the most common serious complication of AOM with clinical findings, including posterior auricular and mastoid erythema, edema and tenderness, proptosis of the auricle, and fever. The diagnosis can often be made clinically; imaging of the mastoid bone with CT is reserved for severe cases or when the diagnosis is unclear. In addition to intravenous antimicrobial therapy, consultation, for the question of myringotomy or other drainage procedure, is recommended.

Table 16.3 Recommended Antibiotics for (Initial or Delayed) Treatment and for Patients Who Have Failed Initial Antibiotic Treatment (AAP/AAFP 2013)

Initial Immediate or Delayed Antibiotic Therapy		Antibiotic Treatment after 48–72 hours of Failure of Initial Antibiotics	
Recommended First-Line Treatment	**Alternative Treatment (PCN Allergy)**	**Recommended First-Line Treatment**	**Alternative Treatment**
Amoxicillin 80–90 mg/kg per day in 2 divided doses	Cefdinir[‡] 14 mg/kg per day in 1 or 2 doses	Amoxicillin-clavulanate* 90 mg/kg per day of amoxicillin component in 2 divided doses	Clindamycin 30–40 mg/kg per day in 3 divided doses, with or without third-generation cephalosporin
Amoxicillin-clavulanate* 90 mg/kg per day of amoxicillin component in 2 divided doses	Cefuroxime[‡] 30 mg/kg per day in 2 divided doses *or* Cefpodoxime[‡] 10 mg/kg per day in 2 divided doses	Ceftriaxone[‡] 50 mg/kg IM or IV daily for 3 days	Failure of second antibiotic: Clindamycin plus a third-generation cephalosporin Tympanocentesis[†] Consult specialist[†]
	Ceftriaxone[‡] 50 mg/kg IM or IV daily for 1 to 3 days		

* May be considered in patients who have received amoxicillin in the previous 30 days or who have the otitis-conjunctivitis syndrome.

[†] Perform tympanocentesis/drainage if skilled in the procedure, or seek a consultation from an otolaryngologist for tympanocentesis/drainage. If the tympanocentesis reveals multidrug-resistant bacteria, seek an infectious disease specialist consultation.

[‡] Cefdinir, cefuroxime, cefpodoxime, and ceftriaxone are highly unlikely to be associated with cross-reactivity with penicillin allergy on the basis of their distinct chemical structures.

IM – intramuscular; IV – intravenous.

Meningitis is a rare complication of AOM, either from bacteremia or direct extension from the middle ear or mastoid space to the dura. Also rare, epidural abscess, subdural abscess, brain abscess, and sigmoid sinus thrombosis may all complicate AOM. Imaging and usually lumbar puncture are indicated for patients with meningeal or other neurologic signs.

Pearls and Pitfalls

1. Pneumatic otoscopy is essential for accurate diagonsis of AOM.
2. AOM should be distinguished from OME.
3. Pain must be assesed and treated; acetaminophen or ibuprofen are effective.
4. The strategy of observation, with initiation of antibioitics only if the patient fails to improve, is reasonable in select patients who have excellent follow-up.

References

Gisselsson-Solen, M. Acute otitis media in children – current treatment and prevention. *Curr. Infect. Dis. Rep.* 2015; 17(5): 476.

Heikkinen, T., Thint, M., and Chonmaitree, T. Prevalence of various respiratory viruses in the middle ear during acute otitis media. *N. Engl. J. Med.* 1999; 340(4): 260–4.

Lieberthal, A. S., Carroll, A. E., Chonmaitree, T., *et al.* The diagnosis and management of acute otitis media. *Pediatrics* 2013; 131(3): e964–99.

Siddiq, S. and Grainger, J. The diagnosis and management of acute otitis media: American Academy of Pediatrics Guidelines 2013. *Arch. Dis. Child. Educ. Pract. Ed.* 2015; 100(4): 193–7.

Subcommittee of Clinical Practice. Guideline for D, Management of Acute Otitis Media in C. Clinical practice guidelines for the diagnosis and management of acute otitis media (AOM) in children in Japan. *Auris Nasus Larynx* 2012; 39(1): 1–8.

Sinusitis

Aaron Kornblith

Introduction and Microbiology

Most cases of rhinosinusitis are viral in etiology, with approximately 2% of episodes being an acute bacterial infection. Bacterial sinusitis is often a secondary complication of viral rhinosinusitis. Common bacterial pathogens are those seen in other infections of the upper airway and include *Streptococcus pneumoniae*, *Haemophilus influenzae*, and *Moraxella catarrhalis*. Anaerobes are less frequently encountered, but play a role in chronic sinusitis and infections extending from a dental source. Invasive fungal sinusitis due to mucormycosis is a rare disease process found in patients with immunosuppression.

Epidemiology

Sinusitis is a common condition for which patients seek medical attention. In the United States, there are more than 30 million patient visits per year pertaining to sinus problems, including allergic rhinitis, viral upper respiratory infections with rhinosinusitis, vasomotor rhinitis, bacterial rhinosinusitis, and nasal polyposis. Sinusitis occurs in patients of all ages, but is more common in adults between the ages of 45 and 74 years. Children with cystic fibrosis are a unique pediatric population at higher risk for sinus disease caused by atypical organisms, especially *Pseudomonas*.

Clinical Features

Sinusitis is categorized by duration of symptoms. Acute sinusitis is defined as symptoms lasting less than 4 weeks' duration. Chronic sinusitis is an infection persisting longer than 12 weeks and subacute sinusitis is defined as 4 to 12 weeks of symptoms. Recurrent acute sinusitis is defined as more than four sinus infections in a year, each with interim resolution (see Tables 17.1 and 17.2).

When evaluating a patient with acute rhinosinusitis, clinicians should use historical and physical exam features to attempt to distinguish viral from bacterial infection. Historical clues are the main way to distinguish viral from bacterial disease, since imaging is often abnormal in both forms. Unfortunately, both viral and bacterial infections present with facial pressure, headache, purulent nasal discharge, smell disturbances, cough, and ear fullness (see Table 17.3). The following suggest a bacterial over viral etiology: persistent symptoms of sinusitis lasting 10 or more days without improvement, onset of severe symptoms or fever accompanied by purulent nasal discharge or facial pain for at least 3 consecutive days, and worsening symptoms following a typical viral upper respiratory infection. Some experts define acute bacterial sinusitis by three cardinal symptoms: purulent nasal drainage, nasal obstruction, and facial pain or pressure. A system of major and minor symptoms has also been proposed (see Table 17.1). Bacterial sinusitis is suggested by the presence of two major factors or one major and one minor factor, or by the presence of pus on nasal examination.

Physical exam findings include swelling, erythema, or edema localized over the involved zygoma or periorbital area. The most important finding to distinguish bacterial from viral disease is the ability of the patient to produce purulent or bloody nasal secretions during the exam, though purulent secretions can occur in viral disease.

History of aspirin sensitivity and asthma may suggest underlying nasal polyps. Similarly, the repetitive abuse of inhaled stimulants may predispose to altered nasal and sinus architecture. On physical examination, the patient's dentition should be checked carefully as a maxillary tooth infection can occasionally be responsible for unilateral maxillary sinusitis.

Differential Diagnosis

It may be difficult to distinguish the different diseases that present with facial, head, or dental pain. Headache syndromes, such as cluster headaches and primary dental disease, should always be considered. Moreover, dental infections may lead

Table 17.1 Major and Minor Sinusitis Factors

Major Factors	Minor Factors
Facial pain/pressure (in conjunction with other nasal symptoms)	Headache
	Halitosis
	Fatigue
Facial fullness	Dental pain
Nasal obstruction	Fever (in non-acute rhinosinusitis)
Nasal discharge/purulence	Cough
Fever (in acute rhinosinusitis)	Ear pressure/fullness

Source: R. M. Rosenfeld, D. Andes, N. Bhattacharyya, *et al.* Clinical practice guideline: adult sinusitis. *Otolaryngol. Head Neck Surg.* 2007; 137(3): S1–31.

Table 17.2 Rhinosinusitis Definitions

Type Rhinosinusitis	Duration	Histrory (See also Table 17.1)
Acute	≤4 weeks	≥2 major factors *or* 1 major factor and 1 minor factor *or* Nasal purulence on exam
Subacute	4–12 weeks	Same
Recurrent acute	≥4 episodes/year, each episode 7–10 days; clears between episodes	Same
Chronic	≥12 weeks	Same. Note: Facial pain in the absence of other nasal symptoms is *not* suggestive of chronic sinusitis!

Source: R. M. Rosenfeld, D. Andes, N. Bhattacharyya, *et al.* Clinical practice guideline: adult sinusitis. *Otolaryngol. Head Neck Surg.* 2007; 137(3): S1–31..

Table 17.3 Cinical Features: Sinusitis Organisms

Organisms	• *Streptococcus sp.* • *Haemophilus influenzae* • *Moraxella catarrhalis* • Anaerobic bacteria • Viruses
Signs and symptoms	• Facial pressure • Headache • Purulent drainage, often unilateral • Otorrhea if perforation of TM has occurred • Smell disturbances
Laboratory and radiographic findings	• Usually not indicated • Refractory sinusitis may require culture-directed therapy • A sinus CT (without contrast) is usually warranted *after* a trial of medical therapy, unless clinical examination suggests an anatomic etiology or a complication of sinusitis, or if there is a diagnostic dilemma
Treatment	• Saline nasal irrigation, best with bulb syringe • Decongestants, oral or topical • Antibiotics • amoxicilin 0.5–1.5 g PO TID × 10–14 days • *or* • amoxicillin/clavulanate 825/125 mg PO BID × 10–14 days • orazithromycin 2 g × 1 dose or 500 mg PO QD × 3 daysorclarithromycin 500 mg PO BID × 14 days Severe, non-responsive or history of recent antibiotic use: levofloxacin 500 mg PO QD × 5–10 days *or* moxifloxacin 400 mg PO QD × 5–10 days • Corticosteroids, in certain circumstances • Surgical treatment if medical treatment fails

CT – computed tomography; TM – tympanic membrane.

to unilateral maxillary sinusitis. Functional obstruction by polyps or other lesions or foreign bodies can cause sinusitis and may be evident on physical examination. A history of seasonal symptoms, associated conjunctivitis, or environmental allergies may suggest allergic rhinitis, while recurrent disease may suggest vasomotor rhinitis.

Allergic fungal sinusitis is usually caused by hypersensitivity to *Aspergillus*. Patients will characteristically have an elevated IgE level, and Charcot–Leyden crystals are noted on pathological examination. Cultures are positive for fungi, and CT imaging demonstrates a unilateral opacification of the involved sinuses, often with a stippled appearance and bone erosion. Treatment includes corticosteroids and surgical debridement. An acute infectious form of *Aspergillus* can also occur.

More important to recognize is invasive fungal rhinosinusitis, which in its acute form is a surgical emergency. It is usually caused by the Mucorales fungi (mucormycosis) and *Aspergillus* patients are often immunocompromised from poorly controlled diabetes, human immunodeficiency virus (HIV), or immunosuppressive therapy, hematologic malignancy, or chemotherapy. Complications include orbital and globe invasion and vision loss, intracranial extension, and death. Emergent evaluation includes advanced imaging of the sinuses, orbit, and brain with CT or MRI and immediate surgical consultation. Treatment includes both operative debridement and antifungal drugs, usually amphotericin.

Laboratory and Radiographic Findings

Radiography is rarely indicated in the initial evaluation of acute sinusitis. Imaging should be obtained in severe disease, such as in elderly, febrile patients, to evaluate for complications and to evaluate chronic infections. Computed tomography (CT) has replaced plain X-rays as the test of choice. CT is sensitive (a normal scan rules out sinusitis), but abnormalities are non-specific (can be seen in asymptomatic patients and viral rhinosinusitis). Findings include mucosal thickening, sinus opacification, and air–fluid levels (see Figure 17.1). Complications of sinusitis such as osteomyelitis and orbital and intracranial abscesses (see below) are best seen with

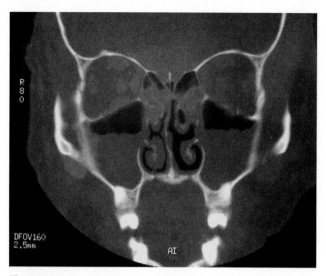

Figure 17.1 Acute maxillary sinusitis on a CT scan coronal image.

addition of IV contrast, or with MRI. Bacterial culture from nasal secretions is unreliable. However, culture-directed medical therapy may be useful in refractory disease. In such cases, endoscopic examination of the nasal passages and sinuses and culture from a sinus aspirate improves the yield of bacterial culture. This procedure has become a mainstay of rhinology practices because the examination can be accomplished with topical anesthesia in the office setting.

Treatment and Prophylaxis

Routine management of suspected acute bacterial sinusitis consists of nasal saline irrigation, oral or topical decongestants (topical or oral), antibiotics, and analgesics. Nasal irrigation is best achieved with a volume of 10 to 20 mL of sterile salt solution, administered via a medical 30 mL syringe or Neti pot, twice per day. The patient must be educated not to use topical decongestants, such as oxymetazoline (Afrin) for more than several days, as prolonged use can lead to rhinitis medicamentosa, in which cessation of the topical decongestant results in rebound inflammation and edema. Non-steroidal anti-inflammatories and acetaminophen are recommended for pain management. Watchful waiting without antibiotics is an option in patients with limited comorbidities and non-severe disease if close follow-up can be arranged. Antibiotic choices are listed in Table 17.3. Intranasal glucocorticoids can be added in cases of suspected underlying allergic rhinitis. Antihistamines are not recommended. Various forms of surgical treatment are used for chronic sinusitis, as well as for locally complicated or invasive disease.

Complications and Admissions Criteria

Complications of sinusitis often stem from local extension into the orbit, surrounding soft tissues, or the central nervous system. Edema of the eyelid, restriction of extraocular movements, neurological symptoms (most often cranial nerve), or vision change should warrant urgent imaging and specialist consultation. Rare complications of sinusitis include

meningitis, epidural abscess, subdural abscess, brain abscess, or isolated cavernous sinus thrombosis. The patient with suspected invasive fungal sinusitis warrants emergent otolaryngologist consultation and treatment. Other indications for immediate imaging and consideration of consultation and admission for parenteral antibiotics include infections in elderly patients and those with poorly controlled diabetes or immunosuppression, presence of high fever, severe pain, or altered mental status.

Pearls and Pitfalls

1. Diagnosis is usually made clinically; CT imaging is reserved for severe or refractory cases.
2. Eyelid edema, vision changes, or cranial nerve involvement may indicate serious complications requiring immediate imaging and consultation.
4. Initial medical therapy includes irrigation, decongestants, and antibiotics.
5. If sinusitis is unresponsive to first-line antibiotics, practitioners can consider broadening coverage, CT imaging. or referral for direct cultures.
6. Sinusitis in the setting of immunosuppression should always prompt consideration of an invasive fungal infection.

References

Bhattacharyya, N. Clinical and symptom criteria for the accurate diagnosis of chronic rhinosinusitis. *Laryngoscope* 2006; 116(Suppl.): 1–22.

Brook, I. The role of bacterial interference in otitis, sinusitis and tonsillitis. *Otolaryngol. Head Neck Surg.* 2005; 133(1): 139–46.

Chandler, J. R., Langenbrunner, D. J., and Stevens, E. R. The pathogenesis of orbital complications in acute sinusitis. *Laryngoscope* 1970; 80(9): 1414–28.

Chow, A. W., Benninger, M. S., Brook, I., *et al.* IDSA clinical practice guideline for acute bacterial rhinosinusitis in children and adults. *Clin. Infect. Dis.* 2012; 54(8): 72.

Fairbanks, D. N. F. *Pocket Guide to Antimicrobial Therapy in Otolaryngology – Head and Neck Surgery*, 12th edn (Washington, DC: American Academy of Otolaryngology, 2005).

Hickner, J. M., Bartlett, J. G., Besser, R., *et al.* Principles of acute antibiotic use for acute rhinosinusitis in adults: background. *Ann. Intern. Med.* 2001; 134(6): 498–505.

Piccirillo, J. R. Acute bacterial sinusitis. *N. Engl. J. Med.* 2004; 351(9): 902–10.

Remmler, D. and Boles, R. Intracranial complications of frontal sinusitis. *Laryngoscope* 1980; 90(11): 1814–24.

Rosenfeld, R. M., Andes, D., Neil, B., *et al.* Clinical practice guideline: adult sinusitis. *Otolaryngol. Head Neck Surg.* 2007; 137(3): S1–31.

Snow, V., Mottur-Pilson, C., and Hickner, J. M. Principles of appropriate antibiotic use for acute sinusitis. *Ann. Intern. Med.* 2001; 134(6): 495.

Wald, E. R., Applegate, K. E., Bordley, C., *et al.* Clinical practice guideline for the diagnosis and management of acute bacterial sinusitis in children aged 1 to 18 years. *Pediatrics* 2013; 132(1): 262–80.

Supraglottitis (Epiglottis)

Chapter 18

Aaron Kornblith

Introduction and Microbiology

Patients with supraglottitis (also referred to as epiglottis) typically present to the acute care setting with complaints of dysphagia, muffled voice, and difficulty handling secretions. However, supraglottitis can be a challenging diagnosis when symptoms are less specific (e.g. isolated odynophagia or fever). It is essential that emergency providers be familiar with the diagnosis and management of supraglottitis because of the potential for rapid progression to complete airway obstruction.

The term supraglottitis is preferred to epiglottitis because it more accurately describes the location of inflammation in the supraglottic larynx, including the epiglottis, arytenoids, and the aryepiglottic folds. The vallecula and tongue base, located superiorly in the oropharynx, may also be affected. Inferiorly, the subglottic structures are rarely affected because the epithelium is more tightly bound at the level of the vocal cords.

Haemophilus influenzae type b (Hib) remains the most common identified organism responsible for supraglottitis. However, with the advent of the Hib vaccine, the overall incidence of supraglottitis, and Hib as a causative organism, has decreased significantly. Most infectious etiologies are bacterial, including non-typeable *Hemophilus*, Streptococci, and *Staphylococcus aureus*, but viral and fungal pathogens also contribute to the overall incidence. Less commonly direct injury such as caustic and thermal injuries may cause supraglottitis.

Epidemiology

In the past, young children made up the majority of cases of supraglottitis (see Chapter 54, Pediatric Respiratory Infections). After introduction of the Hib vaccine, the annual incidence decreased in children. However, the annual incidence in adults has remained steady. Cases still occur in unvaccinated children and those who have not developed immunity after vaccination. Risk factors for development of supraglottitis include diabetes and immunosuppression.

Clinical Features

While the clinical features of supraglottitits change with age, both adult and pediatric patients with supraglottitis are usually febrile and ill-appearing and there may be a history of recent upper respiratory infection. Children commonly present with drooling, prefer to sit upright, and have significant dysphagia. Stridor is more commonly seen in children, and can occur in any phase of the respiratory cycle. Because the airway diameter is smaller, children are much more prone to complete airway obstruction with small increases in swelling, such as can occur during examination of the oropharynx with a tongue blade. The absence of stridor in a child with other indications of supraglottitis may portend imminent airway collapse.

Adult patients typically complain of odonophagia, will be spitting out saliva, and have voice changes described as "muffled" or as a "hot-potato voice." A severe sore throat and a normal-appearing oropharynx, or tenderness localized to the hyoid, should prompt consideration of supraglotitttis. In adults, airway obstruction is a later finding. The progression of symptoms in children is often rapid, occurring over 24 hours, whereas in adults it may be several days (see Table 18.1).

The approach to diagnosis should be guided by the patient's age and clinical status. Visualizing the supraglottic structures is generally required for diagnosis, and the plan for doing so should be coordinated with the plan for airway management. In children, findings of anxiety, respiratory distress, and the tripod position should prompt immediate consultation of an otolaryngologist or anesthesiologist with pediatric expertise, as well as preparation for emergency airway management. In such cases, the goal is to keep the child calm and breathing on their own until the airway can be safely controlled. Gagging or increased anxiety induced by bedside evaluation can potentially provoke airway obstruction and arrest.

In children with mild symptoms, as well as adults, visualization of the larynx, by either fiberoptic or direct visualization is still generally required to rule out the disease, but can often

Table 18.1 Clinical Features: Supraglottitis

Organisms	*Haemophilus* spp.
	Streptococcus pneumoniae
	Streptococcus spp.
	Staphylococcus spp.
	Klebsiella
	Pseudomonas
	Candida
	Viruses
Signs and symptoms	• Ill–appearing patient
	• Drooling
	• Voice change, "hot patato voice"
	• Sore throat
	• Difficulty breathing and/or stridor
Laboratory and radiographic findings	• May have elevated CBC
	• May be rapid *Streptococcus* positive
	• Lateral neck x-ray with thickening of the epiglottis, the "thumb sign," and adjacent aryepiglottics folds
Treatment	• Ampicillin-sulbactam 1.5–3 g IV every 6 hours
	• Cefuroxime 750–1,500 mg IV every 8 hours
	• Ceftriaxone 1–2 g IV every 24 hours
	• Cefotaxime 2 g IV every 4–8 hours
	If PCN allergic:
	Chloramphenicol: 50–100 mg/kg/d IV divided QID

CBC – complete blood count.

be done without controlling the airway first. Laryngoscopy is optimally performed in the operating room with anesthesia and personnel prepared to perform bronchoscopy and/or tracheotomy if necessary. In adult patients, it may in some cases be deemed safe to perform fiberoptic laryngoscopy in the emergency department setting. An adult patient has a larger airway and is often more able to safely tolerate the examination.

Differential Diagnosis

The complaint of a sore throat can be a symptom of many diseases. Supraglottitis can be distinguished from viral laryngotacheitis (croup) by the absence of a "barking" cough. In the largest case series to date, cough was noted in less than 10% of children with supraglottitis, whereas fever and drooling were less common in patients with croup. The differential also includes viral and streptococcal pharyngitis and diptheria. Abscesses of the upper aerodigestive tract, such as a peritonsillar, retropharyngeal, or deep neck abscess, may present in a similar manner to epiglottitis. Ludwig's angina, a necrotizing soft-tissue infection of the sublingual and submental space, will present with elevation of the oral tongue and edema or erythema of submandibular region. Bacterial tracheitis is an uncommon cause of upper airway obstruction that is also life-threatening. Like supraglottitis, tracheitis does not respond to conventional croup therapy, but in contrast to supraglottitis, patients with bacterial tracheitis are able to swallow their oral secretions.

Other disease processes surrounding the epiglottis that may cause thickening include hematoma, cyst, and abscess.

Angioedema may present with stridor and hot-potato voice, though usually without the fever and pain of supraglottitis. Environmental causes include both thermal and chemical injury to the supraglottis.

Laboratory and Radiographic Findings

Diagnosis is made primarily by history and physical exam. Leukocytosis may suggest a bacterial infection and blood cultures will occasionally reveal the etiologic pathogen. Respiratory cultures should be obtained after the airway is secure because of the possibility of worsening respiratory compromise.

Lateral and anteroposterior soft-tissue radiographs may suggest the diagnosis of supraglottitis if there is a classic "thumbprint sign" produced by an edematous epiglottis, or obliteration of the valecula (see Figure 18.1). However, radiographs do not substitute for direct supraglottic visualization for ruling out the disease. Radiographs may also be helpful in differentiating causes of stridor in children (foreign body being a common cause in this population). X-rays should be obtained in a room equipped for emergency airway management rather than in the radiology department. There is little role for CT in the diagnosis of supraglottitis per se, though it is the study for identifying a retropharyngeal abscess.

Point-of-care ultrasound evaluation of the supraglottic space has been described in adults, but its role in diagnosing supraglottitis is yet to be determined.

Treatment and Prophylaxis

Control of the airway, if necessary, and expeditious diagnosis are the first management priorities. Empirical broad spectrum intravenous antibiotics should be administered as soon as the diagnosis is suspected (see Table 18.1). Choice of regimen is optimally dictated by local resistance patterns. Appropriate choices include a combination therapy of a third-generation cephalosporin (e.g. ceftriaxone, cefotaxime) and an antistaphylococcal agent (e.g. clindamycin, vancomycin). Corticosteroids are theoretically beneficial to decrease airway edema; however, there is no prospective evidence of benefit and this therapy remains controversial. If intubation is required, positive end-expiratory pressure should be used since sudden relief of airway obstruction can lead to pulmonary edema.

Complications and Admission Criteria

The most devastating complication is catastrophic airway compromise and death. The main local complication is epiglottic abscess. Associated cellulitis, cervical adenitis, meningitis, and various metastatic complications of bacteremia have all been described.

All patients with suspected or confirmed supraglottitis should be admitted to a monitored setting, typically the intensive care unit, until airway edema improves or they can be safely extubated.

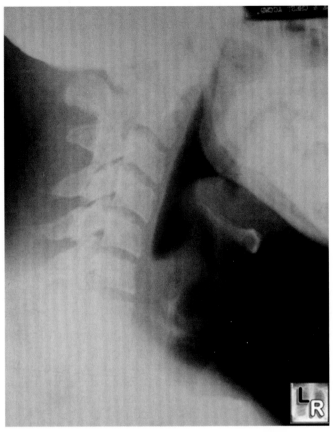

Figure 18.1 Epiglottitis as seen on lateral neck soft tissue X-ray, showing "thumbprint sign" caused by the swollen epiglottis.

Courtesy of Barry Simon, MD.

Pearls and Pitfalls

1. Supraglottitis is an airway emergency that requires providers with expertise in airway management.
2. Supraglottitis should be suspected by history and physical examination.

3. Imaging studies, if needed, are only pursued after the airway is secure.
4. *Haemophilus influenzae* type B vaccination has significantly decreased the incidence of supraglottitis in children.

References

Cantrell, R. W., Bell R. A., and Morioka, W. T. Acute epiglottitis: intubation versus tracheostomy. *Laryngoscope* 1978; 88(6): 994–1005.

Glynn, F. and Fenton, J E. Diagnosis and management of supraglottitis (epiglottitis). *Curr. Infect. Dis. Rep.* 2008; 10(3): 200.

Hung, T. Y., Li, S., Chen, P. S., *et al.* Bedside ultrasonography as a safe and effective tool to diagnose acute epiglottitis. *Am. J. Emerg. Med.* 2011; 29(3): 359.e1.

Fairbanks, D. N. F. *Pocket Guide to Antimicrobial Therapy in Otolaryngology – Head and Neck Surgery*, 12th edn. (Washington, DC: American Academy of Otolaryngology, 2005).

Osborne, R., Avitia, S., Zandifar, H., and Brown, J. Adult supraglottitis subsequent to smoking crack cocaine. *Ear Nose Throat J.* 2003; 82(1): 53–5.

Rodgers, G. K., Galos, R. S., and Johnson, J. T. Hereditary angioedema: case report and review of management. *Otolaryngol. Head Neck Surg.* 1991; 104(3): 394–8.

Shah, R. K., Roberson, D. W., and Jones, D. T. Epiglottitis in the Hemophilus influenzae type B vaccine era: changing trends. *Laryngoscope.* 2004; 114(3): 557.

Somenek, M., Le, M., and Walner, D. L. Membranous laryngitis in a child. *Int. J. Pediatr. Otorhinolaryngol.* 2010; 74(6): 704.

Tibballs, J. and Watson, T. Symptoms and signs differentiating croup and epiglottitis. *J. Paediatr. Child Health* 2011; 47(3): 77.

Chapter

Parotitis

Nisa S. Atigapramoj

19

Outline

Introduction and Microbiology

The parotid glands are two exocrine glands located lateral to the masseter muscle, on the sides of the face and in front of the ear. One of the largest salivary glands, these secrete primarily serous fluid via Stensen's duct which can be found exiting opposite the second upper molar. Inflammation of the glands can be unilateral or bilateral, and can also be acute, chronic, or recurrent. Determining onset, duration of symptoms, and involvement of one or both glands, as well as predisposing factors, can help narrow the differential diagnosis and guide treatment and management.

Possible etiologies of parotid swelling include, but are not limited to, infection, systemic illnesses, tumor, obstruction, and medications. Among the viral causes of parotitis, the mumps virus remains the most common. The mumps virus is an enveloped negative-sense RNA virus belonging to the Paramyxovirus genus. Other viral etiologies include CMV, EBV, Influenza A, Parainfluenza, Adenovirus, and Coxsackievirus. The most common bacterial etiology is *Staphylococcus aureus*, with case reports of MRSA parotitis. Other common bacterial pathogens include oral flora, such as *Streptococcus* species and anaerobes. Gram-negative bacteria, particularly *Haemophilus influenzae* and *Klebsiella pneumonia*, have also been found.

Epidemiology

Prior to the introduction of the live, attenuated measles, mumps, and rubella (MMR) vaccine in 1967, mumps virus infection was the leading cause of acquired parotitis, occurring mostly between winter and spring. With vaccination, in the United States between 2001 and 2005, 200 to 300 cases of mumps were diagnosed annually. In 2010, there were 2,612 reported cases by the Centers for Disease Control. Unvaccinated individuals are particularly at risk for infection, though the majority of outbreak cases have occurred among those who have been vaccinated and not achieved adequate immunity. Additional

risk factors include living in close quarters or crowded environments such as schools and dormitories.

Acute suppurative parotitis tends to occur mostly in the elderly patient population, though there have been reports of it occurring in preterm neonates, as well as those who are dehydrated or have poor oral hygiene.

Clinical Features

Commonly seen in the pediatric patient, mumps parotitis is usually an acute and self-limited disease. In the post-vaccine era, paramyxovirus infection is still the leading cause of viral parotitis. The incubation period is approximately 16 to 18 days (range 12 to 25 days) after exposure. Patients typically present with a non-specific prodrome which includes fever, headaches, myalgias, and generalized malaise (see Table 19.1). In the ensuing days, it is reported that 95% of patients with mumps present with painful, parotid swelling (see Figure 19.1). Parotid gland swelling may last up to 10 days, with complete recovery of all symptoms in a few weeks.

Acute suppurative parotitis is believed to occur when salivary stasis permits retrograde flow of bacteria into Stensen's duct. Suppurative parotitis typically occurs in dehydrated, debilitated patients or in the setting of sialolithiasis (salivary stones). Acute suppurative parotitis is characterized by the sudden onset of pain, unilateral swelling and erythema of the skin overlying the parotid gland. Trismus and dysphagia may also be present. Systemic symptoms may include fever, chills, and also a toxic appearance. Purulent fluid can often be appreciated at the opening of Stenson's duct after gently massaging the cheek.

Chronicity and recurrence of symptoms as well as bilateral involvement suggest a systemic cause for parotitis such as HIV, Sjögren's syndrome, or Juvenile recurrent parotitis.

Differential Diagnosis

Non-infectious etiologies of bilateral parotid enlargement include various autoimmune diseases, particularly Sjögren's

Table 19.1 Clinical Features: Parotitis

	EtiologyEtiology	
Viral	Mumps, CMV, EBV, Influenza A, Parainfluenza, Adenovirus, Coxsackievirus	• Prodrome includes fever and malaise • Uni-/bilateral parotid gland swelling • Anorexia • Clear fluid expressed from Stensen's duct
Bacterial	*Staphylococcus aureus*, gram-negative organisms	• Acute onset of pain • Fever, chills, marked toxicity • Unilateral parotid gland swelling with skin erythema • Purulent discharge from Stensen's duct
Other	HIV, salivary gland stones (sialoadenitis), malnuitition (especially eating disorders), sarcoidosis, Sjögren's syndrome, salivary gland tumors	• Recurrent, bilateral parotitis

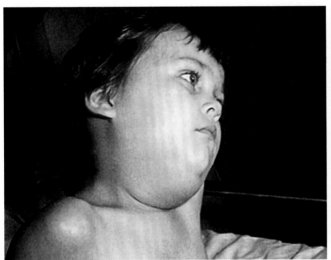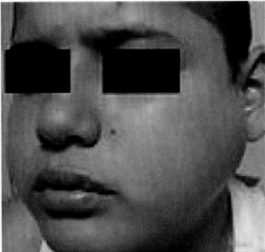

Figure 19.1 Acute mumps parotitis.

syndrome, sarcoidosis, and salivary gland neoplasms. Swelling associated with HIV is often due to lymphoepithelial cysts. Sialoadenitis, obstruction from salivary stones, is usually unilateral and episodic. Malnuitrition in the setting of anorexia nervosa, bulimia, or alcoholism is associated with non-inflammatory salivary gland swelling. Temporal mandibular joint syndrome or isolated bruxism may produce symptoms of bilateral pain that can be mistaken for mumps. Antihistamines and anticholinergics, which reduce salivary flow, may contribute.

Laboratory and Radiographic Findings

Diagnosis of viral parotitis is made by clinical examination. Laboratory studies supportive of mumps demonstrate a leukopenia with lymphocytosis as well as an elevated amylase when parotitis is present. When confirmation is necessary, serology includes positive IgM mumps antibody, a significant rise in IgG titers, or isolation of the virus in specimens.

Imaging modalities for the evaluation of parotitis, particularly to rule out obstruction or abscess in supportive parotitis, include ultrasonography, computed tomography with contrast, and X-ray sialography. X-ray sialography is contraindicated in the acute suppurative stages because it requires dye injection. Magnetic resonance sialography is now available.

Treatment and Prophylaxis

Treatment of parotitis is dependent on the suspected etiology. Initial measures should include analgesia and hydration (oral or intravenous). For sialoadenitis, warm compresses and sialogogues are used, as well as promotion of good oral hygiene.

Treatment of viral parotitis is supportive. When a bacterial infection is suspected, fluids and antibiotics are necessary, and admission and IV antibiotics are generally indicated. Empiric therapy should include an antistaphylococcal agent, such as nafcillin combined with metronidazole or clindamycin. Methicillin-resistant *Staphylococcus aureus* (MRSA) treatment with vancomycin and more advanced gram-negative coverage may be needed in at-risk or immunocompromised patients. Antibiotic therapy can be adjusted once culture results become available. Imaging to evaluate for obstruction and abscess is prudent. Surgical drainage is required for infection with an obstructing salivary stone or for a frank abscess.

The MMR vaccine prevents most cases and complications associated with mumps. Current recommendations are that children receive a first dose of MMR vaccine at ages 12 to

15 months and a second dose at ages 4 to 6 years. Two doses of MMR vaccine are also recommended for students attending colleges and other post-high-school institutions who do not have proof of two prior doses or other evidence of immunity. There may also be consideration for a third MMR dose during an outbreak setting.

Complications and Admission Criteria

Sequelae of mumps parotitis include orchitis and oophoritis. Orchitis can occur in 25% of affected post-pubertal males and is rare in pre-pubescent males, while oophoritis occurs in 5% of post-pubertal females with mumps and is characterized by pelvic pain and tenderness. Additional complications include aseptic meningitis and encephalitis, and rarer incidences of pancreatitis have occurred.

Bacterial parotitis can be complicated by abscess formation or by local extension into surrounding tissues. Rare reported complications involve the facial nerve and jugular venous thrombosis, respiratory obstruction, and osteomyelitis of the facial bone.

Elderly patients with suppurative parotitis should generally be admitted for parenteral antibiotics and hydration. Discharged patients should be followed closely for improvement. Acute mumps parotitis rarely requires admission.

Infection Control

Mumps is transmitted via respiratory droplets, direct contact, or fomites. Viral shedding may occur before clinical symptoms manifest and decreases soon after symptom onset. Current isolation recommendations are for 5 days of droplet precautions.

Perinatal transmission has also been noted; however, most children under 1 year of age are usually protected by maternal antibodies. The best means of prevention is vaccination.

Pearls and Pitfalls

1. Treatment of parotitis is mainly supportive, including hydration and pain control.
2. *Staphylococcus aureus* is the most common bacterial etiology.
3. Consider alternative diagnoses when there is bilateral or recurrent parotitis.
4. MMR vaccination should be encouraged.

References

Al-Dajani, N. and Wootton, S. Cervical lymphadenitis, suppurative parotitis, thyroiditis, and infected cysts. *Infect. Dis. Clin. N. Am.* 2007; 21(2): 523–41.

Baszis, K., Toib, D., Cooper, M., *et al.* Recurrent parotitis as a presentation of primary pediatric Sjogren syndrome. *Pediatrics* 2012; 129(1): e179.

Centers for Disease Control and Prevention, Mumps, retrieved from www.cdc.gov/mumps (last updated May 29, 2015).

Fattahi, T., Lyu, P., and Van Sickels, J. Management of acute suppurative parotitis. *J. Oral Maxillofac. Surg.* 2002; 60(4): 446–8.

McLean, H. Q., Fiebelkorn, A. P., Temte, J. L., *et al.* Prevention of measles, rubella, congenital rubella syndrome, and mumps, 2013: summary recommendations of the Advisory Committee on Immunization Practices (ACIP). *MMWR Morb. Mortal. Wkly. Rep.* 2013; 62(RR04): 1–34.

Pharyngitis and Peritonsillar Abscess

Bradley W. Frazee

Introduction

Sore throat is a very common chief complaint in both adult and pediatric acute care practice, accounting for up to 2% of visits. The diagnosis in the majority of cases is infectious pharyngitis, or tonsillopharyngitis. Most of these infections are viral and require no antimicrobial treatment. However, it is important to correctly identify and treat the subset caused by *S. pyogenes*, usually referred to as group A β-hemolytic *Streptococcus*. Peritonsillar abscess (PTA) also presents as sore throat. It is a relatively common suppurative complication of pharyngitis that in most cases can be safely drained in the emergency department. Finally, acute care providers are advised to always consider several life-threatening infections that can present as sore throat. These include pediatric epiglottitis, croup, bacterial tracheitis, and retropharyngeal abscess, which are covered in Chapter 54; supraglottitis in children and adults, covered in Chapter 18; and deep neck space infections and Lemierre's syndrome, covered in Chapter 21.

Pharyngitis

Epidemiology and Microbiology

Upper respiratory tract infections (URI) lead to roughly 50 million health-care visits per year in the United States, cost more than $40 billion in overall economic impact, and represent the number one reason for outpatient antibiotic prescriptions. Roughly 12 million of these visits are given the final diagnosis of pharyngitis. Pharyngitis occurs more commonly in the winter months in parallel with the rise in respiratory viruses. While only 5 to 15% of pharyngitis in adults is bacterial, roughly 60% of cases are prescribed antibiotics. This fact points to the opportunity that exists for improved evidence-based diagnosis and treatment in the acute care setting.

Leading pharyngitis pathogens are listed in Table 20.1. Group A β hemolytic *streptococcus* (GAS) is the most common and important bacterial pathogen. GAS is more common in children between the ages of 5 and 15 and very uncommon in children less than age 3 and adults over age 45. Antibiotic treatment prevents both suppurative sequelae, such as PTA and otitis media, and the rare non-suppurative sequelae, rheumatic fever and glomerulonephritis. Rheumatic fever is now uncommon in developing countries, complicating less than 1% of GAS pharyngitis cases in children in the United States. Fortunately, GAS has retained its susceptibility to penicillin and other narrow spectrum antibiotics. Other causative bacterial pathogens include *Arcanobacterium*, *Mycoplasma*, and *Chlamydophila* and, in the sexually active population, *N. gonorrhea*. Fusobacterium necrophorum, the oral anaerobe responsible for most cases of Lemierre's syndrome, may be an emerging pharyngitis pathogen among young adults in the United States. Fusobacterium is resistant to macrolide antibiotics. Diptheria is a consideration in developing countries with inadequate vaccination programs.

Viruses cause the majority of pharyngitis. Respiratory viruses predominate, such as rhinovirus, adenovirus, influenza, and coxsackievirus. Many of these present, particularly in pediatric patients, with characteristic clinical syndromes, which are listed in Table 20.1. Epstein–Barr virus (EBV), and occasionally cytalomegalovirus (CMV), are responsible for the mononucleosis syndrome, a major cause of exudative pharyngitis in patients between ages 15 and 24 (see Chapter 60, Fever in the Returning Traveler). Acute HIV infection is one of the most important potential viral etiologies to keep in mind,

Table 20.1 Etiologies of Infectious Pharyngitis

Pathogen	Clinical Syndrome
Bacterial	
Group A β hemolytic *streptococcus* (GAS)	Tonsillopharyngitis, scarlet fever
Group C, G *Streptococcus*	Tonsillopharyngitis
Arcanobacterium haemolyticum	Scarlatiniform rash, pharyngitis
N. gonorrhoeae	Tonsillopharyngitis
Corynebacterium diptheriae	Diptheria
Mixed anaerobes	Vincent's angina
Fusobacterium necrophorum	Tonsillopharyngitis, Lemierre's syndrome, PTA
Francisella tularensis	Oropharyngeal tularemia
Yersinia pestis	Plague
Yersinia enterocolitica	Enterocolitis, pharyngitis
Viral	
Adenovirus	Pharyngoconjunctival fever
HSV-1 and HSV-2	Exudative pharyngitis; anterior oral and lip lesions uncommon
Coxsackievirus	Herpangina and hand foot and mouth disease
Rhinovirus	Non-specific URI
Coronavirus	Non-specific URI
Influenza virus	Influenza
Parainfluenza	Croup, non-specific URI
EBV	Infectious mononucleosis
CMV	CMV mononucleosis
HIV	Primary acute HIV infection
Others	
Mycoplasma pneumoniae	Pneumonitis, bronchitis
Chlamydophila pneumonia	Pneumonia, bronchitis
Chlamydophila psittaci	Psitticosis

GAS – Group A *Streptococcus*; PTA – peritonsillar abscess; EBV – Epstein-Barr virus; CMV – cytomegalovirus.

Reproduced with permission from Oxford University Press. S. Shulman, A. Bisno, H. Clegg, *et al.*, Clinical practice guideline for the diagnosis and management of group A streptococcal pharyngitis: 2012 update by the Infectious Diseases Society of America. *Clin. Infect. Dis.* 2014; 58(10): 1496.

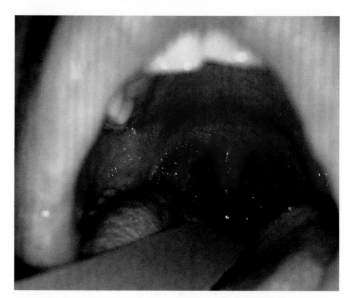

Figure 20.1 GAS Pharyngitis. Typical appearance on oropharynx exam, showing subtle tonsillar exudate and palatal petechiae.

Clinical Features

The clinical findings in pharyngitis range from minor throat pain, odynophagia, and tonsillar erythema in association with a non-specific URI, to massive exudative pharyngitis with high fever, inability to swallow, and airway compromise. Table 20.1 summarizes classic clinical syndromes associated with several pharyngitis pathogens. For example, posterior oropharynx vesicles in a child suggest herpangina, typically due to Coxsackie A virus.

Since GAS is the only pharyngitis pathogen that should be routinely identified and treated, the clinical findings in GAS pharyngitis have been well studied and clearly defined (see

because correct diagnosis can impact both public health and that of the patient.

Table 20.3). These include fever, tonsillar exudate, anterior cervical lymphadenopathy, and lack of cough (see Figure 20.1). Absence of these findings suggests a viral etiology. Paletal petechiae and a scarlatiniform rash (seen in children) are also specific findings. Abdominal pain or vomiting may be the presenting symptoms in young children with GAS.

Mononucleosis, caused predominantly by EBV, often begins with an exudative tonsillitis similar to that of GAS. Symptomatic infection occurs predominantly in patients between the ages of 15 and 24. Lymphadenopathy is typically widespread, and posterior cervical adenopathy is very characteristic. The clinical course, including severe fatigue, can last several weeks, much longer than in GAS infection. Splenomegaly with splenic rupture in males is the most important complication of mononucleosis that acute care physicians should bare in mind.

Differential Diagnosis

The differential diagnosis for sore throat includes all the infectious pharyngitis etiologies listed in Table 20.1. In addition, it is crucial that acute care providers consider the many other potentially life-threatening entities that can present as sore throat. These are listed in Table 20.2. PTA, the most common supportive complication of pharyngitis, is covered below. Pediatric epiglottitis, croup, bacterial tracheitis, and retropharyngeal abscess (RPA) are covered in Chapter 54. Adult supraglottitis is covered in Chapter 18, and deep neck space infections and internal jugular septic thrombophlebitis (Lemierre's syndrome) are covered in Chapter 21. High-risk findings that should prompt consideration of problems other than simple tonsillopharyngitis include the following:

- sitting forward in the "sniffing position" to breath comfortably
- stridor (epiglottitis, airway swelling)
- inability to swallow secretions /drooling
- trismus (deep neck space infection)

- torticollis (retropharyngeal abscess)
- deviated uvula (PTA)
- normal-appearing oropharynx despite sore throat
- midline larynx/hyoid tenderness (epiglottitis/supraglottitis)
- tenderness or swelling overlying the internal jugular (Lemierre's)

Laboratory and Radiographic Findings

There is no role for imaging in the routine evaluation of pharyngitis. However, imaging studies can be used to rule out certain potentially life-threatening non-pharyngitis causes of sore throat. Bedside ultrasound can be used to diagnose PTA (see below). A lateral soft tissue neck X-ray can be used to diagnose epiglottitis and retropharyngeal abscess, in which case it may reveal a thickened epiglottis (thumb print sign) and widened prevertebral space, respectively. Whenever there is a question of deep neck space infection or Lumierre's syndrome, a neck CT scan with contrast should be obtained.

In the case of infectious pharyngitis, blood tests have a limited role. If CBC is obtained, a lymphocyte predominance (>50%) or atypical lymphocytosis should raise suspicion for mononucleosis, which is confirmed with a heterophile antibody test (e.g. Monospot). HIV testing (optimally with a fourth-generation rapid HIV immunoassay) should be obtained when there is any suspicion for acute primary HIV infection.

Etiologic testing in pharyngitis is primarily aimed at identifying GAS pharyngitis for immediate treatment. There is some controversy as to the best diagnostic approach, and guidelines vary. Rapid antigen detection tests (RADT) are the mainstay of diagnostic testing, with throat culture, the criterion standard, serving a secondary role. RADTs have a specificity of 90 to 100% and sensitivity of 70 to 90%. In general, guidelines suggest obtaining RADT as a first line in children older than 3 years of age with a clear-cut pharyngitis (i.e. when pharyngitis is the main, or only, feature of the URI). When the RADT is negative and the suspicion for GAS is high, a throat culture, which is more sensitive than RADT, is recommended. Patients testing positive are treated. A lower threshold for throat culture is warranted in the setting of known exposure to GAS and for pharyngitis occurring in the fall and winter.

Because GAS infection in adults is unusual, and given the test performance characteristics of RADTs, practice guidelines strongly recommend combining a clinical decision rule with a more limited use of RADTs in adults. This approach is outlined in Table 20.3. Throat culture for GAS is not used in adults. It is worth keeping in mind that GAS pharyngitis is generally self-limited and almost never causes serious sequelae in adults. Therefore, in this age group, neither a liberal testing strategy, nor liberal use of antibiotics, is justified.

A throat culture looking for *Fusobacterium necrophorum* can be considered in young adults with prolonged, severe pharyngitis, especially if GAS RADT and heterophile antibody tests are negative. Swabs for rapid nucleic acid amplification tests are use to diagnose suspected *N. gonorrhea* pharyngitis.

Table 20.2 Non-Pharyngitis Causes of Sore Throat

Diagnosis	Clues
Gastroesophageal reflux disease (GERD)	Chest pain
Aortic aneurysm or dissection	Vascular risk factors, wide mediastinum on CXR
Kawasaki disease	Rash
Behçet's disease	Arthritis
Foreign body	Toddler, drooling
Croup	Child, stridor
Peritonsillar abscess	Hot potato voice, deviated uvula
Retropharyngeal abscess	Pediatric age group, torticollis
Deep neck space abscess (e.g. Ludwig's angina)	Trismus, neck swelling, floor of the mouth swelling
Epiglotittis	Drooling, normal-appearing oropharynx, hyoid tenderness
IJ Septic Thrombophlebitis (Lemierre's syndrome)	IJ tenderness, infiltrates on chest X-ray
Cancer	Age, tobacco history
Botulism (e.g. wound botulism)	IDU, diplopia

GERD – gastroesophageal reflux diseases; CXR – chest X-ray; IDU – injection drug use; IJ - internal jugular.

Treatment and Prophylaxis

Treatment of GAS is aimed not only at reducing symptom duration and preventing suppurative complications, but

Table 20.3 Clinical Decision Rule and Testing and Treatment Strategy for GAS in Adults

Clinical Feature	Points	Point Total	Testing and Treatment
Fever	1	≤ 2	No testing; no treatment
Exudate	1		
Anterior cervical lymphadenopathy	1	≥ 3	Test; if positive, treat; if negative, no treatment (nor further testing)
Absence of cough	1		
Optional age factor		Optional treat without testing strategy	
5–15 years	1	4–5	Consider treatment without testing
>45 years	−1		

Testing refers to rapid antigen detection test.

GAS – Group A β hemolytic *Streptococcus*.

Table 20.4 Clinical Features and Treatment: Pharyngitis

Pathogens	Respiratory viruses GAS EBV *F. necrophorum* HIV Others
Signs and symptoms	See Table 20.1 GAS – see Table 20.3 EBV – posterior cervical lymphadenopathy
Laboratory and radiographic findings	GAS – RADT, throat culture EBV – heterophile antibody (Monospot) *F. necrophorum* – throat culture (specify pathogen of interest) *N. gonorrhea* – NAAT HIV – fourth-generation immunoassay
Treatment	**Supportive therapy:** NSAIDs, acetaminophen, aspirin **For severe tonsillitis (marked swelling) may consider:** Dexamethasone 10 mg PO/IV/IM × 1 **Antibiotics in adults:** Penicillin G. benzathine 1.2 million units IM × 1 or Penicillin VK 500 mg PO BID for 10 days or Amoxacillin 500 mg PO BID for 10 days or Cephalexin 500 mg PO BID for 10 days or Clindamycin 300 mg PO TID for 10 days **Antibiotics in children:** If ≤27 kg: Penicillin G. benzathine 600,000 units IM × 1 or If ≤27 kg: Penicillin VK 250 mg PO BID for 10 days or Amoxicillin 25 mg/kg PO BID for 10 days or Cephalexin 25 mg/kg PO BID for 10 days or Clindamycin 10 mg/kg PO TID for 10 days (maximum 300 mg per dose)

at eradicating *Streptococcus* from the oropharynx in order to prevent the non-suppurative complications, rheumatic fever, and glomerulonephritis. Table 20.4 lists antimicrobial treatments for GAS pharyngitis and other bacterial etiologies. Ten days of therapy is generally required for eradication of Streptococcus, though shorter courses of cephalosporins can be used.

Analgesia, and in some instances anti-inflammatory treatment, should be provided for all cases of pharyngitis. Non-steroidal anti-inflammatory drugs (NSAIDs), aspirin, and acetaminophen are the analgesics of choice for pharyngitis, with evidence suggesting NSAIDs may be best. Opioids are rarely indicated. For severe tonsillitis with significant posterior pharyngeal swelling, glucocorticoids seem to hasten improvement and reduce the duration of symptoms.

Dexamethasone 10 mg IM or prednisone 60 mg PO are typically used in adults.

Chronic and recurrent severe tonsillitis in children and adults is sometimes treated with tonsillectomy. Referral and selection of patients involves the primary care physician and surgeon. Long-term prophylactic penicillin therapy to prevent GAS infection is indicated in patients who have had rheumatic fever.

Complications and Admission Criteria

Both suppurative and non-suppurative complications of GAS infection can occur. Suppurative complications that occur predominantly in children include otitis media and cervical lymphadenitis. PTA, an important suppurative complication, is discussed below. Non-suppurative complications of GAS pharyngitis include rheumatic fever, glomerulonephritis, scarlet fever, and pediatric autoimmune neuropsychiatric disorder (PANDAS). Scarlet fever typically occurs at the same time as pharyngitis in children previously exposed to GAS and findings include a "sandpaper" rash and strawberry tongue.

Septic thrombophlebitis of the internal jugular vein (Lemierre's syndrome) is an uncommon but potentially life-threatening suppurative complication of pharyngitis. It can also complicate PTA and other infections of the head and neck. *Fusobacterium necrophorum* is the pathogen classically involved. Lemierre's syndrome is covered in Chapter 21.

Hospital admission is rarely required for infectious pharyngitis itself. Whereas, if there is any suspicion for a complication that could compromise the airway, such as retropharyngeal abscess or supraglottitis, admission and urgent surgical consultation is required.

Peritonsillar Abscess

Peritonsillar abscess, or quincy, is an abscess located in the loose areolar tissue surrounding the palantine tonsils. PTAs are usually unilateral and tend to occur at the superior pole of the tonsil and point into the soft palate anterior to the palatoglossal arch and lateral to the uvula. Even large PTAs are usually located slightly medial and well anterior to the carotid sheath. PTAs usually form as a complication of pharyngitis. Although it can be difficult to differentiate a mature PTA from peritonsillar cellulitis, which precedes it, acute care providers should be adept at distinguishing these infections from routine pharyngitis, since the most important treatment of a PTA is drainage.

Epidemiology and Microbiology

PTAs occur more commonly in adolescents and young adults with an overall incidence of approximately 30 cases per 100,000 population. Previous history of PTA and smoking are risk factors. The most common bacterial pathogens are GAS, other oral Streptococcal species, *S. aureus* and oral anaerobes, particularly *Fusobacterium necrophorum*.

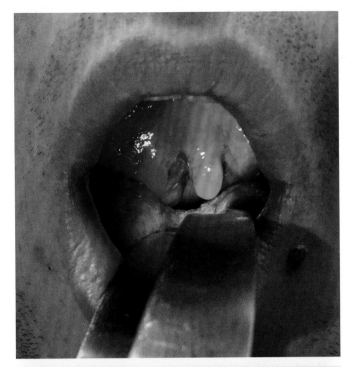

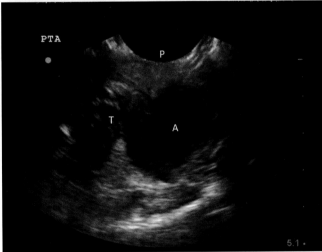

Figure 20.2 Peritonsillar abscess. Oropharynx view showing deviation of uvula leftward, away from the abscess. (A) Intraoral ultrasound showing anechoic abscess cavity adjacent to palatine tonsil (B).

Clinical Features

Patients typically present with a sore throat that has become unilateral and may radiate to the ear. Odynophagia is frequently so severe that the patients are forced to spit out their saliva. A so-called "hot potato voice" is characteristic, though this can also occur in severe tonsillitis and epiglottitis. A history of previous PTA ("throat infection requiring drainage of pus") should be sought. Fever, tachycardia, and signs of dehydration are common, as is marked ipsilateral cervical lymphadenopathy. Examination of the oropharynx will reveal a unilateral erythematous soft palate with deviation of the uvula away from the abscess. Soft palate asymmetry and uvular deviation are key findings (see Figure 20.2). Severe trismus may hamper the examination, and analgesia and sedation may be required in

order to fully visualize the oropharynx. Cases of bilateral PTA have been described.

Differential Diagnosis

The main differential diagnosis includes infectious tonsilopharyngitis, peritonsillar cellulitis, and PTA. All of the other serious causes of sore throat, discussed above under pharyngitis, should be considered.

Laboratory and Radiographic Findings

Blood tests are not routinely required for evaluation of possible PTA. A leukocytosis would be expected on CBC. A lateral soft tissue X-ray of the neck can be obtained if epiglottitis or RPA remain a concern after the physical exam.

In most cases, following physical exam, the main diagnostic issue is distinguishing peritonsillar cellulitis from PTA, and localizing the PTA for drainage. CT scan with contrast is considered the gold standard modality for diagnosing and locating PTAs. Its advantage is that it shows spread to adjacent deep neck spaces, while disadvantages include expense, risk of radiation and contrast nephropathy, and requirement that patients lie supine in an unmonitored setting. Bedside intraoral ultrasound has emerged as a useful alternative to CT, particularly for confirming presence of, and locating, a pus pocket (see Figure 20.2). A high frequency intracavitary probe is used. However, ultrasound is dependent on the skill of the sonographer. Some experts advocate using ultrasound as an adjunct to exam in all cases, while others reserve it for after an unsuccessful aspiration attempt.

Treatment and Prophylaxis

Most experts agree that young children with peritonsillar cellulitis versus PTA should be admitted, treated with parenteral antibiotics, and observed. Treatment of PTA in adults involves drainage, adjunctive antibiotics, and analgesia. There are multiple ways to accomplish each of these. Our preferred approach is as follows (see Table 20.5). Topical lidocaine, delivered by nebulized mist or atomizer, is the most important form of analgesia. For patients that are very anxious and uncooperative, anxiolysis and additional analgesia can be administered and titrated parenterally. Midazolam is a good choice and may partially relieve trismus. Yankauer suction is used to manage secretions, and a laryngoscope with a small Macintosh blade is the best light source (see Figure 20.3). We recommend that cooperative patients hold both of these themselves. We prefer aspiration to incision. This is done with a 10 cc syringe attached to either an 18 gauge needle or 18 or 20 gauge, 3.5 inch spinal needle, which allows the syringe to remain outside the mouth. In either case, the needle guard is cut and replaced so that only 1.5 cm of needle is showing. For blind aspiration, we aspirate at three points in a line along a superior inferior axis, keeping the needle pointed slightly medial of the sagittal plane. After successful drainage, patients should be able to gargle, drink, and take oral medications before discharge.

Adjunctive antibiotics are mandatory and should be active against GAS, *S. aureus*, and anaerobes. Adjunctive glucocorticoids

Table 20.5 Clinical Features and Treatment: Peritonsillar Abscess

Pathogens	GAS Oral *Streptococcus sp.* *F. necrophorum* *S. aureus*
Signs and symptoms	Unilateral pain and odynophagia Fever Unilateral soft palate swelling Uvula deviation
Laboratory and radiographic findings	CT scan with contrast – shows abscess, spread to adjacent spaces, IJ thrombus Bedside intraoral ultrasound – confirms and locates hypoechoic abscess cavity
Treatment	Analgesia and anxiolysis as needed Topical lidocaine mist Aspiration or incision and drainage **Antibiotics:** Oral: Amoxicillin-clavulanate 875/125 mg PO BID × 14 days *or* Clindamycin 300 mg PO QID × 14 days Parenteral: Ampicillin-sulbactam 3 g IV every 6 hours, or Clindamycin 600 mg IV every 8 hours Consider: dexamethasone 10 mg PO/IV/IM × 1

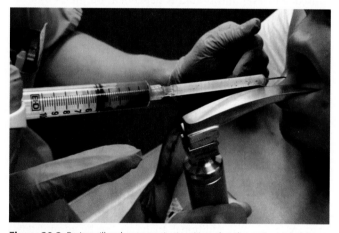

Figure 20.3 Peritonsillar abscess aspiration. Note that the patient is holding the laryngoscope light source and that the plastic sheath on the 20 gauge spinal needle has been trimmed to expose 2 cm of the needle.

are recommended for most patients with PTA, in the same dose as for severe tonsillitis.

Complications and Admission Criteria

There is a long list of potential complications of PTA, all very uncommon. Infection can spread into the adjacent parapharyngeal space and carotid sheath, causing Lemiere's syndrome, nerve involvement, and airway compromise. A ruptured PTA can lead to aspiration pneumonia.

Most adolescents and adults with PTA can be managed as outpatients, with close follow-up. If peritonsillar cellulitis is strongly suspected, initial treatment with antibiotics alone and follow-up in 24 to 48 hours is reasonable. For young children, admission and urgent otolaryngology consultation is recommended.

Pearls and Pitfalls

1. Always consider potentially life-threatening, non-pharyngitis cases of sore throat.
2. Red flags include: preference for the sniffing position, respiratory difficulty, trismus, and a normal-appearing oropharynx.
3. Antibiotics tend to be overused for pharyngitis; in adults, always use a clinical decision rule, and RADT if indicated, to limit the use of empiric antibiotics for GAS.
4. In the right setting, consider *N. gonorrhea* and acute primary HIV infection.
5. Exudative pharyngitis and posterior cervical adenopathy in an adolescent strongly suggests mononucleosis (EBV).
6. Always consider PTA in the setting of unilateral pharyngeal swelling, especially if there is deviation of the uvula.

References

Bulloch, B., Kabani, A., and Tenenbein, M. Oral dexamethasone for the treatment of pain in children with acute pharyngitis: a randomized, double-blind, placebo-controlled trial. *Ann. Emerg. Med.* 2003; 41(5): 601–8.

Cooper, R., Hoffman, J., Bartlett, G., *et al.* Principles of appropriate antibiotic use for acute pharyngitis in adults: background. *Ann. Intern. Med.* 2001; 134: 509–17.

Costantino, T. G., Satz, W. A., Dehnkamp, W., and Goett, H. Randomized trial comparing intraoral ultrasound to landmark-based needle aspiration in patients with suspected peritonsillar abscess. *Acad. Emerg. Med.* 2012; 19(6): 626–31.

Ebell, M. H., Smith, M. A., Barry, H. C., *et al.* The rational clinical examination. Does this patient have strep throat? *JAMA* 2000; 284(22): 2912–18.

Luhmann, J. D., Kennedy, R. M., McAllister, J. D., *et al.* Sedation for peritonsillar abscess drainage in the pediatric emergency department. *Pediatr. Emerg. Care* 2002; 18(1): 1–3.

Shulman, S., Bisno, A., Clegg, H., *et al.* Clinical practice guideline for the diagnosis and management of group A streptococcal pharyngitis: 2012 update by the Infectious Diseases Society of America. *Clin. Infect. Dis.* 2014; 58(10): 1496.

Deep Neck Space Infections

Christopher Hahn and Bradley W. Frazee

Introduction

The oropharynx and neck contain a variety of fascial planes that create a network of potential spaces. These deep neck spaces include the submandibular, peritonsillar, parapharyngeal, retropharyngeal, and prevertebral. If these spaces are seeded by bacteria, infection may travel to vital structures such as the jugular vein, mediastinum, and airway.

This chapter covers several neck space infections. The most important of these is bilateral submandibular space infection, or Ludwig's angina. Peritonsillar abscess and parotitis are covered in Chapter 20 and retropharyngeal space infection (retropharyngeal abscess) in children is discussed further in Chapter 54. Also covered in this chapter is suppurative thrombophlebitis of the internal jugular vein, or Lemierre's syndrome. While relatively uncommon in the post-antibiotic era, infections like Ludwig's angina and Lemierre's syndrome can progress rapidly to life-threatening complications, including airway compromise, mediastinitis, and septicemia. Awareness and thorough understanding of these infections by emergency providers is required for rapid diagnosis and correct management.

Deep Neck Space Infections

Epidemiology and Microbiology

Peritonsillar abscess (see Chapter 20) is typically a complication of pharyngitis, occurs most often in teenagers and young adults, and is by far the most common deep neck space infection. The incidence is estimated to be 30 per 100,000 persons per year. Retropharyngeal abscess is primarily an infection of young children following upper respiratory infections (see Chapter 54, Pediatric Respiratory Infections), though it can occur in adults.

Odontogenic deep neck space infections, like dental caries, are seen in all age groups. The overall incidence has decreased significantly since the widespread use of antibiotics. Prevertebral space infections are typically associated with cervical spine osteomyelitis, paraspinous infection, or esophageal or tracheal instrumentation. Injection drug use (i.e. injecting, or attempting to inject) into neck veins also predisposes to neck infections.

Infections located in the deep structures of the neck are usually caused by bacteria that colonize or infect the oral cavity and upper aerodigestive tract. Dental flora include Streptococcal species, *Corynybacteria Lactobacilis*, and anaerobes such as *Peptostreptococcus*, *Fusobacterium*, *Provetella*, and *Actinomyces*. Increasingly, these organisms produce beta-lactamase. Respiratory flora include *Streptococcus pyogenes*, *Staphylococcus aureus*, and *Haemophilus* species. Very often, deep neck space infections are polymicrobial. Gram-negative rods such as *Klebsiella* and *Pseudomonas aeruginosa* have also been isolated and should be considered in immunocompromised hosts. In prevertebral space infections, which are unique from a microbiologic standpoint, the most common etiologic pathogen is *S. aureus*.

Clinical Features

The clinical features of a particular deep neck space infection reflect the anatomy of the space involved (see Table 21.1). However, these features are both non-specific and often subtle or absent, requiring the clinician to maintain a high index of suspicion.

Parapharyngeal Space

The parapharyngeal space extends from the hyoid bone to the skull base. The space is bound by the peritonsillar space

Table 21.1 Deep Neck Space Infections

Pathogens

Staphylococcus spp.
Streptococcus spp.
Bacteroides
Prevotella
Fusobacterium
Peptostreptococcus
Porphyromonas
Actinomyces
Eikenella
Klebsiella

Signs and symptoms

- Fever and rigors
- Trismus
- Neck swelling
- Sore throat
- Muffled voice
- Neck stiffness
- Odynophagia
- Neck pain
- Dyspnea
- Dysphagia
- Tongue elevation
- Drooling

(separated from it by the superior constrictor muscle), posteriorly by the retropharyngeal space, inferiorly by the carotid sheath and its contents, and medially by the submandibular space. Infection of the parapharyngeal space may be associated with a recent tonsillitis, peritonsillar infection, or dental infection. These precipitating infections are often minor in severity and may resolve by the time infection of the parapharyngeal space develops. In addition to pain, dysphagia, and odynophagia, the patient may also have ipsilateral otalgia, trismus, a muffled voice, and neck stiffness. Parapharyngeal space infections are potentially life-threatening because they can cause airway compromise and rapidly infect adjacent vital structures (see Complications and Admission Criteria, below).

Retropharyngeal Space

Retropharyngeal infections in adults may be odontogenic or develop from pharyngitis or penetrating trauma from a swallowed bone. These infections can be life-threatening as this space communicates with the "danger space," which extends from the base of the skull to the diaphragm and the mediastinum. Sore throat, neck pain, odynophagia, and dysphagia are common presenting signs and symptoms. Neck stiffness due to the irritation of the prevertebral fascia may mimic that of meningitis.

Prevertebral Space

The prevertebral space lies between the vertebral bodies and the prevertebral fascia and extends from the base of the skull to the coccyx. Infections of this space are difficult to diagnose as many patients may not have fever, neck, or back pain or any signs or symptoms of neurologic compromise. Complications of prevertebral space infections include epidural abscess with

paralysis, local destruction and mechanical instability of the spine, and contiguous spread of infection to the psoas muscle sheath leading to psoas muscle abscesses.

Submandibular Space

The submandibular space consists of the sublingual space and the submylohyoid space, which are separated by the mylohyoid muscle. These subdivisions should be conceptually thought of as one unit, however, as they directly communicate posteriorly around the mylohyoid muscle. In patients with suspected submandibular space infection, a thorough dental exam is warranted as odontogenic infections are the most common source. Other less common sources include submandibular sialadenitis, pharyngo-tonsillar infections, traumatic injury, and secondary spread from lateral pharyngeal and parotid space infection.

Ludwig's angina is a specific form of submandibular space infection defined as a bilateral, rapidly progressive cellulitis. It classically presents with erythema and edema under the chin, and induration of the floor of the mouth, which may progress to such an extent that the tongue is displaced posteriorly, potentially resulting in airway obstruction and death (see Figure 21.1). Patients frequently have dysphagia, dyspnea, and difficulty handling secretions. Intubation is challenging because the tongue edema makes it difficult to visualize the vocal folds. Advanced airway techniques such as awake nasal or orotracheal fiberoptic intubation or specialty consultation for surgical airway may be necessary.

Submandibular space infections can present atypically and may meet the classic criteria for Ludwig's angina. Although some degree of neck swelling is almost always seen, other signs and symptoms such as neck pain, dysphagia, odynophagia, dysphonia, dyspnea, fever, and trismus can be absent. Predictors of life-threatening complications include bilateral submandibular involvement, diabetes, and other associated comorbid illness, as well as involvement of the anterior visceral space, which contains the trachea and extends to the superior mediastinum.

Differential Diagnosis

The differential diagnosis associated with deep neck space infections includes other infections of the head and neck such as tonsillitis, sinusitis, and particularly routine dental infections presenting with swelling and trismus. The neck stiffness seen in deep neck space infections that irritate the prevertebral fascia may mimic meningitis. Fever and otalgia can suggest otitis media and otitis externa. Supraglottitis and epiglottitis may also present with drooling, odynophagia, and muffled voice. Trauma from foreign-body ingestion or from injection of illicit drugs may also present with similar symptoms. "Cold" infections such as tuberculosis, and cancer of the neck, may, in some cases, present similarly. Extrapulmonary tuberculosis may rarely present as a deep neck or retropharyngeal abscess.

Laboratory and Radiographic Findings

Diagnosis of deep neck space infections is generally made by physical exam in conjunction with imaging. The constellation

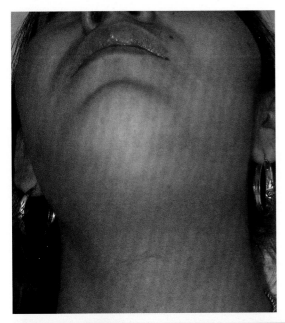

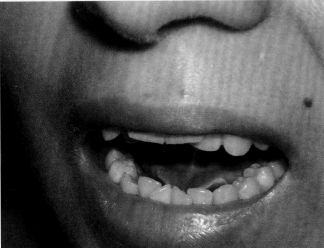

Figure 21.1 Ludwig's angina Submandibular erythema (A); Trismus and indurated, raised floor of the mouth (B).

of signs and symptoms discussed above can point to the particular deep neck space that is likely involved.

Peritonsillar abscess is the one neck space infection that does not require an X-ray, though bedside ultrasound can be useful in many cases (see Chapter 20). In retropharyngeal abscess, plain soft tissue neck X-rays can demonstrate prevertebral swelling. Computed tomography with contrast, however, is the imaging modality of choice in the vast majority of these infections. Although it typically demonstrates a rim-enhancing fluid-filled collection in the affected space, radiologic differentiation between abscess and phlegmon can prove difficult (see Figure 21.1). In early infection, fat stranding and asymmetry in the fascial planes of the neck may be the only findings. Concomitant tonsillitis, sinusitis, dental infection, or evidence of a recent trauma or procedure, may also be noted.

A complete blood count (CBC) may demonstrate a leukocytosis. Blood cultures should be obtained if the patient is febrile. Surgical cultures of the affected fluid may reveal the offending organisms, and subsequent sensitivities may guide antimicrobial selection.

Treatment and Prophylaxis

Infection typically begins as a cellulitis that causes local tissue destruction without formation of a discrete abscess. During this phase, medical therapy with intravenous antibiotics is the primary treatment with the goal of preventing local and systemic spread. As deep neck infections are commonly caused by a mix of pathogens, many of which produce beta-lactamase, broad-spectrum antibiotics with both aerobic and anaerobic coverage is indicated. Appropriate choices include ampicillin–sulbactam or piperacillin–tazobactam. Clindamycin may be considered in patients with penicillin allergy.

Without discrete abscess formation, surgical intervention may be harmful as it can damage natural barriers and allow further spread of infection. Immediate incision and drainage is indicated, however, when there is a well-formed abscess. The procedure is both diagnostic and therapeutic. While peritonsillar abscesses can usually be drained transorally at the bedside in the emergency department or clinic, all other deep neck space abscesses are drained in the operating room. Protection of the airway may require intubation, or even a tracheotomy. Parapharyngeal neck infections and Ludwig's angina are usually drained through the neck in the operating room, sometimes with a concomitant tracheotomy for airway control.

In Ludwig's angina, adjunctive therapy with dexamethasone reduces swelling and may decrease length of hospital stay and need for surgical airway intervention. Intubation is challenging because the tongue edema makes it difficult to visualize the vocal folds, and advanced techniques, such as awake nasal or orotracheal fiberoptic intubation, are often required, or a surgical airway may be necessary.

Complications and Admission Criteria

The most important potential complication is airway compromise. Local complications include necrotizing fasciitis and mediastinitis. Other complications include aspiration pneumonia from impaired swallowing, meningitis, septic shock, and death.

Lemierre's Syndrome

Lemierre's syndrome is septic thrombophlebitis of the internal jugular vein (IJ) with bacteremia, which is often precipitated by a preceding pharyngitis. Lungs, sinuses, middle ear, mastoids, and teeth are less common primary sources of infection. Primary infection gains access to the internal jugular vein by local invasion of the lateral pharyngeal space, which is contiguous with the carotid sheath. The IJ thrombophlebitis commonly leads to metastatic infection, most frequently affecting the lungs, followed by major joints. Much of the literature is in the form of case series that highlight rare presentations involving other organs including the liver, pericardium, brain, muscle, and skin.

Epidemiology and Microbiology

Otherwise healthy adolescents, young adults, and children are most commonly affected, but Lemierre's syndrome has been seen in all age groups. Previously considered a very rare entity, it is now estimated to have an annual incidence of 14.4 and 1.4 per million per year in age groups 15 to 24 and over 40, respectively. Central venous catheters have also been associated with Lemierre's as they provide a nidus for infection.

Fusobacterium necrophorum, a gram-negative anaerobic rod that is part of the normal flora of the oropharynx, is the causative organism in most cases. While development of Lemierre's syndrome is rare, pharyngitis due to *Fusobacterium necrophorum* is relatively common, accounting for 10% of cases in young adults and up to 21% cases of recurrent pharyngitis. The emergence of *Fusobacterium* pharyngitis may account for an apparent rise in Lemierre's syndrome. *Fusobacterium* may be unique in promoting platelet aggregation and thrombosis. Other oropharyngeal flora also have been implicated, including *Eikenella*, Streptococcal species, and *Bacteroides*, and the associated bacteremia is polymicrobial in up to one-third of cases (see Table 21.2).

Clinical Features

Lemierre's syndrome should be considered whenever a patient has prolonged symptoms of pharyngitis or in cases of pharyngitis followed by systemic illness, respiratory complaints, or lateral neck pain. History and physical should focus on head and neck complaints, along with looking for evidence of metastatic infection, primarily in the lungs.

The most common symptom is a sore throat, which may precede other findings by several days and may even resolve before other symptoms develop. Other symptoms include otalgia, dysphagia, dental pain, and neck swelling, which is typically unilateral. As the lungs are the most common site of metastatic infection, patients may present with cough, hemoptysis, dyspnea, and pleuritic chest pain.

Physical exam findings vary and may include signs of pharyngitis/peritonsillar abscess, trismus, and anterior cervical lymphadenopathy. Fever is nearly universal. Neck tenderness and swelling is common, but its absence does not rule out the disease. For unclear reasons, patients with Lemierre's may also be jaundiced. Exam may also reveal evidence of metastatic infection such as pneumonia or less commonly signs of septic arthritis.

Differential Diagnosis

Viral upper respiratory infections also cause sore throat, myalgias, fever, and cough. Identifying Lemierre's syndrome when faced with this constellation can be challenging, though critical to prevent life-threatening complications. Deep space infections of the neck may cause similar symptoms of fever, sore throat, neck pain, and swelling. See Differential Diagnosis for additional diagnoses to consider. In addition, suppurative lymphadenitis and mycotic aneurysms of the carotid artery can cause unilateral neck pain and swelling. Right-sided

Table 21.2 Suppurative Thrombophlebitis of the Internal Jugular Vein (Lemierre's Syndrome)

Pathogens

Fusobacterium necrophorum
Prevotella spp.
Bacteroides spp.
Peptostreptococcus spp.
Propionibacterium spp.
Streptococcus spp.

Signs and symptoms

- Sore throat
- High fever and rigors
- Unilateral anterior neck pain, tenderness, and swelling
- Otalgia
- Dyspnea and cough
- Pleuritic chest pain

Laboratory and radiographic findings

- Blood culture growth of the offending pathogen (most commonly *Fusobacterium necrophorum*)
- Contrast CT demonstrating IJ thrombosis
- Chest X-ray showing nodular opacities, cavitary lesions, or pleural effusion

Treatment

- Ampicillin-sulbactam 3 g IV every 6 hours
- Piperacillin-tazobactam 4.5 g IV every 6 hours
- Clindamycin 600 mg IV every 6–8 hours
- Ertapenem 1 g IV every 24 hours
- Third-generation cephalosporin plus metronidazole (i.e. Ceftriaxone 1 g IV every 24 hours plus metronidazole 500 mg IV every 6–8 hours)
- Add vancomycin if catheter-associated (15–20 mg/kg/dose IV every 8–12 hours, max. 2 g per dose)
- Management of local and metastatic infection
- Anticoagulation and/or surgical intervention should be considered for failure to improve

endocarditis can cause septic pulmonary emboli, while left-sided endocarditis can cause systemic metastatic infection. Pneumonia is a common cause of pleuritic chest pain, cough, fever, and respiratory distress. Non-infectious pulmonary emboli can cause pulmonary infarct, hemoptysis, dyspnea, and pleuritic chest pain.

Laboratory and Radiographic Findings

Other than growth of causative organisms from blood culture, which is critical to the diagnosis, laboratory studies are non-specific in Lemierre's and play little role in making the diagnosis. Due to the high proportion of patients with septic pulmonary emboli, chest x-ray is an important diagnostic study in suspected Lemierre's. Initially, it may demonstrate non-specific nodular infiltrates, which can progress to cavitary lesions with associated pleural effusion. These chest X-ray findings may initially mislead the practitioner toward a diagnosis of pneumonia or right-sided endocarditis. Although ultrasound and MRI can be used to image the IJ thrombus, contrast-enhanced CT imaging showing vein opacification is the preferred modality as it is readily available and able to identify abnormalities in surrounding structures. Fluid culture from a site of metastatic infection, such as arthrocentesis of a septic joint, also may identify the offending pathogen.

Treatment and Prophylaxis

Prolonged therapy with antibiotics is the mainstay of treatment. A total duration of 4 to 6 weeks is necessary in order to adequately penetrate and sterilize the thrombus. Appropriate empiric regimens include ampicillin–sulbactam, piperacillin-tazobactam, clindamycin, or carbapenem monotherapy. A third-generation cephalosporin plus metronidazole is also appropriate. Penicillin monotherapy is not recommended because *Fusobacterium necrophorum* may produce beta-lactamase and a substantial proportion of infections are polymicrobial. In cases of Lemierre's syndrome associated with IJ central venous catheters, the catheter should be removed and antibiotic therapy should include vancomycin to cover MRSA and coagulase negative *S. aureus*.

The use of anticoagulation is controversial, with no controlled trials. Anticoagulation should be considered in cases of thrombus extension or if the patient fails to improve with antibiotic therapy alone. Drainage of adjacent deep neck space abscesses, such as peritonsillar or parapharyngeal abscesses, is often indicated. Internal jugular ligation or excision can be considered in cases of ongoing septic embolization or failure to improve despite appropriate antimicrobial therapy. There are no controlled studies comparing surgical interventions in Lemierre's. Treatment of metastatic infection may require incision and drainage, joint washout, or empyema drainage by thoracentesis or chest tube placement.

Complications and Admission Criteria

Local invasion can lead to deep neck space cellulitis and abscess. As Lemierre's is a right-sided (venous system) infection, metastatic disease most commonly affects the lungs. Less frequently metastatic infection involves the systemic circulation, causing a broad array of complications potentially involving nearly every organ system. Pulmonary complications include lung abscess, pneumonia, empyema, hemothorax, pneumothorax, and acute respiratory distress syndrome (ARDS). Left-sided metastatic infections that have been reported in the setting of Lemierre's syndrome include stroke, meningitis, epidural/subdural abscess, cranial nerve palsies, carotid sheath abscess, hepatic/splenic abscess or infarct, pustular skin lesions, osteomyelitis, gangrene, muscle abscesses, septic arthritis, uveitis, retrobulbar mass, vitreous hemorrhage, septic shock, and death. Clot

extension from the internal jugular vein can also cause cavernous, transverse, lateral, and sigmoid sinus thrombosis.

Pearls and Pitfalls

1. Management of the airway is the first priority.
2. Infections of the floor of the mouth should always raise concern for Ludwig's angina and rapid progression to airway compromise.
3. Lemierre's syndrome should be suspected in cases of prolonged fever and sore throat that fail to respond to standard pharyngitis treatment.
4. Neck stiffness due to infection or irritation of the prevertebral fascia may mimic meningitis.
5. CT with contrast is the imaging study of choice for identification and staging of all deep neck space infections.

References

Boscolo-Rizzo, P. and Da Mosto, M. C. Submandibular space infection: a potentially lethal infection. *Int. J. Infect. Dis.* 2009; 13(3): 327–33.

Eilbert, W. and Singla, N. Lemierre's syndrome. *Int. J. Emerg. Med.* 2013; 6(1): 40.

Marioni, G., Rinaldi, R., Staffieri, C., *et al.* Deep neck infection with dental origin: analysis of 85 consecutive cases (2000–2006). *Acta Oto-Laryngologica* 2008; 128(2): 201–6.

Hagelskjaer, K. L. and Prag, J. Lemierre's syndrome and other disseminated Fusobacterium necrophorum infections in Denmark: a prospective epidemiological and clinical survey. *Euro. J. Clin. Microbiol. Infect. Dis.* 2008; 27(9): 779–89.

Karkos, P. D., Asrani, S., Karkos, C. D., *et al.* Lemierre's syndrome: a systematic review. *Laryngoscope* 2009; 119(8): 1552–9.

Reynolds, S. C. and Chow, A. W. Severe soft tissue infections of the head and neck: a primer for critical care physicians. *Lung* 2009; 187(5): 271.

Smith, J. L., Hsu, J. M., and Chang, J. Predicting deep neck space abscess using computed tomography. *Am. J. Otolaryngol.* 2006; 27(4): 244–7.

Srirompotong, S. and Art-Smart, T. Ludwig's angina: a clinical review. *Eur. Arch. Otorhinolaryngol.* 2003; 260(7): 401–3.

Tan, Z. L., Nagaraja, T. G., and Chengappa, M. M. Fusobacterium necrophorum infections: virulence factors, pathogenic mechanism and control measures. *Vet. Res. Commun.* 1996; 20(2): 113–40.

Wang, L. F., Tai, C. F., Kuo, W. R., and Chien, C. Y. Predisposing factors of complicated deep neck infections: 12-year experience at a single institution. *J. Otolaryngol. Head Neck Surg.* 2010; 39(4): 335–41.

Chapter 22

Dental and Odontogenic Infections

Bradley W. Frazee

Introduction

Infections that arise from the tooth or closely surrounding tissues are referred to as odontogenic. Most dentoalveolar and odontogenic infections are related to dental caries, which is considered the most common chronic infectious disease in the world. These infections range from simple toothache due to pulpitis to severe submandibular and deep neck space infections, which have the potential to compromise the airway. Other complications include tooth loss and infectious endocarditis.

Owing to the often acute onset of severe pain and lack of immediate access to a dentist, these infections are an extremely common problem in acute care medicine, accounting for more than 1% of emergency department (ED) visits in the United States. Practitioners should have a solid understanding of the various types of infections, their initial management, and the complications to look out for. Deep neck space infections, frequently odontogenic in origin, are discussed further in Chapter 21.

Dentoalveolar Infections

Epidemiology, Pathophysiology, and Microbiology

Dentoalveolar infections are common in the general population, afflicting 40% of children by age 6 and 85% by age 17. The incidence approaches 100% by age 45. Fortunately, the

incidence of secondary odontogenic infections has declined with the use of antibiotics, as has their morbidity and mortality. For example, though deep mandibular space abscesses, or Ludwig's angina, still represent 13% of the deep space infections of the neck, their mortality has declined from greater than 50% in the 1940s to approximately 5% currently. Patients with dentoalveolar infections present to the acute care setting with a spectrum of disease ranging from pulpitis to periapical abscesses to deep mandibular space abscesses.

The persistent presence of dental plaque leads to caries and breakdown of the enamel and dentin layers that protect the dental pulp. Once the pulp is exposed, bacteria cause inflammation, termed pulpitis, and subsequent necrosis. The primary pathogen in dental caries and pulpitis is *Streptococcus mutans*, which, in a carbohydrate-rich environment, is both acidogenic and able to survive at a low pH. In pulpitis, infection and inflammation is confined to structures within the tooth canal. Inflammation alone leads to sensitivity, but and once significant swelling occurs within a rigid canal, ischemia ensues and pain becomes spontaneous and more unremitting. Ischemia and necrosis of pulp tissue is referred to as irreversible pulpitis. Thermal, chemical, and traumatic injuries are other causes of pulpitis.

Periapical abscesses are formed as the pulpal abscess erodes out of the tooth canal and decompresses through the apex of the tooth. The abscess may point toward the gingival surface, the alveolar ridge, facial planes of the face, or decompress into oral cavity. Associated periapical periodontitis may lead to loosening of the tooth. Although the initial bacterial pathogen may be *Streptococcus mutans*, mature abscesses are polymicrobial and contain other *Streptoccus* species, *Prevotella*, *Fusobacterium*, *Actinomyces*, and others.

Deep mandibular space infections (also discussed in Chapter 21) are more serious odontogenic infections that occur with decompression of the necrotic dental pulp into the sublingual, submandibular, and submental potential spaces adjacent to the mandible. Infections of the submental space are due to periapical abscesses of the anterior mandibular teeth that decompress below the insertion of the mentalis muscle. Of the three potential spaces, infection of the submental space is the least serious and least likely to communicate with other spaces. Submandibular space and sublingual infections arise from periapical abscesses of the mandibular molars. Submandibular (or submylohyoid) infection occurs when the abscess perforates below the mylohyoid muscle, whereas sublingual infection begins when the abscess perforates above the mylohyoid muscle; however, infection can spread easily between these two potential spaces. Deep mandibular space infections are invariably due to mixed bacteria, including *Streptococcus*, *Actinomyces*, and β-lactamase producing gram-negative anaerobes such as *Bacteroides fragilis* and *Prevotella intermedia*.

Clinical Features

Pulpitis

Pulpitis is the most common type of toothache (see Table 22.1). It is typically accompanied by thermal sensitivity. Spontaneous pain that lasts for minutes to hours or awakens the patient suggests irreversible pulpitis. On physical exam, patients with pulpitis have carious teeth with no more than mild tenderness to percussion. There is no evidence of swelling or fluctuance on the buccal or lingual gingiva.

Periapical Abscess

Patients with a periapical abscess present with pain and thermal sensitivity in a carious tooth that is persistent and well localized. On clinical exam, periapical abscess is distinguished from pulpitis by the presence of exquisite tenderness of the affected tooth to percussion with a tongue blade. The tooth may be loose. The buccal or lingual gingiva supporting the tooth will be swollen and erythematous and may have an area of fluctuance or pointing. There may be mild facial swelling, but significant trismus is uncommon.

Deep Mandibular Space Abscess

Patients with deep mandibular space infections, including the submental, submandibular, and sublingual spaces, may be febrile and have cervical lymphadenopathy. Some degree of trismus and pain with swallowing may be present with any of these, but when severe, these signs suggest submandibular or sublingual space infections.

Patients with submental space infections present with pain and swelling extending from the chin posteriorly to the hyoid bone. Patients should not complain of difficulty breathing, the presence of which suggests the infection has extended posteriorly into the submandibular space.

Submandibular and sublingual infections present with pain and swelling beneath the inferior border of the mandible. Trismus, difficulty swallowing secretions, and drooling are common. These infections present a risk for airway compromise, particularly when the sublingual space is involved and when bilateral. Physical exam reveals submandibular edema extending posteriorly onto the neck. If only the submandibular space is involved the tongue should not be elevated from the floor of the mouth; however, communication with the sublingual space is common. In sublingual space infections, swelling is located under the tongue, so the tongue appears elevated and slightly protuberant between the teeth. Many of these patients have an element of airway compromise and may need emergent airway control, preferably in the operating room.

Ludwig's angina refers to a bilateral necrotizing infection of the sublingual and submandibular spaces, which can descend into the mediastinum (see also Chapter 21). Patients present with pain, trismus, and drooling. They may have difficulty breathing and a preference for the tripod position. Bilateral swelling, brawny induration, and tenderness to palpation over the submandibular space is classically described, along with elevation of the tongue. Palpation of the sublingual mucosa will reveal tense induration of that space. Rapid progression to airway compromise can occur. This life-threatening form of submandibular space infection is discussed further in Chapter 21.

Differential Diagnosis

- Pulpitis is distinguished by mild focal tenderness to tooth percussion and no gingival swelling.
- Periapical abscess is distinguished by significant tenderness to tooth percussion, tooth loosening, gingival swelling, and facial swelling.
- Deep mandibular space infections cause swelling below the jaw; the four types of infections can be distinguished as follows:

  ○ submental infection is distinguished by swelling primarily over the chin without elevation of the tongue or respiratory difficulty
  ○ submandibular infection is distinguished by lack of tongue elevation or respiratory difficulty
  ○ sublingual infection is distinguished by severe trismus and drooling, with elevation of the tongue above the floor of the mouth
  ○ Ludwig's angina is distinguished by bilateral findings, tense edema under the chin, elevation of the tongue, and difficulty breathing

Laboratory and Radiographic Findings

There is little role for blood tests in dentoalveolar infections. Diagnosis is based primarily on imaging, with specialized

Table 22.1 Dentoalveolar Infections: Clinical Features and Treatment

Pathogens	S. mutans	
	S. milleri	
	Other Streptococcus	
	Prevotella species	
	Fusobacterium species	
	Actinomyces	
	Others	
Signs and symptoms	Pulpitis	Cold sensitivity
		Toothache
		Tooth tenderness
	Periapical abscess	Toothache
		Gingival swelling
		Loose tooth
		Facial swelling
	Deep mandibular space infections	Drooling
		Trismus
		Swelling and erythema below mandible
		Elevation of floor of mouth
Radiographic features	Bone lucency on periapical dental X-ray	
	Maxillofacial and neck CT scan with contrast identifies deep mandibular space abscess	
Treatment – pulpitis	Root canal	
	NSAID for analgesia	
	Antibiotics likely not efficacious	
	If antibiotics used:	
	Penicillin VK 500 mg PO TID for 7 days	
Treatment – periapical abscess	Root canal	
	Incision and drainage of pointing abscess	
	Extraction	
	Nerve block	
	NSAID analgesia	
	Antibiotics used for significant cellulitis (facial swelling, trismus):	
	Amoxicillin-clavulanate 500 mg PO TID for 7 days	
	or	
	Clindamycin 300 mg PO QID for 7 days	
Treatment – mandibular space infection	Management by an oral surgeon	
	Surgical drainage of well-formed abscess	
	Ampicillin-sulbactam 3 g IV every 6 hours	
	or	
	Penicillin G 4 million units IV every 6 hours plus metronidazole 500 mg every 8 hours	
	or	
	Clindamycin 600 mg IV every 8 hours	

dental X-rays and CT scanning (see Table 22.1). In pulpitis, dental bite-wing radiographs may show caries invading the pulp. Dental periapical radiographs may demonstrate a bone radiolucency in periapical abscess. As these radiographs are not available in most acute care settings, initial diagnosis is generally made on clinical examination with definitive imaging carried out in a dental clinic.

In deep mandibular space infections, if blood tests are obtained, WBC and ESR and CRP will be elevated. Maxillofacial and neck CT with contrast is required to delineate location and extent of the abscess. Acute care providers should maintain a low threshold for CT scanning in the setting of suspected deep mandibular space infection. However, these patients require careful airway assessment prior to CT.

Treatment and Prophylaxis

Patients presenting to the emergency department for severe, persistent toothache from pulpitis often have irreversible pulpitis, which generally requires endodonic removal of the nerve (root canal) for definitive treatment (see Table 22.1). These patients need semi-urgent referral to a dentist within 48 to 72 hours to prevent further destruction or loss of the tooth. There is no prospective evidence that antibiotics reduce pain duration or tooth loss in pulpitis without evidence of periapical abscess. Nonetheless, some dentists recommend penicillin or clindamycin to cover *Streptococcus mutans* and *Actinomyces* species. Non-steroidal anti-inflammatory agents (NSAIDs) are preferred for analgesia, with judicious use of acetaminophen-opioid agents as needed.

Patients with periapical abscess require incision and drainage. Such pointing abscesses are most often evident in the buccal sulcus. The area can be anesthetized with local infiltration of anesthetic (bupivacaine with epinephrine or mepivicaine) and by placing gauze impregnated with 5% lidocaine jelly over the abscess site. Mandibular teeth can alternatively be anesthetized with an inferior alveolar nerve block. The incision is made down to bone with either an 18-gauge needle or number 15 blade scalpel for larger abscesses. Such abscesses rarely require drain placement. Patients should follow up with a dentist or oral surgeon within 24 hours. Definitive drainage by a dentist is usually achieved through a root canal. Periapical abscesses are generally treated with adjunctive antimicrobials with activity against beta-lactamase producing oral anaerobes. Choices include amoxicillin-clavulanate or clindamycin. The benefit of antibiotics is questionable in uncomplicated abscesses that undergo prompt drainage, but they are strongly indicated for periapical abscesses complicated by systemic signs, trismus or extraoral swelling, or in immunocompromised patients.

Most patients with deep mandibular space abscesses will require operative incision and drainage. A subset with non-severe disease and lacking a well-formed abscess on CT can be successfully treated with parenteral antibiotics alone and close observation on an inpatient basis. Deep mandibular space infections are polymicrobial, typically due to Streptococcal species, anaerobes such as *Bacteroides fragilis*, and fusobacterium. Many isolates are penicillin resistant. As a result, the antibiotics of choice are extended spectrum penicillins, such as ampicillin-sulbactam or penicillin G plus metronidazole. Clindamycin is the drug of choice for penicillin-allergic patients.

Antibiotic prophylaxis to prevent subsequent infectious endocarditis (IE) in the setting of dentoalveolar infection is now recommended for just a limited group of patients with very high risk: those with a prior history of IE; a prosthetic valve; heart transplant with abnormal valve function; and repaired congenital heart disease. Recommended antibiotics for this indication include amoxicillin, clindamycin, and intramuscular ceftriaxone.

Complications and Admission Criteria

All patients with dentoalveolar infections are at increased risk of tooth loss. Patients with irreversible pulpitis or periapical abscess can often have their teeth saved by root canal treatment and placement of a crown. Tooth extraction is sometimes required for advanced periapical abscess. Deep mandibular space infections generally originate from non-salvageable teeth. Osteomyelitis is a potential complication of all dentoalveolar infections, with an incidence ranging from less than 5% in patients with dental caries to 15 to 20% in patients with deep mandibular space infections. Infectious endocarditis is a possible complication of all dentoalveolar infections, and the risk rises further following a procedure that causes additional bacteremia. Other rare complications include sinusitis, cavernous sinus thrombosis, and brain abscess.

Parapharyngeal space infection is a rare but serious potential complication of mandibular dentoalveolar infections, whether periapical abscess or submandibular abscess. Infection of the parapharyngeal space, in turn, can lead to airway obstruction, septic jugular venous thrombophlebitis (Lemierre's syndrome), and involvement of the carotid sheath (see Chapter 21).

Airway compromise is the primary cause of death in patients with deep mandibular space and parapharyngeal infections. The overall mortality rate remains 5 to 10%. Patients with these infections require thorough and serial evaluation of airway status. A significant proportion of these patients require a surgical airway.

Patients with pulpitis and periapical abscess do not require admission unless there is significant associated cellulitis and delayed access to definitive dental care. Almost all patients with deep mandibular space infection will require admission for airway observation, intravenous antibiotic therapy, rehydration, and operative incision and drainage.

Periodontal Infections
Epidemiology, Pathophysiology, and Microbiology

By age 45, approximately 50% of patients have moderate to severe periodontal disease. Risk factors include diabetes, HIV, smoking, injection drug use, and poor oral hygiene. Periodontal infections are typically associated with a history of gingivitis. The persistence of dental plaque causes gingival recession, exposing the cementum and alveolar bone. The hallmark of periodontitis is loss of alveolar bone and integrity of the periodontal ligament below the gum line. In advanced periodontal disease, pockets form around the tooth resulting in periodontal abscess. Necrotizing periodontitis is an acute form of periodontal disease seen in adolescents and young adults that is closely related to acute necrotizing ulcerative gingivitis (see below).

Healthy gingiva has scant bacterial flora, though what is present is primarily *Streptococcus* and *Actinomyces* species. However, as the gingiva becomes diseased, the absolute bacterial count increases and shifts toward anaerobic gram-negative bacilli, particularly *Prevotella intermedia* and spirochetes.

Clinical Features

Patients with periodontal infections present with onset of localized tooth and gum pain and have a history suggestive of gum disease and periodontitis, such as bleeding gums with brushing (see Table 22.2). On physical exam, the gingiva is swollen and erythematous, but the associated teeth are not tender to percussion (unlike a periapical abscess) and may not have caries. The associated teeth may be mobile due to alveolar bone loss. There may also be purulent discharge surrounding the affected teeth. Isolated periodontal disease is usually an incidental finding, because abscesses in the periodontal pocket generally spontaneously drain through the gingival sulcus.

Table 22.2 Periodontal infections and Acute Necrotizing Ulcerative Gingivitis (ANUG): Clinical Features and Treatment

Pathogens	*Actinomyces*	
	Fusobacterium	
	Bacteroides	
	Prevotella	
	Spirochetes	
Signs and symptoms	Gingivitis, periodontitis	Gum pain
		Gingival bleeding
		Gingival swelling and tenderness
		Loose teeth
	ANUG	Fetid breath
		Fever
		Adenopathy
		Pseudomembrane
Radiographic features	Panoramic x-ray and maxillofacial CT may show alveolar bone loss or osteomyelitis	
Treatment	Incision and drainage of periodontal abscess	
	Chlorhexidine gluconate 0.12% mouth rinse	
	plus	
	Amoxicillin–clavulanate 500 mg PO TID,	
	or	
	Clindamycin 300 mg PO TID	
	or	
	Ampicillin–sulbactam 3 g IV every 6 hours	
	or	
	Clindamycin 600 mg IV every 8 hours	
	May consider "Magic Mouthwash" swish and spit up to 4 times per day as needed for comfort	

Laboratory and Radiographic Findings

As with pulpitis and periapical abscess, specialized dental periapical and bitewing radiographs are used to assess for subtle bone loss in periodontal diseases. Since these radiographs are rarely available in the acute care settings, initial diagnosis is made on clinical grounds and further radiographic evaluation can be carried out in a dental clinic.

Treatment

If spontaneous drainage does not occur, a periodontal abscess should be drained as described above for periapical abscess. Since patients with clinically obvious or symptomatic periodontal infection in the acute care setting will typically have severe disease, they should generally be treated with oral amoxicillin–clavulanate or clindamycin, as well as Peridex (chlorhexidine gluconate 0.12%) mouth rinse. Patients require referral to a dentist within 5 to 7 days for periodontal disease or 2 to 3 days for periodontal abscess.

Pericoronitis

Epidemiology and Microbiology

Pericoronitis is a variant of periodontal infection in which the gingiva overlying a tooth becomes inflamed and painful. In children, it can be associated with erupting primary and secondary dentition. In adults, it usually involves gingiva overlying the crown of an impacted third molar, also known as "operculum." A fragment of food can act as a nidus for infection with anaerobic gram-negative bacilli such as *Prevotella intermedia*. *Streptococcus mutans* and *Actinomyces* species can also cause pericoronitis. Inflammation can spread to muscles of mastication, resulting in trismus.

Clinical Features

Patients may report a history of recurrent pain in the region of concern, limited mouth opening, and pain with chewing or swallowing. On physical exam, there is tenderness, edema, and erythema of the operculum overlying a partially erupted tooth. Occasionally, purulent material and a small amount of food can be expressed from under the flap. There may also be generalized swelling and erythema of the adjacent gingiva, reactive cervical lymphadenopathy, and trismus.

Differential Diagnosis

The differential diagnosis for pericoronitis includes periodontal abscess and benign or malignant soft tissue neoplasm.

Laboratory and Radiographic Findings

Panoramic radiograph will most often reveal an impacted third molar with surrounding bone loss. When there are signs of systemic toxicity and severe trismus, CT scan with contrast should be obtained to rule out parapharyngeal abscess.

Treatment

Most cases are mild and only require curettage and irrigation underneath the operculum to remove any purulent material or trapped food, a procedure that can generally be performed with a topical anesthetic alone. Patients should be discharged with chlorhexidine gluconate 0.12% mouth rinse and advised to follow up with a dentist or oral surgeon in 48 to 72 hours. Extraction of the third molar is the definitive treatment for pericoronitis associated with that tooth.

Complications and Admission Criteria

Rarely, patients may have medial extension of the infection into the deep neck spaces (pterygomandibular, lateral pharyngeal, retropharyngeal, submandibular, sublingual) which can lead to airway obstruction. Patients with severe trismus, facial swelling, or systemic signs of toxicity need urgent evaluation by an oral and maxillofacial surgeon for possible admission and treatment with intravenous antibiotics.

Acute Necrotizing Ulcerative Gingivitis

Epidemiology and Microbiology

Acute necrotizing ulcerative gingivitis (ANUG), or Vincent's angina, was relatively unknown until World War I, when approximately 25% of all troops in the European theater were afflicted, thereby leading to the name trench mouth. This rapidly progressive, necrotizing gum inflammation occurs predominantly in young adults and is correlated with stress, smoking, lack of adequate oral hygiene, and immune suppression, particularly HIV. Although ANUG begins in infected gingiva, it rapidly extends to healthy gingival and dental tissue. *Streptococcus* and *Actinomyces* species are the primary initial pathogens, but as the infection evolves and becomes necrotizing, the microbiologic spectrum expands to include anaerobes like *Bacteroides*, *Prevotella*, *Fusobacterium*, and spirochetes (*Treponema vincenti* and *Borrelia* species). Interestingly, most of these pathogens exist as normal oral flora and develop a fulminant form in the stressed patient.

Clinical Features

Patients present with acute onset of malaise, fever, fetid breath, dysphagia, and generalized mouth pain (see Table 22.2). Physical exam is characterized by cervical lymphadenopathy, hyperemic painful gingiva with erosion of the interdental papillae, and the development of a light gray pseudomembrane over the gingival ulcerations.

Differential Diagnosis

Primary herpetic gingivostomatitis can mimick ANUG in its acuity, pain, and lymphadenopathy.

Laboratory and Radiographic Findings

Patients with ANUG may have an elevated WBC and ESR. Panoramic radiographs or maxillofacial CT scan may delineate the degree of alveolar bone destruction.

Treatment

Most patients can be treated with analgesics, oral rehydration, antibiotics, and close follow-up. Some will need admission for underlying immunosuppression and systemic illness. Preferred oral antibiotics include amoxicillin-clavulanate metronidazole and clindamycin, as well as chlorhexidine gluconate 0.12% mouth rinse and good oral hygiene. For those requiring admission, ampicillin-sulbactam or treatment with "Magic Mouthwash," a mild anesthetic solution composed of equal parts antacid, viscous lidocaine, and diphenhydramine, may offer symptomatic relief.

Complications and Admission Criteria

ANUG causes resorption of the alveolar bone, which ultimately leads to loss of otherwise healthy teeth. The incidence of osteomyelitis of the alveolar ridge and mandible in patients with ANUG is 15 to 20%; therefore, a low threshold for admission should be maintained. Patients with ANUG should be admitted for fever, poorly controlled HIV disease, inability to stay adequately hydrated or take oral antibiotics, or poor access to immediate and ongoing dental care.

Pearls and Pitfalls

1. Mandibular dentoalveolar infections can progress to submandibular space infections and airway compromise.
2. Trismus, drooling, and elevation of the tongue are signs of submandibular infection that require immediate airway assessment and management and consultation with an oral surgeon.
3. Periapical or periodontal abscesses that are visible and pointing should be drained in the emergency department.
4. Antibiotics are typically prescribed by acute care practitioners for acute toothache (pulpitis and periapical abscess), though data showing efficacy is lacking; definitive care (root canal or extraction) requires close dental follow-up.
5. Pericoronitis associated with severe trismus or systemic toxicity suggests infection of the parapharyngeal space, which should be evaluated by CT scan with contrast.
6. Acute necrotizing ulcerative gingivostomatitis is unique in that it presents as diffuse mouth pain; in suspected ANUG, test for HIV and maintain a low threshold for admission.

References

Douglass, A. and Douglass, M. Common dental emergencies. *Am. Fam. Physician* 2003; 67(3): 511–16.

Gottlieb, A. and Khishfe, A. Are antibiotics necessary for dental pain without overt infection? *Ann. Emerg. Med.* 2016; 69(1): 128–30.

Keenan, J., Farman, A., Fedorowicz, Z., *et al.* Antibiotics do not reduce toothache caused by irreversible pulpitis. *Evidence-Based Dentistry* 2005; 6(3): 67.

Kurian, M., Mathew, J., Job, A., *et al.* Ludwig's angina. *Clin. Otolaryngol. Allied Sci.* 1997; 22(3): 263–5.

Moyer, G. P., Millon, J. M., and Martinez-Vidal, A. Is conservative treatment of deep neck space infections appropriate? *Head Neck* 2001; 23(2): 126–33.

Siqueira, J. and Roas, I. Microbiology and treatment of acute apical abscesses. *Clin. Microbio. Rev.* 2013; 26(2): 255–73.

23

Infectious Biliary Diseases: Cholecystitis and Cholangitis

Bryan Darger and Rachel L. Chin

Acute Calculous Cholecystitis

Acute pain of biliary origin is a common problem encountered in the acute care setting. Biliary colic, which is self-limited and can be managed in the outpatient setting, can be difficult to differentiate from acute cholecystitis, involving complete cystic duct obstruction and gallbladder wall inflammation, which requires hospitalization. Acute care providers should be well versed in the initial evaluation and management of this common problem. Bedside ultrasound can be used by acute care providers to rapidly confirm or exclude the diagnosis of cholecystitis.

Epidemiology and Microbiology

The prevalence of gallstones in the general population is approximately 10 to 15%, and is higher in people with the following risk factors: female gender, multiparity, obesity, recent pregnancy, hemolytic diseases (e.g. sickle cell disease). Prevalence also increases with age, approaching 30% in patients over 70 years old. Of people with gallstones, 10 to 20% will develop complications such as biliary colic, cholecystitis, cholangitis, or gallstone pancreatitis.

Acute calculous cholecystitis is defined by sustained obstruction of the cystic duct or neck of the gallbladder with gallstones or sludge. In contrast, biliary colic is pain secondary to transient obstruction of the gallbladder. Acute cholecystitis is primarily a localized acute inflammatory process caused by gallbladder obstruction and subsequent distension, though it is managed as an infection. The pathophysiologic role of bacteria in acute cholecystis remains unknown as the recovery of potential bacterial pathogens does not differ significantly between patients with asymptomatic gallstones and those with acute cholecystitis. *Escherichia coli* and *Klebsiella* species are the most common organisms recovered from an acutely inflamed gallbladder; less common species include *Enterobacter* and *Proteus*.

Clinical Features

Although most patients with acute cholecystitis present with right upper quadrant tenderness, few actually present with the classic triad of fever, right upper quadrant pain, and leukocytosis. The pain of acute cholecystitis may radiate to the back and the right shoulder due to secondary irritation of the diaphragm. Acute cholecystitis can be distinguished from biliary colic by constant pain in the right upper quadrant and the presence of Murphy's sign, defined as inspiration limited by pain on palpation of the right upper quadrant. Tenderness is maximal in the epigastrium in approximately 15% of patients. The presence of fever and leukocytosis in the setting of right upper quadrant pain is specific, but not sensitive for acute cholecystitis (see Table 23.1). Recent studies indicate that the presence of Murphy's sign has high sensitivity (97.2%) and positive predictive value (70%). Other less sensitive physical findings include a palpable gallbladder, jaundice, rebound tenderness, and guarding.

Abnormal laboratory findings, which include elevated liver enzymes, hyperbilirubinemia, and elevated alkaline phosphatase levels, are non-specific for acute cholecystitis, but can direct the work-up for other disease processes. In particular, hyperbilirubinemia and elevated alkaline phosphatase levels may suggest choledocholithiasis or Mirizzi's syndrome, in which the common hepatic or common biliary duct is obstructed by a stone impacted in the cystic duct, the neck of the gallbladder, or Hartmann's pouch.

Table 23.1 Clinical Features: Acute Cholecystitis

Signs and symptoms	• Triad of fever, RUQ pain, leukocytosis (present in only 24% of cases) • Nausea/vomiting and postprandial RUQ pain (often following fatty meal) • Predisposition: female gender, multiparity, obesity, recent pregnancy, sickle cell disease • Majority of patients have gallbladder-associated symptoms prior to the development of acute cholecystitis • Diaphragmatic irritation may lead to right shoulder pain • Murphy's sign (inspiratory arrest during deep palpation over the gallbladder) highly sensitive (97.2%), but less specific (48.3%) • Palpable gallbladder is less frequent physical finding; represents body's effort to wall off the inflamed gallbladder • Rebound tenderness and guarding are less commonly found and indicate peritonitis
Laboratory and radiographic findings	• Elevated WBC, variable elevation of alkaline phosphatase, bilirubin, and transaminases • Hyperbilirubinemia and elevated alkaline phosphatase may suggest common bile duct stones or Mirizzi's syndrome • US: gallstones, edema or pericholecystic fluid, sonographic Murphy's sign; sensitivity >92–95% • Biliary scintigraphy: more expensive, but slightly more sensitive; sensitivity >97% • CT scan has minimal role except to exclude other diagnoses • Biliary scintigraphy is less specific in acalculous cholecystitis, and ultrasonography plays a larger role in diagnosis as does percutaneous cholecystostomy

CT – computed tomography; RUQ – right upper quadrant; US, – ultrasound; WBC – white blood (cell) count.

Differential Diagnosis

The differential diagnosis of upper abdominal pain includes gastrointestinal, cardiac, and pulmonary diseases. These diagnoses are not mutually exclusive – for example, cholangitis and pancreatitis can coexist, both secondary to cholelithiasis.

Key features that may help to distinguish acute cholecystitis from biliary colic are:

- constant right upper quadrant pain, lasting >4 to 6 hours
- positive Murphy's sign (sonographic finding is more reliable than physical exam)
- leukocytosis and fever

Other conditions to consider are:
- Gastrointestinal
  - hepatitis
  - acute cholangitis
  - biliary colic
  - perforated ulcer disease
  - dyspepsia
  - appendicitis
  - diverticulitis
  - acute pancreatitis
  - Fitz-Hugh–Curtis syndrome (perihepatitis caused by gonococcal infection)
  - subhepatic or intra-abdominal abscess
  - black widow spider envenomation
- Urological:
  - pyelonephritis
  - nephrolithiasis
  - renal infarct
- Cardiac:
  - acute coronary syndrome
  - myocarditis
  - pericarditis
- Pulmonary:
  - right lower lobe pneumonia
  - pulmonary emboli
  - empyema (other inflammatory pleural effusions)
  - pulmonary infarction

Laboratory and Radiographic Findings

There is no laboratory test that is specific for cholecystitis; however, many tests may be helpful in the confirmation of an infection or inflammatory state (white blood cell count, c-reactive protein), or in assessing the severity of infection and systemic response (platelet count, bilirubin, blood urea nitrogen, creatinine, PT/INR, and arterial blood gas).

Sonography is the preferred initial imaging study to evaluate gallstones and gallbladder pathology due to its high sensitivity for diagnosing acute calculous cholecystitis and accessibility in the emergency setting. Other benefits of ultrasonography include avoiding radiation exposure and comparably lower costs. Prospective trials evaluating the test characteristics of emergency physician-performed bedside ultrasound have shown test characteristics similar to radiology ultrasonography, with sensitivity of 87% and specificity of 82%. Sonographic findings may include the presence of gallstones impacted in the gallbladder neck or cystic duct, positive sonographic Murphy's sign (pain when the gallbladder is palpated by the ultrasound probe), gallbladder distension, gallbladder wall thickening, and pericholecystic fluid (see Figure 23.1). The presence of both gallstones and a sonographic Murphy's sign has a positive predictive value of 92%.

Biliary scintigraphy, otherwise known as hydroxyiminodiacetic acid (HIDA) scan, is a nuclear medicine study used to detect cystic duct obstruction associated with acute cholecystitis. When the diagnosis of acute cholecystitis is in question after sonographic evaluation, especially in the obtunded patient who cannot report pain on palpation, HIDA scan should be obtained. Sensitivity of this study is increased with

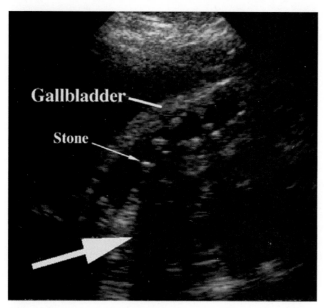

Figure 23.1 Sonographic findings of acute cholecystitis.

the use of morphine, as it increases sphincter of Oddi pressure, causing a more favorable pressure gradient for the radioactive tracer to enter the cystic duct.

Computed tomographic (CT) scan can detect approximately 75% of gallstones. Common findings on CT include gallbladder distension, gallbladder wall thickening, and pericholecystic inflammation and fluid; the last is the most specific finding.

Treatment

Once the diagnosis of acute calculous cholecystitis has been made, the patient should be admitted and evaluated for surgical intervention. A resuscitation phase involves fasting, intravenous hydration, and administration of analgesics and broad-spectrum antibiotics. Acute calculous cholecystitis is primarily an acute inflammatory process that may lead to local or systemic infection. Antimicrobial therapy is standard of care (see Table 23.2). Recommended treatment is a third- or fourth-generation cephalosporin, or a ureidopenicillin with a beta-lactamase inhibitor such as piperacillin-tazobactam. Initial antibiotic therapy should be based on local or institutional bacterial susceptibility patterns of typical gastrointestinal pathogens. There has historically been controversy on the use of opioids for acute calculous cholecystitis because they are thought to induce spasm of the sphincter of Oddi and potentially worsen obstruction; however, there is no clinical evidence to support this, and administration of opioid analgesia is standard.

Definitive therapy for acute calculous cholecystitis is cholecystectomy. Acute cholecystitis was initially considered a relative contraindication for laparoscopic cholecystectomy. However, prospective trials and a Cochrane meta-analysis have since shown that there is no difference in outcomes for patients randomized to early laparoscopic cholecystectomy (defined as within 72 to 96 hours of presentation) compared to those who underwent interval cholecystectomy (6 to 12 weeks after acute

attack). In the early phase of acute inflammation, edematous adhesions are easily separated, whereas later fibrosis can make laparoscopic dissection more difficult. Early intervention also leads to fewer workdays lost and shorter overall hospital stays. The most recent guidelines recommend early laparoscopic cholecystectomy in patients with mild acute cholecystitis, while in patients with moderately severe acute cholecystitis, delayed/ elective laparoscopic cholecystectomy after initial medical treatment with antimicrobial agent is recommended. In non-responders to initial medical treatment, gallbladder drainage should be considered. In patients with severe acute cholecystitis, appropriate organ support in addition to initial medical treatment is necessary. Urgent or early gallbladder drainage is recommended, with elective cholecystectomy performed after resuscitation and antimicrobial therapy to stabilize the patient prior to surgery.

Critically ill patients or those at high risk for surgical complications can be managed successfully with percutaneous cholecystostomy drainage (placement of a catheter into gallbladder). Clinical improvement occurs within 24 hours in 81 to 95% of patients. Ultrasound-guided cholecystostomy can now be done percutaneously by interventional radiologists. Laparoscopic cholecystectomy after cholecystostomy can be safely performed early, within 96 hours after resolution of toxemia, or 8 weeks later on an elective basis. For a minority of patients who remain a high surgical risk because of cardiac, pulmonary, or other system failure, percutaneous cholecystostomy along with percutaneous calculus extraction can be performed, with subsequent removal of the biliary drainage catheter after 6 weeks.

Complications and Admission Criteria

Approximately 15 to 20% of patients with acute calculous cholecystitis deteriorate clinically despite antibiotics and resuscitation, and require emergent cholecystectomy. The risks of conversion to open laparotomy, operative complications, and mortality are higher in this subset of patients.

Complications include gangrenous cholecystitis, gallbladder perforation and peritonitis, gallbladder abscess, gallstone ileus, and emphysematous cholecystitis. Gangrenous cholecystitis is the most common complication of cholecystitis, particularly in older patients, diabetics, or those who delay care. The presence of sepsis is suggestive of gangrene, but gangrene may not be suspected pre-operatively. Perforation of the gallbladder usually occurs secondary to gangrene and may cause a pericholecystic abscess. Less commonly, perforation occurs directly into the peritoneum, leading to generalized peritonitis. A cholecystoenteric fistula may result from erosion of the gallbladder directly into the duodenum, jejunum, or transverse colon. Fistula formation is more often due to long-standing pressure necrosis from stones than to acute cholecystitis. Passage of a gallstone through a cholecystoenteric fistula may lead to the development of mechanical bowel obstruction, usually in the terminal ileum (gallstone ileus). Emphysematous cholecystitis is caused by secondary infection of the gallbladder wall with gas-forming organisms (e.g. *Clostridium perfringens*).

Table 23.2 Therapeutic Recommendations for Acute Cholecystitis

1. Resuscitation

	Intravenous fluids
	Fasting
	Analgesics

Antibiotic therapy	
Often inflammatory and non-infectious, but treated as an infection	**Recommended:**
Bile cultures frequently polymicrobial:	Penicillins:
E. coli	Ampicillin–sulbactam 3 g IV every 6 hours
Klebsiella species	*or*
Enterobacter	Piperacillin–tazobactam 3.375 g IV every 6 hours
Enterococcus	*or*
	Cephalosporins:
	Ceftriaxone 1 g IV every 24 hours
	or
	Cefepime 2 g IV every 12 hours
	plus
	Metronidazole 500 mg IV every 8 hours
	Alternative therapy:
	Fluoroquinolones:
	Ciprofloxacin 400 mg IV every 12 hours
	or
	Levofloxacin 500 mg IV every 24 hours
	plus
	Metronidazole 500 mg IV every 8 hours

2. Intervention

Cholecystectomy	Definitive therapy
	Laparoscopic cholecystectomy recommended within 72 hours of presentation
	Common bile duct exploration may be indicated in patients with persistent hyperbilirubinemia and elevated alkaline phosphatase
Percutaneous cholecystostomy	Recommended for high surgical risk patients
	Followed by elective cholecystectomy when patient is clinically stable
ERCP	Indicated for patients with persistent hyperbilirubinemia
	May be done prior to or after cholecystectomy, if common bile duct exploration is not done at the time of surgery

Factors associated with the development of gangrenous cholecystitis include:

- male gender
- advanced age
- coexisting cardiovascular disease
- diabetes mellitus
- persistent leukocytosis of >15,000/ mm^3 for 24 to 48 hours

Emergent cholecystectomy is required for all of these complications except gallstone ileus, in which the primary surgical goal is to alleviate the obstruction; cholecystoenteric fistulas will usually close spontaneously and subsequent elective cholecystectomy can be done.

The cumulative morbidity of laparoscopic cholecystectomy in the literature is approximately 7%, which is similar to open cholecystectomy, and includes biliary complications such as retained common bile duct stones, a bile leak or fistula, bile duct injury, split and lost gallstones potentially causing intra-abdominal abscesses, cholangitis, and pancreatitis; and non-biliary complications, such as wound infections, bleeding, cardiopulmonary complications, deep vein thrombosis, pulmonary embolism, and bowel perforation due to trocar placement.

Persistent hyperbilirubinemia and elevated alkaline phosphatase levels during resuscitation may indicate choledocholithiasis. Treatment options include intraoperative cholangiography and common bile duct exploration, and pre-operative or post-operative endoscopic retrograde cholangiopancreatography (ERCP) with stone retrieval and/or sphincterotomy.

Special Considerations

Acute Cholecystitis in Pregnancy

Although uncommon in pregnancy, gallstone disease is an important consideration in pregnant women who present with abdominal pain because of the high potential for maternal and fetal morbidity. Pregnant patients with cholecystitis may present with atypical abdominal pain depending on the gestational age of the fetus. Right upper quadrant ultrasound is the ideal diagnostic imaging study to evaluate the gallbladder. Rarely, CT scan may be indicated to evaluate other possible causes of abdominal pain, such as appendicitis, though teratogenicity is a concern and the risks and benefits for the mother and fetus must be considered carefully (see Chapter 58, Fever in Pregnancy, for a full discussion of fetal exposure to diagnostic imaging).

Obstetric and surgical consultants should be contacted early when acute cholecystitis is suspected for specific guidance on further management, such as fetal monitoring, the use of tocolytics and non-teratogenic antibiotics, and discussion of possible surgical intervention. Recent reviews show that laparoscopic cholecystectomy can be performed safely in pregnant women who have refractory biliary symptoms after non-operative management.

Acute Acalculous Cholecystitis

Acute acalculous cholecystitis accounts for 10 to 15% of cases of acute cholecystitis and occurs in severely ill patients, such as those with severe trauma or burns, or with recent major surgery, long-term fasting, total parenteral nutrition, sepsis, diabetes mellitus, atherosclerotic disease, systemic vasculitis, acute renal failure, and acquired immunodeficiency syndrome (AIDS). Acute acalculous cholecystitis is usually a disease of hospitalized patients. The pathophysiology includes gallbladder ischemia, bile stasis or sludge, and local or systemic infection. Presenting symptoms are often vague and non-specific, and diagnosis is especially difficult in non-communicative patients. Diagnostic imaging is similar to that previously described, but has a lower sensitivity for acute acalculous cholecystitis than for acute calculous cholecystitis. Delayed diagnosis and comorbidities contribute to the higher mortality rate of acute acalculous cholecystitis, reported between 10 and 50%, compared to <1% in patients with acute calculous cholecystitis.

Acute Bacterial Cholangitis

Acute cholangitis is a bacterial infection of the biliary tract superimposed on biliary obstruction. The incidence and mortality is higher in the elderly population because of comorbidities and delayed diagnosis. However, early intervention has lowered mortality to less than 1% overall since the year 2000. Current management usually involves a multidisciplinary team of internists, interventional radiologists, gastroenterologists, and surgeons.

Epidemiology and Microbiology

The most common cause of cholangitis in the United States is choledocholithiasis secondary to cholelithiasis. Approximately 6 to 9% of patients with symptomatic gallstone disease in the United States will develop acute cholangitis. In contrast, primary bile duct stones are endemic in Hong Kong and Southeast Asia and the incidence of cholangitis is much higher. Other less common causes of cholangitis include primary malignancies of the bile duct, pancreas, and gallbladder, metastatic disease, benign strictures from bile duct reconstruction and biliary interventions, and sclerosing cholangitis.

Common bile duct stones usually lead to incomplete biliary obstruction and subsequent ascending infection of duodenal bacteria, whereas malignant obstruction is often complete and infection occurs as a result of translocation of bacteria from the portal system. Bile stasis and increased intraluminal pressure in an obstructed biliary system allows for bacterial translocation and multiplication. Translocation occurs at the level of the bile canaliculi; and venous sinusoids, where bile and portal blood are in close proximity. Biliary intervention (ERCP) may also introduce bacteria. The most common pathogens isolated include *E. coli*, *Klebsiella* species, and *Enterococcus*. Anaerobes, such as *Bacteroides* species, are common in polymicrobial infections.

Clinical Features

Acute cholangitis can be a diagnostic challenge (see Table 23.3), and the clinical presentation can range from isolated fever, especially in the elderly, to sepsis. The complete Charcot's triad, defined as fever, right upper quadrant pain, and jaundice, occurs in approximately 50% of patients with cholangitis. Reynolds' pentad, which includes the additional symptoms of hypotension and altered mental status, occurs in only 10 to 30% of patients. Laboratory findings that distinguish cholangitis from acute calculous cholecystitis are hyperbilirubinemia and elevated alkaline phosphatase. One prospective study of 99 consecutive cases of acute cholangitis reported that temperature greater than 39°C, serum bilirubin level greater than 4 mg/dL, and hypotension correlated with severe refractory cases requiring emergent biliary decompression. Risk factors predicting overall poor prognosis include acute renal failure, age older than 50 years, female gender, cirrhosis, cholangitis associated with liver abscess, high malignant biliary stricture, and a history of transhepatic cholangiography. The Tokyo Guidelines, updated in 2013, grade severity of cholangitis as severe, moderate, or mild (see Table 23.4). These severity categories can be used for risk stratification and to guide timing of biliary decompression as discussed below in the Treatment section.

Laboratory and Radiographic Findings

Up to 20 to 30% of patients with acute cholangitis will have positive blood cultures, so these must be obtained immediately in all suspected cases. The diagnosis of acute cholangitis is usually made based on clinical presentation, but imaging studies can evaluate the cause of the obstruction, the degree of biliary dilation, and the presence of other complications, including hepatic abscess. Ultrasonography and CT scan of the abdomen and pelvis are the most common initial studies obtained in the acute setting. Ultrasound has a high sensitivity for gallstones and can detect biliary dilation. Common bile duct diameter greater than 4 mm, with the addition of 1 mm per decade over 40, is considered normal. However, ultrasound has limited ability to evaluate the distal common bile duct and a normal right upper quadrant study does not rule out acute cholangitis. CT scan has been reported to be superior to ultrasound in detecting choledocholithiasis, especially calcified stones, and at specifying the level of obstruction. CT scan also has the advantage of imaging the entire abdomen and evaluating for mass lesions that may be the cause of the obstruction. Magnetic resonance cholangiopancreatography (MRCP), an alternative to the more invasive ERCP, is accurate in defining the biliary anatomy in cases of malignancies or sclerosing cholangitis, but is generally not helpful in the setting of acute cholangitis. ERCP

Table 23.3 Clinical Features: Acute Bacterial Cholangitis

Signs and symptoms	• Diagnostic challenge: spectrum of presentation ranges from fever to sepsis • Charcot's triad: fever, RUQ pain, and jaundice • Reynolds' pentad: Charcot's triad plus hypotension and altered mental status • <10% of patients have previous history of symptomatic gallbladder disease
Laboratory and radiographic findings	• Elevated WBC, alkaline phosphatase, and direct bilirubin; variable elevation in LFTs (may indicate the development of hepatic abscesses) • Ultrasonography is initial imaging study of choice study; very sensitive for gallstones, but limited imaging of distal common bile duct • Normal US does not rule out cholangitis • MRCP provides excellent imaging of biliary anatomy • ERCP is both diagnostic and therapeutic

LFT – liver function test; MRCP – magnetic resonance cholangiopancreatography; RUQ – right upper quadrant; US – ultrasound; WBC – white blood (cell) count.

Table 23.4 Assessment of Acute Cholangitis Severity: Tokyo Guidelines 2013

Severe acute cholangitis (grade III)	Acute cholangitis associated with the onset of dysfunction in at least one of the following organs/systems: • Cardiovascular dysfunction: hyopotension requiring vasopressors • Neurological dysfunction: disturbance of consciousness • Respiratory dysfunction: Pao_1/Fio_2 ratio <300 • Renal dysfunction: oliguria, SCr >2 mg/dL • Hepatic dysfunction: elevated PT/INR >1.5 • Hematological dysfunction: platelet count <100,000/mm^3
Moderate acute cholangitis (grade II)	Acute cholangitis associated with any two of the following conditions: • Abnormal WBC (>12,000, <4,000/mm^3) • High fever (≥39°C) • Age ≥75 years old • Hyperbilirubinemia (total bilirubin ≥5 mg/dL) • Hypoalbuminemia (<lower limit of normal × 0.7)
Mild acute cholangitis (grade I)	Does not meet the criteria of "severe" or "moderate" acute cholangitis at time of initial diagnosis
Urgency of biliary draining	Urgent biliary drainage (<24 hours) is indicated when: (a) obstructive biliary stones are associated with severe or moderate acute cholangitis; or (b) Mild acute cholangitis is not responding to IV antibiotics and fluid resuscitation Early (but not urgent) ERCP (<72 hours) is recommended for patients with mild acute cholangitis who respond to medical therapy

ERCP – endoscopic retrograde cholangiopancreatography; PT/INR – prothrombin time and international normalized ratio; SCr – serum creatinine; WBC – white blood (cell) count.

is potentially both diagnostic and therapeutic, but because of the risk of complications, it should be reserved for patients in whom intervention is likely.

Treatment

Patients diagnosed with acute cholangitis require resuscitation with intravenous fluids, antibiotics, and subsequent biliary decompression (see Table 23.5). Acute cholangitis can result in "pus under pressure"; patients can deteriorate quickly and must be monitored closely for the first 24 to 48 hours. Initial antibiotic therapy should be broad, covering all likely pathogens. Antibiotic recommendations are similar to those for acute cholecystitis and should be based on the cause of obstruction and the patient's prior history of biliary instrumentation. In general, empiric antibiotics should cover enteric gram-negative

bacteria as well as anaerobes. Patients with severe (Grade 3) cholangitis should receive anti-pseudomonal agents (e.g. piperacillin-tazobactam), as this pathogen has been reported in approximately 20% of recent series.

Biliary decompression is usually required for treatment of acute cholangitis, though decompression sometimes occurs spontaneously, and endoscopic retrograde cholangiopancreatography (ERCP) within 72 hours is generally recommended. Approximately 10 to 15% of patients will not respond to medical therapy and supportive measures and will require urgent biliary decompression within 12 to 24 hours of presentation. For patients with severe (grade 3) suppurative cholangitis, with septic shock and end-organ damage, mortality approaches 100% unless prompt endoscopic or surgical treatment of obstruction and drainage of infected bile is carried out. Nonoperative biliary drainage modalities have greatly reduced

Table 23.5 Therapeutic Recommendations for Acute Bacterial Cholangitis

1. Resuscitation	Intravenous fluids Fasting
Antibiotic therapy	Similar to therapy for acute cholecystitis
Frequently polymicrobial Stone disease: *Escherichia coli*, *Klebsiella*, *Proteus*, and *Pseudomonas* Previous biliary interventions: Concern for more resistant bacteria; *Pseudomonas*, *Enterobacter*, *Bacteroides*, *Enterococcus*, and fungus (i.e. *Candida*).	**Recommended:** Penicillins: * Ampicillin-sulbactam 3 g IV every 6 hours *or* Piperacillin-tazobactam 3.375 g IV every 6 hours *or* Cephalosporins: * Ceftriaxone 1 g IV every 24 hours *or* Cefepime 2 g IV every 12 hours *plus* Metronidazole 500 mg IV every 8 hours **Alternative therapy:** Fluoroquinolones: Ciprofloxacin 400 mg IV every 12 hours *or* Levofloxacin 500 mg IV every 24 hours *plus* Metronidazole 500 mg IV every 8 hours
2. Biliary decompression	
Endoscopic drainage Transhepatic drainage Surgical drainage	Includes ERCP with stone extraction and sphincterotomy or stent placement Indicated for patients whose biliary system is not endoscopically accessible Indicated for patients who fail other modalities Higher mortality rates
3. Interval cholecystectomy	Recommended for patients with gallstones because of the 20–25% incidence of recurrent biliary symptoms Done electively when cholangitis has resolved

* These regimens do not provide adequate pseudomonal coverage and should not be used as empiric therapy in patients with severe cholangitis.

mortality as compared to surgical decompression of the biliary tract. Endoscopic decompression consists of cholangiography for diagnosis and stone extraction with optional sphincterotomy or stent placement (see Figure 23.2). The emphasis should be on decompression and not definitive treatment for critically ill patients. Percutaneous decompression can also be effective. Surgical decompression becomes necessary when non-operative drainage has failed. Interval cholecystectomy is recommended after resolution of cholangitis because of the 20 to 25% incidence of recurrent biliary symptoms within 2 years.

Special Considerations

Parasitic Cholangitis

Helminthic biliary infections are prevalent in tropical countries where parasites are endemic and are the second most common cause of cholangitis worldwide. However, with increasing migration and tourism, the incidence in developed countries has increased. Biliary parasites cause damage to the bile ducts by several mechanisms:

* irritating composition of the parasite, parasitic secretions, or eggs
* physical obstruction of the bile ducts

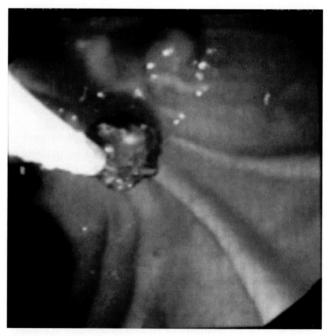

Figure 23.2 Endoscopic drainage and extraction of common bile duct stone.

- induction of biliary stone formation
- introduction of bacteria into the biliary system during migration from the duodenum
- supervening bacterial infection on any of the above

Common biliary parasites include the nematode *Ascaris lumbricoides* and the hermaphroditic trematodes or flukes *Clonorchis sinensis*, *Opisthorchis viverrini* and *felineus*, *Dicrocoelium dendriticum*, and *Fasciola hepatica* and *gigantica*. Infection is transmitted by ingestion of human feces, raw fish, and freshwater plants. Cholangitis is a complication of biliary fluke infections. Patients with biliary ascariasis typically also present with intestinal ascariasis, including symptoms of vomiting, intestinal colic, and/or palpable mass of intestinal worms. *Clonorchis* can cause a chronic infection and may be associated with recurrent pyogenic cholangitis secondary to intrahepatic biliary stone formation. The chronic irritation and inflammation in the bile ducts carries an associated risk of biliary tract malignancies. *Fasciola* is distinguished from the other biliary parasites by its ability to migrate through the duodenal wall into the peritoneal cavity and penetrate the liver. Biliary obstruction in parasitic infection results from the presence of adult flukes and stone formation. The clinical presentation is similar to that of bacterial infection. Diagnosis of parasitic cholangitis is based primarily on identification of eggs in feces and endoscopic evaluation.

Key features that may help distinguish parasitic from bacterial cholangitis are:

- travel to endemic area within the past year
- associated gastrointestinal symptoms
- eosinophilia
- demonstration of eggs in feces or duodenal contents

Treatment modalities for parasitic cholangitis include anthelmintic therapy, endoscopy, and surgery (see Table 23.6). As with other causes of cholangitis, ERCP, with sphincterotomy and parasite and stones extraction, has in large part replaced the surgical approach. Patients with associated acute or chronic cholecystitis from parasite migration into the gallbladder or evidence of obstruction will require cholecystectomy and may require lapoarotomy (see Figure 23.3) for common duct exploration, biliary drainage procedure, or cholecystectomy.

Pearls and Pitfalls

1. Acute cholecystitis is often an inflammatory process without infection, though antibiotics are an important component of treatment.
2. Patients with acute calculus cholecystitis require hospitalization, but definitive cholecystectomy is often delayed.
3. Although it most often occurs in hospitalized patients, consider acalculous cholecystitis in elderly and debilitated patients presenting in the acute care setting.

Table 23.6 Medical Therapy of Parasitic Biliary Diseases

Parasite	Drug
Ascaris	Mebendazole 100 mg PO BID × 3 days
	or
	Pyrantel pamoate 11 mg/kg PO × 1 (maximum dose 1 g)
	or
	Piperazine citrate (not available in the United States)
Clonorchis sinensis	Praziquantel 25 mg/kg PO TID for 2 days
	or
	Albendazole 10 mg/kg/day PO daily × 7 days
	or
	Mebendazole 15 mg/kg PO BID × 30 days
Fasciola hepatica	Triclabendazole 10 mg/kg PO daily × 1–2 days (in the United States, may need special request from the CDC)
	or
	Nitazoxanide 500 mg PO BID × 7 days
	Bithionol (no longer available)

References include World Health Organization and Center for Disease Control and Prevention (CDC).

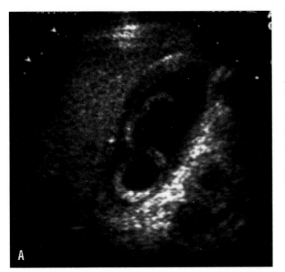
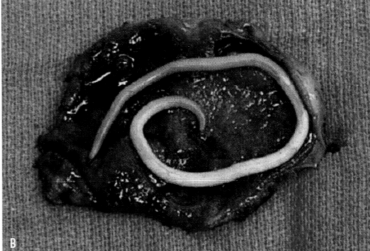

Figure 23.3 Presence of *Ascaris* in the gallbladder by ultrasound and at the time of surgery.

4. Presentation of acute cholangitis ranges from isolated fever to florid sepsis.
5. Normal ultrasonography does not rule out cholangitis.
6. Early decompression of biliary system is indicated for acute cholangitis that does not respond to conservative measures or in patients with evidence of severe cholangitis.
7. Consider parasitic cholangitis in patients who have emigrated from endemic areas.

References

Akyurek, M., Salman, B., Yuksel, O., et al. Management of acute calculous cholecystitis in high-risk patients: percutaneous cholecystostomy followed by early laparoscopic cholecystectomy. *Surg. Laparosc. Endosc. Percutan. Tech.* 2005; 15(6): 315–20.

Bornman, P. C., Van Beljon, J. I., and Krige, J. E. J. Management of cholangitis. *J. Hepatobiliary Pancreat. Surg.* 2003; 10(6): 406–14.

Demehri, F. R. and Hasan, B. A. Evidence-based management of common gallstone-related emergencies. *J. Intensive Care Med.* 2016; 31(1): 3–13.

Fagan, S. P., Awad, S. S., Rahwan, K., et al. Prognostic factors for the development of gangrenous cholecystitis. *Am. J. Surg.* 2003; 186(5): 481–5.

Gigot, J. F., Leese, T., Bereme, T., et al. Acute cholangitis. Multivariate analysis of risk factors. *Ann. Surg.* 1989; 209(4): 435–8.

Glasgow, R. E., Visser, B. C., Harris, H. W., et al. Changing management of gallstone disease during pregnancy. *Surg. Endosc.* 1998; 12(3): 241–6.

Fumihiko, M., Takada, T., Strasberg, S. M., et al. TG13 flowcharts for the diagnosis and treatment of acute cholangitis and cholecystitis. *J. Hepatobiliary Pancreatic Surg.* 2013; 20(1): 47–54.

Gomi, H., Solomkin, J., Takada, T., et al. TG13 antimicrobial therapy for acute cholangitis and cholecystitis. *J. Hepatobiliary Pancreatic Surg.* 2013; 20(1): 60–70.

Gruber, P. J., Silverman, R. A., Gottesfeld, S., et al. Presence of fever and leukocytosis in acute cholecystitis. *Ann. Emerg. Med.* 1996; 28(3): 273–7.

Kimura, Y., Takada, T., Strasberg, S. M., et al. TG13 current terminology, etiology, and epidemiology of acute cholangitis and cholecystitis. *J. Hepatobiliary Pancreatic Sci.* 2013; 20(1): 8–23.

Lai, E. C., Mok, F. P., Tan, E. S., et al. Endoscopic biliary drainage for severe acute cholangitis. *N. Engl. J. Med.* 1992; 326(24): 1582–6.

Lai, P. B. S., Kwong, K. H., Leung, K. L., et al. Randomized trial of early versus delayed laparoscopic cholecystectomy for acute cholecystitis. *Br. J. Surg.* 1998; 85(6): 764–7.

Lo, C. M., Liu, C. I., Fan, S. T., et al. Prospective randomized study of early versus delayed laparoscopic cholecystectomy for acute cholecystitis. *Ann. Surg.* 1998; 227(4): 461–7.

Lowe, S. A. Diagnostic radiography in pregnancy: risks and reality. *Aust. NZ J. Obstet. Gynaecol.* 2004; 44(3): 191–6.

McSherry, C. K., Ferstenberg, H., and Virshup, M. The Mirizzi syndrome: suggested classification and surgical therapy. *Surg. Gastroenterol.* 1982; 1(3): 219–25.

Osman, M., Laustern, S. B., El-Sefi, T., et al. Biliary parasites. *Dig. Surg.* 1998; 15: 287–96.

Paulson, E. K. Acute cholecystitis: CT findings. *Seminars in Ultrasound CT MR* 2000; 21(1): 56–63.

Poon, R. T., Liu, C. L., Lo, C. M., et al. Management of gallstone cholangitis in the era of laparoscopic cholecystectomy. *Arch. Surg.* 2001; 136(1): 11–16.

Singer, A. J., McCracken, G., Henry, M. C., et al. Correlation among clinical, laboratory, and hepatobiliary scanning findings in patients with suspected acute cholecystitis. *Ann. Emerg. Med.* 1996; 28(3): 267–72.

Sung, J. J., Lyon, D. J., Suen, R., et al. Intravenous ciprofloxacin as treatment for patients with acute suppurative cholangitis: a randomized, controlled clinical trial. *J. Antimicrob. Chemother.* 1995; 35(6): 855–64.

Yusoff, I. F., Barkun, J. S., and Barkun, A. N. Diagnosis and management of cholecystitis and cholangitis. *Gastroenterol. Clin. North Am.* 2003; 32(4): 1145–68.

Additional Readings

Indar, A. A. and Beckingham, I. J. Acute cholecystitis. *BMJ* 2002; 325(7365): 639–43.

Lillemoe, K. D. Surgical treatment of biliary tract infections. *Am. Surg.* 2000; 66(2): 138–44.

Mazuski, J. E., Tessier, J. M., May, A. K., et al. The Surgical Infection Society revised guidelines on the management of intra-abdominal infection. *Surg. Infect. (Larchmt.)* 2017; 18(1): 1–76.

Solomkin, J. S., Mazuski, J. E., Bradley, J. S., et al. Diagnosis and management of complicated intra-abdominal infections in adults and children: guidelines by the surgical infection society and the Infectious Disease Society of America. *Clin. Infect. Dis.* 2010; 50(2): 133–64.

Westphal, J. F. and Brogard, J. M. Biliary tract infections: a guide to treatment. *Drugs* 1999; 57(1): 81–91.

Viral Hepatitis

Kavita Radhakrishnan and Michele Tana

Outline

Introduction

A number of viruses primarily infect hepatocytes, though not all cause clinically relevant disease. The classically recognized hepatotropic viruses are the hepatitis A, B, C, D, and E viruses. Of clinically apparent acute and chronic hepatitis, 10 to 20% is cryptogenic in nature and is thought to be caused by as yet unidentified viruses.

Epidemiology and Microbiology

Hepatitis viruses A and E are transmitted via the fecal–oral route, whereas B, C, and D are spread primarily via contact with infected blood or other bodily fluid. Fecal–oral transmission of the A and E viruses is responsible for most acute outbreaks of hepatitis, whereas B and C, though also infrequently the source of acute hepatitis, constitute a major chronic public health burden.

Hepatitis A virus (HAV) infection accounts for approximately 25,000 cases of acute hepatitis annually in the United States, with as many as 40% of the urban population having serologic evidence of past infection. Outbreaks often affect clusters of persons exposed to a single source, such as a food handler or contaminated central water supply. Immigrants from much of Africa, Asia, Latin America, and the Middle East have Hepatitis A immunity, though notably global seroprevalance is decreasing due to rising socioeconomic status, improving water resources, and the availability of vaccination.

Persons infected with hepatitis B virus (HBV) carry the virus in all bodily fluids (blood, breast milk, saliva, semen, and urine). HBV can cause both acute and chronic hepatitis, the latter conferring risk of cirrhosis and hepatocellular carcinoma.

It is estimated that 400 million people worldwide are chronically infected with HBV, with highly endemic regions including Asia, Africa, the Middle East, and much of South America. In these regions, vertical transmission confers a risk of nearly 90% in infants born to mothers with HBe antigen positivity. Horizontal transmission is also highly prevalent via sexual and percutaneous exchange. In the United States, hepatitis B is most common in immigrants from endemic areas and 200,000 to 300,000 new infections occur yearly. Groups at high risk in whom screening is recommended include men who have sexual intercourse with men, pregnant women, persons born in endemic areas and their children, and those who will need immunosuppressive therapy.

Hepatitis C virus (HCV) can also cause both acute and chronic hepatitis. It is estimated that at least 4 million people (1.5%) in the United States have chronic HCV infection. HCV remains the leading cause of chronic liver disease and the most common indication for liver transplantation in the United States. The highest prevalence of HCV is observed among patients with hemophilia, injection drug users, hemodialysis recipients, and Vietnam War veterans. Because the majority of infected persons do not recall or report specific risk factors, the CDC recently broadened screening recommendations such that now all 'baby boomers' or adults born during 1945 to 1965 should receive one-time testing for HCV regardless of HCV risk. Prior to screening of all blood products for HCV, the risk of transmission of HCV by transfusion was 1 in 10 transfusions, but the current estimated risk is 1 in 400,000. The rate of seroconversion from a needle-stick injury from a seropositive source ranges from 1 to 7% in various studies. (See Chapter 57 on Blood or Bodily Fluid Exposure Management and Post-Exposure Prophylaxis for Hepatitis B and HIV.) Sexual and maternal-fetal transmission rates are lower than for HBV.

Hepatitis D virus (HDV) is transmitted parenterally and is dependent on HBV for survival. Estimates of prevalence vary, but approximately 20 million individuals worldwide have evidence of prior exposure to HDV. In a retrospective study of ethnically diverse patients with chronic hepatitis B in London, 8.5% were co-infected with HDV. HDV has no replication machinery of its own and utilizes that of HBV. The virus infects the liver either simultaneously with HBV (co-infection) or in a person chronically infected with the B virus (superinfection). Routes of transmission include intraparenteral drug use and intrafamilial spread. Patients with HBV/HDV coinfection are at risk for increased morbidity and mortality compared to patients monoinfected with HBV.

Hepatitis E virus (HEV) was named for its enteric transmission. It was previously thought to be solely endemic to the developing world, including North Africa, Asia, Central America, and India. Historically, HEV was associated with waterborne transmission after rainy seasons when run-off from rainwater was contaminated by feces. Recently, an increasing number of cases have been reported in non-endemic countries, including France, Germany, and the United States in persons without recent travel to endemic regions. This has led to the discovery of at least four HEV genotypes with genotypes 3 and 4 more prevalent in developed countries and hosted by zoonotic reservoirs, including swine, boar, and deer. Zoonotic transmission has also been recently noted through consumption of raw or undercooked meat from these animals. Intriguingly, the seroprevalence of HEV IgG is fairly common in the United States, with one study of random blood donors demonstrating a proportion of 21.3%, perhaps suggesting that primary infection may be underrecognized. The mortality rate of acute HEV infection is 1 to 2%, but approaches 10 to 30% in pregnant women, with the worst outcomes in the third trimester.

In immunocompromised persons, cytomegalovirus (CMV), Epstein–Barr virus (EBV), or other herpesviridae may cause hepatitis. Other hepatotropic viruses are being investigated, though little clinical disease is attributable to them. These include dengue virus, TT virus, SEN virus, and GB virus (the latter three were named for the patients from whom they were isolated).

Clinical Features

Acute Hepatitis

There are three phases of acute infection: prodrome, jaundice, and convalescence. The *prodrome* follows an incubation period that varies according to the causative hepatitis virus and consists of vague flu-like symptoms: malaise, fatigability, myalgias, pharyngitis, anorexia, nausea, and pyrexia (see Table 24.1). After the 2 to 4 week prodrome, liver enzyme abnormalities develop and may be associated with hyperbilirubinemia or jaundice. During this *icteric phase*, patients may also present with dark urine, light-colored stools, and pruritis. In

Table 24.1 Clinical Features: Acute Hepatitis

Incubation period	Usually 1–4 weeks, may be up to months
Organisms	Hepatitis A, E viruses Hepatitis B, C, D viruses (less common) Drugs and toxins
Signs and symptoms	Prodrome: • Vague "flu-like" symptoms: fever, malaise, fatigability, myalgias, pharyngitis, anorexia, nausea Icteric phase: • jaundice • dark urine • acholic stools • pruritis Convalescence: • clinical improvement • serologic changes
Laboratory and radiologic findings	Mild neutropenia or lymphocytosis Elevated AST and ALT (100s–1,000s units/L) Hyperbilirubinemia (predominantly indirect) Virus-dependent serology (see below) No biliary dilation on ultrasound
Treatment	Supportive – symptom management If not resolving or severe, consider testing for HCV and HBV Careful hygiene to prevent spread

immunocompetent individuals, this will last about a month. *Convalescence* involves gradual clinical improvement and serologic changes (discussed below). Uncomplicated courses of acute HAV and HEV infection tend to present and resolve slightly more rapidly than B, C, and D; resolution of symptoms is generally over by 2 to 3 months for A and E, and 3 to 4 months for other serotypes.

Acute Liver Failure

Acute liver failure is a life-threatening condition, which complicates about 1% of all acute hepatitis. This devastating condition is defined by the presence of hepatic encephalopathy, coagulopathy, and <26 weeks of liver injury in a patient with no known pre-existing liver disease. It is associated with other clinical signs of liver failure, including systemic inflammatory response syndrome (SIRS) and perturbation of glycemic control (see Table 24.2). Without liver transplantation, the mortality rate in patients with acute liver failure is from 50 to 80%. Death can occur within days of onset of encephalopathy and is most commonly due to intracranial hypertension with cerebral edema or sepsis.

Chronic Hepatitis

Of the hepatotropic viruses, only B, C, and D cause chronic infection. The principal long-term sequelae of chronic hepatitis are cirrhosis and hepatocellular carcinoma.

Cirrhosis is a complex condition that can lead to portosystemic hypertension with varix formation, ascites that may be complicated by spontaneous bacterial peritonitis, decreased

Table 24.2 Clinical Features: Acute Liver Failure

Incubation period	Usually 1–4 weeks, may be up to months
Organisms	Hepatitis A, B, and D are most common viral etiologies Drugs and toxins are most common etiology overall
Signs and symptoms	Encephalopathy Coagulopathy Loss of glycemic control Cerebral edema Sepsis
Laboratory and radiologic findings	Elevated AST and ALT (1000s–10,000s units/L) INR ≥1.5
Treatment	ICU admission and supportive care Treatment of the underlying etiology Hemodynamic support Monitor coagulopathy Intracranial pressure monitoring N-Acetylcysteine Consider liver transplantation

INR – international normalized ratio; PT – prothrombin time.

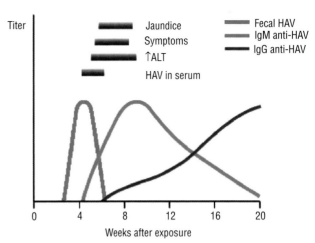

Figure 24.1 Chronology of HAV disease.
Reprinted with permission of The McGraw-Hill Companies from *Current Medical Diagnosis & Treatment* (2007).

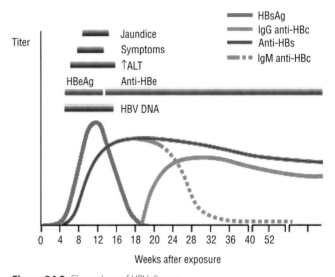

Figure 24.2 Chronology of HBV disease.
Reprinted with permission of The McGraw-Hill Companies from *Current Medical Diagnosis & Treatment* (2007).

protein synthesis, and hepatic encephalopathy. Chronic hepatitis B and cirrhosis of any cause predispose to hepatocellular carcinoma (HCC), a primary malignancy of the liver that can progress in an indolent manner. By the time patients experience pain or recognize increasing abdominal girth, the tumors have typically grown quite large. Therefore, HCC screening with ultrasounds every 6 months is a standard of care for patients with cirrhosis and certain demographic groups with chronic hepatitis B.

Clinical Course by Virus

HAV

HAV has an average incubation period of 30 days, is shed in the feces for 1 to 2 weeks before clinical illness arises, and continues to be infectious during the first week of symptoms. This infection often runs a mild course and the illness is typically subclinical in children, who can spread disease to family members. Complete clinical and laboratory recovery usually occurs by 9 weeks (see Figure 24.1). Although HAV does not cause chronic liver disease, a rare entity known as relapsing hepatitis A has been described, in which patients experience one or two relapses within the first 6 months after the index illness. Fulminant hepatic failure occurs in 1% of cases. The overall fatality rate for acute hepatitis A is 0.1%, but it is significantly greater in the elderly and patients with pre-existing chronic hepatitis B or C.

HBV

HBV has a relatively long incubation period ranging from 6 weeks to 6 months, with an average of 12 to 14 weeks (see Figure 24.2). Manifestation of acute hepatitis B is often insidious, and the majority of cases are minimally symptomatic. In 5 to 10% of patients with acute hepatitis B, a syndrome resembling serum sickness develops, with arthralgias, rash, angioedema, and rarely, proteinuria and hematuria. Acute liver failure occurs in less than 1% of patients. In endemic areas, most cases of HBV infection occur as a result of vertical transmission from an infected mother to an infant at the time of delivery. For the HBV-infected neonate, the risk of developing chronic hepatitis B is greater than 90%, largely because of the lack of immune maturity. In contrast, immunocompetent adults who acquire acute HBV infection develop a chronic infection in only 3 to 8% of cases.

Patients with chronic hepatitis B may present at various phases of infection. They may be positive or negative for the hepatitis B e antigen (HBeAg), and while HBeAg-positive patients tend to have higher viral loads, all viruses are infectious regardless of HBeAg status. The HBV DNA level, ALT level, and other factors such as fibrosis stage and HCC risk are considerations in the decision to initiate antiviral therapy.

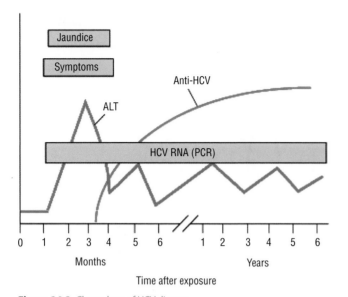

Figure 24.3 Chronology of HCV disease.
Reprinted with permission of The McGraw-Hill Companies from *Current Medical Diagnosis & Treatment* (2007).

Patients with chronic HBV infection are at risk for developing HCC even in the absence of cirrhosis.

HCV

The typical incubation period for HCV infection is 6 to 7 weeks, after which a mild illness may follow, but acute hepatitis C is asymptomatic in 85% of cases (see Figure 24.3). Fulminant hepatic failure is rarely associated with HCV, but 85% of patients acutely infected with HCV will develop chronic hepatitis, and 25 to 35% of those with chronic hepatitis C will develop cirrhosis after an average duration of about 20 years. In contrast to HBV, HCV-associated cirrhosis almost always precedes the development of HCV-associated hepatocellular carcinoma. The annual risk for carcinoma is 1 to 4% for patients with HCV cirrhosis. HCV is implicated in many extrahepatic conditions, including cryoglobulinemia, which may manifest as neuropathy, glomerulonephritis, and arthropathy.

HDV

When acute HDV infection is synchronous with acute HBV ("co-infection"), the nature and severity of illness are similar to isolated acute HBV infection. In acute co-infection, spontaneous clearance of HBV and HDV occurs in 80 to 95% of cases. "Superinfection" occurs when patients with chronic hepatitis B are acutely infected by HDV. Superinfection is more likely to cause acute liver failure (in 2 to 20% of cases, ten times the rate for isolated HBV infection).

HEV

HEV is similar to HAV, in that infection manifests only as acute hepatitis and typically has a milder course in children. The virus has a long incubation period of 2 to 10 weeks, after which a transient macular skin rash may be observed. HEV infection generally lasts 1 to 4 weeks and is self-limited, though associated cholestasis may persist for 2 to 6 months.

Differential Diagnosis

The prodrome of acute viral hepatitis is non-specific and can be difficult to distinguish from other viral syndromes. A clinical history of bodily fluid exposure or food- or water-related infection may support the diagnosis of acute viral hepatitis. Right upper quadrant pain and tenderness are often present in a patient with acute viral hepatitis, prompting consideration of acute cholecystitis and choledocholithiasis.

Non-microbial etiologies of acute hepatitis include autoimmune hepatitis, drugs, and toxins (see Table 24.3). Acute acetaminophen overdose is the most common cause of acute liver failure in the United States. Although 10 grams is usually required to cause acute liver failure, patients with chronic liver disease may develop failure with much smaller doses of acetaminophen (e.g. 3 grams per day over days to weeks).

Laboratory and Radiographic Findings

The basic liver panel includes alanine aminotransferase (ALT), aspartate aminotransferase (AST), total bilirubin, and alkaline phosphatase (ALP). The ALT or AST level in acute viral hepatitis generally ranges from several hundred to a few thousand units/liter. In drug-induced hepatitis, the peak ALT or AST levels may be even higher, sometimes exceeding 10,000 units/liter (U/L). In acute alcoholic hepatitis, the ALT or AST level rarely exceeds 500 U/L, and the AST/ALT ratio is typically >2. Prothrombin time (PT) with international normalized ratio (INR) is the most important laboratory indicator for hepatic dysfunction, whereas the peak level of AST or ALT is of no proven prognostic significance.

The complete blood count (CBC) in viral hepatitis usually reveals a mild degree of neutropenia initially, followed by a mild lymphocytosis. Acute infections may cause reactive thrombocytosis, but many patients with cirrhosis have a low platelet count of less than 120×10^3/mL.

Once the diagnosis of acute viral hepatitis is suspected, specific serologic assays should be obtained to determine the etiology. The HAV IgM antibody becomes detectable about 4 weeks after acute HAV exposure. IgM titer peaks during the first week of clinical illness and disappears by 3 to 6 months, though it may be present for up to a year. HAV IgG becomes detectable about 2 weeks after the IgM and confers long-term immunity. Thus, a positive IgM antibody is a marker of acute infection, whereas positive IgG reflects prior exposure and ongoing immunity.

HBV has more intricate structural characteristics, which allows for multiple serologic assays to determine the nature of infection (see Tables 24.4 and 24.5). Presence of surface antigen (HBsAg) indicates active infection (acute or chronic), whereas antibody against the surface antigen (HBsAb) indicates immunity due to either past infection or vaccination. HBV core antibody IgM can be detected in acute infection, whereas a positive HBV core IgG test reflects previous exposure. HBeAg and HBV DNA are markers of viral replication. They are useful in the evaluation of patients with chronic hepatitis B. Viruses with mutations in the pre-core genomic region are common in the Mediterranean and Far East. These

Table 24.3 Some Common Hepatotoxic Medications

Injury Pattern	Hepatocellular	Cholestatic	Mixed
Lab abnormality	ALT elevation	ALP and bilirubin elevation	ALP and ALT elevation
Medications or classes	Acetaminophen Amiodarone Antiretrovirals Kava kava Ketoconazole SSRIs Statins Isoniazid (INH) Rifampin	Amoxicillin-clavulanate Anabolic steroids Clopidogrel Estrogens Macrolides Phenothiazines TCAs Rifampin	Amitriptyline Carbamazepine Clindamycin Phenytoin Sulfonamides Trazodone Verapamil

ALP – alkaline phosphatase; ALT – alanine aminotransferase; SSRI – selective serotonin reuptake inhibitor; TCA – tricyclic antidepressant.

Table 24.4 HBV Serologic Tests and Interpretations

HBsAg (surface antigen)	*Currently* infected with HBV (acute or chronic)
HBcAb (core antibody)	
IgG	*Past exposure* or false positive test
IgM	Very recent *acute* HBV infection
HBsAb (surface antibody)	*Past* infection with resolution and *immunity*, or vaccination
Markers of viral replication (do these tests only if HBsAg+)	
HBeAg (+)	
HBV-DNA (+)	

Table 24.5 Hepatitis B Viral Serology

	sAg	sAb	cAb	eAg	eAb
Vaccinated	–	+	–	–	–
Acutely infected	+	+/–	IgM	+	–
Chronically infected with active replication	+	–	IgG	+	–
Chronically infected with low replication	+	–	IgG	–	+
Recovery from infection	–	+	IgG	–	+/–
False positive versus remote prior infection	–	–	IgG	–	–

viruses are unable to make HBeAg, but have replicative ability. Thus, patients are HBeAg-negative with detectable HBV DNA.

The presence of HCV antibody does not confer immunity and in association with circulating HCV RNA in the blood reflects active infection. Spontaneous clearance of HCV infection occurs in only 15 to 20% of patients following acute infection; the remaining patients develop chronic HCV infection. Spontaneous clearance of HCV infection, however, confers no protection against reinfection. Serologic conversion or appearance of HCV antibody may take 20 to 150 days (mean 50 days) after acute exposure. Consequently, a negative HCV antibody test during acute hepatitis does not exclude HCV infection. If acute hepatitis C is suspected, reverse transcriptase polymerase chain reaction (RT-PCR) assay should be used to determine the presence of HCV RNA, which becomes detectable 7 to 21 days after acute exposure.

Hepatitis D virus IgM antibody indicates acute infection and IgG reflects prior exposure and chronic immunity. HDV RNA testing is available at select commercial laboratories, but its reliability is debated.

In the immunocompromised patient presenting with acute hepatitis, serologic testing for cytomegalovirus (serum antigen) and Epstein–Barr virus (monospot test) should also be included.

Ultrasound or computed tomography of the abdomen may be helpful in excluding biliary obstruction or gallbladder abnormalities, but their role in evaluating acute hepatitis is generally limited. It is important to remember that gallbladder wall thickening and pericholecystic fluid are non-specific findings in some cirrhotic patients. Liver biopsy is not routinely performed in acute viral hepatitis, because the diagnosis can usually be determined by serologic testing and the results of the liver biopsy rarely change management.

Treatment and Prophylaxis

Acute Liver Failure

In the acute care setting, when a patient presents with hepatitis, recognition of acute liver failure (ALF) is of utmost importance. ALF is defined as evidence of coagulation abnormality (INR ≥1.5) with associated encephalopathy in patients without previously recognized liver disease. While rare, it tends to occur in young patients and is associated with high mortality if not immediately recognized. Management of acute liver failure relies on prompt diagnosis and requires intensive care unit (ICU) admission, consultation with a gastroenterologist, and early referral to a liver transplant center. While the underlying cause is investigated, supportive care and close monitoring of mental status are essential, along with early involvement of transplant hepatologists and surgeons. Further, recent studies have shown that regardless of etiology of ALF, treatment with *N*-acetylcysteine can improve transplant-free survival.

Management and Admission Criteria

Patients with acute hepatitis but without coagulopathy, severe electrolyte derangement, or signs of dehydration can be managed in the outpatient setting with close follow-up. Severe vomiting, diarrhea, or anorexia are indications for inpatient hydration and nutritional support. Elderly patients, those with comorbid medical conditions, and immunocompromised individuals should also be considered for hospitalization because of their diminished functional reserve and greater mortality risk. All clusters or community outbreaks of viral hepatitis are reportable to the department of public health.

Acute Viral Hepatitis

For the majority of patients with acute viral hepatitis, treatment has traditionally been supportive care for the symptomatic patient. More specifically, patients with HAV and HEV have no more specific therapies. In adults with acute HBV infection, the risk for developing chronic hepatitis B is only about 5%. Therefore, even when patients present with significantly elevated transaminases, they can be managed conservatively with close outpatient follow-up unless signs of synthetic dysfunction or encephalopathy are apparent. Whether antiviral therapy using interferon-alpha or nucleic acid analogues is beneficial in otherwise uncomplicated cases of acute HBV infection remains to be demonstrated.

HDV therapies are limited because the virus has no enzymes that are easily targeted by antiviral therapy. Current treatment regimens include interferon-based therapies for 48 weeks, with decreases noted in transaminases. HDV requires addition of a 15 carbon compound (farnesylation) for replication. Ongoing trials are studying the utility of lonafarnib, a farnesyltransferase inhibitor in suppressing HDV RNA.

The recent development of drugs that directly inhibit various key steps in viral replication has lead to the availability of multiple oral HCV treatment regimens. These direct acting antivirals (DAA) have largely replaced interferon-alpha-based treatments. Acutely infected patients are typically followed as outpatients with serial HCV RNA levels and if they do not clear the virus by 6 months, therapy is initiated. Following the advent of DAAs, state-of-the-art treatment for acute and chronic hepatitis C has become a very rapidly evolving field. The American Association for the Study of Liver Diseases and the Infectious Diseases Society of America have created a website with continual updates on HCV treatment recommendations (see www.hcvguidelines.org).

Primary Prophylaxis and Prevention

Primary prophylaxis is the key to prevention, and safe and effective vaccines are now available to prevent viral hepatitis A and B.

Inactivated HAV particles have been manufactured into two commercially available vaccines. A single dose provides 85% immunity for an average of 10 years, but a booster dose at 6 to 12 months increases efficacy to 94%. In recent years, this vaccine has been recommended by the Centers for Disease Control and Prevention for children over 12 months. However, most older children and adults remain unvaccinated, so travelers to developing nations are recommended to vaccinate before the trip. Household contacts of patients with hepatitis A should be treated with a dose of immune globulin to confer passive humoral immunity. This will prevent or attenuate disease in 85% of patients if received either pre-exposure, or post-exposure during the 2- to 6-week incubation phase. However, immune globulin does not incite antibody production, and protection lasts only a few months.

HBV vaccine consists of recombinant surface antigen and confers humoral immunity for subsequent exposure to intact virus. The HBV vaccine series consists of three doses over a period of 6 months (at 0, 1, and 6 months) and produces lasting immunity in >90% of patients. Immunity lasts 10 years, at which point a booster dose is recommended. Hepatitis B immune globulin (HBIg) can attenuate disease severity and, in some cases, offers complete protection against infection as long as it is given within 7 days of exposure.

While treatment of chronic hepatitis B is beyond the scope of this chapter, one noteworthy consideration is HBV reactivation in the setting of immunosuppression. Indeed, it has been found that reactivation of HBV replication occurs in 20 to 50% of patients undergoing immunosuppression or chemotherapy. It is recommended that all patients undergo testing for hepatitis B surface antigen and anti-core antibody prior to starting therapy, and should they be carriers be started on prophylactic antiviral therapy.

HDV immunity can be provided by immunization to HBV because HDV is completely dependent on the presence of HBV for viral replication. No immunizations are currently available for hepatitis C virus.

A recombinant vaccine for HEV (genotype 1) has been developed by researchers in China to prevent HEV infection especially in high-risk groups, including pregnant women and solid organ transplant recipients. This vaccine was tested in more than 100,000 Chinese participants, was found to be safe and effective, and was licensed in China in 2011. A recent study from France demonstrated that ribavirin as monotherapy was effective in treating chronic HEV in post-solid organ transplant patients.

Infection Control

Patients with suspected hepatitis should be treated with strict universal precautions. Those with acute hepatitis should be under contact precautions and be instructed to thoroughly wash their hands, especially following bowel movements.

Pearls and Pitfalls

1. Acute hepatitis can result from hepatotropic viruses A through E, but only B, C, and D cause chronic liver disease.

2. The most serious consequence of acute hepatitis is acute liver failure, defined as severe liver dysfunction, hepatic encephalopathy, and coagulopathy of less than 26 weeks' duration in a patient without known pre-existing liver disease.

3. Hepatic encephalopathy or coagulopathy in a patient with acute viral hepatitis is an ominous sign and should prompt inpatient admission. Acute liver failure necessitates admission to the intensive care unit and immediate referral to a liver transplant center. Clinical condition may deteriorate precipitously and death can occur within days of presentation.

4. In any patient with acute non-viral hepatitis, have a high level of suspicion for ingestion of hepatotoxic drugs. Serum acetaminophen level should be checked in any patient with unexplained elevated liver enzymes.

5. Acetaminophen overdose is the most common cause of acute liver failure in the United States. If diagnosed within the first day, it is treated with *N*-acetylcysteine.

6. Acute viral hepatitis can cause cholestasis and abdominal pain. Ultrasound can help rule out the more common biliary causes of these symptoms.

References

Bernal, W. and Wendon, J. Acute liver failure. *N. Engl. J. Med.* 2014; 370(12): 1170–1.

Cross, T. J., Rizzi, P., Horner, M., *et al.* The increasing prevalence of hepatitis delta virus (HDV) infection in South London. *J. Med. Virol.* 2008; 80(2): 277–82.

Falade-Nwulia, O., Suarez-Cuervo, C., Nelson, D. R., *et al.* Oral direct-acting agent therapy for hepatitis C virus infection: a systematic review. *Annals Intern. Med.* 2017; 166(9): 637–48.

Jacobsen, K. H. and Koopman, J. S. Declining hepatitis A seroprevalence: a global review and analysis. *Epidemiol. Infect.* 2004; 132(6): 1005–22.

Kamal, S. M. Acute hepatitis C: a systematic review. *Am. J. Gastroenterol.* 2008; 103(5): 1283–97; quiz 1298.

Kamar, N., Izopet, J., Tripon, S., *et al.* Ribavirin for chronic hepatitis E virus infection in transplant recipients. *N. Engl. J. Med.* 2014; 370(12): 1111–20.

Khuroo, M. S., Khuroo, M. S., and Khuroo, N. S. Hepatitis E: discovery, global impact, control and cure. *World J. Gastroenterol.* 2016; 22(31): 7030–45.

Lee, W. M., Hynan, L. S., Rossaro, L., *et al.* Intravenous N-acetylcysteine improves transplant-free survival in early stage non-acetaminophen acute liver failure. *Gastroenterology* 2009; 137(3): 856–64, 864 e1.

Lee, W. M., Stravitz, R. T., and Larson, A. M. Introduction to the Revised American Association for the Study of Liver Diseases position paper on acute liver failure 2011. *Hepatology.* 2012; 55(3): 965–7.

Lok, A. S. and McMahon, B. J. Chronic hepatitis B: update 2009. *Hepatology* 2009; 50(3): 661–2.

Polson, J. and Lee, W. M. American Association for the Study of Liver D. AASLD position paper: the management of acute liver failure. *Hepatology* 2005; 41(5): 1179–97.

Price, J. An update on hepatitis B, D, and E viruses. *Top. Antivir. Med.* 2014; 21(5): 157–63.

Renou, C., Afonso, A. M., and Pavio, N. Foodborne transmission of hepatitis E virus from raw pork liver sausage, France. *Emerg. Infect. Dis.* 2014; 20(11): 1945–7.

Romeo, R., Del Ninno, E., Rumi, M., *et al.* A 28-year study of the course of hepatitis Delta infection: a risk factor for cirrhosis and hepatocellular carcinoma. *Gastroenterology* 2009; 136(5): 1629–38.

Smith, B. D., Morgan, R. L., Beckett, G. A., *et al.* Recommendations for the identification of chronic hepatitis C virus infection among persons born during 1945–1965. *MMWR Morb. Mortal. Wkly. Rep.* 2012; 61(RR-4): 1–32.

Terrault, N. A., Lok, A. S. F., McMahon, B. J., *et al.* Update on prevention, diagnosis, and treatment of chronic hepatitis B: AASLD 2018 hepatitis B guidance. *Hepatology.* 2018; 67(4): 1560–99.

Thomas, D. L., Yarbough, P. O., Vlahov, D., *et al.* Seroreactivity to hepatitis E virus in areas where the disease is not endemic. *J. Clin. Microbiol.* 1997; 35(5): 1244–7.

Wedemeyer, H., Yurdaydin, C., Dalekos, G. N., *et al.* Peginterferon plus adefovir versus either drug alone for hepatitis delta. *N. Engl. J. Med.* 2011; 364(4): 322–31.

Zhu, F. C., Zhang, J., Zhang, X. F., *et al.* Efficacy and safety of a recombinant hepatitis E vaccine in healthy adults: a large-scale, randomised, double-blind placebo-controlled, phase 3 trial. *Lancet* 2010; 376(9744): 895–902.

Additional Readings

Davern, T. J. Fulminant hepatic failure in T. M. Bayless and A. M. Diehl (eds.), *Advanced Therapy in Gastroenterology and Liver Disease*, 5th edn. (Ontario: BC Decker, 2006), pp. 629–37.

Pratt, D. S. and Kaplan, M. M. Evaluation of abnormal liver-enzyme results in asymptomatic patients. *N. Engl. J. Med.* 2000; 342(17): 1266–71.

Recommendations for testing, managing, and treating hepatitis C from the American Association for the Study of Liver Diseases and Infectious Diseases Society of America, www.hcvguidelines.org (accessed November 13, 2017).

Peritonitis

Tu Carol Nguyen and Mercedes Torres

Introduction

The tremendous complexity of the abdomen makes diagnosis and treatment of intraperitoneal infection one of the greatest challenges in clinical medicine. Many intra-abdominal infections prompt urgent evaluation and some of these require immediate intervention. These conditions manifest via peritonitis, which is inflammation or infection of the lining of the abdominal cavity. Peritonitis is classified as primary, secondary, or tertiary on the basis of its underlying pathophysiology; the distinction is useful when considering relevant microbiology and treatment. The clinical findings in peritonitis may be diffuse or localized and peritoniteal signs may reflect actual infection within the peritoneal cavity (secondary peritonitis) or just inflammation from a contained underlying infection (such as non-perforated appendicitis).

Primary peritonitis occurs when bacteria seed the peritoneum hematogenously, via indwelling catheters, or by translocation across the intestinal wall. Spontaneous bacterial peritonitis (SBP) and tuberculous peritonitis are examples of this process.

Secondary peritonitis is caused by inflammation and/or infection arising in abdominal organs, as occurs with hollow viscus perforation, biliary tract disease, bowel ischemia, pancreatitis, and pelvic inflammatory disease. The process is generally polymicrobial, but the specific pathogens vary based on the source of infection.

Tertiary peritonitis refers to recurrent or persistent intra-abdominal infection after apparent definitive intervention with antibiotics and drainage.

Epidemiology

The single most common chief complaint for US emergency department (ED) visits is abdominal pain. Although many such patients are suffering from self-limited disease, some require definitive intervention and an error or delay in diagnosis can be disastrous.

The most common cause of primary peritonitis is catheter-related peritonitis, due to a peritoneal dialysis (Tenckhoff) catheter or peritoneovenous shunt.

The most common cause of secondary peritonitis is appendicitis. Lifetime risk of appendicitis in the United States is estimated to be 6 to 7%. Incidence is slightly lower in non-industrialized nations with higher-fiber diets and less use of refined carbohydrates. Although the peak incidence is in the second and third decades of life, appendicitis can occur at any age.

Diverticulitis is another common cause of secondary peritonitis in the United States; incidence is considerably lower in countries with high-fiber diets. One-third of Americans older than age 45, one-half older than age 70, and two-thirds older than age 85 have colonic diverticula. Ten to 25% of these patients develop complications related to their diverticula.

Peptic ulcers are mucosal erosions of the stomach or duodenum that are estimated to affect roughly one in ten people worldwide. In the United States, it has been estimated that, at any given time, 2% of the general population has symptomatic peptic ulcer disease. *Helicobacter pylori* infection (30% prevalence in the United States), alcoholism, and use of non-steroidal anti-inflammatory agents (NSAIDs) are the most common causes of the condition. Between 5 and 10% of patients with an ulcer suffer perforation, and this is fatal in as many as 10% of those affected.

Clinical Features

Primary Peritonitis: Catheter-Related Peritonitis and Spontaneous Bacterial Peritonitis

The most common cause of primary peritonitis is catheter-related peritonitis, due to a peritoneal dialysis (Tenckhoff) catheter or peritoneovenous shunt. Chronic indwelling devices generate peritonitis at a rate of 0.23 episodes per patient per year. Usually a single organism is responsible, with gram-positive cocci – *Staphylococcus aureus* or coagulase negative *Staphylococcus* – in 50%, and gram-negative bacilli – typically *P. aeruginosa* – in 15%. Fungal infections occur infrequently and are attributable to *Candida* species in 80% of cases. Diagnosis is made by analysis of dialysate fluid drawn from the catheter (see below).

Spontaneous bacteria peritonitis (SBP) is a primary peritonitis due to infection of ascites fluid (see Table 25.1). The presence of ascites is a necessary condition for developing such an infection, so this is almost exclusively a disease of patients with liver disease, and less commonly nephrotic syndrome. Translocation of gut bacteria is the initiating event. Phagocyte dysfunction in liver disease and low levels of immunologic proteins in ascites fluid facilitate the infection. The main pathogens are *E. coli*, *Klebsiella* species, and *S. pneumoniae*. The presentation of SBP can be subtle, with abdominal pain absent in more than half of patients with proven SBP. Fever, worsening renal function, nausea, or encephalopathy may be the only presenting symptoms. The diagnosis of SBP is made by ascites fluid analysis (see below). In-hospital mortality for cirrhotic patients with SBP is approximately 25 to 50% and recurrence rates approach 60% at 6 months without prophylaxis.

Secondary Peritonitis

Secondary peritonitis has a more distinct clinical presentation, almost always associated with abdominal pain and tenderness, and often with a history of acute onset. Any process that leads to intraperitoneal contamination or abscess formation can lead to secondary peritonitis, which may be contained to one region of the peritoneal cavity, or widespread. Even without frank intraperitoneal infection, severe inflammation, for example of the appendix, can produce somatic pain and localized signs of peritonitis. Signs of peritonitis include reduced bowel sounds, pain with gentle abdominal wall percussion, muscular rigidity, and rebound tenderness.

Visceral pain is often poorly localized or referred to a site not actually involved in the inflammatory process (see Table 25.2) This is explained by the embryologic migration of nerves and the origin of the gut as a midline structure with symmetric visceral innervation.

The following discussion highlights the most common etiologies of secondary peritonitis: perforated peptic ulcer, appendicitis, diverticulitis, post-operative anastomotic leak, and hepatic and splenic abscess.

Viscus Perforation

Perforated Peptic Ulcer

Peptic ulcers are mucosal erosions of the stomach and duodenum. They are most commonly related to *H. pylori* infection or anti-inflammatory medications. If these ulcers perforate through the submucosa, intraluminal contents can spill freely into the peritoneum (see Table 25.3). Other less common causes

Table 25.1 Clinical Features: Primary Peritonitis

Pathogenesis	Bacterial translocation across bowel or invasion along catheter
Organisms	**Catheter-related:** *Staphylococcus sp.* (66%) Gram-negative rods (33%) **Spontaneous:** *Escherichia coli* (50%) *Streptococcus* spp. (15–20%) *Klebsiella* (10%)
Signs and symptoms	Non-specific: • abdominal pain (<50%) • fever • nausea • catheter-site cellulitis • encephalopathy
Laboratory findings	• Leukocytosis • Catheter-related: fluid WBC >100 cells/mm^3 • SBP: ascites fluid absolute neutrophil count >250 cells/mm^3 • Positive fluid culture

WBC – white blood (cell) count.

Table 25.2 Patterns of Referred Abdominal Pain

Structure	Innervation	Pain
Foregut	T5–T9 roots	Supraumbilical or epigastric
Midgut	T8–T11 roots	Periumbilical
Hindgut	T11–L1 roots	Infraumbilical or pelvic
Diaphragm	Phrenic nerve	Ipsilateral scapula or shoulder

Table 25.3 Clinical Features: Peptic Ulcer Perforation

Pathogenesis	Commonly, *H. pylori* or NSAID use leading to mucosal erosion
Organisms	*Helicobacter pylori* **Peritoneal contamination by:** *Streptococcus* spp. *Lactobacillus* *Candida*
Signs and symptoms	Epigastric/upper abdominal pain: • history of prior episodes • acute onset • unrelenting peritoneal signs
Laboratory and radiographic findings	• Leukocytosis • Subdiaphragmatic air on CXR
Treatment	• Antibiotics (see Treatment section) • Operative closure of perforation • Expectant management if perforation is small and contained

CXR – chest X-ray.

of perforation include trauma, neoplasms, foreign body or corrosive ingestions, or iatrogenic (result of a diagnostic or therapeutic intervention). The spillage of acidic gastric contents,

Table 25.4 Clinical Features: Appendicitis

Pathogenesis	Obstruction by fecalith or swollen lymphatics causing venous congestion leading to ischemia
Organisms	*Bacteroides fragilis* *Escherichia coli* *Enterococcus* (Average of ten organisms isolated)
Signs and symptoms	• Umbilical/right lower abdominal pain • Anorexia (80%) • Nausea (80% – usually without emesis) • Fever
Laboratory and radiographic findings	• Modest leukocytosis (>10,000) • Appendix dilation and wall thickening • Stranding of periappendiceal fat
Treatment	• Antibiotics (see Treatment section) • Appendectomy • Percutaneous drainage of abscess

Table 25.5 Clinical Features: Diverticulitis

Pathogenesis	Unclear; possibly from obstruction of fecal material within colonic diverticula
Organisms	*Bacteroides fragilis* *Escherichia coli* *Enterococcus*
Signs and symptoms	• Left lower abdominal pain (>90%) • Dysuria • Loose bowel movements or constipation • Fever (80%) • Localized peritoneal signs
Laboratory and radiographic findings	• Leukocytosis • Diverticulosis • Free air or pericolonic air pocket • Localized colonic wall thickening/inflammation
Treatment	• Antibiotics • Bowel rest • Percutaneous drainage of abscess • Partial colectomy if recurrent or complicated

bacteria, and fungi into the peritoneum usually causes severe pain and other dramatic findings, and can result in sepsis.

Appendicitis

The appendix is a blind-ended tubular accessory of the cecum that does not have any known physiologic function in humans. When its lumen is obstructed (e.g. by a fecalith), continued mucosal secretion results in increased intraluminal pressure. Progressive increase in this pressure eventually impedes venous outflow, causing congestive ischemia with necrosis and possibly perforation. The typical chronology of symptoms and signs are pain, anorexia, tenderness, fever, and leukocytosis (see Table 25.4). Essentially all patients with appendicitis complain of abdominal pain, 75% in the right lower quadrant, 15% in the periumbilical region, and 10% diffuse. With timely treatment, most cases of appendicitis have a good outcome without peritonitis, but perforation occurs in about 25% of patients and 10% will develop an abscess.

Diverticulitis

Diverticula are small mucosal herniations through intestinal layers in the gastrointestinal wall. True diverticula contain all layers of the gastrointestinal wall and false diverticula or pseudo-diverticula contain only the submucosa and mucosa. Diverticulitis is inflammation of one or more of these diverticula. What triggers diverticulitis remains unclear, but it may be secondary to obstruction from fecal material or undigested food particles that collect in the diverticula, leading to inflammation and infection (see Table 25.5). In Western populations, diverticula are most commonly located in the sigmoid, whereas cecal diverticula are more commonly found in populations of Asian descent. Thus, symptoms are often in the lower left or right abdominal quadrants. At the time of presentation, diverticulitis frequently will have progressed to the point of localized microperforation, and sometimes gross perforation will have occured, with significant leakage of stool into the peritoneal cavity. Bowel habits may be altered, but not uniformly or consistently: painful defecation, constipation, loose stools, dysuria, or urinary retention may occur.

Anastomotic Leaks

Patients who have undergone resections or diversions of the enteric tract are prone to failed healing and leakage at the point of surgical anastomosis. Such anastomotic leaks can manifest within the first days after operation or up to 3 weeks later. Typical timing is between 2 days and 1 week after operation, with a risk of 2 to 16% depending on the type of operation. Anastomotic leaks are more common in patients who are malnourished or immunosuppressed (including chronic steroid users) and also in operations conducted in the setting of active infection. Leakage of enteric contents into the abdomen will produce peritonitis and a clinical syndrome of pain, tenderness, anorexia, and possibly fever and chills.

Solid Organ Abscesses

Liver Abscess

Liver abscesses are classified as pyogenic, amebic, fungal, or hydatid. Worldwide, amebic abscesses are the most common, whereas pyogenic abscesses are more common in the United States (see Table 25.6). *Klebsiella* has emerged as a common pyogenic hepatic abscess pathogen in Asia.

Hepatic abscesses present with right upper quadrant tenderness (70%), fever (>80%), and leukocytosis (75%). There is jaundice in approximately 33% of cases and a positive Murphy's sign in approximately 20%, so imaging is required to differentiate this condition from cholangitis. Overall mortality can be as high as 25% and is increased in patients with malignancy, low albumin (<2.5 g/dL), and multiple abscess foci.

Peripancreatic Abscess

Peripancreatic abscesses are a subacute complication of acute pancreatitis (see Table 25.7). Necrosis of a portion of the gland leaves dying tissue and severe regional inflammation, which can serve as a nidus for infection and abscess formation. *E. coli*

Table 25.6 Clinical Features: Hepatic Abscess

	Pyogenic	Amebic
Pathogenesis	Biliary obstruction or GI infection which spreads via portal vein (15–30% cryptogenic)	Environmentally acquired; invades liver from colon via portal system
Microbes	**Enteric organisms:** *Escherichia coli* *Klebsiella pneumoniae* *Bacteroides* spp. *Enterobacter* 60% polymicrobia Sterile in 15%	*Entamoeba histolytica*
Laboratory and radiographic findings	Majority are right lobed and solitary	Almost uniformly right lobed and solitary
Treatment	• Percutaneous or surgical drainage • Antibiotics	Metronidazole 500 mg PO TID

CT – computed tomography; ELISA – enzyme-linked immunosorbent assay; PO – by mouth.

Table 25.7 Clinical Features: Peripancreatic Abscess

Pathogenesis	Infection of inflamed or necrotic pancreas
Organisms	*Enterobacteriaceae* *Enterococcus* spp. *Staphylococcus* spp. *Candida* spp.
Signs and symptoms	• Fever • Persistent abdominal pain • Persistent anorexia
Laboratory and radiographic findings	• Leukocytosis and fever • Fluid collection along pancreas
Treatment	• Open drainage and necrosectomy • Antibiotics

Table 25.8 Clinical Features: Splenic Abscess

Pathogenesis	• Hematogenous (endocarditis, septic embolization) • Regional infection (intraabdominal) infection
Organisms	*Staphylococci* and *streptococci* (hematogenous) Polymicrobial
Signs and symptoms	• Fever • Left upper quadrant pain
Laboratory and radiologic findings	CT scan shows abscess
Treatment	As for secondary peritonitis

and *Enterococcus* are the most common pathogens, followed by *Staphylococcus*, *Pseudomonas*, and *Candida*; anaerobes are not as prevalent as in other parts of the gastrointestinal tract. Peripancreatic abscesses develop days to weeks after the initial onset of pancreatitis. The symptoms are similar to those of pancreatitis: nausea, vomiting, epigastric pain, and tenderness. Therefore, progression or non-resolution of pancreatitis symptoms (e.g. persistent pain with development of fever or leukocytosis) requires computed tomographic (CT) re-evaluation to rule out abscess formation. However, a necrotic gland does not necessarily indicate infection. Peripancreatic infections carry increased morbidity and mortality and can lead to pancreatic fistulae and hemorrhage from erosion of the gastroduodenal artery.

Splenic Abscess

Splenic abscesses are the least common solid organ abscesses and are associated with high mortality rates (see Table 25.8). These are due to hematogenous spread, typically from endocarditis, or direct extension of infection, but up to 25% are cryptogenic. *Staphylococcus aureus* and *Streptococcal* species are the predominant pathogens. Fever is present in more than 90%

of cases, left upper quadrant pain in 75%, and leukocytosis in 66%. Diagnosis is made by CT scan.

Differential Diagnosis

Abdominal pain is the presenting complaint in an enormous spectrum of disease processes. Work-up of possible peritonitis requires consideration of a complex differential diagnosis. Table 25.9 lists a number of potential causes of peritonitis with historical, exam, or diagnostic findings that can help to distinguish them.

Laboratory and Radiographic Findings

Paracentesis to rule out SBP should be performed in patients with ascites plus abdominal pain, fever, encephalopathy, or evidence of infection without an identifiable source. In the case of known cirrhosis, the fluid need only be sent for cell count, Gram stain, and culture. The presence of greater than 250 neutrophils (ANC)/mm³ is diagnostic of SBP. In the case of an indwelling dialysis catheter, the peritoneal fluid (dialysate) is withrawn and analyzed. A fluid WBC greater than 100 cells/mm³ with greater than 50 neutrophils is diagnostic of peritonitis. A positive fluid culture is also considered diagnostic of

Table 25.9 Differential Diagnosis of Abdominal Pain

Abdominal trauma	History; abdominal wall ecchymosis
Abdominal aortic aneurysm	Pulsatile mass; positive ultrasound; hemorrhagic shock
Adhesive bowel obstruction	Prior operations; lack of air in sigmoid/rectum on KUB; transition zone on CT
Cholecystitis	Gallbladder wall thickening on ultrasound
Constipation	Stool in colon on KUB; impaction on digital rectal
Ectopic pregnancy	Low pelvic pain; elevated beta-HCG
Gastroesophageal reflux	History; relief with antacids and repositioning
Gastritis	Alcoholism; NSAIDs; similar prior episodes
Hepatitis	Constitutional symptoms; history of exposure; ultrasound without evidence of cholecystitis
Hypercalcemia	Vague abdominal pain without tenderness
Incarcerated hernia	Palpable hernia; history of surgery
Inflammatory bowel disease	Prior history; bloody stools; fistulae
Irritable bowel syndrome	Similar prior pain; normal labs and imaging
Ischemic bowel	Acidosis; pain out of proportion to exam; vascular disease; bloody stools; bowel wall thickening or pneumatosis on CT
Ketoacidosis	History of diabetes; hyperglycemia; ketosis
Lymphoma	Visceral or peripheral lymphadenopathy; LDH
Migraine headache	History of migraine; abdominal CT normal
Omental infarction	Clinically similar to appendicitis; CT diagnostic
Ovarian/gonadal torsion	Abdominal pain is referred; primary pain pelvic; ultrasound with poor Doppler flow is diagnostic
Pancreatitis	Amylase or lipase elevation; gland inflammation without abscess on CT
Pelvic inflammatory disease	Tenderness on pelvic exam; normal pelvic ultrasound
Pneumonia	Cough or URI symptoms; chest imaging
Porphyria	Elevated porphyrin levels
Pyelonephritis	Costovertebral tenderness; urinalysis findings
Sickle cell crisis	Sickle disease; dehydration
Tubo-ovarian abscess	Lateralizing pelvic pain; pelvic ultrasound is diagnostic
Typhlitis	Neutropenia; normal appendix but cecal inflammation on CT
Uremia	Vague, diffuse pain with nausea; azotemia
Urolithiasis	Colicky flank pain; microscopic or gross hematuria
Zoster	Rash; dermatomal distribution

HCG – human chorionic gonadotropin; KUB – kidney, ureter, and bladder; LDH – lactate dehydrogenase; NSAID – non-steroidal anti-inflammatory drug; URI – upper respiratory infection.

Table 25.10 Imaging for Acute Abdominal Pain

Modality	Benefits	Limitations
KUB	Rapid, safe, portable Demonstrates bowel obstruction, free air (75%), or constipation	Limited sensitivity for most conditions and may delay ordering other imaging studies
CT	Cross-sectional anatomy Casts "widest net" for abdominal findings	• Possible contrast-induced nephropathy • Requires patient transport • Radiation exposure
US	Safe, portable Can be performed at bedside by acute care providers Most sensitive for biliary and gynecologic pathology and hydronephrosis	• Accuracy dependent on sonologist skill • Not useful for general abdominal survey

primary peritonitis. If a single organism is cultured, SBP is the most likely cause, whereas multiple organisms on Gram stain or culture indicate secondary peritonitis, and the underlying process must be identified.

When investigating the source of abdominal pain, imaging studies are usually required and are sometimes critical (see Table 25.10). The principal modalities are CT and ultrasonography (US). However, plain radiography can be useful early in the work-up to evaluate signs of bowel obstruction, presence of free air, and stool distribution.

CT with intravenous contrast may carry up to a 5% risk of contrast-induced nephropathy (CIN), though this is controversial. Intravenous fluid hydration or sodium bicarbonate prior to the CT, and use of non-ionic low osmolal contrast agents may mitigate the risk of CIN. Oral contrast is recommended in certain settings. If there is any concern for bowel leakage, water-soluble oral contrast should be used to avoid barium peritonitis.

Treatment and Prophylaxis

Management of peritonitis depends on its etiology (see Table 25.11). Therapy for SBP consists of a parenteral cephalosporin for at least 5 days followed by prophylaxis. Prophylaxis with

Table 25.11 Antibiotics for Primary Peritonitis

Spontaneous bacterial peritonitis	Cefotaxime 2 g IV every 8 hours *or* Ceftriaxone 1g IV every 12 hours Nosocomial infection: Piperacillin–tazobactam 3.375 g IV every 6 hours *plus* Vancomycin 15–20 mg/kg/dose IV every 8–12 hours Penicillin allergy: Levofloxacin 500 mg IV daily (only in patients not taking floroquinoline prophylaxis) *or* Vancomycin 15–20 mg/kg/dose IV every 8–12 hours *plus* Aztreonam 2 g IV every 8 hours
Catheter-related peritonitis	Vancomycin 15–20 mg/kg/dose IV every 8–12 hours *plus* Ceftazidime 2 g IV every 8 hours
Prophylaxis	Ciprofloxacin 500 mg PO daily *or* Trimethoprim–sulfamethoxazole 160/800 mg PO daily *or* Norfloxacin 400 mg PO daily
IV – intravenous.	

ciprofloxacin, trimethoprim–sulfamethoxazole, or norfloxacin decreases reinfection rates.

Empiric therapy for peritoneal dialysis catheter-associated peritonitis consists of gram-positive coverage with vancomycin plus an agent with broad gram-negative activity. In some cases, antibiotics may be instilled with the dialysate daily for up to 2 weeks. The regimen should be tailored to culture results as soon as possible.

Secondary peritonitis is treated with empiric antibiotic therapy (see Table 25.12). Diffuse peritonitis requires immediate broad spectrum coverage and evaluation and resuscitation of sepsis. Urgent surgical consultation should be obtained. Simple surgical excision (appendicitis) or CT-guided drainage (diverticular abscess) of the souce of peritonitis may be sufficient in localized infection. Open exploration, peritoneal lavage, and repair are required for diffuse peritonitis (perforated duodenal ulcer, anastomotic leak). If the intraperitoneal contamination is small and contained, antibiotics alone may be used.

When definitive operations are performed, antibiotics are not indicated beyond 24 to 72 hours post-operatively unless an ongoing infection is identified. In patients who undergo catheter drainage, antibiotics are often continued for a predetermined period (5 days to 2 weeks) or as long as pus is draining, which is based on historical practice patterns rather than clinical evidence. Antibiotic prophylaxis has no role in the management of secondary peritonitis.

Infection Control

Peritonitis is not a communicable disease, so special precautions are not required for protection of either the patient or others. Dressings and caps on peritoneal dialysis catheters should be managed in sterile fashion. Otherwise, standard precautions for patient contact are sufficient.

Pearls and Pitfalls

1. Integrate all available information when evaluating abdominal pain, as reliance on only lab studies or radiographs may delay accurate diagnosis and appropriate treatment.

Table 25.12 Antibiotics for Secondary Peritonitis

	Mild or Community-Acquired	**Severe**
Primary treatment	Piperacillin–tazobactam 3.375 g IV every 6 hours *or* Ceftriaxone 1 g IV every 12 hours *plus* Metronidazole 500 mg IV/PO every 8 hours *or* Ertapenem 1 g IV every 24 hours	Piperacillin–tazobactam 3.375 g IV every 6 hours *or* Meropenem 1 g IV every 8 hours *or* Ciprofloxacin 400 mg IV every 12 hours *plus* Metronidazole 500 mg IV every 8 hours
Penicillin-allergic	Ciprofloxacin 400 mg IV every 12 hours *plus* Metronidazole 500 mg PO/IV every 8 hours *or* Moxifloxacin 400 mg IV every 24 hours	Vancomycin 15–20 mg/kg/dose IV every 8–12 hours *plus* Aztreonam 2 g IV every 8 hours *plus* Metronidazole 500 mg IV every 8 hours
IV – intravenous; PO – by mouth.		

2. A history of shifting pain suggests a surgical cause of the acute abdomen.

3. An unremarkable abdominal exam and normal laboratory studies do not rule out peritonitis in an elderly patient with abdominal pain.

4. The use of CT with only IV contrast is sufficient for the diagnosis of most causes of peritonitis.

5. Peritonitis is a process that evolves, so serial abdominal examination is essential.

References

Alabousi, A., Patlas, M. N., Sne, N., and Katz, D. S. Is oral contrast necessary for multidetector computed tomography imaging of patients with acute abdominal pain? *Can. Assoc. Radiol. J.* 2015; 66(4): 318–22.

Barretti, P., Doles, J. V., Pinotti, D. G., and El dib, R. P. Evidence-based medicine: an update on treatments for peritoneal dialysis-related peritonitis. *World J. Nephrol.* 2015; 4(2): 287–94.

Choi, E. J., Lee, H. J., Kim, K. O., et al. Association between acid suppressive therapy and spontaneous bacterial peritonitis in cirrhotic patients with ascites. *Scand. J. Gastroenterol.* 2011; 46(5): 616–20.

Dever, J. B. and Sheikh, M. Y. Review article: spontaneous bacterial peritonitis – bacteriology, diagnosis, treatment, risk factors and prevention. *Aliment Pharmacol. Ther.* 2015; 41(11): 1116–31.

Deshpande, A., Pasupuleti, V., Thota, P., et al. Acid-suppressive therapy is associated with spontaneous bacterial peritonitis in cirrhotic patients: a meta-analysis. *J. Gastroenterol. Hepatol.* 2013; 28(2): 235–42.

Ge, P. S. and Runyon, B. A. The changing role of beta-blocker therapy in patients with cirrhosis. *J. Hepatol.* 2014; 60(3): 643–53.

Glauser, J., Siff, J., and Emerman, C. Emergency department experience with nonoral contrast computed tomography in the evaluation of patients for appendicitis. *J. Patient Saf.* 2014; 10(3): 154–8.

Goel, G. A., Deshpande, A., Lopez, R., et al. Increased rate of spontaneous bacterial peritonitis among cirrhotic patients receiving pharmacologic acid suppression. *Clin. Gastroenterol. Hepatol.* 2012; 10(4): 422–7.

Grabau, C. M., Crago, S. F., Hoff, L. K., et al. Performance standards for therapuetic abdominal paracentesis. *Hepatology* 2004; 40(2): 84–8.

Hill, B. C., Johnson, S. C., Owens, E. K., et al. CT scan for suspected acute abdominal process: impact of combinations of IV, oral, and rectal contrast. *World J. Surg.* 2010; 34(4): 699–703.

Kepner, A. M., Bacasnot, J. V., and Stahlman, B. A. Intravenous contrast alone vs intravenous and oral contrast computed tomography for the diagnosis of appendicitis in adult ED patients. *Am. J. Emerg. Med.* 2012; 30(9): 1765–73.

Kim, D. K., Yoo, T. H., Ryu, D. R., et al. Changes in causative organisms and their antimicrobial susceptibilities in CAPD peritonitis: a single center's experience over one decade. *Perit. Dial. Int.* 2004; 24(5): 424–32.

Loutit, J. Intra-abdominal infections in W. R. Wilson and M. A. Sande (eds.), *Current Diagnosis & Treatment in Infectious Diseases* (New York: McGraw-Hill, 2001), pp. 164–76.

Mandorfer, M., Bota, S., Schwabl, P., et al. Nonselective β blockers increase risk for hepatorenal syndrome and death in patients with cirrhosis and spontaneous bacterial peritonitis. *Gastroenterology* 2014; 146(7): 1680–90.e1.

Nathens, A. B., Curtis, J. R., Beale, R. J., et al. Management of the critically ill patient with severe acute pancreatitis. *Crit. Care Med.* 2004; 32(12): 2524–36.

Ng, K. K., Lee, T. Y., Wan, Y. L., et al. Splenic abscess: diagnosis and management. *Hepatogastroenterology* 2002; 49(44): 567–71.

Ordonez, C. A. and Puyana, J. C. Management of peritonitis in the critically ill patient. *Surg. Clin. North Am.* 2006; 86(6): 1323–49.

Schecter, W. P. Peritoneum and acute abdomen in J. A. Norton, R. R. Bollinger, A. E. Chang, et al. (eds.), *Surgery: Basic Science and Clinical Evidence* (New York: Springer, 2001).

Sersté, T., Melot, C., Francoz, C., et al. Deleterious effects of beta-blockers on survival in patients with cirrhosis and refractory ascites. *Hepatology* 2010; 52(3): 1017–22.

Sigal, S. H., Stanca, C. M., Fernandez, J., et al. Restricted use of albumin for spontaneous bacterial peritonitis. *Gut* 2007; 56(4): 597–9.

Solomkin, J. S., Mazuski, J. E., Bradley, J. S., et al. Diagnosis and management of complicated intra-abdominal infection in adults and children: guidelines by the Surgical Infection Society and the Infectious Diseases Society of America. *Surg. Infect. (Larchmt.)* 2010; 11(1): 79–109.

Sort, P., Navasa, M., Arroyo, V., et al. Effect of intravenous albumin on renal impairment and mortality in patients with cirrhosis and spontaneous bacterial peritonitis. *N. Engl. J. Med.* 1999; 341(6): 403–9.

Soybel, D. I. Acute abdominal pain in W. W. Souba, M. P. Fink, and G. J. Jurkovkich (eds.), *ACS Surgery Principles & Practice* (New York: American College of Surgeons, 2006).

Trikudanathan, G., Israel, J., Cappa, J., and O'Sullivan, D. M. Association between proton pump inhibitors and spontaneous bacterial peritonitis in cirrhotic patients – a systematic review and meta-analysis. *Int. J. Clin. Pract.* 2011; 65(6): 674–8.

Uyeda, J. W., Yu, H., Ramalingam, V., et al. Evaluation of acute abdominal pain in the emergency setting using computed tomography without oral contrast in patients with body mass index greater than 25. *J. Comput. Assist. Tomogr.* 2015; 39(5): 681–6.

Vermeulen, J., Van der harst, E., and Lange, J. F. Pathophysiology and prevention of diverticulitis and perforation. *Neth. J. Med.* 2010; 68(10): 303–9.

Chapter 26

Acute Infectious Diarrhea

Kimberly A. Schertzer and Gus M. Garmel*

Outline

Introduction

Acute diarrhea, defined as the presence of three or more loose stools per day for less than 2 weeks, is generally self-limited and infectious in etiology. In contrast, chronic diarrhea has a duration greater than 3 weeks, is less likely to resolve spontaneously, and is more likely to be mechanical in origin. In general, the pathophysiology of diarrhea is either osmotic, secretory, inflammatory, or mechanical. *Osmotic diarrhea* is the result of poorly absorbed molecules, such as lactulose, that draw water into the intestinal lumen. *Inflammatory diarrhea* occurs when inflammation of the bowel mucosa causes decreased fluid resorption. *Secretory diarrhea* occurs when there is an increased amount of fluid secreted into the bowel lumen, usually secondary to the effects of bacterial enterotoxin or other secretagogues on the mucosa. *Mechanical diarrhea* occurs with increased gut motility, and is often seen in irritable bowel disease or following surgery. Infectious diarrhea encountered in the acute care setting is most often osmotic or inflammatory. The microbiology of infectious diarrhea is discussed below.

Epidemiology

Infectious diarrhea is the second leading cause of mortality worldwide. In the United States, as many as 375 million episodes of diarrheal illness are estimated to occur annually. Recently, diarrheal illness was responsible for 1.5% of all US

emergency department (ED) visits, as well as 1.8 million hospitalizations and 3,100 deaths each year. The CDC has several bulletins and educational campaigns related to diarrheal illnesses following disasters in an attempt to protect the public and health care workers.

Clinical Features

Inflammatory diarrhea tends to cause frequent, small, bloody bowel movements. It is generally associated with fevers, significant abdominal pain, and tenesmus (the frequent urge to have a bowel movement). Large numbers of fecal leukocytes are identified in most cases of inflammatory diarrhea (see Table 26.1).

Non-inflammatory diarrhea tends to be watery, non-bloody, and large volume, often exceeding a liter per day. Although it is generally milder in its course, significant fluid and electrolyte imbalances may occur. Associated nausea, vomiting, and mild abdominal cramping are common, though fever is generally absent. Fecal leukocytes are uncommon.

Differential Diagnosis and Microbiology

Diarrhea may be a presenting sign of primary GI illness (including colitis, inflammatory bowel disease, GI bleed) or AIDS. Although medications (such as excessive cathartic-use antibiotics, chemotherapeutic agents, and less commonly certain antidepressants or lithium) and mechanical factors (such

* The authors wish to acknowledge Jonathan Blum, MD, PhD, Chief of Infectious Diseases, TPMG, Kaiser Santa Clara Medical Center, Santa Clara, CA, for his careful review of and recommendations to this chapter.

Table 26.1 Clinical Features: Acute Infectious Diarrhea

	Pathogen	Signs and Symptoms
Inflammatory	*Campylobacter jejuni* *Clostridium difficile* Enterohemorrhagic and enteroinvasive *Escherichia coli* *Shigella* Non-typhi *Salmonella* *Entamoeba histolytica*	• Bloody • Associated with fever, abdominal pain, and tenesmus • Frequent, small-volume stool • Fecal leukocytes
Non-inflammatory	Rotavirus Norwalk virus Adenovirus *Giardia lamblia* *Cryptosporidium parvum* *Vibrio cholerae* Enterotoxigenic *E. coli*	• Non-bloody • Nausea, vomiting, mild abdominal pain • Watery, large-volume stool

Table 26.2 Viral Diarrheal Illnesses

Pathogen	Key Features	Diagnosis	Treatment
Norovirus and Norwalk-like virus	• Frequent cause of community and cruise ship outbreaks	• Clinical suspicion • PCR	• Supportive
Rotavirus	• Frequently affects children • Peak incidence 3–35 months of age	• Stool enzyme immunoassay and serum antibody tests	• Supportive
Astrovirus	• Frequent cause of US epidemics • Milder clinical symptoms	• Electron microscopy (seldom used)	• Supportive

as lactose intolerance, artificial sweetners, and intestinal disorders like irritable bowel syndrome) may cause acute diarrhea, its origin is usually infectious. Viral etiologies are most common (50 to 70%), followed by bacterial (15 to 20%) and parasitic (10 to 15%). Obtaining a travel history is critical, as it may help to narrow the differential diagnosis in some cases.

Viruses Causing Acute Diarrhea

Viral diarrhea most commonly occurs during winter months as a result of family and community outbreaks of noroviruses or rotavirus (see Table 26.2). Other pathogens include astrovirus, calicivirus, enterovirus, and adenovirus. Incubation periods range from 1 to 3 days, and the resulting illnesses are generally mild and self-limited (typically less than 4 days). Viral diarrhea is characterized by an abrupt onset of abdominal cramps and nausea, followed by diarrhea with or without vomiting. Fever occurs in approximately half the cases, often accompanied by headache, myalgias, and symptoms of upper respiratory infection.

Noroviruses

Currently, noroviruses are the most common cause of gastroenteritis in the United States. Noroviruses are associated with 26% of cases of diarrhea in patients presenting to the ED. Two noroviruses, Norwalk and Norwalk-like virus, are frequently implicated in community outbreaks. They are a common cause of diarrheal outbreaks on cruise ships and in daycare centers. Norovirus has been identified as the responsible agent for as much as 90% of acute diarrheal cases on cruise ships, and it must

be reported when it occurs in this setting. Of the 13.8 million cases of foodborne illness reported in the United States annually, 9.2 million are due to noroviruses. The mode of transmission is predominantly foodborne (37%), followed by person-to-person contact (20%), oysters (10%), and contaminated water (6%).

Rotavirus

Worldwide, rotavirus is the most common cause of severe diarrheal disease in young children and infants. It is thought to be responsible for as many as 20% of the deaths attributed to diarrhea. Rotavirus has a peak incidence between 3 and 35 months of age, though adults may acquire it from their children. It has been implicated in 10% of cases of traveler's diarrhea. Prior illness exposure and immunization may provide protection against severe recurrences. Diagnostic stool enzyme immunoassay and serum antibody tests exist, though they are not generally recommended.

Astrovirus

Astrovirus is associated with 2 to 9% of cases of diarrhea globally. In general, symptoms are similar but milder than those associated with rotavirus, with less nausea, fever, and vomiting. Astrovirus is a frequent cause of US daycare and hospital epidemics.

Bacteria Causing Acute Diarrhea

Campylobacter

Campylobacter now represents the most common cause of bacterial diarrhea in developed countries. It accounts for approximately 1.3 million annual cases in the United States, nearly all due to *Campylobacter jejuni*. The incidence of *Campylobacter*-related diarrhea peaks in late summer and early fall. Spread is most frequently via undercooked poultry, though dogs, cats, and birds have also been identified as reservoirs; person-to-person spread is rare. *Campylobacter* often causes an ileocolitis, which may produce either a watery or hemorrhagic diarrhea. Of patients with *Campylobacter*, more than 50% will have gross or occult blood in their stool. Symptoms include fever, abdominal pain, nausea, and malaise, which may be mistaken for appendicitis or irritable bowel syndrome. The frequency of diarrhea may be dramatic; approximately 20% of individuals with *Campylobacter* diarrhea will have more than fifteen bowel movements daily. Symptoms generally resolve within a week even without antibiotics, though they may persist for 1 to 3 weeks in up to 20% of patients. *Campylobacter* is also the leading cause of traveler's diarrhea in persons visiting South and Southeast Asia.

Complications of *Campylobacter* infection vary according to the age and characteristics of the affected host (see Tables 26.3 and 26.4). Preceding infection with *Campylobacter* has been identified in as many as 40% of patients with Guillain–Barré.

Salmonella

Salmonella accounts for an estimated 1.3 million cases of diarrhea in the United States yearly. It occurs most frequently in the summer and fall months and is commonly implicated in epidemics. The most common serotypes in the United States are *Salmonella enteritidis* and *Salmonella typhimurium*. Transmission is generally foodborne from contaminated poultry, meats, eggs, and milk, though other vectors, such as household pets (especially turtles or lizards), have been identified. Symptoms of *Salmonella* infection include nausea, vomiting, abdominal discomfort (frequently mimicking appendicitis), and occasionally bloody diarrhea. The bacteria usually invade small intestine epithelium, though colonic invasion also occurs. Symptoms generally last from 2 to 24 days. Individuals at the extremes of age (elderly people and children less than 12 months of age) are the highest risk group for salmonellosis. Normal gastric activity effectively kills more than 99.9% of gram-negative bacteria, including *Salmonella*; therefore, patients with raised gastric pH levels through gastrectomy or pharmacologic therapy are at increased risk of *Salmonella* infection.

Salmonellosis has a high rate of complications, including microabscess formation, toxic megacolon, and a notable 2 to 4% rate of bacteremia. Risk factors for the development of these complications include hemolytic or sickle cell anemias, malignancy, steroid use, chemo- or radiation therapy, and acquired immunodeficiency syndrome (AIDS). Elderly patients are less likely to present with classic symptoms of *Salmonella* gastroenteritis, and are at greater risk of developing invasive disease.

Shigella

Shigella infections account for 10 to 20% of bacterial diarrhea in the United States. *Shigella sonnei* accounts for 75% of *Shigella* isolates, and only the *Shigella dysenteriae* strain produces the shiga toxin responsible for serious complications.

Table 26.3 Complications of *Campylobacter* Infection

Population	Complication
Children and young adults	• Appendicitis • Mesenteric adenitis • Toxic megacolon • Pseudomembranous colitis • Cholecystitis
Adults (otherwise healthy)	• Reactive arthritis
Adults with liver disease	• Spontaneous bacterial peritonitis
Infrequent complications	• Hemolytic anemia • Carditis • Encephalopathy • Guillain–Barré syndrome

The inoculum needed to cause infection is extremely small (as low as 200 organisms), with transmission of infection predominately person-to-person or from contaminated food and water supplies. *Shigella* outbreaks are common in nursing facilities, daycare centers, and other institutions. Men who have sex with men are at increased risk for infection with *Shigella flexneri*.

Shigella infections generally begin with fever, fatigue, anorexia, and malaise. This is followed by watery diarrhea that may progress to dysentery, defined as inflammation of the intestine associated with bloody stool and pain. Frequent bowel movements are common; patients may have up to 100 per day in severe cases. Duration of illness ranges from a few days to 1 week. Significant complications include colonic hemorrhage, HUS-TTP (hemolytic uremic syndrome–thrombotic thrombocytopenic purpura), bacteremia, generalized seizures, encephalopathy, and reactive arthritis.

Enterotoxigenic *E. coli* (ETEC)

Enterotoxigenic *E. coli* (ETEC) is the most common cause of traveler's diarrhea worldwide (though *Campylobacter* is more common in South and Southeast Asia). ETEC produces both heat-stabile and heat-labile toxins. It causes a watery diarrhea that is not invasive. Symptoms develop 1 to 3 days following exposure, and may last up to 4 days.

Enteroinvasive *E. coli* (EIEC)

EIEC is similar to *Shigella* infection, though without toxin production. EIEC is marked by fever, predominantly dysenteric diarrhea, and tenesmus. Spread is person-to-person, foodborne, or waterborne.

Enteroaggregative *E. coli* (EAEC)

Responsible for several outbreaks in the United States and industrialized nations, EAEC is also known to cause a persistent chronic diarrhea in children and is an increasingly important pathogen affecting travelers. In some regions of Latin America, it is the second most common bacterial cause of traveler's diarrhea. Transmission is likely foodborne, though exposure does not always result in diarrhea. Symptoms may include watery diarrhea with or without blood or mucus, abdominal pain, nausea, vomiting, fever, and borborygmi. The incubation period ranges from 8 to 18 hours. Duration of symptoms is highly variable, often lasting weeks.

Shiga-Toxin-Producing *Escherichia coli* (STEC), Also Known as Enterohemorrhagic *E. coli* (EHEC)

Shiga-toxin-producing *E. coli* 0157:H7 and related strains (STEC) differs from other forms of *E. coli* in that it produces shiga toxins 1 and 2. These toxins inhibit protein synthesis and cause cell injury and cell death. Most infections occur in the summer and fall months. After an incubation period of 3 to 4 days, STEC causes an initially non-bloody diarrhea that may be followed by a bloody diarrhea after 1 to 3 days. Pre-diarrheal signs include fever, abdominal pain, irritability, fatigue, headache, myalgias, and confusion. There may be severe abdominal pain, pain on defecation, and abdominal tenderness on examination. Patients are generally afebrile on presentation, though they may report a history of fever at symptom onset. STEC infection in children may be mistaken for intussusception, inflammatory colitis, or appendicitis, and, in adults, for diverticulitis, cancer, hemorrhoids, ischemic colitis, or bowel infarction.

A minority of cases of STEC infection will be complicated by the hemolysis and acute renal failure of HUS. In fact, STEC is the most common cause of HUS in the world. There is no correlation between the severity of diarrheal symptoms and the development of HUS, though children younger than 5 years and elderly patients are at increased risk of this complication.

The spread of STEC is primarily foodborne, waterborne, or person-to-person. Outbreaks have been reported in daycare centers. Detection is by culture on a sorbitol–MacConkey's agar, which may not be part of standard stool culture orders at all hospitals. Furthermore, this particular culture only identifies the *E. coli* 0157:H7 strains, which accounts for approximately 50% of STEC cases, and may miss other shiga-toxin-producing *E. coli* strains. For this reason, the CDC recommends assay testing for non-0157:H7 STEC strains simultaneously. Treatment is primarily supportive, consisting of rehydration and time, though patients with HUS may require temporary dialysis. Antibiotics and antimotility agents are contraindicated, as they may increase the likelihood of HUS. Additionally, narcotics and non-steroidal anti-inflammatory agents are not recommended. All cases of STEC require notification and involvement of the health department.

Clostridium difficile

This anaerobic, spore-forming bacillus is a common cause of acute diarrhea among hospitalized patients. Following a disturbance of normal colonic flora, usually due to antibiotics, *C. difficile* enterotoxins A and B interact to cause colitis and pseudomembranes. Nearly all antibiotics have been implicated in the development of *C. difficile* colitis, but the most frequent offenders are clindamycin, cephalosporins, amoxicillin, and flouroquinolones. Amoxicillin is not likely to cause *C. difficile* diarrhea per se, but it contributes to a high incidence in the population because it is used so frequently. Administration of antibiotics within the previous 3 months

is considered a risk factor for the development of *C. difficile* diarrhea. Additional risk factors for symptomatic infection include older age, comorbid illness, current or recent hospitalization (especially with enteral feeding or ICU stay), and elevated gastric pH (use of proton pump inhibitor use). The incubation period is unknown. Initial symptoms typically include a profuse, watery diarrhea, which may progress to bloody diarrhea. This may be accompanied by fever, abdominal cramping, and leukocytosis.

The diagnosis of *C. difficile* is made by detection of the specific toxin through one of several laboratory tests, generally molecular detection (PCR) or antigen testing. Although *C. difficile* diarrhea resolves without treatment in 20% of cases, most clinicians administer oral metronidazole (first line) or oral vancomycin in addition to stopping any potentially responsible antibiotic. The rates of relapse approach 20%. Antimotility agents should be avoided, as they increase the risk of toxic megacolon. Further information about *C. difficile* may be found in Chapter 28.

Yersinia enterocolitica

More common in winter months, *Yersinia* most frequently affects children under 10 years of age. It is found in streams, lake water, and contaminated milk and is transmitted by animals (including dogs, cats, and farm animals). The most common symptom is diffuse, poorly localized abdominal pain, which occurs in up to 84% of cases and may be mistaken for appendicitis. In addition, patients may present with hemorrhagic diarrhea, nausea, vomiting, and arthritis. Laboratory work-up may demonstrate a leukocytosis, elevated ESR, and heme-positive stool. Diagnosis is made with stool cultures on *Yersinia*-selective agar.

Vibrio cholerae and *Non-cholera Vibrios*

Toxigenic *Vibrio cholerae* is infrequent in the United States, with only 35 cases reported between 2010 and 2014. Worldwide incidence is on the rise due to global outbreaks; travelers, outbreak responders, and medical/public health professionals are at increased risk for contracting vibrio-related diarrhea. Most cases occur in individuals returning from travel abroad, or among those ingesting shellfish from the Gulf Coast. *Vibrio cholerae* produces a profuse, "rice water" diarrhea that is severe, acute in onset, and accompanied by significant dehydration. This diarrhea generally lasts 2 to 3 days. Non-cholera *Vibrio* strains, such as *Vibrio parahemolyticus*, are seen more frequently in the United States as a result of contaminated shellfish. *Vibrio vulnificus* has a high complication rate among patients with chronic liver disease. In this population, it frequently causes sepsis and has a mortality rate approaching 50%.

Parasites Causing Acute Diarrhea

In general, parasitic disease tends to be travel-related. Spread is person-to-person or through contact with contaminated food or water. Common offending parasites include *Giardia lamblia*, *Cryptosporidium*, *Isospora belli*, *Cyclospora*, and *Entamoeba*

Table 26.4 Infectious Bacterial Diarrhea

Pathogen	Epidemiologic Settings or Modes of Transmission	Key Features	Diagnosis	Treatment (see Table 26.10)
Campylobacter	• Community acquired • Foodborne	• Frequently from undercooked poultry • Causes an ileocolitis that may produce watery or hemorrhagic diarrhea • Linked to development of Guillain–Barré	• Fecal leukocytes • Stool culture on antibiotic medium	• Supportive • Antibiotics if immunocompromised, high fever, bloody stools, or duration >1 week
Salmonella	• Community acquired • Foodborne	• Foodborne from contaminated poultry, meats, eggs, and milk, and pets • Symptoms may mimic appendicitis • May cause microabscess formation or asymptomatic carrier state	• Stool culture on special agar	• Supportive • Antibiotics for high-risk* patients only
Shigella	• Community acquired • Person-to-person spread	• Causes colonic involvement and mucosal breakdown • Malaise and anorexia are common	• Stool culture	• Antibiotics
Shiga-toxin-producing *E. coli* (STEC)	• Sporadic infection • Community outbreaks • Foodborne (undercooked hamburger, contaminated produce)	• Most patients are afebrile (may report fever at home) • Present with severe abdominal pain and tenderness • Often mistaken for other abdominal illnesses	• Stool culture on sorbitol–MacConkey's agar for 0157:H7 strains • Assay testing for non-0157:H7 strains	• Supportive • Avoid antibiotics as they predispose to HUS-TTP
Clostridium difficile	• Antibiotic use • Nosocomial spread	• Overgrowth of bacteria producing enterotoxins • Highly contagious among hospitalized patients	• PCR • Antigen testing	• Antibiotics • Avoid antimotility agents
Yersinia enterocolitica	• Community acquired • Domestic animals • Foodborne	• Most commonly affects children under 10 years of age • Found in lakes and streams • Most common sign is diffuse, vague abdominal discomfort	• Stool culture on *Yersinia*-selective agar	• Supportive • Antibiotics if enteritis or arthritis present
Vibrio cholerae	• Seafood • Foreign travel	• Acute onset of profound, watery diarrhea • Significant dehydration may occur	• Stool culture	• Supportive • Antibiotics

* High-risk includes immunosuppressed patients, patients at extremes of age, pregnant patients, or patients with cardiac disorders or prosthetic implants.

histolytica (see Table 26.5). In the United States, the most common causes of chronic infectious diarrhea both among immunocompetent and immunocompromised hosts are *Giardia* and *Cryptosporidium*.

Giardia lamblia

Acquisition of *Giardia lamblia* is usually by drinking contaminated lake or stream water. However, spread can also be person-to-person, and *Giardia* is a frequent cause of outbreaks in daycare centers and nursing homes. Although some carriers may be asymptomatic, most develop a chronic, watery diarrhea often associated with mucus. Nausea, abdominal pain, significant and malodorous flatulence, weight loss, and steatorrhea are common.

Cryptosporidium

Cryptosporidium causes an acute, watery diarrhea that resolves spontaneously in 2 to 3 days in immunocompetent adults. However, it is a common cause of chronic diarrhea (4 to 6 weeks) in AIDS patients and immunocompetent children. Symptoms of infection include afebrile diarrhea, fatigue, flatulence, and abdominal pain. *Cryptosporidium* transmission is primarily via water, and outbreaks have occurred from contaminated city water supplies. It is also spread through contact

Table 26.5 Parasitic Diarrheal Illnesses

Pathogen	Key Features	Diagnosis	Treatment
Giardia lamblia	• Watery diarrhea, steatorrhea, flatulence • Acquired from contaminated water and community outbreaks	• Stool ova and parasite testing • EIA (availablility may depend on facility)	• Metronidazole or tinidazole
Cryptosporidium	• Long-term intestinal damage may occur • Fatigue, flatulence, and abdominal discomfort common	• Acid-fast smear of stool samples	• Supportive if immunocompetent • Nitazoxanide in children and in HIV-positive adults
Isospora	• Malaise, headache, and vomiting common • Causes direct cell damage	• Acid-fast stain • Peripheral eosinophilia seen on CBC	• Supportive • Trimethoprim–sulfamethoxazole
Cyclospora cayetanensis	• Causes a watery diarrhea with muscle aches and nausea • Often relapsing episodes • Travel to endemic area is common	• Modified acid-fast smear	• Trimethoprim–sulfamethoxazole
Entamoeba histolytica	• Secretion of toxins causes intestinal ulceration • Complications include liver abscess	• PCR or direct antibody test (availability may depend on facility)	• Metronidazole

CBC – complete blood count; HIV – human immunodeficiency virus.

with livestock and person-to-person, and has been implicated in daycare center outbreaks. Diagnosis is made with a modified acid-fast smear of stool samples.

Isospora

Isospora spread is usually through contaminated water. Predominantly affecting immunocompromised patients, *Isospora* outbreaks have occurred in daycare centers and institutions. Symptoms include watery diarrhea, steatorrhea, headache, fever, malaise, abdominal pain, and vomiting. *Isospora* is difficult to distinguish clinically from *Giardia* infection.

Cyclospora cayetanensis

Travel to an endemic area usually precedes *Cyclospora* infection, which results in a chronic, watery, relapsing diarrhea even in immunocompetent patients. *Cyclospora* is primarily transmitted via contaminated food or water. Diarrhea is typically proceeded by a 1-day prodrome of malaise and fever and other symptoms include abdominal cramping, nausea, and muscle aches. A prolonged watery diarrhea often lasts for several weeks. Diagnosis is by modified acid-fast smear of stool.

Entamoeba histolytica

Entamoeba is primarily a disease of developing countries. In developed countries, it occurs in migrants from endemic areas, returning travelers, and HIV-infected patients. Spread is generally through contaminated water or food. Clinical disease may be asymptomatic, but more commonly manifests as severe bloody diarrhea. Rare complications include peritonitis and development of liver abscesses.

Laboratory and Radiographic Findings

Viruses are the most common causes of acute diarrhea. Most of these are self-limited, requiring only symptomatic treatment.

As a result, ED laboratory work-up is indicated only for specific concerning elements in the history or physical examination.

It is prudent to check serum electrolytes in a patient experiencing profuse diarrhea. In addition, if bloody diarrhea is present, a complete blood count assists in quantifying the amount of blood lost. Bandemia in a toxic-appearing patient suggests an invasive pathogen. Fecal leukocytes indicate colonic inflammation and are neither very sensitive nor specific for acute bacterial infection, though in conjunction with a suggestive clinical history may increase the likelihood of this etiology.

Bacterial stool cultures have limited utility in most patient populations, though they are frequently ordered. Their overall yield is low, with a positive rate reported as low as 1.6%. Cultures should be limited to patients with severe disease and certain comorbidities and risk factors. In addition, there are public health reasons to perform stool cultures in patients in certain occupations, such as those who are food handlers or work in daycare (see Tables 26.6 and 26.7).

Patients with a history of hospitalization or antibiotic use within the previous 3 months should have their stool tested for *C. difficile* toxin. Specifics of this testing (enzymatic vs. PCR) vary by facility. These patients should also be placed on contact isolation. The presentation of *C. difficile* diarrhea or colitis may be delayed for several months after the initial infection with this pathogen. Conscientious handwashing with soap and water is important to prevent spread, as hand-sanitizing gels are generally ineffective against *C. difficile*.

There is no indication to test for ova and parasites in most immunocompetent patients, though testing for parasites is indicated in patients with the risk factors described in Table 26.8.

Radiographs are not typically part of the diagnostic evaluation for patients presenting with acute or chronic diarrheal illnesses. The circumstances to consider imaging

Table 26.6 Indications to Obtain Stool Cultures

Bloody diarrhea (specify concern for *E. coli* 0157:H7)

Fever of 38.5 °C (101.3 °F) or greater

History:

Recent travel to developing countries or to regions with endemic diarrheal illness

Anal intercourse

High-risk employment (food handler, daycare worker, nursing facility worker)

Immunocompromised status

Toxic appearance

Severe diarrheal disease

Extremes of age (<1 year or >65 years)

Consider if:

- Signs of significant dehydration

- Presence of six or more stools in 24 hours

- Diarrhea lasting more than 48 hours

Table 26.7 Diarrheal Illnesses Requiring Health Department Notification (National Standards)

Amebiasis*

Campylobacteriosis*

Cholera, both toxigenic and non-toxigenic strains

Cryptosporidiosis

Cyclosporiasis

Giardiasis

Leptospirosis

Hemolytic uremic syndrome, post-diarrheal

Salmonellosis

Shiga-toxin-producing *Escherichia coli* (STEC)

Shigellosis

Viral hemorrhagic fevers (including Ebola and Marburg virus)

* Notification requirements may vary by state/county.

Based on the 2017 Nationally Notifiable Disease list produced by the Centers for Disease Control and Prevention, wwwn.cdc.gov/nndss/document/NNC_2017_Notification_Requirements_By_Condition_20161108.pdf.

Table 26.8 Indications for Ova and Parasite Testing in the Emergency Department

History of recent travel to mountainous regions or to developing countries

Exposure to groups of infants with diarrhea

History of homosexual activity

AIDS

Chronic diarrhea without previous diagnosis or prior testing

include: potential for foreign body, bowel obstruction, possible mass, pneumatosis intestinalis, perforation, or surgical causes of diarrhea. Computed tomography (CT) should be considered if there is concern for toxic megacolon (a complication of *C. difficile* infection) or pneumatosis intestinalis (air in the bowel wall). Plain film radiographs may be used to exclude free air, bowel obstruction, or radio-opaque foreign bodies when these conditions are possible, though CT imaging will provide more detail and has increased sensitivity and specificity. The risk of radiation-induced malignancy should be considered in younger patients; however, imaging should not be withheld if deemed essential to patient management.

Treatment and Prophylaxis
Fluid Replacement

Dehydrated patients often describe symptoms of dizziness, lightheadedness, and thirst. Clinical signs of dehydration include hypotension, tachycardia, delayed capillary refill, and decreased urine output. Mild to moderate dehydration generally responds well to oral rehydration, and patients should be encouraged to drink fluids containing some glucose and salt. Commercially prepared oral rehydration solutions are recommended over juice or sports drinks. Milk or milk products should be avoided, because a temporary lactase deficiency often accompanies diarrhea. The use of ondanestron in the setting of vomiting with diarrhea has been reported to increase the ability to tolerate oral rehydration, decrease the need for intravenous fluid, and increase overall caregiver satisfaction.

Severe dehydration requires parenteral fluid resuscitation. Normal saline is a reasonable initial option for parenteral hydration of patients with significant dehydration, though close monitoring of electrolytes and hemodynamic status is important. Although controversial, Lactated Ringer's solution may be the crystalloid of choice because it contains both glucose and potassium. One study recommends that the patient's estimated fluid deficit be determined, with 50% replaced in the first hour of treatment. The remainder should be replaced over the subsequent 3 hours, with close observation for signs of hyponatremia (irritability, restlessness, altered mental status or weakness).

Dietary Therapy

Many clinicians continue to recommend the gradual introduction of a limited diet of bananas, rice, applesauce, and toast (BRAT diet), though there is no scientific support for this practice. It is prudent to recommend avoiding caffeine and spicy and fatty foods. In general, fasting and bowel rest is not necessary during acute diarrhea as most nutrients are still absorbed. Early refeeding and oral rehydration therapy have been shown to have better outcomes and shorter duration of diarrhea. Adults should gradually increase their intake of sodium (soups, crackers), potassium (fruit, bananas), and carbohydrates (crackers, rice, bread, pasta) as tolerated.

Antimotility Agents

Antimotility agents (loperamide) slow intraluminal fluid transport and increase intestinal absorption of fluid, decreasing the number of watery stools. They are not recommended in children under 6 years of age or in patients with fever, bloody stools, or immunocompromised status, as they can delay pathogen clearance and increase tissue invasion. In cases of *C. difficile* and *Shigella*, antimotility agents increase the risk of toxic megacolon. In cases of *E. coli* 0157:H7, they have been demonstrated to increase the likelihood of HUS–TTP.

Bismuth Subsalicylate

Bismuth subsalicylate has both an antisecretory effect (salicylate) and antibacterial activity (bismuth). It may have anti-inflammatory properties as well. It has been shown to reduce the frequency of stools in children and decrease the duration of diarrhea by hours in adults. Despite this, current pediatric guidelines do not encourage its use in children because it contains salicylates, which may increase the likelihood of Reye syndrome. It is an appropriate self-treatment agent in adult travelers with mild symptoms of traveler's diarrhea.

Rifaximin

Rifaximin has been studied against other agents as treatment for traveler's diarrhea. Benefit has been demonstrated over placebo. Rifaximin has been suggested when prophylaxis against traveler's diarrhea is indicated. Rifaximin has gained favor over flouroquinolones because of its greater safety and its lower risk of development of *C. difficile* infection and exetended-spectrum beta-lactamase-producing Enterobacteriaceae (ESBL-PE). Rifaximin should not be used if there is clinical suspicion for *Campylobacter*, *Salmonella*, *Shigella*, or other causes of invasive diarrhea. Caution is advised in patients with hepatic impairment.

Probiotics

Probiotics are non-pathogenic bacteria that eliminate or reduce the effects of pathogenic bacteria. Although there are numerous probiotics, most information exists for lactobacilli and bifidobacteria. Studies on probiotic efficacy yield varied results; studies suggest that probiotics may decrease the duration of acute diarrhea by 1 day and the number of stools by 1.5 per day.

Antimicrobial Therapy for Bacterial Diarrhea

The use of antibiotics in acute diarrhea is limited as viral etiologies are four times more common than bacterial. In addition, antibiotics may increase the complication rates of certain infections and, in the emergency setting, it is generally impossible to distinguish between patients harboring pathogens that respond to antibiotics and those in which antibiotics may be contraindicated (see Table 26.9). Moreover, there are increasing concerns about antibiotic resistance and adverse effects of the drugs themselves. For all these reasons, antibiotics should be used judiciously for acute diarrhea.

On the other hand, antibiotics do reduce duration of symptoms by approximately 1 day in patients with severe, bacterial diarrhea. While there are no evidence-based guidelines for selecting patients with acute diarrhea for whom treatment is indicated, it seems reasonable to treat those with the following:

- more than eight stools per day
- diarrhea lasting longer than 1 week

Table 26.9 Role of Antibiotics for Various Pathogens

Pathogens for which antibiotics may be beneficial
Enterotoxigenic *E. Coli* (ETEC) – as self-treatment for traveler's diarrhea
Shigella
Vibrio
Clostridium difficile
Enteroinvasive *E. coli* (EIEC)
Enteroaggregative *E. coli* (EAEC)
Pathogens for which antibiotics are not generally recommended
*Campylobacter**
Enterohemorrhagic *E. coli* (EHEC)* ‡
Salmonella‡ †
Shiga-toxin-producing *E. coli* (STEC)‡

* Offers no benefit.

‡ Increases risk of relapse or other complications.

† Prolongs fecal shedding.

- fever and mucus in stools
- evidence of severe volume depletion
- elderly and immuncompromised patients

Antibiotics generally should be witheld in patients who are afebrile with bloody diarrhea until EHEC has been ruled out.

Antibiotics are not indicated for EHEC infection because they offer no improvement in outcome and are associated with an increased incidence of hemolytic uremic syndrome (see Table 26.10). Some experts recommend *against* starting empiric antibiotics, particularly in bloody diarrhea, until the *absence* of shiga-toxin-producing *E. coli* infection is confirmed by culture. Although no specific clinical trials have explored the use of antibiotics for EIEC, antibiotics are nevertheless recommended, and treatment with antibiotics significantly decreases the duration of illness in enteroaggregative *E. coli* (EAEC). The choice of antibiotics is influenced by local resistance patterns; quinolones and azithromycin are current recommendations as possible therapeutic agents.

Antibiotics are usually not recommended for *Salmonella* infections because they do not reduce symptoms and may prolong the carrier state. However, as up to 4% of these patients will have concomitant bacteremia, antibiotics should be prescribed to anyone who is immunosuppressed, at the extremes of age, pregnant, or has a cardiac disorder, prosthetic implant, or severe diarrhea.

Except in high-risk individuals, such as pregnant women and the immunocompromised, antibiotics are not recommended for *Campylobacter* infection because they offer no benefit. Newborns and infants may require antibiotic treatment if they have persistent fever, bloody diarrhea, diarrhea lasting more than 7 days, volume depletion, or eight or more bowel movements daily. Antibiotics do not alter the course of *Yersinia* infection, though a fluoroquinolone or trimethoprim–sulfamethoxazole (TMP–SMX) is recommended for severe enteritis and complications such as mesenteric adenitis, arthritis, and erythema nodosum. Treatment with

Table 26.10 Antibiotic Therapy for Acute Bacterial Diarrhea

Pathogen	Therapy Recommendation
Campylobacter	Antibiotics only for severe disease or immunocompromised patients Azithromycin 500 mg PO daily × 3 days *or* Ciprofloxacin 500 mg PO twice daily (regional resistance to quinolones is increasing)
Salmonella	Antibiotics only for severe disease, age <1 year or >50, or immunocompromised patients Ciprofloxacin 500 mg PO twice daily (if infection is NOT aquired in Asia) *or* Azithromycin 500 mg PO daily × 7 days (14 days if immunocompromised) if infection acquired in Asia
Shigella	Adults: Ciprofloxacin 750 mg PO daily × 3 days *or* Levofloxacin 500 mg PO daily × 3 days *or* Azithromycin 500 mg PO daily × 3 days (drug of choice for resistant strains) Children: Azithromycin 10 mg/kg/day (max. dose 1 g) once daily × 3 days
Shiga-toxin-producing *E. coli* (STEC)	Supportive therapy WITHOUT antibiotics Increased risk of HUS–TTP with antimicrobial and antimotility treatment
Clostridium difficile	Refer to Chapter 28 in this volume
Yersinia enterocolitica	Antibiotics only for severe disease or immunocompromised patients Ceftriaxone 2 g IV daily (if bacteremic) Gentamicin 5 mg/kg/day IV (if bacteremic) *or* Ciprofloxacin 500 mg PO BID instead of Ceftriaxone (if susceptible)
Vibrio cholerae	Doxycycline 300 mg PO × 1 Children or pregnant adults: Azithromycin 20 mg/kg PO × 1 (maximum is the adult dose of 1 g)
Vibrio parahemolyticus	Generally supportive therapy is best Doxycycline 100 mg PO/IV every 12 hours × 5–7 days
EIEC (enteroinvasive *E. coli*)	Generally supportive therapy is best
EAEC (enteroaggregative *E. coli*)	Usually self-limited, but may benefit patients with HIV Ciprofloxacin 750 mg PO daily × 3 days *or* Ciprofloxacin 500 mg BID × 7 in patients with AIDS
EHEC (enterohemorrhagic *E. coli*)	Antibiotics not recommended

Note: Antibiotic duration may be longer in immunocompromised hosts.

IV – intravenous; PO – by mouth.

Adapted from D. N. Gilbert, H. F. Chambers, G. M. Eliopoulos, M. S. Saag (eds.), *Sanford Guide to Antimicrobial Therapy*, 47th edn (Sperryville, VA: Antimicrobial Therapy, 2017), Kindle edition.

antibiotics decreases mortality and shortens the duration of illness for all patients with *Shigella*. *Vibrio cholerae* recommended treatment is oral doxycycline in adults and azithromycin in children.

Antimicrobial Therapy for Parasitic Diarrhea

Diarrheal illness due to parasites is generally related to travel. Parasitic infection often results in longer periods of diarrhea than viral or bacterial etiologies. Once identified, parasitic organisms typically respond to directed antibiotic therapy, though treatment in immunocompromised hosts is more difficult (see Table 26.11).

Complications and Admission Criteria

Most of the morbidity and mortality associated with acute diarrhea is the result of either dehydration or electrolyte imbalances. It is rare that the infectious nature of acute diarrhea causes problems unless the patient is significantly immunocompromised. Patients with signs of severe dehydration (specifically hypotension or orthostasis) after fluid administration, those unable to maintain a reasonable hydration status, and those with significant metabolic abnormalities due to electrolyte disturbances warrant admission or further observation for IV fluid resuscitation and correction of electrolyte abnormalities. Immunocompromised individuals and those at the

Table 26.11 Therapy for Acute Parasitic Diarrhea

Pathogen	Therapy Recommendation
Giardia	Antibiotic resistance is rare, though treatment failures or relapses are common Tinidazole 2 g PO × 1 *or* Nitazoxanide 500 mg PO BID × 3 days
Cryptosporidium	Antibiotics only for severe disease Nitazoxanide recommended for HIV-negative adults and immunocompetent children Nitazoxanide is NOT approved for immunodeficient patients
Isospora	Immunocompetent adults: TMP-SMX 160/800 mg PO BID × 7–10 days Adults with AIDS: TMP-SMX 160/800 mg PO QID × 3–4 weeks
Cyclospora	Immunocompetent adults: TMP-SMX 160/800 mg PO BID × 7–10 days Adults with HIV/AIDS: TMP-SMX 160/800 mg PO QID × 3–4 weeks (then 1 tab 3 ×/weekly in patients with AIDS)
Entamoeba histolytica (Amebiasis)	Metronidazole 500–750 mg PO TID × 10 days, followed by Iodoquinol 650 mg PO TID × 20 days to clear intestinal cysts
PO – by mouth.	

Table 26.12 Summary of Guideline Recommendations for Evaluation and Treatment of Diarrhea in Immunocompetent Adults (Not Caused by Clostridium Difficile)*

1. Empiric antibiotic therapy is not recommended for community-acquired diarrhea or mild traveler's diarrhea.

2. Severe traveler's diarrhea with fever should be treated with azithromycin, with rare exception.

3. In patients receiving antibiotics for traveler's diarrhea, adjunctive loperamide to decrease duration of diarrhea and increase chance of cure is recommended.

4. Culture-independent methods of stool testing (such as PCR) may be used to identify the etiology in adult patients with dysentery, moderate to severe diarrhea, and symptoms lasting more than 7 days.

5. Persistent diarrhea (14–30 days) should be initially evaluated with culture and/or culture-independent microbiologic testing.

6. Probiotics or prebiotics are not recommended in acute diarrhea in adults, except in cases of post-antibiotic-associated illness.

* Adapted from M. Acree and A. M. Davis, Acute diarrheal infections in adults. *JAMA* 2017; 318(10): 957–8.

extremes of age warrant special consideration for possible admission or additional observation, as do individuals with poor social circumstances.

Infection Control

In general, good hand-washing and hygiene techniques are recommended to control the spread of infection in patients with acute diarrhea. Isolation, especially in cases of patients hospitalized with *C. difficile* or rotavirus, is also recommended to decrease disease transmission. Cases of salmonellosis, shigellosis, and STEC infection should be reported to the Department of Public Health (see Table 26.7). Food handlers and individuals who work with infants and/or the elderly should be kept from work until their diarrhea has resolved. Some health departments require negative stool studies before these employees are allowed to return to work.

A summary of the guideline recommendations for the evaluation and treatment of diarrhea can be found in Table 26.12.

Pearls and Pitfalls

1. Acute care providers should be familiar with current guidelines for management of diarrhea in immunocompetent adults, which are summarized in Table 26.12.

2. Always assess for historical features that may prompt diagnostic testing in the acute care setting, including high-risk sexual behavior, antibiotic use or hospitalization in the preceding 3 months, high-risk employment (e.g. food handlers, day care workers, health care workers who work with high-risk populations), and travel abroad or to mountainous regions.

3. Stool cultures are seldom indicated in cases of acute nonbloody diarrhea, but should be sent in the case of bloody diarrhea, diarrhea with fever, high-risk historical features, extremes of age, toxic appearance, immunocompromised host status, or when diarrhea has been chronic.

4. Studies for ova and parasites are indicated only in patients with AIDS, patients with recent mountain travel, with exposure to groups of young children, and in men with a history of sexual activity with other men.

5. Oral rehydration is recommended in all cases, especially in elderly individuals or travelers with severe, watery diarrhea. Rehydration with intravenous fluids (preferably with Lactated Ringer's solution) for severe fluid losses and electrolyte management constitute the primary treatment in the acute care setting of patients with both acute and chronic diarrhea.

6. Routine antibiotics for community-acquired diarrhea or mild traveler's diarrhea is not recommended. There are risks associated with the use of empiric antibiotics for the treatment of acute diarrhea. Guidelines recommend empiric antimicrobials in travelers with moderate to severe symptoms (such as fever or dysentery) who have a high likelihood of bacterial infection, or when the likelihood of parasitic etiologies is high.

7. Antibiotic treatment of infectious diarrhea in immunocompromised hosts is prescribed for a longer duration.

References

Acree, M. and Davis, A. M. Acute diarrheal infections in adults. *JAMA* 2017; 318(10): 957–8.

Banks, J. B., Sullo, E. J., and Carter, L. Clinical inquiries. What is the best way to evaluate and manage diarrhea in the febrile infant? *J. Fam. Pract.* 2004; 53(12): 996–9.

Beaugerie, L. and Petit, J.-C. Microbial-gut interactions in health and disease. Antibiotic-associated diarrhoea. *Best Pract. Res. Clin. Gastroenterol.* 2004; 18(2): 337–52.

Casburn-Jones, A. C. and Farthing, M. J. G. Management of infectious diarrhoea. *Gut* 2004; 53(2): 296–305.

Colletti, J. E., Brown, K. M., Sharieff, G. Q., *et al.* The management of children with gastroenteritis and dehydration in the emergency department. *J. Emerg. Med.* 2010; 38(5): 686–98.

Danewa, A. S., Shah, D., Batra, P., *et al.* Oral ondansetron management of dehydrating diarrhea with vomiting in children aged 3 months to 5 years: a randomized controlled trial. *J. Pediatr.* 2016; 169: 105–9.e3.

Dennehy, P. H. Rotavirus vaccines: an update. *Curr. Opin. Pediatr.* 2005; 17(1): 88–92.

DuPont, H. L. Persistent diarrhea: a clinical review. *JAMA* 2016; 315(24): 2712–23.

Elmer, G. W. and McFarland, L. V. Biotherapeutic agents in the treatment of infectious diarrhea. *Gastroenterol. Clin. North Am.* 2001; 30(3): 837–54.

Freedman, S. B., Ali, S., Oleszczuk, M., *et al.* Treatment of acute gastroenteritis in children: an overview of systematic reviews of interventions commonly used in developed countries. *Evid.-Based Child Health* 2013; 8(4): 1123–37.

Freeland, A. L., Vaughan, G. H., and Banerjee, S. N. Acute gastroenteritis on cruise ships – United States, 2008–2014. *MMWR Morb. Mortal. Wkly. Rep.* 2016; 65(1): 1–5.

Gendrel, D., Treluyer, J. M., and Richard-Lenoble, D. Parasitic diarrhea in normal and malnourished children. *Fundam. Clin. Pharmacol.* 2003; 17(2): 189–97.

Gilbert, D. N., Chambers, H. F., Eliopoulos, G. M., and Saag, M. S. (eds.), *The Sanford Guide to Antimicrobial Therapy*, 47th edn (Sperryville, VA: Antimicrobial Therapy, 2017).

Goldsweig, C. D. and Pacheco, P. A. Infectious colitis excluding *E. coli* O157:H7 and *C. difficile*. *Gastroenterol. Clin. North Am.* 2001; 30(3): 709–33.

Goodgame, R. W. Viral causes of diarrhea. *Gastroenterol. Clin. North Am.* 2001; 30(3): 779–95.

Gore, J. I. and Surawicz, C. Severe acute diarrhea. *Gastroenterol. Clin. North Am.* 2003; 32(4): 1249–67.

Guerrant, R. L., Van Gilder, T., Steiner, T. S., *et al.* Practice guidelines for the management of infectious diarrhea. *Clin. Infect. Dis.* 2001; 32(3): 331–51.

Huang, D. B., Okhuysen, P. C., Jiang, Z. D., *et al.* Enteroaggregative *Escherichia coli*: an emerging enteric pathogen. *Am. J. Gastroenterol.* 2004; 99(2): 383–9.

Ilnyckyj, A. Clinical evaluation and management of acute infectious diarrhea in adults. *Gastroenterol. Clin. North Am.* 2001; 30(3): 599–609.

Kosek, M., Bern, C., and Guerrant, R. L. The global burden of diarrhoeal disease, as estimated from studies published between 1992 and 2000. *Bull. World Health Organization* 2003; 81(3): 197–204.

Kyne, L., Farrell, R. J., and Kelly, C. P. *Clostridium difficile*. *Gastroenterol. Clin. North Am.* 2001; 30(3): 753–77.

Lee, S. D. and Surawicz, C. M. Infectious causes of chronic diarrhea. *Gastroenterol. Clin. North Am.* 2001; 30(3): 679–92.

Mack, D. R. Probiotics-mixed messages. *Can. Fam. Physician* 2005; 51(11): 1455–7, 1462.

Myer, P. A., Mannalithara, A., Singh, G., *et al.* Clinical and economic burden of emergency department visits due to gastrointestinal diseases in the United States. *Am. J. Gastroenterol.* 2013; 108(9): 1496–507.

Nataro, J. P. and Sears, C. L. Infectious causes of persistent diarrhea. *Pediatr. Infect. Dis. J.* 2001; 20(2): 195–6.

Ramaswamy, K. and Jacobson, K. Infectious diarrhea in children. *Gastroenterol. Clin. North Am.* 2001; 30(3): 611–24.

Ramzan, N. N. Traveler's diarrhea. *Gastroenterol. Clin. North Am.* 2001; 30(3): 665–78.

Riddle, M. S., DuPont, H. L., and Connor, B. A. ACG Clinical Guideline: diagnosis, treatment, and prevention of acute diarrheal infections in adults. *Am. J. Gastroenterol.* 2016; 111(5): 602–22.

Sellin, J. H. The pathophysiology of diarrhea. *Clin. Transplantation* 2001; 15(4): 2–10.

Seupaul, R. A. Diarrhea in S. V. Mahadevan and G. M. Garmel (eds.), *An Introduction to Clinical Emergency Medicine*, 2nd edn (Cambridge University Press, 2012), pp. 279–87.

Sirinavin, S. and Garner, P. Antibiotics for treating salmonella gut infections. *Cochrane Database of Systematic Reviews* 1999, Issue 1, Art. No. CD001167.

Slotwiner-Nie, P. K. and Brandt, L. J. Infectious diarrhea in the elderly. *Gastroenterol. Clin. North Am.* 2001; 30(3): 625–35.

Starr, J. *Clostridium difficile* associated diarrhoea: diagnosis and treatment. *BMJ* 2005; 331(7515): 498–501.

Steffen, R. and Gyr, K. Diet in the treatment of diarrhea: from tradition to evidence. *Clin. Infect. Dis.* 2004; 39(4): 472–3.

Steffen, R., Hill, D. R., and DuPont, H. L. Traveler's diarrhea: a clinical review. *JAMA* 2015; 313(1): 71–80.

Sullivan, A. and Nord, C. E. Probiotics and gastrointestinal diseases. *J. Intern. Med.* 2005; 257(1): 78–92.

Tarr, P. I., Gordon, C. A., and Chandler, W. L. Shiga-toxin-producing *Escherichia coli* and haemolytic uraemic syndrome. *Lancet* 2005; 365(9464): 1073–86.

Tarr, P. I. and Neill, M. A. *Escherichia coli* O157:H7. *Gastroenterol. Clin. North Am.* 2001; 30(3): 735–51.

Thielman, N. M. and Guerrant, R. L. Clinical practice. Acute infectious diarrhea. *N. Engl. J. Med.* 2004; 350(1): 38–47.

Wilhelmi, I., Roman, E., and Sanchez-Fauquier, A. Viruses causing gastroenteritis. *Clin. Microbiol. Infect.* 2003; 9(4): 247–62.

Yates, J. Traveler's diarrhea. *Am. Fam. Physician* 2005; 71(11): 2095–100.

Additional Readings

Gore, J. I. and Surawicz, C. Severe acute diarrhea. *Gastroenterol. Clin. North Am.* 2003; 32(4): 1249–67.

Ilnyckyj, A. Clinical evaluation and management of acute infectious diarrhea in adults. *Gastroenterol. Clin. North Am.* 2001; 30(3): 599–609.

Talan, D., Moran, G. J., Newdow, M., *et al.* Emergency ID NET Study Group. Etiology of bloody diarrhea among patients presenting to United States emergency departments: prevalence of *Escherichia coli* O157:H7 and other enteropathogens. *Clin. Infect. Dis.* 2001; 32(4): 573–80.

Thielman, N. M. and Guerrant, R. L. Clinical practice. Acute infectious diarrhea. *N. Engl. J. Med.* 2004; 350(1): 38–47.

Chapter 27

Diarrhea in HIV-Infected Patients

Michael J. A. Reid and Phyllis C. Tien

Introduction and Microbiology

Diarrhea is an extremely common problem in human immuno-deficiency virus (HIV) positive patients. The list of possible infectious causes is very long and shifts depending on the stage of immunosuppression. At higher CD4 counts, common etiologies include enteric bacterial pathogens such as *Clostridium difficile*, *Salmonella*, *Shigella*, and protozoal diseases such as *Giardia* and *Entamoeba*. With more advanced HIV disease, opportunistic pathogens become more likely, such as cryptosporidia, microsporidia, *Mycobacterium avium* complex disease, and cytomegalovirus virus. Non-infectious causes of diarrhea are also common in this population, particularly medication side effects. In contrast to the evaluation of diarrhea in immunocompetent patients, extensive stool studies play a much larger role in the evaluation of HIV-positive patients. Stool culture, *Clostridium difficile* toxin, ova and parasites, and *Giardia* antigen testing often establish the cause of diarrhea in relatively immunocompetent HIV-positive patients, but in the setting of a CD4 count <200 cells/mm^3, further work-up may be necessary to diagnose opportunistic infections.

Epidemiology

Diarrhea increases in prevalence with lower CD4 counts. More than 50% of patients with a CD4 count below 50 cells/mm^3 will experience at least one episode of diarrhea each year, and in some geographic areas this number approaches 100%. Approximately one-half of patients hospitalized with complications of HIV infection report diarrhea. Diarrhea has been shown to be an independent predictor of death in this population.

Clinical Features

A careful history, including the patient's most recent CD4 count, use of antibiotics, and currently prescribed antiretroviral regimen, often provides diagnostic clues as to the etiology of diarrhea. The duration, frequency, volume, and character of the diarrhea, as well as associated symptoms such as weight loss, fever, and abdominal pain, will help narrow the differential. Patients with bacterial diarrhea will often, though not invariably, present with associated crampy abdominal pain. The lack of associated abdominal pain or other symptoms should suggest viral acute gastroenteritis or medication side effects.

Knowledge of the most recent CD4 count is crucial. In patients with relatively intact immune function, as measured by a current CD4 count greater than 200, viral gastroenteritis and medication side effects account for a majority of cases of acute diarrhea. With decreasing CD4 counts, other pathogens increasingly predominate, and the prevalence of persistent and chronic diarrhea increases several fold (see Differential Diagnosis and Table 27.4).

Likewise, the medication history is also crucial, as is knowledge of which HIV medications are most often associated with diarrhea (see below). Because patients with HIV frequently receive multiple antibiotics, higher rates of both *Clostridium difficile* and small bowel overgrowth are reported. Diarrhea in the setting of recent antibiotic use (within the last 10 weeks) or use of medications that decrease gastric acidity (H2 antagonists and proton pump inhibitors) would raise concern for *Clostridium difficile*. Small bowel overgrowth is characterized by excess growth of mostly gram-negative enteric flora, resulting in chronic diarrhea and malabsorption, culminating in malnutrition and vitamin deficiencies.

An explicit sexual history should be taken, as anal–oral contact increases the risk of certain pathogens, as well as sexually transmitted causes of diarrhea and rectal symptoms. Proctitis due to gonorrhea and chlamydia may be mistaken for colitis. Infections causing enteritis that may be transmitted via a fecal–oral route include *Salmonella*, *Shigella*, *Campylobacter jejuni*, hepatitis A, *Yersinia*, *Giardia lamblia*, *Entamoeba histolytica*, *Cryptosporidium*, and *Herpes simplex*.

A complete social history should also include information about recent travel, dietary changes, pets, water sources, and sick contacts (especially children). If the patient is employed in a food-handling or child-care industry, health department notification may be required. Physical examination should focus on the abdominal exam, noting tenderness, quality of bowel sounds, stool color and guaiac, and any hepatosplenomegaly or masses. The presence of fever and signs of dehydration, such as dry mucous membranes and tachycardia, should be noted. Signs of an invasive pathogen and systemic involvement include fever, severe abdominal cramps, and bloody stools. Patients with long-standing chronic diarrhea often exhibit signs of wasting and malnutrition, though these can result from advanced HIV infection itself. Finally, evaluating the degree of systemic illness is essential to assessing the need for hospital admission.

Fever is generally more common when diarrhea is caused by *Shigella*, *Salmonella*, enteroinvasive *Escherichia coli*, *Campylobacter jejuni*, and CMV, and less common when caused by *Staphylococcus aureus*, *Clostridium perfringens* food poisoning, *Clostridium difficile*, enterotoxigenic *Escherichia coli*, *Escherichia coli* 0157:H7, and *Cryptosporidium*.

Gastrointestinal involvement with Kaposi's sarcoma can cause diarrhea and this should be considered in patients who exhibit cutaneous Kaposi's.

Differential Diagnosis

Diarrhea in HIV-positive patients poses a bigger diagnostic dilemma than it does in an immunocompetent host. HIV patients are susceptible to all the infections that commonly afflict the normal host, as well as a multitude of opportunistic infections that are almost exclusively seen in HIV as well as medication side effects. Moreover, some pathogens that cause mild or self-limiting disease in immunocompetent hosts may cause severe and prolonged disease in the setting of advanced HIV infection.

A useful way to consider the differential diagnosis for diarrhea in an individual infected with HIV is to distinguish acute from chronic diarrhea, and small from large bowel involvement (see Tables 27.1, 27.2, and 27.3). Acute diarrhea is defined as the presence of three or more loose or watery stools per day for less than 2 weeks. Diarrhea is defined as persistent if it has been present between 2 and 4 weeks and is considered chronic when present for 4 weeks or more. Pathogens infecting the small bowel affect the secretory and nutritional absorption functions of the gastrointestinal (GI) tract and typically present with large volumes of watery stool, often accompanied by cramps, bloating, and abdominal gas (see Table 27.1). Severe or prolonged diarrhea may result in dehydration, malnutrition, and weight loss. Large bowel involvement primarily affects water resorptive capacity and typically causes frequent, small-volume diarrhea that may be bloody or mucoid and is often accompanied by pain.

For example, several weeks of voluminous watery diarrhea with cramps, bloating, and nausea in a patient with low CD4 counts would suggest small bowel infection with

Table 27.1 Small Versus Large Bowel Diarrhea

	Symptoms	Common Pathogens
Small bowel	Large volume Watery stool Upper abdominal cramps Bloating Gas Weight loss Malnutrition Dehydration	*Escherichia coli* *Salmonella** Viral (e.g. rotavirus) *Mycobacterium avium* complex *Cryptosporidium** *Giardia lamblia* *Microsporidium** Malabsorption
Large bowel	Small volumes Frequent bowel movements Mucoid or bloody stool Tenesmus Lower abdominal cramps	*Campylobacter jejuni** *Clostridium difficile* Enteroinvasive *E. coli* *Entamoeba histolytica* Gonorrhea *Staphylococcus aureus* *Shigella* *Yersinia* CMV

* May involve both small and large bowel, but typically presents as listed.

Table 27.2 Common Causes of Acute Diarrhea in HIV

Bacterial infections
- **Campylobacter**
- **Clostridium difficile**
- *Escherichia coli*
- **Salmonella**
- **Shigella**
- *Yersinia*
- *Vibrio*

Viral infections
- Adenovirus
- Astrovirus
- **Norovirus**
- **Rotavirus**

Protozoal infections
- *Blastocystis hominis*
- **Entamoeba histolytica**
- **Giardia lamblia**

Other
- Antibiotic-associated diarrhea
- **Antiretroviral-associated diarrhea**

More common entities in **bold**.

Cryptosporidium, *Microsporidium*, *Cystoisospora belli* (formerly *Isospora belli*), or *Giardia*. A recent onset of small-volume diarrhea with hematochezia and tenesmus should raise suspicion for *Shigella* or *Campylobacter* infection of the large bowel, whereas a longer duration of these symptoms suggests colitis from cytomegalovirus (CMV), herpes, or *Clostridium difficile*.

Since the infectious pathogens associated with diarrheal disease in HIV infection vary with the degree of immunosuppression, stratifying patients on the basis of their most recent CD4 count provides another way to structure the differential diagnosis.

For example, watery diarrhea and profound dehydration in a patient with CD4 count of 150 may suggest cryptosporidial infection. In a patient with a CD4 count less than 50 and diarrhea accompanied by fevers and night sweats, *Mycobacterium avium complex* (MAC) or *Mycobacterium tuberculosis* (TB) are possibilities. CMV is another imortant etiology that accounts

Table 27.3 Causes of Persistent and Chronic Diarrhea in HIV

Bacterial and mycobacterial infections
- *Campylobacter jejuni*
- **Clostridium difficile**
- *Escherichia coli*
- *Mycobacterium tuberculosis*
- **Mycobacterium avium complex**
- *Salmonella*
- *Shigella*

Protozoal infections
- **Cryptosporidium**
- *Cyclospora*
- *Cystoisospora belli*
- **Entamoeba histolytica**
- **Giardia lamblia**
- **Microsporidium**

Fungal infections
Candida albicans
Cryptosporosis
Histoplasmosis

Viral infections
- **Cytomegalovirus**
- Herpes
- HIV (AIDS enteropathy)

Other causes
- **Antibiotic, antiretroviral, or other medication effects**
- Functional disorders
- Irritable bowel syndrome
- Inflammatory bowel disease
- Kaposi's sarcoma
- Lymphomas
- Malabsorption
- Pancreatic insufficiency (MAC, CMV, pentamidine, didanosine)
- Small bowel overgrowth

More common entities in **bold**.

Table 27.4 Diarrhea Etiologies According to CD4 Count

CD4 Range	Etiology
CD4 counts >200	• *Clostridium difficile* infection
	• Antiretroviral-associated diarrhea
	• Self-limiting bacterial acute gastroenteritis (AGE)
	• Viral acute gastroenteritis
	• *Giardia lamblia*
	• *Entamoeba histolytica*
	• Self-limiting *Cryptosporidium*
	• *Mycobacterium tuberculosis*
	• Small bowel overgrowth
CD4 counts 50–200	All of the above
	• Invasive/systemic *Salmonella*
	• Invasive bacterial enteritis
CD4 counts <50	All of the above
	• *Mycobacterium avium* complex
	• Chronic and severe *Cryptosporidium* and *Microsporidium*
	• HIV enteropathy
	• CMV colitis

for 5 to 10% of diarrhea in patients with CD4 counts less than 50. Clinical manifestations of CMV colitis include weight loss, anorexia, abdominal pain, debilitating diarrhea, and malaise. Patients with CMV colitis may also experience odynophagia or visual field defects from concomitant esophageal and retinal CMV infection. A retinal exam for CMV is indicated in such cases. Finally, HIV itself infects the gut wall and can cause a chronic diarrheal illness associated with malabsorption and

Table 27.5 Commonly Used Antiretroviral Medications That Can Cause Diarrhea and the Proportion Reporting Diarrhea in Clinical Trials

HIV protease inhibitors:
- Darunavir (8–14%)
- Lopinavir/ritonavir (7–28%)
- Ritonavir (15–68%)

HIV integrase strand transfer inhibitors:
- Dolutegravir (<2%)
- Elvitegravir (7%)
- Raltegravir (<2%)

HIV nucleoside reverse transcriptase inhibitors:
- Abacavir (7%)
- Emtricitabine (9–23%)
- Lamvudine (14–18%)
- Tenofovir (9–16%)
- Zidovudine (8%)

HIV non-nucleoside reverse transcriptase inhibitors:
- Efavirenz (3–14%)
- Etravirine (>2%)
- Nevirapine (<2%)
- Rilpivirine (<2%)

CCR5 antagonists
- Maraviroc (<1%)

Boosting agents
- Cobicistat (<2%)

weight loss. This so-called "HIV enteropathy" is generally seen in very advanced HIV disease (CD4 counts <100). It is a diagnosis of exclusion.

The most common non-infectious causes of diarrhea in HIV-positive patients are medication side effects. Table 27.5 lists commonly used antiretroviral medications and the proportion of patients who reported diarrhea as listed in the pharmaceutical package inserts for the individual antiretroviral drugs. Among the antiretroviral medications, protease inhibitors (especially ritonavir) are the biggest offenders. Because other protease inhibitors as well as nucleoside reverse transcriptase inhibitors are generally used in conjunction with ritonavir, their contribution to the diarrhea may be unclear. Patients will report a temporal association between initiation of the medication and onset of moderate- to low-volume watery diarrhea or loose stools, possibly with abdominal bloating, gas, and discomfort. Abdominal cramps, fever, bloody stool, and dehydration are absent. The diarrhea may wane after 4 to 6 weeks on the medication, but will often persist.

Laboratory Diagnosis and Radiographic Findings

Additional work-up will depend on the patient's immunosuppresion status, severity of diarrhea, and signs of dehydration and wasting on exam. Complete blood count and basic chemistry profile are indicated to evaluate for anemia, leukocytosis, renal impairment, and electrolyte abnormalities. In patients with advanced HIV disease, etiologic diagnosis should always be pursued. Depending on the clinical scenario, the following investigations may be appropriate:

- stool culture and sensitivity (specify cultures for *Escherichia coli* 0157:H7, *Vibrio*, and *Yersinia* if diarrhea is bloody or patient systemically ill)
- guaiac-positive stools in a patient with advanced immunosuppression may suggest mucosal disease such as CMV or HSV proctitis

- stool ova and parasite exam × 3 (order *Cryptosporidium/Microsporidium* separately if CD4 <200)
- *Giardia* enzyme-linked immunosorbent antigen test
- *Clostridium difficile* toxin assay
- stool for leukocytes, occult blood, fecal fat
- serum blood Na, and K for osmotic gap

Initial evaluation should include stool culture and sensitivity and exam for ova and parasites (O&P). Fecal leukocytes may support a diagnosis of bacterial enteritis, but their absence does not rule out infection, and this test therefore has limited utility in the HIV population. Because of the relatively low sensitivity of only one O&P exam (~50%), patients should have follow-up O&P exams on a second and third stool sample.

If the CD4 count is <200, exams for *Microsporidium* and *Cryptosporidium* should also be specifically requested with the O&P exam. Diagnosis of cryptosporidiosis can be made by microscopic identification of the oocysts in stool or tissue with acid-fast staining or direct immunofluorescence, which offers better sensitivity. Immunofluorescence is estimated to be ten times more sensitive than acid-fast staining and is now the gold standard for stool examination. A single stool specimen is usually adequate for diagnosis in individuals with profuse diarrheal illness, whereas repeat stool sampling is recommended for those with milder disease. Recognize that certain pathogens will require upper or lower endoscopy with mucosal aspirate cultures and/or biopsy for diagnosis.

A history of recent antibiotic therapy or hospital admission should always prompt stool collection for *Clostridium difficile* toxin assay. However, this study should be considered in all patients, given the rising prevalence of community-acquired *Clostridium difficile* diarrhea in individuals with no recent antibiotic exposure. All febrile patients should receive blood cultures to rule out bacteremia from *Salmonella* or other enteric bacteria. A separate mycobacterial blood culture should be sent in febrile patients with CD4 count <100 to rule out MAC.

While radiography is generally not indicated, a plain film may show dilated bowel loops suggesting obstruction, free air suggesting perforation, or thumbprinting indicating mucosal edema. Computed tomography (CT) may also show signs of perforation, obstruction, or bowel wall inflammation. CT imaging is also useful to diagnose HIV-related malignancies that could be contributing to diarrhea.

Patients with persistent or chronic diarrhea in whom this initial work-up has not revealed a cause should be referred for endoscopic evaluation. A non-infectious cause, such as medication side effect or irritable bowel syndrome, should also be considered. Colonoscopy or sigmoidoscopy with mucosal biopsy is generally required for diagnosis of CMV colitis. Diagnosis of MAC is usually made by mycobacterial blood culture, though it may only appear in mucosal aspirate. Other diagnoses that may require upper or lower endoscopy with biopsy and/or microbiologic examination of mucosal aspirate include *Microsporidium* and *Cryptosporidium*. Endoscopy is diagnostic in 30 to 70% of cases of pathogen-negative diarrhea. Evidence supports flexible sigmoidoscipy as a first-line screening procedure (80 to 95% sensitive for CMV colitis), followed by colonoscopy and terminal ileoscopy.

Treatment

In patients with CD4 counts >200, the majority of cases of acute diarrhea are self-limiting infections that can be managed conservatively with oral rehydration, symptomatic treatment, and dietary modifications, with early follow-up for results of stool studies. Patients with CD4 counts <200, febrile patients, patients with evidence of systemic involvement, and patients requiring admission for other reasons may be empirically treated with antimicrobials once appropriate specimens have been obtained.

Empiric therapy should be directed at common gram-negative enteric pathogens (e.g. *Salmonella*, *Shigella*, *Yersinia*, *Campylobacter*). An oral fluoroquinolone, such as ciprofloxacin 500 mg BID or levofloxacin 500 mg daily, both for 3 to 5 days, is recommended. Since *Shigella* spp. have shown reduced sensitivity to azithromycin and ciprofloxacin in HIV-positive adults, antimicrobial testing is indicated if *Shigella* is suspected. For *Shigella* isolates that are resistant to both azithromycin and ciprofloxacin, ceftriaxone may be a reasonable parenteral treatment option.

If clinical suspicion for a parasitic infection, such as *Giardia* or *Entamoeba histolytica*, is high, a week of metronidazole 250 to 500 mg TID or a single dose of tinidazole 2 g may be used.

If the patient presents with diarrhea in the setting of recent antibiotic exposure, initiating treatment for *Clostridium difficile* colitis may be appropriate pending the result of the *Clostridium difficile* toxin assay.

Specific therapy that is based on culture results should be initiated as soon as possible. Table 27.6 lists specific antimicrobial therapy, along with characteristic symptoms, for several common pathogens.

Patients presenting to the emergency department with persistent or chronic diarrhea despite treatment for enteric bacteria may be empirically treated with metronidazole or tinidazole for parasites. However, if the stool O&P is negative and symptoms are more consistent with an infectious cause than a medication side effect or irritable bowel syndrome (IBS), these patients should be referred for endoscopy. Both IBS and transient lactose intolerance can follow an acute bacterial gastroenteritis. Finally, local health departments may require notification of positive culture results for certain pathogens (e.g. *Shigella*, gonorrhea), and sexual partner notification may be warranted.

Oral rehydration therapy with balanced electrolytes and glucose should be encouraged in all patients with diarrhea. Intravenous (IV) rehydration is indicated for all patients with moderate to severe dehydration. Further, dietary modification may assist in ameliorating diarrhea. Recommended foods include complex carbohydrates in the form of boiled starches and cereals, such as potatoes, noodles, rice, wheat, and oats, with salt, along with boiled vegetables and lean meats. Soups, crackers, yogurt, and bananas are often well tolerated.

Table 27.6 Clinical Features and Recommended Medications to Treat Diarrhea in HIV-Infected Patients

Organism	Clinical Features	Treatment
Salmonella	Usually food acquired May be invasive and cause sepsis especially in those with a low CD4 count	Ciprofloxacin 500 mg PO BID × 3 days, or ceftriaxone 1–2 g IV daily for up to 2 weeks if evidence of invasive infection (e.g. bacteremia) and 4–6 weeks if CD4 <200
Campylobacter	Possible sexual exposure May be invasive (bloody, fever) with bacteremia/extraintestinal complications in those with CD4 <200	Ciprofloxacin 500 mg PO BID × 3–5 days (2 weeks if bacteremic) *or* Azithromycin 500 mg PO daily × 3–5 days (for quinolone resistance)
Shigella	Possible sexual exposure May be bloody, with fever and upper GI symptoms	Ciprofloxacin 500 mg PO BID × 3–5 days *or* Ceftriaxone 1–2 g daily IV × 3–5 days
Giardia	Gas, bloating, cramps, foul-smelling stools	Metronidazole 250–500 mg PO TID × 7 days *or* Tinidazole 2 g PO × 1
Cystoisospora	Watery, afebrile	Trimethoprim/Sulfamethoxazole 160/800 mg PO QID × 10 days
E. histolytica	Gas, bloating, cramps, foul-smelling stools, may be bloody	Metronidazole 750 mg PO TID × 5–10 days *or* Tinidazole 2 g PO daily × 3–5 days
MAC	Occurs exclusively in low CD4 Fever, weight loss, anemia, night sweats, hepatomegaly, elevated alkaline phosphatase	Azithromycin 500 mg PO three times per week or clarithromycin 500 mg PO BID *plus* Rifabutin 300 mg PO three times per week *plus* Ethambutol 15 mg/kg PO daily indefinitely or until patient is asymptomatic with >12 months of therapy if CD4 >100 for greater than 6 months (treatment should be provided in consultation with specialists and contingent on susceptibility testing) Initiate antiretroviral therapy
C. difficile	Previous antibiotics or hospitalization	Initial episode – mild to moderate disease (WBC <15k and SCr less than 1.5 times premorbid level): • Metronidazole 500 mg PO TID × 10–14 days Initial episode – severe disease (WBC >15k and/or 50% increase in SCr): • Vancomycin 125 mg PO every 6 hours × 10–14 days Initial episode – severe disease with complications (ICU admission due to *C. difficile* disease, toxic megacolon, severe colitis on CT scan, perforation, hypotension, shock) • Vancomycin 500 mg PO every 6 hours × 10–14 days *plus* • Metronidazole 500 mg IV every 8 hours × 10–14 days
Cryptosporidium	Large volumes, nausea/vomiting, cramps, electrolyte imbalance, acidosis in low CD4	Immunocompetent: Nitazoxanide 500 mg PO BID × 3 days CD4 count <100: Nitazoxanide 500 mg PO BID *or* Paromomycin 1 g PO BID plus azithromycin 600 mg PO daily (duration contingent on immune reconstitution after antiretroviral therapy initiation) Initiate antiretroviral therapy
Microsporidium	Watery stools, malabsorption, fever uncommon	Albendazole 400 mg PO BID × 2–4 weeks for initial therapy of intestinal and disseminated microsporidiosis caused by microsporidia other than *E. bieneusi* Initiate antiretroviral therapy
CMV	Occurs exclusively in CD4 <50 Colitis – lower abdominal pain, bright red blood per rectum May coexist with retinitis Requires biopsy for diagnosis	Ganciclovir 5 mg/kg/dose IV every 12 hours (duration about 3–6 weeks contingent on clinical response) Initiate antiretroviral therapy

Lactose-containing foods and high-fat foods should be avoided. Bulking agents such as psyllium may be beneficial.

For symptomatic treatment of patients with chronic diarrhea and in select afebrile patients with acute non-bloody diarrhea, oral antimotility agents such as loperamide (4 mg initially, then 2 mg after each unformed stool, up to 16 mg) or diphenoxylate/atropine (one tablet up to four times per day) may be used. Crofelemer, a botanical agent that blocks chloride secretion and accompanying high-volume water loss, can also be used for the treatment of non-infectious diarrhea in HIV-positive patients receiving antiretroviral therapy. These agents can increase the risk of severe complications in patients with *Clostridium difficile* infection and some other bacterial diarrheas, and should only be used after an initial work-up has been completed.

Patients with advanced HIV disease and infections such as *Cryptosporidium* or MAC may experience severe chronic diarrhea causing dehydration, malnutrition, and weight loss. In these patients, a more aggressive attempt at slowing intestinal motility can include oral tincture of opium or subcutaneous administration of octreotide.

Finally, though antiretroviral medications may worsen diarrhea in patients with infectious causes, many of these infections will prove incurable without sustained treatment of HIV and immune restoration. Antiretroviral medications should be discontinued only as a last resort and in consultation with the prescribing practitioner, as any changes may affect disease resistance patterns and future treatment options.

Complications and Admission Criteria

HIV-infected patients with lower CD4 counts are at higher risk of *Salmonella* bacteremia and septicemia. Complications of *Salmonella* bacteremia in this population include septicemia, pyelonephritis, intra-abdominal abscesses, osteomyelitis, and septic arthritis. Patients with suspected or known *Salmonella* bacteremia should be admitted for treatment with an IV fluoroquinolone, further work-up, and observation. Patients with CD4 counts less than 200 and *Salmonella* bacteremia should be treated for 4 to 6 weeks and, if relapse occurs, should be maintained indefinitely on suppressive fluoroquinolone therapy, such as ciprofloxacin.

Patients with advanced HIV and opportunistic enteric infections (particularly *Cryptosporidium*) can have massive volume loss resulting in hemodynamic compromise, significant electrolyte imbalance (especially hypokalemia), and refractory acidosis from loss of bicarbonate. Such patients will require admission for aggressive IV rehydration, electrolyte repletion, antimotility agents, and correction of acidosis.

Patients with low CD4 counts and chronic diarrhea from conditions such as MAC, *Microsporidium*, *Cryptosporidium*, or HIV enteropathy can develop nutritional, caloric, and vitamin deficiencies. In concert with the catabolic state often seen in advanced HIV, this can result in a state resembling starvation that, in its severe form, will require admission.

Rarely, patients with extensive gastrointestinal Kaposi's sarcoma can experience gastrointestinal hemorrhage. Severe infectious colitis (e.g. *Clostridium difficile*) or infiltrative processes (e.g. lymphoma) can cause perforation.

Admission to the hospital is recommended for patients with:

- CD4 count <200 who have fever and/or signs or symptoms of systemic involvement
- known or suspected bacteremia
- CD4 count <200 and known *Salmonella* infection
- severe dehydration, acidosis, or electrolyte imbalance

Infection Control

Universal blood and bodily fluid precautions are sufficient infection control methods for most pathogens associated with diarrhea in HIV-infected patients. When caring for patients with known *Clostridium difficile* infection, use soap and water for hand hygiene, as alcohol-based hand rubs may not be as effective against spore-forming bacteria. Place these patients in private rooms when available, and use gloves and dedicated equipment for all patient care.

Pearls and Pitfalls

1. Admit patients with CD4 counts <200 and fever or systemic symptoms.
2. Admit patients with severe dehydration, acidosis, or electrolyte imbalance.
3. Chronic diarrhea in patients with CD4 counts >200 is often due to HIV medications.
4. Ova and parasite exam should be sent on three separate stool samples.
5. Remember to consider *C. difficile*.
6. *Salmonella* is more likely to cause sepsis in patients with HIV.
7. In patients with CD4 counts >200, consider viral and common bacterial causes, and medication side effects.
8. In patients with CD4 counts <200, consider *Cryptosporidium*, parasites, and MAC.
9. In patients with severe dehydration, electrolyte disturbances, weight loss and CD4 counts <200, consider *Cryptosporidium*.

References

Angulo, F. J. and Swerdlow, D. L. Bacterial enteric infections in persons infected with human immunodeficiency virus. *Clin. Infect. Dis.* 1995; 21(1): S84–93.

Asmuth, D. M., DeGirolami, P. C., Federman, M., *et al.* Clinical features of microsporidiosis in patients with AIDS. *Clin. Infect. Dis.* 1994; 18(5): 819–25.

Blanshard, C., Francis, N., and Gazzard, B. G. Investigation of chronic diarrhoea in acquired immunodeficiency syndrome. A prospective study of 155 patients. *Gut* 1996; 39(96): 824–32.

Call, S. A., Heudebert, G., Saag, M., and Wilcox, C. M. The changing etiology of chronic diarrhea in HIV-infected patients with CD4 cell counts less than 200 cells/mm^3. *Am. J. Gastroenterol.* 2000; 95(11): 3142–6.

Chen, X. M., Keithly, J. S., Paya, C. V., and LaRusso, N. F. Cryptosporidiosis. *N. Engl. J. Med.* 2002; 346(22): 1723–31.

Cohen, J., West, A. B., and Bini, E. J. Infectious diarrhea in human immunodeficiency virus. *Gastroenterol. Clin. North Am.* 2001; 30(3): 637–64.

Cohen, S. H., Gerding, D. N., Johnson, S., *et al.* Clinical practice guidelines for *Clostridium difficile* infection in adults: 2010 update by the Society for Healthcare Epidemiology of America (SHEA) and the Infectious Diseases Society of America (IDSA). *Infect. Control Hosp. Epidemiol.* 2010; 31(5): 431–55, doi: 10.1086/651706.

Guerrant, R. L., Van Gilder, T., Steiner, T. S., *et al.* Practice guidelines for the management of infectious diarrhea. *Clin. Infect. Dis.* 2001; 32(3): 331–51, doi: 10.1086/318514.

Kearney, D. J., Steuerwald, M., Koch, J., and Cello, J. P. A prospective study of endoscopy in HIV-associated diarrhea. *Am. J. Gastroenterol.* 1999; 94(3): 596–602.

MacArthur, R. D. and DuPont, H. L. Etiology and pharmacologic management of noninfectious diarrhea in HIV-infected individuals in the highly active antiretroviral therapy era. *Clin. Infect. Dis.* 2012; 55(6): 860–7.

Mayer, H. B. and Wanke, C. A. Diagnostic strategies in HIV-infected patients with diarrhea. *AIDS* 1994; 8(12): 1639–48.

Morpeth, S. C. and Thielman, N. M. Diarrhea in patients with AIDS. *Curr. Treat. Options Gastroenterol.* 2006; 9(1): 23–37.

Molina, J. M., Chastang, C., Goguel, J., *et al.* Albendazole for treatment and prophylaxis of microsporidiosis due to Encephalitozoon intestinalis in patients with AIDS: a randomized double-blind controlled trial. *J. Infect. Dis.* 1998; 177(5): 1373–7.

Sanchez, T. H., Brooks, J. T., Sullivan, P. S., *et al.* Bacterial diarrhea in persons with HIV infection, United States, 1992–2002. *Clin. Infect. Dis.* 2005; 41(11): 1621–7.

Sharpstone, D. and Gazzard, B. Gastrointestinal manifestations of HIV infection. *Lancet* 1996; 348(9024): 379–83.

Sherman, D. S. and Fish, D. N. Management of protease inhibitor-associated diarrhea. *Clin. Infect. Dis.* 2000; 30(6): 908–14.

Weber, R., Ledergerber, B., Zbinden, R., *et al.* Enteric infections and diarrhea in human immunodeficiency virus-infected persons: prospective community-based cohort study. Swiss HIV Cohort Study. *Arch. Intern. Med.* 1999; 159(13): 1473–80.

Weber, R., Bryan, R. T., Bishop, H. S., *et al.* Threshold of detection of *Cryptosporidium* oocysts in human stool specimens: evidence for low sensitivity of current diagnostic methods. *J. Clin. Microbiol.* 1991; 29(7): 1323–7.

Additional Readings

Cohen, J., West, A. B., and Bini, E. J. Infectious diarrhea in human immunodeficiency virus. *Gastroenterol. Clin. North Am.* 2001; 30(3): 637–64.

Feasey, N. A., Healey, P., and Gordon, M. A. Review article: the aetiology, investigation and management of diarrhoea in the HIV-positive patient. *Alimentary Pharmacology & Therapeutics* 2011; 34(6): 587–603, PubMed PMID: 21777262.r.

Kaplan, J. E., Benson, C., Holmes, K. K., *et al.* Guidelines for prevention and treatment of opportunistic infections in HIV-infected adults and adolescents: recommendations from CDC, the National Institutes of Health, and the HIV Medicine Association of the Infectious Diseases Society of America. *MMWR Morb. Mortal. Wkly. Rep.* 2009; 58(RR-4): 1–207; quiz CE201-204.

Kearney, D. J., Steuerwald, M., Koch, J., and Cello, J. P. A prospective study of endoscopy in HIV-associated diarrhea. *Am. J. Gastroenterol.* 1999; 94(3): 596–602.

Morpeth, S. C. and Thielman, N. M. Diarrhea in patients with AIDS. *Curr. Treat. Options Gastroenterol.* 2006; 9(1): 23–37.

Rossignol, J. F., Ayoub, A., and Ayers, M. S. Treatment of diarrhea caused by *Cryptosporidium parvum*: a prospective randomized, double-blind, placebo-controlled study of Nitazoxanide. *J. Infect. Dis.* 2001; 184(1): 103–6, doi: 10.1086/321008.

Sanchez, T. H., Brooks, J. T., Sullivan, P. S., *et al.* Bacterial diarrhea in persons with HIV infection, United States, 1992–2002. *Clin. Infect. Dis.* 2005; 41(11): 1621–7.

Weber, R., Ledergerber, B., Zbinden, R., *et al.* Enteric infections and diarrhea in human immunodeficiency virus-infected persons: prospective community-based cohort study. Swiss HIV Cohort Study. *Arch. Intern. Med.* 1999; 159(13): 1473–80.

Clostridium Difficile Infection

Charles Hartis and Nicole Abolins

Introduction and Microbiology

Clostridium difficile infection (CDI), or *Clostridium difficile*-associated diarrhea (CDAD), includes a broad range of clinical syndromes from symptomless carriage to mild diarrhea to toxic megacolon, multi-organ failure, and death. *C. difficile* is primarily responsible for causing a specific type of infectious colitis known as pseudomembranous colitis. Unlike other causes of infectious colitis, CDI is usually associated with antecedent antimicrobial use. The use of antimicrobials alters the normal gastrointestinal flora allowing for the proliferation of *C. difficile*. Although CDI can occur in patients of any age or gender, morbidity and mortality are more increased in the elderly.

C. difficile is an anaerobic, gram-positive, spore-forming bacillus. It produces three pathogenically important exotoxins, toxin A, toxin B and the recently described binary toxin. Incidence, recurrence, and severity of CDI have increased in the past 20 years due, in large part, to the emergence of a new epidemic strain, NAP1/BI/027. This bacterium is now the most common hospital-acquired infectious pathogen, causing 12.1% of all health-care associated infections. This has been linked with a rising incidence of community-associated CDI as well. While the increasing severity and incidence of CDI have spurred research into new treatments, antimicrobial options remain limited.

In the acute care setting, successful management requires obtaining accurate patient and medication history, early symptom recognition, appropriate microbiologic testing, and evaluation of disease severity to guide optimal treatment.

Epidemiology

Clostridium difficile (CD) is the most common cause of infectious antibiotic-associated diarrhea. It may also cause colitis without prior exposure to antibiotics in certain individuals. Annually, there are an estimated 453,000 CDI cases in the United States, causing over 29,000 deaths, adding $3.2 billion in health-care costs. Approximately half of CDI cases are in patients younger than 65 years of age; however, 90% of deaths occur in those older than 65. A recent study showed that 18% of CDI were community acquired, 30% occurred during hospitalization, 24% in long-term care setting, and 24% of cases occurred in the community in patients with recent health-care association. Transmission of CD occurs via the fecal-oral route. Roughly 15% of the general population are asymptomatic carriers of CD. In hospital or long-term care settings, the asymptomatic carriage rate increases to 50%.

The incidence and severity of CDI have increased significantly since 2000. Studies from the late 1990s showed a stable rate of 30 to 40 CDI cases per 100,000 patients. By 2005, this number had risen to 84 cases, and as high as 228 cases per 100,000 patients in those over the age of 65. This increase is thought to be largely due to the emergence of the NAP1/BI/027 strain, first seen in a Canadian epidemic. The NAP1 strain is highly virulent, producing up to 23 times more toxin and leading to a higher mortality (16% vs. 9%) compared to earlier strains. It is distinctly resistant to fluoroquinolones, a trait rarely found in earlier CD strains. It has also been documented to infect certain at-risk populations, such as pregnant women.

Risk factors for CDI include: older age (>65 years), recent antibacterial therapy, immunosuppression, antineoplastic therapy, ICU or prolonged hospital stay, GI surgery or manipulation of the gastrointestinal tract, and gastric acid-reducing therapy. The impact of antibiotics differs by class and spectrum of coverage. Those most strongly associatied with CDI include: clindamycin, fluoroquinolones, cephalosporins, and broad-spectrum beta-lactams. Those less commonly associated with CDI are aminoglycosides, trimethoprim-sulfamethoxazole, tetracyclines, and macrolides. There are reports suggesting that metronidazole and doxycycline may offer protection against CDI.

Table 28.1 Diagnostic Classification of CDI as Defined by the American College of Gastroenterology

	Diagnostic Criteria
Mild	Diarrhea is the only symptom
Moderate	Other symptoms present that do not meet severe/complicated criteria
Severe	Hypoalbuminemia (serum albumin <3 g/dL) and either: - WBC >15,000 cells/mm³ - Abdominal tenderness
Complicated	Any of the following attributable to CDI: - Admission to intensive care unit for CDI - Hypotension with or without required use of vasopressors - Fever ≥38.5 °C - Ileus or significant abdominal distention - Mental status changes - WBC ≥35,000 cells/mm³ or <2,000 cells/mm³ - Serum lactate levels >2.2 mmol/L - End organ failure (mechanical ventilation, renal failure, etc.)
Recurrent CDI	Recurrent CDI within 8 weeks of completion of therapy

Clinical Features

Symptoms of CDI can develop between 5 days and 10 weeks after antibiotic exposure. Voluminous watery diarrhea, often with a characteristic odor, is the hallmark sign of CDI. Other symptoms include anorexia, abdominal pain, and cramping. Fever is present in only about 15% of cases, but is more common in severe cases. Hypotension and shock may also be present in severe cases. Leukocytosis is common, and severe cases may present with extremely elevated WBC counts.

Differential Diagnosis

The differential diagnosis for CDI suspected diarrhea is broad and includes *S. aureus* enterocolitis, *Salmonella*, *Klebsiella*, or *E. coli* infections. Viral and fungal etiologies should be considered as well as non-infectious antibiotic-associated diarrhea.

Laboratory and Radiographic Findings

Blood tests including CBC, metabolic panel, serum albumin, and lactate are important in grading disease severity and determining treatment choice, as outlined in Tables 28.1 and 28.2.

CT scan is recommended in severe disease, and will typically reveal bowel wall thickening. Toxic megacolon, defined as more than 7 cm of colonic dilatation, and bowel perforation are revealed by CT. Endoscopy commonly shows pseudomembranes – a characteristic exudate overlying the colonic mucosa that resembles a second membrane.

In most cases, a positive stool test for CD is necessary to definitively diagnose CDI. The two commonly used laboratory tests are *C. difficile* PCR (polymerase chain reaction) and enzyme immunoassay (EIA) for Toxins A and B and GDH antigen. PCR testing is both more sensitive and specific than EIA and is now considered the preferred test. Other stool tests such as culture, toxigenic culture, and cytotoxin neutralization assay are limited by diagnostic inaccuracies and are rarely used. Serial testing is discouraged, as this is unlikely to improve sensitivity. Retesting patients to determine cure is likewise discouraged, as tests may remain positive in patients whose symptoms have resolved with treatment, resulting in unnecessarily long courses of treatment.

Treatment

Patients with CDI presenting in the acute care setting may be very ill, requiring aggressive fluid resuscitation. Definitive treatment of CDI begins with prompt discontinuation of any inciting antibiotics, if possible. If active infection requires further antimicrobial treatment during CDI, an infectious disease consult may be warranted in order to identify the optimal antimicrobial and duration of treatment. The goal of medication treatment for CDI is eradication of *C. difficile* from the gut, allowing repopulation of normal colonizing flora. Empiric treatment may need to be initiated prior to definitive stool testing. Empiric treatment may need to be initiated prior to definitive stool testing. Drug choice and duration are dictated by severity of disease and whether the case is a recurrence (see Table 28.2). Vancomycin is the mainstay of treatment for CDI. While oral metronidazole has been commonly used, recent guideline changes place it as a second-line agent only for initial episodes. Fidaxomicin is a newer, minimally absorbed macrolide antibiotic targeted at *Clostridia* species. Compared with vancomycin, fidaxomicin is associated with less recurrence. While fidaxomicin remains costly, it has now been elevated as one of the first-line treatments for initial and recurrent CDI. Fulminant episodes (with hypotension, shock, ileus, or megacolon present) should be treated with high dose oral vancomycin and intravenous metronidazole. If ileus present, additional rectal vancomycin may be added.

Recurrences after initial treatment occur in roughly 20% of patients. Following a single recurrence, the risk of further recurrence is 40–65%. Fidaxomicin or vancomycin are also the primary treatment in recurrences, though vancomycin should be given as a prolonged taper or pulse regimen.

For a third or later episode in recurrent CDI, fecal microbiota transplant (FMT) is recommended. This involves purification of human stool and instillation into the gut via endoscope, retention enema, or nasoduodenal tube. Success rates have been reported as high as 91% in patients with multiple recurrences. Limited evidence supports efficacy of FMT in severe CDI. At this time, the Food and Drug Administration in the United States considers FMT an investigational therapy for CDI infections.

Complications and Admission Criteria

Complications of CDI often correlate with disease severity. Mild to moderate disease may cause dehydration and acute renal insufficiency or failure. More severe disease may cause

Table 28.2 Treatment Algorithm with Adults with CBI

Clinical Definition	Supportive Clinical Data	Recommended Treatment
Initial episode, non-severe	White blood cell count <=15,000 cells/ml and serum creatinine <1.5 mg/dl	Vancomycin 125 mg PO QID × 10 days* or Fidaxomicin 200 mg PO BID × 10 days or If above unavailable to patient: Metronidazole 500 mg TID × 10 days
Initial episode, severe	White blood cell count >15,000 cells/ml and serum creatinine ≥1.5 mg/dl	Vancomycin 125 mg PO QID × 10 days* or Fidaxomicin 200 mg PO twice daily × 10 days
Initial episode, fulminant	Hypotension, shock, ileus, megacolon	Vancomycin 500 mg PO QID *plus* Metronidazole IV 500 mg every 8 hours Consider adding vancomycin 500 mg in 100 ml normal saline as a rectal enema every 6 hours
First recurrence		Vancomycin 125 mg PO QID × 10 days (if metronidazole used as the initial treatment) or Vancomycin 125 mg PO pulse/taper† (if vancomycin used initially) or Fidaxomicin 200 mg PO BID × 10 days (if vancomycin used initially)
Second or subsequent recurrence		Vancomycin 125 mg PO pulse/taper† or Vancomycin 125 mg PO QID × 10 days followed by rifaximin 400 mg PO TID × 20 days or Fidaxomicin 200 mg PO BID × 10 days or Fecal microbiota transplant‡

* Patients with slow response to treatment may benefit from 14 days.

† Example vancomycin taper: 125 mg PO QID x 14 days, then BID x 7 days, then daily x 7 days, then every 2–3 days for 2–8 weeks.

‡ Guidelines recommend FMT should not be offered until at least the third episode (second recurrence).

toxic megacolon, bowel perforation, and death. Severe disease may require a partial or total colectomy, thus early surgical consult should be considered for any patients presenting with severe CDI who appear toxic.

There are no consensus admission criteria; however, using the disease severity measures noted above, it is likely that most severe, complicated cases should be admitted. Patients with moderate to severe disease may be admitted based on comorbidities and risk of disease progression.

Infection Control

In the acute care setting, infection control related to CDI may be challenging. The delay in definitive diagnosis of CDI may delay proper precautions. A strong suspicion of CDI should be maintained in any patient with acute diarrhea and recent hospitalization. Further, the rapid turnover of patients in the department may make it difficult to remove environmental contamination between patients. A multidisciplinary approach emphasizing employee best practices as well as optimizing proper environmental cleaning is recommended.

Pearls and Pitfalls

1. *C. difficile* testing should only be done on stool samples that are diarrhea, not formed stool.

2. While metronidazole has historically been used extensively, current guidelines recommend vancomycin or fidaxomicin as first-line agents except in pediatric patients.

3. Severe, complicated disease should be treated with a combination of high-dose enteral vancomycin, IV metronidazole, and possibly rectal vancomycin.

4. Severe, complicated disease should trigger early consultation with gastroenterology and surgery.

5. CDI in patients with pre-existing gastrointestinal conditions (irritable bowel syndrome, inflammatory bowel disease) may be missed; *C. difficile* testing is recommended in patients with inflammatory bowel disease flares.

6. FMT is a highly effective treatment option for patients with multiple recurrences, but may not be available in every facility.

References

Centers for Disease Control and Prevention (CDC). Antibiotic resistance threats in the United States (2013), published online at www.CDC.gov.

Cohen, S. H., Gerding, D. N., Johnson, S., *et al.* Clinical practice guidelines for *Clostridium difficile* infection in adults: 2010 update by the Society for Healthcare Epidemiology of America (SHEA) and the Infectious Diseases Society of America (IDSA). *Infect. Cont. Hosp. Epidemiol.* 2010; 31(5): 431–55.

Johnson, S., Louie, T. J., Gerding, D. N., *et al.* Vancomycin, metronidazole, or tolevamer for *Clostridium difficile* infection: results from two multinational, randomized, controlled trials. *Clin. Infect. Dis.* 2014; 59(3): 345–54.

Kelly, C. P. and LaMont, J. T. *Clostridium difficile* – more difficult than ever. *N. Engl. J. Med.* 2008; 359(40): 1932–40.

Kuijper, E. J., Coignard, B., Tüll, P., *et al.* Emergence of *Clostridium difficile*-associated disease in North America and Europe. *Clin. Microbiol. Infect.* 2006; 12(6): 2–18.

Louie, T. J., Miller, M. A., Mullane, K. M., *et al.* Fidaxomicin versus vancomycin for *Clostridium difficile* infection. *N. Engl. J. Med.* 2011; 364(5): 422–31.

Magill, S. S., Edwards, J. R., Bamberg, W., *et al.* Multistate point-prevalence survey of health care-associated infections. *N. Engl. J. Med.* 2014; 370(13): 1198–208.

McDonald, L. C., Gerding, D. N., Johnson, S., *et al.* Clinical practice guidelines for Clostridium difficile infection in adults and children: 2017 update by the Infectious Disease Society of America (IDSA) and Society for Healthcare Epidemiology of America (SHEA). *Clin. Infect. Dis.* 2018; 66(7): e1–e48.

Surawicz, C. M., Brandt, L. J., Binion, D. G., *et al.* Guidelines for diagnosis, treatment, and prevention of *Clostridium difficile* infections. *Am. J. Gastroenterol.* 2013; 108(4): 478–98, doi: 10.1038/ajg.2013.4.

Tedesco, F. J., Gordon, D., and Fortson, W. C. Approach to patients with multiple relapses of antibiotic-associated pseudomembranous colitis. *Am. J. Gastroenterol.* 1985; 80(11): 867–8.

Zar, F. A., Bakkanagari, S. R., Moorthi, K. M., and Davis, M. B. A comparison of vancomycin and metronidazole for the treatment of *Clostridium difficile*-associated diarrhea, stratified by disease severity. *Clin. Infect. Dis.* 2007; 45(3): 302–7.

Additional Readings

Bakken, J. S., Borody, T., Brandt, L. J., *et al.* Treating *Clostridium difficile* infection with fecal microbiota transplantation. *Clin. Gastroenterol. Hepatol.* 2011; 9(12): 1044–9.

Shin, B. M., Moon, S. J., Kim, Y. S., *et al.* Characterization of cases of *Clostridium difficile* infection (CDI) presenting at an emergency room: molecular and clinical features differentiate community-onset hospital-associated and community-associated CDI in a tertiary care hospital. *J. Clin. Microbiol.* 2011; 49(6): 2161–5, doi: 10.1128/JCM.02330-10.

Chapter 29

Male Genitourinary Infections

Jonathan Schimmel and William D. Binder

Outline

Introduction

The male urinary tract is contiguous with the reproductive organs, so infections arising in the urethra, epididymis, testicle, and prostate often share common symptoms of dysuria, frequency, and urgency. In healthy young or middle-aged men presenting in the acute care setting, these symptoms are usually attributable to sexually transmitted disease (STD), and unlikely to be caused by simple cystitis. This chapter covers male genitourinary infections except for cystitis and pyelonephritis. Chlamydia and gonorrhea are also discussed in Chapter 30.

Urethritis

Epidemiology and Microbiology

Urethritis affects approximately 4 million men in the United States annually. The disorder is often caused by a sexually transmitted infection, and is primarily due to *Neisseria gonorrhoeae* (gonococcal urethritis) or *Chlamydia trachomatis* (non-gonococcal urethritis or NGU). Approximately 575,000 males in the United States were diagnosed in 2013 with either gonorrhea or chlamydia, with peak incidence between 20 and 24 years of age. The actual incidence is likely higher, as up to 90% of male chlamydial infections are asymptomatic.

Other non-gonococcal agents causing urethritis include *Ureaplasma urealyticum*, *Mycoplasma hominis/genitalium*, *Trichomonas vaginalis*, enteric species (if insertive anal intercourse), adenovirus (may also have conjunctivitis), *herpes*

simplex virus (HSV), syphilis (if urethral chancre), papillomavirus (HPV, if urethral condylomata acuminata), or *Candida*. Sterile urethritis can rarely be experienced by those with Behçet's disease.

Mycoplasma genitalium is increasingly recognized as an important cause of NGU. The worldwide rate of infection is 1 to 4% in men and prevalence is higher since carriage may be asymptomatic. Reports suggest that *M. gentalium* is responsible for 15 to 20% of all cases of NGU and up to 25% of nonchlamydial NGU. Its importance as a cause of NGU is second only to *C. Trachomatis*, though some authors suggest it is actually more common. Unfortunately, diagnostic testing for *M. genitalium* is not readily available. The disease should be considered when urethritis is clinically suspected, but sensitive tests for *N. gonorrhea* and *C. Trachomatis* are negative.

Trichomonas vaginalis is a highly prevalent STI that can cause urethritis, though it is frequently asymptomatic in men. Other agents mentioned are either less common, not well studied, or diagnostic testing is not readily available. It should be emphasized that although clues may suggest a particular agent, urethritis tends to present with common symptoms regardless of the specific pathogen.

Risk factors for sexually transmitted urethritis include unprotected intercourse and increasing number of sexual partners, men who have sex with men, geographic location, age, and race/ethnicity. In the United States, rates of gonorrhea and chlamydia are highest in African Americans, followed by American Indians, Native Hawaiians, and Alaska Natives,

Table 29.1 Clinical Features: Urethritis

Organisms	*Neisseria gonorrhoeae* *Chlamydia trachomatis* *Ureaplasma urealyticum* *Mycoplasma hominis/genitalum* *Trichomonas vaginalis* Uncommon: enteric species, adenovirus, HSV, HPV, *Candida*
Incubation period	• Gonococcal: 2–10 days • Chlamydial: 4–12 days
Signs and symptoms	• Dysuria • Urethral discharge • Asymptomatic
Laboratory findings	• Gram stain of urethral discharge with ≥2 WBCs per oil immersion field • First-void urine with positive leukocyte esterase test or microscopy of sediment with ≥10 WBCs per high-power field • Urine NAAT (nucleic acid amplification test) is the test of choice

WBC – white blood (cell) count.

Hispanics, Whites, and finally, Asian men, who have the lowest rate in the United States. Studies suggest that circumcision confers protections from urethritis and other STIs, including HIV, HSV-2, HPV, and syphilis.

Clinical Features

Males with urethritis present with dysuria and/or a urethral discharge. They may give a history of a recent unprotected sexual contact. The presence of a mucoid, mucopurulent, or purulent discharge confirms the diagnosis of urethritis (see Table 29.1). Gonococcal urethritis is typically purulent (see Figure 29.1). Non-gonococcal urethritis is usually mucoid or mucopurulent (see Figure 29.2). Complications of urethritis include urethral scarring and stricture formation, as well as prostatitis. Non-gonococcal urethritis may present with vision loss and polyarthrialgias, a constellation of symptoms known as reactive arthritis (previously Reiter's syndrome).

Differential Diagnosis

The differential diagnosis includes traumatic urethritis (post-instrumentation), cystitis, pyelonephritis, urethral stricture, or urethral foreign body. Urethritis may occur concurrently with neighboring infections, such as epididymitis or prostatitis. Autoimmune causes such as Behçet's disease are rare.

Features that raise the possibility of atypical organisms, urethritis with complications, or non-infectious etiology include:

• systemic signs/symptoms (fever, chills, rash)
• eye and joint complaints
• insertive anal intercourse
• cutaneous lesions of HSV, syphilis, or HPV
• masses or fluctuance along the penile shaft
• recent instrumentation

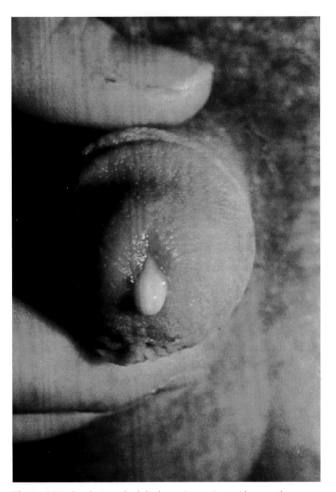

Figure 29.1 Purulent urethral discharge in a patient with gonorrhea. Image courtesy of the Australasian Chapter on Sexual Health Medicine.

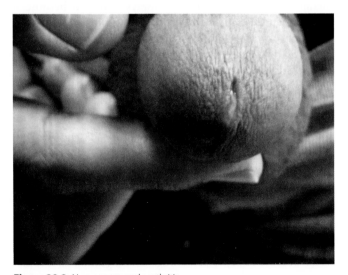

Figure 29.2 Non-gonococcal urethritis. Image Courtesy of Dr. Joseph Engelman, San Francisco City Clinic.

Laboratory Findings

Laboratory diagnosis in men consists of any of the following:

• first-void urine with positive leukocyte esterase test or microscopy of sediment with ≥10 WBCs per high-power field

- gram stain of urethral discharge with ≥5 white blood cells (WBCs) per oil immersion field; sensitivity can be increased if >2 WBCs are used as a cut-off
- positive nucleic acid amplification test (NAAT) on first-void urine (or >20 minutes since last void)

In the typical sexually active young man with symptoms, NAAT (and empiric treatment) is all that is required. Laboratory evaluation should always include both gonorrhea and chlamydia, as co-infection is common. Gram stain of a urethral smear in gonorrhea may reveal WBCs with gram-negative intracellular diplococci. Pyuria without gram-negative diplococci suggests non-gonococcal urethritis (or infection elsewhere in the urinary tract). Other tests include culture, direct immunofluorescence, enzyme immunoassay, or nucleic acid hybridization tests.

Nucleic acid amplification tests (NAAT) performed on first-void urine or urethral swab are the preferred test for confirmation of gonorrhea and chlamydia due to convenience of collection, ease of transport, and high sensitivity and specificity. In men, NAATs have sensitivity and specificity for chlamydia of 84 and 99%, and for gonorrhea of 90 and 99%, respectively.

If urethritis is present and no gonorrhea or chlamydia are detected, consider testing for *T. vaginalis* in geographic areas or populations with high prevalence. The diagnosis can be made by nucleic acid amplification testing or by meatal swabs for wet mount and culture.

Cases of confirmed gonorrhea and chlamydia are required to be reported to local health departments by providers, hospitals, or laboratories.

Treatment and Prophylaxis

While symptoms of urethritis may be self-limited without therapy, antibiotic treatment is always indicated because it reduces transmission, shortens duration of illness, and lowers morbidity. Immediate empiric therapy while confirmatory test results are pending is the recommended approach in the acute care setting, particularly in patients at high risk for STDs or those who may be lost to follow-up. Selected patients who do not meet diagnostic criteria and who have close follow-up may await test results prior to treatment. Treatment in the absence of laboratory confirmation should cover both gonorrhea and chlamydia, since they often coexist.

Gonococcal resistance to the third generation cephalosporin cefixime has increased and this agent is no longer recommended as first-line therapy. Resistance to fluoroquinolones has also increased and this class of antibiotics should no longer be used for initial treatment of urethritis. Although azithromycin and doxycycline are both recommended, azithromycin may be preferred because of better activity against *M. genitalium* and can be given in a directly observed single dose. The current standard regimen is one-time doses of azithromycin 1 g PO plus ceftriaxone 250 mg IM. Even if laboratory testing demonstrates gonorrhea without chlamydia, this regimen should still be given. See Table 29.2 for urethritis therapy recommendations.

All patients diagnosed with an STD should receive counseling about safe sex practices, and should be tested for syphilis and HIV. Those with confirmed gonorrhea, chlamydia,

Table 29.2 Initial Therapy for Urethritis

Patient Category	Therapy Recommendation
Adults	Ceftriaxone 250 mg IM single dose *plus* Azithromycin 1 g PO single dose Persistent or recurrent NGU: Azithromycin 1 g PO single dose (if not used initially) *or* Moxifloxacin 400 mg PO daily for 7 days (if failed azithromycin) For heterosexual men who live in regions where *T. vaginalis* is highly prevalent: Metronidazole 2 g PO single dose *or* tinidazole 2 g PO single dose Suspicion for *M. genitalum* (if failed azithromycin): Moxifloxacin 400 mg PO daily for 7 days *or* Levofloxacin 500 mg PO daily for 7 days *or* Ofloxacin 300 mg po BID for 7 days

If azithromycin cannot be used, substitute doxycycline 100 mg PO BID for 7 days.
If reinfection occurred, the initial regimen may be given again.

or trichomonas should also be followed up in 3 months due to high rates of reinfection.

Expedited partner therapy (EPT) involves providing an additional prescription or medications to the patient so his partner can be treated without direct evaluation. It is preferred that the partner be directly evaluated, but EPT may be considered a reasonable alternative and has been endorsed by the Centers for Disease Control and Prevention (CDC). State laws vary, and we recommend referring to individual state department of public health or the CDC.

Complications and Admission Criteria

Acute complications of urethritis in men include urethral abscess, prostatitis, seminal vesiculitis, epididymitis, proctitis, disseminated gonococcal infection, or reactive arthritis. Consider admission in patients with urethritis who appear ill with any of these complications. Patients with uncomplicated urethritis do not require admission. Long-term complications include urethral scarring with stricture or stenosis, or rarely infertility.

Some men may have persistent discomfort after successful treatment of urethritis. Without objective signs or laboratory confirmation of recurrent or persistent urethritis, avoid re-treating for discomfort or symptoms alone, and consider referral to a urologist.

Infection Control

All sexual partners in the past 60 days of males with urethritis should be referred to a health-care provider for evaluation and treatment, or considered for EPT. Patients should be instructed to refrain from sexual activity until all symptoms have resolved, and until at least 7 days after initiation of therapy.

Epididymitis

Epidemiology and Microbiology

Acute epididymitis is the most common cause of acute scrotal pain in the acute care setting. There are approximately 600,000 cases annually in the United States. The disorder can be either acute or chronic in nature. In sexually active men under 35 years of age, *N. gonorrhoeae* or *C. trachomatis* are the most common causes of bacterial epididymitis. Infection by enteric species may also occur in this age group in patients who practice insertive anal intercourse. In men over the age of 35, *E. coli* and other coliforms, as well as *Pseudomonas*, are statistically more likely the etiology, though sexually transmitted pathogens should still be considered. Rare bacterial causes include brucella, mycobacterium tuberculosis, and mycobacterium marinum. In immunocompromised patients, epididymitis may be secondary to fungi (e.g. candidiasis, blastomycosis, or coccidioidomycosis), or cytomegalovirus.

Non-infectious epididymitis may be due to a post-infectious inflammatory reaction to various pathogens (e.g. mycoplasma pneumonia, adenovirus, enterovirus), or as a manifestation of autoimmune processes including Behçet's disease. Additionally, it may be drug related, such as a side effect of amiodarone.

The proposed mechanism of epididymitis is retrograde movement of infection from the urethra, urinary bladder, or prostate, via the vas deferens. Mechanical causes of urinary reflux predispose patients to infection with urinary coliforms such as *E. coli*. Obstruction and chronic backflow in children can be caused by congenital anomalies such as posterior urethral valves or meatal stenosis. Risk factors in adults include sexual activity, prolonged sitting, prostatic enlargement, urethral stricture, or a chronic indwelling urethral catheter. Surgery or instrumentation are significant risk factors. Men of any age who Valsalva with a full bladder during strenuous activity may also develop epididymitis. Additional risk factors include riding bicycles or motorcycles.

Clinical Features

Epididymitis presents with unilateral scrotal pain that is gradual in onset (see Table 29.3). Pain may begin in the lower abdomen then localize to the scrotum. Urethral symptoms (dysuria, urethral discharge) may precede epididymitis by up to 3 to 4 weeks, may present concurrently, or may be absent. Fever and chills are occasionally present.

Physical exam reveals unilateral testicular tenderness. A prominent and tender epididymis from edema or a reactive hydrocele may be appreciated. Initially, tenderness may localize to the tail of the epididymis, but inflammation often spreads to the entire epididymis and the testicle (epididymo-orchitis). Most cases of epididymitis develop into epididymo-orchitis and, consequently, may be difficult to distinguish from spermatic cord (testicular) torsion. Prehn's sign (relief of pain

Table 29.3 Clinical Features: Epididymitis

Organisms	**<35 years and sexually active:** *Neisseria gonorrhoeae* *Chlamydia trachomatis* **>35 years or prepubescent:** Enteric species **Immunocompromised:** Mycobacteria or fungi
Signs and symptoms	• Unilateral scrotal pain • Dysuria • Urethral discharge
Laboratory and radiologic findings	• Gram stain of urethral discharge with ≥5 WBCs per oil immersion field • First-void urine with positive leukocyte esterase test or microscopy of sediment with ≥10 WBCs per high-power field • Urine NAAT for gonorrhea and chlamydia • Doppler ultrasonography, if obtained for diagnostic uncertainty, may show increased blood flow, decreased vascular resistance, reactive hydrocele, or wall thickening

with scrotal elevation) is characteristic of epididymitis, but is unreliable in distinguishing from torsion.

Symptoms in acute epididymitis are present less than 6 weeks, whereas duration greater than 6 weeks defines chronic epididymitis. This latter condition is further categorized as inflammatory chronic epididymitis, obstructive chronic epididymitis, or chronic epididymalgia. There is a wide differential diagnosis for chronic epididymitis, including trauma, malignancy, autoimmune conditions, or granulomatous disease such as from tuberculosis. These patients should be referred to an urologist.

Differential Diagnosis

The differential diagnosis includes:

- testicular torsion
- torsion of the appendix testis or appendix epididymis
- isolated orchitis
- hydrocele
- spermatocele
- inguinal hernia
- trauma
- testicular cancer
- varicocele (usually asymptomatic, but may cause discomfort)
- several vasculitides, including Kawasaki disease, polyarteritis nodosa, and Henoch–Schönlein purpura (HSP), can present with testicular and epididymal pain

Testicular torsion should be considered in all cases of unilateral testicular pain. Features favoring epididymitis are:

- gradual onset
- prolonged course
- mild to moderate pain
- normal cremasteric reflex
- urine testing supportive of epididymitis/urethritis

Isolated orchitis is generally from a viral process, usually mumps, but rarely other agents. It occurs in 20% of prepubertal males with mumps and should be considered if:

- history of parotitis (orchitis follows parotitis by 3 to 7 days)
- exam shows an enlarged, indurated testicle with a non-tender epididymis

Laboratory and Radiographic Findings

The evaluation for epididymitis is similar to that for urethritis. In the setting of urethral tenderness, the diagnosis is confirmed with one of the following:

- first-void urine with positive leukocyte esterase test or microscopy of sediment with ≥10 WBCs per high-power field
- gram stain of urethral discharge with ≥2 WBCs per oil immersion field
- positive NAAT on first-void urine

Gram stain of urethral discharge should be evaluated, if present, for gram-negative intracellular diplococci suggestive of gonorrhea. Regardless of the result, urine NAAT for gonorrhea and chlamydia should be obtained because co-infection is common. Urine NAATs also help to resolve diagnostic uncertainty, though results will not be immediately available.

The gold standard imaging study for suspected epididymitis is radionuclide scintigraphy; however' this is rarely used in clinical practice since epididymitis is primarily a clinical diagnosis, and ultrasonography is widely available and convenient.

Doppler ultrasonography can help differentiate epididymitis from testicular torsion. Changes consistent with epididymitis include increased blood flow (peak systolic velocity, PSV), decreased vascular resistance, reactive hydrocele, and/or wall thickening. PSV ≥15 has sensitivity and specificity for epididymitis of 89% and 94%, and for orchitis of 84% and 92%, respectively.

If the history, exam, and laboratory findings are consistent with epididymitis, and the concern for torsion is low or torsion has been ruled out, the patient should be treated empirically for epididymitis.

Treatment and Prophylaxis

If epididymitis is suspected based on clinical suspicion and risk factors, empiric therapy should be initiated while awaiting test results (see Table 29.4). If epididymitis is likely due to an STD, the patient should receive ceftriaxone as a single dose plus doxycycline as a 10-day course. If there is concern for enteric species, including from recent genitourinary instrumentation, levofloxacin or ofloxacin can be added. Fluoroquinolone monotherapy can be used in elderly patients without STD risk. Symptoms should improve within 3 days, though complete resolution of discomfort may not occur for weeks. Persistent symptoms despite a full course of antibiotic therapy may be due to unusual organisms, an epididymal abscess or pyocele, reinfection from a partner, or a non-infectious etiology.

If patients are allergic or cannot tolerate one of the recommended antibiotic regimens, consultation with an urologist or

Table 29.4 Epididymitis Empiric Therapy

Patient Category	Therapy Recommendation
Likely due to STD	Ceftriaxone 250 mg IM single dose *plus* Doxycycline 100 mg PO BID × 10 days *or* Azithromycin 1 g PO single dose
Likely due to sexually transmitted chlamydia and gonorrhea and enteric organisms (including men who practice insertive anal sex)	Ceftriaxone 250 mg IM single dose *plus* Levofloxacin 500 mg PO daily for 10 days *or* Ofloxacin 300 mg PO BID for 10 days
Likely due to enteric species (e.g. after instrumentation)	Levofloxacin 500 mg PO daily for 10 days *or* Ofloxacin 300 mg PO BID for 10 days
Adjunctive therapy	• Reduced activity or bed rest • Scrotal elevation and ice • NSAID

NSAID – non-steroidal anti-inflammatory drug.

infectious disease specialist is indicated since alternative therapies have not been well studied. Patients with HIV should receive identical treatment, unless a complication is present.

All patients evaluated for STDs should receive counseling about safe sex practices, and those diagnosed with sexually transmitted epididymitis should be tested for syphilis and HIV. As in urethritis, partners should be evaluated and treated or considered for EPT (see above).

Complications and Admission Criteria

Potential complications include epididymo-orchitis, epididymal or testicular abscess, pyocele, funiculitis, testicular infarction, chronic pain, infertility, Fournier's gangrene, or sepsis.

Most cases can be treated as an outpatient, but consider admission for the following:

- appear toxic with systemic signs/symptoms
- inability to take oral medications
- immunocompromised state

Infection Control

For sexually transmitted epididymitis, patients should refer all partners from the past 60 days for evaluation, or consider EPT. Patients should refrain from sexual activity until all symptoms have resolved, at least 7 days after initiation of therapy.

Acute Bacterial Prostatitis

Epidemiology and Microbiology

The lifetime probability of prostatitis in men approaches 25%. The worldwide prevalence of prostatitis symptoms ranges from 2.2 to 9.7%, and in the United States about 2 million outpatient visits annually are due to prostatitis.

Inflammation and infection of the prostate occurs due to inadequate drainage of prostatic secretions or reflux of urine into the prostatic tissue. Bacterial prostatitis most commonly occurs secondary to a urinary tract infection, which ascends from the urethra to the prostatic ducts, as opposed to an STD. Risk factors include benign prostatic hyperplasia, unprotected anal intercourse, phimosis, urinary tract infection, urethral stricture, urethral catheterization, or instrumentation. Infection can also occur via direct inoculation (prostate biopsy) or through hematogenous spread.

There are four recognized categories of prostatitis recognized by the National Institutes of Health:

(1) acute bacterial (present <3 months)
(2) chronic bacterial
(3) chronic prostatitis/chronic pelvic pain syndrome (further subdivided into inflammatory and non-inflammatory)
(4) asymptomatic inflammatory

While acute bacterial prostatitis accounts for only about 2 to 5% of total cases, it is the most common type to present in the acute care setting and will be the focus of this section. The majority of prostatitis falls into category 3, chronic prostatitis/chronic pelvic pain, accounting for 90 to 95% of cases, but this form is likely less common in the emergency department.

Acute bacterial prostatitis has a bimodal distribution, affecting men aged 20 to 40 years, followed by a second peak in the sixth decade and beyond. The disorder is caused predominantly by *E. coli*, but also *Pseudomonas aeruginosa*, *Klebsiella* spp., *Proteus* spp., *Staphylococcus aureus* or *saprophyticus*, and *Enterococcus* spp. In sexually active men, *N. gonorrhoeae* and *C. trachomatis* are possible causes.

Clinical Features

Acute bacterial prostatitis can generally be diagnosed by history and physical examination. Patients complain of urinary symptoms (dysuria, frequency, and urgency) and pain in the lower abdomen, perineum, or rectum (see Table 29.5). Varying degrees of urinary obstruction can occur, and when present are highly suggestive of the diagnosis. Patients often have systemic symptoms (fever, chills, myalgias) and may present with high fever or toxic appearance.

Digital rectal exam reveals an enlarged, warm, indurated, and exquisitely tender prostate. This exam is valuable in diagnosis and generally considered safe, though prostatic massage and serial prostate exams should be avoided as this can theoretically cause bacteremia. The suprapubic region may be tender from cystitis or acute urinary retention. There may be concurrent epididymo-orchitis.

Differential Diagnosis

The differential diagnosis includes non-bacterial prostatitis, cystitis, proctitis, anal or rectal abscess or fistula.

Laboratory and Radiographic Findings

Mid-stream urinalysis with gram stain and culture should be obtained. Urinalysis typically shows pyuria and bacteriuria.

Table 29.5 Clinical Features and Treatment: Acute Bacterial Prostatitis

Organisms	*Escherichia coli* *Pseudomonas aeruginosa* *Klebsiella* spp. *Proteus* spp. *Staphylococcus aureus/saprophyticus* *Enterococcus* spp.
Signs and symptoms	• Dysuria, frequency, urgency • Abdominal, perineal, rectal pain • Urinary retention • Fever, chills
Laboratory findings	• Pyuria, bacteriuria • Leukocytosis
Treatment	**Outpatient therapy:** Levofloxacin 500 mg PO daily for 6 weeks *or* Ciprofloxacin 500 mg PO BID for 6 weeks *or* TMP–SMX DS one tab. PO BID for 6 weeks **Inpatient therapy:** Levofloxacin 500 mg IV daily *or* Ceftriaxone 1 g IV daily *plus optional* Gentamicin 5 mg/kg/dose IV every 24 hours

If STD suspected, add azithromycin or doxycycline.
TMP – trimethoprim; SMX – sulfamethoxazole; DS – double strength; IV – intravenous.

Antibiotic susceptibilities from culture can be used to guide prolonged antibiotic treatment. In acute bacterial prostatitis, pathogens are almost always isolated from urine, so sterile urine makes this diagnosis unlikely. Additional testing may be indicated in certain situations:

• consider first-void urine NAAT for gonorrhea and chlamydia in sexually active men
• complete blood count for leukocytosis
• inflammatory markers
• blood cultures can be considered in the setting of fever or toxic appearance

Imaging is not routine in the work-up of prostatitis. However, if prostatic abscess is suspected based on palpated fluctuance or treatment failure, a transrectal ultrasound or computed tomographic (CT) scan of the pelvis should be obtained.

Treatment and Prophylaxis

Prostatitis is a clinical diagnosis, and treatment should be started empirically. Strong evidence to guide antibiotic choice does not exist, so treatment should be initiated based on risk factors, then narrowed or modified when culture results become available (see Table 29.5). Oral fluoroquinolone monotherapy is the recommended first-line outpatient treatment, If the patient has received a fluoroquinolone in the past 6 months or if there is high local resistance to fluoroquinolones (consult local antibiogram), then choose an alternative regimen. For patients who warrant inpatient admission, intravenous ceftriaxone, ciprofloxacin, or levofloxacin may be used. An aminoglycoside can be added to this regimen with dosing caution in patients with renal dysfunction.

Adjunctive therapies include bed rest, non-steroidal anti-inflammatory drug, stool softeners, hydration, and sitz baths. Acute urinary obstruction should be relieved by a suprapubic catheter to avoid damaging the edematous prostate or precipitating bacteremia with a Foley catheter.

Complications and Admission Criteria

Complications include sepsis, bladder outlet obstruction with urinary retention (approximately 10% of cases), chronic bacterial prostatitis (approximately 10% of cases), prostatic abscess, or chronic prostatitis/chronic pelvic pain syndrome.

Consider hospitalization and IV antibiotics for any of the following:

- toxic appearance
- elderly patient, multiple comorbidities, or immunosuppressed
- failure of outpatient therapy
- inability to take oral medication

IV antibiotics penetrate the inflamed prostate well and patients tend to respond rapidly. Persistent fever after 48 hours of treatment raises suspicion for prostatic abscess. The duration of therapy for acute prostatitis may need to be continued for up to 6 weeks for severe illness or persistent symptoms.

Pearls and Pitfalls

1. Owing to changing antibiotic resistance patterns, the best current treatment for urethritis is azithromycin 1 g PO plus ceftriaxone 250 mg IM.

2. Consider and test for co-infection with other STDs. Patients and their partners can be referred to an STD clinic or to a primary care provider for testing and counseling for other sexually transmitted infections, including HIV and syphilis.

3. Although epididymitis is more common, testicular torsion, a surgical emergency, must be considered in all patients with acute scrotal pain.

4. Symptoms of epididymitis should improve 1 to 3 days after initiating appropriate therapy. Instruct patients to seek prompt follow-up for persistent or escalating symptoms.

5. Acute bacterial prostatitis can progress to sepsis, and empiric treatment should be started immediately, particularly in toxic-appearing or elderly patients.

6. Failure of antibiotic therapy may be due to unusual organisms (e.g. *Pseudomonas*, *Enterococcus*) or a prostatic abscess, which is diagnosed by transrectal ultrasound or CT.

7. Acute urinary retention due to prostatitis requires a suprapubic rather than Foley catheter, as well as urology consultation.

References

Brede, C. M. and Shoskes, D. A. The etiology and management of acute prostatitis. *Nat. Revi. Urol.* 2011; 8(4): 207–12.

Brown, J. M., Hammers, L. W., Barton, J. W., *et al.* Quantitative Doppler assessment of acute scrotal inflammation. *Radiology* 1995; 197(2): 427–31.

Cazanave, C., Manhart, L. E., and Bebear, C. *Mycoplasma gentalium,* an emerging sexually transmitted pathogen. *Med. et Mal. Infect.* 2012; 42(9): 381–92.

Centers for Disease Control and Prevention. *Sexually Transmitted Disease Surveillance 2013* (Atlanta, GA: US Department of Health and Human Services, 2014).

Centers for Disease Control and Prevention. Sexually transmitted diseases treatment guidelines. *MMWR Morb. Mortal. Wkly. Rep.* 2015; 64(RR-3): 51–3, 60–5, 82–4.

Cook, R. L., Hutchison, S. L., Østergaard, L., *et al.* Systematic review: noninvasive testing for *Chlamydia trachomatis* and *Neisseria gonorrhoeae*. *Ann. of Intern. Med.* 2005; 142(11): 914–25.

Krieger, J. N., Lee, S., Jeon, J., *et al.* Epidemiology of prostatitis. *Int. J. Antimicrob. Agents.* 2008; 31(1): 85–90.

Lipsky, B. A., Byren, I., and Hoey, C. T., Treatment of bacterial prostatitis. *Clin. Infect. Dis.* 2010; 50(12): 1641–52.

Manhart, L. E., Broad, J. M., and Golden, M. R. Mycoplasma genitalium: should we treat and how? *Clin. Infect. Dis.* 2011; 53(3): S129–42.

Pond, M. J., Nori, A. V., Witney, A. A., *et al.* High prevalence of antibiotic-resistant *Mycoplasma gentialium* in nongonococcal urethritis: the need for routine testing and the inadequacy of current treatment options. *Clin. Infect. Dis.* 2014; 58(5): 631–7.

Schewbke, J. R., Rompalo, A., Taylor, S., *et al.* Re-evaluating the treatment of nongonococcal urethritis: emphasizing emerging pathogens – a randomized clinical trial. *Clin. Infect. Dis.* 2011; 52(4): 163–70.

Schofield, C. B. Some factors affecting the incubation period and duration of symptoms of urethritis in men. *B. J. Vener. Dis.* 1982; 58(3): 184–7.

Tobbian, A., Serwadda, D., Quinn, T. C., *et al.* Male circumcision for the prevention of HSV-2 and HPV infections and syphillis. *N. Eng. J. Med.* 2009; 360(13): 1298–309.

Trojian, T. H., Lishnak, T. S., and Heiman, D. Epididymitis and orchitis: an overview. *American Family Physician* 2009; 79(7): 583–7.

Van Howe, R. S. Does circumcision influence sexually transmitted diseases? A literature review. *BJU international* 1999; 83(S1): 52–62.

Wagenlehner, F. M. E., Pilatz, A., Bschleipfer, T., *et al.* Bacterial prostatitis. *World Journal of Urology* 2013; 31(4): 711–16.

Non-Ulcerative Sexually Transmitted Diseases

Jaime Jordan

Chapter 30

Introduction

Sexually transmitted diseases (STDs) are best divided into two major groups: those that cause ulcerative lesions (see Chapter 31, Ulcerative Sexually Transmitted Diseases) and those that do not. Diseases that fall into this latter group include chlamydial infections, gonococcal infections, non-gonococcal urethritis, and human papilloma virus (HPV). Although new tests make diagnosis easier, results are often not available during an acute care visit, and empiric treatment with appropriate follow-up is often the best approach. The CDC recommends a very low threshold for empiric treatment of chlamydia and gonorrhea in high-risk patients (sexually active individuals between the ages of 16 and 25). These infections should almost always be treated in tandem as they are difficult to distinguish clinically and can coexist. Acute care providers should be well versed in the standard treatment regimens for these common STDs. *Trichomonas vaginalis*, a sexually transmitted cause of vulvovaginitis, is covered in Chapter 32.

Chlamydia

Epidemiology and Microbiology

Chlamydia trachomatis is a gram-negative bacterium and an obligate intracellular pathogen. It cannot be isolated with standard culture techniques. Chlamydia is extremely transmissible by sexual contact. It is the most common sexually transmitted bacterial infection in the United States, with an estimated annual incidence of nearly 3 million. It is also one of the most commonly reported to the CDC. In 2013, more than 1.4 million cases were reported. In the United States, it is most common among young people ages 15 to 24. When sexually transmitted, it most commonly causes urethritis in men and cervicitis in women. Co-infection with *N. Gonorrhea* is common.

Clinical Features

In men, *Chlamydia trachomatis* most commonly causes urethritis with dysuria and/or a clear urethral discharge (see

Table 30.1 Clinical Features: Chlamydia

Organism	*Chlamydia trachomatis*
Signs and symptoms	Frequently asymptomatic **Men:** Dysuria and/or clear urethral discharge **Women:** Majority asymptomatic; dysuria, vaginal discharge, spotting
Laboratory findings	• Male genitourinary disease: urine/urethral swabs – nucleic acid amplification test (NAAT) positive for chlamydia *Urine specimen is preferred as it is less invasive and performance is equivalent to urethral specimen* • Female genitourinary disease: urine*/vaginal/cervical swabs – NAATs positive for chlamydia *Vaginal swab is the preferred specimen type*

* NAATs performed on urine sample in female patients may detect up to 10% fewer infections.
NAAT – nucleic acid amplification test.

Table 30.1). In women, *C. trachomatis* typically causes cervicitis. Women may report complaints of dysuria, vaginal discharge, and spotting. However, most chlamydial infections in women are asymptomatic.

Differential Diagnosis

The differential diagnosis for chlamydia includes:
Urethritis:

- *Neisseria gonorrhoeae*
- *Mycoplasma genitalium*
- *Ureaplasma urealyticum*
- adenovirus
- *herpes simplex* virus
- *Trichomonas vaginalis*

Non-infectious causes such as Reiter's syndrome and contact dermatitis from topical preparations or latex condoms should also be considered in the differential diagnosis.
Cervicitis:
C. trachomatis and *N. gonorrhoeae* are the most common causes of acute cervicitis. As mentioned above, non-infectious causes, including contact dermatitis from douches, scented tampons, vaginal creams, or latex condoms, should also be considered.

Treatment

Chlamydia is treated with a single daily dose of oral azithromycin or doxycycline for 7 days (see Table 30.2). Although more expensive and with some documented treatment failures, the single dose of azithromycin can be given during the patient's index visit and ensures compliance with a complete therapeutic course.

Alternative treatment regimens include erythromycin, ofloxacin, levofloxacin, or erythromycin ethylsuccinate.

Complications and Admission Criteria

Patients with chlamydia infections rarely develop complications during the index infection. Women may go on to develop pelvic inflammatory disease (PID); criteria for admitting these patients are listed in the PID section below. Men may develop

Table 30.2 Treatment of Chlamydia Infections

Azithromycin 1 g PO single dose
or
Doxycycline 100 mg PO BID for 7 days
Alternatives:
(all 7-day regimens)
Ofloxacin 300 mg PO BID
or
Levofloxacin 500 mg PO daily
or
Erythromycin base 500 mg PO QID
or
Erythromycin ethylsuccinate 800 mg PO QID
PO – by mouth.

epididymitis and/or orchitis, but rarely require admission. *C. trachomatas* is one of the pathogens associated with reactive arthritis (Reiter's syndrome).

Gonorrhea

Epidemiology and Microbiology

Gonorrhea is caused by the organism *Neisseria gonorrhoeae*, a gram-negative diplococcus. *N. gonorrhea* is a strictly human pathogen that is well adapted for infection of both the male and female genital tracts, and for rapid development of antimicrobial resistance. It is highly infectious and can disseminate beyond the genital tract to other parts of the body. The risk of transmission after a single sexual encounter with a person infected with gonorrhea is around 50%. It is the second most common reported transmissible disease, behind chlamydia, with an estimated 800,000 new infections occuring annually in the United States.

Clinical Features

In men, gonorrhea most commonly causes urethritis characterized by a purulent urethral discharge (see Figure 30.1) and dysuria. Women infected with gonorrhea often have cervicitis, which may present with a mild vaginal discharge, or spotting,

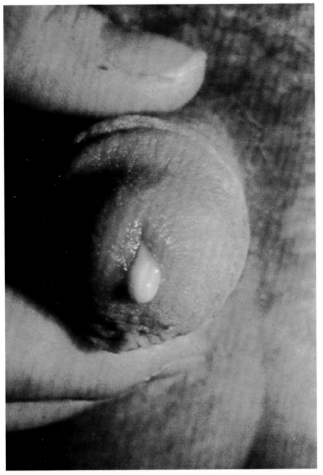

Figure 30.1 Purulent urethral discharge in a patient with gonorrhea. Image courtesy of the Australasian Chapter on Sexual Health Medicine.

particularly after intercourse (see Table 30.3). Gonorrhea may also infect the rectum and pharynx, but patients are often asymptomatic when infection occurs in these areas.

Gonococcal conjunctivitis is a potentially sight-threatening infection. Patients present with a purulent eye discharge and chemosis and may develop corneal ulceration, hypopion, and endophthalmitis. Globe perforation may occur in neglected, inadequately treated, or advanced cases.

Gonorrhea disseminates in 0.5 to 3% of untreated patients. Patients with disseminated gonococcal infection most commonly develop septic arthritis and skin lesions; in rare cases, the infection may cause meningitis and endocarditis. The septic arthritis is usually mono- or oligoarticular, most frequently involving the knee. The skin lesions are commonly described as necrotic pustules on an erythematous base. They occur on the distal extremities and usually total fewer than 20 lesions.

Differential Diagnosis

The differential diagnosis includes:

- Conjunctivitis: other causes including *Staphylococcus, Streptococcus,* and viruses should be considered.
- Gonococcal arthritis: as gonococcal arthritis is a true septic process, not a reactive arthritis, other bacterial causes

including *Staphylococcus aureus* should also be considered. Trauma, rheumatologic conditions, and degenerative joint disease may also cause joint symptoms.

- Gonococcal skin lesions: community-acquired methicillin-resistant *Staphylococcus aureus* infection may cause skin lesions similar to those caused by *N. gonorrhoeae.*

Key features that may help to distinguish gonorrhea from other STDs are:

- presence of a purulent discharge, which may be copious in men with urethritis
- marked chemosis in patients with conjunctival infections
- a single septic knee joint in a sexually active patient should suggest disseminated gonococcal infection

Laboratory Findings

Gram stain may be useful in making the diagnosis in patients with conjunctivitis, or urethritis when there is exudate at the urethral meatus. In men, a gram stain positive for gram-negative intracellular diplococci is more than 99% specific and 95% sensitive in making the diagnosis; however, a negative gram stain does not rule out the diagnosis and further testing is needed in these cases.

As with chlamydia, nucleic acid amplification tests (NAATs) on urine, urethral swabs, and vaginal or cervical swabs can be used to diagnose gonorrhea. Urine testing in men has adequate sensitivity and specificity to make the diagnosis (95 to 97% sensitive, >99% specific) and is preferred to urethral swab testing due to its less invasive nature. In women, NAATs performed on vaginal swab specimens are preferred and have similar sensivity and specificity to cervical samples. Cervical and urine samples may also be utilized. NAATs performed on urine samples in women may detect up to 10% fewer infections. NAATs are the recommended tests for rectal and oropharyngeal gonorrhea and chlamydia, but are not yet cleared by the the FDA. Specimens must be sent to labs that meet specialized regulatory requirements in order to have results reported for patient management. In all cases, NAATs cannot be used to determine organism antibiotic sensitivity, and are not a replacement for cultures if sensitivities are important to patient management or public health.

Treatment

Ceftriaxone as a single-dose regimen can be used to treat uncomplicated gonorrheal infections of the urethra, cervix, or rectum (see Table 30.4). Increased prevalence of quinolone-resistant *Neisseria gonorrhoeae* (QRNG) in the United States has been noted and these drugs are no longer recommended. Cephalosporins have also been noted to have declining effectiveness in the United States, and as such oral cephalosporins are no longer recommended.

Pharyngeal gonorrhea should be treated with ceftriaxone.

Gonococcal conjunctivitis is treated with ceftriaxone. These patients usually should also undergo saline lavage of the infected eye.

Table 30.3 Clinical Features: Gonorrhea

Organism	*Neisseria gonorrhoeae*
Incubation period	Less than 1 week; may be as little as 2 days
Signs and symptoms	**Ophthalmology:** May develop corneal ulceration, hyperopion, and endophthalmitis **Disseminated gonococcal infection:** Septic arthritis and skin lesions; rare cases of meningitis and endocarditis **Genitourinary:** Men: • Dysuria and purulent urethral discharge Women: • Cervicitis • Often infection is asymptomatic • Non-specific symptoms such as a mild vaginal discharge or spotting, particularly after intercourse, may occur
Laboratory findings	• Gram stain positive for gram-negative intracellular diplococci (urethral or conjunctival discharge); negative gram stain does not rule out the diagnosis, and other testing is needed • Male genitoruinary disease: urine/urethral swabs – nucleic acid amplification test (NAAT) positive for gonorrhea *Urine specimen is preferred as it is less invasive and performance is equivalent to urethral specimen* • Female genitourinary disease: urine*/vaginal/cervical swabs – NAATs positive for gonorrhea *Vaginal swab is the preferred specimen type*

* NAATs performed on urine sample in female patients may detect up to 10% fewer infections.

NAAT – nucleic acid amplification test.

Patients with disseminated gonorrhea should be admitted for initial therapy. The recommended regimen is ceftriaxone, 1 g intramuscularly (IM) or intravenously (IV) every 24 hours. Alternative regimens include cefotaxime, ceftizoxime, or spectinomycin.

Complications and Admission Criteria

As with chlamydia, women with untreated gonorrhea may develop PID. Disseminated gonococcal disease can also occur; these patients should usually be admitted as part of their initial treatment. Men may also develop epididymitis and/or orchitis; rarely, these patients are symptomatic enough to need hospitalization.

Non-Gonococcal Urethritis

Epidemiology and Microbiology

While commonly caused by chlamydia and gonorrhea, urethritis may also be caused by *Mycoplasma genitalium*, *Ureaplasma urealyticum*, *Trichomonas vaginalis*, HSV, and adenovirus. These patients present with typical symptoms of urethritis and frequently return for care when initial treatment for chlamydia and gonorrhea does not cure their symptoms (see Table 30.5).

Clinical Features

Patients commonly present with dysuria and/or a urethral discharge and may have been treated for urethritis already.

Differential Diagnosis

The differential diagnosis for non-gonococcal urethritis includes other infectious agents such as chlamydia and gonorrhea, as well as reactive arthritis (Reiter's syndrome) and local irritants.

Laboratory Findings

The diagnosis of NGU is made in patients who have negative gonorrhea testing, and who meet criteria for urethritis.

Diagnostic criteria include:

• mucopurulent or purulent discharge
• gram stain showing 5 or more WBCs per oil immersion field
• positive leukocyte esterase test on first-void urine or specimen that has at least 10 WBCs per high-power field

Treatment

Treatment is either azithromycin 1 g orally once or doxycycline 100 mg orally twice a day for 7 days (if this regimen was not used during an earlier visit). Alternative regimens include erythromycin base, or erythromycin ethylsuccinate, ofloxacin, or levofloxacin for 7 days. Patients who have recurrent or persistent urethritis despite this treatment should receive metronidazole 2 g orally as a single dose, tinidazole 2 g orally as a single dose, or azithromycin 1 g orally as a single dose (if not used for initial treatment).

Complications and Admission Criteria

Complications of this infection are rare.

Pelvic Inflammatory Disease

Epidemiology and Microbiology

Nearly 1 million cases of PID are diagnosed annually in the United States, despite overall decreasing trends. This infection of the upper female genital tract can be caused by several organisms, including *Chlamydia trachomatis*, *Neisseria gonorrhoeae*,

Table 30.4 Treatment of Gonorrheal Infections

Uncomplicated infections of urethra, cervix, or rectum	**Recommended regimen:** Ceftriaxone 250 mg IM* once plus Azithromycin 1 g PO once or Doxycycline 100 mg PO BID for 7 days (azithromycin is preferred) **Alternative regimens:** Only if ceftriaxone is not available: Cefixime 400 mg PO once plus Azithromycin 1 g PO once plus Test of cure in 1 week Severe cephalosporin allergy: Azithromycin 2 g PO once plus Gentamicin 240 mg IM once plus test of cure in 1 week
Uncomplicated pharyngeal infection	Ceftriaxone 250 mg IM single dose plus Azithromycin 1 g PO once or Doxycycline 100 mg PO BID for 7 days (azithromycin is preferred)
Adult conjunctivitis	Consider hospitalization Ceftriaxone 1 g IM/IV every 24 hours Normal saline irrigation
Disseminated gonococcal infection (see Chapter 14, Fever and Rash in Adults)	Strongly consider hospitalization **Recommended regimen:** Ceftriaxone 1 g IM/IV every 24 hours **Alternative regimens:** Cefotaxime 1 g IV every 8 hours or Ceftizoxime 1 g IV every 8 hours Treatment should be continued for 24–48 hours after improvement, at which time therapy may be switched to cefixime 400 mg PO BID to complete at least 1 week of antimicrobial therapy

* In the emergency department, ceftriaxone may be administered intramuscularly or intravenously for STD treatment. Intramuscular injections of ceftriaxone are painful and should be given intravenously at the same dose if access is already available. Intramuscular ceftriaxone should be reconstituted with injectable lidocaine 1% to minimize pain upon injection.

PO – by mouth.

Table 30.5 Clinical Features: Non-Gonococcal Urethritis

Organism	C. trachomatis Mycoplasma genitalium Ureaplasma urealyticum Trichomonas vaginalis HSV Adenovirus
Incubation period	Variable
Signs and symptoms	Dysuria with or without urethral discharge
Laboratory findings	(1) Mucopurulent or purulent discharge; (2) Gram stain showing ≥5 WBCs per oil immersion field; and (3) positive leukocyte esterase test on first-void urine or specimen that shows ≥10 WBCs per high-power field.
Treatment	**Treatment for NGU:** Azithromycin 1 g PO once or Doxycycline 100 mg BID for 7 days **Alternative regimens:** Erythromycin base 500 mg PO QID for 7 days or Erythromycin ethylsuccinate 800 mg PO QID for 7 days or Ofloxacin 300 mg PO BID for 7 days or Levofloxacin 500 mg PO daily for 7 days **Treatment for persistent or recurrent NGU:** Metronidazole 2 g PO single dose or Tinidazole 2 g PO single dose or Azithromycin 1 g PO single dose (if not used for initial treatment)

PO – by mouth; WBC – white blood (cell) count.

Mycoplasma, Ureaplasma, vaginal aerobes, and facultative anaerobes; in fact, infection caused by multiple organisms is common. PID can be a life-altering infection, as complications are common.

Clinical Features

This infection of the female upper genital tract causes a wide array of symptoms (see Table 30.6). Patients may be asymptomatic, have mild symptoms such as pelvic pain and dyspareunia, or have severe illness characterized by peritoneal signs and systemic toxicity. Making the diagnosis of PID is often difficult. The "gold standard" is laparoscopy, but the diagnosis of PID is usually made clinically, based on the following criteria:

- complaints of pelvic or lower abdominal pain (in the absence of another cause e.g. appendicitis) *and*
- cervical motion tenderness, adnexal tenderness, or uterine tenderness

The goal of using this low diagnostic threshold is to identify and treat the mild cases of PID in an attempt to prevent complications, such as chronic pelvic pain, infertility, and ectopic pregnancy.

Differential Diagnosis

Any condition that causes lower abdominal symptoms in women may mimic PID:

- ovarian cysts
- ovarian torsion
- ectopic pregnancy
- appendicitis
- tubo-ovarian abscess
- diverticulitis

Table 30.6 Clinical Features: Pelvic Inflammatory Disease

Organisms	*Chlamydia trachomatis* *Neisseria gonorrhoeae* *Mycoplasma* *Ureaplasma* Vaginal aerobes and facultative anaerobes
Incubation period	Days to years
Signs and symptoms	• Severe cases: fever, abdominal pain, peritoneal signs, systemic toxicity • Mild cases: dyspareunia, pelvic pain, abdominal pain • May be asymptomatic
Laboratory findings	• Laboratory testing may be misleadingly normal • Patients may have an elevated erythrocyte sedimentation rate, peripheral WBC, or C-reactive protein
Treatment	**Outpatient therapy** Regimen A: Ceftriaxone 250 mg IM once *plus* Doxycycline 100 mg PO BID for 14 days *with or without* Metronidazole 500 mg PO BID for 14 days Regimen B: Cefoxitin 2 g IM once *plus* Probenecid 1 g PO once concurrently *plus* Doxycycline 100 mg PO BID for 14 days *with or without* Metronidazole 500 mg PO BID for 14 days Regimen C: Other parenteral third-generation cephalosporin (e.g. cefotaxime 1 g IM once) *plus* Doxycycline 100 mg PO BID for 14 days *with or without* Metronidazole 500 mg PO BID for 14 days **Inpatient therapy** Regimen A: Cefoxitin 2 g IV every 6 hours (or cefotetan 2 g IV every 12 hours) *plus* Doxycycline 100 mg PO or IV every 12 hours Continue for 24–48 hours after improvement Continue doxycycline for a 14-day course total Regimen B: Clindamycin 900 mg IV every 8 hours *plus* Gentamicin* 2 mg/kg IV or IM once as a load, then 1.5 mg/kg/dose IV or IM every 8 hours Continue for 24–48 hours after improvement Then doxycycline 100 mg PO BID or clindamycin 450 mg PO QID to complete 14-day course total

* Gentamicin extended interval dosing is an alternative and may be more convenient.

PO – by mouth; WBC – white blood (cell) count.

Unfortunately, presentation of these conditions may appear clinically to be quite similar; often, further testing such as ultrasound or computed tomographic (CT) scanning may be necessary to make the diagnosis. In clinically unclear cases, laparoscopy may lead to a definitive diagnosis.

Laboratory Findings

The diagnosis is usually made clinically. No single laboratory test is sufficiently sensitive and specific to make the diagnosis

of PID. Laboratory abnormalities may include elevated WBC, sedimentation rate, C-reactive protein, or increased WBCs seen on wet prep. Imaging with transvaginal ultrasound or CT scan is used to identify tubo-ovarian abscess.

Treatment

Treatment of PID aims to cover the most likely pathogens. Oral and parenteral options are available. Please refer to Table 30.6 for specific regimens.

Complications and Admission Criteria

Early complications of this infection are tubo-ovarian abscess and the right upper quadrant pain of perihepatitis (Fitz-Hugh–Curtis syndrome). An evaluation for tubo-ovarian abscess should be undertaken in patients who fail to respond or worsen on standard empirical therapy, as well in any patient with clinically severe PID. The preferred imaging modality, ultrasound versus CT, is institution-dependent. Long-term complications of PID, generally due to scarring of the upper genital tract, include chronic pelvic pain, chronic dyspareunia, infertility, and an increased risk of ectopic pregnancy.

Criteria for admission in the setting of PID include:

- pregnancy
- failure to respond clinically to oral antimicrobials
- inability to complete or tolerate an outpatient oral regimen
- severe illness, nausea and vomiting, or high fever
- concomitant tubo-ovarian abscess
- cases in which other surgical emergencies such as appendicitis cannot be excluded

Human Papilloma Virus

Epidemiology and Microbiology

Human papilloma virus (HPV) is the most common sexually transmitted infection in the United States, with more than 14 million estimated infections annually. Although some infections cause cancer or genital warts (condyloma acuminata), most are asymptomatic or unrecognized. More than 100 types of HPV exist and more than 40 of these can cause genital infection. Whereas types 6 and 11 are most commonly associated with genital warts, others are strongly associated with cervical neoplasia. Between 13 and 18 strains have been characterized as oncogenic, most notably types 16 and 18.

Clinical Features

Most HPV infections are asymptomatic and self-limited. When HPV causes symptoms, patients complain of lesions on the genital mucosa (see Table 30.7). These warts can be flat, papular, or peduncated growths and are found on moist surfaces such as the vulvae, introitus, and cervix, perianally, and on the shaft of the penis (see Figures 30.1 and 30.2). It can also be found anywhere in immunocompromised individuals (see Figure 30.3). Women additionally may have cervical infection manifested by flat warts, seen only on colposcopy.

Differential Diagnosis

Condyloma lata, a skin condition seen in secondary syphilis, and malignancy such as squamous cell carcinoma should be considered in the differential diagnosis.

Laboratory Findings

Anogenital lesions are often highly suggestive of HPV infection, and treatment is frequently based on a clinical diagnosis.

As this is a sexually transmitted disease, evaluation for other sexually transmitted disease is often indicated. Syphilis testing, including dark-field examination, should be considered, as flat condyloma acuminata lesions may resemble those seen with the condyloma lata seen in secondary syphilis.

The most common way to diagnose HPV infection is through screening with routine Pap smears with cytologic testing. Cervical dysplasia or neoplasia should prompt further testing and tissue biopsy may be necessary. HPV DNA testing of cervical scrapings is available and includes HC II (hybrid capture II) and PCR (polymerase chain reaction) testing. Both tests are highly sensitive.

Treatment and Admission Criteria

HPV is treated topically with the goal of eradicating or reducing symptoms. There are many topical options available, and none has been demonstrated to be significantly superior to any other. Multiple treatment applications are required over weeks to months. These treatments may rarely cause local skin reactions and pain.

The two major categories of treatments are immune response modifiers and cytotoxic agents. Immune response modifiers include imiquimod and interferon α, and cytotoxic agents include antiproliferative (podofilox, podophyllin, and 5-fluorouracil) and chemodestructive (salicylic acid, trichloroacetic acid [TCA], and bichloroacetic acid [BCA]) agents.

Surgical treatment may be necessary for extensive lesions or those unresponsive to topical medications. Advantages of surgical therapy include single-treatment regimens with decreased recurrence, though cryosurgery may require multiple sessions to eradicate the lesions.

Complications

The most concerning complication of HPV infection is cervical cancer, particularly its association with high-risk HPV serotypes. Patients with anogenital HPV infection are also at increased risk of developing vaginal and anal carcinoma.

Prevention

In 2006, the FDA licensed an HPV vaccine for use in women aged 9 to 26 years. This vaccine is virtually 100% protective against four HPV types (6, 11, 16, 18), which together are responsible for 70% of cases of cervical cancer and 90% of cases of anogenital warts. The full vaccination series requires three injections over a 6-month period.

Abstinence is the only way to eliminate the risk of transmission of sexually transmitted diseases, but safe sex practices dramatically decrease this risk. Education about barrier protection and safe sex practice is an essential addition to treatment.

Infection Control

Universal precautions should be observed for all patients with sexually transmitted infections. No isolation is required.

Table 30.7 Clinical Features: Human Papilloma Virus

Organism	Human papilloma virus
Signs and symptoms	• Flat, papular, or pedunculated warts on the genitalia or around the anus • Patients often are asymptomatic
Laboratory findings	• Pap smear with cytologic testing is the standard screening procedure, looking for cervical neoplasia • Tissue biopsy may be necessary • HPV DNA testing includes hybrid capture II and polymerase chain reaction testing; both are highly sensitive
Treatment	**Patient-applied:** • Podofilox 0.5% topical solution or gel Apply solution with a cotton swab or gel with a finger. Apply topically to visible genital warts twice a day for 3 days, followed by 4 days of no therapy. This cycle may be repeated, as necessary, for up to four cycles. The total wart area treated should not exceed 10 cm². Total volume of podofilox should be limited to 0.5 mL per day. Demonstrate the proper application technique and identify which warts should be treated. The safety of podofilox during pregnancy has not been established. Do not apply to vaginal mucosa; for external use only. *or* • Imiquimod 5% cream Apply imiquimod cream topically once daily at bedtime, three times a week for up to 16 weeks. The treatment area should be washed with soap and water 6–10 hours after the application. The safety of imiquimod during pregnancy has not been established. Do not apply to vaginal mucosa; for external use only. • Sinecatechins 15% ointment Use a finger to apply a thin layer of ointment topically three times daily until wart resolution (up to 16 weeks). Do not wash off after use. Avoid sexual contact while ointment is on skin. The safety of sinecatechins in pregnancy is not known. Do not apply to vaginal mucosa; for external use only. **Provider-administered:** • Cryotherapy Liquid nitrogen or cryoprobe. Repeat applications every 1–2 weeks. Cryotherapy is safe during pregnancy. *or* • Podophyllin resin 10–25% in a compound tincture of benzoin Apply a small amount topically to each wart and allow to air dry. Treatment can be repeated weekly, if necessary. To avoid the possibility of complications associated with systemic absorption and toxicity: 1. Application should be limited to <0.5 mL of podophyllin or an area of <10 cm² of warts per session, and 2. No open lesions or wounds should exist in the area to which treatment is administered. Some specialists suggest that the preparation should be thoroughly washed off 1–4 hours after application to reduce local irritation. The safety of podophyllin during pregnancy has not been established. Should not be applied to vaginal mucosa; for external use only. *or* • Trichloroacetic acid or bichloroacetic acid 80–90% Apply a small amount topically only to the warts and allow to dry, at which time a white "frosting" develops. If an excess amount of acid is applied, the treated area should be powdered with talc, sodium bicarbonate (i.e. baking soda), or liquid soap preparations to remove unreacted acid. This treatment can be repeated weekly, if necessary. Trichloroacetic acid may be used for internal lesions and during pregnancy. *or* • Surgical removal

Pearls and Pitfalls

1. Patients diagnosed with chlamydia and gonorrhea should refrain from sexual activity during and for 7 days after completion of treatment; treat all partners from the period of 60 days prior to diagnosis.

2. Have a low threshold to treat patients presenting to the acute care setting with symptoms suggestive of chlamydia or gonorrhea. Deferring treatment until the patient has definitive test results may lead to undertreated disease and increased transmission.

3. Any sexually active patient who presents with a single septic joint should be evaluated for disseminated gonococcal infection.

4. Chemosis and purulent eye discharge suggest a gonococcal conjunctivitis. Consider sending a gram stain and culture of the discharge and treat empirically if there is a high suspicion of the infection.

5. Patients who present for care who have been adequately treated for chlamydia and gonorrhea but remain symptomatic should have diagnostic testing to ensure that the patient has urethritis and is treated accordingly.

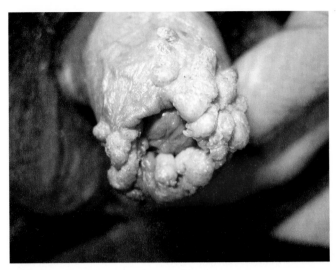

Figure 30.2 Condyloma accuminata on the penis.
Image Courtesy of Dr. Joseph Engelman, San Francisco City Clinic.

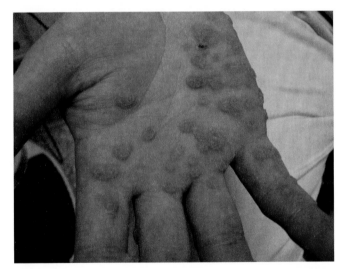

Figure 30.3 Human papilloma virus on the hands in a poorly controlled HIV positive patient.
Image Courtesy of Dr. Joseph Engelman, San Francisco City Clinic.

6. The Centers for Disease Control and Prevention recommend a low clinical threshold to diagnose and treat PID. Failure to do so may put the patient at risk for long-term complications from untreated PID, including chronic pelvic pain, chronic dyspareunia, infertility, and increased risk for ectopic pregnancy.

7. Patients with HPV infections should be referred to a primary care provider who can initiate or continue treatment and monitor the patient's response and follow Pap smears in women with the infection.

8. Patients with HPV should be tested for other sexually transmitted disease as indicated, particularly syphilis, which can also present with skin lesions.

References

Centers for Disease Control and Prevention (CDC). Increase in fluoroquinolone-resistant Neisseria gonorrhoeae among men who have sex with men – United States, 2003 and revised recommendations for gonorrhea treatment. *MMWR Morb. Mortal. Wkly. Rep.* 2004; 53(16): 335–8.

CDC. Sexually transmitted diseases treatment guidelines. *MMWR Morb. Mortal. Wkly. Rep.* 2010; 59(RR-12): 1–110.

CDC. Update to the CDC's sexually transmitted disease treatment guidelines, 2010: oral cephalosporins no longer a recommended treatment for gonococcal infections. *MMWR Morb. Mortal. Wkly. Rep.* 2012; 61(31): 590–4.

CDC. Recommendations for the laboratory based detection of Chlamydia trachomatis and Neisseria gonorrhoeae – 2014. *MMWR Morb. Mortal. Wkly. Rep.* 2014; 63(RR-02): 1–19.

CDC. *Sexually Transmitted Disease Surveillance 2013* (Atlanta, GA: US Department of Health and Human Services, 2014).

Committee on Practice Bulletins – Gynecology. ACOG Practice Bulletin Number 131: Screening for cervical cancer. *Obstet. Gynecol.* 2012; 120(5): 1222–38.

Lau, C.-Y. and Qureshi, A. K. Azithromycin versus doxycycline for genital chlamydial infections: a meta-analysis of randomized clinical trials. *Sex. Transm. Dis.* 2002; 29(9): 497–502.

LeFevre, M. L. U.S. Preventive Services Task Force. Screening for Chlamydia and gonorrhea: U.S. preventive services task force recommendation statement. *Ann. Intern. Med.* 2014; 161(12): 902–10.

Leszczyszyn, J., Lebski, I., Lysenko, L., et al. Anal warts (condylomata acuminata) – current issues and treatment modalities. *Adv. Clin. Exp. Med.* 2014; 23(2): 307–11.

Mehta, S. D., Rothman, R. E., Kelen, G. D., et al. Clinical aspects of diagnosis of gonorrhea and chlamydia infection in an acute care setting. *Clin. Infect. Dis.* 2001; 32: 655–9.

Rousseau, M. C., Pereira, J. S., Prade, J. C., et al. Cervical coinfection with human papillomavirus (HPV) types as a predictor of acquisition and persistence of HPV infection. *J. Infect. Dis.* 2001; 184: 1508–17.

Satterwhite, C. L., Torrone, E., Meites, E., et al. Sexually transmitted infections among U.S. women and men: prevalence and incidence estimates, 2008. *Sex. Transm. Dis.* 2013; 40(3): 187–93.

Westrom, L. *Consequences of Pelvic Inflammatory Disease* (New York: Raven Press, 1992), pp. 100–10.

Chapter 31

Ulcerative Sexually Transmitted Diseases

Jaime Jordan and Joseph Engelman

Introduction

Sexually transmitted diseases (STDs) can be divided into those that cause genital ulcers and those that do not. In North America, ulcerative STDs are most commonly caused by herpes genitalis and syphilis; much rarer causes include lymphogranuloma venereum, chancroid, and granuloma inguinale. Definitive diagnostic tests are not usually available in the acute care setting, and empiric treatment with close follow-up is often the best approach.

Herpes Genitalis

Epidemiology and Microbiology

Genital herpes infection is caused by *herpes simplex* virus (HSV) types 1 and 2. This is by far the most common cause of genital ulcer disease in North America. It is estimated that more than 50 million persons in the United States have the infection, with an annual incidence of more than 775,000. Most US cases are caused by HSV-2, though there is an increasing proportion of anogenital herpes due to HSV-1.

Clinical Features

Herpes genitalis can present with a broad range of symptoms. Serologic testing suggests that many individuals are infected, but are asymptomatic or have minimal symptoms. Symptomatic patients with first-time genital infection and no

prior HSV antibodies, known as primary infection, tend to present with the most severe disease. These very painful lesions may last 2 to 3 weeks unless antiviral therapy is instituted promptly. Acyclovir and valacyclovir are quite safe, relatively inexpensive, and effective if started early, so there are almost no contraindications to immediate start if primary infection is suspected.

Primary infection usually presents in young adults who have avoided infection with either type of herpes virus. Primary herpes is a short incubation process, so patients will typically give a history of recent sexual contact with a new partner. The lesions begin as vesicles that will then ulcerate (see Figure 31.1). Primary lesions are bilateral in distribution, usually quite painful, and will be accompanied by tender bilateral inguinal adenopathy (see Figure 31.2). The patients frequently have sore throat and fever, and may present with aseptic meningitis and urinary retention. Women with genital primary herpes infection and men who have sexual intercourse with men (MSM) with perianal primary infection usually have more symptomatic disease than do heterosexual men with primary genital infection. The diagnosis of primary HSV infection is made clinically at presentation and is typically obvious. There is no adequate point-of-care or send-out testing that will aid in making an immediate diagnosis. Nevertheless, all patients with primary HSV require a polymerase chain reaction (PCR) swab (the preferred test) or culture at first visit to determine viral type. Knowledge of the

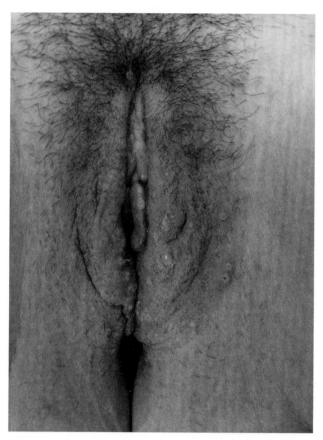

Figure 31.1 New onset herpes in young woman type unknown at first presentation, but bilateral-distribution indicates primary infection.
Image courtesy of Dr. Joseph Engelman, San Francisco City Clinic.

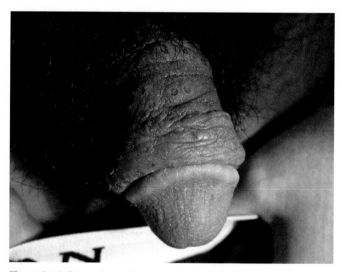

Figure 31.2 Primary herpes lesions on the penis.
Image courtesy of Dr. Joseph Engelman, San Francisco City Clinic.

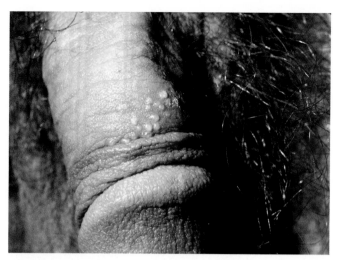

Figure 31.3 Recurrent genital herpes lesions on the penile shaft.
Image courtesy of Dr. Joseph Engelman, San Francisco City Clinic.

is not indicated. If the primary herpes is caused by HSV-2, the patient will be subject to future outbreaks and a high likelihood of asymptomatic viral shedding that would put uninfected sex partners at risk. Suppressive therapy would certainly be an option going forward if the initial PCR/culture results revealed HSV-2 infection. Suppressive therapy would decrease the number of future outbreaks and decrease the risk of asymptomatic anogenital viral shedding.

Patients with primary HSV infection are often in considerable discomfort both physically and emotionally. Many will be angry and depressed and will not comprehend the complexities of their new infection. Therefore, clinicians should discuss immediate treatment options and encourage patients to follow up in 10 to 14 days for test results and a more complete review of their situation. At the follow-up visit, patients will be more comfortable physically and calmer emotionally and will be better equipped to understand their long-term outlook and understand the logic behind the treatment choices.

Patients who already have antibodies to HSV-1 (e.g. those with a history of fever blisters) often have milder symptoms with initial HSV-2 genital infection. While a patient might have localized discomfort, there would not be the same severity of symptoms as seen in primary infection and the vesicles/ulcers would be shorter lived (see Figure 31.3). In this case, PCR/culture would be positive for HSV-2, but antibodies to HSV-2 would not be present, while antibodies to HSV-1 would be present. Patients presenting with recurrent genital HSV-2 tend to have the mildest symptoms of all, with typically mild/moderate localized discomfort or itching. Patients with recurrent HSV-2 outbreaks might not even note the presence of initial vesicles and just present with shallow ulcers or other atypical presentations that might be mistaken for erosions or abrasions. Since recurrences are usually short lived, by the time a patient presents, PCR and/or culture may be negative, but HSV-2 antibody results would be positive and would help confirm the diagnosis. Herpes 1 or 2 can present as herpetic whitlow (see Figure 31.4).

type of HSV responsible for the primary outbreak will allow patients and providers to make more informed decisions about long-term management of genital herpes. If a patient's primary infection is the result of HSV-1, which has a low likelihood of recurrences and a low likelihood of asymptomatic anogenital viral shedding, daily suppressive antiviral therapy

Table 31.1 Clinical Features: Herpes Genitalis

Organisms	*Herpes simplex* virus types 1 and 2
Incubation period	Variable; may be weeks to years
Transmission	Direct sexual contact, including oral genital contact. The infecting partner might be asymptomatic and not known to have HSV infection.
Signs and symptoms	• Systemic symptoms, including fever, myalgias, and sore throat, can occur with primary infection • Vesicles may be noted prior to ulcers • Multiple painful genital ulcers are noted; lesions may coalesce • Bilateral adenopathy may develop, especially in primary infection
Laboratory findings	• Serology may be positive for HSV-1 or HSV-2 • PCR/viral cultures may be positive

PCR – polymerase chain reaction.

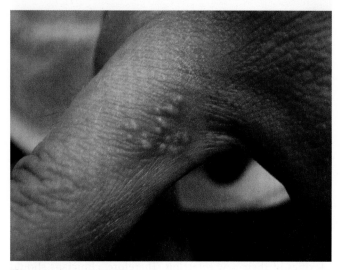

Figure 31.4 Herpetic whitlow.
Image courtesy of Dr. Joseph Engelman, San Francisco City Clinic.

Differential Diagnosis

All of the STDs that cause genital ulcers should be considered in patients presenting with these complaints:

- Syphilis
- chancroid (rare in the United States)
- granuloma inguinale (very rare in the United States)
- lymphogranuloma venereum
- scabies

Non-infectious conditions that can mimic genital herpes include Behçet's syndrome, trauma, contact dermatitis, erythema multiforme, reactive arthritis with genital involvement, psoriasis, fixed drug eruptions, Crohn's disease, and lichen planus.

Key features that may help distinguish herpes from other STDs are:

- systemic symptoms suggest primary genital herpes infection
- multiple painful genital ulcers with a clean base suggest herpes, but may also be seen in patients with chancroid
- recurrences are common and suggest herpes infection, but may also be seen in some other entities (e.g. Behçet's syndrome)

Laboratory and Radiographic Findings

PCR is the preferred laboratory test as it is more sensitive than culture and has become more available. The sensitivity of culture is low, particularly in recurrences or when lesions have begun to heal, so a negative culture does not rule out the disease.

Type-specific serologic testing is available that can aid in the diagnosis of the infection and determine the type of HSV involved. Point-of-care serologic testing is available. False-negative results may occur in the early stages of infection. The presence of serum HSV-2 antibodies is considered diagnostic of anogenital infection.

Serologic testing is recommended in the following patients: (1) those with recurrent or atypical symptoms with negative HSV PCR or cultures; (2) those with a clinical diagnosis of herpes without laboratory confirmation; or (3) those with a partner with genital herpes. The CDC also recommends HSV serologic testing for persons infected with HIV and those at high risk for contracting HIV.

Treatment and Prophylaxis

Primary and recurrent herpes infection can be treated with antiviral agents including acyclovir, famciclovir, and valacyclovir (see Table 31.2). Severe cases (meningitis, severe local disease, urinary retention) require hospitalization and should be treated with intravenous acyclovir.

Complications and Admission Criteria

Viral meningitis occurs in as many as 33% of women and 10% of men with primary genital HSV infection. These patients usually present as their genital lesions are beginning to resolve. Symptoms are typical for viral meningitis, including headache, photophobia, neck pain and stiffness, and fever. Lumbar puncture reveals a leukocytosis with lymphocytic predominance. These patients should generally be admitted for intravenous antiviral treatment. Benign recurrent lymphocytic meningitis, termed Mollaret's meningitis, can follow recurrence of genital HSV by 5 to 7 days.

Primary genital herpes may also be complicated by sacral radiculopathy syndrome, characterized by urinary retention and constipation. These symptoms usually resolve

Table 31.2 Treatment of HSV Infections

Patient Category	Therapy Recommendations
Adults: mucocutaneous	**Genital HSV and proctitis – first clinical episode:** (Duration of therapy 7–10 days, *treatment can be extended if therapy is incomplete after 10 days*) Acyclovir 400 mg PO TID *or* Acyclovir 200 mg PO five times per day *or* Famciclovir 250 mg PO TID *or* Valacyclovir 1 g PO BID **Genital HSV and proctitis – episodic disease:** (Best started at onset of prodrome or first awareness of lesions; all for 5 days unless otherwise noted) Acyclovir 400 mg PO TID *or* Acyclovir 800 mg PO TID for 2 days *or* Acyclovir 800 mg PO BID *or* Famciclovir 125 mg PO BID *or* Famciclovir 1,000 mg PO BID for 1 day *or* Famciclovir 500 mg PO once, then 250 mg BID × 2 days *or* Valacyclovir 500 mg PO BID × 3 days *or* Valacyclovir 1000 mg PO daily **Genital HSV or proctitis – suppressive daily therapy for recurrent disease:** Acyclovir 400 mg PO BID *or* Famciclovir 250 mg PO BID *or* Valacyclovir 500 mg PO daily* *or* Valacyclovir 1,000 mg PO daily **Severe genital HSV or proctitis:** Acyclovir 5–10 mg/kg IV every 8 hours × 5–7 days or until clinical resolution followed by oral therapy to complete a minimum of 10 days; suppressive therapy thereafter, if indicated **Genital HSV in pregnancy:** Acyclovir per above regimen with initial HSV or highly symptomatic recurrent HSV; give IV with life-threatening infection
Immunosuppressed	**Episodic prescription for recurrent infection in HIV-infected patients best started at onset of prodrome or first appearance of lesions.** (All drugs for 5–10 days) Acyclovir 400 mg PO TID *or* Famciclovir 500 mg PO BID *or* Valacyclovir 1,000 mg PO BID **Daily suppressive prescription in HIV-infected patients:** Acyclovir 400–800 mg PO BID to TID *or* Valacyclovir 500 mg PO BID *or* Famciclovir 500 mg PO BID
Antiviral resistant atrains	Foscarnet 40 mg/kg/dose IV every 8 hours until clinical resolution[†]

* Valacyclovir 500 mg once a day might be less effective than other valacyclovir or acyclovir dosing regimens in patients who have very frequent recurrences.

[†] Treatment of resistant strains should be managed in consultation with HIV specialist.

IV – intravenous; PO – by mouth.

spontaneously, though the patients may temporarily need urinary catheterization to aid in voiding and should be admitted for initial management. *Herpes simplex* proctitis and perianal ulcers can occur in men who have sex with men.

Congenital herpes infection is a very serious infection of newborn infants born to women with active herpes infection. The risk of transmission is greatest in women who develop primary infections with HSV-1 or HSV-2 near delivery. Women with genital herpes who become pregnant must tell their obstetrician about their history so they can be followed closely for signs of the infection as they near term. Acyclovir is a category B drug and can be given to pregnant women with primary genital herpes or severe recurrent disease. Women with active recurrent genital herpes should be be offered suppressive therapy at or beyond 36 weeks' gestation.

Infection Control

Patients with active lesions are infectious and should refrain from sexual activity until the lesions resolve. Patients who have no evidence of active lesions, but who have a history of the disease or are serologically positive for HSV, may pass the infection on to sexual partners, even when asymptomatic. In the health-care setting, universal precautions should be observed at all times.

Syphilis
Epidemiology

Compared to herpes genitalis, syphilis is a much less common cause of genital ulcers. Annual reported cases of primary and secondary syphilis in the United States have increased from approximately 7,000 in 2005 to greater than 17,000 in 2013. The estimated annual incidence of the infection in the United States is more than 55,000. Syphilis is more common in patients with lower socioeconomic status, those who abuse drugs, and men who have sex with men, who have accounted for much of the recent increase in incidence.

Clinical Features and Microbiology

Caused by the spirochete *Treponema pallidum*, syphilis progresses through several stages if untreated (see Table 31.3). The primary stage occurs approximately 3 to 4 weeks after inoculation with the spirochete. A chancre, usually painless, develops at the site of inoculation (see Figure 31.5); 25% of patients will develop multiple lesions (greater likelihood in HIV-positive individuals; see Figure 31.6). Oral chancres are rare, but can present on the lips or anywhere inside the oral cavity (see Figures 31.7 and 31.8). After 3 to 6 weeks, the lesion(s) resolves, and the patient becomes asymptomatic. The chancre will be accompanied by a firm, 'rubbery', non-tender localized lymph node. For anogenital chancres, the node would be inguinal or femoral and could be contralateral. For oral lesions, the node will be in the anterior cervical chain and in the rare event of a digital chancre, the ipsilateral epitrochlear node would be involved.

Four to 10 weeks later, the patient may develop symptoms of secondary syphilis. This stage is characterized by a rash, lymphadenopathy, and mucocutaneous lesions such as mucous patches or condyloma lata (see Figure 31.9). The rash begins as a macular rash and rapidly becomes papulosquamous, occurring primarily on the torso (see Figure 31.10); it may also involve the extremities and may involve the palms (see Figure 31.11) and soles. Any scrotal rash could be concerning for syphilis. Secondary syphilis may also present with inguinal lymphadenopathy, epitrochlear adenopathy, and more generalized adenopathy. Patients may develop "moth eaten" alopecia of scalp and eyebrows later in the course of their secondary disease (see Figure 31.12).

Lesions of the mucous membranes (oral cavity, prepuce, labia) are known as mucous patches and the raised, warty-looking lesions on the genitalia and perianal area are known as condyloma lata (see Figures 31.13 and 31.14). All moist lesions are infectious. Even untreated, this stage will resolve to latent disease; latent disease of less than a year's duration is known as early latent and greater than a year is known as late latent.

Table 31.3 Clinical Features: Syphilis

Organism	*Treponema pallidum*
Incubation period	• Primary: 3–4 weeks • Secondary: 7–14 weeks after inoculation • Tertiary: months to years
Transmission	Syphilis may be spread by contact with the primary chancre, mucous patches in the mouth or genitalia, or anogenital condyloma lata
Signs and symptoms	• Primary: usually painless chancre at site of inoculation • Secondary: rash, usually truncal, may involve palms and soles; generalized lymphadenopathy; condyloma lata, mucous patches; may see alopecia in long-standing secondary; auditory and ophthalmic symptoms and signs may occur at any stage, but are more likely to present with secondary and early latent syphilis; eye and ear symptoms should always be sought. • Tertiary: dementia, tabes dorsalis, gummata
Laboratory findings	• Non-treponemal tests (RPR, VDRL): positive suggests disease; may see false positives; should confirm with treponemal test; reactivity of test reflects disease activity • Treponemal tests (TPPA, EIA): specific to spirochete; confirmatory test; usually positive for life; after first infection, reactivity does not correlate with disease activity

RPR – rapid plasma reagin; TPPA – Treponema pallidum particle agglutination; VDRL – venereal disease research laboratory.

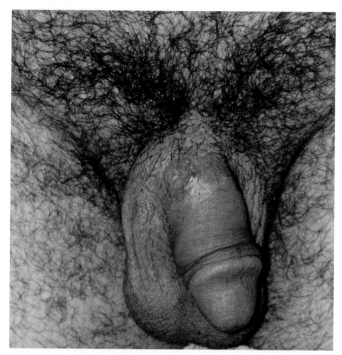

Figure 31.5 Primary syphilis penile chancre.
Image courtesy of Dr. Joseph Engelman, San Francisco City Clinic.

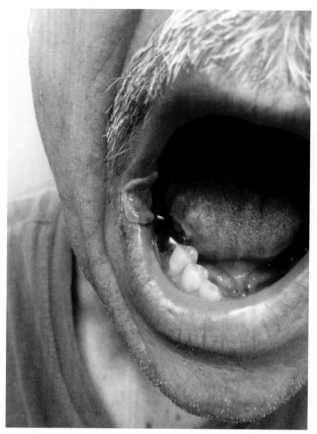

Figure 31.7 Primary syphilis oral chancre.
Image courtesy of Dr. Joseph Engelman, San Francisco City Clinic.

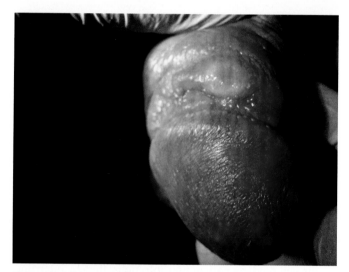

Figure 31.6 Primary syphilis multiple chancres.
Image courtesy of Dr. Joseph Engelman, San Francisco City Clinic.

Latent disease is diagnosed in patients with no physical evidence of early syphilis and a positive syphilis serology. Early latent is grouped with the infectious stages of syphilis, primary and secondary, because 25% of early latent cases will have secondary reactivation and thus become infectious again.

Tertiary syphilis may develop decades after primary infection in up to 25% of untreated patients. In this stage, complications such as aortic root aneurysms, skin gummata, and central nervous system disease can cause severe morbidity. Fortunately, the lesions of late syphilis have become extremely uncommon in the penicillin era – the exception being poorly controlled HIV-infected patients who are at increased risk for

neurosyphilis and whose advancement through stages may be more rapid.

Differential Diagnosis

All of the sexually transmitted diseases that cause genital ulcers should be considered in patients presenting with these complaints:

- herpes genitalis
- chancroid (rare in the United States)
- granuloma inguinale (very rare in the United States)
- lymphogranuloma venereum

Conditions such as Behçet's syndrome, fixed drug eruptions, scabies, pyoderma gangrenosum, and trauma are also in the differential diagnosis.

Key features that may help to distinguish syphilis from other STDs are as follows:

- Patients typically have a single painless genital ulcer. Men who have sexual intercourse with men could have perianal or oral chancres. Any perianal ulcer that is not in the midline (typically anal fissures) should prompt a consideration of primary syphilis. The primary chancre is almost always indurated (it has the same consistency as pinching the tip of one's nose with thumb and forefinger). There will almost always be a localized lymph node that will be firm and nontender. In very early primary syphilis, the lymph node may not yet be present.

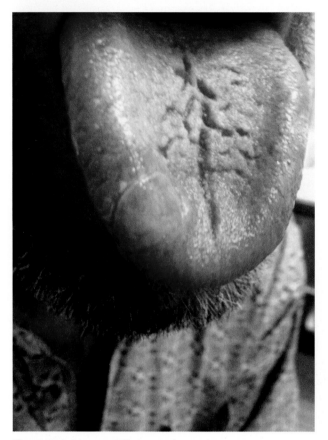

Figure 31.8 Primary syphilis tongue chancre.
Image courtesy of Dr. Joseph Engelman, San Francisco City Clinic.

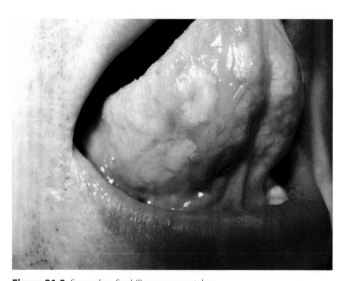

Figure 31.9 Secondary Syphilis mucous patches.
Image courtesy of Dr. Joseph Engelman, San Francisco City Clinic.

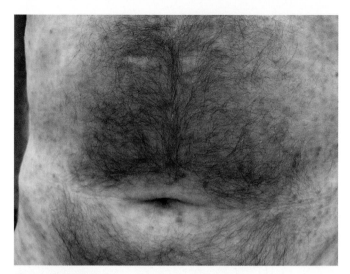

Figure 31.10 Maculopapular rash of secondary syphilis.
Image courtesy of Dr. Joseph Engelman, San Francisco City Clinic.

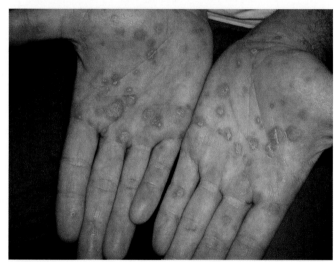

Figure 31.11 Palmar rash due to secondary syphilis.
Image courtesy of Dr. Joseph Engelman, San Francisco City Clinic.

- Do not hesitate to treat immediately if primary syphilis is likely. These patients are often hard to find after they leave the urgent care or ED setting and are highly infectious, thereby putting their sex partners at risk. Many persons with syphilis are coinfected with HIV, thereby increasing the likelihood of HIV transmission as well. Prompt presumptive treatment of this most infectious stage of syphilis will render a patient non-infectious, thereby interrupting the chain of transmission. Since true penicillin allergy is uncommon, there is little downside to rapid treatment of presumptive primary syphilis.
- A truncal papulosquamous rash involving palms and soles. It will be bilaterally symmetrical and will include the palms and soles about 70% of the time. Be sure to examine the skin of the scrotum for annular rash. Any bilaterally symmetrical rash could be secondary syphilis.
- Condyloma lata and/or mucous patches (oral cavity, genitalia, perianal area).
- The rash of secondary syphilis is easily mistaken for pityriasis rosea (PR). Sexually active patients with a rash that looks like pityriasis rosea should be tested for syphilis. There will be a herald patch with PR. A herald patch will be absent in secondary syphilis.

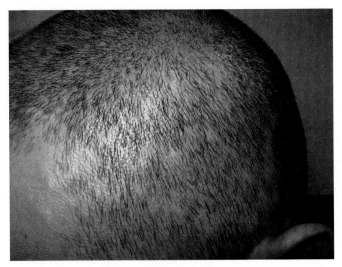

Figure 31.12 Alopecia due to secondary syphilis.
Image courtesy of Dr. Joseph Engelman, San Francisco City Clinic.

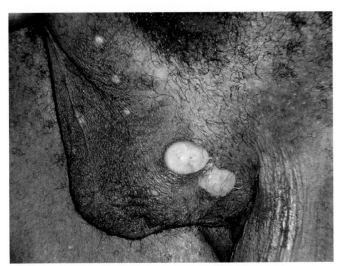

Figure 31.13 Condyloma lata of secondary syphilis on the scrotum.
Image courtesy of Dr. Joseph Engelman, San Francisco City Clinic.

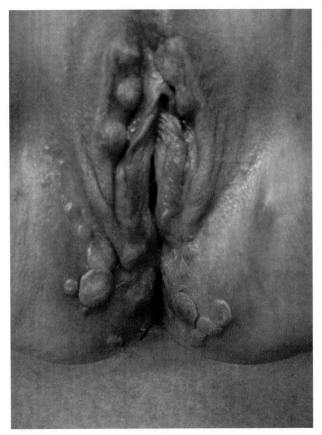

Figure 31.14 Condyloma lata of secondary syphilis on a female genitalia.
Image courtesy of Dr. Joseph Engelman, San Francisco City Clinic.

Laboratory and Radiographic Findings

Darkfield microscopy and direct testing of lesion exudates or tissue for *T. pallidum* are definitive methods for diagnosing moist lesions of early syphilis, though use of these techniques is mostly limited to specialized STD clinics. Thus, in a patient with a genital ulcer suspected to be due to primary syphilis, in most clinical settings the diagnosis is made strictly on clinical grounds and a low threshold is recommended for empiric treatment with penicillin. In early primary syphilis (less than 1 week), the non-treponemal tests, RPR and VDRL, may be negative, but the TPPA becomes positive before the non-treponemal tests, so order the confirmatory test in all cases of primary syphilis.

Serologic testing comprises the main diagnostic methods for secondary, latent, and tertiary syphilis. Both non-treponemal and treponemal tests are available. Non-treponemal tests such as the rapid plasma reagin (RPR) and venereal disease research laboratory (VDRL) assay determine presence and activity of disease, but false positives may occur, and these tests may be falsely negative in early primary syphilis and long-standing latent disease. Because these tests are quantitative and correlate with disease activity, they can be used to monitor response to therapy. Positive non-treponemal tests should be confirmed with a treponemal test, such as the fluorescent treponemal antibody absorbed (FTA), the treponemal pallidum particle agglutination (TP-PA), or the microhemagglutination assay – *Treponema pallidum* (MHA-TP), which is no longer commonly used. These treponemal tests are specific for *T. pallidum*, and the test is usually positive for life. Treponemal test results do not correlate well with disease activity and cannot be used to monitor response to treatment.

In patients with suspected neurosyphilis, cerebrospinal fluid VDRL is typically performed, which is highly specific, but not sensitive. Indications for a lumbar puncture to rule out neurosyphilis include neurologic or ophthalmologic signs or symptoms, other evidence of active tertiary syphilis, or treatment failure.

Treatment and Prophylaxis

Primary syphilis is treated with one dose of benzathine penicillin G (BPG) 2.4 million units intramuscularly as a one-time

Table 31.4 Treatment of Syphilis

Patient Category	Therapy Recommendations
Primary and secondary syphilis	Benzathine penicillin G 2.4 million units IM × 1 PCN allergy (non-pregnant): doxycycline 100 mg PO BID for 14 days Requires well-documented close follow-up
Latent syphilis	**Early latent (<1 year infection duration) (with normal CSF exam, if done):** Benzathine penicillin G 2.4 million units IM × 1 PCN allergy (non-pregnant): Doxycycline 100 mg PO BID × 14 days Requires well-documented close follow-up **Late latent or latent of unknown duration (with normal CSF exam, if done):** Benzathine penicillin G 2.4 million units once weekly for 3 weeks If any dose >2 days late, must recommence prescription from first dose **PCN allergy (non-pregnant):** Doxycycline 100 mg PO BID × 4 weeks
Neurosyphilis	Only penicillin is currently recommended; allergic persons should be desensitized and treated with penicillin. **Recommended:** Aqueous crystalline penicillin G 18–24 million units/day IV, administer as 3–4 million units IV every 4 hours or as continuous infusion × 10–14 days **Alternative:** Procaine penicillin 2.4 million units IM daily *plus* Probenecid 500 mg PO QID for 10–14 days
Syphilis in HIV-infected	Penicillin is the highly preferred regimen for all stages of syphilis in HIV-infected persons Primary, secondary, and latent syphilis: use benzathine penicillin G as for non-HIV persons; PCN-allergic HIV with primary or secondary syphilis: can be treated as allergic HIV-negative person (though *not* the ideal) Alternative non-penicillin treatment for latent syphilis in HIV-infected patients has not been well studied; expert consultation would be advisable Neurosyphilis should be managed as for HIV-negative individuals. Penicillin is the drug of choice, but in penicillin-allergic persons small studies indicate that ceftriaxone 2 g either IM or IV for 10–14 days provides adequate therapy with little risk of cross reactivity
Syphilis in pregnancy	Only penicillin is currently recommended; treatment during pregnancy should be the penicillin regimen appropriate to the stage of syphilis diagnosed; desensitization required for PCN-allergic pregnant patients Some experts recommend a second dose of benzathine penicillin G 2.4 million units IM 1 week after the initial dose for primary, secondary, or early latent syphilis in pregnancy

CSF – cerebrospinal fluid; IM – intramuscular; PCN – penicillin; PO – by mouth.

dose. It is critical to use only benzathine penicillin G, not another formulation or a combination of types of penicillin. Secondary and early latent syphilis are also treated with one dose of benzathine penicillin G 2.4 million units intramuscularly. Patients with late latent syphilis, latent syphilis of unknown duration, or tertiary syphilis *without* neurosyphilis should receive benzathine penicillin G 2.4 million units intramuscularly once a week for 3 weeks. Treat high-risk persons before lab results are available because the patient may not return for results. Neurosyphilis is treated with intravenous aqueous crystalline penicillin G 18–24 million units daily, given as 3 to 4 million units intravenous (IV) every 4 hours or as a continuous infusion for 10 to 14 days. Treatment failure can occur with any regimen and patients should be re-examined both clinically and serologically at 6 months.

Complications and Admission Criteria

Patients with primary and secondary syphilis are managed as outpatients. Neurosyphilis is usually managed in the inpatient setting. Patients infected with HIV may have a more aggressive syphilis infection, and their response to treatment must be monitored closely.

Infection Control

Syphilis may be spread by contact with the primary chancre, mucous patches in the mouth, the skin lesions of secondary syphilis, or genital condyloma lata. Sexual partners of patients diagnosed with syphilis should be evaluated, tested, and treated accordingly. Sexual partners of patients diagnosed with primary, secondary, or early latent syphilis within the last 90 days should be treated presumptively. Partners should also be treated presumptively if serologic data is not available or follow-up is uncertain. Universal precautions should be observed in the health-care setting.

Chancroid
Epidemiology and Microbiology

This ulcerating sexually transmitted disease is caused by *Haemophilus ducreyi*. More common in developing countries,

Table 31.5 Clinical Features: Chancroid

Organism	*Haemophilus ducreyi*
Incubation period	3–5 days; may be as long as 14 days
Transmission	Chancroid is spread by direct contact between infected tissue, typically an ulcer or bubo, and a break in the skin or mucosa as can occur with sex
Signs and symptoms	• Multiple painful genital ulcers • Painful, enlarged, fluctuant inguinal lymph node
Laboratory findings	• Diagnosis usually made clinically • Organism can be cultured, but requires special medium not usually available

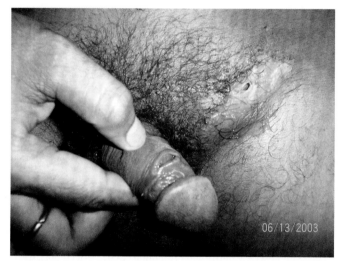

Figure 31.15 Chancroidal ulcer accompanied by ruptured bubo. Image courtesy of Dr. Joseph Engelman, San Francisco City Clinic.

chancroid is rare in the United States, but may occur in sporadic outbreaks. Less than 50 cases are reported to the CDC annually, though this likely underestimates the US incidence because of underreporting and testing challenges. Chancroid is more commonly diagnosed in men, especially if partners include commercial sex workers. Co-infection with syphilis occurs in up to 10% of cases.

Clinical Features

Patients complain of multiple painful genital ulcers within 1 to 2 weeks of primary infection (see Table 31.5); these ulcers may mimic herpes genitalis, but are deeper and more tender and painful. Within a week, up to 40% of patients will develop an inguinal bubo, usually unilateral and frequently painful and fluctuant. These buboes may spontaneously rupture and cause a chronic draining sinus. The combination of painful genital ulcers and fluctuant inguinal lymphadenopathy should raise suspicion for this disease (see Figure 31.15)

Patients with chancroid can transmit the infection until the ulcer heals. The ulcer heals with or without treatment, but treatment speeds healing. Chancroid infection, like other ulcerative STDs, increases risk of HIV transmission and acquisition.

Sites of infection include:

- genitalia: genital ulcer(s)
- inguinal lymph nodes: following small, missed genital ulcer or with genital ulcer
- conjunctivae: autoinoculation from genital source
- fingers: can follow autoinoculation or foreplay

Differential Diagnosis

All of the sexually transmitted diseases that cause genital ulcers should be considered in patients presenting with these complaints:

- syphilis
- *herpes simplex*
- granuloma inguinale
- lymphogranuloma venereum

Conditions such as Behçet's syndrome, fixed drug eruptions, scabies, pyoderma, and trauma are also in the differential diagnosis.

Key features that may help to distinguish chancroid from other STDs are:

- the presence of a painful or fluctuant inguinal lymph node
- multiple, painful genital ulcers; may look very similar to herpes genitalis

Laboratory and Radiographic Findings

The causative organism, *Haemophilus ducreyi*, is fastidious and requires special growth medium for culture. This medium is not commonly available in most microbiology labs, and the diagnosis is usually made clinically. Empiric therapy is simple and inexpensive, and should generally be given if the following diagnostic criteria are positive:

1. The patient has one or more painful genital lesions.
2. The patient has no evidence of *T. pallidum* infection by dark-field examination of ulcer exudates or by a serologic test for syphilis performed at least 7 days after the onset of ulcers.
3. The clinical presentation, appearance of genital ulcers, and, if present, regional adenopathy are typical for chancroid.
4. A test for HSV on the ulcer exudate is negative.

Treatment and Prophylaxis

Recommended treatment for chancroid consists of one of the following: azithromycin, ceftriaxone, ciprofloxacin, or erythromycin base (see Table 31.6).

Buboes should not be incised and drained initally, even if they are very fluctuant. If the bubo appears at risk for spontaneous rupture, needle aspiration of the fluid may help relieve pressure. Buboes that do not respond to antibiotic therapy may require incision and drainage.

Complications and Admission Criteria

The most serious complication of chancroid is scarring of groin lymphatics from lymphadenitis. Patients who present

Table 31.6 Treatment of Chancroid Infections

Patient Category	Therapy Recommendations
Recommended regimen	Azithromycin 1 g PO × 1 *or* Ceftriaxone 250 mg IM × 1 *or* Ciprofloxacin 500 mg PO BID for 3 days *or* Erythromycin base 500 mg PO QID for 7 days
Regimens in pregnancy	Ceftriaxone 250 mg IM × 1 *or* Erythromycin base 500 mg PO QID for 7 days
Treatment in HIV infection	• This group has higher rates of delayed resolution or treatment failure; repeated dosing or longer duration of treatment may be required • Efficacy of azithromycin and ceftriaxone unknown in this group; use only if follow-up is ensured
Management of fluctuant buboes	• Bubo aspiration is simpler and safer than incision and drainage, but reaspiration is often needed; sinus tracts may form • Incision and drainage may be preferred treatment in those not adequately responding to antibiotics alone
Other management considerations	• Follow-up: examine all patients 3–7 days after initiation of treatment. If no clinical improvement: (1) Reassess diagnosis; (2) consider co-infection with another STD or HIV; (3) consider non-compliance; (4) consider antibiotic resistance. • Sex partners: all recent sex partners (within 10 days) should be examined and treated regardless of symptoms. • Candidates for longer treatment and close follow-up: HIV-infected persons; uncircumcised men.

IM – intramuscular; PO – by mouth.

with advanced disease may develop this complication despite appropriate therapy.

Infection Control

This infection is acquired by direct contact with the genital ulcers. All recent sexual partners should be examined and treated regardless of symptoms. Universal precautions should be observed.

Pearls and Pitfalls

1. Viral meningitis is a common complication of primary genital HSV infection.
2. Severe recurrent genital and perirectal HSV-related symptoms are common in HIV-infected patients, especially those with AIDS, and such patients need longer treatment and/or higher doses for episodic mucocutaneous HSV.
3. HSV is the most common identifiable precipitant of erythema multiforme.
4. Consider syphilis in *any* sexually active person with a generalized rash or genital ulcer.
5. Treatment of sex partners is critical to control the spread of syphilis.
6. The genital ulcers of chancroid are similar to, and can easily be mistaken for, those of HSV. Chancroid should be considered in patients with painful genital ulcers and regional adenopathy. Maintain a low threshold for empiric treatment, since definitive diagnostic tests are problematic.
7. Up to 10% of patients with chancroid are co-infected with syphilis; therefore, patients with suspected chancroid *must* also be treated for syphilis.

References

ACOG Practice Bulletin. Clinical management guidelines for obstetrician-gynecologists. No. 82, June 2007. Management of herpes in pregnancy. *Obstet. Gynecol.* 2007; 109(6): 1489–98.

Centers for Disease Control and Prevention (CDC). Brief report: treatment failures in syphilis infections – San Francisco, California, 2002–2003. *MMWR Morb. Mortal. Wkly. Rep.* 2004; 53(9): 197–8.

CDC. *Sexually Transmitted Disease Surveillance 2013* (Atlanta, GA: US Department of Health and Human Services, 2014).

CDC. Sexually transmitted diseases treatment guidelines, 2015. *MMWR Morb. Mortal. Wkly. Rep.* 2015; 64(RR3); 1–137.

Clyne, B. and Jerrard, D. Syphilis testing. *J. Emerg. Med.* 2000; 18(3): 361–7.

Gene, M. and Ledger, W. J. Syphilis in pregnancy. *Sex. Transm. Infect.* 2000; 76(2): 73–9.

Kimberlin, D. W. and Rouse, D. J. Genital herpes. *N. Engl. J. Med.* 2004; 350(19): 1970–7.

Lukehart, S. A., Godornes, C., Molini, B. J., *et al.* Macrolide resistance in Treponema pallidum in the United States and Ireland. *N. Engl. J. Med.* 2004; 351(2): 154–8.

Satterwhite, C. L., Torrone, E., Meites, E., *et al.* Sexually transmitted infections among U.S. women and men: prevalence and incidence estimates, 2008. *Sex. Transm. Dis.* 2013; 40(3): 187–93.

Singh, A. E. and Romanowki, B. Syphilis: review with emphasis on clinical, epidemiological, and some biologic features. *Clin. Microbiol. Rev.* 1999; 12(2): 187–209.

Steiner, I. and Biran, I. Herpes simplex encephalitis. *Curr. Treat. Options Infect. Dis.* 2002; 4: 491–9.

Stephenson-Famy, A. and Gardella, C. Herpes simplex virus infection during pregnancy. *Obstet. Gynecol. Clin. North Am.* 2014; 41(4): 601–14.

Whittington, W. L., Celum, C. L., Cent, A., *et al.* Use of a glycoprotein G-based type-specific assay to detect antibodies to herpes simplex virus type among persons attending sexually transmitted disease clinics. *Sex. Transm. Dis.* 2001; 28(2): 99–104.

Xu, F., Sternberg, M. R., Kottiri, B. J., *et al.* Trends in herpes simplex virus type 1 and type 2 seroprevalence in the United States. *JAMA* 2006; 296(8): 964–73.

Additional Readings

Ernst, A. A., Marvez-Valls, E., and Martin, D. H. Incision and drainage versus aspiration of fluctuant buboes in the emergency department during an epidemic of chancroid. *Sex. Transm. Dis.* 1995; 22(4): 217–20.

Lewis, D. A. Diagnostic tests for chancroid. *Sex. Transm. Infect.* 2000; 76(2): 137–41.

Mutua, F. M., M'imunya, J. M., and Wiysonge, C. S. Genital ulcer disease treatment for reducing sexual acquisition of HIV. *Cochrane Database Syst. Rev.* 2012; (8): 1–36.

Chapter

32

Vulvovaginitis

Jaime Jordan

Introduction

Vulvovaginitis is a common gynocologic problem experienced by most women during their lifetime. It is estimated that symptoms of vulvovaginitis prompt more than 10 million physician visits annually in the United States. Most cases are caused by infectious agents, including anaerobic bacteria such as *Gardnerella vaginalis*, *Trichomonas vaginalis*, and *Candida* species.

Diagnosis of a specific causative organism in patients with vulvovaginitis can be difficult. Although signs, symptoms, and laboratory testing may suggest an organism, significant overlap exists in the specificity and sensitivity of these diagnostic tools.

Bacterial Vaginosis

Epidemiology and Microbiology

Bacterial vaginosis is a common cause of vaginal discharge among women of child-bearing age. The estimated prevalence in the United States among women ages 14 to 49 is more than 21 million. Bacterial vaginosis is caused by proliferation of anaerobic bacteria such as *Gardnerella vaginalis*, *Prevotella species*, *Bacteroides species*, *Mobiluncus species*, *Mycoplasma hominus*, *and Ureaplasma urealyticum*, which replace the usual *Lactobacillus* species found in vaginal flora. Although infection is associated with multiple sexual partners and has a risk profile similar to other sexually transmitted diseases (STDs), women who are not sexually active may acquire this infection; as such, it is not considered an STD. Up to 84% of women with bacterial vaginosis may be symptomless, and men may harbor the organism asymptomatically in the urethra, posing a potential infectious source.

Clinical Features

Symptomatic patients present complaining of a foul or fishy vaginal odor and may have a vaginal discharge. Pruritis, dysuria, and dyspareunia are not typical of bacterial vaginosis. On examination, the vaginal mucosa is not usually inflamed, but there is frequently a thin, homogeneous, gray-white vaginal discharge. The discharge may give off a fishy or foul-smelling odor that is enhanced by mixing with potassium hydroxide. See Table 32.1 for a summary of clinical features.

Laboratory Findings

A vaginal swab should be obtained for gram stain (considered the gold standard diagnostic test) and/or wet preparation. To increase diagnostic accuracy, vaginal fluid should be pH tested.

If a gram stain is not available, diagnosis can be made based on clinical criteria. The Centers for Disease Control and Prevention supports Amsel's diagnostic criteria for bacterial vaginosis, requiring three of the following:

- homogenous, thin, white, discharge that smoothly coats the vaginal walls
- presence of clue cells on microscopic examination
- vaginal fluid pH >4.5
- fishy odor of vaginal discharge before or after the addition of 10% KOH (a positive amine odor test or "whiff" test)

Table 32.1 Clinical Features: Bacterial Vaginosis

Pathogen	**Anaerobic bacteria, including:**
	Gardnerella vaginalis
	Prevotella species, *Bacteroides* species
	Mobiluncus species
	Mycoplasma hominus
	Ureaplasma urealyticum
Signs and symptoms	• Foul or fishy vaginal odor
	• Vaginal discharge; usually thin, gray-white in color
Laboratory findings	• Gram stain showing increase of characteristic bacteria relative to *Lactobacillus*
	• Wet mount positive for clue cells
	• Vaginal fluid pH >4.5
	• May see WBCs on wet mount

WBC – white blood cell.

Treatment

Bacterial vaginosis can be treated with oral or topical antibiotics such as metronidazole or clindamycin (see Table 32.2). Patients taking metronidazole should be instructed to refrain from consuming alcohol until at least 72 hours after taking the last dose of the medication. Probiotic use for treatment and prevention of vaginal infections including bacterial vaginosis has been suggested, but this is still an area of controversy.

All women who meet diagnostic criteria for bacterial vaginosis (BV) and are symptomatic should be treated. Treatment is not recommended for non-pregnant, asymptomatic women. Treatment of asymptomatic pregnant women with bacterial vaginosis is controverserial; consider an obstetrics consult.

Complications

Complications are rare in non-pregnant women. However, bacterial vaginosis during pregnancy is associated with increased risk of adverse pregnancy outcomes, particularly preterm labor.

Infection Control

Treatment of sexual partners does not affect the patient's response to treatment or risk of relapse; therefore, the treatment of sexual partners is not recommended; however, the CDC still recommends that patients abstain from intercourse or use condoms consistently during treatment.

Trichomoniasis

Epidemiology and Microbiology

Trichomoniasis is caused by the flagellated protozoan *Trichomonas vaginalis*. Trichomoniasis is the most common non-viral STD worldwide and is estimated to cause more than 1 million infections annually in the United States. It is commonly co-transmitted with other sexually transmitted pathogens. The infection is found in both men and women.

Table 32.2 Treatment of Bacterial Vaginosis

Patient Category	Therapy Recommendations
Adults: non-pregnant patient	**Recommended regimens:**
	Metronidazole 500 mg PO BID for 7 days
	or
	Metronidazole gel 0.75%, one applicator intravaginally BID for 5 days
	or
	Clindamycin cream 2%, one applicator intravaginally at bedtime for 7 days
	Alternative regimens:
	Tinidazole 2 g PO daily for 2 days
	or
	Tinidazole 1 g PO daily for 5 days
	or
	Clindamycin 300 mg PO BID for 7 days
	or
	Clindamycin ovules 100 g intravaginally once at bedtime for 3 days
Adults: pregnant patient	Metronidazole 500 mg PO BID for 7 days
	or
	Metronidazole 250 mg PO TID for 7 days
	or
	Clindamycin 300 mg PO BID for 7 days

Clinical Features

Most commonly, patients complain of a vaginal discharge which may be described as foul-smelling (see Table 32.3). Up to half of patients complain of dyspareunia. Other common complaints include vulvovaginal pruritis, pain, and dysuria. On exam, the vaginal wall may be diffusely erythematous and the vulva mildly edematous or excoriated. Vaginal discharge is noted in over half of cases and may appear yellow, gray, or yellow-green. The classically described "strawberry cervix" (caused by diffuse punctuate tiny hemorrhages) is seen in only 2% of patients. It is important to remember that women may also be asymptomatic. (Trichomonas infection in men can present as urethritis, though in the majority of cases men are asymptomatic.)

Laboratory Findings

A vaginal (not endocervical) swab should be obtained for wet mount. Because the sensitivity of the wet preparation is 60 to 70% and decreases rapidly with time after sampling, the wet mount should be examined as soon as possible after obtaining the specimen. Point-of-care tests using immunochromatography or nucleic acid probe testing are available, but not widely used. Vaginal culture is a highly sensitive and specific means of making the diagnosis and can be used in suspected cases not confirmed by other testing.

Diagnosis of trichomoniasis is suggested by the following findings:

- profuse, yellow, homogeneous discharge
- strawberry cervix (colpitis macularis)
- vaginal pH greater than 4.5
- motile trichomonads on saline wet mount

Table 32.3 Clinical Features: Trichomoniasis

Pathogen	*Trichomonas vaginalis*
Signs and symptoms	• Vaginal discharge • Vulvovaginal soreness or fullness • Vulvovaginal pruritis • Dyspareunia • Diffuse erythema of vaginal wall • Strawberry cervix
Laboratory findings	• Wet mount demonstrating flagellated protozoa • Vaginal fluid pH >4.5 • Many WBCs on wet mount

WBC – white blood cell.

Table 32.4 Treatment of Trichomoniasis

Patient Category	Therapy Recommendations
Adults: non-pregnant patient	**Recommended regimen:** Metronidazole 2 g PO as a single dose *or* Tinidazole 2 g PO in a single dose **Alternative regimen:** Metronidazole 500 mg PO BID for 7 days
Adults: pregnant patient	Discuss risks and benefits of treatment with patient and her obstetrician **If treatment used:** Metronidazole 2 g PO as a single dose *Note:* Tinidazole is pregnancy category C and its safety in pregnancy has not been well evaluated

Patients taking metronidazole should be instructed to refrain from consuming alcohol until at least 72 hours after taking the last dose of the medication.

Treatment

Recommended treatment by the Centers for Disease Control and Prevention is metronidazole or tinidazole (see Table 32.4).

Complications and Admission Criteria

Vaginal trichomoniasis during pregnancy has been associated with adverse pregnancy outcomes, including premature rupture of membranes, preterm delivery, and low birth weight. Unfortunately, treatment with metronidazole does not appear to decrease this risk, though it may relieve symptoms for the woman and may prevent respiratory or genital infection of the newborn during delivery. Treatment of a pregnant woman with trichomoniasis must include discussion of the risks and benefits of treatment and optimally should involve the patient's obstetrician.

Infection Control

Because trichomoniasis is sexually transmitted, sexual partners should be treated. Patients should avoid sex until they and their sexual partners complete a course of therapy and are asymptomatic.

Candidiasis

Epidemiology and Microbiology

Vulvovaginal candidiasis (VVC) is usually caused by *Candida albicans*, but other *Candida* species and *Torulopsis* species may cause the infection. Candidal species are recognized by the appearance of eliptical, budding yeast, and the ability to produce filamentous forms (hyphae and pseudohyphae).

VVC is a common vaginal infection, but accurate incidence and prevalence is not known. A recent survey in five European countries and the United States found that 29 to 49% of participating women had experienced a health-care provider diagnosed vaginal yeast infection in their lifetime. It predominantly affects menstruating women, being uncommon in prepubertal and post-menopausal women. Important risk factors include diabetes, recent antibiotic use, immunosuppression, and pregnancy. Normal vaginal flora suppress the growth of the organism; symptomatic infection occurs when an imbalance develops, either by suppression of vaginal flora (often caused by the use of antibiotics) or by overgrowth of the yeast (as seen in patients with diabetes). VVC is not sexually transmitted, though it may coexist with another sexually transmitted infection.

Clinical Features

The most common presenting complaint is vulvovaginal itching, which may be severe and can lead to excoriation (see Table 32.5). Vaginal pain or burning is common. Vaginal discharge may not be a prominent complaint, and a change in odor is not typical. Dysuria (caused by urine passing over irritated and raw genital tissue) is common, as is dyspareunia. On examination, the vulvae and vaginal walls are erythematous and may be edematous. Excoriations may be seen from scratching due to the intense pruritis. Vaginal discharge, when present, is typically white and may have a curd-like, cottage cheese appearance.

Patients with VVC are classified as either uncomplicated or complicated. Uncomplicated VVC is defined as (1) sporadic or infrequent, (2) mild-to-moderate, (3) likely to be due to *Candida albicans*, and (4) occurring in an immunocompetent host. Complicated VVC is defined as (1) recurrent, (2) severe, (3) caused by non-*albicans* species, or (4) occurring in patients who are pregnant, debilitated, or immunocompromised (including those with diabetes or renal disease).

Laboratory Findings

A vaginal swab should be obtained for wet preparation, and a gram stain may also be ordered. Wet mount examination with KOH, which tends to dissolve other cellular elements, may show yeast and pseudohyphae. Vaginal pH is typically normal (<4.5). Inflammatory cells are minimal in CVV, so large numbers of white cells suggests another cause or co-infection. Culture should be considered in patients with signs

Chapter 32: Vulvovaginitis

Table 32.5 Clinical Features: Candidiasis

Pathogens	*Candida albicans* Other *Candida* species *Torulopsis* species
Signs and symptoms	• Vulvovaginal pruritis, soreness, edema, erythema • Vulvovaginal excoriations • Dysuria • Dyspareunia • Discharge, usually white, sometimes curd-like
Laboratory findings	• Presence of hyphae or pseudohyphae on KOH prep. • Normal vaginal pH (<4.5) • Few WBCs on wet mount

WBC – white blood cell.

Table 32.6 Treatment of Vulvovaginal Candidiasis

Patient Category	Therapy Recommendations
Adults: uncomplicated	**Oral agent:** Fluconazole 150 mg PO once **Intravaginal agents*:** Clotrimazole 1% cream, one applicatorful intravaginally for 7 days *or* Miconazole 2% cream, one applicatorful intravaginally for 7 day
Adults: complicated	**Severe VVC:** Fluconazole 150 mg PO every 72 hours × 2–3 doses *or* Topical azole therapy for 7–14 days **Recurrent VVC:** Fluconazole 150 mg PO every 72 hours × 2–3 doses *followed by* Fluconazole 150 mg PO once weekly for 6 months *or if unable to take fluconazole* Topical azole therapy induction followed by maintenance therapy up to 6 months may also be used **VVC in pregnancy:** Only use topical intravaginal azole agents for 7 days

* Many different topical azole agents and preparations exist. Consult individual drug package insert for treatment dosing, duration, and contraindications.

or symptoms highly suggestive of candidiasis with a negative wet mount.

The following findings suggest the diagnosis of VVC:
- scant to moderate white, clumped vaginal discharge adherent to vaginal walls
- vaginal pH less than 4.5
- yeast and/or pseudohyphae on wet prep/gram stain
- negative whiff test
- vaginal and/or vulvar erythema/pruritic

Treatment

Up to 20% of women may be colonized with *Candida* species, so asymptomatic women found to have yeast on wet prep or Pap smear do not warrant treatment. Most patients with VVC will respond to a short or long course of oral or topical therapy (see Table 32.6) depending on whether they have uncomplicated or complicated disease. Many patients may prefer the convenience of a one-time oral dose of fluconazole, though clinical efficacy is similar between topical antifungals and oral fluconazole. In general, topical treatments have fewer systemic side effects and provide faster relief than oral fluconazole. Severe VVC, with extensive erythema, edema, and excoriation, should be treated with a longer course of antifungals. Pregnant patients should be treated only with intravaginal topical azole agents for 7 days.

Complications

Vaginal culture is indicated in complicated VVC, as conventional antimycotic therapies are not as effective against the non-*albicans Candida* species and other yeast. These patients often need a longer course of therapy, and referral to a primary care physician or gynecologist is recommended for close follow-up and additional therapy as needed.

Infection Control

Vulvovaginal candidiasis is not usually acquired through sexual contact, so treatment of sexual partners is not recommended. If the patient has recurrent infections, however, treatment of the sexual partners should be considered.

Differential Diagnosis of Vulvovaginitis

The main differential diagnosis includes the infectious causes of vulvovaginitis discussed in this chapter, summarized in Table 32.7. In sexually active women, the first priority is to diagnose, and in many cases empirically treat, cervicitis from chlamydia or gonorrhea. Non-infectious causes include contact vulvovaginitis (from douches, vaginal creams, scented tampons, sexual aids, latex), local inflammatory response to an intravaginal foreign body, atrophic vaginitis, and invasive carcinoma of the cervix.

Pearls and Pitfalls

1. Symptomatic pregnant women meeting diagnostic criteria for bacterial vaginosis should be treated.
2. Pregnant patients with trichomoniasis can be treated with a single dose of 2 g of metronidazole after a discussion of the risks and benefits of treatment; however, tinidazole is contraindicated.
3. Intravaginal creams and suppositories are oil-based and may weaken diaphragms and condoms that contain latex; other forms of birth control should be used during treatment with these agents.
4. Vulvovaginal candidiasis may be the first symptom of diabetes.

Table 32.7 Summary of Clinical Features of Vulvovaginitis

	Bacterial Vaginosis	Trichomoniasis	Vulvovaginal Candidiasis
History:			
Vaginal discharge	20%	50–75%	50%
Vaginal itching	10%	25–50%	50%
Foul odor	50%	10–25%	Rare
Dyspareunia	Rare	50%	Common
Lower abdominal pain	No	5–10%	No
Dysuria	10–20%	25%	Common
Exam:			
Vulvar erythema/edema	Not common	10–30%	Common
Vaginal erythema	Not common	20–75%	Common
Vaginal discharge present	70%	50–75%	Most; not all
Color of vaginal discharge	Gray; yellow	Yellow-green	White
Odor	45%	Rare	Rare
Diagnostic testing:			
pH >4.5	Yes	Yes	No
WBCs	++	+++	No
Clue cells	Yes	No	No
Trichomonads	No	Yes	No
Yeast forms	No	No	Yes
Sexually transmitted?	No	Yes	No
Treat sexual partners?	No	Yes	No

References

Borges, S., Silva, J., and Teixeira, P. The role of lactobacilli and probiotics in maintaining vaginal health. *Arch. Gynecol. Obstet.* 2014; 289(3): 479–89.

Center for Disease Control and Prevention (CDC). Sexually transmitted diseases treatment guidelines, 2015. *MMWR Morb. Mortal. Wkly. Rep.* 2015; 64(3): 1–140.

CDC. Bacterial vaginosis (BV) statistics, www.cdc.gov/std/bv/stats.htm (accessed September 1, 2016).

Fethers, K. A., Fairley, C. K., Hocking, J. S., *et al.* Sexual risk factors and bacterial vaginosis: a systematic review and meta-analysis. *Clin. Infect. Dis.* 2008; 47(11): 1426–35.

Foxman, B., Muraglia, R., Dietz, J. P., *et al.* Prevalence of recurrent vulvovaginal candidiasis in 5 European countries and the United States: results from an internet panel survey. *J. Low. Genit. Tract. Dis.* 2013; 17(3): 340–5.

Guise, J. M., Mohan, S. M., Aickin, M., *et al.* Screening for bacterial vaginosis in pregnancy. *Am. J. Prev. Med.* 2001; 20(3): 62–72.

Hager, W. D. Treatment of metronidazole-resistant Trichomonas vaginalis with tinidazole. *Sex. Transm. Dis.* 2004; 31(6): 343–5.

Hainer, B. L. and Gibson, M. V. Vaginitis: diagnosis and treatment. *Am. Fam. Physician* 2011; 83(7): 807–15.

Holley, R. L., Richter, H. E., Varner, R. E., *et al.* A randomized, double-blind clinical trial of vaginal acidification versus placebo for the treatment of symptomatic bacterial vaginosis. *Sex. Transm. Dis.* 2004; 31(4): 236–8.

Kane, B. G., Degutis, L. C., Sayward, H. K., and D'Onofrio, G. Compliance with the Centers for Disease Control and Prevention recommendations for the diagnosis and treatment of sexually transmitted diseases. *Acad. Emerg. Med.* 2004; 11(4): 371–7.

Klebanoff, M. A., Schwebke, J. R., Zhang, J., *et al.* Vulvovaginal symptoms in women with bacterial vaginosis. *Obstet. Gynecol.* 2004; 104(2): 267–72.

Koumans, E. H., Sternberg, M., Bruce, C., *et al.* The prevalence of bacterial vaginosis in the United States, 2001–2004; associations with symptoms, sexual behaviors, and reproductive health. *Sex. Transm. Dis.* 2007; 34(11): 864–9.

Mashburn, J.. Vaginal infections update. *J. Midwifery Womens Health* 2012; 57(6): 629–34.

Rathod, S. D. and Buffler, P. A. Highly-cited estimates of the cumulative incidence and recurrence of vulvovaginal candidiasis are inadequately documented. *BMC Womens Health* 2014; 14(1): 43.

Satterwhite, C. L., Torrone, E., Meites, E., *et al.* Sexually transmitted infections among US women and men:prevalence and incidence estimates, 2008. *Sex. Transm. Dis.* 2013; 40(3): 187–93.

Schwebke, J. R. Bacterial vaginosis. *Curr. Infect. Dis. Rep.* 2000; 2(1): 14–17.

Chapter

33

Adult Septic Arthritis

Robert Goodnough and Christopher Fee

Introduction and Microbiology

Septic arthritis refers to a bacterial infection within a synovial joint. It is most commonly the result of hematogenous spread and seeding of the synovium. Less frequent causes of septic arthritis include complications from joint aspirations or injections, penetrating trauma, and extension from an adjacent osteomyelitis. Bacterial invasion of a joint causes activation of a potent host immune inflammatory response, which results in the production of proteolytic enzymes that destroy the extracellular cartilage matrix of the affected joint. Septic arthritis is considered a medical emergency because permanent joint damage from this inflammatory response can occur within days. Prosthetic joint infections are discussed in Chapter 39.

Approximately half of septic arthrits cases are caused by *Staphylococcus aureus*, a large proportion of which are MRSA in contemporary case series. Other etiologic pathogens include Streptococcal species, *Neiseria gonorrhoea*, and various gram-negative coliform species.

Epidemiology

Populations at increased risk for septic arthritis include individuals older than 80 years of age, those with osteo-arthritis or rheumatoid arthritis, those with prior joint surgery, and those on corticosteroids or with human immunodeficiency virus (HIV)/acquired immunodeficiency syndrome (AIDS). Individuals with diabetes mellitus or other chronic medical conditions such as renal disease, cirrhosis, granulomatous disease, or malignancy are also at increased risk. Pediatric septic arthritis is covered in Chapter 53. Limited single center studies have demonstrated estimates of prevalence of septic arthritis is between 8 and 27% in those presenting with a swollen joint to acute care facilities with an in-hospital mortality rate for septic arthritis ranging from 7 to 15%.

Clinical Features

Septic arthritis typically presents with erythema, swelling, tenderness, and warmth of the affected joint (see Figure 33.1). The patient will display decreased and painful range of motion of the affected joint (see Table 33.1). Signs and symptoms of inflammation may be less pronounced in those who are immunosuppressed. The knee joint is the most commonly affected joint (representing approximately 50% of all cases), followed by the hip, shoulder, wrist, and ankle, in descending order of frequency. Septic arthritis of the sacroiliac joint and the sternoclavicular joint may be seen in intravenous drug users.

Differential Diagnosis

Key features that may help to distinguish septic arthritis from other arthropathies are:

- single joint involvement
- acute onset of severe pain, swelling, heat, and erythema
- inability to perform active range of motion or bear weight
- severe pain with passive range of motion
- fever and tachycardia
- gonococcal arthritis occurs in young otherwise healthy sexually active adults with a female preponderance and may occur in conjunction with other signs of disseminated gonococcal disease: migratory polyarthritis, tenosynovitis, and vesicopapular skin lesions (see Chapter 30); ultimately, it is critical to note that none of the above features will allow a clinician to rule in or rule out a septic arthritis without joint aspiration

Other conditions to consider include:

- acute exacerbation of chronic arthritis (e.g. rheumatoid), though a high index of suspicion should be maintained
- viral arthritis
- crystal-induced arthritis (gout or pseudogout)
- reactive arthritis

Table 33.1 Adult Acute Septic Arthritis

Pathogens	*Staphylococcus aureus* (including MRSA) is most common *Streptococcus* spp. *N. gonorrhea* Gram-negative rods
Clinical features	• Warmth, erythema, painful range of motion and effusion of affected joint • Fever and malaise
Laboratory and radiographic findings	• WBC, ESR, and CRP are usually elevated, but are unreliable markers for acute diagnosis • Blood cultures are positive in up to 50% • Radiographs may show underlying trauma, soft-tissue swelling, joint effusion, foreign body, or subcutaneous gas • Infected joint fluid may appear purulent, opaque, with variable viscosity; typically >50,000 WBC/mm^3, >90% PMNs • Synovial fluid lactate, if available; >10 mmol/L indicative of bacterial septic arthritis
Differential diagnosis	• Gout • Pseudogout • Viral arthritis (often polyarticular) • Reactive arthritis • Inflammatory arthritis • Transient synovitis • Bursitis • Trauma • Hemarthrosis
Treatment	• Hold antibiotics until joint aspiration is performed for synovial fluid culture • Emergent drainage (surgical versus repeat bedside aspiration) in conjunction with an orthopedic consultant • Empiric IV antibiotics after arthrocentesis Vancomycin 15–20 mg/kg/dose IV every 8–12 hours *plus** Ceftriaxone 1 g IV every 24 hours *or* Ciprofloxacin 400 mg IV every 12 hours

* Gram-negative empiric coverage should be considered if infection is associated with trauma, injection drug use, immunosuppression, or if Gram stain reveals gram-negative bacilli.

CRP – C-reactive protein; ESR – erythrocyte sedimentation rate; IV – intravenous; MRSA – methicillin-resistant *Staphylococcus aureus*; PMNs – polymorphonuclear neutrophil leukocytes; WBC – white blood (cell) count.

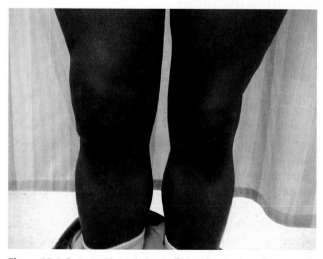

Figure 33.1 Patient with a right knee effusion showing loss of contour of patella and effusion extending into the suprapatellar pouch of joint.

Permission granted to use this image by Dr. Charlie Goldberg and Dr. Jan Thompson (co-creators of the website from the University of California, San Diego).

Key clinical questions that help to diagnose septic arthritis are:

• age greater than 80
• history of immunosuppression (diabetes, rheumatoid arthritis, HIV)
• injection drug use
• joint prosthesis

Complicating the distinction between septic arthritis and other causes of monoarticular arthritis is the fact that septic arthritis frequently occurs after seeding of a pre-existing joint effusion due to conditions such as rheumatoid arthritis or gout. Ultimately, it is critical to note that none of the above features will allow a clinician to rule in or rule out septic arthritis without joint aspiration.

Laboratory and Radiographic Findings

The definitive diagnosis of septic arthritis relies upon culturing the causative organism from the synovial fluid of the affected joint. Antibiotics have been shown to substantially decrease culture yields and should be withheld until aspiration is performed. Therefore, timely arthrocentesis is crucial in all cases of suspected septic arthritis. Synovial fluid should be sent for aerobic and anaerobic culture and, depending on the clinical situation, for mycobacterial, fungal, and gonococcal culture.

If quantity allows, synovial fluid should also be sent for cell count and examined by polarized light microscopy for negative (gout) and positive (pseudogout) birefringement crystals. Synovial fluid culture is positive in approximately 90% of non-gonococcal septic arthritis cases, and gram stain is positive in less than 50%. A synovial fluid cell count of greater than 50,000/mm^3 is the classic cut-off for the diagnosis of septic arthritis, with polymorphonuclear neutrophil (PMNs) of at least 90%. However, many studies have shown that synovial fluid leukocyte counts less than 25,000/mm^3 are common, particularly in immunocompromised patients and MRSA infections. One diagnostic marker that has shown promise is synovial fluid lactate. Multiple studes have shown it to have both a high positive likelihood ratio (confirms the diagnosis) and a low negative likelihood ratio (rules out the diagnosis) when set to a diagnostic cut-off value of >10mm/L.

Besides obtaining joint fluid, radiographs of the affected joint(s) should generally be obtained to assess for associated osteomyelitis, pre-existing disease, and foreign bodies. Two sets of blood cultures should be obtained in all patients being evaluated for septic arthritis. The white blood cell count (WBC) and erythrocyte sedimentation rate (ESR) may be elevated. C-reactive protein (CRP) is usually elevated to greater than 100 mg/L and the CRP level can be used to track the response to therapy.

Treatment and Prophylaxis

The treatment of septic arthritis involves early drainage of the purulent joint effusion and treatment with appropriate antibiotics. Empiric antibiotics should include coverage for methicillin-resistant *Staphylococcus aureus* (MRSA), which was shown to be a common etiology in a small case series. There is controversy regarding the best method of drainage for septic arthritis – serial arthrocentesis versus surgical incision and drainage, which can be arthroscopic or by arthrotomy. The approach will depend in large part on the preference of the orthopedic consultant. Empiric antibiotics that cover gram-positive bacteria including MRSA, typically vancomycin, should be administered as soon as possible following diagnostic joint aspiration and blood cultures. Gram-negative coverage is added in the setting of gram-negative bacilli on Gram stain, trauma, injection drug use, or immunosuppression. See Table 33.1.

Complications and Admission Criteria

All patients with suspected septic arthritis should be admitted. Septic arthritis should be considered a surgical emergency requiring urgent orthopedic consultation and either surgical or bedside drainage to prevent destruction of the articular cartilage. Treatment delay is correlated with morbidity and mortality. The main complication of septic arthritis is progressive joint destruction and decreased function. Other complications can stem from underlying bacteremia and endocarditis. Elderly and immunosuppressed patients and those with underlying rheumatoid arthritis have a worse prognosis related to the infection itself. Reported mortality from septic arthritis ranges from 8% to as high as 15%.

Box 33.1 Standard Emergency Department Evaluation for Septic Arthritis

1. Synovial fluid for:
   - gram stain
   - cell count and differential
   - culture (aerobic, anaerobic, gonococcal, fungal, mycobacterium)
   - crystal analysis
   - consider synovial fluid lactate level
2. Blood samples for:
   - ESR
   - CRP
   - WBC
   - blood culture
3. Radiographs of affected joint

Pearls and Pitfalls

1. Antibiotics should be held until joint aspiration is performed and blood cultures are drawn.
2. Aspiration with a large-bore (18 gauge) needle utilizing sterile technique is the most important diagnostic test to perform and should be part of the initial evaluation of a suspected septic joint.
3. High index of suspicion should be maintained in patients with a history of immunocompromise or chronic arthritis.
4. Gram stain of synovial fluid may be negative in up to half of cases and should not be relied on to rule out septic arthritis.
5. Synovial fluid cell counts may be less than 25,000/mm^3.

References

Carpenter, C. R., Schuur, J. D., Everett, W. W., and Pines, J. M. Evidence-based diagnostics: adult septic arthritis. *Acad. Emerg. Med.* 2011; 18(8): 781–96.

Frazee, B. W., Fee, C., and Lambert, L. How common is MRSA in adult septic arthritis? *Ann. Emerg. Med.* 2009; 54(5): 695–700.

Goodman, S. B., Chou, L. B., and Schurman, D. J. Management of pyarthrosis in M. W. Chapman (ed.), *Chapman's Orthopedic Surgery* (Philadelphia, PA: Lippincott Williams & Wilkins, 2001), pp. 3561–75.

Manadan, A. M. and Block, J. A. Daily needle aspiration versus surgical lavage for the treatment of bacterial septic arthritis in adults. *Am. J. Ther.* 2004; 11(5): 412–15.

Margaretten, M. E., Kohlwes, J., Moore, D., and Bent, S. Does this adult patient have septic arthritis? *JAMA* 2007; 297 (13): 1478–88.

Shah, K. Spear, J, Nathanson, L. A., *et al.* Does the presence of crystal arthritis rule out septic arthritis? *J. Emerg. Med.* 2007; 32(1): 23–6.

Shirtliff, M. E. and Mader, J. T. Acute septic arthritis. *Clin. Microbiol. Rev.* 2002; 15(4): 527–44.

Smith, J. W., Chalupa, P., and Hasan, M. S. Infectious arthritis: clinical features, laboratory findings and treatment. *Clin. Microbiol. Infect.* 2006; 12(4): 309–14.

34

Diabetic Foot Infections

Tamara John and Melinda Sharkey

Introduction and Microbiology

A diabetic foot infection (DFI) is defined as any inframalleolar infection in a person with diabetes mellitus. Most DFIs arise from diabetic foot ulcers. Diabetic foot ulcers occur in the setting of compromised protective sensation due to peripheral neuropathy. Immune deficiency and arterial insufficiency, which is often present in diabetic patients, further compromise the ability to fight off infection and heal an ulcer. This combination of inadequate blood flow, compromised immune function, and the absence of pain due to the diabetic neuropathy can result in serious infection.

All diabetic foot ulcers should be treated as chronic wounds that will not heal on their own. Intervention, including debridement, application of special dressings and pressure reduction/offloading, are mandatory. It is also critical that infected diabetic foot ulcers be recognized and treated promptly because they represent the biggest risk factor for non-traumatic amputations in diabetic patients. Approximately one in five diabetic foot ulcers results in lower extremity amputation.

Acute infections are usually monomicrobial, whereas chronic infections are polymicrobial. *Staphylococcus aureus* and beta-hemolytic *Streptococcus* (especially group B) are most common. *Staphylococcus aureus* is most virulent. Chronic wounds may contain *Enterococcus*, *Enterobacteriaceae*, anaerobes and gram-negative rods, including *Pseudomonas aeruginosa*. Previous treatment or hospitalization may predispose to resistant organisms such as methicillin-resistant *S. aureus* (MRSA) or vancomycin-resistant *Enterococcus* (VRE).

Epidemiology

Diabetic foot infections account for the largest number of diabetes-related hospital bed days. In the United States alone, about 82,000 limb amputations are performed annually in

those with diabetes, and an amputation in a diabetic patient is associated with a 5-year mortality rate between 39 and 68%. Lavery *et al.* studied 1,666 diabetic patients and found a 56-fold increase in risk of hospitalization and a 155-fold increase in risk of amputation among diabetics who developed foot infections.

Clinical Features

Purulent secretions, necrotic tissue, and signs of inflammation including pain, redness, warmth, tenderness, and induration indicate infection of a diabetic foot ulcer (see Figure 34.1 and Table 34.1). Atherosclerosis can markedly decrease blood flow to the lower extremities and therefore inhibit healing of diabetic foot ulcers. All patients seen in the acute care setting with diabetic foot ulcers should undergo a basic peripheral vascular exam including palpation of the peripheral pulses and measurement of the ankle brachial index in each leg. An ankle brachial index is calculated by dividing the blood pressure in the calf of the affected foot by the blood pressure in the upper extremity. An ankle brachial index of 1 is normal. Patients with an ankle-brachial index (ABI) of less than 0.9 require evaluation by a vascular surgeon.

Probing of bone in the depths of an infected diabetic foot ulcer has been shown to strongly correlate with the presence of underlying osteomyelitis and should be done on initial assessment using a sterile metal instrument or the wooden end of a sterile cotton swab. Bone detected on probing has been shown to be 66% sensitive and 85% specific for underlying osteomyelitis. If bone is probed, other tests to diagnose osteomyelitis are unnecessary, though radiographs (three views of the foot) should be done to assess the extent of bony involvement.

A classification system created by the International Working Group on the Diabetic Foot and Infectious Disease Society of

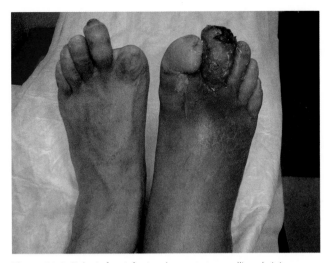

Figure 34.1 Diabetic foot infection demonstrates swelling, draining purulence, necrotic tissue, and associated cellulitis of the dorsum of the foot. Permission granted to use this image by Dr. Charlie Goldberg and Dr. Jan Thompson (co-creators of the website from the University of California, San Diego).

America (IDSA) assists in categorizing the severity of disease and helps guide diagnosis, treatment, and prognosis of DFIs:

- **Uninfected:** Foot ulcers that lack purulence or other signs of infection. Antibiotics are not indicated.
- **Mild:** Infections of skin and superficial soft tissues requiring the presence of two or more manifestations of inflammation (e.g. erythema, pain, warmth, or induration) and if present, <2 cm of erythema around ulcer. There should be no associated systemic inflammation.
- **Moderate:** Local infection with >2 cm of erythema around the ulcer or involvement of deeper tissues including muscle, tendon, joint, and/or bone. No systemic inflammatory signs are present.
- **Severe:** Infected ulcers that are accompanied by systemic inflammation manifested by ≥ two of the following: fever >38 or <36°C, HR >90, RR>20 or $PaCO_2$<32 mm Hg, WBC >12,000 or <4,000 cells/uL or ≥ 10% immature (band) forms.

Utility of the IDSA classification system has been prospectively validated. There is a statistically significant correlation between the defined severity of infection and risk of amputation, anatomic level of amputation, and need for hospitalization. Patients with mild infections do not require hospitalization and are unlikely to develop osteomyelitis or require amputations, whereas those with more severe disease will require more aggressive medical and surgical care.

Differential Diagnosis

Key features that may help to distinguish diabetic foot osteomyelitis from acute Charcot arthropathy are:

- presence of ulcer with signs of infection
- elevated white blood cell count (WBC) (erythrocyte sedimentation rate [ESR] may be elevated in both conditions)
- systemic inflammatory response is more indicative of infection

- typical radiographic appearance of Charcot arthropathy: dorsal dislocations of toes and midfoot, metatarsophalangeal joint destruction, metatarsal stress fractures, flattened arch, destruction of talus, cuneiform, or cuboid bones
- combined technetium-99 bone scan and indium-labeled leukocyte scan may improve specificity
- magnetic resonance imaging (MRI) cannot distinguish bone edema due to neuroarthropathy from osteomyelitis

Laboratory and Radiographic Findings

If there is clinical evidence of infection, a bacterial culture should be obtained prior to empiric antibiotic administration. Generally, superficial wound swabs are not considered reliable and deep-tissue cultures via biopsy or curettage after wound irrigation and debridement are desirable. Consequently, if the patient is not systemically infected and will be taken in a timely manner for formal irrigation and debridement, it is better to hold antibiotics until deep tissue cultures can be obtained intraoperatively. Mild, acute infections in a patient not recently treated with antibiotics are sometimes treated empirically.

Laboratory tests should include complete blood count with differential, ESR, C-reactive protein (CRP), basic chemistry panel, hemoglobin A1C, prealbumin, and urine microalbumin. Recent studies found that CRP has the highest sensitivity and specificity for distinguishing mild from uninfected ulcers. A lactate level should be sent in patients who are febrile or appear toxic.

Prealbumin is a marker for short-term evaluation of nutrition status and is important because malnutrition is associated with impaired wound healing. Microalbuminuria is used for early detection of diabetic nephropathy, but is also a significant risk factor for foot ulcers.

Radiographic imaging of the infected foot is required because presence of osteomyelitis will affect surgical planning. Plain radiographs (anteroposterior, lateral, and oblique views) of the involved foot are sufficient in the majority of cases to assess for bony involvement and to look for foreign bodies and gas. The radiographic triad of osteomyelitis includes demineralization, periosteal reaction, and bony destruction, but these findings may not be evident for up to 2 weeks after infection. If the diagnosis of osteomyelitis is in question, other imaging modalities can be utilized. MRI has emerged as the advanced imaging modality of choice; it is very sensitive, but not specific in diagnosing osteomyelitis. MRI will clearly show edema and hyperemia of the bone, but this may also be caused by surrounding soft-tissue infection and not by infection of the bone itself. Technetium radionuclide bone scans also suffer from poor specificity. Combining technetium scans with indium white blood cell scans can reduce the false positive rate.

Treatment

When signs of systemic toxicity are present, the patient should be assessed for sepsis and resuscitated, hyperglycemia should be controlled, and comorbidities treated. The need for hospitalization depends on the severity of the infection.

Table 34.1 Clinical Features: Diabetic Foot Infections

Pathogens	*Staphylococcus aureus* (including MRSA)
	Beta-hemolytic *Streptococcus* (especially group B) *Enterococcus* (VRE has been described)
	Enterobacteriaceae
	Anaerobes
	Gram-negative rods (including *Pseudomonas aeruginosa*)
Signs and symptoms	• Foot ulcer
	• Purulent secretion
	• Redness, warmth, swelling, induration, and/or pain and tenderness
	• If severe, systemic toxicity possible
Laboratory and radiographic findings	• Plain radiographs show osteomyelitis as demineralization, periosteal reaction, and bony destruction after 2 weeks
	• MRI highly sensitive for bone edema
	• ESR and CRP are elevated
	• Severe hyperglycemia and electrolyte imbalance in severe cases
Treatment	**Clinically uninfected wounds:**
	• No antibiotic therapy
	• Wound care
	• Off-loading of ulceration
	Empiric therapy for mild to moderate infection:
	• Thorough debridement
	• Wound care
	• Off-loading of ulceration
	and:
	MSSA
	Cephalexin 500 mg PO QID for 10–14 days
	or
	Dicloxacillin 500 mg PO QID for 10–14 days
	or
	Clindamycin 300 mg PO TID for 10–14 days
	or
	Amoxicillin-clavulanate 875/125 mg PO BID for 10–14 days
	MRSA
	Doxycycline 100 mg PO BID for 10–14 days
	or
	Trimethoprim/sulfamethoxazole 160/800 mg PO BID for 10–14 days
	Empiric antibiotics for severe infection:
	Vancomycin 10–15 mg/kg/dose IV every 8–12 hours
	plus
	Ertapenem 1 g IV daily
	or
	Piperacillin-tazobactam 4.5 g IV every 8 hours (pseudomonas coverage)

CRP – C-reactive protein; ESR – erythrocyte sedimentation rate; IV – intravenous; MRI – magnetic resonance imaging; MRSA – methicillin-resistant *Staphylococcus aureus*.

Initial antibiotic therapy is usually empiric, in which case the choice of antibiotic depends on the severity of the infection. Few clinical trials of antibiotic therapy for diabetic foot infection have been published; however, the regimen should generally be consistent with guidelines published by the Infectious Diseases Society of America. Broad-spectrum intravenous antibiotics are indicated for severe, extensive, or chronic infections and should include activity against gram-positive cocci. Coverage for methicillin-resistant *Staphylococcus aureus* (MRSA) is generally required. Empiric treatment with oral antibiotics that cover the most frequent pathogens is often sufficient for cure in mild and moderate infections.

It is important to note that in the past few decades, a major problem with treating diabetic foot infections has been the increased rate of isolation of antibiotic resistant pathogens, particularly MRSA, and to a lesser degree glycopeptide intermediate, *S. aureus*, vancomycin-resistant enterococci, extended-spectrum beta-lactamase, or carbapenamase-producing gram-negative bacilli, and highly resistant strains of *P. aeruginosa*.

Indications for amputation include necrotizing fasciitis, gas gangrene, extensive soft-tissue loss, or critical ischemia (ABI <0.5). Urgent amputation is reserved for those cases in which extensive necrosis or life-threatening infection is present. Undrained pus will not respond to antibiotics alone and pus under pressure can cause sepsis and should be drained promptly. Mild infections can be observed to determine the efficacy of medical therapy and to await demarcation of the boundary between necrotic and viable tissue. In the case of dry gangrene, waiting for the necrotic portion to autoamputate is a

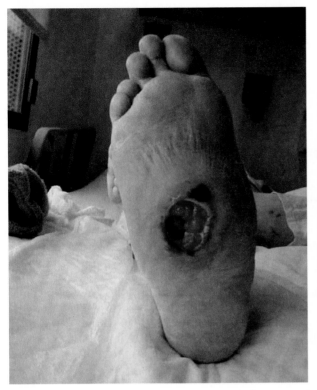
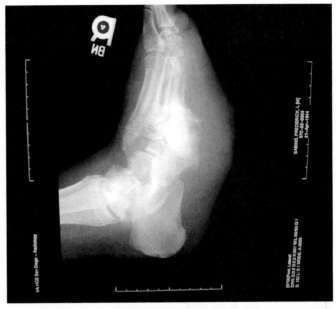

Figure 34.2 Photograph and corresponding radiograph of a patient with neuropathic arthropathy of the foot showing a typical rocker-bottom foot with an associated plantar ulcer. The plain radiograph shows severe bony destruction through the tarsal-metatarsal joint.

Permission granted to use this image by Dr. Charlie Goldberg and Dr. Jan Thompson (co-creators of the website from the University of California, San Diego).

reasonable option. A dry and adherent heel eschar should not be debrided unless it appears to be the source of infection.

Special Considerations

Osteomyelitis

Diagnosis of osteomyelitis in the diabetic foot can be difficult, and the optimal treatment remains controversial. Osteomyelitis causes impaired wound healing and may act as a focus for recurrent infection. As the size and depth of an ulcer increases, the likelihood of underlying bone infection increases as well. The forefoot is most commonly affected. The presence of osteomyelitis signifies a greater likelihood of surgery, including amputation, and longer duration of antibiotics. Osteomyelitis in patients with diabetic foot is usually the result of contiguous spread from a soft tissue focus. The most common causative pathogen is *S. aureus*, including MRSA. *Enterobacteriaceae* are more common than *Pseudomonas* species. However, antimicrobial selection should be based on culture results whenever possible.

Charcot Arthropathy

Diabetes is the most common cause of neuropathic arthropathy (Charcot arthropathy), a non-infectious condition in which joint destruction occurs secondary to lack of protective sensation. Diagnosis is often clinical, especially in the early stages. In acute Charcot neuroarthropathy, the foot is warm, edematous, and markedly erythematous. Patients will demonstrate a sensory and autonomic neuropathy and may or may not complain of pain. The exact mechanism of progressive joint destruction has yet to be understood. In the foot, neuro-arthropathy can affect the forefoot, the midfoot, and the hindfoot. Most commonly, Lisfranc's joint (tarsal-metatarsal joint) is affected. Patients with neuroarthropathy need to be followed closely and treated carefully because the associated foot deformities result in a particularly high risk of developing severe diabetic foot ulcers (see Figure 34.2).

Complications and Admission Criteria

According to the 2012 IDSA Clinical Practice Guidelines for the diagnosis and treatment of diabetic foot infections, admission is indicated for:

- all patients with severe infection determined by the IDSA classification system
- selected patients with a moderate infection + complicating features (e.g. severe peripheral artery disease, lack of home support)
- any patient unable to comply with an appropriate outpatient treatment regimen for psychological or social reasons

Pearls and Pitfalls

1. Not all diabetic foot ulcers are infected.
2. Infection may be more extensive than the initial appearance because of spread among foot compartments, along the deep plantar space, or along the tendon sheaths.

3. Palpable dorsalis pedis and posterior tibial pulses generally indicate adequate perfusion.

4. Caution must be used when interpreting ABIs in the presence of arterial calcification, which is suggested by ABIs of >1.3.

5. Suspect underlying osteomyelitis when an ulcer does not heal after 6 weeks of appropriate wound care.

6. Visible or easily palpated bone within an ulcer is likely to be complicated by osteomyelitis.

7. A sausage toe deformity, resulting from soft-tissue inflammation and underlying bony changes, is also highly suggestive of osteomyelitis.

8. Superficial wound cultures have no utility in directing antibiotic therapy and should not be performed. For osteomyelitis, deep tissue and bone cultures are necessary to direct treatment. If patient is clinically stable, antibiotics should be held until such cultures are obtained.

References

Brem, H. B., Sheehan, P., Rosenberg, H. J., *et al.* Evidence-based protocol for diabetic foot ulcers. *Plast. Reconstr. Surg.* 2006; 117(7): 193S–209S.

Grayson, M. L., Gibbons, G. W., Balogh, K., *et al.* Probing to bone in infected pedal ulcers: a clinical sign of underlying osteomyelitis in diabetic patients. *JAMA* 1995; 273(9): 721–3.

Guyton, G. P. and Saltzman, C. L. The diabetic foot: basic mechanisms of disease. *J. Bone Joint Surg.* 2001; 83: 1083–96.

Lavery, L. A., Armstrong, D. G., Murdoch, D. P., *et al.* Validation of the Infectious Disease Society of America's diabetic foot infection classification system. *Clin. Infect. Dis.* 2007; 44(4): 562–5.

Lipsky, B. A., Berendt, A. R., Cornia, P. B., *et al.* Infectious Diseases Society of America clinical practice guideline for the diagnosis and treatment of diabetic foot infections. *Clin. Infect. Dis.* 2012; 54(12): e132–73.

Lipsky, B. A., Berendt, A. R., Deery, H. G., *et al.* Diagnosis and treatment of diabetic foot infections. *Clin. Infect. Dis.* 2004; 39(7): 885–910.

Richard, J. L., Lavigne, J. P., and Sotto, A. Diabetes and foot infection: more than double trouble. *Diabetes/Metabolism Res. Rev.* 2012; 28(1) 46–53.

Roberts, A. D. and Simon, G. L. Diabetic foot infections: the role of microbiology and antibiotic treatment. *Sem. Vasc. Surg.* 2012; 25(2): 75–81.

Spichler, A., Hurwitz, B. L., Armstrong, D. G., and Lipsky, B. A. Microbiology of diabetic foot infections: from Louis Pasteur to "crime scene investigation." *BMC Medicine* 2015; 13(1): 2.

Uckay, I., Gariani, K., Pataky, Z., and Lipsky, B. A. Diabetic foot infections: state-of-the art. *Diabetes, Obesity & Metabolism* 2014; 16(4): 305–16.

Chapter 35

Hand Infections: Fight Bite, Purulent Tenosynovitis, Felon, and Paronychia

Michael Kohn

Introduction

Our hands are our mechanical interface with the world, so they are frequently injured and exposed to infection. This chapter starts by covering two true hand emergencies: fight bite and purulent tenosynovitis. Information on the frequency of these problems in the emergency department is impossible to come by because they do not have specific ICD-9 diagnosis codes, but they put the patient at risk for lasting disability and are important to diagnose and treat appropriately. Acute paronychia and felon are also discussed. These are bacterial infections of, respectively, the dorsal and palmar surfaces of the fingertip. Felon is roughly one-tenth as common as paronychia, but more serious. Lastly, herpetic whitlow is discussed, primaily to distiguish it from paronychia and felon, because it is not a bacterial infection and does not require drainage or antibiotics.

Fight Bite

The most notorious of all non-venomous bite wounds is the fight bite. As the name implies, this injury occurs when the subject punches an adversary in the teeth, lacerating the dorsum of one or more metacarpal-phalangeal (MCP) joints (see Figure 35.1). Other names for this injury, such as "morsus humanus" or "clenched fist injury," have been proposed,

though "fight bite" is more descriptive and widely used. The fight bite is more prone to infection than other animal bites because of the location of the bite and the typical delay in treatment rather than due to the mix of organisms in the human mouth. Common fight bite infections include cellulitis, subcutaneous abscesses, septic MCP joint, and purulent tenosynovitis. In the pre-antibiotic era, fight bite infections commonly necessitated finger and occasionally arm amputations.

Epidemiology and Microbiology

Fight bite infections are usually polymicrobial and often involve *Streptococcus* species, *Staphylococcus* species, *Eikenella*, and oral anaerobic bacteria. The first two fight-bite patients reported in the medical literature were described by William H. Peters in 1911. He was primarily concerned with culturing mouth organisms, specifically Fusobacteria, from the infected wounds. Various other studies emphasizing the symbiosis of spirochetes and fusiform organisms in fight bites appeared afterwards. In 1930, Michael L. Mason and Sumner L. Koch published a 34-page study of fight bites emphasizing the importance of the anatomy of the injured area in determining the spread of infection. In 1983, Schmidt identified *Eikenella corrodens*, a microaerophilic gram-negative rod, as an important etiologic agent in fight bite infections.

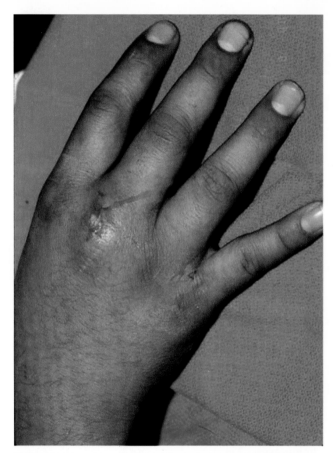

Figure 35.1 Examples of fight bite. Also known as a "clenched fist injury," this serious injury typically is characterized by a laceration on the dorsal metacarpal-phalangeal joint.

Courtesy of Dr. Alan Bindiger.

Clinical Features

Clinicians should be suspicious of a fight bite in any laceration over the dorsal MCP joint, particularly in young male patients (see Table 35.1). Exploration of the skin wound and examination of the extensor hood (with the MCP flexed) are essential to determine whether the joint capsule has been violated. Sometimes adequate visualization of the extensor hood requires extension of the skin wound.

Differential Diagnosis

Fight bites should be distinguished from occlusive bites (which are somewhat less prone to infection) and other hand lacerations (which are substantially less prone to infection).

Key features that distinguish fight bite from typical hand lacerations are:

- polymicrobial and more prone to infection
- progression of infection because of delayed diagnosis and treatment
- high suspicion of human bite based on location over the dorsal MCP

Radiographic Findings

An X-ray may reveal air or even a piece of tooth in the MCP joint.

Table 35.1 Clinical Features: Fight Bite (Clenched Fist Injury)

Organisms	*Streptococcus* (predominantly *S. anginosus*) *Staphylococcus* species *Eikenella* Oral anaerobes
Signs and symptoms	Laceration over the dorsal MCP joint Examine with MCP flexed for laceration of the extensor hood
Laboratory and radiographic findings	X-ray may reveal air or a retained tooth in the MCP joint
Treatment	**Uninfected, extensor hood intact:** Thorough irrigation, no sutures Prophylaxis: Amoxicillin-clavulanate 875/125 mg PO BID × 5 days *or* Ciprofloxacin 500 mg PO BID *plus* Clindamycin* 450 mg PO TID, both × 5 days **Uninfected, extensor hood violated:** Irrigation of joint, splinting, prophylactic antibiotics Admission or next-day follow-up by hand surgeon **Infected:** Usually requires admission for joint wash-out and parenteral antibiotics Ampicillin-sulbactam 3 g IV every 6 hours *or* Ciprofloxacin 400 mg (500 mg) IV (PO) every 12 hours *plus* Metronidazole 500 mg IV/PO every 8 hours

* *E. corrodens* is uniformly resistant to clindamycin, so clindamycin must be used in combination with another antibiotic.

IV – intravenous; PO – by mouth.

Treatment and Prophylaxis

Antibiotic recommendations for prophylaxis and treatment of fight bite infections are based on the susceptibilities of the common infectious agents: *Streptococcus* species (especially *S. anginosus*), *Staphylococcus aureus*, and *Eikenella*. The choice is between a single beta-lactam–beta-lactamase inhibitor drug such as amoxicillin–clavulanate or a combination of clindamycin with either penicillin, a second- or third-generation cephalosporin, or a fluoroquinolone. Although it is effective against methicillin-resistant *S. aureus* (MRSA), clindamycin alone is never adequate therapy, as *E. corrodens* is uniformly resistant to clindamycin.

An uninfected fight bite that does not violate the extensor hood should be irrigated thoroughly under pressure and dressed open (no closure by suture, adhesive strips, or glue). There is no evidence regarding prophylactic antibiotics in this situation. Although a short, 3- to 5-day course of antibiotics might be justifiable, thorough irrigation and precautions to return for signs of infection are more important.

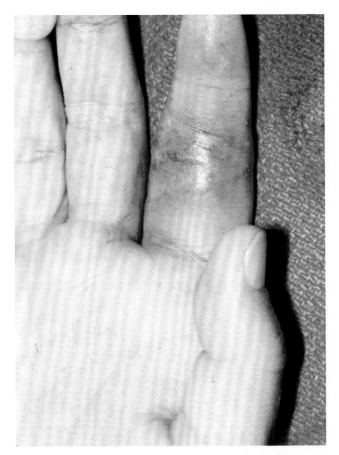

Figure 35.2 Purulent flexor tenosynovitis of the index finger of the right hand.

Courtesy of Dr. Alan Bindiger.

Complications and Admission Criteria

An uninfected fight bite that does violate the extensor hood requires thorough irrigation of the joint, splinting, prophylactic antibiotics, and either admission or next-day follow-up. Prophylactic antibiotics should be administered. A hand surgeon usually manages treatment.

An infected fight bite almost always requires hospitalization for intravenous antibiotics and potential surgical debridement.

Purulent Tenosynovitis

An important element of the surgical anatomy of the hand is that the deep and superficial flexors to the digits run through delicate tendon sheaths and utilize a complex system of tissue pulleys. Repairing damage to these sheaths and pulleys requires magnification and the controlled, sterile environment of the operating room. In contrast, the extensor tendons to the digits do not run through sheaths, and damaged extensors may be repaired in the emergency department (ED). That is why the palm and dorsum of the hand are sometimes referred to as the "OR side" and the "ER side," respectively.

Purulent tenosynovitis is a bacterial infection within one of the flexor tendon sheaths (see Figure 35.2). The inoculum comes from a puncture wound or laceration to the palmar surface of the hand or finger and spreads rapidly throughout the tendon sheath.

Microbiology

As with all skin infections resulting from lacerations or puncture wounds, the primary bacterial pathogens are *Staphylococcus aureus*, *Streptococcus*, and anaerobes.

Clinical Features

Patients with purulent tenosynovitis present with a painful swollen digit any time from hours to weeks after a palmar wound (see Table 35.2). Kanavel's four cardinal signs of purulent tenosynovitis are as follows:

1. slightly flexed finger posture
2. symmetrical swelling
3. pain on passive extension
4. tenderness along flexor tendon sheath

These findings distinguish purulent tenosynovitis from the less serious localized subcutaneous abscess.

Differential Diagnosis

Purulent tenosynovitis can be distinguished from less serious localized subcutaneous abscess by Kanavel's signs mentioned above.

Acute inflammatory reactions to insect bites and stings may present similarly, but can usually be identified by history.

Radiographic Findings

Point-of-care ultrasound (POCUS) shows promise in identifying or ruling out fluid collected around the flexor tendon, but the evidence is limited to two case reports and a four-case series.

Treatment

Prior to the epidemic of community-acquired methicillin-resistant *S. aureus* (MRSA), appropriate empiric antibiotic therapy included the following options: first-generation cephalosporin (e.g. cefazolin); antistaphylococcal penicillin (e.g. nafcillin); and beta-lactam–beta-lactamase inhibitor (e.g. ampicillin-sulbactam).

The increasing prevalence of MRSA in skin and soft tissue infections now mandates the addition of vancomycin and clindamycin. These infections are best managed by a hand surgeon and usually require surgical intervention, to irrigate the tendon sheath and obtain cultures to guide antibiotic therapy.

Complications and Admission Criteria

Patients with purulent tenosynovitis require hospitalization. In early, apparently mild infections, intravenous antibiotics and close observation may suffice. If the infection does not improve within 24 hours of antibiotic treatment, or if the infection is already established or advanced, surgery is required.

Table 35.2 Clinical Features: Purulent Tenosynovitis

Organisms	*Staphylococcus aureus* (methicillin resistance increasing in the community) *Streptococcus pyogenes* (group A) Anaerobes
Signs and symptoms	**Kanavel's signs:** • slightly flexed finger posture • symmetrical swelling • pain on passive extension • tenderness along flexor tendon sheath
Laboratory and radiographic findings	This is a clinical diagnosis requiring operative irrigation of the tendon sheath, at which time cultures should be obtained
Treatment	Hospital admission and operative irrigation of the tendon sheath; antibiotic therapy should be guided by operative cultures **Empiric IV antibiotics (no MRSA):** Ampicillin-sulbactam 3 g IV every 6 hours **Empiric IV antibiotics (MRSA):** Vancomycin 15–20 mg/kg/dose IV every 8–12 hours *plus* Ampicillin-sulbactam 3 g IV every 6 hours *Or, if penicillin allergy:* Ciprofloxacin 400 mg IV every 12 hours *and* Metronidazole 500 mg IV every 8 hours

IV – intravenous; MRSA – methicillin-resistant *Staphylococcus aureus*; PO – by mouth.

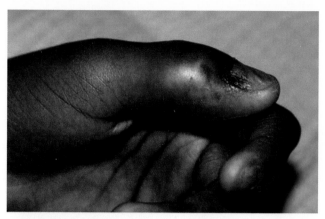

Figure 35.3 Acute paronychia of the left thumb. Courtesy of Dr. Alan Bindiger.

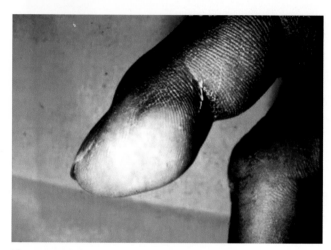

Figure 35.4 Felon. Courtesy of Dr. Alan Bindiger.

Acute Paronychia and Felon

Acute paronychia, a bacterial infection of the skin eponychia folds that hold the nail plate in place, is the most common of hand infections (see Figure 35.3). A felon is a painful and potentially disabling infection of the fingertip pulp that can progress to tissue necrosis and osteomyelitis of the distal phalanx (see Figure 35.4). Except in the very early stages, pus occupies the closed space formed by the fibrous septae of the fingertip.

Microbiology

As with purulent tenosynovitis, the infection in both paronychia and felon results from a break in the skin, and the common organisms are *S. aureus* (increasingly methicillin resistant), *Streptococcus* species, and anaerobes.

Clinical Features

The tenderness, erythema, and edema of the felon are all limited to the volar pad of the distal phalanx (see Table 35.3). In contrast, the paronychia is limited to the dorsal side of the fingertip. Sometimes, there is visible pus under the nail plate. Paronychia and felon are occasionally found together.

Differential Diagnosis

Acute paronychia should be distinguished from chronic paronychia as described below, and from herpetic whitlow, as incision and drainage of herpetic whitlow is contraindicated (see section below).

Chronic paronychia is inflammation of the nail folds of greater than 6 weeks' duration:

- rarely seen in the ED
- results from repeated exposure of hands to water and irritants
- commonly caused by *Candida albicans*
- treat by avoiding exposure to water and irritants
- topical steroids or antifungals also helpful

Treatment

Early incision and drainage is the mainstay of treatment for both felon and paronychia. For a felon, a simple, lateral longitudinal incision is usually adequate. Occasionally, bilateral incisions and passage of a through-and-through wick or drain is necessary. For a paronychia, adequate drainage may be obtained by simply elevating the edge of the eponychia. If subungual pus is present, the clinician should resect a longitudinal section of the nail plate on the side of the paronychia. Recently, authors have discouraged use of systemic antistaphylococcal antibiotics for both paronychia and felon in immunocompetent patients without osteitis unless refractory to surgical drainage. Some

Table 35.3 Clinical Features: Felon and (Acute) Paronychia

Organisms	*Staphylococcus aureus* *Streptococcus* spp. Anaerobes
Signs and symptoms	**Felon (volar pad of distal phalanx):** Tenderness Erythema Tense edema **Paronychia (skin folds around the fingernail):** Tenderness, erythema, edema Fluctuance Look for subungual pus (pus under the nail plate)
Laboratory/radiographic findings	In long-standing felon, X-ray may reveal osteomyelitis of the distal phalanx
Treatment	Primary treatment is incision and drainage **Felon:** Single lateral longitudinal incision with placement of gauze wick or, occasionally, bilateral longitudinal incisions with placement of a through-and-through wick or drain **Paronychia:** No subungual pus – elevate the skin fold, drain, and place a small wick Subungual pus – remove a longitudinal section of the nail plate to drain and maintain drainage **Antibiotics**: Less important than drainage and may be unnecessary in immunocompetent patients without osteitis unless refractory to simple drainage Must consider MRSA: Clindamycin 450 mg PO TID *or* TMP-SMX one to two DS tabs. PO BID If MRSA unlikely: Cephalexin 500 mg PO QID *or* Dicloxacillin 500 mg PO QID *or* Amoxicillin-sulbactam 875/125 mg PO BID

DS – double strength; PO – by mouth; SMX – sulfamethoxazole; TMP – trimethoprim.

have likened treating a simple paronychia with oral antibiotics to "killing a fly with a cannon."

Complications and Admission Criteria

Felon has the potential to become a serious bacterial infection that can progress to osteomyelitis of the distal phalanx and even to sepsis requiring hospitalization.

Herpetic Whitlow

Herpetic whitlow is a *herpes simplex* infection of the finger that can be confused with a paronychia or felon.

Epidemiology and Microbiology

In children, herpetic infections of the hand are exclusively due to *herpes simplex* type 1 autoinoculation from the mouth during an episode of gingivostomatitis. In adults, herpetic whitlow is caused by either *herpes simplex* type 1 or type 2. Herpes simplex type 2 infections occur more frequently in women and are associated with a history of genital herpes. As with other herpes infections, herpetic whitlow can recur after the primary infection. The occurrence of herpetic whitlow in dentists,

anesthetists, nurses, and others with occupational exposure to oral secretions has decreased in recent years.

Clinical Features

Herpetic whitlow that involves the fingertip may be distinguished from felon or paronychia by the presence of vesicles, and a serous crusting, rather than purulent, discharge. The simultaneous presence of cold sores, or a history of previous similar infections, can also make the diagnosis. Although rarely done, a Tzanck smear of the discharge may show multinucleated giant cells. Herpetic whitlow can be associated with lymphangitic streaking up the forearm and swollen epitrochlear or axillary nodes, which may be mistaken as an indication of bacterial infection.

Differential Diagnosis

Distinguish from felon or paronychia by:

- presence of vesicles
- serous, crusting, rather than purulent, discharge
- simultaneous presence of cold sores
- history of previous similar infections

237

Table 35.4 Clinical Features: Herpetic Whitlow

Organism	*Herpes simplex* type 1 or 2
Signs and symptoms	Vesicles
	Serous, crusting, not purulent, discharge
	Often associated with perioral cold sores
Laboratory findings	Although rarely done, Tzanck smear may show multinucleated giant cells
Treatment	Condition is self-limited, but severe cases may be treated with:
	Acyclovir 400 mg PO TID × 7 days
PO – by mouth.	

Treatment

It is important to distinguish herpetic whitlow from felon or paronychia, because herpetic whitlow should not be incised and drained. Although the infection is usually self-limited, treatment with oral acyclovir is indicated for severe acute cases. In patients with frequent, painful recurrences, maintenance acyclovir therapy may ultimately be necessary.

Complications

Herpetic whitlow can recur after the primary infection.

Pearls and Pitfalls

1. Suspect a fight bite in any knuckle laceration. Make sure to inspect the extensor hood, even if it requires extending the wound. Never close a fight bite.
2. *E. corrodens* is uniformly resistant to clindamycin, so clindamycin alone is never adequate treatment for a fight bite.
3. Purulent tenosynovitis is a true hand emergency requiring admission and consultation of a hand surgeon.
4. Distinguish herpetic whitlow from felon and paronychia by the presence of vesicles, a clear and crusting rather than purulent discharge, the simultaneous presence of cold sores, or a history of recurrent infections.

References

Boland, F. Morsus humanus. *JAMA* 1941; 116(2): 127–31.

Boles, S. D. and Schmidt, C. C. Pyogenic flexor tenosynovitis. *Hand Clin.* 1998; 14(4): 567–78.

Bowling, J. C., Saha, M., and Bunker, C. B. Herpetic whitlow: a forgotten diagnosis. *Clin. Exp. Dermatol.* 2005; 30(5): 609–10.

Gill, M. J., Arlette, J., and Buchan, K. Herpes simplex virus infection of the hand. A profile of 79 cases. *Am. J. Med.* 1988; 84(1): 89–93.

Kanavel, A. B. *Infections of the Hand; a Guide to the Surgical Treatment of Acute and Chronic Suppurative Processes in the Fingers, Hand, and Forearm*, 7th edn. (Philadelphia, PA: Lea & Febiger, 1939).

Karanas, Y. L., Bogdan, M. A., and Chang, J. Community acquired methicillin-resistant *Staphylococcus aureus* hand infections: case reports and clinical implications. *J. Hand Surg. [Am.]* 2000; 25(4): 760–3.

Mason, M. and Koch, S. Human bite infections of the hand. *Surg. Gynecol. Obstet.* 1930; 51(5): 591–625.

Peters, W. Hand infection apparently due to *Bacillus fusiformis. J. Infect. Dis.* 1911; 8: 455–62.

Rockwell, P. G. Acute and chronic paronychia. *Am. Fam. Physician* 2001; 63(6): 1113–16.

Schmidt, D. R. and Heckman, J. D. *Eikenella corrodens* in human bite infections of the hand. *J. Trauma* 1983; 23(6): 478–82.

Welch, C. Human bite infections of the hand. *N. Engl. J. Med.* 1936; 215: 901–5.

Additional Readings

Clark, D. C. Common acute hand infections. *Am. Fam. Physician* 2003; 68(11): 2167–76.

Franko, O. I. and Abrams, R. A. Hand infections. *Orthop. Clin. North Am.* 2013; 44(4): 625–34.

Giladi, A. M., Malay, S., and Chung, K. C. A systematic review of the management of acute pyogenic flexor tenosynovitis. *J. Hand Surg. Eur.* 2015; 40(7): 720–8.

Handley, N. and Unger, A. Antibiotic overuse and paronychia: a teachable moment. *JAMA Intern. Med.* 2016; 176(1): 19–20.

Pierrart, J., Delgrande, D., Mamane, W., *et al.* Acute felon and paronychia: antibiotics not necessary after surgical treatment. Prospective study of 46 patients. *Hand Surg. Rehabil.* 2016; 35(1): 40–3.

Shoji, K., Cavanaugh, Z., and Rodner, C. M. Acute fight bite. *J. Hand Surg. Am.* 2013; 38(8): 1612–14.

Open Fractures

Robert Goodnough and Melinda Sharkey

Introduction

Open fractures occur when the involved bone and surrounding soft tissues communicate with the outside environment because of a traumatic break in the overlying skin. Many open fractures are a result of high-energy trauma and are associated with severe soft-tissue injury. Lower energy open fractures occur when the skin break is caused by an "inside-out" injury, sometimes called a "poke-hole." This occurs when a fractured end of the bone penetrates the overlying skin.

Staphylococcus aureus is the predominant pathogen that is isolated from osteomyelitis following an open fracture. MRSA is particularly common in those requiring operative fixation. Other relatively common pathogens include coagulase-negative *Staphylococcus*, *Streptococcus* species, *Enterococcus*, and gram-negative organisms. *Pseudomonas aeruginosa* causes osteomyelitis following a plantar puncture wound with an associated minor foot fracture. Fungi, including mucormycosis species, can follow open wounds from a natural disaster involving wood and buiding material projectiles. *Acinetobacter baumannii* has been associated with combat casualties of the lower extremities.

Epidemiology

Fractures represent a major public health problem. The lifetime risk of fracture up to the age of 65 years is one in two, and every year 1 in 118 people younger than 65 years of age sustains a fracture. Approximately 2% of all fractures and dislocations are open.

Clinical Features

Open fractures can be classified according to the Gustilo–Anderson classification system. Although Gustilo–Anderson classification is widely used, it shows poor inter-observer agreement. The gold standard remains an assessment in the operating room. However, it is important that acute-care physicians be comfortable in Gustilo–Anderson classification as the

type of open fracture correlates with prognosis and complication rates, and can guide initial management (see Figures 36.1, 36.2, and 36.3).

Differential Diagnosis

Key clinical questions that may help in the diagnosis of open fractures are:

- Is an open fracture the source of visible bleeding?
- How large is the wound and how severe is the soft-tissue damage?
- Are the joints above and below affected?
- What is the neurovascular status of the affected limb?
- Does the wound contain a foreign body?

Treatment and Prophylaxis

The rate of infection despite antibiotic administration in type I fractures ranges from 0 to 2%, in type II fractures from 2 to 10%, and in type III fractures from 10 to 50%. Administration of antibiotics for open fractures should not be thought of as a prophylactic measure, but rather as a treatment measure. All open fractures are contaminated with bacteria. Delay in administration of antibiotics beyond 3 hours increases the risk of infection.

Proper management of open fractures includes the following steps:

- careful examination of the involved limb
- injury classification (Gustilo–Anderson)
- immediate antibiotic administration
- tetanus prophylaxis
- wound management
- fracture stabilization
- attention to patient analgesia
- immediate orthopedic consultation

There is a lack of evidence to support targeted versus broad spectrum antibiotic therapy. Moreover, changing patterns of

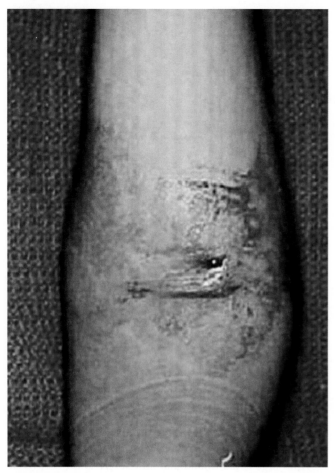

Figure 36.1 Photographic example of a grade I open fracture of the elbow that shows a small, less than 1 cm, skin opening and minimal soft soft-tissue damage.

Photograph from the Orthopedic Trauma Association website, www.ota.org.

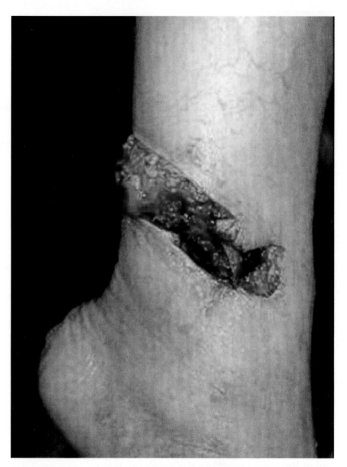

Figure 36.2 Photographic example of a grade II open fracture of the distal tibia with a >1 1 cm skin opening, with moderate to severe soft soft-tissue damage, but adequate soft soft-tissue coverage of bone.

Photograph from the Orthopedic Trauma Association website, www.ota.org.

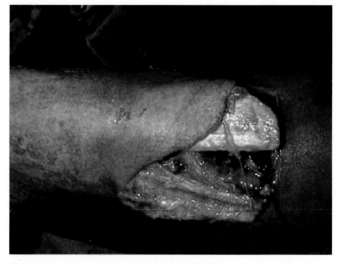

Figure 36.3 Photographic example of a grade III open fracture of the tibia. Notice the >11 cm skin break, as well as extensive soft soft-tissue injury, including periosteal and muscle stripping from bone.

Photograph from the Orthopedic Trauma Association website, www.ota.org.

antibiotic resistance hamper development of strict antibiotic guidelines. Early discussion with the orthopedic consultant and tailoring antibiotic choice to the wound appearance and degree of contamination is critical.

In general, patients with types I and II open fractures should at least receive a first-generation cephalosporin to cover gram-positive bacterial contamination. Alternative single agent choices for types I and II open fractures include quinolones or clindamycin, keeping in mind that quinolones may be detrimental to healing in type III fractures.

For a type III fracture, an aminoglycoside, to cover gram-negative bacteria, is added to the first-generation cephalosporin. For elderly patients or those with renal insufficiency, quinolones, aztreonam, or third-generation cephalosporins can be used in place of an aminoglycoside for gram-negative coverage.

A fracture that occurs in a highly contaminated environment should additionally be treated with penicillin or clindamycin to cover *Clostridium perfringens*.

In addition to antibiotic administration, initial management should include wound irrigation with sterile saline and application of a sterile dressing. The extremity should then be splinted to increase patient comfort and to limit further damage to soft tissue, and radiographs should be obtained. In addition, a complete neurovascular exam of the injured extremity as well as an exam for compartment syndrome should be performed.

Table 36.1 Gustilo–Anderson Classification of Open Fractures

Fracture Type	Soft-Tissue Injury	Bone Injury	Antibiotics[*]
Type I	<1 cm skin opening, minimal soft-tissue damage	Simple transverse or short oblique fracture	Cefazolin 2 g IV every 8 hours Alternative: Clindamycin 900 mg IV every 8 hours
Type II	>1 cm skin opening, moderate to severe soft-tissue damage but adequate bone coverage	Transverse and oblique fractures, minimal comminution	
Type III >10 cm skin break with extensive soft-tissue injury, often with a severe crushing component and fracture pattern consistent with a high-energy mechanism			
Type IIIA	Limited periosteal stripping, bone coverage usually adequate	Segmental fractures, highly comminuted fractures	Cefazolin 2 g IV every 8 hours and Gentamicin 5 mg/kg/dose IV every 24 hours Alternative: Clindamycin 900 mg IV every 8 hours and Gentamicin 5 mg/kg/dose IV every 24 hours
Type IIIB	Extensive periosteal and muscle stripping from bone, usually severe contamination	Segmental fractures, highly comminuted fractures	
Type IIIC	Any open fracture associated with vascular injury requiring surgical repair	Variable	

* Penicillin G 2–4 million units IV every 4 to 6 hours or clindamycin 900 mg IV every 8 hours should be added for highly contaminated wounds (i.e. those occurring in a farmyard) to cover *Clostridium perfringens*. Gentamicin dosing may need to be adjusted with renal dysnfuction.

IV – intravenous.

After initial acute treatment, the patient will need to be taken to the operating room for formal irrigation and debridement of the wound and fixation of the fracture.

Ultimately, increased risk of infection is associated with delay to antibiotics and delay in admission to an inpatient service that manages orthopedic trauma. In general, open fractures should undergo definitive operative care within 6 hours (the so-called "6-hour rule"), though there is limited evidence showing higher rates of infection when operation is delayed. It is important to regard these injuries as surgical emergencies with a time-sensitive approach to antibiotic administration and definitive surgical service consultation.

Complications and Admission Criteria

In general, all patients with open fractures should be admitted to a center that is familiar with orthopedic trauma for operative management. Complications of open fractures include the following: compartment syndrome, vascular injury, osteomyelitis, loss of function, and non-union.

Pearls and Pitfalls

1. Antibiotics should be initiated immediately on recognition of an open fracture.
2. Following identification and initial irrigation, the wound should be covered with a sterile dressing and repeat examinations avoided.
3. The joint above and below should be examined and imaged to rule out adjacent fractures.
4. Open fractures are often high-energy injuries with increased risk of neurovascular injury and/or compartment syndrome.

5. Bleeding in the presence of underlying fracture should be considered an open fracture until proven otherwise.

References

Gustilo, R. B. and Anderson, J. T. Prevention of infection in the treatment of one thousand and twenty-five open fractures of long bones. *J. Bone Joint Surg.* 1976; 58(4): 453–8.

Gustilo, R. B., Mendoza, R. M., and Williams, D. N. Problems in the management of type III (severe) open fractures: a new classification of type III open fractures. *J. Trauma* 1984; 24(8): 742–6.

Hoff, W. S., Bonadies, J. A., Cachecho, R., and Dorlac, W. C. East Practice Management Guidelines Work Group: update to practice management guidelines for prophylactic antibiotic use in open fractures. *J. Trauma & Acute Care Surg.* 2011; 70(3): 751–4.

Kim, P. H. and Leopold, S. S. Gustilo-Anderson classification. *Clin. Orthop. & Related Res.* 2012; 470(11): 3270–4.

O'Brien, C. L., Menon, M., and Jomha, N. M. Controversies in the management of open fractures. *Open Orthop. J.* 2014; 8(1): 178–84.

Patzakis, M. J., Harvey, J. P., and Ivler, D. The role of antibiotics in the management of open fractures. *J. Bone Joint Surg.* 1974; 56(3): 532–41.

Patzakis, M. P. and Wilkins, J. Factors influencing infection rate in open fracture wounds. *Clin. Orthop.* 1989; 243: 36–40.

Rodriguez, L., Jung, H. S., Goulet, J. A., *et al.* Evidence-based protocol for prophylactic antibiotics in open fractures: improved antibiotic stewardship with no increase in infection rates. *J. Trauma & Acute Care Surg.* 2014; 77(3): 400–8.

Zalavras, C. G. and Patzakis, M. J. Open fractures: evaluation and management. *J. Am. Acad. Orthop. Surg.* 2003; 11(3): 212–19.

Chapter

37

Osteomyelitis

Melinda Sharkey

Introduction and Microbiology

Adult osteomyelitis is an infectious inflammatory disease of bone, often of bacterial origin. Early diagnosis, antibiotic therapy, and often surgical management can control and even eradicate bone infection. Causative organisms vary depending on the portal of entry (direct inoculation versus hematogenous seeding) and the associated health status of the patient. Osteomyelitis, particularly chronic osteomyelitis, can be very difficult to treat and long-term arrest of infection and prevention of re-activation rather than cure is often the goal of treatment. Osteomyelitis of the spine is covered in more detail in Chapter 40.

Staphylococcus aureus is the most common pathogen in osteomyelitis overall, and MRSA osteomyelitis is now common, particlularly in the post-operative setting. Patients with chronic medical conditions are especially prone to infection with gram-negative organisms, including *Pseudomonas aeruginosa*, as well as by fungi and atypical mycobacteria. Salmonella osteomyelitis in sickle cell disease patients is well described. Osteomyelitis of the foot in diabetics tends to be polymicrobial and this entity is covered in Chapter 34.

Epidemiology

Osteomyelitis in adults often arises after open fracture, orthopedic surgical procedures, or in the setting of diabetic foot ulcers. Hematogenous osteomyelitis is less common, but increases in incidence with increasing age and often manifests as vertebral osteomyelitis. Patients with increased susceptibility to osteomyelitis include those with sickle cell disease, chronic granulomatous disease, diabetes mellitus, and human immunodeficiency virus (HIV)/acquired immunodeficiency syndrome (AIDS).

Clinical Features

The most common route of infection is direct inoculation due to injury or bony surgery. Hematogenous osteomyelitis secondary to bacteremia is usually a single organism infection, whereas direct penetration may involve multiple organisms. *S. aureus* is the causative organism in most cases of osteomyelitis.

The inflammatory process causes tissue necrosis and destruction of bony structure. Infection also obliterates vascular channels to the periosteum and intramedullary bone, leading to ischemia and areas of necrotic cortical bone, or sequestra. These sequestra are the hallmark of chronic osteomyelitis. Surviving periosteum forms new bone, called an involucrum, which encases the dead bone. Draining sinuses form when purulence tracks to the skin surface through irregularities in the involucrum.

Presentation can vary from an open wound with exposed bone or a draining sinus to swelling and tenderness without any skin changes (see Table 37.1). In acute osteomyelitis, defined as less than 6 weeks from onset of infection, patients may present with fevers, chills, and night sweats indicating intermittent or persistent bacteremia. With progression to a chronic phase, patients complain of chronic pain and drainage with or without low-grade fevers. Probing to bone with the wooden end of a sterile cotton applicator can detect osteomyelitis at the base of diabetic foot ulcers.

Differential Diagnosis

- tumor
- pathologic fracture or impending pathologic fracture
- traumatic fracture or stress fracture
- septic arthritis
- inflammatory arthritis
- gout
- reactive bone marrow edema

Laboratory and Radiographic Findings

The white blood cell count (WBC) is usually elevated in acute but not chronic osteomyelitis. The erythrocyte sedimentation

Table 37.1 Clinical Features: Osteomyelitis

Organisms	Hematogenous osteomyelitis: *S. aureus* Direct penetration: multiple organisms
Signs and symptoms	**Acute osteomyelitis:** Fever, chills, pain, swelling, drainage from surgical wound or open fracture site, night sweats **Chronic osteomyelitis:** Draining sinus, pain, low-grade fevers
Laboratory and radiologic findings	• WBC may be normal in chronic cases; ESR and CRP are elevated • Blood culture may identify organism in acute osteomyelitis • Plain radiographs lag by 2 weeks and show soft-tissue swelling, periosteal thickening and elevation, and focal osteopenia • MRI can differentiate between involvement of bone and soft tissue; affected areas appear as low signal on T1 and high signal on T2 • Technetium- 99 bone scan shows increased uptake within 48 hours • Deep bone biopsy is necessary to identify causative organism in chronic osteomyelitis
Treatment	• Surgical drainage, debridement, dead space management, and possible soft tissue coverage **Empiric antibiotics:** Vancomycin (for MRSA) 15–20 mg/kg/dose IV every 8–12 hours (serum trough levels should be 15–20) *plus* Piperacillin/tazobactam 4.5 g IV every 6 hours *or* Levofloxacin 750 mg IV/PO daily **Antibiotics for known MSSA infections:** Nafcillin 2 g IV every 6 hours *or* Cefazolin 2 g IV every 8 hours Modify host factors as necessary (smoking cessation, improved nutrition, and diabetes management)

CRP – C-reactive protein; ESR – erythrocyte sedimentation rate; IV – intravenous; MRI – magnetic resonance imaging; MRSA – methicillin-resistant *Staphylococcus aureus*; WBC – white blood (cell) count.

rate (ESR) and C-reactive protein (CRP) are elevated in both acute and chronic cases. The CRP is more specific, but should not be used alone to rule out osteomyelitis. The WBC, ESR, and CRP should be measured at initial evaluation and followed to track response to treatment.

Identification of the causative pathogen with a positive culture is the most important diagnostic step. Blood cultures can obviate the need for more invasive bone cultures and are more likely to be positive in acute and hematogenous osteomyelitis and in diseases involving the spinal column. In most cases of chronic osteomyelitis, sampling of affected bone or deep soft tissue will likely be required. Unless the patient is acutely ill, antibiotics should not be given until operative or deep-tissue specimens are obtained. Sinus tract and cutaneous wound cultures do not reliably predict the organisms responsible for the underlying bone infection.

Plain radiographs are often used to screen for osteomyelitis. Radiologic evidence of osteomyelitis is apparent 2 weeks after the start of infection: the earliest radiographic changes are soft-tissue swelling, periosteal thickening or elevation, and focal osteopenia (see Figures 37.1 and 37.2). Magnetic resonance imaging (MRI), which has a high sensitivity and specificity for detection of osteomyelitis, should be performed for suspicious cases and is useful for evaluating the bone and surrounding soft tissue. Edema appears dark on the T1-weighted sequence and bright on T2 (see Figure 37.3). Plain radiographs showing osteomyelitis of the boney spine should be followed immediately by MRI to assess for spinal canal and spinal cord involvement (see Figure 37.3). Computed tomographic (CT) scan defines a sequestrum and soft tissue abnormalities well, and can be used for surgical planning.

Nuclear modalities are useful in the setting of metallic hardware, though similarity between osteomyelitis and other causes of bone inflammation limits specificity. Technetium-99 bone scans are positive within 48 hours of infection (see Figure 37.4).

Indium-labeled white blood cell scan is positive in 80% of cases of acute osteomyelitis. Positron emission tomography and three-phase bone scans are also used for diagnosis and the choice of nuclear modality is institution-dependent.

Standard emergency department evaluation for osteomyelitis includes:

- radiographs
- complete blood count (CBC), ESR, CRP
- blood cultures
- MRI if radiographs unclear
- nuclear medicine studies if MRI not possible or extent of involvement unknown

Treatment

Acute osteomyelitis is usually treated by targeted intravenous antibiotics for 4 to 6 weeks. The specific antibiotic regimen should be based on culture results. Placement of a peripherally inserted central catheter may be required for administration of intravenous antibiotics at home (e.g. vancomycin, nafcillin).

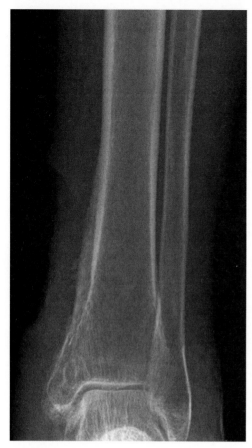

Figure 37.1 AP radiograph of the left ankle in a patient with a chronic ulcer over the medial ankle with underlying chronic osteomyelitis of the medial malleolus and medial distal tibia. Note the periosteal elevation and osteopenia.

A course of oral antibiotics may be given following completion of intravenous antibiotics. Clinical response as well as laboratory markers, such as CRP, are used to monitor treatment response.

Definitive treatment of chronic or refractory acute osteomyelitis requires drainage of the abscess and debridement of all devitalized tissue and obliteration of dead space. Management of large bony and soft tissue defects may require complex and staged reconstructive surgery. The surgical therapy is combined with tailored antibiotic therapy, and when possible, correction of host comorbidities: poor nutrition status, smoking, poorly controlled diabetes, and vascular compromise.

Complications and Admission Criteria

Admission is generally necessary for initial diagnostic evaluation, identification of organism, and initiation of antibiotic therapy in patients presenting with a suspected bone infection.

Special Considerations

- Sickle cell disease: it can be difficult to differentiate acute bone infarct from osteomyelitis, so early cultures may be important. The most common pathogens in sickle cell patients are *S. auerus* followed by *Salmonella* spp.

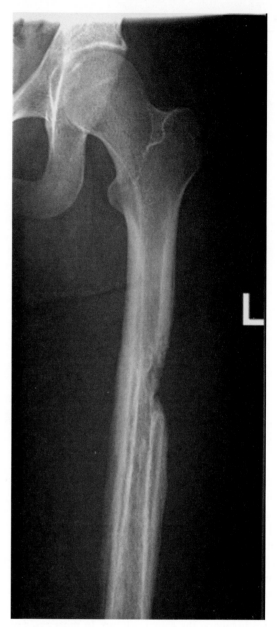

Figure 37.2 AP radiograph of a patient with osteomyelitis of the left femur.

- Injection drug users are susceptible to hematogenous osteomyelitis. In this population, the typical locations for infection are the spine, as well as unusual locations in the axial skeleton like the clavicle and pubis. Causative organisms include *S. aureus*, *S. epidermidis*, gram-negative rods, and *Candida* spp.
- Pressure ulcers are a common problem in debilitated and immobilized patients. Non-healing cutaneous ulcers may indicate an underlying bone infection. Definitive diagnosis requires a positive bone culture and pathological examination demonstrating inflammatory cells in bone marrow tissue. While prevention is the ultimate goal, treatment for osteomyelitis from pressure ulcers consists of a 6- to 8-week course of antibiotics followed by delayed flap coverage.

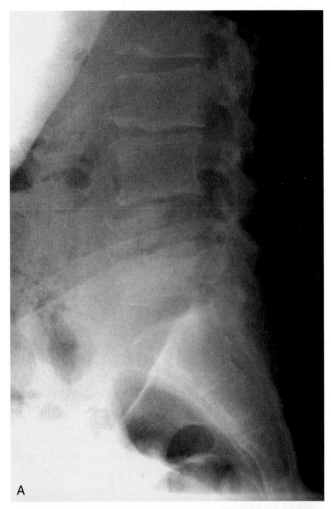

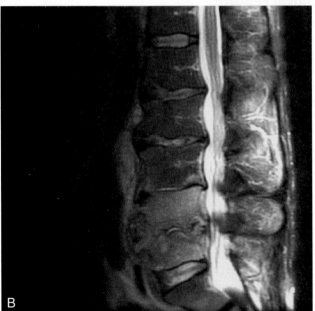

Figure 37.3 Bacterial osteomyelitis of the lumbar spine. Lateral plane radiograph (A) demonstrates destruction of the L4 and L5 vertebral bodies and disk spaces. Sagittal T2-weighted MRI from the same patient (B).

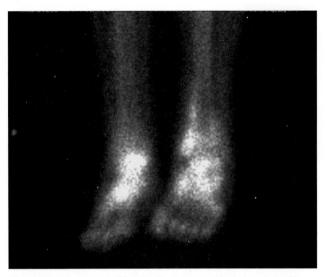

Figure 37.4 Bone scan of the distal lower extremities in a patient with osteomyelitis showing increased uptake in the left medial malleolus and distal tibia compared to the right ankle. This bone scan corresponds to the radiographs in Figure 37.1.

Pearls and Pitfalls

1. Withhold antibiotics until cultures are obtained if the patient is clinically stable.
2. Sinus tract cultures and wound swabs are unreliable.
3. Surgical debridement is usually necessary for chronic and often acute osteomyelitis.

References

Calhoun, J. H. and Manring, M. M. Adult osteomyelitis. *Infect. Dis. Clin. N. Am.* 2005; 19(4): 765–86.

Darouiche, R. O., Landon, G. C., Klima, M., *et al.* Osteomyelitis associated with pressure sores. *Arch. Intern. Med.* 1994; 154(7): 753–8.

Forsberg, J. A., Potter, B. K., Cierny, G., 3rd, *et al.* Diagnosis and management of chronic infection. *J. Am. Acad. Orthop. Surg.* 2011; 19(1): S8–19.

Gustilo, R. B., Gruninger, R. P., and Tsukayama, D. T. *Orthopaedic Infection: Diagnosis and Treatment* (Philadelphia, PA: Saunders, 1989).

Lazzarini, L., Mader, J. T., and Calhoun, J. H. Osteomyelitis in long bones. *J. Bone Joint Surg. Am.* 2004; 86-A(10): 2305–18.

Lew, D. P. and Waldvogel, F. A. Osteomyelitis. *Lancet* 2004; 364(9431): 369–79.

Mouzopoulos, G., Kanakaris, N. K., Kontakis, G., *et al.* Management of bone infections in adults: the surgeon's and microbiologist's perspectives. *Injury* 2011; 42(5): S18–23.

Plantar Puncture Wounds

Bradley W. Frazee

Introduction

Puncture wounds to the plantar surface of the foot are a common and seemingly innocuous injury that have the potential for serious complications. While relatively minor abscesses and cellulitis are the most common infectious complications, these injuries have gained notoriety because they may also result in osteomyelitis – which can present in a delayed fashion in otherwise healthy patients. Deep-seeded infections are related to both the puncture mechanism, which can innoculate bone, joint, and tendon located near the skin surface with bacteria, as well as the frequent introduction of foreign material such as soil, rubber, cotton fibers, and pins.

The microbiology of plantar puncture wound infections includes common skin infection pathogens, particularly *Staphylococcus aureus* (the most common isolate) and β-strepotococcus species, as well as *Pseudomonas auruginosa* in the case of osteomyelitis. Systematic case series all pre-date the emergence of community-associated MRSA, but it is reasonable to assume that MRSA now accounts for a high proportion of *S. aureus* infections following plantar puncture wounds.

Epidemiology

Puncture wounds of the foot are a common problem encountered by the acute care provider. In one study, puncture wounds made up 0.8% of all pediatric emergency department visits. There is a seasonal variation, with the highest incidence seen from May through October when children go barefoot and people engage in more outdoor activities. The majority of these injuries are caused by nails (98%). Of the remaining cases, a wide variety of other objects have been described, including wood, toothpicks, glass, plastic, rock, bones, coral, straw, bullets, wire, and sewing needles.

Among plantar puncture wounds presenting for medical evaluation, approximately 5 to 10% have an associated infection, mostly subcutaneous abscesses and cellulitis. Osteomyelitis and septic arthritis complicate less than 2%.

Risk factors for infection include delay to presentation beyond 24 hours and persistent symptoms beyond 48 hours, missed foreign body, puncture through an athletic shoe, puncture overlying the metatarsal heads and calcaneous, and immunospression. It is thought that sweaty athletic shoes and socks may harbor *Pseudomonas*. In a series of pediatric osteomyelitis cases, the mean time to diagnosis was 2 weeks, with a range of 6 days to 16 months. Diabetic neuropathy, which leads to unnoticed injury, presents a high risk for advanced and serious infection (see Chapter 34, Diabetic Foot Infections).

Clinical Features

The evaluation of plantar puncture wounds should include assessment for historical factors that increase the risk of infection, as well as a careful physical exam focused on discovering an occult foreign body, which may be radiolucent (see Table 38.1). Factors that should increase the suspicion for infection include the following:

- time elapsed since injury and duration of symptoms; delayed presentation and persistent symptoms beyond 48 hours suggest there may be a foreign body or early infection
- material and length of the penetrating object
- environment in which injury occurred (e.g. barnyard, aquatic)
- type of shoe worn
- presence of constitutional symptoms, including fever, chills, vomiting
- comorbidities, including diabetes, human immunodeficiency virus (HIV), long-term steroid use, peripheral vascular disease, asplenia, or transplanted organs

The best approach to the physical exam is to lay the patient prone with the knee bent 90 degrees with the foot near eye level of the examiner. Under a bright light, the wound should be carefully examined for subtle evidence of purulence and explored for foreign body. Judicious use of lidocaine with epinephrine can allow more extensive exploration with a sharp instrument in a relatively bloodless field.

Table 38.1 Clinical Features: Plantar Puncture Wound Infection

Common organisms	**Cellulitis:** *Staphylococcus aureus* (most common) Beta-hemolytic *Streptococcus* **Osteomyelitis in non-diabetic patients:** *Pseudomonas aeruginosa* (>90%) **Osteomyelitis in diabetic patients:** *Staphylococcus aureus* or polymicrobial
Signs and symptoms	• Antalgic (abnormal) gait • Warmth, erythema, tenderness, swelling surrounding puncture site • Wound drainage • Fever, chills, vomiting, tachycardia if systemic involvement
Laboratory and radiographic findings	• WBC may be elevated • ESR, CRP may be elevated • Superficial wound swabs are not recommended • Plain x-rays can reveal fracture or foreign body • MRI to evaluate for suspected osteomyelitis • Ultrasound can reveal and localize a non-radiopaque foreign body and abscess

CRP – C-reactive protein; CT – computed tomography; ESR – erythrocyte sedimentation rate; WBC – white blood (cell) count.

Retained foreign body occurs in 3% of all plantar puncture wounds and may or may not be associated with infection at the time of presentation. Depending on the footwear, the entry of a sharp object into the foot can carry with it particles of dirt, grass, sock, and rubber sole or other shoe material. Broken needles or pins are the culprits in 30% of cases. Foreign bodies may act as a continued nidus of infection and inflammation, preventing proper healing, or may cause persistent discomfort and difficulty with ambulation. The spectrum of infection can span from wound-related cellulitis to abscess, to osteomyelitis and septic arthritis (see Chapter 12, Bacterial Skin and Soft-Tissue Infections, Chapter 33, Adult Septic Arthritis, Chapter 65, Sepsis, and Chapter 37, Osteomyelitis). Osteomyelitis may be preceded by a period of clinical improvement and it may occur despite prophylactic antibiotics. Drainage and fluctuance may be subtle. Frank cellulitis, lymphangitis, and fever or other signs of systemic infection are uncommon.

Laboratory and Radiographic Findings

Blood tests are not needed to evaluate most plantar puncture wounds that present early or with just a superficial wound infection. If symptoms have been present for more than 48 hours with risk factors, then complete blood count (CBC) with differential, erythrocyte sedimentation rate (ESR) and/or C-reactive protein (CRP) should be obtained. A normal CRP or ESR, however, does not rule out osteomyelitis or other significant infection. Blood cultures should be obtained for fever or significant suspicion of osteomyelitis. Superficial swabs for Gram stain and culture are not recommended; however, deep specimens taken after incision and drainage may be useful. Foot joint aspiration and bone biopsy, obtained intraoperatively,

are the gold standard for diagnosis of osteomyelitis and septic arthritis.

Plain radiographs should routinely be obtained for plantar puncture wounds. Plain films can rule out fracture and radiopaque foreign body and may reveal signs of osteomyelitis in cases of delayed or return presentation. However, they will miss non-radiopaque foreign bodies and osteomyelitis in the acute phase. All metal fragments and most glass fragments will appear on plain X-ray, but wood or plastic may not. Computed tomography (CT) is more sensitive for small foreign bodies and abscesses. Magnetic resonance imaging (MRI) is the most sensitive modality for detecting deep abscess, osteomyelitis, or septic arthritis and should be considered in all patients presenting with prolonged or recurrent symptoms or an elevated CRP or ESR. Bedside ultrasound can be used to localize non-radiopaque foreign bodies, such as thorns and splinters, and abscesses, facilitating removal and drainage.

Failure to obtain radiographic evaluation is the most frequent cause of missed foreign body. Indications for removal of foreign bodies include location near or into bone, joint, or neurovascular structures, infection, or persistent symptoms. Fluoroscopy is the current imaging method of choice to assist with removal of radiopaque foreign bodies.

Treatment and Prophylaxis

Although there is no current consensus on the appropriate treatment for plantar puncture wounds, initial treatment for all puncture wounds should include the following:

- Wound care: Cleansing with soap and water and debridement of non-viable tissue flaps should be performed for all wounds.
- Varying recommendations exist regarding more aggressive treatment such as coring the wound. These interventions can be painful and difficult to perform, but may be worthwhile in deep wounds with gross contamination. High pressure irrigation is controversial as it may contaminate surrounding tissues.
- Foreign body removal: Once detected, most foreign bodies should be removed to reduce the risk of infection and persistent pain. Risks of removal of foreign bodies must be taken into consideration according to location and characteristics of object.
- Tetanus immunization: Plantar puncture wounds should be treated as highly tetanus-prone. *Clostridium tetani* spores are ubiquitous in soil and puncture wounds constitute an oxygen-poor environment (see Chapter 10, Tetanus).
- Antibiotics: Wounds with signs of infection at the time of presentation should be treated with antibiotics. Following plantar puncture wound, the most common cellulitis pathogen is *Staphylococcus aureus* and the most common osteomyelitis pathogen is *Pseudomonas aeruginosa*. *P. aeruginosa* should be suspected in patients with a history of a nail puncture wound through a tennis shoe. One study showed that cases of cellulitis or osteochondritis following a nail puncture wound were successfully treated with intravenous

Table 38.2 Treatment of Plantar Puncture Wounds

Treatment	• Meticulous exam for subtle signs of infection or occult foreign body
	• Wound care, including debridement and irrigation
	• Foreign body removal
	• Tetanus immunization
	• Antibiotic prophylaxis not recommended for clean wounds in immunocompetent patients
	• No data on prophylactic antibiotic choice or duration. *Staphylococcus*, *Streptococcus*, or *Pseudomonas* coverage for contaminated or deep wounds or immunocompromised patients may prevent complications
	Cellulitis*:
	• 7 days of therapy with oral *Staphylococcus* and *Streptococcus* coverage with or without additional antipseudomonal coverage
	***Staphylococcus* and *Streptococcus* coverage:**
	• Cephalexin 500 mg PO QID for non-purulent cellulitis, if purulent drainage or abscess, add TMP-SMX DS one to two tabs. PO BID
	or
	Clindamycin 450 mg PO QID
	Additional antipseudomonal coverage:
	• Ciprofloxacin 750 mg PO BID
	Early bone involvement (osteochondritis)*:
	• Ciprofloxacin 750 mg PO BID for 14 days
	Osteomyelitis:
	Cefepime 2 g IV every 12 hours
	or
	Ciprofloxacin 400 mg IV every 12 hours
	or
	Piperacillin-tazobactam 4.5 g IV every 6 hours
	Antibiotic therapy should be directed by surgical/bone culture as there is significant pseudomonal resistance in each locality; treat for 4 to 6 weeks.

* In limited studies, oral therapy of 750 mg BID was preceded by 24 hours of IV ciprofloxacin coupled with surgical intervention.

PO – by mouth; TMP-SMX DS – trimethoprim-sulfamethoxazole double-strength tablet.

(IV) ciprofloxacin for 24 hours in conjunction with surgical intervention followed by oral ciprofloxacin (750 mg BID) for 7 to 14 days. However, fluoroquinolone-resistant *P. aeruginosa* is increasingly common and fluoroquinolones are generally not recommended for children. In such cases, there is no appropriate oral antibiotic therapy; alternative therapies are IV ceftazidime or IV cefepime. The use of prophylactic antibiotics in uncomplicated plantar puncture wounds is controversial and there are no controlled studies on this practice. Widespread use of prophylactic antibiotics is not recommended. The decision to prescribe prophylactic antibiotics should take into account the nature of the wound, as well as patient risk factors for infection. Prophylactic antibiotics should be considered in the case of gross contamination, wounds overlying the metatarsal heads or calcaneous, or wounds presenting after 24 hours with persistent symptoms. A quinolone with Stapylococcal activity taken for 3 to 5 days is the most commonly recommended regimen.

• Follow-up care: Regardless of whether prophylactic antibiotics are used, all plantar puncture wounds are at high risk for delayed infection. Patients should undergo mandatory 48-hour follow-up, as well as be counseled carefully on signs of delayed infection.

Complications and Admission Criteria

Complications of plantar puncture wounds include cellulitis, abscess, septic arthritis, osteomyelitis, and necrotizing soft-tissue infections (particularly in diabetics). Infections are commonly associated with retained foreign body. Diabetic patients with wounds through a rubber-soled shoe or overlying the metatarsal heads or calcaneous are at increased risk of osteomyelitis. These patients typically present with persistent symptoms of pain and/or drainage 1 week or more after injury, but external signs of infection may be absent.

Pearls and Pitfalls

1. A meticulous physical exam to search for and remove radiolucent foreign bodies such as cotton fibers and rubber is rcommended in all cases.
2. Plain X-rays should be routinely obtained to assess for fracture and radioopaque retained foreign body.
3. Symptoms present beyond 48 hours should prompt consideration of blood tests such as ESR and CRP and advanced imaging, to assess for osteomyelitis and occult abscess or retained foreign body.
4. Delayed infectious complications may occur despite correct initial care, so all patients should receive careful follow-up instructions.

References

Baldwin, G. and Colbourne, M. Puncture wounds. *Pediatr. Rev.* 1999; 20(1): 21–3.

Chachad, S. and Kamat, D. Management of plantar puncture wounds in children. *Clin. Pediatr.* 2004; 43(3): 213–16.

Chisholm, C. D. and Schlesser, J. F. Plantar puncture wounds: controversies and treatment recommendations. *Ann. Emerg. Med.* 1989; 18(12): 1352–7.

Gasink, L. B., Fishman, N. O., Weiner, M. G., *et al.* Fluoroquinolone-resistant *Pseudomonas aeruginosa*: assessment of risk factors and clinical impact. *Am. J. Med.* 2006; 119(6): 526.e19–25.

Lavery, L. A., Walker, S. C., Harkless, L. B., *et al.* Infected puncture wounds in diabetic and non-diabetic adults. *Diabetes Care* 1995; 18(12): 1588–91.

Raz, R. and Miron, D. Oral ciprofloxacin for treatment of infection following nail puncture wounds of the foot. *Clin. Infect. Dis.* 1995; 21(1): 194–5.

Schwab, R. A. and Powers, R. D. Conservative therapy of plantar puncture wounds. *J. Emerg. Med.* 1995; 13(3): 291–5.

Prosthetic Joint Infections

Elisabeth Giblin and Scott C. Sherman

Introduction and Microbiology

Prosthetic joint infection is a feared complication of total joint replacement surgery and occurs as a result of bacterial contamination of the implant surface. It can occur at any point after the initial operation and is characterized by a slow, indolent course that usually results in a delay in diagnosis. Diagnosis and treatment are difficult, and eradication by non-operative means is rare if not impossible. The consequences of misdiagnosis are substantial and may lead to unnecessary surgery in the case of a false positive. Delays in diagnosis can make control of the infection more difficult and necessitate removal of the prosthesis, which entails prolonged immobilization and delayed reimplantation.

Prosthetic joint infections are typically classified according to time of onset from arthroplasty. The bacteriology varies for each type. Early onset infections occur less than 3 months from initial arthroplasty. They are typically caused by virulent organisms acquired during implantation, such as *S. aureus* and gram-negative bacteria, and may be polymicrobial. Delayed onset infections are defined as occurring 3 to 12 months after surgery. They are caused by less virulent organisms acquired during implantation, such as coagulase-negative *Staphylococci*, *Enterocci*, and *Propionibacterium acnes*. Late-onset infections occurring more than 12 months after surgery are usually caused by hematogenous spread from the oral cavity, skin, or gastrointestinal or urinary tract infection. The most common pathogens in this setting include *S. aureus*, beta hemolytic streptococci, and gram-negative bacteria.

Epidemiology

In the United States in 2010, there were 719,0000 total knee and 332,000 total hip arthroplasties with an incidence that is expected to continue to rise. Prosthetic joint infection is an uncommon complication, affecting 1 to 3% of total joint replacements. Infection most frequently affects the knee, followed by the hip. The cost to the US health-care system to treat joint infections was estimated at $566 million in 2009 and projected to reach $1.62 billion by 2020.

Clinical Features

Presenting symptoms are variable for each patient and dependent on the time course of the infection and the immune status of the patient (see Table 39.1). Pain and decreased range of motion of the joint are common. Drainage is also quite suggestive of infection if it is present in the first few weeks postoperatively. Fever, while helpful in making the diagnosis, is often absent and should not be relied upon. Other symptoms include swelling, erythema, and warmth surrounding the joint or an effusion. The presence of a sinus tract between the joint and skin is suggestive of a chronic infection. Risk factors for infection include a history of revision, poor wound healing, obesity, immunosuppressive medications, diabetes, rheumatoid arthritis, and malignancy.

Differential Diagnosis

Key features that distinguish prosthetic joint infection from other conditions are:

- pain localized to joint
- elevated erythrocyte sedimentation rate (ESR) and CRP
- effusion, decreased range of motion (variable)
  Other conditions to consider are:
- aseptic loosening
- post-operative hematoma
- implant failure
- periprosthetic fracture

Key clinical questions that help to distinguish post-operative joint infection are:

- is the ESR or CRP elevated?
- is there a history of trauma?

Table 39.1 Clinical Features: Prosthetic Joint Infection

Organisms	*S. aureus* and *S. epidermidis* most common
Signs and symptoms	• Severe joint pain with decreased range of motion • Swelling/effusion • Warmth/erythema • Persistent post-operative pain, swelling • Draining sinus tract
Laboratory and diagnostic findings	• CRP usually elevated • Plain radiographs usually normal or non-specific • Synovial fluid white cell count elevated (10,000–50,000/mL) • Nuclear medicine studies show increased signal
Treatment	• Do not give empiric antibiotics unless absolutely necessary (in order to ensure accurate surgical cultures) • Surgical incision and drainage with retention of implants if <6 weeks' symptoms • IV culture-guided antimicrobials are given for at least 4 weeks, often followed by oral suppresive therapy

CRP – C-reactive protein; IV – intravenous.

- has the patient had persistent post-operative pain?
- is the patient less than 6 weeks post-operative?

Laboratory and Radiographic Findings

The ESR and CRP have important roles in the evaluation of the painful prosthetic joint. An elevated CRP greater than 3 months after surgery should raise concern for infection. Sensitivity and specificity of ESR greater than 30 mm/hr have been reported to be 82% and 85%, and for CRP greater than 10 mg/L, 96% and 92%. A normal ESR and CRP makes prosthetic joint infection unlikely.

Plain radiographs usually appear normal, but should be obtained routinely to rule out wear, osteolysis, or fracture. When present, radiographic findings are non-specific and include periosteal reaction, scattered osteolysis, or bone resorption.

Joint aspiration employing sterile technique is the usual diagnostic technique and should be part of the early evaluation. It can be performed at bedside for superficial joints such as the knee, but may require fluoroscopic guidance for deep joints such as the shoulder and hip. Unlike native joints, prosthetic joint aspiration should always be done in consultation with an orthopedic surgeon. Gram stain has poor sensitivity. Sensitivity of bacterial culture ranges from 50 to 93% and is greatly reduced if antibiotics have been administered. Synovial fluid cell counts of 10,000 to 50,000 leukocytes/mL are suggestive of an infection, but no strict threshold exists.

Nuclear studies are frequently used to detect infection or loosening of the implants. Although sensitive, they are not specific. The physician should be aware that the technetium-99

bone scan may remain abnormal for up to 1 year post-operatively. Indium-111 tagged white blood cell scan is an alternative nuclear study, but takes 2 days to perform.

Standard tests to order for evaluation of prosthetic joint infections are:

- ESR and CRP
- joint aspiration
- plain radiographs
- nuclear medicine studies

Treatment and Prophylaxis

Treatment of prosthetic joint infection is operative. Unless clinically necessary because of sepsis, antibiotics should not be given until joint fluid or operative cultures can be obtained, and optimally not until a pathogen has been isolated. Suppression of established infection with chronic antibiotics is reserved for only severely debilitated patients who are unable to tolerate additional surgery, as attempts at suppression only lead to more extensive and resistant infection. At surgical incision and debridement, retention of implants may be considered if symptoms have been present for less than 6 weeks. Better outcomes have been reported when incision and drainage are performed early. In the United States, the preferred treatment for prosthetic joint infection is two-stage revision arthroplasty. All implants are removed and replaced with antibiotic-impregnated cement, followed by 6 weeks of intravenous antibiotics. Reimplantation is attempted after eradication of infection is confirmed.

Complications and Admission Criteria

Complications include:

- early implant failure
- persistent infection precluding retention of implants due to delayed diagnosis or intervention

Admission is indicated for bacteremia or sepsis.

Pearls and Pitfalls

1. ESR and CRP are useful in evaluation of the painful joint arthroplasty.
2. Empiric antibiotics should not be given until a surgical culture has been obtained.
3. Surgical incision and drainage should be performed as early as possible if attempting to retain implants.
4. Painful joint arthroplasty must be approached with a high index of suspicion for infection and should include evaluation by an orthopedic surgeon.

References

Bauer, T. W., Parvizi, J., Kobayashi, N., and Krebs, V. Diagnosis of periprosthetic infection. *J. Bone Joint Surg. Am.* 2006; 88(4): 869–82.

Della Valle, C. J., Zuckerman, J. D., and Di Cesare, P. E. Periprosthetic sepsis. *Clin. Orthop.* 2004; 420: 26–31.

Hanssen, A. D. and Spangehl, M. J. Treatment of the infected hip replacement. *Clin. Orthop.* 2004; 420: 63–71.

Kurtz, S. M., Ong, K. L., Lau, E., *et al.* Prosthetic joint infection risk after TKA in the Medicare population. *Clin. Orthop. Relat. Res.* 2010; 468(1): 52–6.

Larsson, S., Thelander, U., and Friberg, S. C-reactive protein (CRP) levels after elective orthopedic surgery. *Clin. Orthop.* 1992; 275: 237–42.

Tande, A. and Patel, R. Prosthetic joint infections. *J. Clin. Microbiol. Rev.* 2014; 27(2): 302–45, http://cmr.asm.org/content/27/2/302.full.pdf.

Zimmerli, W., Trampuz, A., and Ochsner, P. E. Prosthetic-joint infections. *N. Engl. J. Med.* 2004; 351(16): 1645–54.

Chapter

40

Spine Infections

Scott C. Sherman and Elena Strunk

Vertebral Osteomyelitis

Introduction

Pyogenic infections of the spine are most frequently caused by hematogenous spread. Other possible mechanisms are direct inoculation and local extension from a contiguous infection. Involved structures may include the vertebral body, intervertebral disk, spinal canal, or surrounding soft tissues. Because it is an uncommon disease, diagnosis of vertebral body osteomyelitis is often delayed, and late diagnosis may result in collapse of the vertebral body, kyphosis, and spinal instability that can lead to neurologic compromise.

Epidemiology and Microbiology

The spine is involved in 2 to 4% of all cases of osteomyelitis, with the lumbar region most frequently involved. The incidence of vertebral osteomyelitis has been increasing in recent years, thought to be due to an aging population. Vertebral osteomyelitis is most common in patients older than 50 years of age, though increasing incidence has been noted in younger patients who inject drugs. Risk factors include advanced age, intravenous drug use, recent urinary tract infection, trauma, or any immunocompromised state due to steroid use, malignancy, chronic illness, or liver disease.

Gram-positive organisms are responsible for the majority of cases, with *Staphylococcus aureus* reported as the causative organism in greater than 50% of cases. Vertebral infection by *Escherichia coli* and *Proteus* has been associated with preceding urinary tract infection, and infection by *Pseudomonas* has been reported in injection drug users. Diabetes mellitus or penetrating trauma may increase susceptibility to

anaerobic infection. Patients with sickle cell anemia are at risk for *Salmonella* osteomyelitis. *Staphylococcus epidermidis* and *Streptococcus viridans* cause infections characterized by an indolent course.

Clinical Features

Patients complain of axial back pain, insidious in onset and worsened by motion, which is constant and unrelieved by rest (see Table 40.1). Pain may be present for over 3 months and the patient may complain that it is unremitting and worse at night. Fever is not reliably present. The presentation is usually subacute or chronic in nature. On physical examination, the most common finding is exquisite tenderness to palpation of the affected area due to paraspinal muscle spasm. However, in contrast to those with simple musculoskeletal pain, patients with vertebral osteomyelitis will have percussion tenderness over the involved spinous process, with a sensitivity of 86% and specificity of 60%. Neurologic symptoms are uncommon on initial presentation. The earliest sign of spinal cord involvement is often clonus in the ankle.

Differential Diagnosis

Other conditions to consider are:

- epidural abscess
- neoplasm or metastatic disease
- osteoporotic vertebral compression fracture

Key features that may help to distinguish pyogenic vertebral osteomyelitis from tuberculous osteomyelitis are:

- history of recent travel or residence in tuberculosis-endemic areas

Table 40.1 Clinical Features: Vertebral Osteomyelitis

Incubation period	Weeks to months
Organisms	*Staphylococcus aureus* (most common)
	E. coli
	Proteus
	Pseudomonas
	Salmonella
	Staphylococcus epidermidis
	Streptococcus viridans
	Bartonella quintana
	Mycobacterium tuberculosis
	Histoplasma capsulatum
Signs and symptoms	Back pain
	Tenderness to palpation
	Loss of motion
	Pseudoscoliosis
	Fever (unreliable)
Laboratory and diagnostic findings	ESR and CRP elevated
	Plain radiographs show changes at 2–3 weeks. Initial osteolysis of the vertebral body may progress to disk space narrowing, end plate sclerosis, and vertebral body collapse
	MRI with gadolinium contrast shows hypointense signal on T1-weighted images and hyperintense signal on T2-weighted images within the vertebral body or disk
	Core needle biopsy
Treatment	Hold antibiotics until biopsy, unless absolutely necessary
	Cefazolin 2 g IV every 8 hours
	or
	Nafcillin 2 g IV every 6 hours
	or
	Vancomycin (for MRSA coverage) 15–20 mg/kg/dose IV every 8–12 hours with target trough 15–20 mg/L

CRP – C-reactive protein; ESR – erythrocyte sedimentation rate; IV – intravenous; MRI – magnetic resonance imaging; MRSA – methicillin-resistant *Staphylococcus aureus*.

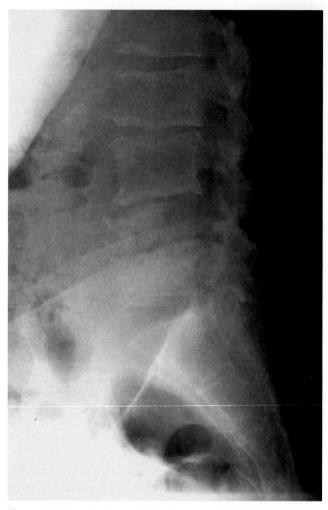

Figure 40.1 Lateral radiograph of the lumbar spine demonstrating destruction of the L4 and L5 vertebral bodies and intervening disk space from bacterial osteomyelitis.

- relative intervertebral disk space sparing in tuberculous osteomyelitis
- thoracic region involvement more frequent in tuberculous osteomyelitis

Laboratory and Radiographic Findings

Leukocytosis is usually absent, but the erythrocyte sedimentation rate (ESR) and C-reactive protein (CRP) are elevated in many cases. Blood cultures should be obtained, but are positive in only 40 to 60% of cases, though the yield may be better during febrile episodes. A purified protein derivative (PPD) test should be ordered along with an anergy test to rule out tuberculous osteomyelitis.

Plain radiographs should be part of the initial evaluation. Findings such as osteolysis of the vertebral body are non-specific and first appear 2 to 3 weeks after infection. Disk space narrowing and adjacent end plate sclerosis characterize more advanced disease that, if left untreated, progresses to eventual collapse of the vertebral body with local kyphosis (see Figure 40.1).

Magnetic resonance imaging (MRI) is the imaging study of choice in spinal infections because of its very high sensitivity, specificity, and accuracy. Osteomyelitis appears as areas of hypointense signal on T1-weighted images and hyperintense signal on T2-weighted images within the vertebral body or disk. Gadolinium contrast enables earlier detection as well as improving specificity (see Figure 40.2). Technetium-99 bone scan is highly sensitive, but because of its poor specificity should be limited to those cases in which MRI is contraindicated.

Core needle biopsy is essential because identification of the organism guides all future treatment. Biopsy should be performed under fluoroscopic or computed tomographic (CT) guidance. Yields as high as 70 to 100% have been reported, though more commonly it is lower, especially with non-*Staphylococcus* species. Because antibiotics have been shown to significantly decrease the yield rate, whenever possible they should be held until biopsy unless the patient is septic, critically ill, or develops a neurologic deficit. In cases where therapy has already been initiated, antibiotics should be held for 2 weeks

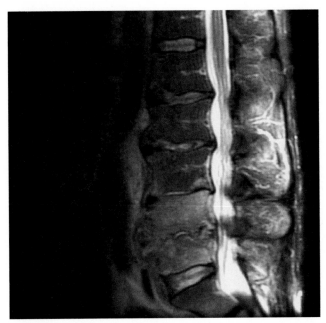

Figure 40.2 Sagittal T2-weighted MRI of the lumbar spine demonstrating destruction of the L4 and L5 vertebral bodies and the intervening disk space from bacterial osteomyelitis. The MRI corresponds to the plain radiograph in Figure 40.1.

prior to biopsy to maximize the likelihood that an organism will be isolated.

Treatment and Prophylaxis

The goals of treatment are to identify the organism and eradicate the infection, while maintaining spinal stability and a normal neurologic status. When patients are neurologically intact, non-operative treatment is successful in the majority of cases. However, patients are often debilitated and have significant comorbidities that contribute to a mortality rate as high as 5 to 15%. During the course of treatment, neurologic status must be carefully monitored. Intravenous antibiotics are administered for a minimum period of 6 to 8 weeks, usually 3 months. The duration of treatment is ultimately dictated by the patient's clinical progress.

Surgery is indicated when an open biopsy is necessary in order to identify an organism. Indications for surgical debridement also include clinically significant sepsis, failure of non-operative treatment, cord compression with neurologic deficit, and spinal deformity or instability. Non-operative treatment is deemed to have failed if symptoms, inflammatory markers, and imaging studies do not improve after 1 month of therapy. Surgical treatment most commonly consists of anterior debridement and fusion.

Special Considerations

Tuberculous Osteomyelitis of the Spine

Pott's disease is characterized by an indolent course with less severe back pain, longer duration of symptoms, and absence of fever. The spine is involved in more than 50% of tuberculous infections of bone. Patients are usually immigrants from

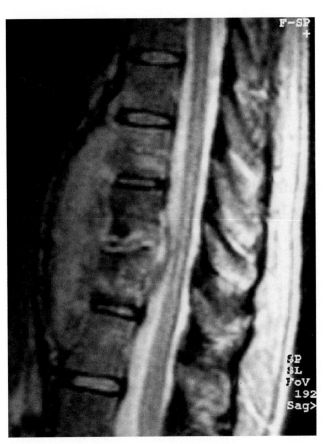

Figure 40.3 Sagittal MRI of the spine of a patient with tuberculosis of the spine. Notice the well-defined large anterior soft-tissue abscess. From: J. Griffith, S. M. Kumta, P. C. Leung, *et al.*, Imaging of musculoskeletal tuberculosis: a new look at an old disease. *Clin. Orthop.* 2002; 398: 32–9.

countries where the disease is endemic. Plain radiographs may show vertebral body destruction with relative sparing of the disk space, kyphosis, and a large soft-tissue mass with calcifications that is considered pathognomonic. MRI findings include a well-defined abscess with spreading anteriorly to adjacent levels (see Figure 40.3). The lesion may be confused with tumor. Treatment is with oral antibiotics consisting of isoniazid, rifampin, ethambutol, and pyrazinamide for the first 2 months, followed by a regimen based on sensitivities, usually isoniazid and rifampin, for an additional 8 to 10 months. Treatment may last up to 2 years. Surgery is indicated in the presence of a progressive kyphotic deformity or neurologic compromise (see Chapter 47, Tuberculosis).

Post-Operative Infection

Post-operative infections are becoming increasingly common as more spinal procedures are performed. Rates are historically higher than other orthopedic procedures. The most common organisms are *Staphylococcus aureus* and *Streptococcus epidermidis*. Instrumented fusion and staged surgery have been identified as independent risk factors. The most common presentation occurs during the second post-operative week, with wound discharge and dehiscence. Treatment is surgical irrigation and debridement with primary or delayed closure.

Complications and Admission Criteria

Complications include:

- collapse of vertebral body causing kyphotic deformity
- neurologic compromise
- extension of infection to adjacent structures
- bacteremia and sepsis

Admission is generally necessary, to perform a biopsy, identify the organism, and initiate intravenous antibiotic therapy.

Epidural Abscesses

Introduction

An epidural abscess usually develops in association with vertebral osteomyelitis. It can cause neurologic injury through mechanical compression of the neural elements and ischemic thrombosis of the spinal cord. In the presence of a neurologic deficit, it is considered a surgical emergency requiring urgent decompression. A delay in diagnosis can have devastating consequences, including permanent paraplegia.

Epidemiology

Epidural abscesses are estimated to occur in 0.2 to 2 cases per 10,000 hospital admissions and have been increasing over the past decade. Peak incidence is the sixth and seventh decade of life with a 2:1 male predominance. The lumbar spine is usually the affected region. *S. aureus* accounts for approximately 70% of epidural abscesses, followed by *Streptococcus* species, with 7% of cases.

Clinical Features

Presentation can be highly variable, and immunocompromised patients should be approached with a high index of suspicion. Patients usually present with a neurologic deficit and unremitting back pain that is not relieved by rest. Most are febrile. Symptoms progress from localized back pain and radiculopathy to motor weakness, bowel or bladder incontinence, and eventually complete paralysis. Physical examination should include assessment of perineal sensation and anal sphincter tone. A post-void residual urinary volume greater than 100 to 200 mL is indicative of retention. Straight leg raise maneuver may elicit radicular pain. Diminished reflexes are an early neurologic sign, with progression to hyperreflexia, clonus, and positive Babinski response (up-going toes). Risk factors for epidural abscess include any immunocompromised state secondary to diabetes mellitus, renal disease, alcoholism, human immunodeficiency virus (HIV), cancer, chronic steroid use, or sepsis; intravenous drug use; obesity; and trauma. Additional risk factors include recent spinal surgery or epidural injection.

Differential Diagnosis

Other conditions to consider are:

- vertebral osteomyelitis
- intra-abdominal or retroperitoneal abscess

Table 40.2 Clinical Features: Epidural Abscess

Organisms	*S. aureus* (most common)
	Streptococcus species
	After spinal procedure:
	S. aureus
	Coagulase-negative *Staphylococci*
	Gram-negative bacilli (including *Pseudomonas*)
	Aspergillus (after steroid injections)
	Immunocompromised host:
	Candida species
	Aspergillus species
	Cryptococcus neoformans
	Nocardia asteroids
	Mycobacterium tuberculosis
	Other mycobacteria
Signs and symptoms	Fever (60–80%)
	Focal vertebral pain
	Tenderness to percussion
	Radicular pain or paresthesias along involved nerve roots
	Evidence of spinal cord compression: motor weakness, bowel or bladder dysfunction, sensory changes, paralysis (possible depressed respiratory function if cervical cord involved)
Laboratory and diagnostic findings	Elevated WBC, ESR, and CRP
	Plain radiographs may show evidence of osteomyelitis
	MRI with gadolinium will demonstrate ring-enhancing lesion in epidural space with or without osteomyelitis
Treatment	Immediate broad-spectrum antibiotics
	Vancomycin 15–20 mg/kg IV every 8–12 hours *plus*
	Piperacillin-tazobactam 4.5 g IV every 6 hours
	Or, if penicillin allergy:
	Aztreonam 2 g IV every 8 hours
	Emergent surgical decompression

IV – intravenous; WBC – white blood (cell) count.

- cauda equina syndrome
- epidural hematoma
- disk herniation
- meningitis
- neoplasm
- cord infarction
- acute viral flaccid paralysis: West Nile virus, enterovirus 71

Laboratory and Radiographic Findings

Elevated white blood cell count, ESR, and CRP are common. Blood cultures may yield the organism in 60% of patients.

Plain radiographs should be assessed for evidence of vertebral osteomyelitis. MRI with gadolinium contrast is the study of choice and should be obtained emergently if epidural abscess is suspected. With addition of contrast, the abscess will appear as a ring-enhancing lesion and can be delineated from the neural elements (see Figure 40.4). Standard laboratory tests to order for epidural abscess are:

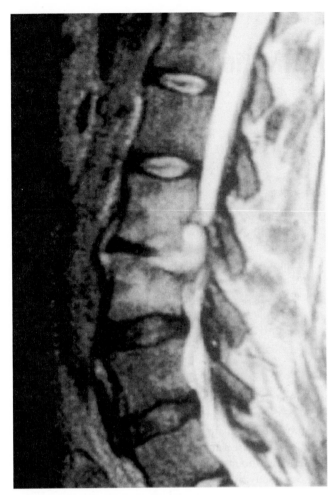

Figure 40.4 Sagittal MRI of the spine of a patient with an epidural abscess.

- white blood cell count (leukocytosis)
- ESR and CRP
- MRI with gadolinium

A proposed clinical decision guideline to increase the diagnostic accuracy for spinal epidural abscess suggests obtaining an emergent MRI in patients with spine pain and either:

- progressive neurologic deficits or
- fever, risk factors, static neurologic deficits, or radicular pain *and* elevated ESR or CRP

Treatment

Diagnosis of an epidural abscess should be followed immediately by the administration of broad-spectrum antibiotics with activity against *Staphylococcus* and *Streptococcus* with additional coverage for gram-negative organisms if there is a history of immune suppression. If neurologic compromise is present, treatment includes emergent surgical decompression and drainage of the abscess. Surgery is followed by long-term antibiotic therapy with at least 4 weeks of intravenous antibiotics. In patients with no neurologic deficit, percutaneous drainage of the epidural abscess has been reported to have good results. However, no neurologic recovery is expected in patient with paraplegia present for greater than 12 hours.

Complications and Admission Criteria

Complications and admission criteria include:

- cauda equine syndrome: paraplegia, sexual dysfunction, and bowel and bladder incontinence
- bacteremia and sepsis

Pearls and Pitfalls

1. Diagnosis of vertebral osteomyelitis is often delayed.
2. Antibiotics should be held until core needle biopsy is performed unless clinically necessary.
3. Neurologic status must be closely monitored over the course of antibiotic therapy.
4. The earliest sign of spinal cord involvement is ankle clonus.
5. Collapse of the vertebral body and local kyphosis seen in advanced disease may be confused for osteoporotic vertebral compression fracture.
6. Neurologic deficits at the initial presentation are only present in 30% of patients with spinal epidural abscess.
7. Permanent neurologic sequelae are common if the disease is allowed to progress without treatment.
8. Normal inflammatory markers (ESR and CRP) help exclude the diagnosis.
9. Lumbar puncture is contraindicated if epidural abscess is suspected.

References

An, H. S. and Seldomridge, J. A. Spinal infections: diagnostic tests and imaging studies. *Clin. Orthop.* 2006; 444: 27–33.

Bluman, E. M., Palumbo, M. A., and Lucas, P. R. Spinal epidural abscess in adults. *J. Am. Acad. Orthop. Surg.* 2004; 12(3): 155–63.

Davis, D. P., Salazar, A., Chan, T. C., *et al.* Prospective evaluation of a clinical decision guideline to diagnose spinal epidural abscess in patients who present to the emergency department with spine pain. *J. Neurosurg. Spine* 2011; 14(6): 765–70.

Della-Giustina, D. Evaluation and treatment of acute back pain in the emergency department. *Emerg. Med. Clin. N. Am.* 2015; 33(2): 311–26.

Fang, A., Hu, S. S., Endres, N., *et al.* Risk factors for infection after spinal surgery. *Spine* 2005; 30(12): 1460–5.

Kehrer, M., Pedersen, C., Jensen, T. G., *et al.* Increasing incidence of pyogenic spondylodiscitis: a 14-year population-based study. *J. Infect.* 2014; 68(4): 313–20.

Pradilla, G., Nagahama, Y., Spivak, A. M., *et al.* Spinal epidural abscess: current diagnosis and management. *Curr. Infect. Dis. Rep.* 2010; 12(6): 484–91.

Swanson, A. N., Pappou, I. P., Cammisa, F. P., *et al.* Chronic infections of the spine: surgical indications and treatments. *Clin. Orthop.* 2006; 444: 100–6.

Tay, B. K., Deckey, J., and Hu, S. S. Spinal infections. *J. Am. Acad. Orthop. Surg.* 2002; 10(3): 188–97.

Tompkins, M., Panuncialman, I., Lucas, P., *et al.* Spinal epidural abscess. *J. Emerg. Med.* 2010; 39(3): 384–90.

Weinstein, M. A., McCabe, J. P., and Cammisa, F. P., Jr. Postoperative spinal wound infection: a review of 2,391 consecutive index procedures. *J. Spinal Disord.* 2000; 13(5): 422–6.

Chapter

41

Conjunctival and Corneal Infections

Michelle Y. Peng and Saras Ramanathan

Introduction

Infections to the surface of the eye are common, and the consequences of misdiagnosis or delayed referral may be severe; therefore, familiarity with basic anatomy and presentations of these infections is crucial to the acute care provider. The conjunctiva is a well-vascularized, clear membrane that both envelops the anterior portion of the globe and wraps underneath the eyelids (see Figure 41.1). The conjunctiva, along with the tear film, provides a physical and immunologic barrier against microbes and can produce an antimicrobial environment when activated.

Just deep to the conjunctiva is the vascularized episclera, and beneath this the sclera, which lies just over the choroid. The choroid and the episclera provide oxygen to the poorly vascularized sclera.

The cornea itself is subject to inflammation, which can be due to non-infectious causes (non-infectious keratitis) or infectiou s causes (infectious keratitis, from bacteria, viruses, or fungi).

Conjunctivitis

Epidemiology and Microbiology

Conjunctivitis accounts for 1% of all primary care consultations and affects persons of all races. Its annual incidence is approximately 135 cases per 10,000 population. Adenovirus is the most common pathogen in children, followed by *S. pneumoniae*, *S. aureus*, and *Moraxella catarrhalis*. In adults, the most common bacterial pathogens include *S. aureus*, *H. influenzae*, *S. pneumoniae*, and *Moraxella* species.

Clinical Features

Inflammation of the conjunctiva or conjunctivitis is a common diagnosis and is separated into three categories: bacterial, viral,

and allergic (see Figure 41.2). While the patient will commonly present with red eye and discharge, the clinical history may also contribute greatly to the diagnosis (see Table 41.1).

In the acute care setting, a slit lamp examination of the eye is preferable, though not necessary, in suspected uncomplicated conjunctivitis. A careful pen light exam can suffice in ruling out a corneal opacity (which suggests keratitis). Visual acuity should be assessed.

Differential Diagnosis

- subconjunctival hemorrhage (history of trauma)
- dry eye syndrome
- blepharitis (inflammation of lid margins, sensation of grittiness)
- episcleritis (sectoral inflammation)
- scleritis (accompanied by dull ache, inflammation of deep scleral vessels, bluish discoloration of sclera)

Laboratory Findings

Cultures should be performed in all cases of neonatal conjunctivitis as *Neisseria* and chlamydia species may be present. Culture is otherwise not needed to confirm the diagnosis, except in the instance of chronic, recurrent, or severe disease. In these cases, Gram stain and culture may be useful.

Treatment and Prophylaxis

As a general rule, all contact lens wearers diagnosed with any ocular complaint should discontinue contact lens use until seen by an ophthalmologist. Suspected conjunctivitis is difficult to differentiate from bacterial keratitis in contact lens wearers, and should generally be treated with an anti-pseudomonal topical antibiotic, typically a fluoroquinolone.

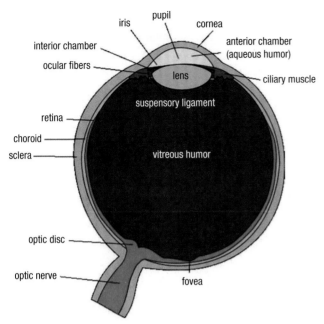

Figure 41.1 Eye anatomy. From http://en.wikipedia.org/wiki/Image:Schematic_diagram_of_the_human_eye_with_English_annotations.svg (accessed November 20, 2017), created by Erin Silversmith (August 30, 2006). Permission is granted to copy, distribute, and/or modify this document under the terms of the GNU Free Documentation License, Version 1.2 or any later version published by the Free Software Foundation; with no invariant sections, no front-cover texts, and no back-cover texts. A copy of the license is included in the section entitled "GNU Free Documentation License."

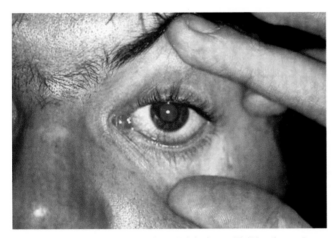

Figure 41.2 Conjunctivitis. From http://phil.cdc.gov/Phil/details.asp, Centers for Disease Control and Prevention/Joe Miller, 1976.

Viral conjunctivitis generally requires only supportive care, though topical antihistamines or decongestants as well as cool compresses and artificial tears may provide symptomatic relief.

Allergic conjunctivitis, if mild, may also be treated with artificial tears and cool compresses. If more severe, topical or systemic antihistamines may be considered. Avoidance of the underlying provoking substance will also improve the conjunctivitis.

Bacterial conjunctivitis may be self-limited, though antibiotic treatment will reduce the duration of symptoms by 2 to 5 days.

Complications and Admission Criteria

Hyperacute bacterial conjunctivitis (e.g. purulent discharge that reaccumulates after being wiped away) should raise concern for *Neisseria* species, especially *N. gonorrhoeae* (see Figure 41.3), which can be rapidly sight-threatening with corneal infection, scarring, and perforation, as well as other systemic sequelae. Evaluate for coexisting urethritis and cervicitis, though its absence does not exclude *Neisseria* conjunctivitis. Suspicion of this diagnosis necessitates immediate consultation with an ophthalmologist, and patients should receive intramuscular or intravenous ceftriaxone or cefotaxime. Patients should also undergo copious irrigation of purulent material.

In addition, more than 30% of patients with gonococcal conjunctivitis have coexisting chlamydial infection, thus concern for gonococcus should initiate empiric treatment for both infections. Isolated chlamydial infection may present with concomitant asymptomatic urogenital infection. This diagnosis may also be confirmed with direct fluorescent antibody staining or polymerase chain reaction (PCR) of conjunctival smears. Most clinicians, however, treat both empirically and do not routinely send for conjunctival smears for PCR. Coexisting chlamydial infection is treated with systemic antibiotic therapy such as azithromycin or doxycycline.

Keratitis

Epidemiology and Microbiology

Infectious keratitis (see Figures 41.4 and 41.5) is one of the most common preventable causes of blindness worldwide, and may be due to bacterial, viral, or fungal etiologies. There are an estimated 30,000 cases of bacterial keratitis annually in the United States alone. The most frequent risk factor in the United States is contact lens use, and is correlated with overnight wear, as well as days worn without removal. *Staphylococci* and gram-negative rods (*Pseudomonas*) were shown to be the most commonly isolated organisms. HSV keratitis, with a prevalence of 150 per 100,000 population, deserves attention because it has a high recurrence rate (~60% within 20 years). About 10 to 20% of patients will have recurrence within 1 year.

Non-infectious keratitis may present similarly and is due to mechanical (lid defects), neurologic (neurotrophic keratitis), immunologic (collagen vascular disease, sarcoidosis, rheumatoid arthritis, systemic lupus erythematosis), dermatologic (erythema multiforme, ocular rosacea), and traumatic (chemical, thermal injury; foreign bodies) causes.

Clinical Features

A detailed history is particularly relevant in the setting of keratitis. Risk factors that should be specifically sought out in the history include:

- contact lens practices (type of lens, solution, wear schedule, personal hygiene, swimming, hot tub use)
- previous ocular history, including HSV/VZV keratitis, previous bacterial keratitis, trauma, previous ocular history

Table 41.1 Clinical Features: Conjunctivitis

	Bacterial	Viral	Allergic
Predisposing factors	Neonates – vaginal delivery, inadequate prenatal care Children – contact with an affected individual; bacterial otitis media, sinusitis, pharyngitis, oculogenital spread from sexual abuse Adults – contact with affected individual; oculogenital spread; infection or abnormality of lid and its structures; immunosuppression; trauma	Exposure to affected individual (particularly in school setting); prior herpes infection; trigger for reactivation such as stress, acute illness, ultraviolet exposure, or trauma	History of environmental allergies or other atopic disease (eczema)
Signs and symptoms	Unilateral or bilateral Characterized by thick, purulent discharge throughout the day	Unilateral or bilateral (often sequential) – conjunctival injection, watery discharge, mild mucous Often preauricular lymphadenopathy	Bilateral – distinguished by itchiness, watery mucoid discharge Otherwise symptoms may be similar to those of viral conjunctivitis Patients may have history of other seasonal allergies or atopy
Organisms	*Chalmydia trachomatis* *Staphylococcus aureus* (more common in adults) *Streptococcus pneumoniae* *Haemophilus influenzae* *Moraxella catarrhalis* *Neisseria* (see Pearls and Pitfalls for further discussion)	Most common is adenovirus (many different strains), *herpes simplex* virus,* and picornavirus	No organisms involved; can be caused by perfume, cosmetics, drugs, other irritants

* Usually causes keratitis, but can cause conjunctivitis alone.

Table 41.2 Initial Therapy

Patient Category		Therapy Recommendation
Neonates	Chlamydia Gonococcus	• Erythromycin 50 mg/kg/day PO given in four divided doses for 14 days • Cefotaxime 100 mg/kg IM/IV × 1
Adults	Allergic Viral Bacterial	• Artificial tears, cool compresses • Oral antihistamines, allergen avoidance • Over-the-counter topical antihistamines/decongestants* • Artificial tears, most cases do not require antiviral treatment • Typically self-limited in immunocompetent patients, may consider topical therapy with: Erythromycin 0.5% opthalmic ointment 1 cm ribbon into affected eye(s) QID × 5 days Contact lens wearers should be covered for *Pseudomonas*: Ofloxacin 0.3% opthalmic drops: 1–2 drops into affected eye(s) × 5 days

* Decongestants should not be used long term as they can cause rebound hyperemia.

- other systemic medical conditions, immune status, systemic medications, history of drug-resistant infections
- current and recently used ocular medications

Contact-lens-related keratitis suggests a bacterial etiology. Herpes or varicella-zoster infection, particularly in the V1 distribution, should raise the specter of viral keratitis, as should an immunocompromised state. Trauma with plant material, ocular surface disease, and topical steroid use predispose patients to fungal infections. Table 41.3 summarizes the clinical features of keratitis.

Suspected keratitis generally warrants a full ophthalmologic exam with a slit lamp and consultation with an ophthalmologist. Visual acuity must be assessed. If photophobia is severe, ophthalmoplegic drops may be required prior to examination with a bright light. A corneal opacity is diagnostic of keratitis. Flourescein exam is used to evaluate for a corneal defect and dendrites. An associated hypopyon may be seen in the anterior chamber.

Depending on the type of keratitis, there may be distinguishing features. For example, varicella-zoster virus (VZV) and HSV keratitis are characterized with fluorescein exam by branching dendritic epithelial lesions and terminal bulbs at the tips of dendrite branches. VSV lesions typically have a fine and lacy appearance, with linear defects in epithelium; HSV lesions are described as "thick and ropy," with an epithelium that is elevated and appears "painted on."

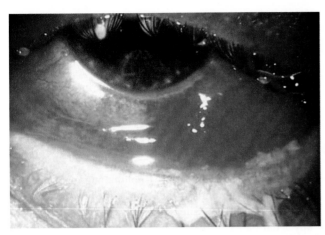

Figure 41.3 Gonorrheal conjunctivitis. From http://phil.cdc.gov/Phil/details.asp, Centers for Disease Control and Prevention, 1977.

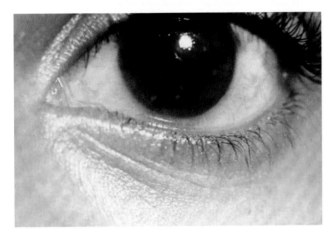

Figure 41.4 Keratitis. From http://phil.cdc.gov/Phil/details.asp, Centers for Disease Control and Prevention/Susan Lindsley, VD, 1973.

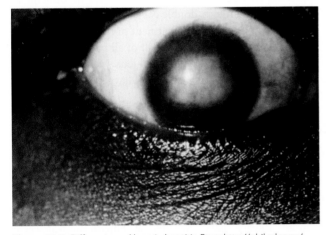

Figure 41.5 Diffuse stromal haze in keratitis. From http://phil.cdc.gov/Phil/details.asp, Centers for Disease Control and Prevention/Susan Lindsley, VD, 1973.

Table 41.3 Clinical Features: Keratitis

Organisms	**Bacteria:** *Staphylococcus aureus* *Staphylococcus epidermidis* *Streptococcus pneumoniae* and other *Streptococcus* spp. *Pseudomonas aeruginosa* (most common in soft contact lens wearers) Enterobacteriaceae (including *Proteus*, *Enterobacter*, and *Serratia*) **Viral:** *Herpes simplex* (HSV) Varicella–zoster (VZV) Epstein–Barr (EBV) Cytomegalovirus (CMV) Adenovirus **Fungal:** Filamentous fungi: *Fusarium Aspergillus Candida*
Signs and symptoms	Pain, redness, discharge, foreign body sensation, blurred vision, and photophobia Other accompanying signs of infectious keratitis visualized with a slit lamp may include: • Eyelid inflammation • Conjunctival edema, purulent discharge • Corneal epithelial defects, stromal infiltrates • Anterior chamber reaction, hypopyon
Laboratory and radiographic findings	No laboratory confirmation required; cultures should be taken in the setting of symptoms refractory to treatment or large central corneal infiltrates

- blepharitis – a disorder of the eyelids only
- conjunctivitis – should be limited to the conjunctiva only; no corneal infiltrate
- scleritis and episcleritis – scleral inflammation without corneal involvement
- uveitis – usually bilateral red eye, without corneal involvement
- non-infectious infiltrates – extended contact lens wear, systemic inflammatory disorders

Onchocerciasis ("river blindness") is endemic in many countries in Africa and is an infection from the parasite *Onchocerca volvulus*, transmitted by the black fly. The skin findings of dryness and depigmentation, along with subcutaneous nodules containing the worms, usually precede the ocular findings. The microfilariae can be identified within the skin and sometimes visualized in the anterior chamber. Blindness is caused by corneal inflammation and scarring. Treatment is one dose of ivermectin (150 micrograms/kg by mouth [PO]) and should be continued yearly.

In developing countries, there should also be a low threshold for suspicion of mycobacterial causes of keratitis (non-tuberculous mycobacteria such as *M. fortuitum* and *M. chelonae*, as well as *M. tuberculosis*).

Differential Diagnosis

Keratitis may have a similar presentation to a number of eye disorders, but there are ways to distinguish it from others based on a thorough history and physical:

Laboratory Findings

The diagnosis of bacterial keratitis, typically in a contact lens wearer, is based on history and physical and does not require laboratory confirmation. The majority (~95%) of cases of bacterial keratitis resolve with initial treatment. However, cases involving large central corneal infiltrates and those that do not respond promptly to treatment should undergo gram stain and culture with urgent ophthalmologic follow-up. Viral etiologies – HSV, VZV, Epstein–Barr virus (EBV), and cytomegalovirus (CMV) – may be diagnosed initially by history and physical, but corneal smears are recommended and can be sent for enzyme-linked immunosorbent assay (ELISA) antibodies, viral culture, or polymerase chain reaction. Situations involving unusual exposures such as vegetable matter or exposure to hot tubs suggest involvement of more atypical organisms and require culture, gram stain, and immediate referral.

Treatment and Prophylaxis

Duration of therapy depends on clinical response. Generally, an improvement in pain, discharge, stabilization of corneal infiltrate, and improved injection and edema should be seen within 48 hours or the treatment regimen should be adjusted.

In general, topical monotherapy with first-generation fluoroquinolones (e.g. ciprofloxacin, ofloxacin, levofloxacin) have been the mainstay of treatment, as they cover gram-negative bacteria, but patients at higher risk for gram-positive infection should be treated with a newer fluoroquinolone such as gatifloxacin or moxifloxacin. In the setting of severe infection, a regimen of cefazolin and tobramycin should be utilized, both of which should be in fortified doses (see Table 41.4). Systemic antibiotics are rarely used, as they achieve a low concentration within the avascular cornea. They should be provided, however, when the integrity of ocular structures have been violated (e.g. corneal perforation).

Viral keratitis generally does not always require treatment. *Herpes simplex* keratitis should be cared for by an ophthalmologist. Treatment generally consists of oral antiviral medication with or without topical antiviral drops. Patients with recurrent episodes may be given long-term prophylaxis.

Although steroids decrease the amount of inflammation and corneal precipitate, as a general rule, acute care providers should avoid prescribing steroid eye drops. In some cases (e.g. fungal and herpetic keratitis), steroids can exacerbate the infection, which can result in blindness.

Complications and Admission Criteria

A first-time diagnosis of keratitis does not require admission. However, patients who fail to respond to treatment and who have a high risk of visual loss should be referred urgently to an ophthalmologist for further care. Delayed diagnosis can be associated with rapidly progressing keratitis, with destruction of the cornea within 1 to 2 days. Additionally, patients with extenuating social situations such as a history of medical noncompliance should be admitted for treatment in order to prevent visual compromise.

Neonates suspected of having congenital HSV (80% of which is HSV-2 because it is transmitted from maternal genitalia) should be admitted. These patients require systemic antivirals.

Major complications of keratitis include:

- formation of scar tissue and neovascularization
- uneven healing of stroma that results in irregular astigmatism
- corneal perforation, potential loss of globe and vision
- acute retinal necrosis, particularly in the cases of VZV and HSV keratitis

Pearls and Pitfalls

1. For neonates, conjunctivitis ("ophthalmia neonatorum" within the first month of life) from either *N. gonorrhoeae* (usually 3 to 4 days after birth) or *C. trachomatis* (usually 7 days after birth) can be transmitted during passage through the birth canal. Neonatal conjunctivitis can lead to corneal ulceration and perforation, and can be associated with other localized or disseminated infections. *C. trachomatis* more commonly causes conjunctivitis in a neonate.

2. A red eye accompanied by high-risk findings, such as decreased visual acuity, a fixed pupil, corneal opacity, or photophobia, indicates that a more thorough evaluation for other retinal, neurological, or inflammatory etiologies should be undertaken.

3. Aminoglycoside ointment and drops should generally be avoided, as they can damage the corneal epithelium and, after multiple days of use, cause a reactive keratoconjunctivitis.

4. Topical vasoconstricting agents can cause rebound hyperemia with prolonged use. Antihistamine eyedrop formulations sometimes contain vasoconstricting agents. Patients should be advised not to use such medications for longer than 2 weeks.

5. One in five cases of fungal keratitis can be complicated with bacterial co-infection. Clinically, they can be difficult to distinguish; therefore, double coverage is warranted.

6. Have a low threshold for treatment of bacterial keratitis in contact lens wearers. Almost half of all patients diagnosed with bacterial keratitis are contact lens wearers.

7. Surgical procedures such as LASIK have made fungal etiologies more common in keratitis.

References

Acyclovir for the prevention of recurrent herpes simplex virus eye disease. Herpetic Eye Disease Study Group. *N. Engl. J. Med.* 1998; 339(5): 300–6.

Ahmed, I., Ai, E., Chang, E., and Luckie, A. Ophthalmic manifestations of HIV (University of California at San Francisco, HIV Insite, January 2006), available at http://hivinsite.ucsf.edu/InSite?page=kb-00&doc=kb-04–01–12 (accessed September 15, 2016).

American Academy of Ophthalmology Cornea/External Disease Panel. Preferred Practice Pattern® Guidelines. Conjunctivitis (San Francisco, CA: American Academy of Ophthalmology, 2013), available at www.aao.org/ppp (accessed November 20, 2017).

Cheng, K. H., Leung, S. L., Hoekman, H. W., *et al.* Incidence of contact-lens-associated microbial keratitis and its related morbidity. *Lancet* 1999; 354(9174): 181–5.

Table 41.4 Initial Therapy for Keratitis

Patient Category	Therapy Recommendation
Adults	**Bacterial keratitis:** • Commercially available topical fluoroquinolones: Ciprofloxacin 0.3% Gatifloxacin 0.5% Levofloxacin 0.5% Moxifloxacin 0.5% Ofloxacin 0.3% *or* Tobramycin (9–14 mg/mL) alternating with fortified cefazolin (50 mg/mL) – for severe, multi-organismal infections. Should be used in conjunction with an ophthalmologist. May not be available commercially and will need specialized pharmacy compounding. • Systemic antibiotics – should be used in conjunction with an ophthalmologist **Viral keratitis:** • HZV/VZV: Acyclovir 400 mg PO five times daily, for 7 days *or* Valacyclovir 500 mg PO BID, for 7 days • Herpes zoster ophthalmicus (HZO) and disseminated disease: Acyclovir 800 mg PO five times daily × 7 days *or* Valacyclovir 1,000 mg PO TID × 7 days **Fungal keratitis[‡]:** Natamycin 5% 1 drop into affected eye every 2 hours *plus* Voriconazole 400 mg PO BID × 1, then 200 mg PO BID
Children	**Bacterial keratitis:** Treatment generally follows that of adults **Viral keratitis:** • HSV[*] or VZV[†]: Systemic acyclovir: • <3 months: 20 mg/kg/dose IV every 8 hours; ≥3 months: 10 mg/kg/dose IV every 8 hours; **Fungal keratitis[‡]:** Treatment generally follows that of adults
Pregnant women	**Bacterial keratitis:** Treatment generally follows that of non-pregnant adults with the caveat that fluoroquinolone eye drops should be avoided when possible **Viral keratitis:** Treatment generally follows that of non-pregnant adults with the caveat that all systemic antiviral medications are pregnancy category B; all should be administered judiciously **Fungal keratitis[‡]:** Antifungals listed above in non-pregnant adults are pregnancy category C; all should be administered with caution
Immunocompromised	Same as for non-immunocompromised persons and children, but be aware that they may have a more fulminant and prolonged course of keratitis. IV antivirals are not needed for HIV patients with keratitis, with the exception of those who have acute retinal necrosis, uveitis, or cranial nerve involvement. If these infections are suspected (in HIV and non-HIV patients), ophthalmologic consult should be obtained urgently.

[*] If congenital HSV disease is suspected, these patients should be admitted and given systemic acyclovir therapy (see Complications and Admission Criteria).

[†] Systemic corticosteroids also seem to reduce the short-term symptoms of pain, though the long-term post-herpetic neuralgia has not been definitively shown. Because of this, and the risk of further suppressing the immune system, only patients who have low risk of immunocompromise and who are in severe pain should be considered for this therapy.

[‡] Should only be used in conjunction with ophthalmologist; oral antifungals may also be recommended along with topical antifungals depending on response. *DO NOT USE TOPICAL OR ORAL STEROIDS WITH FUNGAL INFECTIONS.*

HIV – human immunodeficiency virus; IV – intravenous.

Galindez, O. A., Sabates, N. R., Whitacre, M. M., *et al.* Rapidly progressive outer retinal necrosis caused by varicella zoster virus in a patient with human immunodeficiency virus. *J. Infect. Dis.* 1996; 22(1): 149–51.

Goldstein, D. A. and Tessler, H. H. Episcleritis, Scleritis, and other scleral disorders in M. Yanoff, J. S. Duker, J. J. Augsburger, *et al.* (eds.), *Ophthalmology* (St. Louis. MO: Mosby, 2004), pp. 512–18.

Green, M., Apel, A., and Stapleton, F. Risk factors and causative organisms in microbial keratitis. *Cornea* 2008; 27(1): 22–7.

Jacobs, D. S. Conjunctivitis. *UpToDate*, available at www.uptodate .com/contents/conjunctivitis (accessed November 20, 2017).

Keay, L., Edwards, K., Naduvilath, T., *et al.* Microbial keratitis predisposing factors and moribidy. *Ophthalmology* 2006; 113(1): 109–16.

McLeod, S. L. Infectious keratitis in M. Yanoff, J. S. Duker, J. J. Augsburger, *et al.* (eds.), *Ophthalmology* (St. Louis. MO: Mosby, 2004), pp. 466–91.

Morrow, G. L. and Abbot, R. L. Conjunctivitis. *Am. Fam. Physician* 1998; 57(4): 735–46, available at www.aafp.org/afp/980600ap/ carter.html (accessed November 20, 2017).

Rietveld, R. P., ter Riet, G., Bindels, P. J., *et al.* Predicting bacterial cause in infectious conjunctivitis: cohort study on informativeness of combinations of signs and symptoms. *BMJ* 2004; 329(7459): 206–10.

Rose, P. W., Harnden, A., Brueggemann, A. B., *et al.* Chloramphenicol treatment for acute infective conjunctivitis in children in primary care: a randomised double-blind placebo-controlled trial. *Lancet* 2005; 366(9479): 37–43.

Sellitti, T. P., Huang, A. J., Schiffman, J., and Davis, J. L. Association of herpes zoster ophthalmicus with acquired immunodeficiency syndrome and acute retinal necrosis. *Am. J. Ophthalmol.* 1993; 116(3): 297–301.

Sheikh, A. and Hurwitz, B. Antibiotics versus placebo for acute bacterial conjunctivitis. *Cochrane Database Syst. Rev.* 2006; 2: CD001211.

Smith, A. F. and Waycaster, C. Estimate of the direct and indirect annual cost of bacterial conjunctivitis in the United States. *BMC Ophthalmol.* 2009; 9: 13.

Tullo, A. B. Clinical and epidemiological features of adenovirus keratoconjunctivitis. *Trans. Ophthalmol. Soc. UK* 1980; 100: 263–7.

Periocular Infections

Kareem Moussa and Saras Ramanathan

Introduction

The eyelid is the first line of defense for the eye. An understanding of the anatomy, structure, and function of the various components of the eyelid is necessary for the proper diagnosis and management of periocular infections and mimickers of periocular infections, some of which may be life-threatening conditions.

A cross section of the eyelid shows that the eyelid is composed of four basic structures (see Figure 42.1). From anterior to posterior, these structures are: skin, orbicularis oculi, tarsus, and conjunctiva. The skin of the eyelid is the thinnest of the entire body and has no subcutaneous fat layer. It also serves as a physical barrier against infection. The orbicularis oculi muscle, innervated by the facial nerve, narrows the palpebral fissure, the space between the upper and lower eyelids, when it contracts. Patients with seventh nerve palsies are at increased risk of corneal exposure and corneal infections due to paresis of the orbicularis oculi muscle and decreased eyelid closure (see Chapter 41, Conjunctival and Corneal Infections). The tarsus, a dense connective tissue that provides structural support to the eyelid, is immediately posterior to the orbicularis oculi muscle. Another muscle, the levator palpebrae muscle, inserts into the superior border of the tarsus. Deriving its innervation from the oculomotor nerve, the levator palpebrae muscle elevates the eyelid. The posterior surface of the eyelid is lined by conjunctiva, a vascularized, transparent mucous membrane, with a key protective role mediating both passive and active immunity.

Superior to the tarsus in the upper eyelid is the orbital septum, a dense fibrous sheath that functions as a barrier between the eyelid and the orbit.

Additional clinically relevant structures of the eyelid include the eyelashes, glands of Zeis, and meibomian glands. There are approximately 100 eyelashes in the upper eyelid, and 50 in the lower eyelid, originating just anterior to the tarsus, and forming two to three rows. The glands of Zeis are modified sebaceous glands associated with eyelash follicles. The meibomian glands are modified sebaceous glands located within the tarsus. They synthesize and secrete lipids, an essential component of the tear film. There are approximately 25 meibomian glands in the upper eyelid and 20 in the lower eyelid. As discussed later in this chapter, infectious and non-infectious processes commonly involve the meibomian glands and the glands of Zeis.

The anatomy of the lacrimal drainage system is intricately tied to that of the eyelid (see Figure 42.2). An understanding of the anatomy of the lacrimal system is crucial to properly differentiate among the various infections that can arise within this system. Drainage of tears begins within the puncta, which are located at the posterior edge of the medial upper and lower eyelids, at the junction of the eyelash-bearing (lateral five-sixths) and non-eyelash-bearing (medial one-sixth) eyelid. The natural flow of tears is into the puncta, through the canaliculi, which pass vertically from the lid margin for 2 mm, then turn medially and pass horizontally for 8 mm, and empty into the lacrimal sac, which is approximately 10 to 12 mm long

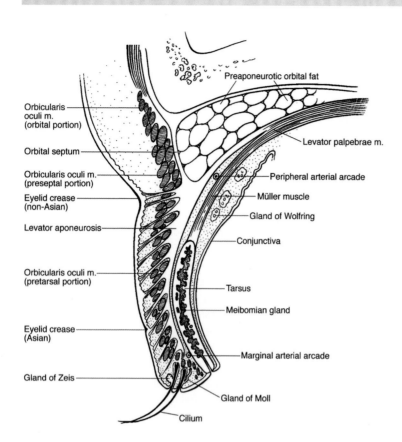

Figure 42.1 Cross section of the upper eyelid.
Permission for use obtained from American Academy of Ophthalmology, San Francisco, CA.

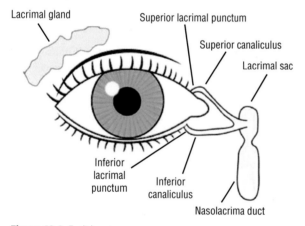

Figure 42.2 Eyelid anatomy.
Adapted from drawing by Felipe Micaroni Lalli.

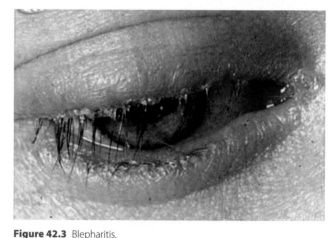

Figure 42.3 Blepharitis.
Courtesy of Professor J. Wollensak, Atlas of Ophthalmology, www.atlasophthalmology.com.

and lies in the lacrimal fossa between the anterior and posterior lacrimal crests. Tears then travel down the nasolacrimal duct, approximately 12 to 18 mm long, and pass by the valve of Hasner, a mucosal fold at the distal end of the nasolacrimal duct, to empty through the inferior nasal meatus, below the inferior turbinate. Obstructions of this delicate system can lead to infection.

Blepharitis

Epidemiology and Microbiology

Blepharitis (see Figure 42.3) is a common cause of ocular irritation. It is usually bilateral, and affects women more than men. It typically presents between the ages of 40 and 50 years old, and is more common in those with fair skin. Blepharitis can be divided into anterior blepharitis and posterior blepharitis. There is often overlap between the two, and poor correlation between signs and symptoms can make management challenging.

Anterior blepharitis is an inflammatory process involving the bases of the eyelashes. It may be infectious (typically due to *Staphylococcus aureus*) or non-infectious (seborrheic). Patients with seborrheic blepharitis often have seborrheic dermatitis that may involve the scalp and nasolabial folds.

Posterior blepharitis is caused by dysfunction of the meibomian glands. While the exact mechanism is unknown, bacterial lipases may result in the formation of free fatty acids, which increase the melting point of the lipids synthesized by the meibomian glands and prevent its expression from the glands, leading to instability of the tear film and ocular irritation.

Clinical Features

Table 42.1 summarizes the clinical features of blepharitis. Differentiating between the different types of blepharitis is difficult; fortunately, it is typically not necessary for management purposes.

Table 42.1 Clinical Features: Blepharitis

Organisms	*Staphylococcus aureus* *Coagulase-negative staphylococcus*
Signs and symptoms	• usually bilateral and intermittent symptoms • inflamed eyelid margins • eyelid itching, burning, or soreness • mild foreign-body sensation • crusting and debris of eyelid margins, especially on awakening • with or without misdirection or loss of eyelashes • with or without conjunctival injection • with or without swollen eyelids • with or without light sensitivity
Laboratory and radiographic findings	There are no specific laboratory tests or radiographic findings for blepharitis. It is possible to do a microbial culture of the eyelid by swabbing the eyelashes, but this is usually not necessary.

Differential Diagnosis

Blepharitis is usually fairly straightforward to diagnose. However, a broad initial differential can avoid misdiagnosis:

- Orbital cellulitis is distinguished from blepharitis by the presence of more systemic symptoms, tender sinuses, and sometimes limited extraocular movements.
- Squamous cell, basal cell, or sebaceous cell carcinoma of the eyelid are rare, but can be missed in those diagnosed with chronic blepharitis; biopsy in these cases can be helpful.
- Viral or bacterial conjunctivitis usually affects the conjunctiva more than the eyelid itself.
- Dry eye syndrome often is associated with blepharitis.
- Chalazia (chronic granulomatous, inflammatory lesions) are painless when palpated.
- Ocular *herpes simplex* usually presents as a painful red eye and will manifest dendrites on fluorescein staining.
- *Herpes zoster ophthalmicus* entails inflammation of the conjunctiva and/or cornea and less of the eyelid itself.
- Molluscum contagiosum is characterized by dome-shaped, umbilicated shiny nodules on the eyelid that are usually non-tender.
- Crab lice (infestation with *Phthirus pubis*) may also be in other places on the body.

Treatment and Prophylaxis

Eyelid hygiene is extremely important (e.g. washing eyelids and eyelashes with diluted baby shampoo, eyelid cleanser) (see Table 42.2). Clean, warm compresses at the onset of symptoms may limit severity. Those with dry eyes can be given artificial tears (e.g. hypromellose 0.3%). Many cases

Table 42.2 Treatment of Blepharitis

Patient Category	Therapy Recommendations
Adults: preferred choices	• **Warm compresses.** Apply warm compresses to the eyelids for several minutes to soften adherent scurf or discharge and warm meibomian gland secretions. The warm compress may consist of a clean cloth soaked in hot tap water, or a bag of rice or gel pack heated in a microwave. The compress should not be too hot as it may burn the thin eyelid skin. Vertical massage of the eyelid may help with meibomian gland secretion expression. • **Eyelid cleansing.** Gently cleanse the eyelashes using diluted baby shampoo or commercially available eyelid cleansers using a pad, cotton ball, cotton swab, or clean fingertip. • Once- or twice-daily compresses and massage, as well as regular eyelid cleansing (daily or several times weekly) is generally adequate for symptomatic control. • A **topical antibiotic ointment** such as bacitracin or erythromycin can be applied topically to the eyelid margins one or more times daily, or at bedtime, for a few weeks. For those unresponsive to these ointments, metronidazole gel is an alternative treatment. The frequency and duration of treatment depends on the severity of disease and response to treatment. • **Tetracyclines** have been shown to decrease bacterial lipase production and demonstrated efficacy in the treatment of meibomian gland dysfunction. Oral doxycycline or minocycline 100 mg can be given daily, to be tapered to 40 to 50 mg daily after clinical improvement is noted (usually 2–6 weeks). Alternatively, oral erythromycin (250–500 mg daily) or azithromycin (250–500 mg, one to three times a week, or 1 g per week for three weeks) may be used. Treatment can be intermittently discontinued and restarted based on the severity of symptoms and medication tolerance. • **Omega 3-fatty acid supplementation** (two 1,000 mg capsules three times a day) has been shown to improve symptoms in some patients. • A brief course of **topical corticosteroid** such as fluorometholone twice daily may help improve symptoms. Referral to an ophthalmologist is indicated in such cases, as topical steroids can have adverse effects, such as intraocular pressure elevation. • **Artificial tears** may improve symptoms in cases of aqueous tear deficiency. If artificial tears are used more than four times per day, non-preserved tears should be used to avoid preservative toxicity.

PO – by mouth.

Table 42.3 Clinical Features: Chalazia and Hordeola

Organisms	**Chalazia:** No organisms (sterile) **Hordeola:** *Staphylococcus aureus* Coagulase-negative *Staphylococcus*
Signs and symptoms	Hordeola tend to present more acutely and more painful than chalazia. Otherwise, both present as visible, palpable, subcutaneous nodules, often with swelling and/or tenderness.
Laboratory and radiographic findings	Not indicated unless there is concern for a malignant process masquerading as a chalazion. Chalazion biopsy reveals lipogranulomatous inflammation.

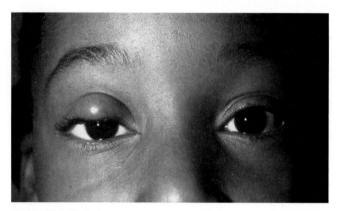

Figure 42.4 Chalazion.
Permission for use obtained from American Academy of Ophthalmology, San Francisco, CA.

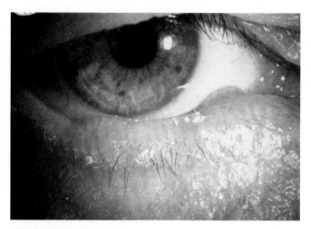

Figure 42.5 Hordeolum.
Courtesy of Professor J. Wollensak, Atlas of Ophthalmology, www.atlasophthalmology.com.

of blepharitis will resolve without antibiotic (topical or systemic) treatment.

Chalazia and Hordeola

Epidemiology and Microbiology

Chalazia (see Figure 42.4) and hordeola (see Figure 42.5) present as cystic masses involving the eyelid. A chalazion is a focal area of inflammation within the eyelid due to an obstructed meibomian gland or gland of Zeis. Chalazia are sterile. A hordeolum is an infection of a meibomian gland (also called "inernal hordeolum") or gland of Zeis (also called "external hordeolum"). The most common pathogen is *Staphylococcus aureus*.

Chalazia and hordeola can present at any age. They are more commonly encountered in patients with meibomian gland disease and rosacea. It is prudent not to misdiagnose sebaceous cell carcinoma as a recurrent chalazion, as they may present similarly. If there is any doubt, the lesion should be biopsied.

Clinical Features

Table 42.3 summarizes the clinical features of chalazia and hordeola.

Differential Diagnosis

- preseptal cellulitis tends to be more diffuse and less nodular; a hordeolum can evolve into a preseptal cellulitis

- sebaceous cell carcinoma can be mistaken for a recurrent chalazion
- pyogenic granuloma is a benign lesion often associated with prior trauma or surgery

Treatment and Prophylaxis

Most chalazia and hordeola will resolve with medical management:

- Warm compresses with massage over the lesion four times daily for 10 minutes.
- If there is drainage, consider a topical antibiotic such as bacitracin or erythromycin ointment twice daily. Oral doxycycline 100 mg twice daily can also be considered for its antibacterial and anti-inflammatory effect.
- If a hordeolum evolves into a preseptal cellulitis, treat with systemic antibiotics as discussed later in this chapter.
- If medical management fails, refer to an ophthalmologist for consideration of incision and curettage of the lesion. For a persistent chalazion, a steroid injection can also be considered (0.2 to 1.0 mL of triamcinolone 40mg/mL).

Dacryocystitis

Epidemiology and Microbiology

Dacryocystitis (see Figure 42.6) is an inflammation of the lacrimal sac. It can be either congenital or acquired. Congenital

Table 42.4 Clinical Features: Dacryocystitis

Organisms	Usually due to streptococci (including *Streptococcus pneumoniae*) or *Staphylococcus aureus*
Signs and symptoms	• Pain, swelling, and erythema over inner aspect of lower eyelid • Commonly presents in adults as periorbital cellulitis • Excessive tearing • With or without fever • Tenderness in medial canthal region
Laboratory and radiographic findings	As in many of these disorders, this is a clinical diagnosis. Other laboratory or imaging modalities may be used to rule out other diseases (e.g. CT scan for mass as a cause of dacryocystitis).

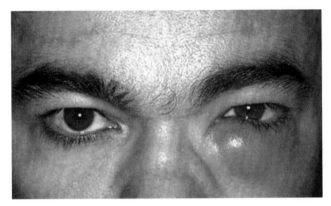

Figure 42.6 Dacryocystitis.
Courtesy of Professor Georg Michelson, Atlas of Ophthalmology, www.atlasophthalmology.com.

dacryocystitis is related to the embryogenesis of the lacrimal excretory system. The lower end of the nasolacrimal duct (valve of Hasner) is the last to canalize. Approximately 20% of neonates have excess tearing due to delayed canalization; however, spontaneous resolution occurs in over 90% of cases within the first year of life. Neonates with an imperforate valve of Hasner are at increased risk of developing nasolacrimal duct obstruction and subsequent dacryocystitis.

Acquired dacryocystitis in adults is also usually secondary to nasolacrimal duct obstruction, which is typically idiopathic, but can be due to malignancy. Those at higher risk for acquired dacryocystitis include females, those with flatter noses and narrower faces, and age greater than 40. African Americans seem to have a low risk of dacryocystitis.

Dacrocystitis is usually caused by Streptococcal species, *S. aureus* and *S. epidermidis*.

Clinical Features

Table 42.4 summarizes the clinical features of dacryocystitis.

Differential Diagnosis

• Dacryocystocele is an enlargement of a non-inflamed lacrimal sac due to nasolacrimal duct obstruction secondary to an imperforate valve of Hasner.
• Canaliculitis typically presents as unilateral tearing with chronic mucopurulent conjunctivitis. There is no nasolacrimal sac distention or inflammation. Often, concretions consisting of sulfur granules can be expressed on canalicular massage. Canaliculitis is frequently caused by *Actinomyces israelii*.
• Chalazion.
• Orbital or preseptal cellulitis.
• Ethmoid sinusitis.
• Consider congenital encephalocele in a neonate and lacrimal sac tumor in an adult if there is involvement above the medial canthus.

Treatment and Prophylaxis

Obtain a gram stain and culture of any discharge to help guide antibiotic therapy. Afebrile adults and children can be managed as outpatients with appropriate antibiotics (see Table 42.5). Febrile, ill-appearing patients should be admitted for IV antibiotics. Consider probing and irrigation after the infection resolves. Do not irrigate the lacrimal system during an acute infection. This can be considered if medical management fails and requires referral to an ophthalmologist. Adults often require surgical correction following resolution of the infection (dacryocystorhinostomy).

Complications and Admission Criteria

Patients who are febrile and appear acutely ill should be hospitalized for IV antibiotics and possible surgical management as mentioned above. Dacryocystitis can progress to orbital cellulitis and has been reported to lead to orbital abscess as well as cavernous sinus thrombosis.

Periorbital and Orbital Cellulitis
Epidemiology and Microbiology

Orbital and periorbital (or preseptal) cellulitis are commonly encountered problems in the acute care setting. Periorbital cellulitis arises from minor skin trauma, insect bites, and underlying sinusitis and dacrocystitis, and less commonly from bacteremia. Consequently, the common pathogens are *S. aureus*, beta-hemolytic streptococci, and *S. pneumoniae*. Methicillin-resistant *S. aureus* (MRSA) has emerged as a causitive pathogen. Orbital cellulitis is usually due to underlying sinusitis and the common pathogens are *S. aureus*, *Streptococcus pyogenes*, and pneumococcus. *Streptococcus anguinosus*, an oral commensal, was a common isolate in a recent case series. Fungal pathogens (*Mucormycosis* and others) are the cause of highly aggressive orbital cellulitis in immunocompromised adults.

Table 42.5 Treatment of Dacryocystitis

Patient Category	Therapy Recommendations
Adults	**Mild disease, afebrile:** Augmentin 875/125 mg PO BID for 7 days *or* Clindamycin 300 mg PO TID for 7 days **Acutely ill or febrile:** • Hospitalization and IV antibiotics Ceftriaxone 1 g IV every 24 hours *plus* Vancomycin 15–20 mg/kg/dose IV every 8–12 hours
Children	**Mild disease, afebrile:** Amoxicillin/clavulanate 45 mg/kg/day of amoxicillin component PO in two divided doses for 7 days *or* Clindamycin 10 mg/kg/dose PO TID for 7 days **Acutely ill or febrile:** • Hospitalization and IV antibiotics Vancomycin 15 mg/kg/dose IV every 6 hours *plus* Cefotaxime 50 mg/kg/dose IV every 8 hours Infectious disease consultation
Adults and children	• Apply warm compresses and massage to the medial canthal region QID. • Administer pain medication. • Topical antibiotic drops can be used in addition to systemic therapy, but their use alone is not adequate. • Antibiotic treatment choice should be guided by culture results. • A treatment course of 7–10 days is usually sufficient.

Table 42.6 Clinical Features: Periorbital and Orbital Cellulitis

	Periorbital (Preseptal)	Orbital (Postseptal)
Etiology	Trauma, bacteremia	Sinusitis
Organisms	**Trauma:** *Staphylococcus aureus* (including MRSA) Group A *Streptococcus* **Bacteremia:** *Streptococcus pneumoniae*	*Streptococcus pneumoniae* *Staphylococcus aureus* Group A *Streptococcus* Anaerobes Fungi, including mucormycosis (*Haemophilus influenzae* no longer predominant in post-vaccination era)
Mean age	<2 years	12 years
Clinical findings	• Erythema and induration of periorbital tissues • Tenderness of periorbital tissues • Generally less toxic-appearing (unless bacteremic)	Same symptoms as periorbital cellulitis, but may also have: • proptosis • conjunctival edema or chemosis • ophthalmoplegia • decreased visual acuity • increased intraocular pressure • headache

Periorbital cellulitis is much more common than orbital cellulitis. Both periorbital and orbital cellulitis are more prevalent in children than adults, with incidence of periorbital cellulitis peaking in younger children (3 to 36 months of age).

Clinical Features

Table 42.6 summarizes the clinical features that distinguish these two disorders from each other. Distinguishing periorbital cellulitis from orbital cellulitis is difficult. At times, periorbital cellulitis may appear worse than orbital cellulitis, as in Figure 42.7 (periorbital cellulitis caused by a mucormycosis fungal infection in an immunosuppressed patient) and Figure 42.8 (orbital cellulitis caused by *Staphylococcus aureus*).

Differential Diagnosis

Other diagnoses to consider besides orbital and periorbital cellulitis are:

• cavernous sinus thrombosis: usually accompanied by headache and, in later stages, by severe gaze palsies and other eye findings

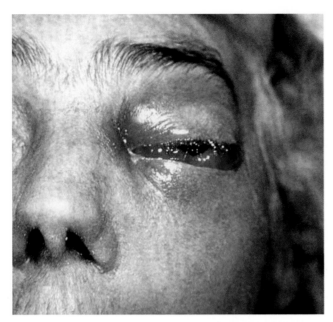

Figure 42.7 Periorbital cellulitis caused by mucormycosis.
From http://phil.cdc.gov/Phil/details.asp, Centers for Disease Control and Prevention/Dr. Thomas F. Sellers/Emory University, 1960.

- neoplasms (e.g. neuroblastoma, rhabdomyosarcoma, retinoblastoma): typically less systemic symptoms
- endocrinopathies (e.g. thyroid ophthalmopathy): usually less erythema, swelling, and tenderness
- hordeolum/blepharitis: generally confined to eyelid margin
- conjunctivitis: normally confined to conjunctiva and less periorbital erythema and swelling

Other presentations of rare disorders include:

- orbital pseudotumor
- periocular dermoid cyst
- granulomatosis with polyangiitis

Laboratory and Radiographic Findings

There are no definitive laboratory tests for periorbital and orbital cellulitis. Blood cultures are generally recommended in the pediatric population, where up to one-third of patients may have positive cultures, as well as in febrile adults. Cultures of eye secretions may be confusing because of contaminants; in general, such cultures should not be used to narrow antibiotic therapy, but rather to identify possible antibiotic-resistant organisms. The most specific cultures are from sinus contents or abscess material if surgically drained.

Because most cases of periorbital and orbital cellulitis occur in children, the decision to proceed with imaging is generally based on clinical exam. In children where vision cannot be accurately assessed, the threshold for imaging should be lowered. Furthermore, even if orbital involvement seems certain on exam, imaging may help direct surgical drainage.

High-resolution CT scanning is considered modality of choice to distinguish periorbital from orbital cellulitis, as well as to evaluate other competing diagnoses. Axial and coronal

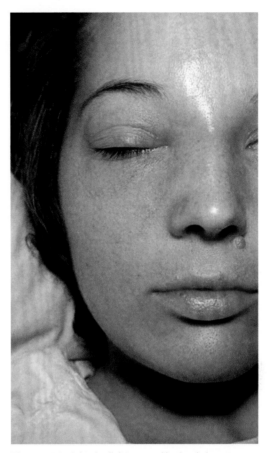

Figure 42.8 Orbital cellulitis caused by *Staphylococcus aureus*.
From http://phil.cdc.gov/Phil/details.asp, Centers for Disease Control and Prevention/Dr. Thomas F. Sellers/Emory University, 1963.

views are necessary: the former to evaluate for brain abscess in the parenchyma, and the latter for any subperiorbital processes. Magnetic resonance imaging (MRI) can also be used, but is less available and more difficult to perform in the pediatric population because it requires a longer imaging time.

Orbital ultrasonography is also used in some institutions, but is extremely operator dependent. This modality is useful for sequential follow-up of abscesses and in children where the sedation necessary for CT or MRI is contraindicated.

Treatment and Prophylaxis

Although children with periorbital cellulitis were previously hospitalized for observation, the trend is toward outpatient management with close follow-up for patients who do not appear toxic. There are a number of suggested regimens that target the usual causative pathogens, including MRSA, with duration of treatment for 7 to 10 days as shown in Table 42.7.

All patients with suspected orbial cellulitis are treated with IV antibiotics for 1 week (or until afebrile and clinically improved). Patients with periorbital cellulitis who are less than 1 year of age or toxic-appearing should be treated for orbital cellulitis. There is limited data regarding the optimal duration of therapy, and the most conservative recommendation is for outpatient antibiotics for 2 to 3 weeks after clinical improvement

Table 42.7 Treatment and Prophylaxis for Periorbital and Orbital Cellulitis

Patient Category	Therapy Recommendations
Adults: preferred choices	**For periorbital cellulitis:** Clindamycin 300 mg PO TID *or* TMP/SMX DS one to two tabs. PO BID *plus* Amoxicillin 875 mg PO BID *or* Amoxicillin/clavulanate 875 mg PO BID *or* Cefpodoxime 400 mg PO BID *or* Cefdinir 300 mg PO BID **For orbital cellulitis:** • For empiric treatment or polymicrobial infection: Vancomycin 15–20 mg/kg/dose IV every 8–12 hours *plus* Piperacillin-tazobactam 4.5 g IV every 6 hours *or* Ceftriaxone 2 g IV every 24 hours (every 12 hours if intracranial extension is suspected) *or* Cefotaxime 2 g IV every 4 hours
Children: preferred choices	**For periorbital cellulitis:** Clindamycin 30–40 mg/kg/day PO in three to four equally divided doses, not to exceed 1.8 g per day *or* TMP/SMX 8–12 mg/kg/day of the TMP component PO divided every 12 hours *plus* Amoxicillin 45–100 mg/kg/day PO in divided doses every 12 hours (higher dosing for severe infection) *or* Amoxicillin/clavulanate 45–90 mg/kg/day of the amoxicillin component PO divided every 12 hours (higher dosing for severe infection) *or* Cefpodoxime 10 mg/kg/day PO divided every 12 hours in those 12 years of age or younger; 400 mg PO every 12 hours in those older than 12 years of age *or* Cefdinir 7 mg/kg/dose PO twice daily (maximum daily dose 600 mg) **For orbital cellulitis:** • For empiric treatment or polymicrobial infection: Vancomycin 15 mg/kg/dose IV every 6 hours *plus* Piperacillin-tazobactam 80 mg/kg/dose of the piperacillin component IV every 6 hours, maximum of 4 g per dose *or* Ceftriaxone 50 mg/kg/dose IV every 24 hours (twice per day if intracranial extension is suspected), maximum 2 g per dose *or* Cefotaxime 50 mg/kg/dose IV every 6 hours, maximum 2 g per dose
Pregnant women	Same as for non-pregnant adults, as all recommended drugs in the table are pregnancy category B. The only exception is for MRSA coverage, where vancomycin is pregnancy category C. In cases where MRSA is highly suspected and/or culture results identify MRSA, the risks of a spreading orbital cellulitis would warrant use of vancomycin, but recommendation is to consult infectious disease service as well.
Immunocompromised	Same as for non-immunocompromised persons and children, but awareness that other infections (particularly fungal causes) could be present as well. Initial treatment would be the same, but additional fungal cultures should be sent if fungal causes are suspected and then treated with amphotericin B.

DS – double strength; IV – intravenous; MRSA – methicillin-resistant *Staphylococcus aureus*; TMP/SMX – trimethoprim–sulfamethoxazole.

from intravenous antibiotics, though many clinicians may choose not to prescribe such a long duration of therapy.

Failure to respond to IV antibiotics warrants repeat imaging and possible surgical drainage.

Complications and Admission Criteria

Any patient with suspected orbital cellulitis should be admitted for IV antibiotics and observation. Complications include subperiostial abscess, orbital abscess, extraorbital extension, including cavernous sinus thrombosis and brain abscess, and blindness. Untreated orbital cellulitis can be fatal in up to 17% of patients and lead to blindness in the affected eye of approximately 20% of patients. With proper treatment of orbital cellulitis, the rate of visual loss is still 3 to 10% and mortality 1 to 2%. Permanent vision loss can occur from orbital cellulitis by two mechanisms: (1) increased intraorbital pressure causing damage to the optic nerve; or (2) direct extension of infection into the optic nerve. Cavernous sinus thrombosis is a potential complication and can be distinguished from orbital cellulitis by cranial MRI.

Pearls and Pitfalls

1. Perform a complete examination of the globe, especially the conjunctiva and cornea, for ocular *herpes simplex* or *herpes zoster ophthalmicus*.
2. Beware of recurrent blepharitis or chalazia that do not respond to treatment. An occult malignancy could be the cause.
3. Congenital dacryocystitis in neonates should be treated aggressively because the orbital septum is not fully formed and extension of the infection can lead to brain abscesses and sepsis. This condition can also be associated with amniotocele (when amniotic fluid is retained in the lacrimal sac because of an obstructed nasolacrimal duct) and requires probing of the duct.
4. Severe cases of dacryocystitis can manifest by pupillary dysfunction due to increased intraorbital pressure and its effects on pupillomotor fibers in the orbit.
5. Orbital cellulitis should be strongly considered in the setting of pupillary dysfunction, diplopia, or loss of peripheral vision.
6. Squamous, basal, and sebaceous cell cancers can sometimes be misdiagnosed as chronic dacryocystitis.
7. Consider fungal (e.g. *Mucormycosis*, *Aspergillus*) orbital cellulitis in immunosuppressed adults, which can be lethal.
8. Patients with altered level of consciousness and ocular infections should be evaluated for meningitis and intracranial abscess formation, which can be extensions of orbital cellulitis.

References

American Academy of Ophthalmology. *Blepharitis Preferred Practice Patterns* (San Francisco, CA, 2013).

American Academy of Ophthalmology. *Basic and Clinical Science Course: Orbit, Eyelids, and Lacrimal System* (San Francisco, CA, 2014).

Bowling, B. and Kanski, J. J. *Clinical Ophthalmology: A Systematic Approach*, 7th edn. (London: Elsevier, 2011).

Carter, S. R. Eyelid disorders: diagnosis and management. *Am. Fam. Physician* 1998; 57(11): 2695–702, available at www.aafp.org/afp/980600ap/carter.html (accessed November 20, 2017).

Frith, P., Gray, R., MacLennan, A. H., *et al.* (eds.). *The Eye in Clinical Practice*, 2nd edn. (London: Blackwell Science, 2001).

Gerstenblith, A. T. and Rabinowitz, M. P. *The Wills Eye Manual: Office and Emergency Room Diagnosis and Treatment of Eye Disease*, 6th edn. (Philadelphia, PA: Lippincott Williams and Wilkins, 2012).

Givner, L. B. Periorbital versus orbital cellulitis. *Pediatr. Infect. Dis. J.* 2002; 21(12): 1157–8.

Howe, L. and Jones, N. S. Guidelines for the management of periorbital cellulitis/abscess. *Clin. Otolaryngol. Allied Sci.* 2004; 29(1): 725–8.

Hurwitz, J. J. The lacrimal drainage system in M. Yanoff, J. S. Duker, J. J. Augsburger, *et al.* (eds.), *Ophthalmology* (St. Louis, MO: Mosby, 2004), p. 764.

Liu, C., Bayer, A., Cosgrove, S. E., *et al.* Clinical practice guidelines by the Infectious Diseases Society of America for the treatment of methicillin-resistant Staphylococcus aureus infections in adults and children. *Clin. Infect. Dis.* 2011; 52(3): e18–55.

Nageswaran, S., Woods, C. R., Benjamin, D. K., Jr., *et al.* Orbital cellulitis in children. *Pediatr. Infect. Dis. J.* 2006; 25(8): 695–9.

Sobol, S. E., Marchand, J., Tewfik, T. L., *et al.* Orbital complications of sinusitis in children. *J. Otolaryngol.* 2002; 31(3): 131–6.

Chapter 43

Infections of the Uvea, Vitreous, and Retina

Greg Bever and Saras Ramanathan

Introduction

The uvea lies between the corneoscleral layer of the eye and the retina, and is composed of anterior (iris and ciliary body) and posterior (choroid) structures (see Figure 43.1). The general term "uveitis" most commonly refers to *anterior* uveitis, which includes iritis and inflammation of other structures of the anterior chamber. Extension of the inflammation to the ciliary body is termed iridocyclitis. If inflammation is located in the vitreous humor, it is sometimes termed *intermediate* uveitis. Inflammation of posterior uveal tract is termed *posterior* uveitis. This includes choroiditis, retinitis, and chorioretinitis. Endophthalmitis is an infection throughout the globe involving the vitreous humor (see Figure 43.1).

Although uveitis is often associated with non-infectious systemic diseases (e.g. vasculitides), this chapter focuses on infectious causes of uveitis. While the definitive diagnosis and management of infectious uveitis is beyond the scope of most acute care providers, it is important to be able to distinguish these deep-seated and sight-threatening infections from more routine and superficial problems such as conjunctivitis and corneal abrasion.

Uveitis and Retinitis

Epidemiology and Microbiology

The annual incidence of uveitis is about 40 new cases per 100,000, with anterior uveitis accounting for approximately 75% of cases. Most of these new cases present initially to the acute care setting.

Most cases of anterior uveitis are idiopathic or related to systemic disease. Among infectious cases, etiologic pathogens include: *herpes simplex* virus (HSV), varicella-zoster virus (VZV), cytomegalovirus (CMV), Lyme disease, syphillis, and tuberculosis.

Similarly, posterior uveitis of infectious origin can be caused by many different agents. One of the most common causes of such chorioretinal infiltrates is toxoplasmosis (see Figure 43.2). Although patients with acquired immunodeficiency syndrome (AIDS) are particularly susceptible to ocular toxoplasmosis due to reactivation, normal hosts with a history of exposure to cats or eating undercooked meats can also develop ocular toxoplasmosis. Ocular toxoplasmosis may occur in infants via vertical transmission from mothers who are infected during pregnancy. In ocular toxoplasmosis, parasites accumulate primarily on the retina and can spread to the choroid and sclera.

Another important cause of infectious posterior uveitis is CMV (see Figure 43.3). It is rare in immunocompetent patients and its presence should prompt testing for human immunodeficiency virus (HIV), as it usually occurs in HIV patients with low CD4 counts (e.g. fewer than 50 cells/mL). With wide use of combination antiretroviral therapy (ART), the incidence of CMV retinitis has dramatically decreased. Immune recovery uveitis related to anti-CMV immunity may occur in some patients following the initiation of ART.

Clinical Features

Most patients with anterior uveitis will present with a red eye. Chorioretinitis presents with visual changes with or without eye pain. The evaluation should always begin with an assessment of visual acuity. In general, patients with eye complaints associated with photophobia, decreased visual acuity, or pain that is not relieved by anesthetic drops should undergo a slit lamp exam. Direct fundoscopy can be used in the acute care

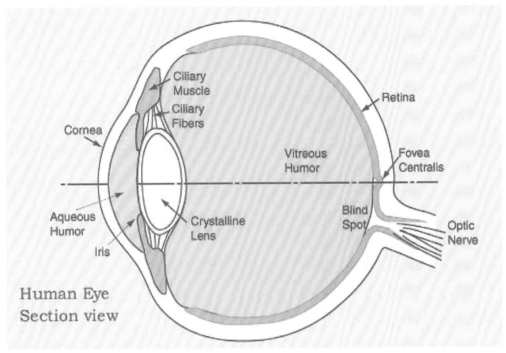

Figure 43.1 Illustration of eye anatomy.
From http://commons.wikimedia.org/wiki/Image:Eyesection.gif; Sathiyam2k, Illustration of human eye, not copyrighted.

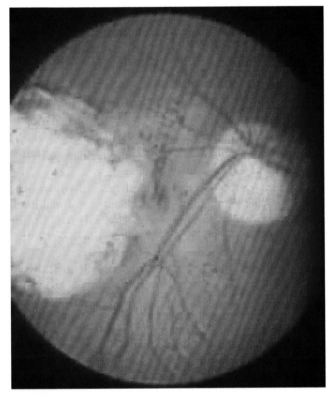

Figure 43.2 Severe chorioretinitis from *Toxoplasmosis gondii*.
From www.dpd.cdc.gov/dpdx/HTML/ImageLibrary/Toxoplasmosis_il.htm.

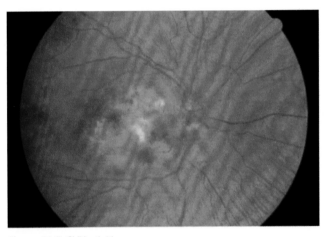

Figure 43.3 CMV retinitis.
National Eye Institute, National Institutes of Health, Ref. No. EDA07, www.flickr.com/photos/nationaleyeinstitute/7544815070/in/album-72157646474384400/.

Differential Diagnosis

Other conditions to consider (often described as "masquerade syndromes" for uveitis) are:

- giant retinal tears
- ocular ischemic syndrome
- leukemia
- lymphoma
- ocular melanoma
- pigmentary dispersion syndrome
- retinoblastoma

setting to detect chorioretinitis lesions. Since the majority of cases of uveitis are associated with systemic disesase, a complete history and physical exam looking for clues to systemic illness is essential (see Table 43.1).

Table 43.1 Causative pathogens and Clinical Features: Infectious Uveitis and Retinitis

Pathogens	**Bacterial**:
	Atypical mycobacteria
	Brucellosis
	Bartonella henselae (cat scratch disease)
	Mycobacterium leprae (leprosy)
	Borrelia burgdorferi (Lyme disease)
	Propionibacterium
	Treponema pallidum (syphilis)
	Mycobacterium tuberculosis
	Viral:
	Cytomegalovirus
	Epstein–Barr virus
	Herpes simplex virus
	Varicella-zoster virus
	Human T-cell leukemia virus
	Mumps virus
	Rubeola virus
	Vaccinia virus
	HIV
	West Nile virus
	Ebola virus
	Fungal:
	Aspergillus
	Blastomycosis
	Candida spp.
	Coccidioides
	Cryptococcus
	Histoplasma
	Sporotrichosis (*Sporothrix schenckii*)
	Parasitic (protozoan/helminthic):
	Toxoplasmosis gondii
	Acanthamoeba
	Cysticercosis
	Onchocerciasis
	Pneumocystis carinii
	Toxocariasis
Signs and symptoms	**Anterior uveitis:**
	• pain
	• redness
	• photophobia
	• ciliary flush (ring of red at corneal limbus)
	• white blood cells and "flare" (haze caused by extravasated plasma proteins) in anterior chamber
	Posterior uveitis:
	• Blurred vision, usually painless and without photophobia
	• typically no conjunctival redness
	• macular edema
	• perivascular retinal exudates
	• choroidal and retinal inflammatory lesions

Key features that may help to distinguish anterior uveitis from conjunctivitis, keratitis, and episcleritis are:

- "ciliary flush," or perilimbal (the intersection of the sclera and cornea) injection
- photophobia

- white blood cells and flare in the anterior chamber
- deep pain (where conjunctivitis, and episcleritis may have some irritation, uveitis is typically described as a "deeper pain")

Laboratory Findings

Uveitis is a clinical diagnosis that should be made in conjunction with an ophthalmologist who can perform a detailed eye exam and follow the patient over time. When an infectious etiology is suspected, other clinical manifestations of the disease may help make the diagnosis (e.g. pulmonary tuberculosis or signs of HIV infection). Testing for tuberculosis exposure and serologic testing for syphilis and connective tissue disease is often appropriate, and generally will be directed by the consultant.

Treatment and Prophylaxis

Treatment for non-infectious uveitis (e.g. topical steroids and cycloplegia) differs from that of infectious uveitis. Infectious uveitis should be treated with the general systemic treatment of the underlying infection (e.g. tuberculosis, syphilis, HSV, VZV, and CMV). In many cases, there is good ocular penetration from the systemic medication and no local ocular antimicrobial treatment is required. In immunocompromised patients, uveitis may be due to chronic infections such as toxoplasmosis, syphilis, tuberculosis, coccidioidomycosis, and histoplasmosis. Ophthalmologists should be closely involved in the management of these patients to monitor for resolution of ocular findings.

Complications and Admission Criteria

As a general rule, the diagnosis of uveitis/retinitis does not require admission, though exceptions include:

- acute retinal necrosis (ARN)
- rapidly progressive outer retinal necrosis (RPORN)
- associated systemic illness requiring inpatient treatment (e.g. syphilis and IV penicillin)

ARN (see Figure 43.4) must be diagnosed by an ophthalmologist and can be identified by the triad of multifocal peripheral retinitis, vitritis, and occlusive retinal vasculitis. The etiology of ARN is viral (HSV, VZV, or rarely CMV). Treatment should include intravenous antiviral agents such as acyclovir.

RPORN (see Figure 43.5) is a variant of ARN that should be considered in immunosuppressed patients (e.g. HIV, bone marrow transplant). Patients may have only a simple complaint of decreased vision (usually bilateral) and be without pain, redness, or appreciable intraocular inflammation. Many of these patients have a history of cutaneous zoster, as VZV is the most common etiology. RPORN can cause retinal disintegration involving the central vision (macula) and requires immediate high-dose antiviral therapy as well as maintenance therapy from an ophthalmologist.

Endophthalmitis

Acute bacterial endophthalmitis is a vision-threatening condition and must be managed as an emergency. Since most cases occur in the setting of previous ocular surgery, these infections

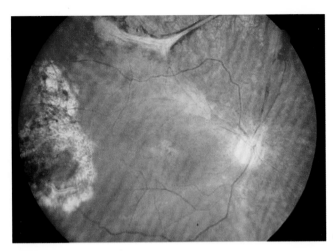

Figure 43.4 Acute retinal necrosis.
Courtesy of Michael Morley, MD (Ophthalmic Consultants of Boston).

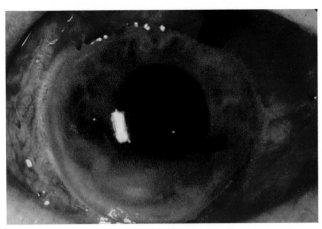

Figure 43.6 Endophthalmitis.
Courtesy of Michael Morley, MD (Ophthalmic Consultants of Boston).

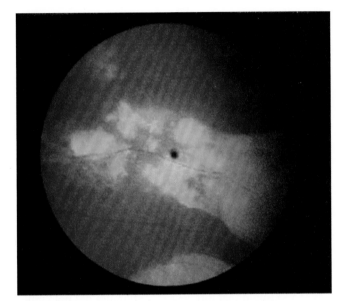

Figure 43.5 Rapidly progressive outer retinal necrosis.
Courtesy of Michael Morley, MD (Ophthalmic Consultants of Boston).

are commonly diagnosed and managed by ophthalmologists. But endophthalmitis can also be caused by ocular trauma and bacteremia, and acute care providers should be familiar with the clinical features of these infections.

Epidemiology and Microbiology

Most cases of endophthalmitis (see Figure 43.6) are bacterial and present acutely. Rarely, fungi may cause endophthalmitis, but viruses and parasites do not. The clinical outcome depends both on the virulence of the infecting organism and on the speed with which appropriate therapy is initiated.

In the United States, the most common form of endophthalmitis is acute endophthalmitis after cataract surgery. Cataract surgery involves entering the anterior chamber with instruments and can, on occasion, result in disruption of the vitreous humor during surgical manuevers. Endophthalmitis is a relatively infrequent complication of cataract surgery (less than 0.1% of cases in some studies), but, because of the large number of cataract operations performed (more than 2 million per year in the United States), it is an important clinical problem. The infection occurs within the first six post-operative weeks and 75% of cases present within 1 week of surgery. Most cases are caused by gram-positive bacteria, with coagulase-negative *Staphylococci* being the leading pathogen. Risk factors for this infection include diabetes, blepharitis, wound leak after surgery, and complicated surgical course (e.g. a torn posterior capsule or iris prolapse).

Endophthalmitis can complicate penetrating globe injury, particularly with retained foreign body. This type of endophalmitis has a particularly fulminant course and is most commonly caused by *Bacillus cereus*. One study showed 45% of eyes end up with vision of hand motions (HM) or worse.

Other types of endophalmitis include the following:

- endogenous, from seeding of the eye during bacteremia (risk factors include history of bacteremia or fungemia, endocarditis, abdominal abscesses, meningitis, illicit injection drug use, immunosuppresion, and indwelling catheters)
- chronic pseudophakia-related endophthalmitis (often due to *Propionibacterium acnes* and involving a biofilm plaque within remnant lens capsule)
- bleb-related (infection of a "filtering bleb," which is an intentional surgical window created in the sclera to treat severe glaucoma)
- post-intravitreal injection (following injection of steroids or anti-vascular endothelial growth factor medication for conditions such as exudative macular degeneration or diabetic macular edema)

Clinical Features

In the acute care setting, any patient presenting with eye complaints in the setting of recent ophthalmologic surgery should be considered to have endophthalmitis until proven otherwise.

Table 43.2 Causative pathogens and Clinical Features: Endophthalmitis

Pathogens	**Bacterial:**
	Coagulase-negative *Staphylococci* (most common etiology in acute post-operative cases)
	Staphylococcus aureus
	Streptococcus spp. (more common in post-intravitreal injection cases)
	Gram-negative organisms (e.g. *Pseudomonas*)
	Other gram-positive organisms (e.g. *Enterococcus*)
	Fungal:
	Candida albicans
	Aspergillus
	Fusarium
Signs and symptoms	• decreased visual acuity
	• eye pain (though possible with minimal pain)
	• conjunctival injection
	• hypopyon
	• eyelid edema
	• anterior chamber cell and flare on slit lamp
	• periphlebitis
	• vitritis
	• corneal edema

Table 43.2 summarizes the most important clinical features of endophthalmitis.

Differential Diagnosis

In the early post-operative period, it is important to distinguish endophthalmitis from toxic anterior segment syndrome (TASS), which is associated with the sterilization of surgical instruments or with the irrigating solution used during cataract surgery. Features of TASS that distinguish it from endophthalmitis include: onset on the first post-operative day (endophthalmitis usually takes a few days to manifest), lack of vitritis, less pain, and diffuse limbus to limbus corneal edema. Because these distinguishing features are not always reliable, any post-operative inflammation must be approached with a high index of suspicion for infectious etiologies.

Laboratory and Radiographic Findings

As in most ocular disease, the diagnosis of endophthalmitis is made by physical exam. Leukocytosis is not a reliable predictor of serious disease. A "B-scan" (ultrasound of the eye) can show increased vitreous echogenicity and/or retinochoroidal thickening, but these findings are not diagnostic. Aqueous or vitreous samples can be taken by an ophthalmologist to obtain cultures that may help direct therapy, though negative cultures do not exclude the diagnosis. A vitreous specimen provides more reliable culture results than an aqueous specimen; one study found that 48% of cases with a negative aqueous culture showed microbial growth in vitreous culture. In the setting of possible penetrating ocular trauma, ocular CT can be invaluable in identifying occult globe penetration and intraocular foreign body, which if unrecognized can lead rapidly to endophthalmitis. In the case of suspected endogenous endophthalmitis due to bacteremia or fungemia, blood cultures should be obtained.

Table 43.3 Initial Therapy for Endophthalmitis

Patient Category	Therapy Recommendation
Adults	**Bacterial**:
	• Vitrectomy or aspiration of vitreous
	• Vitreous injection of antibiotics
	• Vancomycin 1 mg/0.1 mL
	plus
	• Ceftazidime 2.25 mg/0.1 mL (or, rarely, amikacin 0.4 mg/0.1 mL)
	• Vitreous injection of steroids (dexamethasone 0.4 mg/0.1 mL) is controversial
	Fungal:
	• Vitrectomy or aspiration of vitreous
	• Vitreous injection of antifungal agents
	• Amphotericin B 5 mcg or 10 mcg/0.1 mL
	or
	• Voriconazole 100 mcg/0.1 mL
	• Systemic antifungals for at least 4–6 weeks
	• Fluconazole 800 mg PO (loading), then 400–800 mg PO daily
	or
	• Voriconazole PO/IV 400 mg BID × 2 doses (loading), then 300 mg PO BID
	• Amphotericin B has poor ocular penetration, but can be used in cases of resistence
Children and pregnant women	Treatment generally follows that of non-pregnant adults (always done in conjunction with an ophthalmologist). Not all treatment is well documented or tested in this population because of its rarity of occurrence, but benefits are understood to be greater than risks.

Treatment

Needle aspiration of the vitreous gel or surgical vitrectomy, as well as intravitreal antibiotics, are the traditional mainstays of treatment (see Table 43.3). The use of intravitreal steroids is controversial. The landmark Endophthalmitis Vitrectomy Study (EVS) found that intravenous antibiotics did not confer any significant benefit to either "tap (vitreous aspiration for culture) and inject (intravitreal injection of antibiotics)" or vitrectomy with intravitreal antibiotics. The study also found that for presenting visual acuity of hand motion (HM) or better, "tap and inject" in clinic was sufficent treatment. However, if the presenting visual acuity was light perception (LP) or worse, there was a benefit to immediate surgical intervention with vitrectomy (and administration of intravitreal antibiotics at the time of surgery). Although the EVS trial included patients specifically with acute post-operative endophthalmitis, the conclusions drawn from this study are often extrapolated to endophthalmitis cases of other etiologies.

Complications and Admission Criteria

• All patients with suspected endophthalmitis require emergent ophthalmology consult and possible admission if the diagnosis is confirmed.

• Endophthalmitis is an emergency, as undiagnosed and untreated cases often result in loss of vision; even some cases that have been treated promptly will be left with compromised vision.

Pearls and Pitfalls

1. Uveitis, infectious and non-infectious, is often associated with systemic illness.
2. The redness of simple conjunctivitis usually spares the limbus, whereas the presence of "ciliary flush" is suggestive of uveitis.
3. Photophobia is a symptom that points more toward uveitis than conjunctivitis.
4. Endophthalmitis should be high on the differential for any eye complaint in a patient who has had recent cataract surgery, especially during the first post-operative week.
5. If a foreign body is suspected in association with the globe trauma, there should be a low threshold for obtaining a CT scan.
6. Any patient with prior filtering glaucoma surgery (e.g. trabeculectomy or tube shunt) that presents with signs and symptoms of infectious conjunctivitis should be evaluated by an ophthalmologist and treated aggressively to prevent progression to bleb-related endophthalmitis.

References

Cetinkaya, S., Dadaci, Z., Aksoy, H., *et al.* Toxic anterior-segment syndrome (TASS). *Clin. Ophthalmol.* 2014; 8: 2065–9.

Durand, M. L. Bacterial endophthalmitis. *UpToDate*, available www.uptodate.com (accessed January 15, 2016).

Durand, M. L. and Kauffman, C. A. Epidemiology, clinical manifestations, and diagnosis of fungal endophthalmitis. *UpToDate*, available at www.uptodate.com (accessed January 16, 2016).

Gerstenblith, A. T., Rabinowitz, M. P., Barahimi, B. I., *et al.* (eds.). *The Wills Eye Manual: Office and Emergency Room Diagnosis and Treatment of Eye Disease*, 6th edn. (Philadelphia, PA: Lippincott Williams & Wilkins, 2012).

Pappas, P. G., Kauffman, C. A., Andes, D. R., *et al.* Clinical practice guidelines for the management of candidiasis: 2016 update by the Infectious Diseases Society of America. *Clin. Infect. Dis.* 2016; 62(4): 1–50.

Results of the Endophthalmitis Vitrectomy Study. A randomized trial of immediate vitrectomy and of intravenous antibiotics for the treatment of postoperative bacterial endophthalmitis. Endophthalmitis Vitrectomy Study Group. *Arch. Ophthalmol.* 1995; 113(12): 1479–96.

Van Gelder, R. N. and Margolis, T. P. Ebola and the ophthalmologist. *Ophthalmology* 2015; 122(11): 2152–4.

Vaziri, K., Schwartz, S. G., Kishor, K., *et al.* Endophthalmitis: state of the art. *Clin. Ophthalmol.* 2015; 9: 95–108.

Community-Acquired Pneumonia

Bradley W. Frazee, Christopher Fee, and Rachel L. Chin

Introduction and Microbiology

Community-acquired pneumonia (CAP) is defined as an infection of the pulmonary parenchyma, acquired in the community. The definition of CAP excludes patients who are hospitalized, have been hospitalized in the 14 days prior to the onset of symptoms, or who reside in long-term care facilities, including nursing homes. While this chapter focuses on CAP in immunocompetent adults, it will also touch on health-care-associated pneumonia (HCAP). See Chapter 45, HIV-associated Respiratory Infections, for a discussion of pulmonary infections in immunocompromised patients, and Chapter 54, Pediatric Respiratory Infections, for a discussion on pediatric pulmonary infections.

Streptococcus pneumoniae remains the most important CAP bacterial pathogen, accounting for 5 to 13% of inpatient cases and an even higher proportion of the deaths from CAP. Current *S. pneumoniae* resistance to both to penicillins and macrolides, as well as the possibility of future widespread resistance to fluoroquinolones, drives current recommendations for empiric therapy. The risk factors for infection with drug-resistant *S. pneumoniae* include significant medical comorbidities and use of antimicrobials within the prior 3 months.

The so-called atypical bacterial causes of CAP, those that cannot be seen on gram stain or cultured on typical media, include *Mycoplasma pneumoniae, Chlamydophila* (formerly chlamydia) *pneumoniae,* and *Legionella pneumophila. M. pneumoniae* and *C. pneumoniae* are common causes of CAP in ambulatory patients younger than 50. Although generally less severe, pneumonia caused by *M. pneumoniae* and *C. pneumoniae* may be difficult to distinguish on clinical grounds. *Legionella,* by contrast, can cause severe pneumonia and is associated with outbreaks linked to contaminated water sources, such as hot tubs, swimming pools, or air conditioning systems. A urinary antigen test for *Legionella* serogroup 1 (responsible for ~70 to 80% of cases) is available. Many treatment guidelines include antibiotics active against

atypical bacteria (macrolide/azalide, doxycycline, and fluoroquinolones) for all empiric CAP therapy. *Haemophilus influenzae* and *Moraxella catarrhalis* are relatively common causes of CAP in elderly patients, smokers, and patients with chronic obstructive pulmonary disease (COPD).

Pneumonia caused by enteric gram-negative organisms and occuring in community-dwelling individuals, while relatively uncommon, is important to identify, because such organisms may be multidrug resistant and immediate broad spectrum antibiotic therapy appears to reduce mortality. The category health-care-associated pneumonia (HCAP) has been developed to identify patients presenting from the community who are at risk for multidrug-resistant organisms due to extensive health-care contact. HCAP is defined by presence of any of the following patient risk factors: hospitalization for 2 or more days within the last 90 days; residence in nursing or other long-term care facility; receiving hemodialysis within 30 days; receiving home infusion therapy, wound care, or chemotherapy; or having a co-habitating family member with a known multidrug-resistant pathogen. Important multi-drug resistant organisms (MDROs) in this category include *Klebsiella pneumoniae, Escherichia coli* and *Pseudomonas aeruginosa,* and methicillin-resistant *Staphylococcus aureus* (MRSA). Recent experience indicates that identifying HCAP in the ED and treating all such patients empirically for MDRO pneumonia has likely led to overly liberal use of very broad-spectrum antibiotics. Upcoming guidelines are expected to recommend a narrower set of risk factors for identifying community-dwelling patients at risk for MDRO pneumonia.

Staphylococcus aureus pneumonia occurs not only in those with HCAP, but also following influenza virus infection, which increases susceptiblity to this pathogen. MRSA now accounts for roughly half of cases, and has been associated with a more severe, necrotizing form of pneumonia. Oral anaerobes are associated with aspiration pneumonia and lung abscess. Respiratory viruses, such as influenza rhinovirus and respiratory syncytial virus (RSV), are a very common cause of CAP, together accounting for up to 23% of adult cases requiring hospitalization. Viral pneumonia may be clinically indistinguishable from bacterial pneumonia. Tuberculosis and fungal pneumonia (e.g. coccidioidomycosis and histoplasmosis) and atypical bacteria (e.g. *Nocardia* and *Actinomyces*), though typically indolent in onset, may be mistaken for bacterial pneumonia and should remain on the differential diagnosis when faced with clinical CAP that does not respond to antibiotic therapy. Despite advances in diagnostic testing, no causative organism can be identified in about up to 62% of CAP cases.

Epidemiology

CAP is the leading cause of death from infectious disease in the United States and the eighth leading cause of death overall. It accounts for approximately 1 million hospitalizations. Mortality rates are less than 1 to 5% in the outpatient setting, but as high as 12% in hospitalized patients. The incidence of CAP is highest in the winter months and important risk factors include increasing age, smoking, and alcholism.

Bacterial CAP is not generally thought of as a contagious or transmissible infection. In most cases, it involves inoculation of the normally sterile pulmonary parenchyma by the patient's own oropharyngeal flora. A notable exception is *Mycoplasma pneumoniae*, which can be transmitted among close contacts by droplet spread, resulting in case clusters among young people. Also, colonization with drug-resistant *S. pneumoniae* strains can spread among close contacts, such as within families, day care centers, and nursing homes, and outbreaks of pneumococcal

pneumonia occasionally occur in these settings. Furthermore, primary infection with *Mycobacteria tuberculosis*, which is highly transmissible, can present clinically as CAP.

Clinical Features

Common clinical features of CAP include productive cough, fever, pleuritic chest pain, and dyspnea (see Table 44.1). Gastrointestinal symptoms, including nausea, vomiting, and diarrhea, may be prominent. Mental status changes can be seen, particularly in the elderly, and indicate a worse prognosis. Chest pain occurs in 30% of cases, chills in 40 to 50%, and rigors in 15%. Because of the rapid onset of symptoms, most individuals seek medical care within a week of infection.

On physical examination, approximately 80% of patients are febrile, though fever may be absent, especially in the elderly. A respiratory rate above 24 breaths/minute is noted in 45 to 70% of patients and may be the most sensitive sign in the elderly. Tachycardia is common. Careful chest examination usually reveals rales or evidence of consolidation, but this can easily be missed. Oxygen saturation is often decreased, though patients with good cardiopulmonary reserve can maintain normal saturation with significant disease, and normal pulse oximetry by no means excludes pneumonia. At the same time, oxygen saturation as low as 90 to 92% is well tolerated by otherwise healthy patients, and this finding alone does not mandate hospital admission. (See Complications and Admission Criteria, below.)

No constellation of signs and symptoms has been found to predict with certainty whether or not a patient has pneumonia. Nonetheless, in non-elderly patients with normal vital signs

Table 44.1 Clinical Features: Community-Acquired Pneumonia

Pathogens	**Common, with these bacteria covered in most treatment regimens:**
	Streptococcus pneumoniae
	Mycoplasma pneumoniae
	Chlamydophilae (formerly chlamydia) *pneumoniae*
	Legionella pneumophila
	Haemophilus influenzae
	Moraxella catarrhalis
	Respiratory viruses
	Less common, predominantly occur in special at-risk populations:
	Enteric gram-negative bacteria
	Pseudomonas aeruginosa
	Staphylococcus aureus
Signs and symptoms	Cough, sputum production, dyspnea, pleurisy, GI symptoms, altered mental status
	Fever, tachypnea, low oxygen saturation, rales or evidence of consolidation
Laboratory and radiographic findings	Chest X-ray demonstrates an infiltrate
	Blood count: leukocytosis; left shift (bands); leukopenia is associated with severe disease
	Lactate: level >2 mmol/L is associated with severe disease
	Blood cultures (obtain two sets prior to antibiotics in patients requiring ICU hospitalization, meeting criteria for HCAP [i.e. at risk for drug-resistant bacteria], those meeting criteria for severe sepsis or septic shock [see Chapter 65, Sepsis], and those typically excluded from CAP treatment guidelines [i.e. immunosuppressed, solid organ transplant recipients, children]) positive in 5–14%
	Sputum culture and gram stain (obtain in most patients requiring hospitalization and all intubated patients)
	Legionella urinary antigen test (obtain in severe disease)
	Pneumococcal urinary antigen test
	Rapid antigen tests for influenza virus (during outbreaks)

GI – gastrointestinal; ICU – intensive care unit.

Box 44.1 Uncommon Causes of Cough and Infiltrate on Chest X-Ray

Uncommon infectious causes of pneumonia:
- tuberculosis (HIV infection, foreign born)
- fungal infections (e.g. coccidioidomycosis and histoplasmosis)
- *Pneumocystis* (human immunodeficiency virus [HIV] infection)
- *Bordetella pertussis* (chronic cough; normal chest x-ray)
- hantavirus pulmonary syndrome (most often in rural southwestern United States)
- *Coxiella burnetti* (Q fever; bioterrorism)
- anthrax (bioterrorism)
- plague (bioterrorism)
- tularemia (bioterrorism)

Non-infectious causes of cough and abnormal chest x-ray:
- malignancy
- pulmonary hemorrhage
- pulmonary edema
- interstitial lung disease

and no abnormal findings on chest auscultation, radiographic pneumonia is very unlikely. In such patients, a chest X-ray may not be necessary to exclude CAP.

Finally, it is critical to recognize the clinical features, such as respiratory rate above 30, which are correlated with severe CAP and worse prognosis. These features are enumerated under Complications and Admission Criteria, below.

Differential Diagnosis

Among ambulatory patients with acute cough and signs and symptoms of infection, often the main differential diagnosis is between acute bronchitis (almost always viral) and CAP (defined by an infiltrate on chest X-ray). However, less common but serious diagnoses can easily be mistaken for CAP (see Box 44.1).

Laboratory and Radiographic Findings

The presence of an infiltrate on plain chest radiograph is considered the "gold standard" for the diagnosis of CAP, when clinical features are supportive. Acute care practitioners should maintain a low threshold for obtaining a chest X-ray to assess for possible CAP. The radiographic appearances of CAP include lobar consolidation, interstitial infiltrates, cavitation, and pleural effusion. False-negative results are possible and may be due to dehydration or presentation within the first 24 hours of infection. Correlation between a particular chest X-ray finding and certain pathogens is not reliable. Multilobar involvement and large parapneumonic effusion are associated with a worse prognosis and generally require hospitalization. Chest computed tomographic (CT) scan is more sensitive than chest X-ray for small infiltrates, occult multilobar involvement, adenopathy, and effusion, but there is no evidence that routine CT scanning improves management or outcome. In many cases, chest X-ray is the only diagnostic test required in the evaluation of CAP.

Leukocytosis with a left shift is the major blood test abnormality found in CAP, though it is neither sensitive nor specific. Leukopenia (white blood cell [WBC] count less than 4,000 cells/mm^3) can also occur and connotes a worse prognosis. In addition to complete blood count, thorough severity assessment requires serum chemistries, serum lactate, and an assessment of oxygenation and mental status.

Diagnostic tests to determine the etiologic organism in CAP may include sputum Gram stain and culture, blood cultures, urinary antigen tests, and PCR on respiratory specimens. Etiologic testing is rarely indicated in outpatients because empiric treatment is almost always successful. In one study of more than 700 ambulatory patients with CAP treated with empiric antibiotics, only 1% required hospitalization due to failure of the outpatient regimen.

Performing etiological testing in all hospitalized patients, though controversial, is widely recommended. While such tests may not change initial acute care management, results can be crucial to later management and are important for public health surveillance. In general, the more severe the pneumonia, the more likely that sputum and blood cultures will lead to a change in management. Blood cultures prior to antibiotics are recommended in those patients with the following additional factors:

- requiring ICU hospitalization
- cavitary lesions
- leukopenia
- active alcohol abuse
- chronic severe liver disease
- asplenia (anatomic or functional)
- positive pneumococcal urinary antigen test results
- pleural effusion
- meeting HCAP criteria (e.g. those at risk for drug-resistant organisms)
- excluded from CAP treatment guidelines (e.g. immunosuppressed, solid organ transplant recipients, children)
- meeting criteria for severe sepsis or septic shock (see Chapter 65, Sepsis)

Sputum studies are reserved for patients with cavitary lesions, pleural effusion, structural lung disease, those able to produce a good expectorated specimen, those who have failed outpatient therapy, and those with severe pneumonia requiring ICU admission.

Urine antigen assays are available for the diagnosis of *Legionella* serogroup 1 and *S. pneumoniae* infection. These tests are recommended in cases of severe CAP. With their high specificity and a turnaround time of less than 1 hour, they offer the possibility of rapid etiologic diagnosis and often remain positive even when specimens are collected after antibiotic therapy is started.

Real-time PCR for influenza, performed on nasopharyngeal specimens, is recommended during flu season, particularly in patients requiring hospitalization. A positive test for influenza has a number of implications: in patients ill enough to require admission for CAP, it should prompt antiviral therapy; establishing the diagnosis is important for epidemiologic purposes; it has hospital infection control implications; and it might reduce unnecessary antibiotic use.

Treatment and Prophylaxis

Numerous resources are available to assist in the selection of initial antibiotic therapy for CAP in outpatients and hospitalized patients (see Tables 44.2 and 44.3). However, frequently-updated, hospital-specific treatment recommendation-based on, local bacterial susceptibility data, are preferred. Treatment guidelines are based on the principles (listed in Box 44.2).

Beta-lactam and macrolide/azalide-resistant *S. pneumoniae* is a significant problem in the United States, with resistance rates around 25% for both antibiotic classes. Recent antibiotic therapy with any drug from a class is a major risk factor for resistance to that class. Comorbidities, advanced age, immunocompromise, and having a child in day care also increase the risk of a drug-resistant strain. Fluoroquinolone resistance remains less than 5% in most regions of the United States, and limiting use of fluoroquinolones is recommended in an effort to prevent a future rise in resistance to this class. CAP treatment guidelines aim to tailor the empiric regimen according to risk for drug-resistant *S. pneumoniae*, while minimizing use of fluouroquinolones.

Administering antibiotics as soon as possible to patients requiring hospitalization remains a paramount goal in the ED management of CAP. This is particularly true of those patients meeting criteria for severe sepsis or septic shock in whom prompt antibiotic administration is associated with a reduced mortality. How rapidly the chest x-ray is obtained and interpreted and blood cultures drawn is an important determinant of time to first antibiotic dose.

An important means of reducing morbidity and mortality from CAP is appropriate use of pneumococcal vaccines in target populations (see Table 44.4), as well as widespread use of the annual influenza vaccine.

Box 44.2 General principles of CAP treatment

- Initial antibiotic selection in the acute care setting is always empiric (versus pathogen-directed).
- Antibiotic selection begins with categorizing the patient with regard to severity and site of care (outpatient, hospital ward, ICU).
- For outpatient therapy (see Table 44.2), antibiotics with activity against drug-resistant *S. pneumoniae* are necessary only in patients at risk, based on comorbidities and recent (within 3 months) antibiotic use.
- For inpatient therapy (see Table 44.3), activity against drug-resistant *S. pneumoniae* is always provided.
- All antibiotic regimens ensure activity against atypical pathogens.
- Patient exposures that indicate health-care-associated pneumonia (HCAP) generally mandate empiric treatment of multidrug-resistant pathogens; such broad spectrum activity is not provided in standard CAP regimens.
- Activity against *S. aureus* (MRSA) and anaerobes is reserved for patients at increased risk.
- Consider drug allergy history and pregnancy status.
- Rapid administration of empiric antibiotics for those patients meeting criteria for severe sepsis or septic shock is associated with reduced mortality.

Table 44.2 Initial Therapy for Outpatient: Community-Acquired Pneumonia

Patient Category	Therapy Recommendation
Adults: previously healthy and no use of antimicrobials within the previous 3 months Presence of comorbidities such as chronic heart, lung, liver, or renal disease; diabetes; alcoholism; malignancies; asplenia; immunosuppressive drugs; use of antimicrobials within the previous 3 months (an alternative from a different class should be selected); or exposures indicating health-care-associated pneumonia†	**A macrolide or doxycycline:** Azithromycin 500 mg PO on day 1, then 250 mg PO daily for days 2–5, or 2 g (sustained release) PO × 1 *or* Clarithromycin XR 1 g PO daily or 500 mg PO BID × 7 days *or* Doxycycline 100 mg PO BID × 7–10 days **A respiratory fluoroquinolone or a beta-lactam plus a macrolide*:** Levofloxacin 750 mg PO daily × 5 days *or* Moxifloxacin 400 mg PO daily × 7 days *or* Amoxicillin-clavulanate 875/125 mg PO BID *plus* Azithromycin 500 mg PO daily × 3 days *or* Azithromycin 2 g PO × 1 *or* Clarithromycin XR 1 g PO daily × 7 days *or* Clarithromycin 500 mg PO BID × 7 days
Pregnant women	Same as for non-pregnant adults, except avoid doxycycline and fluoroquinolones

* In communities where pneumococcal macrolide resistance rates exceed 25%, choose a fluouroquinolone.

† Hospitalization within the last 30 days; residence in nursing or other long-term care facility; receiving hemodialysis; receiving IV therapy, wound care, or chemotherapy.

PO – by mouth.

Table 44.3 Initial Therapy for Inpatient: Community-Acquired Pneumonia

Patient Category	Therapy Recommendation
Adults: non-ICU	**A respiratory fluoroquinolone or a beta-lactam plus a macrolide:** Ceftriaxone 1 g IV every 24 hours *plus* Azithromycin 500 mg IV every 24 hours *or monotherapy with:* Levofloxacin 750 mg IV every 24 hours *or* Moxifloxacin 400 mg IV every 24 hours
ICU patients	**A beta-lactam plus either a respiratory fluoroquinolone or azithromycin (same doses as for non-ICU patients):** Ceftriaxone 1 g IV every 24 hours *plus* Azithromycin 500 mg IV every 24 hours *or* a respiratory fluoroquinolone *plus consider*, if MRSA risk factors[†] Vancomycin 15–20 mg/kg/dose IV every 8–12 hours, with MRSA risk factors
Health-care-associated pneumonia* (at risk for drug-resistant enteric gram-negative pathogens, such as *Pseudomonas* suspected CA-MRSA Infection[†])	**Antipseudomonal beta-lactam:** Piperacillin-tazobactam 4.5 g IV every 6 hours *or* Cefepime 2 g IV every 8 hours *plus* either a respiratory fluoroquinolone *or* Gentamicin or tobramycin 5 mg/kg/dose IV every 24 hours *plus (in all cases)* Azithromycin 500 mg IV every 24 hours (for non-fluoroquinolone regimens) *plus* Vancomycin 15–20 mg/kg/dose IV every 8–12 hours
Suspected influenza (and symptoms present <48 hours or requiring hospitalization)	Add oseltamivir 75 mg PO BID × 5 days

[†] MRSA risk factors: cavitary lesion; consistent gram stain; health-care-associated pneumonia; injection drug use; prior influenza.

* Patient risk factors indicating health-care-associated pneumonia: hospitalization within the last 90 days; residence in nursing or other long-term care facility; receiving hemodialysis; receiving IV therapy, wound care, or chemotherapy; co-habitation with a person with known drug-resistant pathogen.

IV – intravenous; PO – by mouth. CA-MRSA–community-acquired methicillin-resistant *staphylococcus aureus*.

Adapted from L. A. Mandell, R. G. Wunderink, A. Anzueto, *et al*. Infectious Diseases Society of America/American Thoracic Society consensus guidelines on the management of community-acquired pneumonia in adults. *Clin. Infect. Dis.* 2007; 44(2): S27–72.

Table 44.4 Recommendation for Vaccine Prevention of Community-Acquired Pneumonia

Factor	Pneumococcal vaccine
Route of administration	IM injection of pneumococcal conjugate vaccine (PCV13)
Recommended groups	All persons ≥65 years of age High-risk persons 2–64 years of age
Specific high-risk indications for vaccination	Chronic cardiovascular, pulmonary, renal, or liver disease; diabetes mellitus; CSF leaks; alcoholism; asplenia; immunocompromising conditions/medications; Native Americans and Alaska natives; long-term care facility residents
Revaccination schedule	Revaccination with pneumococcal polysaccharide vaccine (PPSV23) after 1 year

CSF – cerebrospinal fluid; IM – intramuscular.

Adapted from L. A. Mandell, R. G. Wunderink, A. Anzueto, *et al*. Infectious Diseases Society of America/American Thoracic Society consensus guidelines on the management of community-acquired pneumonia in adults. *Clin. Infect. Dis.* 2007; 44(2): S27–72 and CDC Guidelines.

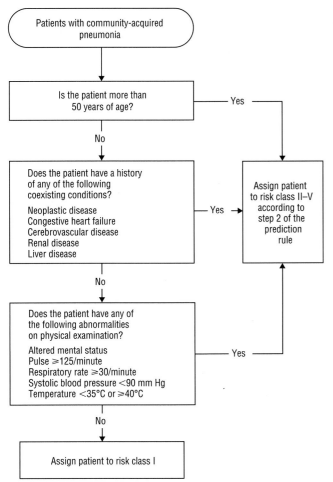

Figure 44.1 Pneumonia Severity Index. Identifying patients in risk class.
Reprinted from M. J. Fine, T. E. Auble, D. M. Yealy, *et al.*, A prediction rule to identify low-risk patients with community-acquired pneumonia. *N. Engl. J. Med.* 1997; 336(4): 243–50. Copyright 1997 Massachusetts Medical Society. All rights reserved.

Table 44.5 PSI-Based Mortality Prediction for Community-Acquired Pneumonia

Class	Points	Mortality	Disposition
1	<51	0.1%	Outpatient
2	51–70	0.6%	Outpatient
3	71–90	0.9%	Inpatient briefly vs. outpatient
4	91–130	9.5%	Inpatient
5	>130	26.7%	Inpatient, possible ICU

Complications and Admission Criteria

A critical task of the acute care provider in evaluating CAP is to correctly assess need for hospitalization. Hospital admission is costly and can lead to further iatrogenic complications, so inappropriate admission must be minimized. Furthermore, practitioners must recognize signs of occult severe disease requiring ICU level care. The pneumonia severity index (PSI) (see Figure 44.1 and Table 44.5) and CURB-65 score (see Tables 44.6 and 44.7) provide an objective means to assess prognosis and aid in disposition and treatment decisions.

Table 44.6 The CURB-65 Severity Assessment Tool

Confusion
Urea (BUN ≥7 mmol/L or approximately ≥20 mg/dL)
Respiratory rate ≥30 breaths/min.
Blood pressure (SBP <90 mm Hg or DBP ≤60 mm Hg)
65 years old or greater
One point is assigned for each CURB-65 criteria that is present.

BUN – blood urea nitrogen; DBP – diastolic blood pressure; SBP – systolic blood pressure.

Table 44.7 CURB-65 Score and Mortality Prediction

Score	30-Day Mortality Rate	Patient Disposition
0–1	1.5%	Outpatient
2	9.2%	Outpatient vs. brief inpatient
3–5	22%	Inpatient; consider ICU if 4 or 5 points

The PSI is based on age, comorbidities, vital sign abnormalities, and laboratory and chest X-ray findings. Non-elderly patients without major comorbidities or major vital sign abnormalities are assigned to class 1 without the need for blood tests (see Figure 44.1). For patients not satisfying PSI class 1 criteria, a scoring system based on 22 clinical and laboratory elements is used to assign patients to classes 2 to 5 (point scoring system- not shown). Classes 1 and 2 have a 30-day mortality of 0.1% and 0.6%, respectively, and are usually candidates for outpatient management. Class 3 is associated with a 0.9 to 2.8% mortality, suggesting that hospitalization is appropriate, and classes 4 and 5 are associated with 8.2 to 9.3% and 27 to 31.1% mortality and thus almost always require admission (see Table 44.5). Performance of the PSI in determining prognosis has been validated in more than 50,000 patients and, when used consistently by practitioners, leads to a decreased CAP hospitalization rate without adversely affecting outcome. It is important to recognize that the PSI has limitations and should contribute to, but not supersede, physician judgment. Reasons to hospitalize patients assigned to classes 1 to 3 include the following: poor oxygenation (SpO$_2$ <90), pleural complications, psychosocial issues (psychiatric illness, alcoholism, poor home situation); inability to take antibiotics by mouth; and patient preference.

The CURB-65 severity assessment tool, published by the British Thoracic Society, is attractive because it is simple to remember and can be calculated using a bedside assessment plus a blood urea nitrogen level (see Table 44.6). However, it is not as well studied or validated as the PSI. The CURB-65 tool may be particularly useful in identifying patients who require ICU admission, such as those with a score of 3, 4, or 5, in whom the hospital mortality is 17%, 41%, and 57% respectively (see Table 44.7).

Additional signs of severe pneumonia that do not appear in the PSI or CURB-65 indexes are multilobar disease evident on chest X-ray, severe hypoxemia, leukocytosis in excess of 20 cells/mm^3 or leukopenia (<4 cells/mm^3), and elevated serum lactate. A reasonable practice is to send a serum lactate in any CAP patient in whom blood cultures are drawn. A lactate level greater than 2 mmol/L in this setting indicates likely tissue hypoperfusion from sepsis, need for aggressive resuscitation, and consideration of ICU-level care.

The major complications of CAP that may require ED intervention are ventilatory failure, sepsis syndrome, and pleural complications. Parapneumonic effusion is present in 20 to 40% of CAP requiring hospitalization, and empyema complicates 5 to 7% of cases. Diagnostic thoracentesis is recommended for an effusion measuring greater than 10 mm on lateral decubitus chest x-ray, and pleural fluid should be obtained prior to administering antibiotics, if possible. Indications for definitive drainage are complex, but pleural fluid with a pH less than 7.2 is the best single indicator. The extent to which practitioners are involved in managing pleural complications of CAP will depend greatly on the practice setting, but diagnostic thoracentesis can be rapidly and safely performed in the ED with ultrasound guidance.

Special Considerations – Pneumonia in Nursing Home Residents

Among the patient factors indicating HCAP, residence in a long-term care facility (LTCF) is undoubtedly the most frequently encountered. Not only are such patients at increased risk for multidrug-resistant pathogens requiring expanded empiric antibiotic coverage, but pneumonia can present atypically in this population. Pneumonia is up to ten times more common in LTCF residents, compared to elderly patients in the community. Factors associated with an increased risk of pneumonia include older age, immobility, difficulty swallowing, inability to take oral medications, and presence of a feeding tube. Diagnosis can be very difficult in this population because localizing signs such as cough are often absent and chest x-ray interpretation may be hampered by chronic changes, dehydration, and patient positioning. Elevated respiratory rate may be the best early sign. Pathogens responsible for pneumonia in LTCF residents include *S. aureus* (including MRSA), multidrug-resistant gram-negative bacteria, and *Legionella*. Recommended empiric regimens generally combine an antipseudomonal beta-lactam plus an antipseudomonal fluoroquinolone. Vancomycin or linezolid is added if there is a high local incidence of MRSA. Acute hospitalization, which is costly and associated with decreased quality of life and functional status, is usually, but not invariably, necessary in LTCF residents diagnosed with pneumonia. Return to the nursing home for further treatment, after blood cultures and a dose of parenteral antibiotic, may be considered in those who can eat and drink, have relatively normal vital signs (e.g. respiratory rate <30), and adequate oxygenation.

Pearls and Pitfalls

1. Chest X-ray is required for the diagnosis of CAP in the acute care setting.
2. A normal chest X-ray in a well-appearing immunocompetent young patient with respiratory symptoms usually signifies bronchitis that does not require antibiotics.
3. A normal chest X-ray in an ill-appearing or elderly patient could signify a false-negative test for CAP, but should prompt a search for other sources of fever or respiratory symptoms.
4. Chest X-ray opacities may be caused by serious non-infectious problems (such as heart failure) and uncommon infectious diseases (such as tuberculosis or fungi) that may masquerade as CAP.
5. Clinical features and radiographic changes do not help to identify the etiologic pathogen in CAP.
6. Initial antibiotic therapy in the acute care setting is almost always empirical, dictated by disease severity, recent antibiotic use, and comorbidities.
7. Careful and structured severity assessment (using the pneumonia severity index or CURB-65 score) is recommended in order to reduce unnecessary hospitalization and to identify occult severe CAP.
8. Microbiologic tests to determine etiology, such as blood cultures, are generally reserved for patients who are at risk for drug-resistant pathogens and require hospitalization.

References

Centers for Disease Control and Prevention (CDC). Use of 13-valent pneumococcal conjugate vaccine and 23-valent pneumococcal polysaccharide vaccine among adults aged ≥65 years: recommendations of the Advisory Committee on Immunization Practices (ACIP). *MMWR Morb. Mortal. Wkly. Rep.* 2014; 63(37): 822–5.

CDC. Intervals between PCV13 and PPSV23 vaccines: recommendations of the Advisory Committee on Immunization Practices (ACIP). *MMWR Morb. Mortal. Wkly. Rep.* 2015; 64(34): 944–7.

Ferrer, R., Martin-Loeches, I., Phillips, G., *et al.* Empiric antibiotic treatement reduces mortality in severe sepsis and septic shock from the first hour: results from a guideline-based performance improvement program. *Crit. Care Med.* 2014; 42(8): 1749–55.

Fine, M. J., Auble, T. E., Yealy, D. M., *et al.* A prediction rule to identify low-risk patients with community-acquired pneumonia. *N. Engl. J. Med.* 1997; 336(4): 243–50.

Jain, S., Self, W. H., Wunderink, R. G., *et al.* Community-acquired pneumonia requiring hospitalization among U.S. adults. *N. Eng. J. Med.* 2015; 373(5): 415–27.

Kennedy, M., Bates, D. W., Wright, S. B., *et al.* Do emergency department blood cultures change practice in patients with pneumonia? *Ann. Emerg. Med.* 2005; 46(5): 393–400.

Lim, W. S., van der Eerden, M. M., Laing, R., *et al.* Defining community acquired pneumonia severity on presentation to hospital: an international derivation and validation study. *Thorax* 2003; 58(5): 377–82.

Loeb, M., Carusone, S. C., Goeree, T., *et al.* Effect of a clinical pathway to reduce hospitalizations in nursing home residents with pneumonia: a randomized controlled trial. *JAMA* 2006; 295(21): 2503–10.

Mandell, L. A., Wunderink, R. G., Anzueto, A., *et al.* Infectious Diseases Society of America/American Thoracic Society consensus guidelines on the management of community-acquired pneumonia in adults. *Clin. Infect. Dis.* 2007; 44(2): S27–72.

Marie, T. J., Lau, C. Y., Wheeler, S. L., *et al.* A controlled trial of a critical pathway for treatment of community-acquired pneumonia. CAPITAL Study Investigators. Community-acquired pneumonia intervention trial assessing levofloxacin. *JAMA* 2000; 283(6): 749–55.

Metlay, J. P., Kapoor, W. N., and Fine, M. J. Does this patient have community-acquired pneumonia? Diagnosing pneumonia by history and physical examination. *JAMA* 1997; 278(17): 1440–5.

Musher, D. M. and Thorner, A. R. Community-acquired pneumonia. *N. Engl. J. Med.* 2014; 371(17): 1619–28.

Shapiro, N. I., Howell, M. D., Talmor, D., *et al.* Serum lactate as a predictor of mortality in emergency department patients with infection. *Ann. Emerg. Med.* 2005; 45(5): 524–8.

Chapter 45

HIV-Associated Respiratory Infections

Rachel Greenblatt and Laurence Huang

Introduction

Pulmonary disease is a significant cause of morbidity and mortality in HIV-infected individuals and is a frequent cause of emergency department visits. The differential diagnosis of HIV-associated pulmonary disease is broad and includes both infectious and non-infectious conditions. Infectious causes range from minor (e.g. viral upper respiratory infection) to life-threatening (e.g. *Pneumocystis* pneumonia [PCP]). This chapter focuses on the three most important and common respiratory infections in HIV-infected patients: bacterial pneumonia, PCP, and tuberculosis. The pathogens that cause bacterial pneunonia (whether community-associated [CAP] or health-care-associated) in HIV-infected patients are essentially the same as in immunocompetent hosts, with *Streptococcus pneumonieae* predominating. These bacterial pathogens are discussed in detail in Chapter 44. PCP is caused by the fungus *Pneumocystis jirovecii* (formerly considered a parasite and named *P. carinii*), which causes clinical pneumonia almost exclusively in immunocompromised individuals. Pulmonary tuberculosis is also discussed in detail in Chapter 47. Other important infectious etiologies include respiratory viruses and cytomegalovirus, the endemic fungal infections, as well as crypotococcus, *Toxoplasma gondii*, the atypical mycobacteria, and others (see Table 45.1).

In the current combination antiretroviral therapy (cART) era, HIV-infected patients are increasingly presenting with non-infectious pulmonary diseases, including chronic obstructive pulmonary disease (COPD), asthma, pulmonary fibrosis, lung cancer, and pulmonary hypertension.[1] Pulmonary kaposis sarcoma, previously common, is rarely seen now. Although the list of potential diseases may seem overwhelming, an understanding of the most commonly encountered infections and their characteristic presentations will help narrow the differential diagnosis.

Epidemiology

Respiratory infections are more common in HIV-infected patients at all CD4 levels than in HIV-uninfected individuals. The spectrum of pulmonary disease for HIV-infected patients has dramatically changed with the use of cART. However, of the more than 1 million people who are infected with HIV living in the United States, only 81.9% have been diagnosed and only 65.8% are linked to care, so there will continue to be patients presenting with the "classic" complications of HIV and AIDS even in the era of cART.[2] PCP remains the most common AIDS-defining pulmonary infection in the United States,[3] though it is responsible for a declining proportion of hospitalizations and deaths.[4] The proportion of pulmonary infections secondary to bacterial pneumonia has increased despite an overall decrease in total number of cases, and is currently the most common cause of respiratory infection in patients with HIV. Rates of bacterial infection are between five- and 25-fold higher in HIV-infected patients than in non-HIV-infected populations.[5] Globally, *Mycobacterium tuberculosis* (TB) pneumonia is the most common cause of death in HIV-infected individuals.[6] HIV-infected patients who have latent TB infection face a 10% *per year* risk of progressing from latent to active TB compared to an approximately 10% *lifetime* risk in non-HIV-infected individuals.[7]

Clinical Features

The clinical and radiographic presentations of common HIV-associated pulmonary infections overlap. The goal of the

Table 45.1 List of Important HIV-Associated Pulmonary Infections and Common Non-Infectious Pulmonary Diseases

Infections:

Bacterial pneumonia

	Streptococcus pneumonia
	Heamophilus influenzae
	Staphylococcus aureus
	Gram-negative bacilli
	Legionella pneumophila

Mycobacteria

	M. tuberculois
	M. avium complex
	Others

Atypical bacteria

	Nocardia
	Actinomyces

Viruses

	Respiratory viruses (e.g. influenza)
	Cytomegalovirus

Parasites and helminths

	Toxoplasma gondi
	Strongyloides

Fungi

	Pneumocystis jirovecii
	Histoplasma capsulatum
	Coccidioidis immitis
	Blastomycis dermatiditis
	Aspergillus species
	Cryptococcus neoformans

Cancer:

	Kaposis sarcoma
	Lymphoma
	Lung cancer
	Metastasis

Other:

	Lymphocitic interstitial pneumonia

history and physical is to narrow the differential diagnosis, recognize constellations of particular symptoms and signs, and guide diagnostic testing and therapy.

All of the HIV-associated pulmonary diseases can present with cough, shortness of breath, and decreased exercise tolerance. There are some characteristic presentations that may point to a particular diagnosis (see Table 45.1). Purulent sputum is typically associated with bacterial bronchitis or pneumonia, whereas a dry, non-productive cough is typically associated with PCP.[8] The duration of symptoms can also be useful in differentiating between infections. Bacterial pneumonia characteristically presents with an acute onset over 3 to 5 days, whereas PCP and TB present with a more indolent course over weeks. Although patients with any pulmonary infection may complain of pleuritic chest pain, persistent and severe pleuritic pain should raise the suspicion for

a pneumothorax, particularly in patients with cysts and pneumatoceles secondary to PCP.[9]

The presence of extrapulmonary symptoms must also be noted, because these can be related to a primary pulmonary infection and suggest a unifying diagnosis. A chronic history of constitutional symptoms such as night sweats and weight loss is common with TB infection. Lymphadenopathy, abdominal complaints, and organomegaly (hepatomegaly, splenomegaly) suggest infiltrative, disseminated, granulomatous infection such as TB, non-tuberculous mycobacteria, or endemic fungal disease such as histoplamosis or coccidioidomycosis. New-onset confusion, headache, or focal neurologic findings may indicate both neurologic and pulmonary involvement by *Cryptococcus neoformans* or *Toxoplasma gondii*. However, isolated pneumonia in cryptococcal disease is rare.[10] Visual complaints, odynophagia, and respiratory symptoms may herald concurrent cytomegalovirus (CMV) retinitis, esophagitis, and pneumonitis, in which case, biopsy of a peripheral lymph node, lumbar puncture, or dilated funduscopic examination may yield the correct diagnosis.

It must be emphasized that more than one infectious agent may present simultaneously in HIV-infected patients. Occasionally, patients will have characteristics of dual respiratory infection with distinctive symptoms suggestive of both a bacterial process and PCP or TB. For example, a patient who develops a cough productive of purulent sputum over several days may also complain of several weeks of fevers and dyspnea. Such a patient may have bacterial pneumonia superimposed on PCP. In these cases of suspected dual infection, empiric treatment for both processes is appropriate pending diagnostic testing.

A thorough physical examination with emphasis on cardiopulmonary findings will help the acute care physician narrow the differential diagnosis. Patients with HIV-associated pulmonary infections are typically febrile, tachycardic, and tachypneic. The presence of hypotension may indicate bacterial sepsis requiring urgent evaluation and management. A decreased oxygen saturation is often noted and is a common and appropriate indication for admission. If outpatient management is being considered, post-ambulation pulse oximetry should be checked, because some patients will manifest a decrease in oxygen saturation only after exertion; patients with post-ambulation desaturatation usually require admission.

The pulmonary examination should focus on the presence and characterization of focal or diffuse findings. Patients with bacterial pneumonia will often have a focal lung examination suggestive of lobar consolidation with or without an accompanying pleural effusion. In contrast, patients with PCP typically have diffuse findings, with bilateral rales the most frequent finding. Of note, it is common for patients with PCP to have a normal lung examination. The presence of diffuse wheezes or decreased breath sounds can suggest an exacerbation of asthma or COPD. The unilateral absence of breath sounds may suggest a pneumothorax in a patient complaining of pleuritic chest pain.

The remainder of the physical examination can also be helpful in assessing a patient's underlying immune status as well as the etiology of the respiratory symptoms. PCP, bacterial pneumonia, and occasionally TB are often the initial HIV-identifying illnesses in patients who are unaware of their HIV infection. Oropharyngeal thrush is a common finding in such patients. Lymphadenopathy may suggest disseminated mycobacterial or fungal disease. Common skin findings include sebbhoreic dermatitis, Kaposi's sarcoma (KS), or molluscum-like lesions consistent with disseminated cryptococcosis. A fundoscopic exam can reveal viral, fungal, or mycobacterial infections.

Laboratory and Radiographic Findings

The CD4 count is essential in formulating a differential diagnosis in HIV-infected patients with respiratory symptoms. In cases where the patient is unaware of a recent CD4 count, the total lymphocyte count can be obtained rapidly and serve as a surrogate marker, helping to estimate the degree of immune suppression. In studies in resource-limited settings, a total lymphocyte count below 1,200 cells/mm³ has a high positive predictive value for a CD4 count below 200 cells/mm³.[11] It is important to note that acute illness can suppress the CD4 count below the true baseline value, and a repeat CD4 count after resolution of the acute illness may be indicated.

A room-air arterial blood gas (ABG) should be drawn in any patient with mild to moderate respiratory compromise or suspected PCP. A PaO_2 ≤70 mm Hg or an alveolar-arterial oxygen gradient ≥35 mm Hg is an indication for adjunctive corticosteroid treatment in PCP. Serum lactate dehydrogenase (LDH) is another laboratory test that may have utility in PCP. The LDH is elevated in ~93% of patients with PCP, and the degree of elevation correlates with prognosis.[12] Serial LDH values can help assess severity and progression of illness; however, elevated LDH levels can be seen in other pulmonary diseases and are therefore non-specific. In addition to these and other more common laboratory tests (e.g. complete blood count and metabolic panels), an electrocardiogram should be obtained to evaluate for cardiac disease as a potential etiology of respiratory symptoms (see Table 45.2).

All HIV-infected patients who present with a suspected pulmonary infection should have two sets of blood cultures drawn in the ED prior to initiating antibiotic therapy. This recommendation is consistent with both the Infectious Diseases Society of America (IDSA) and the American Thoracic Society (ATS) guidelines for management of community-acquired pneumonia and with the Guidelines for Prevention and Treatment of Opportunistic Infections in HIV-Infected Adults and Adolescents. *Streptococcus pneumoniae* bacteremia is more common in patients with HIV, particularly in those with low CD4 count. HIV-infected patients who are injection drug users are another population that should always have blood cultures. Positive blood cultures with subsequent antibiotic susceptibility testing will help guide appropriate antimicrobial therapy.

If a bacterial respiratory infection is suspected in a patient requiring hospitalization, a sputum sample should be sent for gram stain and culture.[13] Sputum studies can also be considered in HIV-infected patients being treated for CAP in the outpatient setting, especially if an unusual pathogen such as *Pseudomonas aeruginosa* is suspected, which generally is not covered by standard outpatient oral antimicrobial therapy.[14] Urine and serum *Histoplasma* polysaccharide antigen and cryptococcal antigen are useful in aiding in the diagnosis of histoplasmosis and cryptococcal pneumonia respectively.

Sputum should also be sent for PCP and acid-fast bacilli (AFB) in most cases. Patients with PCP alone (without a superimposed bacterial pneumonia) usually have a non-productive cough, and are unable to produce a spontaneously expectorated sputum sample. In these cases, sputum induction using nebulized hypertonic saline should be performed if available. Sputum induction has a sensitivity of 55 TO 90% for PCP, with the higher sensitivities resulting from concentration of the sputum specimen and staining with direct fluorescent antibodies specific for human *Pneumocystis*.[15] In patients suspected of having TB, expectorated or induced sputum for AFB should be collected daily for 2 to 3 consecutive days while the patient is in respiratory isolation. The sensitivity of sputum AFB smears for *M. tuberculosis* ranges from 50 to 60% and can approach 90% in those patients with disseminated disease. Three negative AFB smears do not rule out active TB, but the likelihood of airborne transmission to other patients and health-care providers is significantly decreased. GeneXpert, a real-time PCR, can confirm diagnosis quickly with 90% sensitivity and 99% specificity and identify rifampicin resistance.[16]

There are caveats to sputum collection for PCP and AFB. Patients who are recently diagnosed with PCP and have undergone a complete course of treatment may continue to have positive sputum stains for PCP despite resolution of infection. This can make it difficult to distinguish between recurrent or inadequately treated PCP and a new infectious process.[17] Likewise, a positive sputum AFB smear can be due to colonization or infection by non-tuberculous mycobacteria such as *Mycobacterium avium* complex (MAC) rather than *M. tuberculosis* infection. Nevertheless, a positive AFB smear mandates appropriate infection control and treatment measures until a definitive diagnosis is made.

Chest Imaging

Although each of the common HIV-associated pulmonary infections has characteristic chest radiograph (CXR) findings, overlap in appearance does occur. A basic approach to interpretation of the CXR includes the following assessment: (a) "normal" or "abnormal"; if abnormal, (b) pattern of disease (e.g. alveolar, interstitial/reticular, or nodular); and (c) distribution of disease (e.g. unilateral or bilateral, focal or diffuse); and associated findings (e.g. pleural effusion, mediastinal or hilar adenopathy, pneumatocele, or cavitation). Because HIV-infected patients may present with multiple respiratory infections over the course of their HIV infection and may have residual radiographic findings from prior infections or underlying pulmonary conditions, it is critical to compare the current radiograph against the most recent prior radiographs.

Table 45.2 Clinical Features: HIV-Associated Pulmonary Infections

Clinical Features	Bacterial Pneumonia	*Pneumocystis* Pneumonia	Tuberculosis
Organisms	*Streptococcus pneumoniae* *Haemophilus* species Gram negatives and anaerobes (predisposing factors: alcohol use, aspiration, cigarette smoking)*	*Pneumocystis jirovecii*	*Mycobacterium tuberculosis*
Signs and Symptoms	• Cough with purulent sputum • Fever, chills, rigors • Acute onset, symptoms <1 week	• Non-productive cough • Exertional dyspnea • Fever • Gradual onset, symptoms >1 week • Crackles and rhonchi common, but normal exam in 50% of cases	• Cough • Fever, night sweats, malaise • Weight loss • Gradual onset, symptoms >2 weeks • Lymphadenopathy
Laboratory and radiographic tests	• Any CD4 count • Elevated WBC • Chest radiograph: focal alveolar consolidation, with or without associated pleural effusion	• CD4 count: <200 cells/μL • Widened alveolar-arterial gradient (>35 mm Hg difference) • Elevated 1–3- β-d-glucan • Elevated serum LDH • Chest radiograph: interstitial or granular pattern • HRCT: ground-glass opacities	• Any CD4 count • Chest radiograph: alveolar pattern (often with cavitation), miliary pattern, nodules, intrathoracic adenopathy, pleural effusion

* Boyton 2005; Feikin *et al.* 2004.
HRCT – high-resolution computed tomography; LDH – lactate dehydrogenase; WBC – white blood (cell) count.

Characteristic findings in bacterial pneumonia are similar to those in the HIV-uninfected population, with focal, lobar, or segmental alveolar infiltrates predominating (see Figure 45.1). In contrast, *Haemophilus influenzae* pneumonia seems to have a higher likelihood of presenting with an interstitial pattern that mimics PCP,[18] whereas *Pseudomonas aeruginosa* and *Staphylococcal aureus* both more often present with cavitation.

The characteristic radiograph in PCP shows bilateral, diffuse interstitial, reticular, or granular opacities (see Figure 45.2). The findings are unilateral or asymmetric in a small proportion. PCP presents with thin-walled cysts or pneumatoceles in 10 to 20% of cases or these can develop over the course of treatment. Pneumatoceles vary in size and in number from single to innumerable. They place the patient at increased risk for pneumothorax. A normal CXR or one with focal lobar consolidation does not rule out PCP. PCP should remain high on the differential diagnosis in an HIV-infected patient with a CD4 count less than 200 cells/μL who is hypoxemic and febrile and who has a normal chest radiograph. Intrathoracic adenopathy and pleural effusions, however, are rare in PCP, and these findings should prompt a search and treatment for an alternate or coexisting process.[19]

Like PCP, *M. tuberculosis* can present with a variety of radiographic findings. The specific pattern seen often correlates with the patient's degree of immune suppression, so knowledge of the most recent CD4 count is helpful. TB developing early in the course of HIV infection typically presents with a pattern of classic reactivation disease, with cavitating infiltrates in the upper lung zones (see Figure 45.3). TB developing in the later stages of HIV infection (i.e. low CD4 count) often presents with middle and lower lung zone infiltrates or with other findings of primary infection such as adenopathy or pleural effusion, and

less frequently presents with cavitation (see Figure 45.4). This radiographic picture can imitate a bacterial pneumonia. HIV-infected patients with active pulmonary TB may also have a normal CXR, though this is rare, and a high degree of suspicion must be maintained.[20]

Oftentimes in the ED, CXRs are obtained in HIV-infected patients who have no specific pulmonary complaints. In one study of such patients found to have an abnormal CXR (i.e. nodular disease or adenopathy), 26% had TB and 17% had non-tuberculous mycobacteria. For this reason, patients with HIV with suppressed CD4 counts and abnormal CXRs should undergo further work-up or close follow-up.[21]

Chest computed tomography (CT) has become an important modality for evaluating HIV-infected patients with pulmonary symptoms because of its high sensitivity for the detection of early pulmonary disease. Patients with PCP and a normal chest radiograph will have diffuse or patchy areas of ground-glass opacity on high-resolution CT (see Figure 45.5).[22] Whereas the presence of ground-glass opacity is non-specific, its absence strongly argues against a diagnosis of PCP. Lymphadenopathy is a common CT finding in patients with negative CXRs and pulmonary symptoms, and is most often due to typical and atypical mycobacterial disease, bacterial pneumonia, and lymphoma.[23]

Differential Diagnosis

When evaluating HIV-infected patients with respiratory symptoms, one must consider both infectious and non-infectious causes of cough, dyspnea, and hypoxia (see Table 45.1). Exacerbations of underlying asthma or COPD are common. HIV-associated cardiomyopathy or pulmonary arterial

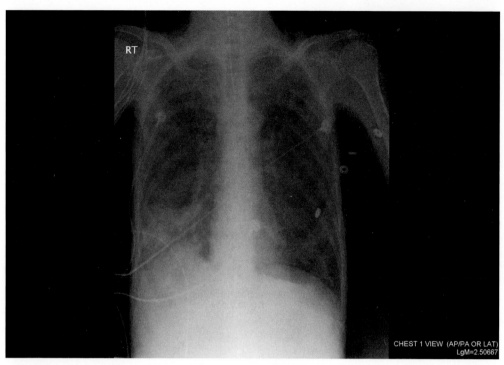

Figure 45.1 Chest radiograph of an HIV-infected patient, CD4 count less than 200 cells/μL, with lobar consolidation from *S. pneumoniae*. This patient was also found to have *S. pneumoniae* bacteremia, meningitis, and *Staphylococcus aureus* bacteremia.

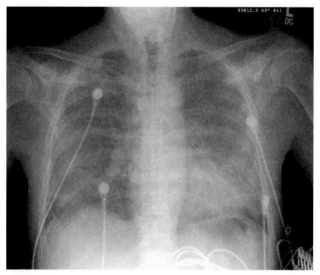

Figure 45.2 Chest radiograph of an HIV-infected patient, CD4 count less than 200 cells/μL, demonstrating the bilateral, reticular pattern characteristic of PCP.

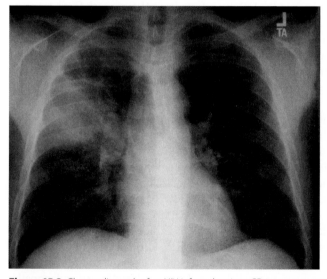

Figure 45.3 Chest radiograph of an HIV-infected patient, CD4 count greater than 200 cells/μL, revealing right upper lobe infiltrate with areas of cavitation. Sputum AFB stain was positive and multiple sputum AFB cultures grew *Mycobacterium tuberculosis*.

Courtesy of L. Huang, MD, used with permission.

hypertension are important diagnoses to consider in a patient with suggestive findings on examination (e.g. elevated jugular venous pressure and rales) and CXR (e.g. cardiomegaly and pulmonary edema).

Infectious and non-infectious causes of pulmonary disease in HIV-infected patients often can be distinguished with a thorough history, physical examination, and basic diagnostic tests. Patients with both common and uncommon pulmonary infections typically complain of fever, cough (with or without purulent sputum, blood-tinged sputum, or frank hemoptysis), dyspnea, night sweats, fatigue, decreased exercise tolerance,

and weight loss of varying duration. The most common pulmonary infections leading to an ED visit and admission are bacterial pneumonia followed by PCP, both of which are significantly more common than the next most common diagnoses: TB, pulmonary KS (associated with human herpes virus-8 [HHV-8]), and various fungal infections.

Pulmonary KS can mimic acute infection and oftentimes presents with dyspnea, non-productive cough, fever, and hemoptysis.

A patient's social and travel history can be a clue to undiagnosed HIV as well as to the likelihood of a particular pulmonary infection. Social questions should include a history of potential HIV risk factors (men who have sexual intercourse with men, injection drug use, or sex for drugs or with sex workers). Since many cases of TB in HIV-infected patients are newly acquired as opposed to reactivation, it is important to ask about potential TB exposure, such as recently being in a health-care setting, prison, homeless shelter, or recent immigration from an endemic country. Recent conversion to a positive tuberculin skin test (PPD), defined in HIV-infected persons as induration of 5 mm or greater, is important. The probability of presenting with fungal pneumonia is associated with living in or traveling to endemic areas. Histoplasmosis is common in the Mississippi River Valley and coccidioidomycosis in the southwest United States, but patients can present with reactivation disease, so a thorough travel history is important. Certain respiratory diseases are associated with a particular mode of HIV transmission. KS is almost exclusively seen in men who have sex with men, whereas TB and bacterial pneumonia are more common in injection drug users.

CD4 Count and Prior Respiratory Infection History

Knowing the patient's most recent CD4 count, as well as any prior history of opportunistic infections (OIs), is essential to narrowing the differential diagnosis. The CD4 count is still an excellent indicator of an HIV-infected patient's susceptibility to opportunistic respiratory infections (see Table 45.3). The patient's use and adherence to cART and OI prophylaxis should also be noted.

Some pulmonary infections, such as bacterial pneumonia and TB, can occur at any CD4 count, but both are more frequent and have a higher complication rate as the CD4 count declines. At low CD4 counts, the risk of bacteremia and disseminated TB increases. Most opportunistic respiratory infections occur predominantly at a CD4 count less than 200 cells/μL. At this CD4 level, PCP and cryptococcal pneumonia enter the differential diagnosis. At a CD4 count less than 100 cells/μL, pulmonary KS, *Toxoplasma gondii*, and *Pseudomonas aeruginosa* pneumonia can be seen. When the CD4 count drops below 50 cells/μL, the endemic fungi (e.g. *Histoplasma*

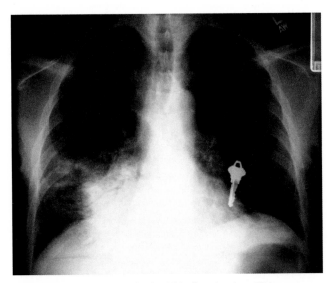

Figure 45.4 Chest radiograph of an HIV-infected patient, CD4 count less than 200 cells/μL, revealing right lower lung consolidation with air bronchograms. Sputum AFB cultures grew *Mycobacterium tuberculosis* that was mono-rifampin resistant. In this case, the solution to the diagnosis of TB was knowledge of the patient's CD4 count and an understanding that TB can present in this manner in such an individual.

Courtesy of L. Huang, MD, used with permission.

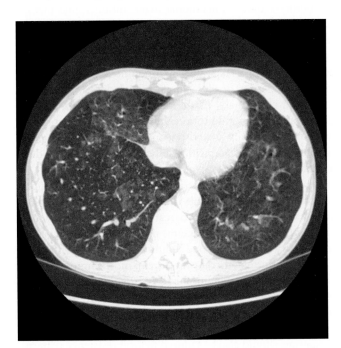

Figure 45.5 Chest CT scan of an HIV-infected patient, CD4 count less than 200 cells/μL with ground-glass opacities characteristic of PCP.

Chest radiograph characteristically shows bilateral opacities in a central or perihilar distribution, and typical findings include nodules, diffuse parenchymal lesions, lymphadenopathy, and pleural effusions. Typical skin lesions of KS are usually but not invariably present, and diagnosis is aided by bronchoscopy.[24]

Initiation of antiretroviral therapy can trigger new respiratory symptoms. Be aware of timing of cART administration, as immune reconstitution syndrome, a paradoxical worsening of symptoms related to recovery of the immune system, could be contributing.

Table 45.3 Standard Acute Care Evaluation for HIV-Infected Patients with Suspected Pulmonary Infection

All patients:
- CD4 count (if unknown or last value >6 months ago)
- Complete blood count with differential and metabolic panel
- Chest radiograph (PA and lateral)
- Electrocardiogram

Selected patients:
- Room-air arterial blood gas (if patient has mild to moderate respiratory compromise or if PCP is suspected)
- Serum LDH (if PCP is suspected)
- Sputum Gram stain and culture (if bacterial pneumonia is suspected)
- Blood cultures (two sets prior to antibiotic administration if bacterial pneumonia is suspected)
- Serum cryptococcal antigen (if CD4 count <200 cells/μL)

PA – posteroanterior.

capsulatum, Coccidioides immitis), *Aspergillus* species, CMV, and non-tuberculous mycobacteria become considerations. These CD4 count cut-offs should serve as a general guideline, because exceptions can occur.

Unfortunately, patients presenting to the acute care setting may not have had a recent CD4 count. Total lymphocyte count can be used as a rough indicator of T-cell level. Oropharyngeal thrush (e.g. candidiasis) is a good clinical marker of suppressed immune function; history of thrush increases the risk of subsequent PCP.

Many of the HIV-associated OIs recur. Recurrent bacterial pneumonia (e.g. two or more episodes in a 12-month period) is an AIDS-defining illness.[25] Patients with a history of PCP and fungal infections (cryptococcosis, coccidioidomycosis, and histoplasmosis) are also at high risk for recurrent illness, especially if they fail to take secondary prophylaxis or maintenance therapy. Therefore, acute care physicians should always ask about a prior history of pulmonary infections.

HIV-infected patients, especially those with the lowest CD4 counts, may develop an OI despite the use of antimicrobial prophylaxis. CD4 counts and adherence to OI prophylaxis should serve only as a general guide as to which pulmonary infections are most likely to occur in a patient.

Treatment

Since the symptoms, physical findings, and radiographic appearance of the most common HIV-associated pulmonary infections are non-specific and overlap, definitive diagnosis is rarely possible in the acute care setting. Therefore, it is usually necessary to begin empiric therapy before a definitive diagnosis has been made. Empiric therapy is entirely appropriate, provided that the appropriate studies for definitive diagnosis have been initiated and follow-up is ensured.

Selecting appropriate initial treatment depends on the patient's history, physical examination, CD4 count, and results of imaging studies. Because the most common causes of HIV-associated pulmonary infection are bacterial pneumonia and PCP, empiric therapy for one or both is often implemented.

In most cases, empiric treatment for bacterial community-acquired pneumonia is recommended. A typical patient with bacterial pneumonia may present with a CD4 count greater than 200 cells/μL, a chest radiograph with a non-cavitating focal, segmental, or lobar infiltrate, and a history of 3 to 5 days of fevers, rigors, and cough productive of purulent sputum. Given this constellation of findings, the probability of bacterial pneumonia is significantly higher than that of PCP or TB, and empiric therapy for bacterial pneumonia alone would be appropriate pending further diagnostic testing (see Tables 45.4 and 45.5). Other factors favoring bacterial pneumoia include focal findings on lung examination, leukocytosis, and a history of cigarette smoking, intravenous drug use, or prior bacterial pneumonia. Even if the CD4 count is less than 200 cells/μL, if the CXR shows a focal alveolar infiltrate and other findings are consistent with bacterial pneumonia, empiric treatment for common bacterial pathogens alone is reasonable.

Table 45.4 Differential Diagnosis of Respiratory Infections in HIV and AIDS

Any CD4 count	• Bacterial pneumonia (most commonly *S. pneumoniae* or *H. influenzae*) • *M. tuberculosis* pneumonia (TB)
CD4 <200 cells/μL	• *Pneumocystis* pneumonia (PCP) • *Cryptococcus neoformans* pneumonia • Bacterial pneumonia complicated by bacteremia • Extrapulmonary or disseminated TB
CD4 <100 cells/μL	• *Pseudomonas aeruginosa* pneumonia • *Toxoplasma gondii* pneumonia • Pulmonary Kaposi's sarcoma (usually associated with mucocutaneous involvement)
CD4 <50 cells/μL	• *Histoplasma capsulatum* or *Coccidioides immitis* pneumonia, usually associated with disseminated disease • Cytomegalovirus pneumonia, usually associated with disseminated disease • *Mycobacterium avium* complex pneumonia, usually associated with disseminated disease • *Aspergillus* species pneumonia

The ATS and IDSA guidelines for management of community-acquired pneumonia make antimicrobial therapy recommendations that can be used as a guide for HIV-infected patients as well. For outpatient treatment of patients with immunosuppressing conditions such as HIV, guidelines recommend monotherapy with a respiratory fluoroquinolone (e.g. moxifloxacin or levofloxacin) or a β-lactam (e.g. high dose amoxicillin or amoxicillin-clavulanate) plus a macrolide. In general, a hospitalized patient with mild to moderate respiratory compromise should be treated with an anti-pneumococcal β-lactam (e.g. ceftriaxone, cefotaxime, ampicillin-sulbactam) plus a macrolide or monotherapy with a respiratory fluoroquinolone.

For patients with severe respiratory compromise or patients requiring intensive care unit (ICU) admission, combination therapy with an anti-pneumococcal β-lactam (e.g. ceftriaxone, cefotaxime, ampicillin-sulbactam) plus either azithromycin or a respiratory fluoroquinolone should be instituted, with a goal of providing optimal therapy for the two most commonly identified causes of lethal pneumonia (*S. pneumoniae* and *Legionella* species). For penicillin-allergic patients, a respiratory fluoroquinolone and aztreonam are recommended. Vancomycin or linezolid should be added if MRSA is suspected. These recommendations should also be tailored to local resistance patterns, where this information is available.

In cases where the clinical scenario suggests a bacterial pneumonia, but TB is still on the differential, we recommend avoiding the use of fluoroquinolones until TB has been ruled either in or out. There is a higher prevalence of multidrug-resistant TB in HIV-infected patients, and fluoroquinolones are becoming a mainstay of TB therapy. All efforts must be made to prevent the development of fluoroquinolone resistance in multidrug-resistant TB.[26]

If the CD4 count is 200 cells/μL or less, the CXR reveals bilateral interstitial, reticular, or granular opacities, the LDH is elevated, and the patient describes a subacute onset of fevers,

Table 45.5 Management of Respiratory Infection in Patients with HIV/AIDS and CD4 Count (Known or Suspected) Less than 200 cells/μL

Acute Symptoms (<1 Week)	
Normal CXR	• Symptomatic treatment for URI • Arrange follow-up with primary provider • If symptoms persist or progress, consider repeat chest radiograph or high resolution CT to evaluate for PCP
Abnormal CXR	• Bacterial pneumonia > PCP, TB • Consider admission for antibiotics and further evaluation for PCP or TB if risk factors present (e.g. prior PCP, homeless) or mixed clinical picture (e.g. non-productive cough, severe dyspnea that are more suggestive of PCP)
Chronic Symptoms (>1 Week)	
Normal CXR or Interstitial Infiltrate	**Non-productive cough:** • PCP > bacterial pneumonia, TB • Evaluate for PCP (and possibly TB) with induced sputum, bronchoscopy • Empiric treatment for PCP while awaiting diagnostic testing **Productive cough:** • Mixed clinical picture: consider empiric treatment for both bacterial pneumonia and PCP while awaiting further diagnostic testing
Alveolar infiltrate	**Non-productive cough:** • Mixed clinical picture: consider empiric treatment for both bacterial pneumonia and PCP while awaiting further diagnostic testing **Productive cough:** • Bacterial pneumonia > PCP or TB • Consider treatment with antibiotics for bacterial pneumonia and further evaluation for PCP and TB

CXR – chest x-ray; URI – upper respiratory infection.

dyspnea, and dry cough, PCP is the most likely diagnosis. Empiric therapy with trimethoprim-sulfamethoxazole and corticosteroids (for PaO$_2$ ≤70 mm Hg on room air or alveolar-arterial oxygen gradient ≥35 mm Hg) should be initiated while arranging for sputum induction or bronchoscopy to diagnose PCP.

In reality, it is quite common for patients to present with features of both a bacterial pneumonia and PCP (e.g. subacute onset of fevers, but cough productive of purulent sputum). Therefore, it is reasonable to begin empiric therapy for both bacterial pneumonia and PCP while awaiting further testing to arrive at a definitive diagnosis. As the CD4 count declines below 200 cells/μL, the number of possible diagnoses increases. However, bacterial pneumonia and PCP still remain the two most common etiologies.

Admission Criteria

A patient who has an established primary care provider, a CD4 count greater than 200 cells/μL, and normal ambulatory pulse oximetry, who is suspected to have bacterial pneumonia, can usually be discharged home on appropriate empiric antibiotic therapy with close follow-up. Clinical predictors including CURB-65 score or the pneumonia severity index should be used as with non-HIV infected patients to aid decisions about admission.

Patients with CD4 count less than 200 cells/μL and history or imaging studies suspicious for PCP or TB should generally be admitted for diagnostic work-up. If outpatient diagnostic testing (sputum induction and potentially bronchoalveolar lavage) can be arranged in an expedited manner, discharge can be considered. However, patients with a presumed diagnosis of PCP should not be discharged without a plan to establish a definitive microbiologic diagnosis (see Table 45.6).

Isolation and Infection Control

The transmission of infectious respiratory disease between HIV-infected patients and to health-care workers (HCWs) in the hospital is a significant concern. Tuberculosis is of particular concern. The clinical and radiographic presentation of pulmonary TB in the setting of HIV is often atypical. An active cough, as well as certain medical procedures (e.g. endotracheal intubation, sputum induction, and bronchoscopy), increase the burden of airborne bacilli and thus infectious risk. All suspected cases of TB must be placed in respiratory isolation (preferably negative pressure respiratory isolation). Appropriate precautions, including use of N-95 face masks, should be implemented until three separate sputum specimens have been examined and are negative for AFB.

Pearls and Pitfalls

1. In a patient with HIV and respiratory symptoms, the differential diagnosis is broad and includes both infectious and non-infectious causes, which may be related or unrelated to underlying HIV infection.

2. A patient's CD4 count, history of prior OI, and adherence to cART and OI prophylaxis are essential in helping to narrow the differential diagnosis.

3. *M. tuberculosis* and bacterial pneumonia can occur at any CD4 count.

4. The two most common HIV-associated pulmonary infections are bacterial pneumonia and PCP; history, physical examination, and chest radiograph findings are often helpful in differentiating between these two infections.

5. While the classic CXR finding in PCP is a diffuse, bilateral interstitial infiltrate, it can also manifest as a focal air-space opacity or a normal CXR; pleural effusion is very unusual.

Table 45.6 Treatment of Common HIV-Related Pulmonary Infections

Infection	Preferred Therapy	Alternative Therapies and Other Issues
Pneumocystis jiroveci pneumonia (PCP)	TMP/SMX: 15–20 mg TMP/kg/day PO divided every 8–12 hours (not acutely ill and PaO2>70 mm Hg) *or* TMP/SMX: 15–20 mg TMP/kg/day IV/PO divided every 6–12 hours Total duration 21 days *and* Prednisone 40 mg PO BID days 1–5, 40 mg PO daily days 6–10, then 20 mg PO daily days 11–21, if PaO$_2$ ≤70 mm Hg at room air or alveolar-arterial O$_2$ gradient ≥35 mm Hg	Primaquine 30 mg PO daily and clindamycin 900 mg IV every 8 hours or clindamycin 450 mg PO QID *or* Dapsone 100 mg PO daily and TMP 5 mg/kg PO TID *or* Atovaquone 750 mg PO BID *or* Pentamidine 4 mg/kg IV daily
Mycobacterium tuberculosis	See Chapter 47 for TB treatment regimens	Urgent initiation of TB therapy in the ED is rarely necessary Consultation with infectious disease specialist or pharmacist recommended because of multiple drug interactions between TB therapy and cART; prescribe pyridoxine (vitamin B6) 50 mg PO daily to decrease risk of neuropathy
Bacterial Pneumonia	See Chapter 44 for pneumonia treatment regimens	Minimize use of fluoroquinolones unless there is no suspicion of TB; quinolones should be reserved for treatment of drug-resistant TB and in TB patients with liver disease; empiric *Pseudomonas aeruginosa* coverage should be included for patients with HCAP, or those with CD4 count <100, history of *Pseudomonas aeruginosa* infection, or neutropenia; if community-acquired MRSA is possible, add vancomycin or linezolid

cART – highly active antiretroviral therapy; IV – intravenous; PO – by mouth; SMX – sulfamethoxazole; TMP – trimethoprim.

Table 45.7 Indications for Admission for HIV-Infected Patients with Suspected Pulmonary Infection

High risk for clinical deterioration CURB-65 score: 0–1: treat as an outpatient 2–3: hospitalize or watch closely as an outpatient 4–5: hospitalize*	CURB-65 score (1 point for each): • Confusion • Urea >20 mg/dL • Tachypnea with respiratory rate ≥30 breaths per minute • Hypotension with systolic blood pressure persistently <90 mm Hg after initial fluid resuscitation • Age ≥65 *or* Consider use of pneumonia severity index Consider admission if: • Hypoxia with O$_2$ sat. <92%, decreased PaO$_2$, elevated alveolar-arterial oxygen gradient, or requiring supplemental oxygen • Decreased exercise tolerance with limited ability to perform independent daily activities • General ill appearance • Coexisting medical or psychiatric disease that potentially increases severity of pulmonary infection or decreases likelihood of outpatient treatment adherence • Marginal social situation (e.g. homeless, substance abuser)
Potential for infection transmission	• Any patient with suspected active tuberculosis and with risk of transmission to other individuals at place of residence
Other	• Inability to provide appropriate follow-up (e.g. no primary care provider) • Inability to schedule necessary diagnostic testing (e.g. sputum induction, bronchoscopy)

* Lim *et al.* 2003.

6. Fever, hypoxemia, dry cough, and a normal chest radiograph in a patient with CD4 count below 200 cells/μL is highly suggestive of PCP. Further evaluation is recommended with HRCT, sputum induction, or bronchoscopy.

7. Indolent fevers, night sweats, and weight loss in a patient with either diffuse lymphadenopathy or a cavitary or miliary pattern on CXR is highly suggestive of infection with TB or endemic fungi.

8. When considering need for admission, remember that rapid definitive diagnosis is important, particularly in the case of PCP or TB, and is often difficult to accomplish on an outpatient basis.

References

Afessa, B., Green, W., Chiao, J., and Frederick, W. Pulmonary complications of HIV infection: autopsy findings. *Chest* 1998; 113(5): 1225–9.

Boyton, R. J. Infectious lung complications in patients with HIV/AIDS. *Curr. Opin. Pulm. Med.* 2005; 11(3): 203–7.

Buchacz, K., Baker, R. K., Palella, F. J., et al. AIDS-defining opportunistic illnesses in US patients, 1994–2007: a cohort study. *AIDS Lond. Engl.* 2010; 24(10): 1549–59.

Centers for Disease Control and Prevention. 1993 revised classification system for HIV infection and expanded surveillance case definition for AIDS among adolescents and adults. *JAMA* 1993; 269(6): 729–30.

Chuck, S. L. and Sande, M. A. Infections with Cryptococcus neoformans in the acquired immunodeficiency syndrome. *N. Engl. J. Med.* 1989; 321(12): 794–9.

Corbett, E. L., Watt, C. J., Walker, N., et al. The growing burden of tuberculosis: global trends and interactions with the HIV epidemic. *Arch. Intern. Med.* 2003; 163(9): 1009–21.

Cordero, E., Pachón, J., Rivero, A., et al. Usefulness of sputum culture for diagnosis of bacterial pneumonia in HIV-infected patients. *Eur. J. Clin. Microbiol. Infect. Dis.* 2002; 21(5): 362–7.

Da Silva, R. M., Teixeira, P. J. Z., and Da Silva Moreira, J. The clinical utility of induced sputum for the diagnosis of bacterial community-acquired pneumonia in HIV-infected patients: a prospective cross-sectional study. *Braz. J. Infect. Dis.* 2006; 10(2): 89–93.

Estébanez-Muñoz, M., Soto-Abánades, C. I., Ríos-Blanco, J. J., and Arribas, J. R. Updating our understanding of pulmonary disease associated with HIV infection. *Arch. Bronconeumol.* 2012; 48(4): 126–32.

Feikin, D. R., Feldman, C., Schuchat, A., and Janoff, E. N. Global strategies to prevent bacterial pneumonia in adults with HIV disease. *Lancet Infect. Dis.* 2004; 4(7): 445–55.

Gold, J. A., Rom, W. N., and Harkin, T. J. Significance of abnormal chest radiograph findings in patients with HIV-1 infection without respiratory symptoms. *Chest* 2002; 121(5): 1472–7.

Greenberg, S. D., Frager, D., Suster, B., et al. Active pulmonary tuberculosis in patients with AIDS: spectrum of radiographic findings (including a normal appearance). *Radiology* 1994; 193(1): 115–19.

Hall, H. I., Frazier, E. L., Rhodes, P., et al. Differences in human immunodeficiency virus care and treatment among subpopulations in the United States. *JAMA Intern. Med.* 2013; 173(14): 1337–44.

Hidalgo, A., Falcó, V., Mauleón, S., et al. Accuracy of high-resolution CT in distinguishing between Pneumocystis carinii pneumonia and non-Pneumocystis carinii pneumonia in AIDS patients. *Eur. Radiol.* 2003; 13(5): 1179–84.

Hirschtick, R. E., Glassroth, J., Jordan, M. C., et al. Bacterial pneumonia in persons infected with the human immunodeficiency virus. Pulmonary Complications of HIV Infection Study Group. *N. Engl. J. Med.* 1995; 333(13): 845–51.

Huang, L., Schnapp, L. M., Gruden, J. F., et al. Presentation of AIDS-related pulmonary Kaposi's sarcoma diagnosed by bronchoscopy. *Am. J. Respir. Crit. Care Med.* 1996; 153(4 Pt. 1): 1385–90.

Huang, L. and Stansell, J. D. AIDS and the lung. *Med. Clin. North Am.* 1996; 80(4): 775–801.

Jasmer, R. M., Gotway, M. B., Creasman, J. M., et al. Clinical and radiographic predictors of the etiology of computed tomography-diagnosed intrathoracic lymphadenopathy in HIV-infected patients. *J. Acquir. Immune Defic. Syndr. 1999* 2002; 31(3): 291–8.

Kanmogne, G. D. Noninfectious pulmonary complications of HIV/AIDS. *Curr. Opin. Pulm. Med.* 2005; 11(3): 208–12.

Kaplan, J. E., Benson, C., Holmes, K. K., et al. Guidelines for Prevention and Treatment of Opportunistic Infections in HIV-Infected Adults and Adolescents: recommendations from CDC, the National Institutes of Health, and the HIV Medicine Association of the Infectious Diseases Society of America. *MMWR Morb. Mortal. Wkly. Rep.* 2009; 58(RR-4): 1–207; quiz CE1–4.

Kennedy, C. A. and Goetz, M. B. Atypical roentgenographic manifestations of Pneumocystis carinii pneumonia. *Arch. Intern. Med.* 1992; 152(7): 1390–8.

Lim, W. S., van der Eerden, M. M., Laing, R., et al. Defining community acquired pneumonia severity on presentation to hospital: an international derivation and validation study. *Thorax* 2003; 58(5): 377–82.

Moreno, S., Martinez, R., Barros, C., et al. Latent Haemophilus influenzae pneumonia in patients infected with HIV. *AIDS Lond. Engl.* 1991; 5(8): 967–70.

Obirikorang, C., Quaye, L., and Acheampong, I. Total lymphocyte count as a surrogate marker for CD4 count in resource-limited settings. *BMC Infect. Dis.* 2012; 12: 128.

O'Donnell, W. J., Pieciak, W., Chertow, G. M., et al. Clearance of Pneumocystis carinii cysts in acute P carinii pneumonia: assessment by serial sputum induction. *Chest* 1998; 114(5): 1264–8.

Smith, R. L., Yew, K., Berkowitz, K. A., and Aranda, C. P. Factors affecting the yield of acid-fast sputum smears in patients with HIV and tuberculosis. *Chest* 1994; 106(3): 684–6.

Stansell, J. D., Osmond, D. H., Charlebois, E., et al. Predictors of Pneumocystis carinii pneumonia in HIV-infected persons. Pulmonary Complications of HIV Infection Study Group. *Am. J. Respir. Crit. Care Med.* 1997; 155(1): 60–6.

Taylor, Z., Nolan, C. M., and Blumberg, H. M. American Thoracic Society, Centers for Disease Control and Prevention, Infectious Diseases Society of America. Controlling tuberculosis in the United States. Recommendations from the American Thoracic Society, CDC, and the Infectious Diseases Society of America. *MMWR Morb. Mortal. Wkly. Rep.* 2005; 54(RR-12): 1–81.

Turner, D., Schwarz, Y., and Yust, I. Induced sputum for diagnosing Pneumocystis carinii pneumonia in HIV patients: new data, new issues. *Eur. Respir. J.* 2003; 21(2): 204–8.

Zaman, M. K. and White, D. A. Serum lactate dehydrogenase levels and Pneumocystis carinii pneumonia. Diagnostic and prognostic significance. *Am. Rev. Respir. Dis.* 1988; 137(4): 796–800.

Additional Readings

Centers for Disease Control and Prevention. Guidelines for the prevention and treatment of opportunistic infections in HIV-infected adults and adolescents: recommendations from CDC, the National Institutes of Health, and the HIV Medicine Association/Infectious Diseases Society of America. *MMWR Morb. Mortal. Wkly. Rep.* 2009; 58(RR-4): 1–207.

Crothers, K., Morris, A., and Huang, L. Pulmonary complications of human immunodeficiency virus infection in R. J. Mason, V. C. Broaddus, T. Martin, *et al.* (eds.), *Murray and Nadel's Textbook of Respiratory Medicine* (Philadelphia, PA: Elsevier, 2010), pp. 1914–50.

Mandell, L. A., Wunderink, R. G., Anzueto, A., *et al.* Infectious Diseases Society of America/American Thoracic Society consensus guidelines on the management of community acquired pneumonia in adults. *Clin. Infect. Dis.* 2007; 44(2): S27–72.

Notes

1 Kanmogne 2005.
2 Hall *et al.* 2013.
3 Buchacz *et al.* 2010.
4 Kanmogne 2005.
5 Afessa *et al.* 1998; Hirschtick *et al.* 1995.
6 Corbett *et al.* 2003.
7 Taylor *et al.* 2005.
8 Stansell *et al.* 1997.
9 Huang and Stansell 1996.
10 Chuck and Sande 1989.
11 Obirikorang *et al.* 2012.
12 Zaman and White 1988.
13 Cordero *et al.* 2002.
14 Kaplan *et al.* 2009.
15 Turner *et al.* 2003; Smith *et al.* 1994.
16 Estébanez-Muñoz *et al.* 2012.
17 O'Donnell *et al.* 1998.
18 Moreno *et al.* 1991.
19 Kennedy and Goetz 1992.
20 Greenberg *et al.* 1994.
21 Gold *et al.* 2002.
22 Hidalgo *et al.* 2003.
23 Jasmer *et al.* 2002.
24 Huang *et al.* 1996.
25 CDC 1993.
26 Taylor *et al.* 2005.

Chapter

46

Influenza

Asim A. Jani and Timothy M. Uyeki*

Introduction and Microbiology

Influenza is an acute respiratory disease caused by infection with human influenza viruses that are transmitted primarily by droplets expelled during coughing and sneezing. Influenza type A and B virus infections can cause substantial human disease and mortality worldwide. Patients can present with different signs and symptoms depending upon host factors such as age, underlying chronic disease, immune function, and complications associated with influenza. Seasonal winter influenza epidemics in temperate countries can substantially impact the emergency department (ED), but travelers may present with influenza illness acquired in other countries year-round. Rarely, the emergence of a novel influenza A virus can lead to a influenza pandemic.

Influenza viruses are single-stranded negative-sense RNA viruses of the family *Orthomyxoviridae*. Of four known types of influenza viruses, three types (A, B, and C) are known to infect humans, but only type A and B viruses are associated with seasonal epidemics worldwide. The genome contains eight gene segments that code for 11 proteins, including the two main surface glycoproteins, hemagglutinin (HA) and neuraminidase (NA). Type A viruses are further classified into subtypes based on their HA and NA proteins. Currently circulating human influenza A virus subtypes include A (H1N1) pdm09 and A (H3N2) viruses. Human influenza viruses bind to and replicate primarily in epithelial cells of the upper respiratory tract, though infection of lower respiratory tract tissues can occur.

Influenza viruses are evolving continuously through a process called "antigenic drift" in which random point mutations in the HA gene result in changes to the HA surface protein.

Minor changes in the genetic composition of influenza viruses can create new virus strains. Humoral immunity is based largely upon strain-specific HA antibodies and is reduced in young children, immunosuppressed and immunocompromised, and elderly persons, and wanes over time. In addition to waning immunity, antigenic drift is the reason that influenza virus strain surveillance must be conducted worldwide year-round and vaccine strains must be updated each year. Because of this and waning immunity, annual influenza vaccination is needed.

"Antigenic shift" is the emergence of a novel influenza A virus in humans. While most instances of antigenic shift represent sporadic zoonotic infections with an influenza A virus of animal origin, if the novel influenza A virus acquires the ability for sustained human-to-human transmission, a pandemic of variable severity can result. This can occur through direct mutation from an influenza A virus circulating among birds or pigs (such as the H1N1 virus that caused the 1918–1919 "Spanish flu" pandemic resulting in an estimated 20 to 100 million deaths worldwide, or the H1N1pdm09 virus that caused the 2009 pandemic that resulted in an estimated 200,000 respiratory deaths globally) or through genetic reassortment between human and avian influenza A viruses. The natural reservoir for nearly all influenza A virus subtypes is in wild aquatic ducks and geese; a small number of new subtypes have been identified in bats. The 1957–1958 "Asian influenza" H2N2 and 1968–1969 "Hong Kong influenza" H3N2 pandemic viruses originated through genetic reassortment between human influenza A and low pathogenic avian influenza A viruses. Once a pandemic influenza A virus emerges, in subsequent years, it continues to circulate among humans as a seasonal influenza A virus and evolves through antigenic drift.

---

* Disclaimer: The findings and conclusions in this report are those of the authors and do not necessarily represent the official position of the Centers for Disease Control and Prevention.

Box 46.1 Persons at High Risk for Developing Complications from Influenza

- children aged <5 years, but especially those aged <2 years
- adults aged ≥65 years
- pregnant women up to 2 weeks post-partum
- residents of nursing homes and other long-term care facilities
- American Indians and Alaska Natives
- persons with certain chronic medical conditions
  ○ asthma
  ○ neurological and neurodevelopment conditions (including disorders of the brain, spinal cord, peripheral nerve, and muscle such as cerebral palsy, epilepsy [seizure disorders], stroke, intellectual disability [mental retardation], moderate to severe developmental delay, muscular dystrophy, or spinal cord injury)
  ○ chronic lung disease (such as chronic obstructive pulmonary disease [COPD] and cystic fibrosis)
  ○ cardiac disease (e.g. congenital heart disease, congestive heart failure, coronary artery disease)*
  ○ hematologic disorders
  ○ endocrine disorders (e.g. diabetes mellitus)
  ○ renal disease
  ○ hepatic disease
  ○ metabolic disorders (such as inherited metabolic disorders and mitochondrial disorders)
  ○ immunosuppression due to medical conditions (e.g. HIV) or treatment (chemotherapy, radiation, chronic corticosteroid use)
  ○ persons aged <19 years receiving long-term aspirin therapy
  ○ extreme obesity (BMI ≥40)

* Excludes isolated hypertension.

Epidemiology

Seasonal influenza epidemics of unpredictable and variable severity occur during winter months in temperate climates of the Northern (October to April) and Southern (May to September) Hemispheres. In temperate climates, communities may experience high influenza activity for 6 to 8 weeks, though influenza virus infections may occur for several weeks longer. Attack rates are usually highest in schoolchildren with high rates of visits to outpatient clinics and EDs. In the United States each year, there was an estimated average of more than 200,000 hospitalizations, and between 3,400 and 49,000 deaths attributable to influenza and its complications during 1976 to 2007. The variability in the severity of seasonal influenza epidemics is highlighted by the range in estimated number of medical visits (4.3 to 16.7 million), hospitalizations (140,000 to 710,000), and deaths (12,000 to 56,000) attributable to influenza each year in the United States from 2010 to 2016. Those at highest risk for complications from influenza are young children, persons with chronic underlying conditions (e.g. cardiopulmonary diseases, immunosuppression), pregnant women, and the elderly (see Box 46.1).

In tropical and subtropical countries, influenza activity can occur year-round and may increase during cooler temperature months or rainy seasons. Worldwide, influenza outbreaks with high attack rates can occur at any time, especially among nursing home residents, children at boarding schools and camps, and travelers in large organized tour groups such as cruise ship passengers. Thus, a returned traveler from any part of the world presenting to an acute care setting with acute respiratory illness at any time of year should be evaluated for possible influenza, including when influenza activity is low in the local community.

Clinical Features

Following infection of the upper respiratory tract, the incubation period is generally 2 days, with a range of 1 to 4 days. Most infected children and adults shed influenza virus in the upper respiratory tract beginning one day prior to symptom onset and continuing for 4 to 5 days. Young infants can shed influenza viruses for 1 to 3 weeks and immunosuppressed or immunocompromised persons can shed viruses for longer periods. Persons with pneumonia and respiratory failure may have ongoing influenza viral replication in the lower respiratory tract after viral shedding is not detectable in upper respiratory tract specimens.

Signs and symptoms of influenza vary by age, immune function, underlying conditions, and whether complications are present. Uncomplicated influenza in older children and adults is typically characterized by abrupt onset of high fever and other systemic symptoms – chills, myalgias, fatigue, malaise, and headache; and respiratory symptoms such as non-productive cough, non-exudative pharyngitis, rhinorrhea, and nasal congestion (see Tables 46.1 and 46.2). Adults may complain of chest pain. While fever is typical, it is not always present, and immunosuppressed persons and elderly, in particular, may not manifest fever with influenza. Influenza virus is a common pathogen identified among adults admitted to the hospital with a diagnosis of community-acquired pneumonia.

Table 46.1 Signs and Symptoms of Uncomplicated Influenza in Patients without Underlying Conditions

	Infants and Young Children	School-Age Children	Adults	Elderly
Fever (subjective and objective)	Often high fever; or fever alone	+	+	Absent or low grade
Chills		+	+	+
Headache		+	+	+
Rhinorrhea	+	+	+	+
Nasal congestion	+	+	+	+
Sore throat		+	+	+
Myalgia		+	+	+
Cough, non-productive		+	+	+
Chest discomfort or pain		+	+	+
Abdominal pain		+		
Vomiting			+	
Diarrhea	+	+		
Malaise		+	+	+
Fatigue		+	+	+

+ may be present.

Table 46.2 Clinical Features of Uncomplicated Influenza

Incubation period	Generally 2 days, range 1–4 days
	Viral shedding occurs the day prior to onset of clinical symptoms and continues for 4–5 days in most persons (longer in infants and immunosuppressed persons)
Signs and symptoms*	Initially, systemic symptoms predominate
	• Fever (duration 3 days, range 2–8 days) and non-productive cough
	• Chills, malaise, headache, myalgias, sore throat, rhinorrhea, nasal congestion, anorexia
	Symptoms can last 1–3 weeks depending on baseline health status
	• Cough, fatigue, and malaise
Laboratory and radiologic findings	WBC often normal (unless invasive bacterial co-infection is present)
	Sputum Gram stain unremarkable
	CXR usually normal in uncomplicated influenza

* Differs by age and underlying conditions. Young infants may have fever without respiratory symptoms, young children may have abdominal pain and diarrhea, adults may complain of chest pain and vomiting, elderly may not always have fever.

CXR – chest x-ray; WBC – white blood (cell) count.

Young infants can present with high fever and a "sepsis-like" syndrome without respiratory findings. Gastrointestinal symptoms (diarrhea) can occur in young children and are more common with influenza B, while schoolchildren may occasionally complain of abdominal pain. Mild illness and asymptomatic infection can occur. There is a wide range of clinical complications associated with influenza (see Table 46.3), especially in persons who are at higher risk of developing complications from influenza (see Box 46.1).

The clinical diagnosis of influenza is challenging because the signs and symptoms of uncomplicated influenza overlap with those caused by infection with many co-circulating pathogens (respiratory viruses, atypical bacteria, or fungi). In general, high fever and cough are frequently associated with influenza. A clinical diagnosis is most accurate during peak community influenza activity. Since influenza vaccination is of variable effectiveness – depending on the match in any given year between circulating virus strains and the influenza vaccine virus strains, as well as on host factors – a history of current season influenza vaccination does not exclude a diagnosis of influenza. Influenza vaccine effectiveness is lowest in elderly and infants due to reduced immune function.

Differential Diagnosis

The differential diagnosis of uncomplicated acute influenza-like illness in a patient without underlying conditions includes infection with:

- respiratory viruses (influenza viruses, parainfluenza viruses, respiratory syncytial virus, rhinoviruses, adenoviruses, human metapneumovirus, non-SARS coronarviruses, bocavirus, enteroviruses)
- atypical bacteria (*Legionella pneumophila*, *Mycoplasma pneumoniae*, *Chlamydia pneumoniae*)
- community-acquired bacteria (e.g. *Streptococcus pneumoniae*, *Hemophilous influenzae*, *Bordetella pertussis*)

Fungal (*Histoplasma*, *Cryptococcus*, *Coccidioides*) and parasitic causes of influenza-like illness are less common. Rare human

Table 46.3 Clinical Complications Associated with Influenza

Infants and young children:

Fever without respiratory complication, "sepsis-like syndrome"

Otitis media

Bronchiolitis

Croup

Reactive airway disease

Pneumonia

Myocarditis, pericarditis

Rhabdomyolysis

Febrile seizures

Encephalopathy and encephalitis

Invasive bacterial infection (sepsis, pneumonia, MRSA, MSSA, *Streptococcus pneumoniae*, Group A *Streptoccoccus*, *Haemophilus influenzae*)

Reye syndrome (with aspirin use)

Sudden death (may be related to cytokine dysregulation)

Exacerbation of chronic disease

School-age children:

Bronchitis

Sinusitis

Reactive airway disease

Pneumonia

Myocarditis, pericarditis myocardial infarction

Myositis (bilateral gastrocnemius, soleus)

Rhabdomyolysis

Encephalopathy and encephalitis

Invasive bacterial infection (sepsis, pneumonia, MRSA, MSSA, *Streptococcus pheumoniae*, Group A *Streptococcus*, *Haemophilus influenzae*)

Reye syndrome (with aspirin use)

Toxic shock syndrome

Sudden death (may be related to cytokine dysregulation)

Exacerbation of chronic disease

Adults:

Bronchitis

Sinusitis

Reactive airway disease

Pneumonia

Myocarditis, pericarditis myocardial infarction

Myositis

Rhabdomyolysis

Invasive bacterial infection (sepsis, pneumonia, MRSA, MSSA, *Streptoccoccus pneumoniae*, Group A *Streptococcus*, *Haemophilus influenzae*)

Toxic shock syndrome

Exacerbation of chronic disease

Elderly patients:

Pneumonia

Invasive bacterial infection (sepsis, pneumonia, MRSA, MSSA, *Streptococcus pneumoniae*, Group A *Streptococcus*, *Haemophilus influenzae*)

Myositis

Exacerbation of chronic disease

Special groups – pregnant women:

Dehydration

Table 46.3 (cont.)

Pneumonia

Cardiopulmonary disease

Special groups – immunocompromised, immunosuppressed

Infectious and non-infectious complications associated with influenza observed in immunocompetent persons are possible

MRSA – methicillin-resistant *Staphylococcus aureus*; MSSA – methicillin-sensitive *Staphylococcus aureus*.

infection with other infectious agents such as *Bacillus anthracis*, *SARS-associated Coronavirus*, *Middle East Respiratory Syndrome Coronavirus* (*MERS–CoV*) and novel influenza A viruses (avian influenza A viruses [e.g. H5N1, H7N9], variant influenza A viruses of swine-origin [H1N1v, H1N2v, H3N2v]) can present initially with influenza-like illness, but a good history, including recent travel and exposure to animals (e.g. poultry, pigs, camels) or sick contacts, and radiographic and laboratory testing results, can help to distinguish the features of these uncommon pathogens from illness caused by seasonal influenza A and B viruses. Immunocompromised and immunocompetent patients can present with influenza-like illness caused by opportunistic pathogens such as *Mycobacterium tuberculosis* or fungi. The medical history, a history of similar acute respiratory illnesses in household members, exposure history, and a travel history may be very helpful in formulating the differential diagnosis.

Laboratory and Radiographic Findings

In patients with influenza, the peripheral blood WBC may reveal leukopenia and lymphopenia, but it may also be normal or slightly elevated. Transaminases may be mildly elevated.

Chest X-ray is an important diagnostic test for risk stratification in suspected influenza. In a patient with fever and cough, chest X-ray is the best way to distinguish community-acquired pneumonia from uncomplicated influenza. The chest X-ray is usually normal in patients with uncomplicated influenza. Primary influenza pneumonia typically produces bilateral interstitial infiltrates and opacities, with or without consolidation. Influenza can also be complicated by bacterial pneumonia, in which case the chest X-ray can show single or multiple, lobar or cavitary infiltrates. In general, patients with a clinical syndrome suspicious for influenza (including high fever) and an abnormal chest X-ray, whether consistent with influenza pneumonia or secondary bacterial pneumonia, should undergo a careful evaluation for possible hospital admission (see Complications and Admission Criteria, below).

Influenza virus infection can be confirmed by a variety of testing methods of which molecular assays are the most accurate. If results are properly interpreted, testing can inform clinical management (see Table 46.4). It is important to obtain the appropriate respiratory specimens during the period of highest influenza viral shedding. In the acute care setting, the best clinical specimens are nasopharyngeal or nasal swabs or aspirates that are collected as close to illness onset as possible, and ideally within 4 days after fever onset. Patients presenting with

Table 46.4 Tests Available for Detection of Influenza Viruses in Respiratory Specimens

Influenza Tests*	
Rapid diagnostic test (antigen detection)†	• Enzyme immunoassay (utilizes monoclonal antibodies against influenza viruses) or immunofluorescence assay • Can yield results within 15 minutes • Can differentiate between influenza A and B virus infection • Sensitivity 10–70%, Specificity 90–99% compared to RT-PCR or viral culture ➢ False-negative results can occur during peak influenza activity ➢ False positive results can occur during low influenza activity • Most rapid influenza diagnostic tests are point-of-care assays approved for use in the patient's room
Immunofluorescence (antigen detection)	• Direct (DFA) or indirect (IFA) fluorescent antibody staining (uses monoclonal antibodies against influenza viruses) • Can yield results in 2–4 hours • Can differentiate between influenza A and B virus infection • Requires fluorescent microscope ➢ Moderately high sensitivity, high specificity compared to RT-PCR or viral culture
Molecular assays (nucleic acid detection)‡	• Molecular assays include rapid molecular assays, other nucleic acid detection assays, cartridge-based multi-pathogen assays, and conventional and real-time RT-PCR • Rapid molecular assays can yield results within 15–30 minutes ➢ High sensitivity, high specificity • Some commercially available molecular assays can yield results in 70–80 minutes ➢ High sensitivity, high specificity • Conventional and real-time RT-PCR assays may yield results in 4–8 hours or longer ➢ Very high sensitivity and specificity
Viral culture	• Considered a "gold standard" influenza test • Tissue cell culture requires 2–10 days • Shell vial cell culture requires 1–3 days

* Collect nasopharyngeal and nasal swab or aspirate specimens as close to illness onset as possible (within 4 days) for all tests. Interpretation of all influenza test results are influenced by the prevalence of circulating influenza viruses in the population tested (how much influenza activity is occurring). Serological testing for seasonal influenza A and B virus antibodies required paired acute and convalescent serum, cannot inform clinical management, and is not recommended.

† Some assays utilize an analyzer reader device. The US FDA has reclassified these devices to require higher sensitivity and specificity.

‡ The main differences among the molecular assays are the time to produce results and sensitivity to detect influenza viral nucleic acid. Some assays require a device to perform nucleic acid amplification and detection.

RNA – ribonucleic acid; RT-PCR – reverse-transcription polymerase chain reaction.

pneumonia more than 4 to 5 days after illness onset should also have lower respiratory tract specimens tested for influenza viruses.

Tests that are most useful for the acute care setting include rapid influenza diagnostic tests (RIDTs), rapid molecular assays, and other molecular assays, if timely results are available. Rapid influenza diagnostic tests are antigen detection screening tests that can yield results within 15 minutes and include tests that only detect influenza A viral antigens; tests that detect, but do not distinguish between influenza A and B viral antigens; and tests that detect and distinguish between influenza A and B viral antigens. To properly interpret results, physicians should understand the limitations of RIDTs. While RIDTs have high specificity (90 to 99%), their sensitivities are only low to moderate (10 to 70%) compared to RT-PCR or viral culture, so false-negative results can occur frequently during influenza season. The most important factor influencing the accuracy of RIDTs (in terms of post-test probability) is how prevalent influenza activity is among the patient population being tested. Positive test results are most likely true positive and negative results more likely falsely negative during peak community influenza activity.

Recently, rapid molecular influenza assays are available that can produce results within 15–30 minutes. These rapid molecular assays and other molecular assays can detect and distinguish between influenza A and B viruses in respiratory specimens and have higher sensitivities than RIDTs; therefore, false-negative results are less frequent. Some influenza molecular assays are available that can produce results in approximately 70 to 80 minutes with high sensitivity and high specificity.

Persons who received intranasally administered live attenuated influenza virus (LAIV) vaccine can shed virus in the nasal passages for 7 days after vaccination and may test positive by rapid tests and other influenza tests if tested within 7 days of LAIV vaccination. However, LAIV vaccine was not recommended in the United States during the 2016–2018 seasons.

A diagnosis of laboratory-confirmed influenza in a patient who is stable enough to be discharged can reduce length of stay in the ED, reduce inappropriate antibiotic use, and reduce costs by avoiding the need for additional laboratory tests. Current information on influenza tests is available at the Centers for Disease Control and Prevention (CDC) influenza website.

Treatment

Antiviral treatment of uncomplicated influenza with a neuraminidase inhibitor drug (oral oseltamivir, inhaled zanamivir,

Table 46.5 Recommended Antivirals for Influenza*

ANTIVIRALS	Oseltamivir	Zanamivir	Peramivir
Route	Oral	Oral inhalation	Intravenous
Activity	Influenza A and B	Influenza A and B	Influenza A and B
Treatment 5 days' duration	**<1 year old:** 3mg/kg/dose PO BID **≥1 year old:** ≤15 kg: 30 mg PO BID >15–23 kg: 45 mg PO BID >23–40 kg: 60 mg PO BID >40 kg: 75 mg PO BID **Adults:** 75 mg PO BID	**≥7 years old:** 10 mg (two inhalations of 5 mg each) BID	**2–12 years old:** 12 mg/kg dose, up to 600 mg maximum, IV over 15–30 minutes × 1 dose **>13 years old:** 600 mg dose IV over 15–30 minutes × 1 dose
Prophylaxis	**≥3 months:** Same as treatment dose, but only once daily	**≥5 years old:** 10 mg (two inhalations of 5 mg each) once daily	Not approved
Primary adverse effects	Nausea, vomiting	Bronchospasm	Diarrhea

* Amantadine and rimantidine are no longer recommended in the United States for treatment of influenza A because of high resistance rates. Physicians should consult the package insert for each antiviral medication for drug interactions, contraindications, adverse events, and dosage – especially for pediatric patients. Dosage adjustment for oseltamivir or peramivir is needed for reduced creatinine clearance or dialysis.

or intravenous peramivir) **is recommended as soon as possible** for outpatients of all ages who are considered to be at **high-risk of complications** from influenza (see Box 46.1). In addition, all patients with progressive disease and all hospitalized patients with suspected or laboratory-confirmed influenza should be treated as soon as possible without waiting for laboratory testing results (see Table 46.5). Meta-analyses of observational studies suggest that antiviral treatment is most beneficial when started soon after illness onset, and can reduce the risk of severe complications and death from influenza, compared to late treatment or no antiviral treatment.

Patients with uncomplicated influenza who are not in a high-risk group and who present within 48 hours of illness onset may also receive antiviral treatment based upon clinical judgment. Randomized trials indicate that early initiation of antiviral treatment can decrease the signs and symptoms of influenza by approximately 1 day compared to placebo, and can reduce the occurrence of moderate complications such as otitis media, sinusitis, and the need for antibiotic treatment of lower respiratory tract disease. The main drug-related adverse events are the following: oral oseltamivir is associated with nausea and vomiting; and inhaled zanamivir is associated with bronchospasm and is not recommended for persons with underlying airway disease. Otherwise, treatment of uncomplicated influenza is supportive. Antiviral treatment of influenza A with amantadine or rimantadine is not recommended due to the high frequency of resistance to these drugs. Latest antiviral treatment recommendations are available at the CDC influenza website.

Patients who are being discharged or their parents and their families should be cautioned about possible complications of influenza. Aspirin (salicylic acid) and salicylate-containing products are contraindicated in patients aged <18 years because of the risk of Reye syndrome.

In addition to antiviral treatment, supportive management of mild to moderate complications can be done on an outpatient basis with good follow-up. Treatment of patients with exacerbation of underlying conditions should focus upon stabilization of chronic disease.

Complications and Admission Criteria

Minor to moderate complications of influenza may not require hospital admission, but severe complications can be life-threatening and require hospitalization (see Table 46.3). Minor to moderate complications include otitis media in young children, and sinusitis and bronchitis in children and adults. School-age children can experience very painful bilateral myositis of the soleus and gastrocnemius muscles and may refuse to walk, and bronchiolitis and croup in young children may also require hospitalization.

Viral pneumonia is more likely to occur in elderly persons, pregnant women, and patients with chronic cardiovascular or chronic pulmonary disease. Chest X-rays can reveal rapid progression from bilateral interstitial infiltrates to ARDS. Influenza A(H1N1)pdm09 virus infection can progress rapidly to severe viral pneumonia within a few days without bacterial co-infection. However, secondary bacterial pneumonia can develop shortly after the onset of influenza illness or after uncomplicated influenza symptoms are resolving. The most common invasive bacterial pathogens associated with co-infection with influenza viruses include *Streptococcus pneumoniae*, *Staphylococcus aureus*, Group A Streptococcus (*S. pyogenes*), and *Hemophilus influenzae*. Fulminant progression and high fatality occurs with *Staphylococcus aureus*, especially with invasive methicillin-resistant (MRSA) infections. A less well-recognized severe complication associated with influenza is meningitis from *Neisseria meningitidis* co-infection or during recovery from influenza.

Neurological complications of influenza are more common in young children than adults. Febrile and complex seizures may occur. Fulminant and severe influenza-associated acute encephalopathy and encephalitis (with unremarkable CSF findings) occur shortly after illness onset and can result in severe disability and death. Post-infectious encephalopathy and demyelinating syndrome can occur approximately 1 to 2 weeks after onset of influenza. Reye syndrome, characterized by hypoglycemia, hyperammonemia, and encephalopathy, is associated with aspirin use, and may follow influenza onset by 1 to 2 weeks; it can also occur with influenza B more commonly than influenza A without exposure to salicylates.

Other severe extrapulmonary complications of influenza include toxic shock syndrome, myocarditis, myocardial infraction and pericarditis. Severe rhabdomyolysis may result in myoglobinuria and renal failure. Hypotension and hypothermia have also been reported in pediatric influenza patients with fatal outcomes. A sepsis-like syndrome without respiratory findings may occur in young infants with influenza. Multiorgan failure (respiratory and renal failure, with or without refractory shock) can occur within 1 week of illness onset.

Exacerbation of chronic underlying diseases is common with influenza. Influenza can precipitate worsening of cardiopulmonary disease such as congestive cardiac failure and coronary artery disease, chronic obstructive pulmonary disease, and asthma. Persons with neurological diseases that limit breathing or clearance of secretions are at high risk of respiratory complications, including pneumonia.

Unstable patients should be hospitalized, including for severe dehydration, hypotension, respiratory distress (hypoxia, hypoxemia, pneumonia), prolonged seizures, encephalopathy or encephalitis, severe myositis, rhabdomyolysis, myocarditis/pericarditis, invasive bacterial infections, sepsis, and exacerbation of underlying chronic conditions.

Special Groups

Pregnant women may experience severe dehydration and cardiopulmonary complications with influenza. Elderly persons may present with malaise and altered mental status without predominant respiratory symptoms, but have high rates of influenza complications such as pneumonia. Elderly nursing home residents are at particularly high risk for pneumonia and death from influenza. Immunocompromised persons may experience a variety of severe complications (e.g. pneumonia) from influenza requiring hospitalization.

Infection Prevention and Control

Infection prevention and control of influenza in the acute care setting is focused upon reducing the risk of influenza among health-care personnel and prevention of nosocomial transmission. All health-care personnel should receive annual influenza vaccination. Triage in the acute care setting should rapidly separate persons with influenza-like illness from others. Patients with suspected influenza should be isolated or cohorted if possible. Strict adherence to hand hygiene and standard respiratory hygiene/cough protocols should be emphasized. Standard, contact, and droplet precautions should be followed for patients with suspected influenza. The latest recommendations on infection prevention and control for seasonal influenza in health-care settings, including long-term care facilities, and influenza vaccination are available at the CDC website.

Vaccination

Annual influenza vaccination is recommended for all persons aged ≥6 months, and especially persons at high risk for complications from influenza, their household contacts and caregivers, and for all health-care personnel. Several kinds of influenza vaccines (trivalent or quadrivalent; standard dose, high-dose, egg-derived, tissue cell-culture derived, recombinant, adjuvanted; inactivated or live-attenuated) are available. Each year, the influenza vaccine virus strains [influenza A (H1N1)pdm09, A (H3N2), and influenza B] may be updated based upon global strain surveillance data. Live attenuated influenza virus vaccine for intranasal administration was approved in the United States for non-pregnant individuals aged 2 to 49 years without underlying chronic comorbidities, but was not recommended during the 2016–2018 seasons. Influenza vaccine effectiveness in preventing illness and hospitalization is generally moderate, but is lower in very young children and elderly persons, and when significant antigenic drift in circulating strains distinct from vaccine strains occurs. However, a recent study reported >50% effectiveness at preventing death among children aged 6 months to 17 years with underlying high-risk conditions and 65% among those without high-risk conditions. Acute care physicians should not discount the possibility of influenza in persons who have received influenza vaccine.

Pearls and Pitfalls

- Close follow-up of influenza patients who are discharged from the ED is critical. Patients and family members must be educated that complications of influenza can develop and that further medical care may be needed for worsening symptoms.
- Elderly patients with influenza may not have fever and can present with confusion or altered mental status without typical respiratory symptoms. Such patients can progress rapidly to viral pneumonia.
- The best way to prevent influenza is to receive annual influenza vaccination. Health-care workers can transmit influenza virus to co-workers and to patients, but this can be prevented by annual influenza vaccination and strict adherence to infection prevention and control precautions.
- Do not exclude the possibility of influenza in a patient who received current season influenza vaccination. Influenza vaccination is generally of moderate effectiveness for multiple reasons (including decreased immunogenicity in young and elderly; antigenic drift).
- To reduce the risk of Reye syndrome, aspirin and salicylate-containing products should not be given to persons aged <18 years.
- If invasive bacterial co-infection is suspected, empiric antibiotic treatment should consider covering MRSA until antimicrobial susceptibility data are available. Fulminant disease progression and death can occur after a brief influenza

illness and co-infection with invasive *Streptococcus pneumoniae*, *methicillin-sensitive Staphylococcus aureus*, MRSA, or *Group A Streptococcus*.

- Exacerbation of underlying chronic conditions is common with influenza, including cardiopulmonary diseases.
- Influenza is unpredictable and the timing of peak activity, severity of circulating virus strains, predominant strains in the future, geographical spread, and occurrence of the next pandemic cannot be determined.
- Because influenza viruses are dynamic, and new therapies and vaccines are under development, emergency physicians should consult the latest information on influenza, diagnostic testing, antiviral treatment, and influenza vaccines and recommendations of the Advisory Committee on Immunization Practices from websites of the CDC, the Infectious Diseases Society of America (IDSA), and the World Health Organization (WHO).

References

Babcock, H. M., Merz, L. R., and Fraser, V. J. Is influenza an influenza-like illness? Clinical presentation of influenza in hospitalized patients. *Infect. Control Hosp. Epidemiol.* 2006; 27(3): 266–70.

Brankston, G., Gitterman, L., Hirji, Z., *et al.* Transmission of influenza A in human beings. *Lancet Infect. Dis.* 2007; 7(4): 257–65.

Bridges, C. B., Kuehnert, M. J., and Hall, C. B. Transmission of influenza: implications for control in health care settings. *Clin. Infect. Dis.* 2003; 37(8): 1094–101.

Call, S. A., Vollenweider, M. A., Hornung, C. A., *et al.* Does this patient have influenza? *JAMA* 2005; 293(8): 987–97.

Centers for Disease Control and Prevention (CDC). Estimates of deaths associated with seasonal influenza – United States, 1976–2007. *MMWR Morb. Mortal. Wkly. Rep.* 2010; 59(33): 1057–62.

CDC, Clinical Description & Lab Diagnosis of Influenza, www.cdc.gov/flu/professionals/diagnosis/index.htm (accessed November 21, 2017).

CDC, Disease burden of influenza, www.cdc.gov/flu/about/disease/burden.htm (accessed November 21, 2017).

CDC, Influenza antiviral medications: summary for clinicians, www.cdc.gov/flu/professionals/antivirals/summary-clinicians.htm (accessed November 21, 2017).

CDC, Prevent seasonal flu, www.cdc.gov/flu/protect/vaccine/index.htm (accessed November 21, 2017).

CDC, Prevention strategies for seasonal influenza in healthcare settings, www.cdc.gov/flu/professionals/infectioncontrol/healthcaresettings.htm (accessed November 21, 2017).

CDC, www.cdc.gov/flu/about (accessed November 21, 2017).

Dawood, F. S., Chaves, S. S., Pérez, A., *et al.* Emerging Infections Program Network. Complications and associated bacterial coinfections among children hospitalized with seasonal or pandemic influenza, United States, 2003–2010. *J. Infect. Dis.* 2014; 209(5): 686–94.

Dobson, J., Whitley, R. J., Pocock, S., and Monto, A. S. Oseltamivir treatment for influenza in adults: a meta-analysis of randomised controlled trials. *Lancet* 2015; 385(9979): 1729–37.

Flannery, B., Reynolds, S., Blanton, L., *et al.* Influenza vaccine effectiveness against pediatric deaths: 2010–2014. *Pediatrics* 2017; 139(5), published online April 3, 2017.

IDSA, Influenza, www.idsociety.org/Influenza/ (accessed November 21, 2017).

Kash, J. C. and Taubenberger, J. K. The role of viral, host, and secondary bacterial factors in influenza pathogenesis. *Am. J. Pathol.* 2015; 185(6): 1528–36.

Little, P., Stuart, B., Hobbs, F. D., *et al.* An internet-delivered handwashing intervention to modify influenza-like illness and respiratory infection transmission (PRIMIT): a primary care randomized trial. *Lancet* 2015; 386(10004): 1631–9.

Monto, A. S., Gravenstein, S., Elliott, M., *et al.* Clinical signs and symptoms predicting influenza infection. *Arch. Int. Med.* 2000; 160(21): 3243–7.

Muthuri, S. G., Venkatesan, S., Myles, P. R., *et al.* Effectiveness of neuraminidase inhibitors in reducing mortality in patients admitted to hospital with influenza A H1N1pdm09 virus infection: a meta-analysis of individual participant data. *Lancet Respir. Med.* 2014; 2(5): 395–404.

Napolitano, L. M., Angus, D. C., and Uyeki, T. M. Critically ill patients with influenza A(H1N1)pdm09 virus infection in 2014. *JAMA* 2014; 311(13): 1289–90.

Poehling, K. A., Edwards, K. M., Weinberg, G. A., *et al.* The underrecognized burden of influenza in young children. *N. Engl. J. Med.* 2006; 355(1): 31–40.

Randolph, A. G., Vaughn, F., Sullivan, R., *et al.* Pediatric Acute Lung Injury and Sepsis Investigator's Network and the National Heart, Lung, and Blood Institute ARDS Clinical Trials Network. Critically ill children during the 2009–2010 influenza pandemic in the United States. *Pediatrics* 2011; 128(6): e1450–8.

Thompson, W. W., Shay, D. K., Weintraub, E., *et al.* Influenza-associated hospitalizations in the United States. *JAMA* 2004; 292(11): 1333–40.

Uyeki, T. M. Preventing and controlling influenza with available interventions. *N. Engl. J. Med.* 2014; 370(9): 789–91.

Walsh, E. E., Cox, C., and Falsey, A. R. Clinical features of influenza A virus infection in older hospitalized persons. *J. Am. Geriatr. Soc.* 2002; 50(9): 1498–503.

Wong, K. K., Jain, S., Blanton, L., *et al.* Influenza-associated pediatric deaths in the United States, 2004–2012. *Pediatrics* 2013; 132(5): 796–804.

World Health Organization, Influenza, www.who.int/influenza/en/ (accessed November 21, 2017).

Additional Readings

Abraham, M. K., Perkins, J., Vilke, G. M., and Coyne, C. J. Influenza in the emergency department: vaccination, diagnosis, and treatment: clinical practice paper approved by American Academy of Emergency Medicine Clinical Guidelines Committee. *J. Emerg. Med.* 2016; 50(3): 536–42.

Bonner, B. B., Monroe, K. W., Talley, L. I., *et al.* Impact of the rapid diagnosis of influenza on physician decision-making and patient management in the pediatric emergency department: results of a randomized, prospective, controlled trial. *Pediatrics* 2003; 112(2): 363–7.

Dugas, A. F., Valsamakis, A., Atreya, M. R., *et al.* Clinical diagnosis of influenza in the ED. *Am. J. Emerg. Med.* 2015; 33(6): 770–5.

Dugas, A. F., Valsamakis, A., Gaydos, C. A., *et al.* Evaluation of the Xpert Flu rapid PCR assay in high-risk emergency department patients. *J. Clin. Microbiol.* 2014; 52(12): 4353–5.

Kourtis, A. P., Read, J. S., and Jamieson, D. J. Pregnancy and infection. *N. Eng. J. Med* 2014; 370(23): 2211–18.

Kwong, J. C., Schwartz, K. L., Campitelli, M. A., *et al.* Acute myocardial infarction after laboratory-confirmed influenza infection. *N. Engl. J. Med.* 2018; 378(4): 345–53.

Malosh, R. E., Martin, E. T., Heikkinen, T., *et al.* Efficacy and safety of oseltamivir in children: systematic review and individual patient data meta-analysis of randomized controlled trials. *Clin. Infect. Dis.* 2017; doi: 10.1093/cid/cix1040.

Merckx, J., Wali, R., Schiller, I., *et al.* Diagnostic accuracy of novel and traditional rapid tests for influenza infection compared with reverse transcriptase polymerase chain reaction: a systematic review and meta-analysis. *Ann. Intern. Med.* 2017; 167(6): 394–409.

Ploin, D., Gillet, Y., Morfin, F., *et al.* Influenza burden in febrile infants and young children in a pediatric emergency department. *Pediatr. Infect. Dis. J.* 2007; 26(2): 142–7.

Chapter 47

Tuberculosis

Robert Blount, Payam Nahid, and Adithya Cattamanchi

Introduction and Microbiology

Mycobacterium tuberculosis is a large, non-motile, curved rod that causes the vast majority of human tuberculosis cases. *M. tuberculosis* and three very closely related mycobacterial species (*M. bovis*, *M. africanum*, and *M. microti*) all cause tuberculous disease, and they comprise what is known as the *M. tuberculosis* complex. *M. tuberculosis* is an obligate aerobe, accounting for its predilection to cause disease in the well-aerated upper lobes of the lung. However, *M. tuberculosis* can persist in a dormant state for many years even with a limited oxygen supply. The organisms also persist in the environment and are resistant to disinfecting agents.

Mycobacterium species are classified as acid-fast organisms because of their ability to retain certain dyes when heated and treated with acidified compounds. Humans are the only known reservoir of infection.

Epidemiology

Tuberculosis has surpassed human immunodeficiency virus (HIV) as the leading cause of death related to an infectious disease. Nearly one-third of the world's population is infected with *Mycobacterium tuberculosis*. In 2013, the World Health Organization (WHO) estimated there were 9 million new cases of tuberculosis and 1.5 million deaths due to the disease.

HIV-infected persons are approximately 30 times more likely to develop active tuberculosis compared to those not infected with HIV. Whereas the average person infected with *Mycobacterium tuberculosis* has a 10% lifetime chance of developing active disease, immunocompromised patients can have their risk jump to that same percentage *annually*. Tuberculosis is the leading cause of death among HIV-infected persons, accounting for 25% of worldwide deaths in this group.

Drug resistance is of increasing concern, particularly among high-risk populations such as persons born in countries with high rates of drug resistance and those with a prior history of tuberculosis treatment. Multidrug-resistant tuberculosis (MDR-TB), defined as *Mycobacterium tuberculosis* resistant to at least isoniazid and rifampin (the two most powerful antituberculosis drugs), accounted for approximately 5% of new tuberculosis cases worldwide in 2013. Extensively drug-resistant tuberculosis (XDR-TB), defined as MDR-TB with additional resistance to a fluoroquinolone and at least one injectable second-line antituberculosis drug, has been documented in every country surveyed.

In the United States, following a resurgence in the 1980s, the incidence of tuberculosis has been declining since 1993 and is currently at an all-time low, with only 9,582 cases of active tuberculosis reported in 2013. However, the rate of decline has slowed since 2000. In addition, wide disparities persist with immigrants, minority groups, and people living in poverty being disproportionately affected. In 2013, 65% of active tuberculosis cases reported in the United States were in foreign-born persons. African Americans, Hispanics, American Indians, and Alaska Natives were more than seven times more likely to have active tuberculosis in 2013 compared with Whites, while Asians were 27 times more likely to have active tuberculosis compared to Whites. In 2013, MDR-TB accounted for 1.4% of active tuberculosis cases tested for drug susceptibility in the United States, with 89.5% of MDR-TB cases arising in foreign-born populations.

Tuberculosis cases develop either through exogenous infection with rapid progression to clinical illness or through endogenous reactivation of latent infection. In the developing world, where the burden of disease is high, the majority of new cases arise from transmission through contact with active cases of tuberculosis. In low-incidence countries, the majority of new cases arise from reactivation of latent infection. Molecular epidemiologic data from low-incidence countries has shown that up to 90% of all tuberculosis cases are due to reactivation of latent infection. Thus, identification and treatment of persons with latent infection is a major priority.

Pathogenesis and Risk Factors

The development of tuberculosis can be thought of as a two-phase process: the acquisition of *M. tuberculosis* infection and the subsequent development of active tuberculosis. Infection occurs when a susceptible individual is exposed to a person with active tuberculosis. The most common route of transmission is inhalation of aerosolized particles of approximately 1 to 5 μm generated when a person with active disease coughs. In heavily exposed individuals, there is a 30% chance of infection; it is estimated that as few as five viable bacilli delivered to a terminal alveolus can cause infection.

In the majority of cases, infected patients with an intact immune system will experience few or no symptoms after the initial exposure. Both innate and adaptive host defense mechanisms prevent active disease in most persons, but are unable to eliminate the tubercle bacilli, leading to a "latent" infected state. Although little is known about this pathologic state, histopathological animal model studies have demonstrated that granulomas are formed through the sensitized immune response at approximately 4 weeks: lymphocytes surround the initial macrophage and neutrophil responders to the mycobacterial infection, and sequester the bacilli. Some bacilli may escape this initial immune response and disseminate to organs outside of the lungs producing other latent foci of infection. Mycobacteria have also been shown to adapt to the immune response through decreased metabolism and develop resistance to hostile environmental elements, which may help explain how latent bacteria can remain viable for decades.

Approximately 3 to 5% of immunocompetent individuals will bypass a latent infection and develop active tuberculosis within 1 year of becoming infected, with an additional 3 to 5% progressing to active tuberculosis within their lifetime after a prolonged latent infection. Thus, 90% of infected, healthy persons will never develop clinical manifestations of tuberculosis.

The likelihood of developing active tuberculosis is related to both host and environmental factors. HIV infection is clearly the strongest risk factor for the development of active tuberculosis. The annual risk of developing active tuberculosis is 5 to 8% and the lifetime risk is 20% or greater in HIV-infected persons with a positive tuberculin skin test. The likelihood of disseminated disease is also increased in this population. In the United States, 20% of extrapulmonary tuberculosis cases are in HIV-infected patients, and 50% of tuberculosis infections in HIV patients have extrapulmonary foci. In addition, active tuberculosis has also been shown to accelerate the course of HIV infection.

Other conditions associated with impaired cell-mediated immunity also increase the risk of tuberculosis. Examples include nutritional deficiencies, hematologic malignancies, chemotherapy, and treatment with tumor necrosis factor alpha (TNF-alpha) inhibitors. Conditions such as diabetes mellitus and uremia are also associated with increased risk. Inhaled air pollutants and toxins also increase the risk of tuberculosis. Cigarette smoking, for instance, has a well-documented association with active tuberculosis and worse treatment outcomes. Pulmonary silicosis also increases the risk of tuberculosis, presumably because of the effects of silica on alveolar macrophage function. In addition to associated medical conditions and environmental exposures, age has a marked effect on the development of tuberculosis. The elderly and young children are at increased risk for developing tuberculosis and disseminated disease. The majority of child cases occur between the ages of 1 and 4, with one in four infections manifesting as extrapulmonary. Children under 4 years of age are more likely to experience hematogenous dissemination of mycobacteria and are at an increased risk of tubercular meningitis.

Clinical Features

Current guidelines recommend targeted screening of persons at high risk for the development of active tuberculosis. The guidelines emphasize that a decision to screen implies a decision to treat if the screening test is positive. Screening should be performed in those with increased risk of recent infection (e.g. contacts of active tuberculosis cases, recent immigrants from high burden countries, and health-care personnel) and in populations where TB transmission is ongoing (e.g. homeless persons). Screening should also be performed in those at highest risk of progression to active TB, including persons with HIV infection or receiving immunosuppressive therapy. Other groups at high risk of progression to active TB (e.g. persons with diabetes, tobacco smokers, infants and young children) should be considered for screening, particularly if there is any risk of TB exposure.

General Manifestations of Tuberculosis

The clinical presentation of tuberculosis varies tremendously depending on the affected site or sites of disease, the effectiveness of host defense mechanisms in containing the infection,

Table 47.1 Clinical Features: Tuberculosis

Incubation period	Variable
Organism	*Mycobacterium tuberculosis*
Signs and symptoms	• Cough is the most common symptom • Night sweats, fever, malaise, and weight loss • Hemoptysis and pleuritic chest pain
Laboratory and radiographic findings	• Laboratory studies are often normal • There may be anemia, leukocytosis, leukopenia, or hyponatremia • **Acute primary TB CXR** – middle or lower lung infiltration with ipsilateral hilar lymphadenopathy • **Reactivation TB CXR** – upper lobe infiltration or cavitation are present unilaterally or bilaterally or in a miliary pattern • **Advanced HIV CXR** – cavitation rare; lower lung or diffuse infiltration with intrathoracic lymphadenopathy • **Young children** – cavitation rare; intrathoracic lymphadenopathy with occasional lower lung infiltration
CXR – chest X-ray.	

and the presence of associated diseases (see Table 47.1). The systemic symptoms associated with active tuberculosis include fever, night sweats, malaise, anorexia, and weight loss. Fever is the most common systemic complaint, occurring in approximately 35 to 80% of cases. The systemic symptoms are thought to be mediated by the production of cytokines, particularly TNF-alpha, in response to the presence of *M. tuberculosis* antigens.

The systemic manifestations of tuberculosis may be obscured or modified by the presence of associated conditions including alcohol and drug abuse, HIV infection, diabetes, and chronic kidney disease. Additionally, children under 5 years of age are more likely to have subtle or atypical clinical presentations. For unclear reasons, neuropsychological changes such as depression and hypomania have also been reported in association with active tuberculosis. As these factors may obscure typical presenting symptoms, a high index of suspicion is often necessary to make the diagnosis of tuberculosis.

Pulmonary Tuberculosis

Pulmonary involvement is the most common manifestation of tuberculosis, occurring in approximately 80% of cases.

Cough is the most common symptom and may initially be non-productive. As the disease progresses and tissue necrosis occurs, the cough typically becomes productive. Hemoptysis is common with more extensive involvement. Pleuritic chest pain may result from inflammation of lung parenchyma adjacent to a pleural surface, pleural effusion, or an empyema. Physical findings are non-specific and generally not helpful in distinguishing tuberculosis from other pulmonary infections. Crackles can be heard in areas of pulmonary involvement, and bronchial breath sounds may indicate areas of consolidation.

Extrapulmonary Tuberculosis

Extrapulmonary involvement is more common in young children and HIV-infected persons. Following initial infection with *M. tuberculosis* in the lung, failure to contain the infection can result in hematogenous dissemination of bacilli and the establishment of latent foci of infection in almost any organ of the body. Extrapulmonary disease occurs in approximately

15% of active tuberculosis cases and can involve virtually any organ system. Common sites of extrapulmonary infections include lymph nodes (granulomatous lymphadenitis, which is often painless and can be with or without fever), pleura (pleural effusion causing shortness of breath and pleuritic chest pain), genitourinary tract, joints, and bones (most classically spinal osteomyelitis, or Pott's disease). Life-threatening disease involving the meninges, brain parenchyma, and pericardium can occur.

Depending on the site of involvement, patients with extrapulmonary tuberculosis may present with painless lymphadenopathy, abdominal pain, dysuria, monoarticular joint swelling, back pain, headache, cranial nerve impairments, altered mental status, focal neurological symptoms, or seizures, in addition to or instead of cough. Very rarely, tuberculosis can present acutely as bacteremia or sepsis.

Latent Tuberculosis Infection

Latent tuberculosis infection is a clinical condition characterized by evidence of prior *M. tuberculosis* infection and lack of clinical or radiological signs of active tuberculosis. Consequently, persons with latent tuberculosis infection are asymptomatic and have normal chest radiographs. The only evidence of tuberculosis infection is an immune response to tuberculosis antigens demonstrated through a tuberculin skin test or through interferon gamma release assays.

Differential Diagnosis

The differential diagnosis of tuberculosis is broad and depends on the suspected site of infection.

There are no key features that can reliably distinguish tuberculosis from other pulmonary infections. The following can be suggestive of tuberculosis, but their absence does not rule out the diagnosis:

• CXR is typically abnormal (except in HIV-infected persons) and classically shows upper-lobe thick-walled cavitation with surrounding consolidation
• symptoms are subacute to chronic and are usually constitutional in nature

- patients typically have demographic characteristics that place them at risk for tuberculosis

  Other conditions to consider are as follows:
- other bacterial pneumonia may cause cavitary pulmonary lesions (e.g. *Staphylococcus aureus*, gram-negative rods, and anaerobes)
- other mycobacterial pneumonias (e.g. *M. kansasii*)
- carcinoma (e.g. squamous cell, melanoma, sarcoma)
- autoimmune disease (granulomatosis with polyangiitis, sarcoidosis)
- septic emboli

Laboratory and Radiographic Findings

Although laboratory studies are often normal, there are a few non-specific abnormalities that may be associated with active tuberculosis. The most common hematologic abnormalities in tuberculosis are an elevation in the peripheral blood leukocyte count and anemia, which occur in 10% of patients without bone marrow involvement. Anemia is more common in advanced or disseminated infection. Other reported hematologic abnormalities include leukopenia and elevations in the peripheral blood monocyte and eosinophil counts. Hyponatremia is a fairly common metabolic effect of tuberculosis, occurring in up to 11% of patients in one report.

Radiographic Features

The chest radiograph is abnormal in nearly all cases of pulmonary tuberculosis. One exception is with HIV-related pulmonary tuberculosis in which up to 11% of chest radiographs have been reported to be normal.

In acute primary tuberculosis, chest radiography commonly shows middle or lower lung zone infiltrates with ipsilateral hilar lymphadenopathy. Atelectasis may be seen because of airway compression. Cavitation may occur if the primary process persists (progressive primary tuberculosis).

In reactivation tuberculosis, abnormalities are typically present in the upper lobe of one or both lungs. The most common sites of involvement are the apical and posterior segments of the right lung and the apical-posterior segment of the left lung. Involvement of the anterior segment alone is rare. Cavitation secondary to destruction of lung tissue is often present. The development of a fibrotic scar with loss of lung parenchymal volume and calcification is seen with healing of tuberculous lesions. A miliary pattern of involvement may be seen when a tuberculous focus erodes into lymph or blood vessels allowing for dissemination of tuberculous bacilli.

In HIV-infected persons, particularly those with advanced disease, cavitation is less common and lower lung zone or diffuse infiltrates along with intrathoracic lymphadenopathy are more often seen.

Although recognition of the classic findings in primary and reactivation tuberculosis remains important, the time from acquisition of infection to development of clinical disease may not reliably predict the radiographic appearance of tuberculosis.

Latent Tuberculosis Infection

The tuberculin skin test or an interferon gamma release assay can be used for diagnosis of latent tuberculosis infection. The tuberculin skin test demonstrates a delayed-type hypersensitivity reaction to purified protein derivative (PPD), a crude mixture of mycobacterial antigens. The test is performed by the Mantoux method – intradermal injection of 0.1 mL (five tuberculin units) of PPD typically on the volar surface of the forearm. Reading of the test is conventionally done after 48 to 72 hours, but may be delayed up to 1 week.

Reaction size is determined by measuring the diameter of induration and is recorded in millimeters. Recommended cut-offs for a positive test vary with the population being tested (see Table 47.2).

- **Highest risk persons** (immunodeficient states and contacts of tuberculosis cases) have the lowest cut-off of 5 mm.
- **Intermediate-risk persons** (health-care workers, residents of correctional facilities or nursing homes, homeless persons, and children <4 years old) have a cut-off of 10 mm.
- **Low-risk persons** (routine job screening) have the highest cut-off of 15 mm and in general should not be tested.

Although widely used, the tuberculin skin test has problems with both specificity and sensitivity. False positive results are seen in populations with high background rates of nontuberculous mycobacterial infections and bacille Calmette–Guérin (BCG) vaccination. False-negative tests are seen in HIV infection and in other conditions of decreased cell-mediated immunity.

There are currently two FDA-approved interferon gamma release assays for the diagnosis of latent tuberculosis infection: the QuantiFERON-TB Gold In-Tube® assay and the T-SPOT.TB® assay. Unlike the tuberculin skin test, these assays are performed on blood specimens and therefore do not require patient follow-up for interpretion of results. Test results can be available within 24 hours, and cut-offs for positive test results are the same regardless of the population being tested. According to CDC guidelines, either the tuberculin skin test or an interferon gamma release assay can be used to diagnose latent tuberculosis infection in most situations, with the exception that interferon gamma release assays are preferable in those who have received the BCG vaccine and in those who are unlikely to follow up for tuberculin skin test reading and interpretation.

Microbiologic Diagnosis: Pulmonary Tuberculosis

The definitive diagnosis of pulmonary tuberculosis is most often made through the isolation of *M. tuberculosis* in sputum culture or by one of three FDA-approved rapid nucleic acid amplification tests (Xpert MTB/Rif®, Enhanced Amplified Mycobacterium Tuberculosis Direct Test®, or Amplicor Mycobacterium Tuberculosis Test®). Current CDC guidelines recommend that a minimum of three sputum specimens should be collected for smear and culture at least 8 hours apart during the initial evaluation of suspected cases of pulmonary tuberculosis, and at least one sputum specimen should also be

Table 47.2 Criteria for Positive Tuberculin Skin Test

Reaction ≥5 mm of Induration	Reaction ≥10 mm of Induration	Reaction ≥15 mm of Induration
1. HIV-infected persons 2. Recent contact with a person having active TB disease 3. Fibrotic changes on chest radiograph consistent with prior TB 4. Patients with organ transplants and other immunosuppressed patients (receiving the equivalent of ≥15 mg/day of prednisone for 1 month or more, or taking TNF-alpha antagonists)	1. Recent immigrants (i.e. within the last 5 years) from high-prevalence countries 2. Injection drug users 3. Residents and employees of high-risk congregate settings, including health-care facilities, prisons and jails, long-term care facilities, and homeless shelters 4. Mycobacteriology laboratory personnel 5. Persons with silicosis, diabetes mellitus, chronic renal failure, hematologic disorders (e.g. leukemias and lymphomas), other specific malignancies (e.g. carcinoma of the head or neck and lung), weight loss of >10% of ideal body weight, gastrectomy, and jejunoileal bypass 6. Children <4 years of age and all children exposed to adults in high risk categories	1. Persons with no TB risk factors

Adapted from: Centers for Disease Control and Prevention, Tuberculin skin testing (October 2011), available at www.cdc.gov/tb.

submitted for nucleic acid amplification testing from patients with suspected pulmonary tuberculosis for whom rapid receipt of results would impact patient management or tuberculosis control activities.

In patients who are not producing sputum, several options exist. The most effective is sputum induction by inhalation of nebulized 3 to 7% hypertonic saline. Sputum induction is well tolerated, inexpensive, and has a similar sensitivity to bronchoalveolar lavage. Pulmonary secretions containing tuberculous bacilli are frequently swallowed and can be recovered from the gastric contents. In young children who cannot voluntarily expectorate sputum, early morning sampling of gastric contents via a nasogastric tube is often performed, though sputum induction has been shown to be safe and to have a yield comparable to or better than gastric lavage even in children as young as 1 month old. Fiberoptic bronchoscopy is often the next diagnostic modality if sputum inductions are negative or cannot be performed.

The diagnosis of pulmonary tuberculosis can also be made clinically in the absence of positive cultures, though this approach does not allow for the determination of drug susceptibility and is not standard of care. In a high-risk patient, resolution or improvement of radiographic changes following antituberculosis chemotherapy is sufficient to make the diagnosis of pulmonary tuberculosis and to necessitate a complete course of therapy. In general, a clinical response should be seen within 2 months of initiating treatment.

Microbiologic Diagnosis: Extrapulmonary Tuberculosis

The diagnosis of extrapulmonary tuberculosis is challenging. Sites of infection may be difficult to access and often contain relatively few bacilli. The cornerstone of diagnosis remains isolation of tuberculous bacilli from suspected sites of infection. Multiple samples from all affected sites should be sent for culture to maximize the diagnostic yield for both smear and culture analysis. If possible, fluid from the suspected site of infection should be aspirated – it takes 5,000 to 10,000 mycobacteria

bacilli per mL for detection with a smear; some more sensitive culture methods can detect as few as ten bacilli per mL. Surgical procedures are often needed to obtain adequate tissue samples. Cerebrospinal fluid (CSF) analysis will often show a neutrophilic predominance, mononuclear cells, a low glucose level, and a remarkably high protein level in mycobacterial meningitis. According to WHO guidelines, Xpert MTB/Rif® is the preferable initial diagnostic test for CSF specimens given the importance of establishing a rapid diagnosis, and can also be used to test other non-respiratory specimens (lymph nodes and other tissues), though data is currently limited.

Treatment

The treatment of active tuberculosis and latent infections is reviewed in Tables 47.3 and 47.4. National evidence-based guidelines for the treatment of tuberculosis and latent infections have been published in joint statements by the American Thoracic Society, Infectious Diseases Society of America, and the Centers for Disease Control and Prevention (CDC).

General Principles

The goals of antituberculosis therapy include achieving cure without relapse of disease, stopping transmission of *M. tuberculosis*, and preventing the emergence of drug-resistant strains. Tuberculosis treatment differs from that of many other infectious diseases in that the responsibility for ensuring treatment completion lies with the treating clinician. For each individual patient, special consideration should be given to the specific clinical and social context in which tuberculosis treatment is being administered.

Directly observed therapy (providing medications and watching the patient swallow them) is recommended for all patients and has been shown to increase compliance and completion of therapy. Tuberculosis is generally treated through public health agencies because of the significant infrastructure and cost of administering directly observed therapy. Active tuberculosis should never be treated with a single drug,

Table 47.3 Recommended Dosages for First-Line Antituberculosis Drugs Used for Initial Treatment in Children and Adults

Drug	Type of Administration	Dosage Frequency*		
		Daily	2 days/week†	3 days/week†
Isoniazid	Oral, intramuscular, or intravenous			
Children		10 mg/kg	20–30 mg/kg	–
Adults		5 mg/kg	15 mg/kg	15 mg/kg
Maximum		300 mg	900 mg	900 mg
Rifampin	Oral or intravenous			
Children		10–20 mg/kg	10–20 mg/kg	–
Adults		10 mg/kg	10 mg/kg	10 mg/kg
Maximum		600 mg	600 mg	600 mg
Rifabutin	Oral			
Adults		5 mg/kg	5 mg/kg	5 mg/kg
Maximum		300 mg	300 mg	300 mg
Pyrazinamide	Oral			
Children		15–30 mg/kg	50 mg/kg (2 g max)	–
Adults		25 mg/kg	50 mg/kg	35–40 mg/kg
Maximum		2 g	4 g	3 g
Ethambutol	Oral			
Children		15–20 mg/kg (1 g max)	50 mg/kg (2.5 g max)	–
Adults		15–25 mg/kg	50 mg/kg	25–30 mg/kg
Maximum		1,600 mg	4,000 mg	2,400 mg

* Doses per weight are based on ideal body weight. Children weighing >40 kg should receive adult doses.

† Must be administered by directly observed therapy only.

Source: Adapted with permission from the American Medical Association. H. M. Blumberg, M. K. Leonard, Jr., and R. M. Jasmer, Update on the treatment of tuberculosis and latent tuberculosis infection. *JAMA* 2005; 293(22): 2776–84.

and a single drug should never be added to a failing regimen because of the risk of acquiring drug resistance. Thus, multidrug therapy is always required.

The efficacy of treatment should be monitored by obtaining sputum for acid-fast bacillus (AFB) smear and culture at least monthly until two consecutive cultures are negative. Cultures should always be obtained after 2 months of treatment because positive cultures at this stage predict a high risk of relapse and mandate prolongation of therapy. Drug susceptibility testing should be performed on the initial culture and again if cultures remain positive after 3 months of treatment.

Tuberculosis treatment with combination chemotherapy can be complicated by both mild and serious adverse reactions (see Table 47.5). Mild adverse reactions can generally be managed with conservative therapy aimed at controlling symptoms, whereas with more severe reactions the offending drug or drugs must be discontinued. Managing serious adverse reactions frequently necessitates expert consultation. Although it is important to recognize the potential for adverse effects, first-line drugs should not be discontinued without adequate justification.

Treatment of Drug-Susceptible Disease

Tuberculosis treatment is generally divided into two phases: the initiation (bactericidal) phase, which lasts 2 months, and the

continuation phase, which lasts 4 to 7 months for patients with drug-susceptible disease (see Figure 47.1). Antituberculosis treatment should be administered following bacteriologic confirmation of tuberculosis or empirically when there is a high clinical suspicion for disease prior to culture confirmation and, in certain cases, prior to the availability of AFB smear microscopy results. Treatment is generally initiated with an empiric four-drug regimen consisting of isoniazid, rifampin, ethambutol, and pyrazinamide. Recommended dosages and dosing schedules for first-line antituberculosis medications are shown in Table 47.3.

A special warning is needed about the use of fluoroquinolones in empirically treating infections in the acute care setting. Fluoroquinolones are active against *M. tuberculosis* and are important second-line agents in patients that have drug-resistant tuberculosis or cannot tolerate first-line agents. To minimize the potential development of fluoroquinolone-resistant tuberculosis, this class of medication should be avoided in patients in whom tuberculosis is part of the differential diagnosis and in whom a trial of empiric antibiotics is planned.

Treatment of Latent Tuberculosis Infection

There are several drug regimens available for the treatment of latent tuberculosis infection (LTBI). Prior to initiating

Table 47.4 Treatment of Latent Tuberculosis Infection

Drug Regimen	Duration	Oral Dose	Dosing Frequency
Isoniazid	9 months	Adults: 5 mg/kg Children: 10–20 mg/kg Maximum dose: 300 mg	Daily
		Adults: 15 mg/kg Children: 20–40 mg/kg Maximum dose: 900 mg	Twice weekly*
	6 months†	Adults: 5 mg/kg Maximum dose: 300 mg	Daily
		Adults: 15 mg/kg Maximum dose: 900 mg	Twice weekly*
Rifampin	4 months	Adults: 10 mg/kg Children: 10–20 mg/kg Maximum dose: 600 mg	Daily
Isoniazid and rifapentine	3 months	Adults and Children ≥ 12 years **Isoniazid:** 15 mg/kg (900 mg maximum) **Rifapentine:** 10–14 kg: 300 mg 14.1–25 kg: 450 mg 25.1–32 kg: 600 mg 32.1–50 kg: 750 mg >50 kg: 900 mg	Once weekly*

* Therapy must be directly observed when given twice weekly or weekly.

† Therapy for 6 months not recommended in children.

Table 47.5 Monitoring Recommendations and Adverse Reactions for First-Line Antituberculosis Drugs

Medication	Monitoring	Adverse Reactions
Isoniazid	• No routine monitoring • Hepatic enzymes if pre-existing liver disease, HIV infection, or pregnancy	• Hepatic enzyme elevation, hepatitis, and fatal hepatitis • Peripheral neuropathy and CNS effects • Increased phenytoin levels • Lupus-like syndrome
Rifampin	• No routine monitoring • Check for drug interactions	• Pruritis with or without rash (typically self-limited) • Nausea, anorexia, abdominal pain • Flu-like syndrome • Hepatotoxicity • Orange discoloration of bodily fluids (sputum, urine, sweat, tears) • Drug interactions due to induction of hepatic microsomal enzymes
Rifabutin	• Similar to rifampin	• Hematologic toxicity such as neutropenia • Uveitis • Orange discoloration of bodily fluids • Polyarthralgias • Pseudo-jaundice (skin discoloration with normal bilirubin) • Hepatotoxicity
Pyrazinamide	• Hepatic enzymes if pre-existing liver disease or when used with rifampin for latent tuberculosis treatment • Serum uric acid measurements serve as a surrogate marker for compliance	• Hepatotoxicity • Hyperuricemia, gouty arthritis • Polyarthralgia (usually responds to non-steroidal anti-inflammatory agents) • Nausea, vomiting, abdominal discomfort • Transient morbilliform rash (usually not an indication for discontinuation)
Ethambutol	• Monthly color and acuity vision check	• Decreased visual acuity or decreased red-green color discrimination (dose related) should prompt immediate and permanent discontinuation • Rash

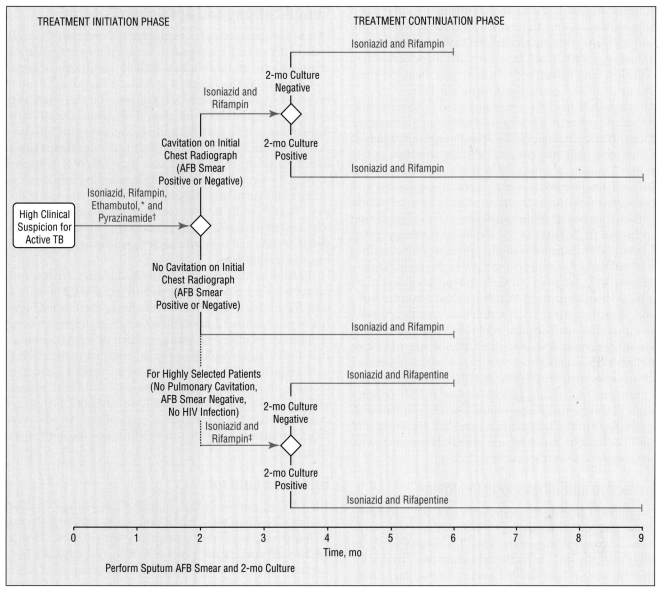

TREATMENT INITIATION PHASE

TREATMENT CONTINUATION PHASE

Time, mo

Perform Sputum AFB Smear and 2-mo Culture

Figure 47.1 Treatment algorithm for drug-susceptible pulmonary tuberculosis. In patients with suspected drug-susceptible tuberculosis, treatment is initiated with isoniazid (INH), rifampin (RIF), pyrazinamide (PZA),† and ethambutol (ETH)* for the initial 2 months of therapy. Further treatment decisions are based on the presence of cavitation on the initial chest radiograph and the results of repeat AFB smear and culture performed after the initial 2 months of drug treatment. Treatment is continued with INH and RIF for a total of 6 months when cavitation was not present on the initial chest radiograph and when cavitation was present, but the repeat tuberculosis culture is negative after the initial 2 months of therapy. The continuation phase should be extended 3 months (total treatment duration 9 months) if cavitation was present on the initial chest radiograph and the repeat tuberculosis culture is positive. In highly selected patients (HIV negative, no cavitation on chest radiograph, negative sputum AFB smears performed after the initial 2 months of therapy), treatment with once-weekly INH and rifapentine‡ can be considered as an alternative to INH and RIF.

* ETH may be discontinued when results of drug susceptibility testing indicate no drug resistance.

† PZA may be discontinued after it has been taken for 2 months.

‡ Rifapentine should not be used in patients who have HIV and tuberculosis or in patients with extrapulmonary tuberculosis.

Source: Reproduced with permission from the American Medical Association. H. M. Blumberg, M. K. Leonard, Jr., and R. M. Jasmer, Update on the treatment of tuberculosis and latent tuberculosis infection. *JAMA* 2005; 293(22): 2776–84.

treatment for latent infection, it is important to exclude the presence of active tuberculosis. Isoniazid (INH) can be given as a single drug for either 9 months or 6 months in duration (see Table 47.4). The 9-month regimen is preferred over 6 months, as it is more efficacious if adhered to. INH can be given as a single daily dose (300 mg for adults, 5 to 10 mg/kg for children) or twice weekly (15 mg/kg) when therapy is directly observed.

Hepatotoxicity and peripheral neuropathy are the major adverse events associated with INH therapy. Asymptomatic elevations in liver enzymes are relatively common, but the rate of symptomatic hepatitis is low (1 to 3 per 1,000 persons treated). Alcohol consumption has been shown to significantly increase the risk of INH-induced hepatitis. Routine monitoring of liver enzymes is not currently recommended except for patients who are HIV-infected, pregnant, or taking other hepatotoxic medications and those with chronic liver disease and alcohol abuse. Patients predisposed to the development of peripheral neuropathy (such as patients with diabetes mellitus, malnutrition, renal failure, and HIV infection) should be given pyridoxine 25 to 50 mg/day concurrently with INH.

Although INH has been the mainstay of LTBI treatment, shorter-course regimens are being used increasingly. In a recent randomized controlled trial, combination therapy with isoniazid and rifapentine, administered as 12 directly observed weekly doses over 3 months, was found to be non-inferior to 9 months of daily self-administered isoniazid in select populations and was associated with higher treatment completion rates (82.1% completion compared to 69.0% completion in the isoniazid-only group [p<0.001]). Subjects in the combination therapy group were more likely to experience adverse events necessitating drug discontinuation (4.9% compared to 3.7% in the isoniazid-only group [p=0.009]), but were less likely to experience confirmed drug-related hepatotoxicity (0.4% compared to 2.7% in the isoniazid-only group [p<0.001]). This regimen is currently approved for use in healthy non-pregnant adults, HIV-infected persons not on antiretrovirals, and children 12 years of age and older. In addition to this combination regimen, a 4-month regimen of rifampin is an acceptable alternative to INH based on experience with this regimen in treating patients exposed to INH-resistant TB cases. A clinical trial demonstrated that it is well tolerated, with very low rates of hepatotoxicity, and has higher rates of treatment completion than 9 months of INH. However, data on efficacy compared to INH are currently lacking.

HIV Infection and Tuberculosis Treatment

The treatment of patients co-infected with HIV and *M. tuberculosis* is complicated by overlapping toxicity profiles of some medications and complex drug interactions. The optimal timing of initiating anti-retroviral medication in patients being treated for tuberculosis has not been clearly established. Drug interactions resulting in altered serum drug levels are common between anti-retroviral and antituberculosis medications. Updated guidelines, specific interactions, and dosage recommendations for most anti-retroviral medications are published by the CDC at www.cdc.gov/tb/topic/tbhivcoinfection/default.htm.

Treatment of Extrapulmonary Tuberculosis

Extrapulmonary tuberculosis is treated with the same drug regimens as pulmonary tuberculosis. Treatment duration is 6 months for every site except the meninges. Meningeal tuberculosis should be treated for a minimum of 9 to 12 months. The addition of systemic corticosteroids is recommended for the treatment of pericardial and meningeal tuberculosis only. However, data showing a significant decrease in morbidity or mortality with corticosteroids are limited, particularly in HIV-infected patients.

Drug-Resistant Tuberculosis

Treatment of drug-resistant tuberculosis is complex and should only be done in consultation with an expert.

Complications and Admission Criteria

One of the most serious complications of untreated tuberculosis is the risk of transmission in the community. Clinical complications of tuberculosis include progressive hypoxia and dyspnea as the infection spreads in the lungs. Rapidly progressive shortness of breath and pleuritic chest pain may indicate pneumothorax or pleural effusion. Occasionally, hemoptysis can be massive and require emergent intervention. Dissemination of infection may occur during the initial infectious phase or may represent progression of untreated or partially treated infections. Life-threatening infection can occur in the form of meningitis, pericarditis, and spinal disease. Death results in approximately 40 to 60% of patients who are left untreated. Most importantly, failure to promptly detect, isolate, and treat persons with pulmonary tuberculosis can lead to outbreaks.

Because of the potential public health risk, persons with suspected tuberculosis should generally be admitted to the hospital for further evaluation. Notable exceptions include low-risk persons who are housed, do not reside in congregate living facilities, do not live with young children or immunocompromised persons, are willing to remain confined in their homes until evaluation for active tuberculosis is completed, and have access to appropriate medical follow-up. In addition, patients who have progressive disease while on adequate therapy, are unable to care for themselves as outpatients, or who have failed community-based treatment efforts may require hospital admission.

Infection Control

The CDC recommends that all health-care settings establish a tuberculosis infection control program to minimize the risk of health-care-associated tuberculosis transmission. Risk to health-care workers and patients results predominantly from contact with patients with unsuspected or undiagnosed tuberculosis. *M. tuberculosis* is transmitted in airborne particles 1 to 5 μm in size that are generated when persons with pulmonary or laryngeal tuberculosis cough, sneeze, shout, or sing. The droplets are carried by normal air currents and can remain airborne for prolonged periods and spread throughout a room or even a building if they access a central ventilation system. Thus, effective control measures include immediate isolation of persons with suspected pulmonary tuberculosis, use of respiratory isolation rooms (negative pressure ventilation room with a minimum of 6 to 12 air exchanges per hour with an approved exhaust filtration mechanism), appropriate use of airborne infection precautions during contact with suspected cases, decontamination of patient care areas following triage of suspected cases, and both routine monitoring and post-exposure evaluation of health-care staff.

The risk of tuberculosis transmission in health-care settings varies according to the specific setting, tuberculosis prevalence in the community, effectiveness of tuberculosis control measures, and the characteristics of the specific exposure. Patients with cough, cavitary disease, or positive AFB smears and those undergoing aerosol-generating procedures (sputum induction, bronchoscopy) are more likely to be infectious. Tuberculosis transmission is also increased when the exposure occurs in a small, enclosed setting and when inadequate ventilation fails to dilute or remove infectious droplet nuclei. Any person with suspected tuberculosis should immediately be placed in an airborne infection isolation room, when available. Airborne infection precautions should immediately be instituted, including the use of appropriately fitted respiratory masks for all persons entering the room. Both respiratory isolation and airborne precautions can be discontinued if another diagnosis explaining the clinical syndrome is confirmed, or if the patient has three consecutive negative AFB sputum smear results collected at least 8 hours apart (at least one specimen should be an early-morning specimen). The duration of respiratory isolation and airborne precautions can potentially be shortened with diagnostic strategies that incorporate rapid nucleic acid amplification tests.

Pearls and Pitfalls

1. All patients with respiratory complaints should be asked about signs and symptoms of tuberculosis disease, history of tuberculosis exposure or infection, and medical conditions that increase the risk of tuberculosis.

2. Tuberculosis should be considered in any patient with unexplained cough greater than 2 weeks in duration, unintentional weight loss, hemoptysis, night sweats, or characteristic radiographic findings. The diagnosis should also be considered in immunosuppressed patients with any respiratory or systemic complaints.

3. Any person with suspected tuberculosis should immediately be placed in an airborne infection isolation room. Airborne infection precautions should include the use of appropriately fitted respiratory masks for all persons entering the room.

4. The standard diagnosis of pulmonary tuberculosis involves submitting at least three sputum specimens for AFB smear and culture. Additionally, at least one sputum specimen should be submitted for rapid nucleic acid amplification testing in situations where rapid receipt of results would impact patient management or tuberculosis control activities.

5. If the suspicion of tuberculosis is high, combination chemotherapy using one of the recommended regimens may be initiated before AFB smear and nucleic acid amplification testing results are known.

6. If AFB smears and nucleic acid amplification testing are negative and suspicion for active tuberculosis is low, treatment can be deferred until the results of mycobacterial cultures are known and a comparison chest radiograph is available (usually within 2 months). This approach requires that the patient have adequate follow-up.

7. Fluoroquinolones are important second-line agents for the treatment of tuberculosis. To minimize the potential for development of fluoroquinolone-resistant tuberculosis, this class of medication should be avoided in patients in whom tuberculosis is part of the differential diagnosis and in whom a trial of empiric antibiotics for other reasons is planned.

8. A negative tuberculin skin test or interferon gamma release assay does not rule out active tuberculosis.

References

Alami, N. N., Yuen, C. M., Miramontes, R., *et al.* Trends in tuberculosis – United States, 2013. *MMWR Morb. Mortal. Wkly. Rep.* 2014; 63(11): 229–33.

Blumberg, H. M., Burman, W. J., Chaisson, R. E., *et al.* American Thoracic Society/Centers for Disease Control and Prevention/Infectious Diseases Society of America: treatment of tuberculosis. *Am. J. Respir. Crit. Care Med.* 2003; 167(4): 603–62.

Blumberg, H. M., Leonard, M. K., Jr., and Jasmer, R. M. Update on the treatment of tuberculosis and latent tuberculosis infection. *JAMA* 2005; 293(22): 2776–84.

Cattamanchi, A., Hopewell, P. C., Gonzalez, L. C., *et al.* A 13-year molecular epidemiological analysis of tuberculosis in San Francisco. *Int. J. Tuberc. Lung Dis.* 2006; 10(3): 297–304.

Centers for Disease Control and Prevention (CDC), Division of Tuberculosis Elimination. Latent tuberculosis infection; a guide for primary health providers (April 2013), www.cdc.gov/tb/publications/ltbi/treatment.htm (accessed November 22, 2017).

CDC. Updated Guidelines for the Use of Nucleic Acid Amplification Tests in the Diagnosis of Tuberculosis. *MMWR Morb. Mortal. Wkly. Rep.* 2009; 58(1): 7–10.

Chiang, C. Y., Slama, K., and Enarson, D. A. Associations between tobacco and tuberculosis. *Int. J. Tuberc. Lung Dis.* 2007; 11(3): 258–62.

Hass, D. W. and Des Prez, R. M. Tuberculosis and acquired immunodeficiency syndrome: a historical perspective on recent developments. *Am. J. Med.* 1994; 96(5): 439–50.

Havlir, D. V. and Barnes, P. F. Tuberculosis in patients with human immunodeficiency virus infection. *N. Engl. J. Med.* 1999; 340(5): 367–73.

Horsburgh, C. R., Jr. and Rubin, E. J. Latent tuberculosis infection in the United States. *N. Engl. J. Med.* 2011; 364(15): 1441–8.

Jensen, P. A., Lambert, L. A., Iademarco, M. F., *et al.* Guidelines for preventing the transmission of *Mycobacterium tuberculosis* in health-care settings, 2005. *MMWR Morb. Mortal. Wkly. Rep.* 2005; 54(17): 1–141.

Mayosi B. M., Ntsekhe M., Volmink J. A., *et al.* Interventions for treating tuberculous pericarditis. *Cochrane Database Syst. Rev.* 2002; 4: CD000526.

Mayosi, B. M., Ntsekhe, M., Yusuf, S., *et. al.* Prednisolone and *Mycobacterium indicus pranii* in tuberculous pericarditis. *N. Engl. J. Med.* 2014; 371(12): 1121–30.

Menzies, D., Long, R., and Schwartzman, K. Adverse events with 4 months of rifampin therapy or 9 months of isoniazid therapy for latent tuberculosis infection: a randomized trial. *Ann. Intern. Med.* 2008; 149(10): 689–97.

Nahid, P. and Daley, C. L. Prevention of tuberculosis in HIV-infected patients. *Curr. Opin. Infect. Dis.* 2006; 19(2): 189–93.

Prasad, K. and Singh, M. B. Corticosteroids for managing tuberculous meningitis. *Cochrane Database Syst. Rev.* 2008; 1: CD002244.

Sterling, T. R., Villarino, M. E., Chaisson, R. E., *et al.* Three months of rifapentine and isoniazid for latent tuberculosis infection. *N. Engl. J. Med.* 2011; 365(23): 2155–66.

Trenton, A. J. and Currier, G. W. Treatment of comorbid tuberculosis and depression. Primary care companion. *J. Clin. Psychiatry* 2001; 3(6): 236–43.

Woolwine, S. C. and Bishai, W. R. Overview of the pathogenesis of tuberculosis from a cellular and molecular perspective in L. B. Reichman and E. S. Hershfield (eds.), *Tuberculosis: A Comprehensive International Approach*, 3rd edn. (New York: Informa Healthcare, 2006), pp. 101–12.

World Health Organization. Tuberculosis fact sheet (October 2014), swww.who.int/mediacentre/factsheets/fs104/en/ (accessed November 22, 2017).

World Health Organization. Xpert MTB/RIF assay for the diagnosis of pulmonary and extrapulmonary TB in adults and children: Policy update 2013, www.who.int/tb/publications/2014/en/ (accessed November 22, 2017).

Additional Readings

Davies, P. D. O., Gordon, S. B., and Davies, G. (eds.), *Clinical Tuberculosis*, 5th edn. (Boca Raton, FL: CRC Press, Taylor & Francis Group, 2014).

Nahid, P., Pai, M., and Hopewell, P. C. Advances in the diagnosis and treatment of tuberculosis. *Proc. Am. Thorac. Soc.* 2006; 3(1): 103–10.

Perez-Velez, C. M. and Marais, B. J. Tuberculosis in children. *N. Engl. J. Med.* 2012; 367(4): 348–61.

Raviglione, M. C. (ed.), *Reishman and Hershfield's Tuberculosis: A Comprehensive International Approach*, 3rd edn. (New York: Informa Healthcare, 2006).

Zumla, A., Raviglione, M., Hafner, R., and von Reyn, F. Tuberculosis. *N. Engl. J. Med.* 2013; 368(8): 745–55.

Lower Urinary Tract Infection in Adults

Fredrick M. Abrahamian

Outline

Introduction and Microbiology

Symptomatic acute lower urinary tract infection (UTI), also known as acute cystitis, can be divided into complicated and uncomplicated infections. In uncomplicated lower UTI, there are no signs and symptoms of upper UTI such as fever, chills, or flank pain. Uncomplicated lower UTI is a common diagnosis in healthy, young, non-pregnant, immunocompetent females with normal renal function and no underlying structural defects in urinary anatomy.

Lower UTI is considered complicated in the setting of a functional abnormality of the urinary tract (e.g. neurogenic bladder), anatomic abnormality of the urinary tract (e.g. urethral stricture), immunosuppression, pregnancy, indwelling urinary catheter use, or recent urinary tract instrumentation. Moreover, lower UTIs in men are generally considered complicated.

Uncomplicated infections do not require extensive diagnostic tests and can be effectively treated with short-term antimicrobial regimens. Complicated infections often require additional diagnostic tests, are treated with longer duration antimicrobial therapy, and may have a higher risk of treatment failure and complications.

The infecting organism in lower UTI generally arises from enteric flora that colonizes the patient's perineum and urethra. In uncomplicated UTIs, *Escherichia coli* is responsible for the majority of infections. Other organisms may include *Klebsiella* species, *Proteus mirabilis*, and *Staphylococcus saprophyticus*. Complicated infections may be due to the same or more resistant strains of the organisms causing uncomplicated UTIs, or unusual pathogens such as *Pseudomonas aeruginosa*.

Epidemiology

UTI affects half of all women at least once during their lifetime, and during any given year, 11% of women report having had a UTI. The incidence increases with age and sexual activity. The prevalence of UTI in otherwise healthy adult males younger than age 50 is less than 1%. In this population, the symptoms of dysuria or urinary frequency are usually due to sexually transmitted infections (STIs). In men older than 50, the incidence of lower UTI increases dramatically because of enlargement of the prostate and associated urinary retention or instrumentation of the urinary tract. UTIs in men are considered complicated because most of them occur in association with other conditions such as STIs, nephrolithiasis, urologic anatomic abnormalities (e.g. prostate hypertrophy), prostatitis, or urinary tract instrumentation.

The incidence of lower UTI in women has been shown to increase as a result of the following risk factors: increased frequency of intercourse in the past month; spermicide or diaphragm use; a new sexual partner within the past 12 months; and occurrence of first UTI at 15 years of age or younger. Among elderly women living in long-term care facilities, the risk of lower UTI increases with age and debility, especially in those with conditions associated with impaired voiding or poor perineal hygiene.

Clinical Features

Symptoms of lower UTI can include dysuria, urinary frequency, hematuria, urgency, and suprapubic discomfort (see Table 48.1). A symptom of dysuria and frequency in women

Table 48.1 Clinical Features: Lower Urinary Tract Infection in Adults

Organisms	**Uncomplicated infections:** *Escherichia coli* is responsible for the majority of infections. Other organisms may include: *Klebsiella* species *Proteus mirabilis* *Staphylococcus saprophyticus* **Complicated infections:** May be due to the same or more resistant strains of the organisms causing uncomplicated UTIs, or unusual pathogens such as *Pseudomonas species*
Signs and symptoms	Dysuria, urinary frequency, hematuria, urgency, and suprapubic discomfort
Laboratory findings	**Urine dipstick:** Positive leukocyte esterase and nitrite test **Urine microscopy:** Presence of pyuria and bacteriuria **Urine culture:** Isolation of ≥10³ CFU/mL of a single uropathogen
Antimicrobial treatment	**Acute uncomplicated lower UTI:** Local *E. coli* resistance to TMP-SMX <20%: TMP-SMX DS (160/800 mg) one tab. PO BID × 3 days *or* Nitrofurantoin 100 mg PO BID × 5 days *or* Fosfomycin 3 g PO × 1 If *E. coli* resistance to TMP-SMX ≥ 20%: Nitrofurantoin 100 mg PO BID × 5 days *or* Ciprofloxacin 500 mg PO BID × 3 days *or* Levofloxacin 500 mg PO daily × 3 days *or* Fosfomycin 3 g PO × 1 **Lower UTI in pregnancy:** Cephalexin 500 mg PO QID × 7 days *or* Amoxicillin–clavulanate 875/125 mg PO BID × 7 days **Complicated lower UTI:** Ciprofloxacin 500 mg PO bid × 7 days *or* Levofloxacin 500 mg PO daily × 7 days **Complicated lower UTI and fluoroquinolone allergy:** Amoxicillin–clavulanate 875/125 mg PO BID × 10–14 days *or* Cephalexin 500 mg PO QID × 10–14 days *or* TMP/SMX DS (160/800 mg) one tab. PO BID × 14 days

CFU – colony-forming units; DS – double strength; PO – by mouth; TMP/SMX – trimethoprim-sulfamethoxazole; UTI – urinary tract infection.

without vaginal discharge or irritation increases the pre-test probability of lower UTI. The presence of symptoms similar to those of a prior lower UTI also increases the probability of infection.

Lower UTI can also be associated with mild back pain due to referred pain from the bladder. However, moderate-to-severe back pain or costovertebral angle tenderness, especially when associated with fever or vomiting, is indicative of an upper UTI.

Differential Diagnosis

Other conditions to consider include:

- pyelonephritis
- vaginal infections (e.g. bacterial vaginosis, *Trichomonas vaginitis*, candidiasis)
- pelvic inflammatory disease
- genital herpes infection
- non-infectious causes (e.g. trauma, irritant, allergy)
- prostatitis, orchitis, epididymitis, urethritis, benign prostatic hypertrophy
- urolithiasis
- pregnancy
- ovarian cyst or torsion
- appendicitis, inflammatory bowel disease, diverticular disease, bladder carcinoma
- abdominal aortic aneurysm

Key features that may help to distinguish lower UTIs are:

- symptoms of dysuria and frequency in women without vaginal discharge or irritation increase the pretest probability of lower UTI

- moderate-to-severe back pain or costovertebral angle tenderness, especially when associated with fever and vomiting, is indicative of an upper UTI
- uncomplicated cystitis is rare in men. Voiding symptoms in sexually active men are usually due to urethritis from a sexually transmitted pathogen rather than cystitis; whereas in older men, bacterial cystitis usually signifies obstructive urethritis from prostate hypertrophy, and is often accompanied by prostatitis or epididymitis

Laboratory Findings

Urine Collection Methods

The initial step in the diagnosis of a UTI is the careful collection of urine for urinalysis and potentially a urine culture. In most adults, the midstream voiding specimen is adequate. Catheterization is indicated if the patient cannot void spontaneously, is too ill or immobilized to provide an adequate specimen, is unable to follow instructions, is extremely obese, or has copious vaginal discharge. Regardless of the collection method, any study of urine must be performed soon after collection. Urine specimens that are allowed to sit become alkaline, with subsequent dissolution of the cellular elements and multiplication of bacteria.

Urine Dipstick

Pyuria, as indicated by a positive leukocyte esterase dipstick test, is found in the vast majority of patients with UTI. Urine dipstick testing for leukocyte esterase has shown a sensitivity of 62 to 98% and a specificity of 55 to 96%. However, low-level pyuria (6 to 20 white blood cells [WBCs] per high-power field [hpf] microscopy on a centrifuged specimen) can be associated with false-negative leukocyte esterase dipstick test results.

A positive result on the nitrite test is highly specific for UTI (>90%) due to members of the family *Enterobacteriaceae*, such as *E. coli* and *Proteus* species. However, it is an insensitive screening test, as only less than 50% of patients with UTI have a positive nitrite test result. In general, the performance characteristics of leukocyte esterase and nitrite tests in detecting bacteriuria are better at high colony counts than at lower colony counts.

Urine Microscopy

The initial diagnosis of a UTI is confirmed if pyuria and bacteriuria are detected on a microscopic examination of the urine. The definition of pyuria varies based on the laboratory counting technique. Pyuria defined as more than ten WBCs/mm^3 by hemocytometer or more than five WBCs/hpf by centrifuge, and microscopy has generally been found to be over 80% sensitive and specific for UTI. The sensitivity of the finding of pyuria appears to be decreased with low bacterial count infections, and specificity appears to be less among women who also have vaginal symptoms. The presence of visible bacteria on microscopic examination increases the specificity to 85 to 95%.

Urine Culture

The traditional reference standard for diagnosing UTI is defined as the isolation of at least 10^5 colony-forming units (CFU)/mL of a single uropathogen. However, one-third to one-half of the cases of acute cystitis are characterized by low bacterial concentration (10^2 to 10^4 CFU/mL), which has been termed the *urethral syndrome*. It has been postulated that women with a traditionally negative urine culture (<10^5 CFU/mL) have infection localized to the urethra. Recent studies have shown that using a definition of at least 10^3 CFU/mL has the best combination of sensitivity (95%) and specificity (85%) for diagnosing acute UTI in symptomatic patients.

Uncomplicated lower UTIs can be treated empirically without the need to perform a urine culture. A urine culture is recommended in complicated infections. Cultures are also warranted in women whose symptoms either do not resolve with therapy, or recur within 2 to 4 weeks after the completion of treatment.

Asymptomatic Bacteriuria

The prevalence of asymptomatic bacteriuria (ABU) varies with age, sex, and the presence of genitourinary abnormalities (e.g. healthy, pre-menopausal women: <5%; post-menopausal women aged 50 to 70 years: 2.8 to 8.6%; pregnant women: 2 to 10%; diabetic women: 9 to 27%). Rates of ABU in elderly women and men living in long-term care facilities are 25 to 50% and 15 to 40%, respectively. ABU is very common in patients with long-term indwelling catheter use.

The diagnosis of ABU is based on the results of a urine culture, and not the presence of pyuria or bacteriuria on initial microscopy. For women, bacteriuria is defined as two consecutive voided urine specimens with isolation of the same bacterial strain in quantitative counts of at least 10^5 CFU/mL. For men, a single, clean-catch voided urine specimen with one bacterial species isolated in a quantitative count of at least 10^5 CFU/mL identifies bacteriuria. A single catheterized urine specimen with one bacterial species isolated in a quantitative count of at least 10^2 CFU/mL identifies bacteriuria in women or men.

Treatment

Uncomplicated Lower UTI

The treatment of choice for uncomplicated lower UTI includes nitrofurantoin or trimethoprim/sulfamethoxazole (TMP/SMX), whereas the fluoroquinolones (e.g. ciprofloxacin, levofloxacin) are reserved as alternate second-line agents. Current recommendations are to avoid TMP/SMX as the first-line empiric agent of choice when local resistance of *E. coli* to TMP/SMX is 20% or greater.

Most uncomplicated lower UTIs can be managed with a short course of antibiotic therapy. Three days of therapy has been shown to be equivalent in efficacy to longer durations of treatment (i.e. 7 or 10 days) in studies of TMP/SMX and ciprofloxacin for uncomplicated lower UTIs. Other options for therapy can include nitrofurantoin for 5 days or fosfomycin as a single dose. In comparison to longer durations of treatment with TMP/SMX or fluoroquinolones, single-dose therapy is less effective against eradicating bacteriuria. Oral beta-lactams (e.g. cefpodoxime) are inferior to fluoroquinolones and best used when alternate therapies are not appropriate.

Patients with moderate-to-severe dysuria may also benefit symptomatically from the use of phenazopyridine. A potential but rare side effect of phenazopyridine is a hemolytic reaction in patients with glucose-6-phosphate dehydrogenase deficiency.

Complicated Lower UTI

Short-course antimicrobial regimens are not suitable for the treatment of complicated lower UTIs. Uncomplicated or complicated infections due to *S. saprophyticus* should also be treated with at least 7 days of antimicrobial therapy. In general, for complicated infections, fluoroquinolones (e.g. ciprofloxacin, levofloxacin) prescribed for a duration of 7 days are considered first-line agents. Second-line agents can include oral cephalosporins, amoxicillin-clavulanate, or TMP-SMX for 10 to 14 days.

Lower UTI in Pregnancy

In pregnant women, options for antimicrobial therapy are more restricted because of the potential adverse effects of the drugs on the fetus. Oral cephalosporins are considered safe in pregnancy and are commonly used for the treatment of lower UTI in pregnant women. Nitrofurantoin is also widely used, though case control studies suggest a slight increased risk of teratogenicity. TMP-SMX should be avoided in early pregnancy and within 2 weeks of expected delivery date (because of a theoretical increased risk of neonatal hyperbilirubinemia). The quinolones are contraindicated in pregnancy because of adverse effects on fetal bone and cartilage development.

Asymptomatic Bacteriuria

Antimicrobial treatment of ABU during pregnancy decreases the significant 20 to 30% risk of pyelonephritis and the frequency of low-birth-weight infants and preterm delivery. The recommended duration of therapy is 3 to 7 days. Patients should be instructed to follow up for periodic screening for bacteriuria after completion of therapy.

Treatment of ABU is not recommended in pre-menopausal, non-pregnant women, diabetic women, elderly institutionalized residents of long-term care facilities, and patients with an indwelling urethral catheter.

Complications and Admission Criteria

The majority of women with uncomplicated lower UTIs have improvement of their symptoms within 72 hours after the initiation of antimicrobial therapy. Complications of lower UTI include progression to pyelonephritis and papillary necrosis; however, these complications and long-term adverse effects are rare, even in women with frequent recurrences. Recurrence of infection within a few months can be observed in 10 to 20% of women, which may be due to the original strain or a new strain.

Failure of resolution of symptoms should raise the possibility of the improper antimicrobial choice, presence of resistant or unusual organism, or incorrect working diagnosis. Urine cultures are recommended in cases of recurrent UTI.

Symptomatic infections in the elderly, immunocompromised patients, and in those with indwelling catheters may carry a higher risk of complications, which can include progression to upper UTI.

Patients with isolated lower UTIs are stable by definition, with no evidence of systemic toxicity, and can be managed on an outpatient basis. The presence of vomiting and fever are clues to an upper UTI.

Pearls and Pitfalls

1. Avoid fluoroquinolones (e.g. ciprofloxacin, levofloxacin) as first-line therapy for uncomplicated lower UTIs.
2. Obtain urine culture in complicated infections.
3. The diagnosis of ABU is based on results of culture, not the presence of pyuria or bacteriuria.
4. Patients with moderate-to-severe dysuria may benefit symptomatically from the use of phenazopyridine.
5. ABU during pregnancy should be treated with a course of antimicrobial therapy.

References

Barber, A. E., Norton, J. P., Spivak, A. M., *et al*. Urinary tract Infections: current and emerging management strategies. *Clin. Infect. Dis.* 2013; 57(5): 719–24.

Gupta, K., Hooton, T. M., and Stamm, W. E. Increasing antimicrobial resistance and the management of uncomplicated community-acquired urinary tract infections. *Ann. Intern. Med.* 2001; 135(1): 41–50.

Hooton, T. M. Recurrent urinary tract infection in women. *Int. J. Antimicrob. Agents* 2001; 17(4): 259–68.

Hooton, T. M. and Stamm, W. E. Diagnosis and treatment of uncomplicated urinary tract infection. *Infect. Dis. Clin. North Am.* 1997; 11(3): 551–81.

Nicolle, L. E. Urinary tract infection in long-term care facility residents. *Clin. Infect. Dis.* 2000; 31(3): 757–61.

Reid, G. Potential preventive strategies and therapies in urinary tract infection. *World J. Urol.* 1999; 17(6): 359–63.

Ronald, A. R. and Harding, G. K. Complicated urinary tract infections. *Infect. Dis. Clin. North Am.* 1997; 11(3): 583–92.

Scholes, D., Hooton, T. M., Roberts, P. L., *et al*. Risk factors for recurrent urinary tract infection in young women. *J. Infect. Dis.* 2000; 182(4): 1177–82.

Additional Readings

Bent, S., Nallamothu, B. K., Simel D. L., *et al*. Does this woman have an acute uncomplicated urinary tract infection? *JAMA* 2002; 287(20): 2701–10.

Grigoryan, L., Trautner, B. W., and Gupta, K. Diagnosis and management of urinary tract infections in the outpatient setting. *JAMA* 2014; 312(16): 1677–84.

Gupta, K., Hooton, T. M., Naber, K. G., *et al*. International clinical practice guidelines for the treatment of acute uncomplicated cystitis and pyelonephritis in women: a 2010 update by the Infectious Disease Society of America and the European Society for Microbiology and Infectious Diseases. *Clin. Infect. Dis.* 2011; 52(5): e103–20.

Hooton, T. M. Uncomplicated urinary tract infection. *N. Engl. J. Med.* 2012; 366(11): 1028–37.

Nicolle, L. E., Bradley, S., Colgan, R., *et al.* Infectious Diseases Society of America guidelines for the diagnosis and treatment of asymptomatic bacteriuria in adults. *Clin. Infect. Dis.* 2005; 40(5): 643–54.

Wilson, M. L. and Gaido, L. Laboratory diagnosis of urinary tract infections in adult patients. *Clin. Infect. Dis.* 2004; 38(8): 1150–8.

Pyelonephritis in Adults

Fredrick M. Abrahamian

Introduction and Microbiology

Acute pyelonephritis, an upper urinary tract infection (UTI), describes a clinical syndrome characterized by bacteriuria associated with fever, flank pain or tenderness, and lower UTI symptoms (e.g. frequency, urgency, dysuria). Uncomplicated infections are generally thought of in healthy, non-pregnant females aged 18 to 40 years, without underlying comorbidities, structural defects in urinary anatomy, or renal dysfunction.

Risk factors for complicated infection include extremes of age, male gender, anatomic or functional abnormality of the urinary tract, presence of foreign body within urinary tract (e.g. urinary catheter), urinary tract obstruction, immunosuppressed state, pregnancy, history of urinary tract instrumentation, or the presence of an unusual or resistant organism.

The organism that is responsible for the vast majority of uncomplicated and complicated cases of acute pyelonephritis is *Escherichia coli* (see Table 49.1). Uncomplicated infections may also be due to *Proteus mirabilis*, *Klebsiella* species, and enterococci. The microbiologic etiologies of complicated infections, in addition to *E. coli*, may also include *Proteus mirabilis*, *Klebsiella* species, enterococci, *Pseudomonas aeruginosa*, *Enterobacter*, and rarely *Staphylococcus aureus*. Recurrent infections place the patient at a higher risk of harboring a resistant organism as the cause of infection. In men with prostatitis, gram-negative enteric organisms (e.g. *E. coli*) are the most frequent cause; however, *Neisseria gonorrhoeae* and *Chlamydia trachomatis* may also be culprits (especially in younger patients). In those with acquired immunodeficiency syndrome, the prostate may be the focus of *Cryptococcus neoformans*.

Epidemiology

Pyelonephritis is a commonly diagnosed condition in the emergency department. There are approximately 250,000 cases of acute pyelonephritis annually occurring in the United States,

and it is estimated that 30% of these patients are hospitalized. The prevalence of disease is greater in women than men. Men are at a higher risk of infection if they are uncircumcised, have enlarged prostates resulting in urinary stasis, participate in insertive rectal intercourse, or have undergone recent urologic instrumentation or surgery.

Other populations at risk for acute pyelonephritis include those with urinary catheters, spinal cord injury, neurogenic bladder, or fistulae involving the bladder or ureters, or those who have undergone renal transplantation. Pregnant women, especially during the second trimester, are also at a higher risk for pyelonephritis because of hormonally induced changes in the urinary system. Potential complications of acute pyelonephritis during pregnancy include premature labor and low-birth-weight infant delivery.

Clinical Features

Clinically, acute pyelonephritis presents as a combination of fever, chills, flank pain, or costovertebral angle tenderness in association with urinary frequency, dysuria, or hematuria. The spectrum of disease can range from mild illness to fulminant septic shock. The pain associated with pyelonephritis can occasionally present at atypical locations such as the epigastric region or right or left upper abdominal quadrants. Voiding symptoms may be absent in a significant proportion of young women with confirmed pyelonephritis.

The presentation of pyelonephritis is particularly challenging in the elderly, where it can often present with any one of a number of symptoms, including abdominal pain, altered mental status, or sepsis syndrome. Fever in this population may be low-grade or absent.

UTI in older men should raise suspicion for acute prostatitis. The clinical presentation of acute prostatitis is similar to pyelonephritis and includes symptoms of UTI (e.g. frequency, urgency, dysuria), fever, chills, and perineal and low back pain. On physical examination, the prostate gland is swollen and

Table 49.1 Clinical Features: Acute Pyelonephritis in Adults

Organisms	The organism that is responsible for the vast majority of uncomplicated and complicated cases of acute pyelonephritis is *Escherichia coli*. Uncomplicated infections may also be due to: *Proteus mirabilis* *Klebsiella* species Enterococci The microbiologic etiology of complicated infections, in addition to the above organism may also be: *Pseudomonas aeruginosa* *Enterobacter* species *Staphylococcus aureus* (rare)
Signs and symptoms	Fever, chills, flank pain, or costovertebral angle tenderness in association with urinary frequency, dysuria, or hematuria
Laboratory findings	**Urine dipstick:** Positive leukocyte esterase and nitrite test **Urine microscopy:** Presence of pyuria and bacteriuria **Urine culture:** Isolation of $\geq 10^3$ CFU/mL of a single uropathogen

tender and bladder outlet obstruction may result in urinary retention.

Differential Diagnosis

Other conditions to consider include:

- nephrolithiasis with or without infection
- pelvic inflammatory disease, ovarian cyst, or torsion
- ectopic pregnancy
- acute prostatitis
- renal abscess, carcinoma
- abdominal pathology (e.g. pancreatitis, abdominal aortic aneurysm)
- renal artery stenosis or vein thrombosis
- pulmonary pathology (e.g. pneumonia)

Key features that may help distinguish pyelonephritis are:

- bacteriuria associated with fever, vomiting, flank pain or tenderness, and lower urinary tract symptoms (e.g. frequency, urgency, and dysuria)
- sudden-onset colicky back and flank pain associated with nausea and vomiting should raise suspicion for nephrolithiasis

Laboratory Findings

The laboratory diagnosis of acute pyelonephritis is based primarily on the results of urinalysis and urine culture. UTI is confirmed if pyuria and bacteriuria are detected on a microscopic examination of the urine. Pyuria, commonly defined as >10 white blood cells (WBC)/mm³ in a urine specimen, is present in the majority of symptomatic patients. The majority of patients will exhibit positive urine cultures. Urine culture specimens should be obtained prior to the initiation of antibiotic therapy.

In uncomplicated infections, blood culture results seldom differ from urine culture results and rarely lead to a change in antimicrobial therapy. Discrepancies between blood and urine cultures are often due to contamination by skin flora. Similar findings have also been demonstrated in pregnant patients with pyelonephritis. Blood cultures are best reserved for patients with complicated infections or when the source of fever is unclear.

Common imaging modalities utilized in the emergency department to evaluate renal pathology include ultrasound and computed tomographic (CT) scan. Most cases of acute pyelonephritis do not require radiographic evaluation. Imaging may provide insight as to the cause of the symptom in patients with an uncertain diagnosis. Renal ultrasound demonstrates hydronephrosis with high sensitivity. Additionally, renal or extrarenal abscesses and distal hydroureter (e.g. ureterovesical or uteropelvic junction) can be visualized by ultrasound.

Helical CT scan is considered the imaging modality of choice for definitive assessment of most types of renal pathology. Unenhanced CT of the abdomen and pelvis is an appropriate imaging study for the evaluation of urinary stones. In addition, CT scan can demonstrate hydroureter at all levels, hydronephrosis, and the precise location of gas and abscess. Contrast-enhanced CT scan delineates renal and perinephric abscesses and shows abnormalities in renal perfusion (e.g. renal infarction from renal artery occlusion or renal vein thrombosis).

Treatment

The choice of initial empiric antimicrobial therapy should be directed toward the most likely microbiologic etiology (see Table 49.2). Most uncomplicated infections can be managed on an outpatient basis with a 7-day course of a fluoroquinolone (e.g. ciprofloxacin, levofloxacin).

Other options for therapy include trimethoprim-sulfamethoxazole double strength (TMP/SMX-DS), amoxicillin-clavulanate, or oral cephalosporins for 14 days. Increasing *E. coli* resistance to commonly used drugs for the treatment of UTI (e.g. fluoroquinolones, TMP-SMX) is a concern. In the United States, approximately 30% of *E. coli* is currently resistant to ampicillin and amoxicillin.

Intravenous antimicrobial therapy for patients requiring hospitalization may include a fluoroquinolone (e.g. ciprofloxacin, levofloxacin), ceftriaxone, piperacillin-tazobactam, ertapenem, or doripenem. A combination therapy may include ampicillin and an aminoglycoside (e.g. gentamicin).

Table 49.2 Initial Empiric Therapy for Acute Pyelonephritis in Adults*

Therapy Recommendation

Outpatient therapy:

Ciprofloxacin 500 mg PO BID × 7 days

or

Levofloxacin 750 mg PO daily × 5 days

or

Amoxicillin–clavulanate 875/125 mg PO BID × 14 days

or

TMP-SMX DS (160/800 mg) 1 tab. PO BID × 14 days

Inpatient therapy (× 14 days):

Ciprofloxacin 400 mg IV every 12 hours

or

Levofloxacin 750 mg IV every 24 hours

or

Ceftriaxone 1 g IV every 24 hours

or

Ertapenem 1 g IV every 24 hours

or

Piperacillin–tazobactam 3.375 g IV every 6 hours

or

Ampicillin–sulbactam 3 g IV every 6 hours

---

* The choice of initial empiric antimicrobial therapy is best directed toward the most likely microbiologic etiology and knowledge of local susceptibility patterns.

DS – double strength; IV – intravenous; PO – by mouth; TMP-SMX – trimethoprim-sulfamethoxazole.

The recommended duration of therapy for hospitalized patients is 14 days.

The quinolones are contraindicated in pregnancy because of adverse effects on fetal bone and cartilage development. Inpatient therapy for pyelonephritis during pregnancy may include a third-generation cephalosporin (e.g. ceftriaxone). Oral therapy can include cephalexin or amoxicillin–clavulanate.

Acute prostatitis responds well to oral antimicrobial therapy. Fluoroquinolones, TMP-SMX, and cephalosporins have good penetration into prostatic tissue. The duration of therapy is 2 to 4 weeks. Complications of acute prostatitis can include prostatic abscess formation and should be suspected in patients failing antimicrobial therapy. The diagnosis can be made by CT scan or transrectal ultrasonography. Treatment usually involves surgical drainage because antimicrobial therapy alone may not be sufficient for cure.

If sexually transmitted infections (e.g. *N. gonorrhoeae* and *C. trachomatis*) are suspected as the cause of prostatitis, treatment should include ceftriaxone and doxycycline. Fluoroquinolones are no longer recommended for the treatment of gonococcal infections and associated conditions such as pelvic inflammatory disease in the United States.

Treatment of UTI in the presence of an indwelling catheter includes removal of the catheter if possible, as well as intravenous antimicrobial therapy directed against *Enterobacteriaceae*, *Pseudomonas aeruginosa*, and enterococci. Suggested monotherapy includes ciprofloxacin, levofloxacin, piperacillin-tazobactam, doripenem, imipenem, or meropenem. Combination therapy may include ampicillin and gentamicin. Cephalosporins and ertapenem should be avoided because they are not active against enterococci. The initial recommended duration of antimicrobial therapy for catheter-associated UTI is 7 days.

Complications and Admission Criteria

The majority of patients with acute pyelonephritis will have improvement of their symptoms within 72 hours after the initiation of antimicrobial therapy. Failure to improve should raise the possibility of an inappropriate antimicrobial choice, the presence of a resistant or unusual organism, or an incorrect working diagnosis (e.g. nephrolithiasis is commonly misdiagnosed as pyelonephritis). Treatment failure may also be due to the presence of complications such as urinary obstruction, papillary necrosis, intrarenal or perinephric abscess formation, or emphysematous pyelonephritis.

The clinical presentation of intrarenal or perinephric abscess can be similar to pyelonephritis. Predisposing factors to abscess formation include urinary tract obstruction due to calculi and diabetes mellitus. *E. coli* and other gram-negative enteric bacilli are usually the causative microbiologic agents. *Staphylococcus aureus* may also be a culprit, often from hematogenous seeding (i.e. staphylococcal bacteremia and/or endocarditis). In about 30% of patients with perinephric abscess, the urinalysis is normal, and 40% have sterile urine cultures. The diagnosis is often suspected in patients who do not respond to initial antimicrobial therapy within 48 hours. Ultrasound and CT scan are both capable of demonstrating the abscess. Emergency department management involves the initiation of intravenous broad-spectrum antibiotics and urologic consultation for definitive surgical drainage (e.g. percutaneous or open surgical drainage).

Emphysematous pyelonephritis is a severe necrotizing form of infection that results in the formation of gas in the renal parenchyma and collecting tissues. It is a rare condition that is generally seen in the setting of diabetes with poor glycemic control. It is most often associated with *E. coli*, *Klebsiella*, and *Proteus* species. While the presentation can be non-specific and similar to pyelonephritis, these patients are often very sick on presentation. CT scan of the abdomen and pelvis is the best imaging modality for the evaluation of emphysematous pyelonephritis. The precise localization of gas allows differentiation of emphysematous pyelonephritis from other potential sources such as emphysematous pyelitis, perinephric emphysema, or abscess. Early surgical intervention (e.g. drainage or nephrectomy) in combination with broad-spectrum antibiotics has been shown to decrease mortality from emphysematous pyelonephritis. Emergency department management involves the initiation of intravenous broad-spectrum antibiotics and urologic consultation for definitive surgical management.

Xanthogranulomatous pyelonephritis is a rare, severe suppurative reaction to chronic renal infection in which dead renal tissue is replaced by granulomas. Predisposing factors include urinary obstruction by tumor or calculi, renal ischemia, dyslipidemia, diabetes, and an immunocompromised state. It is more common in women, with the peak incidence between the fifth and seventh decades. Common microbiologic culprits include *Proteus* species and *E. coli*. The presentation can be non-specific and similar to pyelonephritis. The CT scan may show low-attenuation masses with destruction of the renal parenchyma and possibly the presence of a staghorn calculus. The ultimate diagnosis requires biopsy, and treatment includes partial or complete nephrectomy.

Indications for hospitalization in patients with acute pyelonephritis include hemodynamic instability, persistent vomiting or inability to tolerate fluids, and the presence of complications (e.g. urinary tract obstruction, emphysematous pyelonephritis). In addition, pregnant patients are also best managed as inpatients because of the higher risk of complications. If deemed appropriate for outpatient therapy, these patients require close follow-up.

Pearls and Pitfalls

1. The pain associated with acute pyelonephritis can occasionally present at atypical locations such as the epigastric region or right or left upper abdominal quadrants.
2. Urinary tract infection in older men should raise suspicion for acute prostatitis.
3. Urine culture should be performed on patients with acute pyelonephritis.
4. In uncomplicated infections, blood culture results seldom differ from urine culture results or lead to a change in antimicrobial therapy.
5. Treatment failure may be due to the presence of complications such as urinary obstruction or abscess formation.

References

Hill, J. B., Sheffield, J. S., McIntire, D. D., *et al.* Acute pyelonephritis in pregnancy. *Obstet. Gynecol.* 2005; 105(1): 18–23.

Hooton, T. M. Uncomplicated urinary tract infection. *N. Engl. J. Med.* 2012; 366(11): 1028–37.

Liu, H. and Mulholland, S. G. Appropriate antibiotic treatment of genitourinary infections in hospitalized patients. *Am. J. Med.* 2005; 118(7A): 14–20S.

Scholes, D., Hooton, T. M., Roberts, P. L., *et al.* Risk factors associated with acute pyelonephritis in healthy women. *Ann. Intern. Med.* 2005; 142(1): 20–7.

Sheffield, J. S. and Cunningham, F. G. Urinary tract infection in women. *Obstet. Gynecol.* 2005; 106(5 Pt. 1): 1085–92.

Song, E. K. and Zwanger, M. Xanthogranulomatous pyelonephritis. *J. Emerg. Med.* 2001; 21(1): 63–4.

Talan, D. A., Klimberg, I. W., Nicolle, L. E., *et al.* Once daily, extended release ciprofloxacin for complicated urinary tract infections and acute uncomplicated pyelonephritis. *J. Urol.* 2004; 171(2 Pt. 1): 734–9.

Velasco, M., Martinez, J. A., Moreno-Martinez, A., *et al.* Blood cultures for women with uncomplicated acute pyelonephritis: are they necessary? *Clin. Infect. Dis.* 2003; 37(8): 1127–30.

Additional Readings

Gupta, K., Hooton, T. M., Naber, K. G., *et al.* International clinical practice guidelines for the treatment of acute uncomplicated cystitis and pyelonephritis in women: a 2010 update by the Infectious Disease Society of America and the European Society for Microbiology and Infectious Diseases. *Clin. Infect. Dis.* 2011; 52(5): e103–20.

Hooton, T. M., Bradley, S. F., Cardenas, D. D., *et al.* Diagnosis, prevention, and treatment of catheter-associated urinary tract infection in adults: 2009 international clinical practice guidelines from the Infectious Diseases Society of America. *Clin. Infect. Dis.* 2010; 50(5): 625–63.

Sandberg, T., Skoog, G., Hermansson, A. B., *et al.* Ciprofloxacin for 7 days versus 14 days in women with acute pyelonephritis: a randomized, open-label and double-blind, placebo-controlled, non-inferiority trial. *Lancet* 2012; 380(9840): 484–90.

Chapter

50

Fever in the Newborn

Maureen McCollough

Introduction and Microbiology

The neonate is defined as a newborn infant less than 4 weeks old, and fever in this age group as a temperature greater than 100.4 °F or 38 °C. Because the clinical exam is limited and because of the high risk of serious bacterial infection in this age group, it is recommended that all febrile neonates must be admitted for a sepsis work-up and empiric antibiotic therapy.

Neonatal infections are unique, in that transmission of organisms can occur transplacentally during gestation and can present early on or be delayed by months or longer. Vertical transmission can occur in utero or during delivery. Infections can be acquired from family members or hospital personnel. The newborn immune system is immature, increasing the susceptibility to infection. Other disease processes such as hyaline membrane disease may complicate infectious presentations. Finally, the presentation of infectious diseases in neonates is variable, often with subtle signs and symptoms.

Group B streptococcus and *Escherichia coli* are the most common bacterial cause of neonatal sepsis in the United States. *Listeria monocytogenes*, *Klebsiella*, enterococcus, non-group D alpha hemolytic strep, and non-typeable *Haemophilus influenzae* are other bacterial causes. Viral causes include herpes simplex virus (sometimes with no symptoms in the mother), influenza, enterovirus (coxsackie and echoviruses), and adenovirus (typically with liver and CNS involvement). Microbiology is discussed further under the clinical features of specific types of infection.

Epidemiology

Neonates who are less than 2 weeks old who present to the Emergency Department (ED) have a particularly high incidence of serious illness with 10 to 33% requiring hospital admission. The most common diagnoses in admitted neonates include respiratory infections, sepsis, dehydration, congenital heart disease, bowel obstruction, hypoglycemia, and seizures.

The incidence of serious bacterial infections such as bacteremia, urinary tract infections, or meningitis is highest in the neonatal age group compared to older infants. The overall incidence in published studies is as high as 20% or even higher in ill-appearing or hyperpyrexic neonates (temperatures >40 °C). In neonates, serious bacterial infections such as urinary tract infections are often as common as viral infections.

Clinical Features

Fever in the newborn period is defined as greater than 100.4 °F or 38 °C. Furthermore, while the differential for an ill-appearing young infant is broad, any ill-appearing young infant should be considered septic until proven otherwise, regardless of temperature. "Early onset" sepsis occurs within hours or a few days of birth and is often associated with perinatal risk factors. "Late onset" sepsis usually occurs after 1 week of age, develops more gradually, and is more commonly associated with community-acquired organisms.

Undressing the baby to look for signs of poor perfusion or petechiae is important, though the clinical signs of sepsis may be subtle. Lethargy, irritability, or decreased oral intake is common. Other clinical features include apnea, tachypnea, cyanosis, respiratory distress, tachycardia, bradycardia, jaundice, pallor, vomiting, diarrhea, temperature instability (high or low), abdominal distension, or ileus. It is not uncommon for septic newborns to be unable to mount a febrile response.

Well-appearing febrile neonates are common. Most neonatal visits to the acute care setting will be an otherwise healthy-appearing newborn with fever. Despite a non-toxic appearance, fever in the neonatal period must be taken seriously as other signs of serious bacterial illness may be subtle and a thorough work-up for a source is still indicated. Bundling of the neonate in clothes or blankets may cause an elevation of the skin temperature, but is very rarely a cause of a rectal temperature

>38 °C. And fever >38.5 °C should never be considered secondary to bundling. Neonates with a reported fever per rectum at home but afebrile upon presentation should still be considered at risk.

The past medical history for a neonate is obviously limited, but must include both prenatal and postnatal risk factors. The mother may have had serological screens for *Treponema pallidum*, rubella, and hepatitis B virus. Cultures may have been taken for group B streptococci, herpes simplex, *Neisseria gonorrhoeae*, or chlamydia. Prenatal infections that can be transmitted transplacentally include syphilis, rubella, cytomegalovirus (CMV), parvovirus B19, human immunodeficiency virus (HIV), varicella zoster, *Listeria monocytogenes*, *Borrelia burgdorferi*, and toxoplasmosis (see Chapter 58, Fever in Pregnancy). Vertically transmitted organisms (colonizing the birth canal) include group B streptococci, gonococci, *Listeria monocytogenes*, *E. coli*, chlamydia, genital *Mycoplasma*, and herpes and enteroviruses.

The evaluation of a neonate who appears critically ill requires a physical examination looking for sources of infection such as herpes lesions or omphalitis (see Table 50.1). Herpes may present as a disseminated infection involving multiple organ systems, or encephalitis with or without a rash, or less commonly as a disease localized to the skin, eyes, or mouth. If lesions are found, they will usually appear on the birth "presenting" portion of the baby. If the child was delivered head first, thoroughly examine the scalp for lesions, especially where a fetal scalp electrode may have been inserted.

The fontanelle of a newborn should be flat. A depressed fontanelle can indicate dehydration; a full fontanelle can suggest meningitis. The umbilical area should be examined for signs of omphalitis, a true medical emergency. Redness at the area of the umbilical cord should be considered an early sign of omphalitis. Omphalitis, a mixed gram-positive and gram-negative infection, can spread hematogenously or directly into the peritoneum.

In a male infant who has been circumcised, the penis should be examined for signs of infection. Urinary tract infections account for most of the serious bacterial infections in neonates with rates higher in males, especially uncircumcised males, hyperpyrexic infants, and those with more prolonged illness. Neonatal urinary tract infection (UTI) often presents with non-specific signs and symptoms, such as vomiting, diarrhea, irritability, or jaundice.

Respiratory infections are a significant cause of fever or illness in neonates. Pneumonia in the first week of life (less than 7 days since birth) is most commonly due to group B *Streptococcus*, but may also be caused by *Escherichia Coli*, *Listeria monocytogenes*, or *Klebsiella pneumoniae*. If pneumonia is accompanied by eye discharge, chlamydia testing is imperative. Other organisms causing pneumonia in young neonates include herpes simplex virus, cytomegalovirus, adenovirus, treponema pallidum, and *Mycobacterium tuberculosis*. Pneumonia in neonates greater than age 7 days old may also be caused by respiratory syncytial virus (RSV), *Streptococcus pneumoniae*, *Staphylococcus aureus*, or type B and non-typeable *Haemophilus influenzae*.

Signs of neonatal pneumonia include tachypnea, retractions, grunting, rales, wheezing, cyanosis, and respiratory distress or overt respiratory failure. Other associated symptoms include fever, feeding difficulty, or irritability. RSV can cause bronchiolitis and may present with apnea. Chlamydia often presents in a non-febrile, well-appearing infant with cough. Neonatal pertussis commonly presents with apnea, cyanosis, and post-tussive vomiting. Serious sequelae such as ventricular fibrillation or seizures may develop.

Otitis media is another febrile illness that can be difficult to diagnose in neonates because the tympanic membranes are difficult to visualize. In up to one-third of infants in the first month diagnosed with otitis media, the etiological organisms are *Escherichia coli*, *Klebsiella pneumoniae*, *Pseudomonas aeruginosa*, and group B *Streptococcus*.

Differential Diagnosis

The most common sources of bacterial infections in neonates are meningitis, bacteremia, urinary tract infections, and pneumonia, though the non-infectious differential of an ill-appearing neonate is broad and includes some disease processes unique to the neonatal period. The mnemonic S-S-I-C-C-C-F-I-T describes possible etiologies of critical illness in the neonate (see Box 50.1).

Neonatal seizures will often present with tonic or clonic movements or autonomic repetitive movements such as blinking, lip smacking, or bicycling. Inborn errors of metabolism and congenital adrenal hyperplasia present with altered mental status, vomiting, and dehydration. Congenital adrenal hyperplasia will produce electrolyte imbalances, including hyponatremia and hyperkalemia. Neonates with central nervous system (CNS) hemorrhage often exhibit altered mental status, vomiting, and bulging fontanelles. Congenital heart disease presenting emergently in the neonatal period is often due to closure of the ductus arteriosus. Infants with structural lesions requiring a patent ductus arteriosus for blood flow will develop sudden cyanosis or shock. Prostaglandin E1, a potent vasodilator, is vital to their survival. Toxin ingestion may be accidental or intentional (such as mistaking other powders for formula, or giving baking soda to alleviate colic). Volvulus occurs secondary to congenital malrotation of the intestine and is a surgical emergency. Volvulus may present rather benignly with vomiting and irritability, but will soon progress to altered mental status and shock as the bowel infarcts. Surgery is the only treatment.

Laboratory and Radiographic Findings

The work-up of a febrile neonate in the ED (see Table 50.2) includes evaluation of blood, urine, cerebrospinal fluid (CSF), and stool if indicated by symptoms. Recent studies have attempted to establish whether a viral process (such as RSV bronchiolitis or influenza A diagnosed by rapid bedside test) can explain the fever in a well-appearing neonate and obviate the need for a complete work-up for bacterial infection. For example, in one study, in infants younger than 28 days with fever and positive RSV testing, there were no cases of

Table 50.1 Clinical Features: Neonatal Fever

	Organisms	Signs and Symptoms	Laboratory and Radiologic Findings
Meningitis	**Bacterial**: Group B *Streptococcus* *Listeria* *Escherichia coli* *Klebsiella* *Enterococcus* Non-group D alpha-hemolytic strep *Haemophilus influenzae* **Viral:** Herpes simplex Enterovirus Adenovirus	• Fever • Apnea, tachypnea, cyanosis, respiratory distress • Tachycardia, bradycardia • Jaundice, pallor • Vomiting, diarrhea, abdominal distension, or ileus • Hyper- or hypothermia	• CSF Gram stain – bacteria • CSF WBC <20/mm³ normal • CSF protein 20–170 mg/dL normal • CSF glucose 34–119 mg/dL normal • Consider herpes if CSF shows pleocytosis, predominance of RBCs or high protein; PCR is >95% sensitive for herpes in CSF; may also be isolated by viral culture
Bacteremia	Group B *Streptococcus* *Listeria* *Escherichia coli* *Klebsiella* *Enterococcus* Non-group D alpha-Hemolytic strep *Haemophilus influenzae*	• Fever • Irritability • Apnea, tachypnea, cyanosis, respiratory distress • Tachycardia, bradycardia • Jaundice, pallor • Vomiting, diarrhea, abdominal distension, or ileus • Hyper- or hypothermia	• Positive blood culture • Serum markers are too insensitive to rule out bacteremia
Otitis media	*Escherichia coli* *Klebsiella pneumoniae* *Pseudomonas aeruginosa* Group B *Streptococcus*	Tympanic membranes can be difficult to visualize	No laboratory or radiographs
Pneumonia	**At birth:** Group B *Streptococcus* Herpes simplex virus CMV Adenovirus *Treponema pallidum* *Listeria* *Mycobacterium tuberculosis* **After birth (>24 hours later):** Group B *Streptococcus* *Escherichia coli* *Klebsiella pneumoniae* *Ureaplasma Urealyticum* **After 7 days:** RSV *Streptococcus pneumoniae* *Staphylococcus aureus* *Haemophilus Influenzae* type B and non-typeable *Bordetella pertussis*	• Fever • Apnea • Tachypnea, grunting, rales, wheezing, cyanosis, respiratory distress or overt failure • RSV – apnea, wheezing, tachypnea, difficulty feeding; more severe in premature or infants with underlying cardiac or pulmonary disease • Hypotension, sepsis, meningitis, especially group B *Streptococcus* • Feeding difficulty, irritability • Chlamydia often presents with an afebrile well-appearing infant with cough; conjunctivitis may be present • Pertussis – often no catarrhal stage of sneezing and congestion; often no paroxysmal cough or whoop; more often tachypnea, apnea, cyanosis, gagging, feeding difficulty, post-tussive vomiting; rarely ventricular fibrillation, seizures, subarachnoid hemorrhage, rectal prolapse, hernias, dehydration	Chest X-ray: usually diffuse bilateral granular or patchy infiltrates RSV may show hyperinflation, peribronchial cuffing, interstitial infiltrates, or atelectasis Chlamydia may show bilateral interstitial infiltrates with hyperinflation Pertussis may show perihilar infiltrates and atelectasis; possible pneumothorax and pneumomediastinum Laboratory tests are generally unhelpful for the diagnosis of pneumonia Rapid RSV or pertussis nasopharyngeal testing can be useful Pertussis does not commonly produce lymphocytosis
Omphalitis	Mixed gram-positive, and gram-negative	Redness surrounding the umbilical cord	No laboratory or radiographs
Urinary tract infection	*Escherichia coli* Other gram-negative bacilli *Enterococcus* spp.	• Fever • Irritability • Apnea, tachypnea, cyanosis, respiratory distress • Tachycardia, bradycardia • Jaundice, pallor • Vomiting, diarrhea, abdominal distension, or ileus • Hyper- or hypothermia	Urinalysis alone is insufficient to rule out a UTI
Rash/lesions	Herpes simplex virus	May be disseminated and present as encephalitis with or without lesions	Tzanck smear of lesion may show multinucleated giant cells Direct fluorescent antibody testing of air-dried smear may be more sensitive

CSF – cerebrospinal fluid; PCR – polymerase chain reaction; RBC – red blood cell; WBC – white blood (cell) count.

Box 50.1 Differential Diagnosis for the Critically Ill-Appearing Neonate in the Emergency Department: *S-S-I-C-C-C-F-I-T* mnemonic

S – Sepsis

S – Seizures

I – Inborn errors of metabolism or other metabolic disorders

C – CNS bleed

C – Congenital adrenal hyperplasia

C – Congenital heart disease

F – Formula mix-ups

I – Intestinal disasters, e.g. volvulus, incarcerated hernia

T – Toxins, including any herbs, teas, or powders such as baking soda given to infants for ailments such as colic, spitting up, or constipation

CNS – Central nervous system.

Table 50.2 Work-up of Febrile Neonates in the Emergency Department

CBC (other serum markers such as CRP may be included, but are not diagnostic)

Blood culture

Urinalysis

Urine culture

Stool culture if applicable

CSF for cell count, glucose, protein, Gram stain, and culture

Chest x-ray if indicated

RSV swab if indicated

Pertussis swab if indicated

Rapid influenza A test (not yet accepted as standard practice to rule out the need for a full work-up in a febrile neonate)

CBC – complete blood count; CRP – C-reactive protein; CSF – cerebrospinal fluid.

Serum markers' sensitivity and specificity will also increase the longer the duration of illness. Other markers, such as an elevated interleukin-6, procalcitonin, or tumor necrosis factor alpha level, are also not sensitive enough to obviate the need for a work-up in a febrile neonate. Given the lack of predictive value of serum markers, they should not be used to decide on cessation of a septic work-up of a febrile neonate, patient admission, or administration of antibiotics.

Because the signs of meningitis can be very subtle or non-existent in some neonates, a lumbar puncture (LP) is indicated not only in a septic or ill-appearing infant, but also in well-appearing febrile neonates. The infant should be placed in a sitting or lateral non-flexed position to minimize the development of hypoxia during the LP. Placing the infant on a pulse oximeter during the procedure also minimizes the risk of an unrecognized hypoxia. If the infant is critically ill, the risk of apnea increases, and it may be better to delay the LP, obtain blood cultures, administer antibiotics, and then examine the CSF at a later time when the infant is more clinically stable. If the CSF has many white blood cells (WBCs) or a predominance of red blood cells without organisms on Gram stain, herpes meningitis should be considered. A polymerase chain reaction (PCR) assay on CSF for herpes simplex virus is more than 95% sensitive.

A urinalysis is insufficient to rule out a UTI in very young infants. Young infants often cannot mount an inflammatory response in the bladder. A positive bacterial nitrite response also is not sensitive as it requires the urine to be held within the bladder for a period of time; in general, this does not occur in neonates. For these reasons, a culture must be sent along with a urinalysis. Because a bag specimen can often result in false-positive growth, a catheterized specimen is recommended. Urine latex agglutination testing for group B *Streptococcus* is available, but has limited sensitivity.

For newborns with signs of lower respiratory tract disease or complaints of apnea or a brief resolved unexplained event (BRUE), a nasopharyngeal swab should be sent for RSV by immunoassay or PCR, and for pertussis by direct fluorescent antibody (DFA) test or enzyme-linked immunoassay (ELISA) test. If conjunctivitis with discharge is present in a newborn with pneumonia, the eye secretions should be tested for *Chlamydia trachomatis* using DFA, ELISA, or culture. Blood cultures are positive in a minority of neonates with bacterial pneumonia, but are often positive in neonates with urinary tract infections.

Chest radiographs may show diffuse bilateral granular or patchy infiltrates. RSV often causes hyperinflation, peribronchial cuffing, interstitial infiltrates, or atelectasis on x-ray. *Chlamydia trachomatis* typically causes bilateral interstitial infiltrates with hyperinflation, and *Bordetella pertussis* infection may result in perihilar infiltrates, atelectasis, pneumothorax, and pneumomediastinum.

Treatment and Prophylaxis

The evaluation of a critically ill-appearing neonate who presents to the ED begins with placement of a cardiac monitor, pulse

meningitis, though the difference in the rate of meningitis between the RSV-positive and RSV-negative groups was not statistically significant. In addition, the overall rate of serious bacterial infections (or SBI, including UTI, bacterial enteritis, bacteremia, and bacterial meningitis) in infants <28 days old was high at 13%, and still significant at 10% in the RSV-postive group. If rapid viral diagnostic tests such as RSV or influenza are to be used in the ED, the particular sensitivity and positive predictive value of these tests and the overall prevalence of SBI in the relevant age group must be taken into account. Although these rapid viral studies have proven to be useful in the management of older febrile infants, further studies are needed to determine whether positive, rapid bedside viral tests can mitigate the need for a complete septic work-up in a febrile neonate.

More recently, serum markers have been evaluated as early indicators of neonatal sepsis. Unfortunately, they all lack the sensitivity and specificity to rule out sepsis in the febrile neonate in the ED. For neonatal sepsis, an abnormal C-reactive protein (CRP), the most readily available of the newer serum markers, is 75% sensitive and 86% specific; while an immature neutrophil (band) to total neutrophil ratio above 0.2 is 60 to 90% sensitive and 70 to 80% specific for diagnosing neonatal sepsis.

oximeter, assessment of vital signs including blood pressure, and bedside testing for blood glucose. Blood pressure is often a forgotten vital sign in very ill-appearing young infants. A systolic blood pressure below 60 mm Hg is considered abnormal. Neonates may be hypothermic or hyperthermic when septic. The temperature of the undressed neonate should be rechecked periodically because young infants have difficulty maintaining their temperature as a result of their large body surfaces. For this reason, consider radiant warming for hypothermic and even normothermic neonates.

Intubation may be necessary if a high-flow oxygen mask is not sufficient to reverse hypoxia. The infant's work of breathing must also be considered when deciding whether or not to intubate. High-flow nasal cannula oxygen delivery has been evaluated in small studies for young infants with respiratory distress due to lower respiratory infections such as bronchiolitis. If intubation is required, uncuffed endotracheal tubes are recommended for neonates. Intravenous lines are often hard to establish in young infants, especially when they are ill, dehydrated, or in extremis. Scalp veins can be used to deliver both fluid boluses and medications. Commercial devices are also available that use infrared technology to aid in establishing intravenous lines. An intraosseous (IO) line or an umbilical vein line can be used if no intravenous lines can be established. Young infants have a limited ability to maintain normal glucose; therefore, frequent bedside measurement of serum glucose is mandatory. Blood glucose concentrations below 40 mg/dL are considered abnormal in neonates. Because bedside glucose tests can be inaccurate, it is often recommended that levels below 50 mg/dL mandate intervention consisting of 5 mL/kg bolus of intravenous D10.

If saline boluses are required, begin with 10 mL/kg at a time and reassess. Maintenance fluids can be sustained with D5¼NS at 4 mL per kg per hour while in the ED. Packed red blood cells, platelets, or fresh frozen plasma should be administered in 10 mL/kg dosages. Communication with a neonatal or pediatric intensive care unit early on is important to expedite the transfer of the critically ill neonate. Ampicillin 50 mg/kg per dose IV every 8 to 12 hours (covering *Streptococcus*, *Listeria*, some *Enterococcus*) plus cefotaxime 50 mg/kg per dose IV every 8 to 12 hours (offers additional gram-negative coverage) is often recommended for empiric treatment of febrile neonates. Ampicillin and gentamicin are another alternative combination. Gentamicin is nephrotoxic and ototoxic with prolonged administration, and doses and frequencies should be adjusted for gestational age and weight.

If herpes simplex meningitis is suspected, acyclovir should be initiated. A high suspicion for herpes meningitis is warranted if (a) CSF has high WBC or high protein or predominance of red blood cells (RBCs) but no organisms, or (b) CSF pleocytosis is present with vesicular rash on infant, seizures, focal neurological signs, pneumonitis or hepatitis, or a maternal history of genital herpes.

Admission is warranted for all neonates with evidence of lower respiratory tract infection or wheezing consistent with bronchiolitis, as the risk of apnea is significant. Evaluation should focus on work of breathing and oxygen requirement of the infant. Supportive care includes suctioning, oxygen, and possibly intubation. Neither inhaled beta-agonists nor epinephrine or systemic steroids have been shown to be useful; these therapies may be useful, however, in infants with a strong family history of atopic disease or asthma.

Ampicillin plus either gentamicin or cefotaxime is indicated for neonatal pneumonia. Chlamydia can be treated with a macrolide. Pertussis treatment with macrolides or trimethoprim-sulfamethoxazole may be effective only during the coryza stage.

Complications and Admission Criteria

All febrile neonates should be admitted to the hospital regardless of appearance. Correct hypothermia, hypovolemia, hypoglycemia, and other electrolyte abnormalities early. If the child is ill-appearing or if a bacterial source for the fever has been established, antibiotics should be administered in the ED. Emergency physicians should also have a low threshold for administering empiric antibiotics to febrile neonates.

Pearls and Pitfalls

1. All emergency departments should be prepared to care for all critically ill infants and children, which includes having the correct pediatric equipment.
2. Emergency providers should know the range of normal vital signs, findings on physical exam, and laboratory parameters in neonates; this will allow for identification of those at risk for serious illness.
3. Be aware that infants are at risk for both perinatal and community-acquired infections during the first month of life.
4. Febrile neonates are at high risk for meningitis, bacteremia, and UTIs, and therefore a complete septic work-up is always indicated in infants less than 4 weeks of age.
5. Septic young infants may present with very subtle signs such as tachypnea or decreased feeding.
6. Admission to the hospital with intravenous antibiotics is strongly advised for any neonate presenting with a fever.

References

American Academy of Pediatrics, Subcommittee on Diagnosis and Management of Bronchiolitis. Diagnosis and management of bronchiolitis. *Pediatrics* 2006; 118(4): 1774–93.

Anbar, R. D., Richardson-de Corral, V., and O'Malley, P. J. Difficulties in universal application of criteria identifying infants at low risk for serious bacterial infection. *J. Pediatr.* 1986; 109(3): 483–5.

Bonsu, B. K. and Harper, M. B. Utility of the peripheral blood white blood cell count for identifying sick young infants who need lumbar puncture. *Ann. Emerg. Med.* 2003; 41(2): 206–14.

Bressan, S., Andreola, B., Cattelan, F., *et al.* Predicting severe bacterial infections in well-appearing febrile neonates: laboratory markers accuracy and duration of fever. *Pediatr. Infect. Dis. J.* 2010; 29(3): 227–32.

Carstairs, K. L., Tanen, D. A., Johnson, A. S., *et al.* Pneumococcal bacteremia in febrile infants presenting to the emergency department before and after the introduction of heptavalent pneumococcal vaccine. *Ann. Emerg. Med.* 2007; 49(6): 772–7.

Caviness, A. C., Demmler, G. J., Almendarez, Y., *et al.* The prevalence of neonatal herpes simplex virus infection compared with serious bacterial illness in hospitalized neonates. *J. Pediatr.* 2008; 153(2): 164–9.

Cheng, T. L. and Partridge, J. C. Effect of bundling and high environmental temperature on neonatal body temperature. *Pediatrics* 1993; 92(2): 238–40.

Gerdes, J. S. Diagnosis and management of bacterial infections in the neonate. *Pediatr. Clin. North Am.* 2004; 51(4): 939–59.

Griffin, M. P., Lake, D. E., and Moorman, J. R. Heart rate characteristics and laboratory tests in neonatal sepsis. *Pediatrics* 2005; 115(4): 937–41.

Grijalva, C. G., Poehling, K. A., Edwards, K. M., *et al.* Accuracy and interpretation of rapid influenza tests in children. *Pediatrics* 2007; 119(1): e6–11.1.

Hoppe, J. E. Neonatal pertussis. *Pediatr. Infect. Dis. J.* 2000; 19(3): 244–7.

Hsiao, A. L., Chen, L., and Baker, M. D. Incidence and predictors of serious bacterial infections among 57- to 180-day-old infants. *Pediatrics* 2006; 117(5): 1695–701.

Kadish, H. A., Loveridge, B., Tobey, J., *et al.* Applying outpatient protocols in febrile infants 1–28 days of age: can the threshold be lowered? *Clin. Pediatr.* 2000; 39(2): 81–8.

Levine, D. A., Platt, S. L., Dayan, P. S., *et al.* Risk of serious bacterial infection in young febrile infants with respiratory syncytial virus infections. *Pediatrics* 2004; 113(6): 1728–34.

Malk, A., Hui, C. P. S., Pennie, R. A., and Kirpalani, H. Beyond the complete blood cell count and C-reactive protein. *Arch. Pediatr. Adolesc. Med.* 2003; 57(6): 511–16.

Milesi, C., Boubal, M., Jacquot, A., *et al.* High-flow nasal cannula: recommendations for daily practice in pediatrics. *Ann. Intensive Care* 2014; 4: 29.

Poland, R. and Watterberg, K. Sepsis in the newborn. *Pediatr. Rev.* 1993; 14(7): 262–3.

Sadow, K. B., Derr, R., and Teach, S. J. Bacterial infections in infants 60 days and younger. *Arch. Pediatr. Adolesc. Med.* 1999; 153(6): 611–14.

Scarfone, R. J. Controversies in the treatment of bronchiolitis. *Curr. Opin. Pediatr.* 2005; 17(1): 62–6.

Smitherman, H. F., Caviness, A. C., and Macias, C. G. Retrospective review of serious bacterial infections in infants who are 0 to 36 months of age and have influenza A infection. *Pediatrics* 2005; 115(3): 710–18.

Stanley, R., Pagon, Z., and Bachur, R. Hyperpyrexia among infants younger than 3 months. *Pediatric. Emerg. Care* 2005; 21(5): 291–4.

Tipple, M. A., Beem, M. O., and Saxon, E. M. Clinical characteristics of the afebrile pneumonia associated with *Chlamydia trachomatis* infection in infants less than 6 months of age. *Pediatrics* 1979; 63(2): 192–7.

Willwerth, B. M., Harper, M. B., and Greenes, D. S. Identifying hospitalized infants who have bronchiolitis and are at high risk for apnea. *Ann. Emerg. Med.* 2006; 48(4): 441–7.

Zorc, J. J., Levine, D. A., Platt, S. L., *et al.* Clinical and demographic factors associated with urinary tract infection in young febrile infants. *Pediatrics* 2005; 116(3): 644–8.

Additional Readings

American College of Emergency Physicians (ACEP) Pediatric Committee. Clinical policy for children younger than three years presenting to the emergency department with fever. *Ann. Emerg. Med.* 2003; 42(4): 530–45.

American Heart Association (AHA). 2005 guidelines for cardiopulmonary resuscitation (CPR) and emergency cardiovascular care (ECC) of pediatric and neonatal patients: pediatric advanced life support. *Pediatrics* 2006; 117(5): e1005–28.

Millar, K. R., Gloor, J. E., Wellington, N., and Joubert, G. Early neonatal presentations to the pediatric emergency department. *Pediatr. Emerg. Care* 2000; 16(3): 145–52.

The Febrile Child

Paul Ishimine

Introduction

Fever is one of the most common chief complaints in children who present to the emergency department. Most febrile children will have infectious causes for their fever, and while most of these children have benign viral illnesses, a subset of these children will have more serious underlying infections.

Even though fever is a common presenting complaint in the emergency department, there is no standard approach to evaluation and management that applies to all patients and to all practice settings, rather the approach will vary widely depending on many factors. These include limitations of the history and physical examination and differing level of risk acceptance among parents and physicians, as well as the changing epidemiology of serious bacterial infections, new and evolving diagnostic tests, and expert consensus. The challenge for the acute care provider faced with a febrile child is to identify the patient at high risk for serious underlying infection, while limiting unnecessary testing and treatment.

Because immune function, likely pathogens, and exam findings vary significantly depending on the age of the patient, risk assessment of febrile children is stratified by age. This categorization schema oversimplifies the heterogeneous level of risk for patients both within and among age groups, but because previous research has used arbitrary age cut-offs for study populations, this categorization continues to serve as the foundation for organizing the approach to the febrile young child. This chapter focuses on febrile neonates (0 to 28 days), infants, and toddlers up to 24 months of age without an obvious focus of infection. Chapter 50 covers the febrile neonate in more detail.

Epidemiology

Neonates are at particularly high risk for serious bacterial infection (SBI), including bacteremia, meningitis, pneumonia, urinary tract infections (UTIs), bacterial gastroenteritis, and osteomyelitis (see Chapter 50). About 12% of all febrile neonates presenting to emergency departments (ED) have SBI. The most common types of bacterial infection in this age group are UTIs, and the predominant bacterial pathogen is *Escherichia coli*. Group B *Streptococcus* is another frequent cause of SBI. Conversely, only a small percentage of neonates are infected with *Streptococcus pneumonia*. *Listeria monocytogenes*, once thought to be a significant pathogen in this population, is rarely found in febrile neonates. Neonates are also at higher risk for significant sequelae from common viral infections (e.g. herpes simplex virus meningitis).

The epidemiologic landscape in older infants and toddlers has changed dramatically since the introduction of pneumococcal conjugate vaccines (PCVs). As with infants, the most commonly identified bacterial infections in these older children are urinary tract infections, which are most commonly caused by *E. coli*.

Streptococcus pneumoniae had been the dominant cause of serious invasive disease in young children. Bacteremia and pneumonia were most often due to pneumococcus. In 2000, a heptavalent pneumococcal conjugate vaccine (PCV7) was introduced, which provided protection against the seven most common pneuomococcal serotypes, leading to a significant reduction in invasive pneumococcal disease. A new pneumococcal conjugate vaccine covering 13 serotypes (PCV13) was licensed in 2010, adding coverage for six additional serotypes. Early epidemiologic data demonstrates further declines in the rates of invasive pneumococcal disease with PCV13 vacination. While the full vaccination regimen is a four-dose series (given at 2, 4, 6, and 12–15 months of age), significant protection is conferred with two doses of this vaccine.

E. coli bacteremia is now more common than pneumococcal bacteremia in children younger than 12 months and is almost always associated with a concomitant UTI. *Salmonella* causes 1 to 7% of bacteremia in children in this age group, and the relative contribution of *Salmonella* as a cause of bacteremia is believed to be increasing as pneumococcal disease becomes less common. Although the majority of patients with *Salmonella* bacteremia have gastroenteritis, 5% had occult bacteremia. Meningococcal infections are infrequent, with an incidence rate of 2.7 per 100,000 infants, but are associated with high rates of morbidity and mortality. Usually, these patients appear ill, though 12 to 16% of patients with meningococcal disease have unsuspected infection.

Clinical Features

While there are fluctuations in the normal body temperature, the most commonly accepted definition of fever is a temperature of 38.0 °C (100.4 °F). Rectal thermometry is the current reference standard for outpatient temperature measurement because this method most accurately reflects core body temperature. Subjective determination of fever by caretakers at home is a moderately accurate predictor of true fever, and a patient with a fever measured rectally at home should undergo the same evaluation as if this measurement were obtained in the acute care setting.

The characteristics of a patient's fever have marginal utility in predicting serious bacterial infection. Hyperpyrexia (temperature ≥40 °C) may be associated with increased rates of serious bacterial infection, especially in young children. However, the relationship between height of fever and bacterial infection in older infants and toddlers is less clear. The duration of fever does not predict whether a child has occult bacteremia, and response to antipyretic medications does not distinguish between bacterial and viral causes of fever. While bundling a young child may increase the skin temperature, this does not increase the core temperature. Teething does not cause fever.

An assessment of the child's overall appearance is important. If a febrile child is irritable, lethargic, or poorly interactive, a comprehensive evaluation, followed by antibiotic treatment and hospitalization are indicated, regardless of age or risk factors. The physical examination may reveal a focal infection, and decrease the need for additional testing. Febrile patients with clinically recognizable viral conditions (e.g. croup, varicella, stomatitis) or viral infections confirmed by laboratory testing have lower rates of bacteremia than patients with no obvious source of infection. However, while the physical examination can be informative, neonates and young infants may have serious bacterial infections that are not readily identifiable on physical exam.

Differential Diagnosis

The complete list of differential diagnoses in the febrile child is extremely long. Fever is most commonly caused by infections. Focal bacterial infections include those of the ears, eyes, sinuses, pharynx, and surrounding tissues; the brain and meninges; the cardiac, pulmonary, gastrointestinal, and urogenital systems; and the musculoskeletal, dermatological, and lymphatic systems. Children may also have bacteremia. Less commonly, patients can have parasitic or fungal infections. Non-infectious causes of fever in a child must also be considered and include autoimmune disease such as juvenile idiopathic arthritis, systemic lupus erythematosus, serum sickness, and inflammatory bowel disease; Kawasaki disease; malignancies; neurologic lesions and seizures; and thyroid dysfunction. Exogenous etiologies of fever include vaccine reactions, environmental heat exposure, and toxic ingestions.

Laboratory and Radiographic Findings

Ancillary studies are utilized to supplement information gathered from the history and physical examination. Because the history and physical examination tends to be less reliable in younger children, laboratory and radiographic studies are more frequently obtained in this group of patients when compared with older children.

In febrile neonates, a comprehensive evaluation for sepsis is indicated, including blood cultures, urinalysis and urine culture, and cerebrospinal fluid (CSF) analysis and culture (see Chapter 50). A peripheral white blood cell count (WBC) is often ordered, but this is neither sensitive nor specific for bacterial infection. Although various options for rapid testing for UTIs exist (e.g. urine dipstick, standard urinalysis, enhanced urinalysis), no rapid test detects all cases of UTI, and urine cultures must be sent in all of these patients. Urine should be collected by bladder catheterization or, if necessary, suprapubic aspiration, because bag urine specimens are associated with unacceptably high rates of contamination. Chest X-rays are indicated in the presence of respiratory symptoms, and stool analyses are indicated in the presence of diarrhea. The presence of signs suggestive of viral illness does not negate the need for a full diagnostic evaluation. The indications for herpes simplex virus (HSV) testing in neonates are controversial, but HSV testing should be considered in any ill-appearing neonate or neonates with risk factors or exam findings suggestive of HSV, such as primary maternal HSV infection at time of delivery; prolonged rupture of membranes at delivery; the use of fetal scalp electrodes; skin, eye, or mouth lesions; and seizures.

The approach to febrile young infants between the ages of 1 and 2 months is more controversial. Traditional approaches to the febrile young infant have advocated a full sepsis evaluation, consisting of a complete blood count, blood culture, urinalysis, urine culture, and CSF analysis in these children (e.g. "Philadelphia Criteria," "Boston Criteria"). Common fever management guidelines incorporate the peripheral WBC, which is usually considered abnormal if the count is above 15,000/mm^3 or below 5,000/mm^3 or if the band-to-neutrophil ratio is above 0.2. If any of these tests are abnormal, patients receive broad-spectrum antibiotic treatment and are admitted.

The need for lumbar puncture (LP) in these febrile young infants is controversial. In one study, 50% of pediatric EDs with clinical practice guidelines for the evaluation of febrile infants aged 28 to 56 days recommended selective CSF testing in this age group. Typically, an abnormal peripheral WBC is used to identify a patient requiring LP.

The urine is considered abnormal if the urine dipstick is positive for nitrite or leukocyte esterase, if there are five or more WBCs per high-power field (HPF) on microscopy, or if there are organisms seen on gram stain of unspun urine. Additional symptom-directed testing in this 1- to 3-month-old group should include fecal leukocytes and stool cultures for diarrhea, and chest X-rays for signs of pulmonary disease.

For older children, the approach to diagnostic testing can be more selective. The widespread use of PCV has lowered the rates of bacteremia significantly. The incidence of true positive blood cultures in children who present to the emergency department is less than 1%, with the rate of contaminated blood cultures exceeding that of true positives. Surrogate tests for predicting bacteremia are inaccurate. In particular, there is poor correlation between the peripheral WBC count and bacteremia in patients with pneumococcal, E. coli, and meningococcal bacteremia. Although the full PCV series requires four doses, significant protection is provided by a minimum of two doses, and so routine blood testing is generally unwarranted in children who have received at least two PCV vaccinations.

UTIs are common sources of fever in young children. Risk factors for UTI include young age, uncircumcised status, female sex (girls are at higher risk for UTIs compared to circumcised boys in all age categories), and non-black race. Urine testing is generally indicated in girls and uncircumcised boys younger than 2 years with at least one risk factor for UTI (history of UTI, temperature >39 °C, fever without other apparent source, ill appearance, suprapubic tenderness, fever lasting for more than 24 hours, or non-black race). Circumcised boys younger than 2 years without suprapubic tenderness and with no more than three risk factors for UTI (temperature ≥39 °C, fever without other apparent source, fever lasting longer than 24 hours, or non-black race) have a probability of UTI of ≤2%.

Rapid urine tests have very good sensitivity for detecting UTIs. The enhanced urinalysis (≥10 WBC/HPF or bacteria on Gram stained, uncentrifuged urine) or a standard urinalysis (combination of ≥10 WBC/HPF and bacteriuria) are good screening tests. A urine dipstick test which is positive for either leukocyte esterase or nitrites has a sensitivity of 88%. However, because no rapid screening test detects all UTIs, urine cultures should be ordered in all patients in whom a urinalysis is sent.

The diagnosis of pneumonia in young children can be difficult. Physician assessment of pneumonia based on history and physical exam findings is only moderately correlated with the radiographic diagnosis of pneumonia. The role of pulse oximetry in detecting pneumonia is unclear. A chest X-ray should be obtained in febrile children if there are physical examination findings suggestive of pneumonia, such as hypoxemia, significant respiratory distress, or an abnormal lung examination. Unfortunately, while chest X-ray is often considered the gold standard for diagnosing pneumonia, there is considerable variability in the interpretation of X-rays among pediatric radiologists and radiographic findings cannot be used to reliably distinguish between bacterial and non-bacterial causes of pneumonia.

Febrile infants with viral infections have lower rates of concomitant bacterial infections. Most studies of rapid viral testing include testing for respiratory syncytial virus (RSV) or influenza. Febrile infants have significantly lower rates of bacterial infections if they have positive RSV or influenza tests. Most concomitant bacterial infections are urinary tract infections. Only limited data exists for febrile neonates, but these

studies have found no difference in SBI rates in neonates who were virus test positive compared with those who were virus test negative.

Treatment and Prophylaxis

Because of the high rate of serious bacterial infections in neonates, all febrile neonates should receive broad-spectrum antibiotics. Typically, these patients are treated with a third-generation cephalosporin, commonly cefotaxime (ceftriaxone is not recommended for neonates with jaundice because of the concern for inducing unconjugated hyperbilirubinemia). Although ampicillin has traditionally been given to treat infections with Listeria monocytogenes, the incidence of Listeria infection in neonates is extremely low. Indications for empiric treatment with acyclovir are controversial; while some clinicians treat all febrile neonates ≤21 days of age, others reserve the use of acyclovir for those patients at high risk of HSV infection (see above).

For 1- to 2-month-old infants who have abnormal tests or who look ill, antibiotic therapy and hospitalization is warranted. Empiric ceftriaxone is commonly used for this age group. Additional antibiotics should be considered in select circumstances. Patients with findings suspicious for meningitis should receive vancomycin and higher doses of ceftriaxone. Although some studies suggest that patients in this age group with UTIs may be treated on an outpatient basis, there are no large prospective studies that demonstrate the safety of this approach.

The use of ceftriaxone prior to discharge for full-term, well-appearing 1- to 2-month-old infants with no laboratory or CSF abnormalities is acceptable, but so is the practice of withholding antibiotics in these low-risk patients. Patients who do not undergo lumbar puncture in the ED, however, should not receive antibiotics, as this will confound the evaluation for meningitis if the patient is still febrile on follow-up examination. Close follow-up must be ensured prior to discharge for all patients.

For children 3 months of age and older, antibiotics are generally reserved for treatment of clinically apparent or documented infections. UTIs are the most common serious bacterial infections. The empiric regimen should be tailored to local antibiotic susceptibility data, but reasonable choices include cefixime or cephalexin for 7 to 14 days.

Although most pneumonia in children is viral, the etiology is difficult to determine based on laboratory and radiographic studies. Therefore, patients with infiltrates on chest radiographs should be treated with antibiotics, usually amoxicillin. Treatment duration is typically 7 to 10 days, though there is limited data on optimal duration. Recommendations for empiric pneumonia treatment may change with declining rates of pneumococcal pneumonia.

Complications and Admission Criteria

All febrile neonates, regardless of test results, should be hospitalized. Febrile young infants between 1 and 2 months of age who have abnormal laboratory studies should be hospitalized

Table 51.1 Antibiotic Treatment

	Therapy Recommendations
Empiric antibiotic therapy	Neonates*: Ampicillin 50 mg/kg/dose IV every 8–12 hours *plus* Cefotaxime 50 mg/kg/dose IV every 8–12 hours Acyclovir 20 mg/kg/dose IV every 8–12 hours Young infants (if given): Ceftriaxone 50 mg/kg/dose IV/IM daily Older infants: Empiric antibiotic therapy generally not indicated
Pneumonia	Amoxicillin: 90 mg/kg/day PO divided into three daily doses for 7–10 days
Urinary tract infection (antibiotic choice should be tailored to local epidemiology)	Cefixime: 8 mg/kg/day divided every 12–24 hours for 7–14 days *or* Cephalexin: 50–100 mg/kg/day PO divided into four doses for 7–14 days
Meningitis*	Cefotaxime (neonates*) 100–200 mg/kg/day IV divided every 6–12 hours (use smaller doses and longer intervals for small neonates) *or* Ceftriaxone[†] 50 mg/kg/dose IV every 12 hours *plus* Vancomycin: 15 mg/kg/dose IV every 6 hours Acyclovir: 10–15 mg/kg/dose IV every 8 hours (if HSV encephalitis suspected)

* Neonatal dosing and frequency must be adjusted for weight, postnatal age, and gestational age; consult institutional guidelines for specific dosing recommendations.

[†] Ceftriaxone generally not recommended in neonates.

HSV – herpes simplex virus; PO – by mouth.

as well. Conversely, most children older than 2 months of age can be discharged with close outpatient follow-up.

Patients who return with positive blood cultures should be re-examined, and if they are ill-appearing, should undergo repeat blood cultures, LP, intravenous antibiotics, and hospital admission. Patients with pneumococcal bacteremia who are afebrile on repeat evaluation and who appear well can be followed on an outpatient basis after repeat blood cultures and antibiotics. The treatment and disposition for well-appearing children with *Salmonella* bacteremia is less clear, but patients with meningococcal bacteremia should be hospitalized for parenteral antibiotics pending results of repeat blood cultures.

Infection Control

Universal precautions should be maintained. No isolation is required.

Pearls and Pitfalls

1. All febrile neonates require a full sepsis evaluation, parenteral antibiotics, and hospital admission.
2. Febrile young infants (1–2 months of age) need blood and urine testing. CSF testing should be strongly considered. If results of these tests are normal, the child looks well, and close follow-up can be ensured, these children may be discharged. Parenteral antibiotics are optional prior to discharge. For patients with abnormal peripheral white blood cell counts or urinary tract infections, antibiotic treatment and hospitalization is generally indicated.

3. Older children (>2–24 months) who otherwise look well require only selective testing. Generally, circumcised boys younger than 6 months of age, uncircumcised boys younger than 12 months old and girls younger than 2 years old who have fever without source require urinalysis and urine cultures.
4. Children who have received at least two pneumococcal conjugate vaccine (PCV) doses generally do not require blood testing.

References

American Academy of Pediatrics Subcommittee on Urinary Tract Infection. Urinary tract infection: clinical practice guideline for the diagnosis and management of the initial UTI in febrile infants and children 2 to 24 months. *Pediatrics* 2011; 128(3): 595–610.

Aronson, P. L., Thurm, C., Williams, D. J., *et al.* Association of clinical practice guidelines with emergency department management of febrile infants </=56 days of age. *J. Hosp. Med.* 2015; 10(6): 358–65.

Baker, M. D., Avner, J. R., and Bell, L. M. Failure of infant observation scales in detecting serious illness in febrile, 4- to 8-week-old infants. *Pediatrics* 1990; 85(6): 1040–3.

Baker, M. D., Bell, L. M., Avner, J. R. The efficacy of routine outpatient management without antibiotics of fever in selected infants. *Pediatrics* 1999; 103(3): 627–31.

Biondi, E., Evans, R., Mischler, M., *et al.* Epidemiology of bacteremia in febrile infants in the United States. *Pediatrics* 2013; 132(6): 990–6.

Bonsu, B. K. and Harper, M. B. Utility of the peripheral blood white blood cell count for identifying sick young infants who need lumbar puncture. *Ann. Emerg. Med.* 2003; 41(2): 206–14.

Bradley, J. S., Byington, C. L., Shah, S. S., *et al.* The management of community-acquired pneumonia in infants and children older than 3 months of age: clinical practice guidelines by the Pediatric Infectious Diseases Society and the Infectious Diseases Society of America. *Clin. Infect. Dis.* 2011; 53(7): e25–76.

Byington, C. L., Enriquez, F. R., Hoff, C., *et al.* Serious bacterial infections in febrile infants 1 to 90 days old with and without viral infections. *Pediatrics* 2004; 113(6): 1662–6.

Caviness, A. C., Demmler, G. J., Swint, J. M., and Cantor, S. B. Cost-effectiveness analysis of herpes simplex virus testing and treatment strategies in febrile neonates. *Arch. Pediatr. Adolesc. Med.* 2008; 162(7): 665–74.

Greenhow, T. L., Hung, Y. Y., and Herz, A. M. Changing epidemiology of bacteremia in infants aged 1 week to 3 months. *Pediatrics* 2012; 129(3): e590–6.

Greenhow, T. L., Hung, Y. Y., Herz, A. M., *et al.* The changing epidemiology of serious bacterial infections in young infants. *Pediatr. Infect. Dis. J.* 2014; 33(6): 595–9.

Hassoun, A., Stankovic, C., Rogers, A., *et al.* Listeria and enterococcal infections in neonates 28 days of age and younger: is empiric parenteral ampicillin still indicated? *Pediatr. Emerg. Care* 2014; 30(4): 240–3.

Hsiao, A. L., Chen, L., and Baker, M. D. Incidence and predictors of serious bacterial infections among 57- to 180-day-old infants. *Pediatrics* 2006; 117(5): 1695–701.

Kuppermann, N., Malley, R., Inkelis, S. H., and Fleisher, G. R. Clinical and hematologic features do not reliably identify children with unsuspected meningococcal disease. *Pediatrics* 1999; 103(2): E20.

Levine, D. A., Platt, S. L., Dayan, P. S., *et al.* Risk of serious bacterial infection in young febrile infants with respiratory syncytial virus infections. *Pediatrics* 2004; 113(6): 1728–34.

Long, S. S., Pool, T. E., Vodzak, J., *et al.* Herpes simplex virus infection in young infants during 2 decades of empiric acyclovir therapy. *Pediatr. Infect. Dis. J.* 2011; 30(7): 556–61.

MacNeil, J. R., Bennett, N., Farley, M. M., *et al.* Epidemiology of infant meningococcal disease in the United States, 2006–2012. *Pediatrics* 2015; 135(2): e305–11.

Shaikh, N., Morone, N. E., Lopez, J., *et al.* Does this child have a urinary tract infection? *JAMA* 2007; 298(24): 2895–904.

Tsai, M. H., Huang, Y. C., Chiu, C. H., *et al.* Nontyphoidal Salmonella bacteremia in previously healthy children: analysis of 199 episodes. *Pediatr. Infect. Dis. J.* 2007; 26(10): 909–13.

Additional Readings

Alpern, E. and Henretig, F. Fever in G. Fleisher, S. Ludwig, R. G. Bachur, *et al.* (eds.), *Textbook of Pediatric Emergency Medicine*, 6th edn. (Philadelphia, PA: Lippincott Williams & Wilkins, 2010), pp. 265–75.

Baker, M. D., Bell, L. M., and Avner, J. R. Outpatient management without antibiotics of fever in selected infants. *N. Engl. J. Med.* 1993; 329(20): 1437–41.

Baskin, M. N., O'Rourke, E. J., and Fleisher, G. R. Outpatient treatment of febrile infants 28 to 89 days of age with intramuscular administration of ceftriaxone. *J. Pediatr.* 1992; 120(1): 22–7.

Dagan, R., Powell, K. R., Hall, C. B., and Menegus, M. A. Identification of infants unlikely to have serious bacterial infection although hospitalized for suspected sepsis. *J. Pediatr.* 1985; 107(6): 855–60.

Chapter 52

Fever and Rash in the Pediatric Population

Catherine Marco, Janel Kittredge-Sterling, and Rachel L. Chin

Introduction

Fever and rash in the pediatric population is a common symptom complex. Many etiologies of fever and rash occurring in both adults and pediatrics are discussed in Chapter 14, Fever and Rash in Adults, including rickettsial infections, viral infections such as measles and rubella, and drug hypersensitivity reactions. Several specific etiologies specifically occurring in pediatric patients are discussed in this chapter, including non-specific viral exanthems, roseola infantum, erythema infectiosum, varicella zoster infection, meningococcal infection, staphylococcal scalded skin syndrome, and Kawasaki disease.

An appropriate history is helpful in establishing the correct diagnosis causing fever and rash. Important historical features should be sought (see Table 52.1).

The physical examination can also be essential for establishing the correct diagnosis. General appearance and vital signs should be recorded and addressed if unstable. The skin should be examined thoroughly, under adequate lighting. Information regarding the lesions should be documented.

Epidemiology

One study demonstrated that in the pediatric population, 72% of cases of fever and rash were caused by viruses, and 20% were caused by bacteria. Viral exanthems may be caused by enteroviruses, adenoviruses, echovirus, and numerous others. Infections with enteroviruses often peak in summer and fall months.

Non-Specific Viral Exanthems

Non-specific viral exanthems occur with increased frequency in the pediatric population. A variety of enteroviruses may cause a symptom complex including fever, malaise, gastrointestinal complaints, meningitis, and rash (see Table 52.2). The enterovirus exanthem typically is non-specific widespread maculopapular eruption, though petechiae, mimicking meningococcal infection, may be seen. Petechiae have been also been reported with coxsackievirus A9, echovirus 9, coxsackievirus A4, B2–5, and echovirus 3, 4, and 7 infections.

Roseola Infantum

Roseola infantum (also known as exanthema subitum or sixth disease) is caused by human herpes virus-6 and human herpes virus-7, and is typically spread by saliva (see Table 52.3). The incubation period is 1 to 2 weeks and most cases occur in spring and early fall. Children between 6 months and 3 years of age are most commonly affected.

Fever often precedes the exanthem. The febrile child usually appears well and is playful. Cervical lymphadenopathy, pharyngeal erythema with or without exudates, and otitis media may occur. The exanthem typically appears after fever resolution (hence the term "roseola subitum"). The rash typically begins on the trunk and spreads upward to the neck and proximal extremities. The exanthema is often pink and blanching, and may be macular, papular, or maculopapular (see Figure 52.1). Berliner's sign may be seen, with palpebral and periorbital edema, resulting in the appearance of "heavy eyelids."

Table 52.1 Focused History and Physical Exam in Pediatric Patients with Fever and Rash

History:
- duration of symptoms
- associated symptoms (e.g. fever, headache, gastrointestinal symptoms, pruritus)
- evolution of lesions
- distribution
- history of animal or arthropod bites
- exacerbating and relieving factors (e.g. environmental exposures, foods, medications)
- medical history, occupational history, sexual history, medications, illicit drug history, travel, and allergies

Examination:
Type of lesions, size, color, secondary findings (e.g. scale, excoriations), and distribution.
Primary lesions should be identified and may include the following:
- *Macules* are flat lesions defined by an area of changed color (e.g. blanchable erythema).
- *Papules* are raised, solid lesions <5 mm in diameter.
- *Plaques* are lesions >5 mm in diameter with a flat, plateau-like surface.
- *Nodules* are lesions >5 mm in diameter with a more rounded configuration.
- *Wheals* (urticaria, hives) are papules or plaques that are pale pink and may appear annular (ring-like) as they enlarge; classic (non-vasculitic) wheals are transient, lasting only 24–48 hours in any defined area.
- *Vesicles* (<5 mm) and *bullae* (>5 mm) are circumscribed, elevated lesions containing fluid.
- *Pustules* are raised lesions containing purulent exudates. Vesicular processes such as varicella or herpes simplex may evolve to pustules.
- *Non-palpable purpura* is a flat lesion that is due to bleeding into the skin. If <3 mm in diameter the purpuric lesions are termed *petechiae*. If >3 mm, they are termed *ecchymoses*. *Palpable purpura* is a raised lesion that is due to inflammation of the vessel wall (vasculitis) with subsequent hemorrhage.
- An *ulcer* is a defect in the skin extending at least into the upper layer of the dermis.
- *Eschar* is a necrotic lesion covered with a black crust.
Secondary lesions may include:
- scale
- crust
- fissure
- erosions
- ulcer
- scar
- excoriation
- infection
- pigment changes
- lichenification
Color may be:
- normal
- erythematous
- violaceous
- hyperpigmented
- hypopigmented
Patterns of lesions should be established as:
- single
- grouped
- scattered
- linear
- annular
- symmetric
- dermatomal
- central or peripheral
- along Blaschko's lines (specific linear skin patterns thought to be of embryonic origin, usually forming a "V" shape over the spine and "S" shapes over the chest, stomach, and sides)

The diagnosis is made clinically. Therapy is supportive and should include antipyretics and oral hydration.

Erythema Infectiosum

Erythema infectiosum was first recognized in 1889 and was termed *fifth disease* because of its position among the other common childhood exanthems in the chronologic order in which they were first recognized (following measles, scarlet fever, rubella, and Dukes' disease). Caused by the virus parvovirus B19, erythema infectiosum is common in childhood, with peak rates between the ages of 5 and 14 years. Transmission of the virus occurs via respiratory droplets.

Table 52.2 Clinical Features: Non-Specific Viral Exanthems

Organisms	Enterovirus Coxsackievirus A9 Echovirus 9 Coxsackievirus A4, B2–5 Echovirus 3, 4, and 7 Adenovirus, RSV Parainfluenza 1, 2, and 3 Influenza A, B Cytomegalovirus Epstein–Barr Parvovirus B19
Signs and symptoms	• Fever • Non-specific maculopapular eruption • Petechiae • Nausea, vomiting, diarrhea • Malaise
Laboratory findings	• No laboratory testing necessary • Lymphocytosis may be present
Treatment	• Hydration (oral or intravenous) • Antipyretic agents • Antipruritic agents • Instructions for caregivers, including warning signs of severe infection

RSV – respiratory syncytial virus.

Table 52.3 Clinical Features: Roseola Infantum

Organisms	Human herpes virus-6 Human herpes virus-7
Incubation period	1–2 weeks
Signs and symptoms	• Febrile child usually appears well and is playful. • Cervical lymphadenopathy, pharyngeal erythema with or without exudates, and otitis media may occur. • The exanthem appears after fever resolution. • The rash typically begins on the trunk and spreads upward to the neck and proximal extremities. • The exanthema is often pink and may be macular, papular, or maculopapular. • Palpebral and periorbital edema (Berliner's sign) is common.
Laboratory findings	• Not recommended. Clinical diagnosis.
Treatment	Therapy is supportive and should include antipyretics and oral hydration.

Many cases (up to 20%) are asymptomatic. Following an incubation period of 4 to 14 days, a prodromal phase may include low-grade fever, headache, pharyngitis, myalgias, nausea, diarrhea, and joint pain (see Table 52.4). Skin findings include erythema of cheeks, the result of coalescent erythematous papules ("slapped cheek" appearance; see Figure 52.2). Approximately 2 days after the onset of the facial erythema, the typical lacy reticular extremity rash appears and usually fades in 6 to 14 days. An enanthema may also be seen, with erythema of the tongue and pharynx, and macules on the buccal

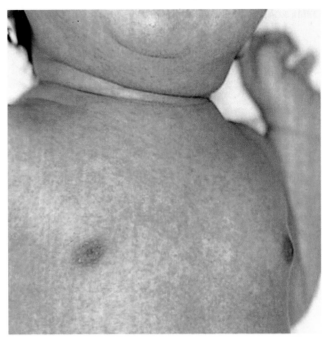

Figure 52.1 Roseola.
Photograph source: www.derm101.com, with permission.

mucosa and palate. Arthralgias or arthritis may be seen in 10% of affected children, typically involving large joints. Arthritis may last up to 3 weeks.

Significant complications of parvovirus B19 infection may occur in the immunocompromised, the fetus, and patients with hemoglobinopathies. Among immunocompromised patients, including human immunodeficiency virus (HIV) infection, congenital immunodeficiencies, acute leukemia, organ transplants, and lupus erythematosus, or in infants younger than 1 year old, parvovirus B19 may cause a serious prolonged chronic anemia resulting from persistent lysis of red-blood-cell (RBC) precursors. Administration of intravenous immune globulin (IVIG), which contains pooled, neutralizing anti-B19 antibody, has been used successfully in immunodeficient patients.

If infected during pregnancy, parvovirus B19 infection may result in vertical transmission to the fetus, causing infection of erythroid precursors and extensive hemolysis, leading to severe anemia, tissue hypoxia, high-output heart failure, and generalized edema (hydrops fetalis). Most reported fetal losses secondary to parvovirus B19 have occurred in the first trimester of pregnancy (see Chapter 58, Fever in Pregnancy).

Among patients with chronic hemolytic anemias, transient aplastic crisis manifested by anemia, reticulocytopenia, and RBC aplasia may result. Aplastic crisis may also be seen in patients with hereditary spherocytosis, sickle-cell disease, glucose-6-phosphate dehydrogenase (G6PD) deficiency, pyruvate-kinase deficiency, iron deficiency, and the thalassemias.

Management of patients with erythema infectiosum includes supportive care with antipyretics, oral hydration, and antipruritic agents, if needed. There are no published timing

Table 52.4 Clinical Features: Erythema Infectiosum

Organism	Parvovirus B19
Incubation period	Defined by days prior to appearance of rash; ranges from 4 to 15 days.
Signs and symptoms	**Skin:** erythema infectiosum (fifth disease): facial erythema ("slapped cheek"), circumoral pallor (18 days after infection); reticular rash (trunk and limbs). **Bone marrow:** transient aplasia (patients with thalassemia, hemolytic anemia); chronic pure red cell aplasia (immunosuppressed, especially HIV, transplant, sickle cell); hemophagocytic syndrome (immunocompromised). **Fetus:** Hydrops fetalis (pregnant with acute infection: risk ~1.6%; highest between 11 and 23 weeks gestation); anemia; thrombocytopenia. **Other:** CNS (encephalopathy); liver (hepatitis); heart (myocarditis).
Laboratory findings	Laboratory testing not indicated in uncomplicated cases. IgM (85%+ with erythema infectiosum or aplastic crisis; turns negative within 3 months); IgG (2 weeks post-infection; lifelong); PCR most sensitive (*not* diagnostic alone). Giant pronormoblasts blood/BM suggests diagnosis.
Treatment	In uncomplicated cases: supportive care (hydration, antipyretics). NSAIDs for arthropathy; blood products for transient aplasia; weekly US for infected pregnant women; cordicentesis and intrauterine transfusions for hydrops fetalis. **Immunosuppressed treatment regimen:** Chronic pure red cell aplasia: Immune globulin 0.4 g/kg/day IV for 5 days or 1 g/kg/day for 2–3 days; may need to repeat monthly

CNS – central nervous system; NSAID – non-steroidal anti-inflammatory drug; PCR – polymerase chain reaction; US – ultrasound.

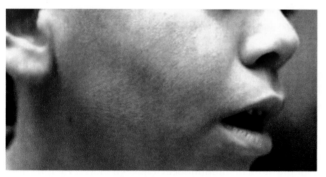

Figure 52.2 Erythema infectiosum.

Photograph source: Centers for Disease Control Public Health Image Library, http://phil.cdc.gov/Phil/publicdomain.asp.

recommendations for returning to school or day care. Typically, the onset of the facial rash corresponds with a decrease in contagion.

Additional therapies may be indicated for complicated cases. Patients with chronic hemolytic anemias who develop transient aplastic crisis (pallor, weakness, and lethargy) may require blood transfusion. Pregnant women with signs or symptoms suggestive of B19 infection or known recent exposure to infected contacts should have serum B19 IgM and IgG titers drawn. If maternal infection is identified, serial fetal ultrasounds should be performed to evaluate for hydrops fetalis.

Varicella Zoster

Varicella zoster (chickenpox) is a clinical disease caused by the varicella-zoster virus (VZV), a double-stranded DNA virus and a member of the Herpesviridae family. VZV is the agent that causes both varicella (chickenpox) and herpes zoster (shingles). Varicella infections have been rare in the United States since the widespread administration of the varicella vaccine beginning in 1995. Varicella infections are more prevalent in temperate climates and are common during March, April, and

May. Although children rarely develop zoster, it may be seen in children who are immunosuppressed, such as those with HIV infection, immunosuppressive drugs, or cancer. Varicella is contagious, with an estimated 80 to 90% transmission rate among household contacts. Transmission occurs by way of direct contact with infected vesicular fluid and inoculation by airborne transmission.

Acute varicella among young, healthy, non-pregnant patients typically follows a benign, self-limiting disease course. Prior to the appearance of the rash, a 1- to 2-day prodrome may occur, with headache, malaise, and fever (see Table 52.5). Children may present with the rash and fever simultaneously. The typical exanthem of varicella begins on the head, spreads centripetally, extending to the extremities. The rash typically occurs in three stages, beginning with macules, evolving to papules, and then to vesicles on an erythematous base, commonly described as "dewdrop on a rose petal" (see Figure 52.3). After the vesicles have formed, they may develop to pustules that later crust and scab. New crops of vesicles may form during the ensuing days. Complications of varicella may include skin bacterial superinfection, neurologic complications, pneumonia, encephalitis, asymptomatic transient hepatitis, thrombocytopenia, ophthalmologic keratitis, anterior uveitis, and death.

After the resolution of primary varicella, the latent virus lies dormant in ganglia, most commonly the thoracic and trigeminal ganglia. The reactivation of VZV appears in one or more ganglia as herpes zoster (shingles). A prodrome of burning, pain, itching, or tingling may precede the skin lesions. The vesicles are distributed along a dermatome and may persist for up to 4 weeks. Significant morbidity may occur in elderly patients, including post-herpetic neuralgia, with persistent pain and dysesthesia. The disease course may be more severe in immunocompromised patients, with involvement of multiple nerve roots or, rarely, disseminated visceral disease. Ocular manifestations of VZV may include herpes zoster ophthalmicus, affecting the areas distributed by the ophthalmic division of

Table 52.5 Clinical Features: Varicella Zoster

Organism	Varicella zoster virus
Incubation period	1–2 weeks
Signs and symptoms	• Prodrome: fever, malaise • 1–2 days later: rash • Three phases: macules, papules, vesicles • Lesions crust and scab • Lesions appear in crops; often all three phases are seen simultaneously in the same patient
Laboratory findings	Not indicated. Clinical diagnosis.
Treatment	Therapy is supportive and should include antipyretics, antipruritics, and oral hydration.

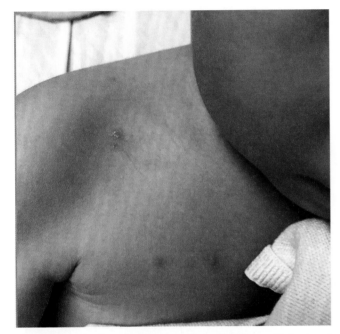

Figure 52.3 Varicella zoster infection. An immunized 3-year-old, developed scattered lesions after exposure to chicken pox in daycare. The picture shows varied stages of lesions with classic vesicular forms as well as crusted forms and early vesicles.
Photo Courtesy of Israel Green-Hopkins MD.

the trigeminal nerve. Herpes zoster virus (HZV) ophthalmicus may result in chronic ocular inflammation, visual loss, tissue scarring, and debilitating pain. Ocular manifestations should be considered if Hutchinson's sign is present, with skin involvement of the tip of the nose (see Chapter 41, Conjunctival and Corneal Infections). Herpes zoster oticus may present with devastating otalgia, associated with vesicular involvement of the external ear canal and pinna. Ramsey Hunt syndrome occurs when herpes zoster oticus produces a facial paralysis (VII) (see Chapter 15, Otitis Externa). The onset of pain in and around the ear, mouth, and face may precede the rash for hours to days.

The varicella vaccine, a live attenuated vaccine, was approved in 1995 for use in the United States. The administration of this vaccine has reduced the incidence of varicella, as well as the incidence of varicella-related hospitalizations. The efficacy of the vaccine is estimated to be 70 to 90%. The vaccine is administered between 12 and 15 months of age. Children receive a booster shot at 4 to 6 years of age. Children older than 6 but younger than 13 years who have not received the vaccine, or had chickenpox, can get the vaccine with the two doses given at least 3 months apart.

Treatment of varicella is generally supportive and should include antipruritics, skin hygiene, antipyretics, and adequate oral hydration. The use of antiviral agents (acyclovir, famciclovir, valacyclovir) has not been proven to decrease the complication rate in healthy children. Therefore, the use of these agents is typically reserved for newborns, preterm infants, children older than 13 years of age, and adults. If antiviral therapy is used, it should be initiated within 24 to 48 hours from the onset of the rash. Intravenous acyclovir is recommended for the immunocompromised patient to reduce the incidence of dissemination and shorten the disease course. Antiviral agents should be administered for all patients with herpes zoster, within 3 days of the appearance of the skin lesions. Steroids may reduce the incidence of post-herpetic neuralgia, if administered within 72 hours of the appearance of lesions.

Meningococcal Infection

Meningococcal infection is caused by the organism *Neisseria meningitidis*. Meningococcal disease typically manifests as three syndromes: meningitis (50.2%), bacteremia (37.5%), or bacteremic pneumonia (9.2%). Infection is typically transmitted by respiratory tract secretions.

Meningococcal disease typically affects healthy children and adolescents, and may result in significant morbidity and mortality. Infection is fatal in approximately 10% of cases. Approximately 800 to 1,200 cases are reported annually in the United States.

Immunization against meningococcal infection is recommended for groups at increased risk for infection, including adolescents and persons at risk for exposure.

Four vaccines are licensed in the United States and provide protection against four (A, C, W, and Y) and two (C and Y) serogroups. Vaccines that protect against serogroup B meningococcal disease (MenB) have recently been licensed by the Food and Drug Administration (FDA) for use in the United States and approved for use in persons aged 10 to 25 years: MenB-FHbp (Trumenba, Wyeth Pharmaceuticals, Inc.) and MenB-4C (Bexsero, Novartis Vaccines). MenB vaccine should either be administered as a three-dose series of MenB-FHbp or a two-dose series of MenB-4C. The two MenB vaccines are not interchangeable; the same vaccine product must be used for all doses. Seven outbreaks of serogroup B meningococcal disease have occurred on college campuses since 2009 (range = 2 to 13 cases), resulting in 41 cases and 3 deaths.

Early symptoms typically occur 3 to 7 days after exposure and may include fever, malaise, arthralgias, nausea, and vomiting. 10% of cases may present with Waterhouse-Friderichsen syndrome, which is shock with intracutaneous hemorrhage. Cutaneous findings of macules, papules, vesicles, or petechiae and purpura may be present.

Table 52.6 Clinical Features: Staphylococcal Scalded Skin Syndrome

Organisms	*Staphylococcus aureus*
Incubation period	Unknown
Signs and symptoms	• Fever: >38.9°C; hypotension: SBP <90 in adults or orthostatic hypotension • Rash: diffuse macular erythroderma; desquamation: palms and soles usually involved, 1–2 weeks after onset of illness • Perioral hyperemia and conjunctivitis • Intraoral mucous membranes are spared
Laboratory findings	• None indicated • Blood cultures and skin biopsy may be performed in cases of uncertain diagnosis
Treatment*	Nafcillin 25 mg/kg/dose IV every 6–8 hours (neonates), or 25–50 mg/kg/dose IV every 6 hours for older children *followed by* Dicloxacillin 12.5 mg/kg/dose PO QID **Alternative treatment:** Clindamycin 10 mg/kg/dose IV every 8 hours *plus* Vancomycin 15 mg/kg/dose IV every 6 hours for MRSA Some favor linezolid instead of vancomycin if MRSA is a concern, mainly because of protein synthesis inhibition Avoid corticosteroids as these can worsen immune function Supportive case or ICU monitoring

* Pediatric dosing provided. Do not exceed maximum adult doses.

IV – intravenous; SBP – systolic blood pressure.

The diagnosis should be suspected clinically in the ED setting and treated promptly. Confirmatory tests may include blood cultures, CSF cultures, or skin scrapings.

Rapid administration of antibiotics is essential to improve outcomes. Empiric therapy should be instituted to cover bacterial etiologies of meningitis and may include a third generation cephalosporin, such as ceftriaxone or cefotaxime, plus vancomycin. Alternative antibiotics may include penicillin G, chloramphenicol, fluoroquinolones, or aztreonam. Dexamethasone should also be considered for suspected or proven meningitis.

Staphylococcal Scalded-Skin Syndrome

The staphylococcal scalded-skin syndrome (SSSS; Ritter's disease) is a generalized form of bullous impetigo and is caused by the dissemination of *Staphylococcus aureus* exfoliative toxins. These toxins will cause disruption to layers of the epidermis resulting in fragile, tense bullae which oftentimes are no longer intact on presentation. In infants, this disease entity is termed "pemphigus neonatorum." SSSS is most common in patients under 2 years of age. Mortality is typically less than 5%.

Patients often have fever, irritability, and skin tenderness (see Table 52.6). Cutaneous findings include diffuse erythema, flaccid blisters, and superficial skin sloughing (see Figure 52.4). Nikolsky's sign (the superficial layers of skin slipping free from the lower layers with slight pressure) is positive. Affected infants often have conjunctivitis; mucous membranes are not involved, but may appear hyperemic.

The diagnosis is usually made clinically. It may be confirmed by a positive staphylococcal culture. SSSS may appear clinically very similar to toxic epidermal necrolysis, though toxic epidermal necrolysis (TEN) is more commonly seen in adults or older children as a drug reaction. A skin biopsy can be performed to differentiate, but is often not required as the diagnosis can be made clinically.

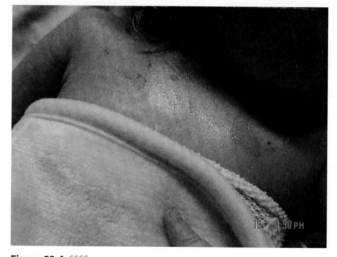

Figure 52.4 SSSS.
Photograph courtesy of David C. Brancati, DO.

Management should include an intravenous antistaphylococcal antibiotic, such as nafcillin or dicloxacillin. Alternatives may include clindamycin plus oxacillin, or vancomycin, if methicillin-resistant *S. aureus* (MRSA) is suspected and/or prevalent in the community. Supportive care should include hydration, skin care with the use of emollients to improve barrier function, and temperature regulation. Supportive care, wound care, and burn or intensive care unit (ICU) admission may be indicated.

Kawasaki Disease – Mucocutaneous Lymph Node Syndrome

Kawasaki disease (mucocutaneous lymph node syndrome) is an acute febrile vasculitis, specifically of small- and medium-sized

Table 52.7 Clinical Features: Kawasaki Disease

Acute stage (days 1–11)	• Sudden onset of fever above 38.5°C and lasts for 1 week or longer and does not respond to antipyretic treatment • An extremely irritable child • Red eyes (bilateral conjunctival injection) • Dry, red, and cracked lips with possible bleeding • Intensely red and spotty tongue, described as a strawberry tongue • Hands and feet that are red and swollen, so much so that child refuses to walk • Rashes that involve the trunk, arms, and legs, which usually appear within 5 days after onset of fever. The rashes may appear in several forms and can be itchy. Often prominent in the perineum and groin. • Enlarged lymph glands • Abnormal liver test • Heart complications in the first stage may include myocarditis and pericarditis
Subacute stage (days 11–21)	• Fever, rash, and enlarged lymph nodes have usually resolved by this stage. A persistent fever may result in a less favorable outcome because of a greater risk of heart complications. • Persistent irritability, poor appetite, and conjunctival injection (red eyes) • Peeling of skin of the fingertips and toes begins • Thrombocytosis (increased number of platelet particles in the blood) may develop, with the platelet count topping 1 million (normal range 150–400,000). This increases chance of blood clots. • Arthritis and arthralgia (muscle and joint aches) may occur • Heart problems (aneurysms or ballooning of blood vessels) may develop during this stage
Convalescent stage (days 21–60)	• Clinical signs begin to disappear and laboratory test results return to normal • Most significant clinical finding that persists through this stage is that coronary artery aneurysms (ballooning of blood vessels to and from the heart) continue to enlarge. This may lead to rupture of the blood vessels, heart attack, and death.
Late effects/chronic stage	• During the first year or two after the illness, coronary aneurysms heal and the amount of coronary artery dilation can become less (amount of healing depends on the amount of damage) • Vessel walls will never return to normal as thickening of these walls occurs during the healing process • Aneurysms formed during an episode of Kawasaki disease are of lifetime significance as these may be the cause of heart disease in adulthood

blood vessels throughout the body and, of particular concern, the coronary arteries.

Kawasaki disease is one of the most common vasculidities of childhood. It is seen in infants and young children. Of cases, 80% occur in children younger than 4 years of age; the peak age is between 1 and 2 years. The disease is very uncommon in children older than 14 years old or adults. It is more common in boys than girls. Although cases of Kawasaki disease have been reported in children of all ethnic origins, the highest incidence remains in children of Asian descent, especially Japanese. Annually, ~5,000 children are hospitalized for Kawasaki disease in the United States.

The disease typically occurs in winter and spring and is usually self-limiting, resolving spontaneously without treatment within 2 to 4 weeks. However, 15 to 20% of cases will have complications such as damage to coronary arteries, leading to myocardial infarction and heart failure.

Clinical features are characterized by three phases (see Table 52.7). The acute febrile period (phase I) is manifested by the abrupt onset of fever, >38.5 °C lasting approximately 12 days, typically poorly responsive to antipyretics. Symptoms of diarrhea, arthritis, and photophobia may be present. In the subacute phase (phase II), desquamation, thrombocytosis, arthritis, arthralgias, and carditis may be present. This phase may last 30 days. There is a high risk for sudden death during this phase of the illness if illness has gone untreated. During the convalescent phase (phase III), which occurs within 8 to 10 weeks after the onset of the illness, most signs of the illness have resolved; mortality drops significantly during this phase.

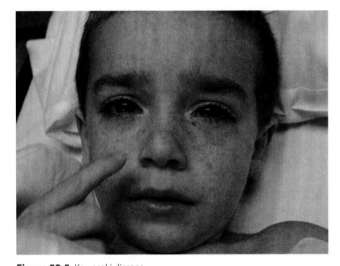

Figure 52.5 Kawasaki disease.
Photograph courtesy of David C. Brancati, DO.

During phase I, erythematous skin changes are first detected by perineal erythema and desquamation. Lesions and desquamation will then be noticed on the palms and soles and typically appear 1 to 3 days after the onset of the fever. Within 2 days, the blotchy, erythematous, macular lesions spread to the extremities and trunk. Non-exudative injected conjunctivae, seen in approximately 90% of patients, may be present for 1 to 3 weeks (see Figure 52.5). Diffuse oropharyngeal erythema with "strawberry" tongue is often present.

Table 52.8 Kawasaki Disease: Treatment

Treatment	**Acute phase:**
	Immune globulin 2 g/kg/dose IV × 1
	plus
	Aspirin 80–100 mg/kg/day PO divided every 6 hours until the patient has been afebrile for several days*
	Subacute and convalescent phases:
	Aspirin 1–5 mg/kg/dose PO once daily for as long as 6–8 weeks†

* Some clinicians recommend the use of high-dose aspirin therapy until day 14 of illness.

† Aspirin can be discontinued after 6 to 8 weeks if all echocardiograms show no evidence of coronary artery abnormalities. If coronary artery abnormalities are detected, low-dose aspirin therapy should be continued indefinitely.

The diagnosis is typically based on clinical findings. Liver function tests may be elevated. Leukocytosis, thrombocytosis, and an elevated CRP may be seen. The erythrocyte sedimentation rate (ESR) is elevated during phase II and returns to normal in phase III. Pyuria may be seen on urinalysis. Electrocardiography (ECG) may show PR and QT prolongation or acute ST/T wave changes.

Coronary aneurysms present in 25% of cases and may be diagnosed by echocardiography or coronary angiography. For epidemiologic surveillance, the CDC defines a case of KS as illness in a patient with fever of 5 or more days' duration (or fever until the date of administration of intravenous immunoglobulin if it is given before the fifth day of fever), and the presence of at least four of the following five clinical signs:

- rash
- cervical lymphadenopathy (at least 1.5 cm in diameter)
- bilateral conjunctival injection
- pral mucosal changes
- peripheral extremity changes

Patients whose illness does not meet the above KS case definition but who have fever and coronary artery abnormalities are classified as having atypical or incomplete KS.

Management of Kawasaki disease includes hospital admission, high dose IVIG (2 g/kg IV as a single dose) therapy, and aspirin therapy (80 to 100 mg/kg/day) (see Table 52.8). Treatment with IVIG within the first 10 days of illness reduces the prevalence of coronary artery aneurysms fivefold compared with children not treated with IVIG.

Steroids have not been shown to improve outcomes. Early cardiology evaluation is important to identify and treat possible coronary artery involvement.

Differential Diagnosis

The differential diagnosis of fever and rash in the pediatric population is broad. Some of the potential diagnoses that should be considered include:

- Bacterial and rickettsial infections:
  - meningococcal disease
  - SSSS
  - Rocky Mountain spotted fever
  - scarlet fever
  - toxic shock syndrome
- Viral infections:
  - varicella zoster infection
  - measles
  - rubella
  - non-specific viral exanthema
  - roseola
  - erythema infectiosum
  - pityriasis rosea
  - infectious mononucleosis
- Drug hypersensitivity reactions
- Systemic and connective tissue disorders:
  - erythema multiforme
  - toxic epidermal necrolysis
  - erythema nodosum
  - systemic lupus erythematosus
  - Kawasaki disease
  - juvenile rheumatoid arthritis
  - Schönlein–Henoch purpura
  - malignancies

Laboratory and Radiographic Findings

Many laboratory tests are discussed above with specific diagnoses. In general, patients with fever and rash should be evaluated using an adequate physical examination and, in selected cases, complete blood count, platelet count, serologic tests, skin biopsy, or cultures of blood or skin lesions.

Complications and Admission Criteria

Many pediatric patients with fever and rash can be safely discharged home, following appropriate physical and laboratory evaluation, if the patient is clinically stable, with normal vital signs; if the diagnosis is considered relatively benign and no specific inpatient therapy is indicated; and if there is adequate home care and follow-up arrangements have been made.

Certain patients should often be managed as inpatients, including patients with immunosuppression, systemic bacterial infections, sepsis, unstable vital signs, or those lacking appropriate home resources or medical follow-up.

Infection Control

Pediatric patients with fever and rash often do not have a definitive diagnosis made while in the emergency department. Thus, patients presenting with fever and rash should be considered contagious. Standard precautions should be used when treating patients with fever and rash.

Close contacts of possible cases of meningococcal disease (including household contacts, child-care contacts, and health-care providers) should undergo prophylactic treatment with rifampin (600 mg by mouth [PO] BID for four doses), ceftriaxone (250 mg intramuscular [IM]), or ciprofloxacin (500 mg PO).

Pearls and Pitfalls

1. Consider life-threatening infections, specifically meningococcal infection, in pediatric patients presenting with fever and rash.
2. Administer antibiotics early, even if the definitive diagnosis is not established.
3. Admit patients with possible life-threatening conditions or uncertain diagnosis.

References

American Heart Association Committee on Rheumatic Fever, Endocarditis, and Kawasaki Disease. Diagnostic guidelines for Kawasaki disease. *Am. J. Dis. Child.* 1990; 144(11): 1218–19.

Biesbroeck, L. and Sidbury, R. Viral exanthems: an update. *Dermatologic Therapy* 2013; 26(6): 433–8.

Burns, J. C. The riddle of Kawasaki disease. *N. Engl. J. Med.* 2007; 356(7): 659–61.

Centers for Disease Control and Prevention (CDC). Parvovirus B19 and fifth disease, www.cdc.gov/parvovirusB19/fifth-disease.html (accessed 18 August 2016).

CDC. Prevention and control of meningococcal disease: recommendations of the Advisory Committee on Immunization Practices (ACIP). *MMWR Morb. Mortal. Wkly. Rep.* 2013; 62(RR02): 1–22.

CDC. Kawasaki syndrome, www.cdc.gov/kawasaki/ (accessed 18 August 2016).

CDC. Recommended immunization schedule for persons aged 0 through 18 years, www.cdc.gov/vaccines/schedules/hcp/imz/child-adolescent-shell.html (accessed 18 August 2016).

CDC. Use of serogroup B meningococcal vaccines in adolescents and young adults: recommendations of the Advisory Committee on Immunization Practices, 2015. *MMWR Morb. Mortal. Wkly. Rep.* 2015; 64(41): 1171–6.

Chen, M. T. Clinical manifestations of varicella-zoster virus infection. *Dermatol. Clin.* 2002; 20(2): 267–82.

Cunha, B. A. Rocky Mountain spotted fever revisited. *Arch. Intern. Med.* 2004; 164: 221–3.

Dajani, A. S., Taubert, K. A., Takahashi, M., *et al.* Guidelines for long-term management of patients with Kawasaki disease. Report from the Committee on Rheumatic Fever, Endocarditis, and Kawasaki Disease, Council on Cardiovascular Disease in the Young, American Heart Association. *Circulation* 1994; 89: 916–22.

Diaz, P. S. The epidemiology and control of invasive meningococcal disease. *Pediatr. Infect. Dis. J.* 1999; 18(7): 633–4.

Duke, T. and Mgone, C. S. Measles: not just another viral exanthem. *Lancet* 2003; 36(9359): 763–73.

Frickhofen, N., Abkowitz, J. L., Safford, M., *et al.* Persistent B19 parvovirus infection in patients infected with human immunodeficiency virus type 1: a treatable cause of anemia in AIDS. *Ann. Intern. Med.* 1990; 113(12): 926–33.

Gardner, P. Clinical practice: prevention of meningococcal disease. *N. Engl. J. Med.* 2006; 355(14): 1466–73.

Goodyear, H. M., Laidler, P. W., Price, E. H., *et al.* Acute infectious erythemas in children: a clinico-microbiological study. *Br. J. Dermatol.* 1991; 124(5): 433–8.

Heegaard, E. D. and Brown, K. E. Human parvovirus B19. *Clin. Microbiol. Rev.* 2002; 15(3): 485–505.

Metry, D. and Katta, R. New and emerging pediatric infections. *Dermatol. Clin.* 2003; 21(2): 269–76.

Newburger, J. W., Sleeper, L. A., McCrindle, B. W., *et al.* Randomized trial of pulsed corticosteroid therapy for primary treatment of Kawasaki disease. *N. Engl. J. Med.* 2007; 356: 663–76.

Norbeck, O., Papadogiannakis, N., Petersson, K., *et al.* Revised clinical presentation of parvovirus B19-associated intrauterine fetal death. *Clin. Infect. Dis.* 2002; 35(9): 1032–8.

Patel, G. K. and Finlay, A. Y. Staphylococcal scalded skin syndrome: diagnosis and management. *Am. J. Clin. Dermatol.* 2003; 4(3): 165–75.

Pollard, A. J., Britto, J., Nadel, S., *et al.* Emergency management of meningococcal disease. *Arch. Dis. Child.* 1999; 80(3): 290–6.

Rotbart, H. A., McCracken, G. H., Whitley, R. J., *et al.* Clinical significance of enteroviruses in serious summer febrile illnesses of children. *Pediatr. Infect. Dis. J.* 1999; 18: 869–74.

Stanley, J. R. and Amagai, M. Pemphigus, bullous impetigo, and the staphylococcal scalded-skin syndrome. *N. Engl. J. Med.* 2006; 355(17): 1800–10.

Stone, R. C. and Micali, G. A. Schwartz RA: roseola infantum and its causal human herpesviruses. *Int. J. Dermatol.* 2014; 53(4): 397–403.

Thomas, S. L. and Hall, A. J. What does epidemiology tell us about risk factors for herpes zoster? *Lancet Infect. Dis.* 2004; 4(1): 26–33.

Tunkel, A. R., Hartman, B. J., Kaplan, S. L., *et al.* Practice guidelines for the management of bacterial meningitis. *Clin. Infect. Dis.* 2004; 39(9): 1267–84.

Young, N. and Brown, K. Mechanisms of disease: parvovirus B19. *N. Engl. J. Med.* 2004; 350(6): 586–97.

Additional Readings

Cherry, J. D. Viral exanthems. *Curr. Probl. Pediatr.* 1983; 13(6): 1–44.

Mancinci, A. Exanthems in childhood: an update. *Pediatr. Ann.* 1998; 27(3): 163–70.

McCann, D. J., Nadel, E. S., and Brown, D. F. Rash and fever. *J. Emerg. Med.* 2006; 31(3): 293–7.

Shulman, S. T., De Inocencio, J., and Hirsch, R. Kawasaki disease. *Pediatr. Clin. North Am.* 1995; 42(5): 1205–22.

Pediatric Orthopedic Infections

Cordelia W. Carter and Melinda S. Sharkey

Introduction

The annual incidence of bone and joint infections in children is estimated to be 8 in 100,000 in children in high-income countries. Most cases occur during the first decade of life, with half in children younger than 5 years old. *Staphylococcus aureus* is the causative organism in up to 90% of cases, followed by *Streptococcus* species. Methicillin-resistant *Staphylococcus aureus* (MRSA) is an important pathogen in both community- and health-care-associated disease. If not promptly recognized and treated, these orthopedic infections can lead to significant morbidity in children. Acute care providers should be well versed in the recognition and initial management of these common infections. A coordinated multidisciplinary team approach to definitive treatment can result in favorable outcomes.

Osteomyelitis in Children

Osteomyelitis is an infection of the bone most commonly caused by bacteria. In children, acute osteomyelitis is primarily hematogenous in origin and is often seen in otherwise healthy children. Historically, acute osteomyelitis in children was associated with high mortality rates of 20 to 50%. Heightened awareness and advances in treatment have improved outcomes.

Epidemiology and Microbiology

In the United States, osteomyelitis in children is relatively uncommon. The annual incidence is estimated to be 1 in 5,000 in children younger than 13 years old. Most cases occur during the first decade of life, with half of cases in children younger than 5 years old. Boys are more commonly affected than girls. The majority of cases are hematogenous in origin and classically the infection begins at the metaphysis. High-risk groups include immunocompromised children such as those with sickle cell disease, those receiving chemotherapy, and those with asplenia. For the most part, the microbiology of osteomyelitis and septic arthritis are similar and are considered together here as bone and joint infections. *Staphylococcus aureus* is the predominant organism in bone and joint infections, followed by beta hemolytic streptococci. *S. pneumonia* has declined as a cause of childhood osteomyelitis since the introduction of the pneumococcal vaccine, though it is still an important pathogen to consider in certain high-risk groups, such as asplenic patients. Similarly, the implementation of the *H. influenza* type B vaccine has led to a marked decline in gram-negative infections overall. *Kingella kingae*, while difficult to detect in culture, has effectively replaced *H. influenzae* as a significant cause of musculoskeletal infections in children. *Salmonella* species occur in children with sickle cell disease. *Brucella*, *M. tuberculosis*, and *Salmonella* are more common in developing countries. *Bartonella henselae* osteomyelitis occurs in the setting of cat exposure.

Since the early 2000s, bone and joint infections have increasingly been caused by community-associated methicillin-resistant *Staphylococcus aureus* (CA-MRSA). The emergence of CA-MRSA has led to more severe and difficult to treat infections, and increased complication rates and utilization of hospital resources. The most widespread clone of MRSA, USA 300, carries a gene for Panton–Valentine–leukocidin (PVL), a

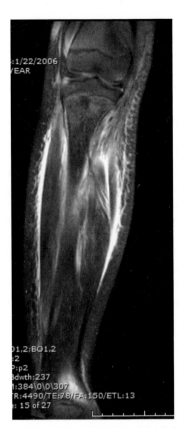

Figure 53.1 MRI T2 image of the leg of a 7-year-old girl who presented a week after falling off her bike onto her left knee with leg pain, swelling, fever, and hemodynamic instability. MRI shows tibial osteomyelitis with associated subperiosteal abscess, myositis, and extensive subcutaneous edema. MRSA was isolated. She required multiple surgical debridements.

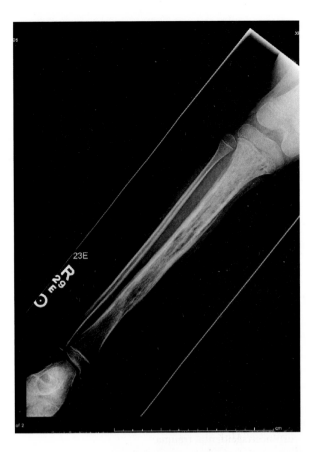

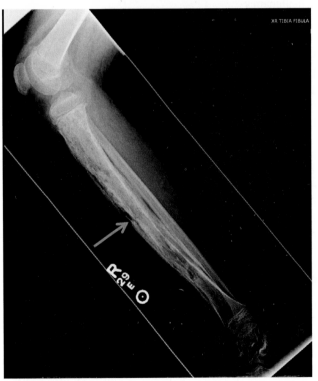

Figure 53.2 AP and lateral radiographs of the tibia of same 7-year-old patient 2 months after initial treatment. Extensive destructive bony changes throughout the diaphysis and metaphysis, as well as diffuse periosteal reaction and a non-displaced pathologic fracture of the diaphysis (arrow) are apparent.

cytotoxin that is associated with tissue destruction. Children who present with musculoskeletal infections due to CA-MRSA are more likely to require admission to the intensive care unit (ICU); to develop associated deep venous thrombosis (DVT) and septic pulmonary emboli; and to require multiple surgical debridements than children with infection due to another pathogen (see Figures 53.1 and 53.2).

Age is another epidemiologic factor to consider in the evaluation and treatment of children with bone and joint infections. Neonates less than 1 month old commonly develop infections due to group B *Streptococcus*. *Neisseria gonorrhoeae* may also cause infections in neonates exposed perinatally, as well as septic arthritis in older patients who are sexually active.

Clinical Features

Presenting signs and symptoms of osteomyelitis include increasing pain and limited use of the affected limb, fever, and possibly redness, swelling, and warmth. Most children present with acute symptoms and are often systemically ill (see Table 53.1). A preceding history of (usually minor) trauma is present 30% of the time. Acute hematogenous osteomyelitis is usually localized to a single site, with the metaphyses of the long bones of the lower extremities most commonly involved.

Table 53.1 Clinical Features and Initial Evaluation: Osteomyelitis in Children

Organism	• *S. aureus* most common
Signs and symptoms	• Fever • Limited use of extremity • Localized pain, swelling, erythema, warmth • Single site (multiple sites in neonates) • Concomitant septic arthritis
Laboratory and radiographic evaluation	• WBC, ESR, CRP, basic chemistry • Blood cultures • X-ray: bone changes present at ~1–2 weeks • MRI with and without contrast: critical to obtain early

CRP – C-reactive protein; ESR – erythrocyte sedimentation rate; MRI – magnetic resonance imaging;; WBC – white blood (cell) count.

Differential Diagnosis

The clinical presentation of osteomyelitis can be variable and non-specific. A wide range of conditions must be considered, including trauma, systemic disease, and malignancy. Other conditions to consider are:

- soft-tissue infection (cellulitis, pyomyositis)
- septic arthritis (patients can present with osteomyelitis and associated septic arthritis)
- fracture/non-accidental trauma
- malignancy
- sickle-cell-associated pain crisis and bone infarct

Laboratory and Radiographic Evaluation

Blood should be sent for complete blood count (CBC), basic chemistries, erythrocyte sedimentation rate (ESR), and C-reactive protein (CRP). Blood cultures should be drawn prior to starting antibiotics.

Plain radiographs should be performed on every patient. The first appreciable sign of infection is soft-tissue swelling, which appears within 48 hours of infection, followed by new periosteal bone formation within 5 to 7 days and osteolysis at 10 to 14 days. Early magnetic resonance imaging (MRI) with and without gadolinium contrast is an important part of the work-up and allows precise delineation of the site and extent of infection, including any abscesses that may require surgical drainage.

Treatment

Treatment is often non-operative in uncomplicated osteomyelitis. After blood cultures are drawn, initial empiric IV antibiotic treatment should begin. The regimen should cover methicillin-sensitive *S. aureus* (MSSA) and MRSA (see Table 53.4). Clinical response to antibiotics as well as the MRI findings (presence of deep bone or subperiosteal abscesses) will guide the decision for surgical debridement.

Complications and Admission Criteria

All patients with suspected osteomyelitis should be admitted to the hospital for continued clinical and laboratory evaluation, adjustment of antibiotics based on culture results, and possible surgical debridement.

Most children with osteomyelitis do well. Complications include chronic osteomyelitis, associated septic arthritis with joint damage, pathologic fracture, and abnormal bone growth.

Septic Arthritis in Children

Introduction

Septic arthritis is the presence of infection in a closed joint space. It is usually the result of a bacterial infection, though other organisms (e.g. fungus) may also cause intra-articular infection. Any joint may be affected by septic arthritis; the most commonly involved joints in children are the hip and knee. The usual route of infection is hematogenous. Additionally, septic arthritis may result from direct extension into the joint space from adjacent osteomyelitis. Joints that have an intra-articular metaphysis (e.g. the hip, shoulder, ankle, and elbow) are more likely to be affected in this way, as the infection may breach the metaphyseal periosteum and enter the joint. Local trauma and direct innoculation are other possible causes of intra-articular infection.

Septic arthritis is traditionally described as an isolated clinical entity. However, as the epidemiology of pediatric musculoskeletal infection evolves, it has become increasingly common for septic arthritis to be present as part of a more complicated osteoarticular infection, often involving adjacent bone and soft tissue with resultant associated osteomyelitis, pyomyositis, and abscess formation. Septic arthritis – with or without associated areas of infection – is one of the true "orthopedic emergencies." A delay in treatment of septic arthritis may have devastating consequences, including rapid cytokine-mediated articular cartilage damage and irreparable joint destruction.

Epidemiology and Microbiology

Septic arthritis occurs with approximately the same frequency as osteomyelitis. In the newborn period, septic arthritis is associated with invasive procedures and catheters. Predisposing factors in children include immunodeficiency and underlying arthritis, such as juvenile idiopathic arthritis, but septic arthritis usually occurs in children who are otherwise healthy. It is more common in boys. The microbiology of septic arthritis in children mirrors that of osteomyelitis and is covered in that section above.

Clinical Features

Children with septic arthritis typically present with the acute onset of fever and malaise with a painful, warm, and swollen joint (see Table 53.2). A review of systems may reveal recent changes, including irritability, decreased appetite, and lethargy. Because movement of the affected joint is painful, patients with septic arthritis will avoid loading and motion of the joint. In cases of septic arthritis affecting the lower extremities, children may limp or refuse to bear weight altogether. Children with infection of the upper extremities may preferentially use the unaffected upper extremity ("pseudoparalysis").

Table 53.2 Clinical Features and Evaluation: Septic Arthritis in Children

Organism	• S. aureus most common
Signs and symptoms	• Fever • Obvious effusion in superficial joints • Erythema, warmth, and limited motion of joint
Laboratory and radiographic evaluation	• WBC, ESR, CRP • Blood cultures • X-rays • Aspirate of joint fluid for cell count, Gram stain, and culture

CRP – C-reactive protein; ESR – erythrocyte sedimentation rate; WBC – white blood (cell) count.

Table 53.3 Differential Diagnosis for Pediatric Septic Arthritis

Traumatic	• Fracture • Other musculoskeletal injury (e.g. muscle strain) • Non-accidental trauma
Inflammatory	• Transient synovitis • Juvenile inflammatory arthritis • Post-infectious arthritis • Reactive arthritis
Infectious	• Adjacent osseous or soft-tissue infection (e.g. iliopsoas abscess, femoral osteomyelitis) • Viral arthritis • Lyme arthritis (Borreliosis) • Tuberculosis
Other musculoskeletal conditions	• Legg-Calvé-Perthes disease • Slipped capital femoral epiphysis (SCFE) • Pigmented villonodular synovitis (PVNS) • Tumor
Non-musculoskeletal conditions	• Appendicitis • Pyelonephritis • Genitourinary infections

Physical examination findings include fever and in more advanced infections, tachycardia and even hypotension, may be present. Children with septic arthritis usually appear ill. Children with septic hip arthritis may preferentially hold the lower extremity in a flexed, abducted, and externally rotated position. Children with infections of the upper extremities may "splint" the affected arm by holding it protectively near the body. Inspection of the affected joint reveals effusion and erythema. Palpation demonstrates warmth and tenderness. Attempts to perform passive range-of-motion of an affected joint are met with resistance, as this is exquisitely painful when the joint is acutely infected. Physical examination should encompass the entire limb of interest. Attempted passive motion of the hip, knee, and ankle in a limping child is imperative and examination of the unaffected side may be useful for comparison.

Differential Diagnosis

The differential diagnosis for septic arthritis includes traumatic, inflammatory, and infectious etiologies that may mimic joint infection in their clinical presentation (see Table 53.3).

It may be difficult to differentiate transient synovitis of the hip from septic arthritis because the presenting symptoms are quite similar. Accurate diagnosis is imperative, because while the treatment for transient synovitis of the hip is observation and anti-inflammatory medication, the treatment for septic arthritis is prompt surgical drainage combined with antibiotic therapy in an effort to prevent joint destruction. One useful algorithm for determining the likelihood of septic arthritis in a child with a painful hip has been described by Kocher et al. This algorithm uses the following four criteria (i.e. the "Kocher criteria") to predict the likelihood that septic arthritis exists: (1) inability to bear weight; (2) ESR >40mm/hour; (3) history of fever (temperature >38.5°C); and (4) WBC >12,000 cells/mm³. The chances of septic hip arthritis being present with one of these predictors present is <3%; when two predictors are present, this increases to 40%, and when three of the four predictors are present, the likelihood of septic arthritis is >93%. Subsequent modifications to this predictive algorithm have demonstrated that a CRP > 2 mg/dL is also highly predictive of septic arthritis.

Laboratory and Radographic Findings

Blood tests to order in suspected musculoskeletal infection include a complete blood count (CBC,) erythrocyte sedimentation rate (ESR), C-reactive protein (CRP), and blood cultures. In Lyme-endemic areas, titers for *Borrelia burgdorferi* should also be sent. Because septic arthritis is typically treated by surgical drainage, adolescent females with a suspected musculoskeletal infection should undergo routine pregnancy screening. Patients with septic arthritis will typically have elevated white blood cell counts (WBCs) and elevated inflammatory markers (ESR, CRP). Blood cultures are positive in up to 40% of cases.

Patients with an obvious joint effusion should undergo aspiration prior to initiation of antibiotic treatment to optimize the chances of recovering the causative organism and tailoring antibiotic treatment according to pathogen susceptibility. Aspiration of deeper joints with suspected infection (e.g. the hip) may be done under ultrasound guidance. The color and consistency of the aspirated fluid should be documented and the fluid should be sent for analysis, gram stain, and culture. Fluid cell counts of >50,000 WBCs/mm³ are highly suggestive of infection, especially if the percentage of polymorphonuclear leukocytes (PMNs) is >75%. A positive gram stain is also considered diagnostic for the presence of intra-articular infection.

Plain radiographs of the affected limbs and/or joints are part of routine evaluation for pediatric musculoskeletal infection. In the hip, the presence of an effusion may be detected by asymmetric widening of the joint space. Radiographic findings in the setting of acute joint infection may be subtle or even non-existent, but other etiologies of pain, including fracture and tumor, may be elucidated with plain radiographs.

Ultrasound is quickly becoming the standard of care for evaluation of suspected hip infection in children. It is also useful to evaluate the elbow and ankle. The fact that ultrasound is portable, non-invasive, and is performed without radiation contributes to its great clinical utility. Additionally, once the presence of an effusion has been confirmed, ultrasound-guided joint aspiration may be performed.

Finally, magnetic resonance imaging (MRI) performed with intravenous contrast has become an important tool in the evaluation of pediatric musculoskeletal infection as the growing presence of increasingly virulent bacteria (most notably, CA-MRSA) has resulted in more aggressive infections involving joints, bones, and soft tissues. MRI is therefore helpful both diagnostically and for surgical planning.

Treatment

A multidisciplinary team of health-care providers (orthopedic surgeons, radiologists, anesthesiologists, and emergency care providers) should be involved as early as possible in the care of suspected septic arthritis in a child. Invasive procedures such as joint aspiration or surgical irrigation and debridement should be performed in a coordinated fashion. The definitive treatment of septic arthritis is prompt surgical incision and drainage combined with antibiotic therapy. All patients with a suspected joint infection should therefore remain NPO (nil per OS) in anticipation of surgical intervention. Once joint aspiration and blood cultures have been obtained, broad-spectrum intravenous antibiotic should be initiated. Antibiotic choice should be made based upon the patient's age and likely causative organisms, as well as upon local epidemiologic patterns of infection and antibiotic resistance. Enlisting the help of infectious disease specialists can be helpful in determining the best choice of antibiotic, as well as defining the route of administration and duration of antibiotic therapy. An adaptation of one recently published guideline for the empiric treatment of pediatric musculoskeletal infection is shown below in Table 53.4.

Complications and Admission Criteria

Because septic arthritis is a "surgical emergency," all patients with septic arthritis should be admitted to the hospital. Unfortunately, biomechanical sequelae of some kind, such as joint laxity or restriction, occur in up to 25% of children with septic arthritis, even with prompt treatment.

Special Considerations

Lyme Arthritis

The clinical presentation and symptoms of pediatric Lyme arthritis may closely mimic those of of septic arthritis. Additionally, there may be a significant overlap in the laboratory values of patients with both septic and Lyme arthritis, which further complicates the clinical picture. For example, in a study of 20 children with Lyme arthritis of the hip, Bachur *et al.* reported peripheral WBC values as high as 22,000/mm³; CRP values as high as 7.3 mg/dL; ESR values as high as 94 mm/hour; and cell counts from the joint aspirate as high as 158,000 cells/mm³ – values all highly suggestive of septic arthritis. For patients who live in areas of the country where Lyme disease is prevalent, Lyme titers should be promptly sent, as surgical treatment is not indicated for Lyme arthritis.

Table 53.4 Suggested Guidelines for the Empiric Antibiotic Treatment of Pediatric Musculoskeletal Infection

- Neonates* (<1 month)
  - Ampicillin/sulbactam
    plus
  - Gentamicin (may be added for high-risk neonates)
- Infants (1–3 months)
  - Vancomycin
    - 15 mg/kg/dose IV every 6 hours
    plus
  - Ceftriaxone
    - 50 mg/kg/dose IV every 12 hours
- Children and adolescents
  - First-generation cephalosporin if prevalence of MSSA in community >90%
  - Antistaphylococcal penicillin if prevalence of MSSA in community >90%
  - Clindamycin 10 mg/kg/dose IV every 6 hours if prevalence of MRSA in community ≥10% and prevalence of clindamycin-resistant *S. aureus* <10%
    or
  - Vancomycin 15 mg/kg/dose IV every 6 hours if prevalence of MRSA in community ≥10% and prevalence of clindamycin resistant *S. aureus* ≥10%
    plus
  - Rifampin
    - 10 mg/kg/day IV/PO divided every 12 hours

* Neonatal dosing and frequency must be adjusted for weight, postnatal age, and gestational age; consult institutional guidelines for specific dosing recommendations.

Modified from Copley 2009 and Peltola and Pääkkönen 2014.

Neonatal Musculoskeletal Infections

Neonates should be considered separately because of the significant morbidity and poor outcomes associated with the septic arthritis and osteomyelitis in this high-risk population. Affected infants are usually systemically ill. Presentation may be subtle and include pseudoparalysis, anorexia, irritability, or lethargy. The incidence is estimated to be 1 to 3 of every 1,000 neonatal intensive care unit admissions. Because of their immature immune systems, neonates are vulnerable to infections caused by group B *Streptococcus* and gram-negative rods with involvement at multiple sites. Temperature and WBC may remain normal, causing a delay in diagnosis, and ESR and CRP are similarly unreliable.

Diskitis

Diskitis is an uncommon infection of the intervertebral disk and adjacent end plates. Affected children are usually younger than 5 years, and the lumbar spine is most frequently involved. *Staphylococcus aureus* is the most common bacterial isolate. Young children may have difficulty localizing their pain. Radiographs show disk space narrowing after about 1 week. Treatment is admission for antibiotics and bracing.

Sickle Cell Disease

Because of their increased susceptibility to infections of all kind, including osteoarticular infections, patients with sickle cell disease deserve special consideration. Patients with sickle cell disease and osteoarticular infections present with similar symptoms as otherwise healthy patients: pain, swelling, fever, and tenderness. However, such symptoms can masquerade as a sickle cell painful crisis. Similarly, they will have elevated WBC and markers of inflammation, including ESR. While *S. aureus* remains the most common pathogen isolated, children with sickle cell disease are uniquely susceptible to osteoarticular infections caused by the *Salmonella* species.

Pearls and Pitfalls

1. MRI with and without contrast is the gold standard in the detection of osteomyelitis, as well as to delineate the location and extent of infection and guide the need for surgical treatment, and should be obtained early in suspected cases.
2. Initial empiric antibiotic therapy should target *Staphylococcus aureus*, including MRSA.
3. Because the metaphyseal regions of the proximal humerus, proximal femur, distal tibia, and distal humerus are intra-articular, osteomyelitis in these sites is prone to concomitant septic arthritis.
4. Children with septic arthritis usually will not tolerate attempted passive range-of-motion of the affected joint.
5. The "Kocher criteria" – (1) inability to bear weight; (2) ESR >40mm/hour; (3) history of fever; and (4) WBC >12,000 cells/mm^3 – may be used to help distinguish septic arthritis of the hip from transient synovitis.
6. Fever (temperature >38.5 ˚C) and elevated CRP (>2 mg/dL) may be the best clinical predictors of the presence of septic arthritis.
7. Ultrasound-guided hip aspiration can be performed safely in the acute care setting for patients with suspected septic arthritis of the hip.
8. Lyme arthritis may closely mimic septic arthritis.

References

Bachur, R. G., Adams, C. A., and Montreaux, M. C. Evaluating the child with acute hip pain ("irritable hip") in a Lyme endemic region. *J. Pediatr.* 2015; 166(2): 407–11.

Caird, M. S., Flynn, J. M., Leung, Y. L., *et al.* Factors distinguishing septic arthritis from transient synovitis of the hip in children. A prospective study. *JBJS* 2006; 88(6): 1251–7.

Chambers, J. B., Forsythe, D. A., Bertrand, S. L., *et al.* Retrospective review of osteoarticular infections in a pediatric sickle cell age group. *J. Pediatr. Orthop.* 2000; 20(5): 682–5.

Copley, L. A. Pediaric musculoskeletal infection: trends and antibiotic recommendations. *J. Am. Acad. Orthop. Surg.* 2009; 17(10): 618–26.

Early, S. D., Kay, R. M., and Tolo, V. T. Childhood diskitis. *J. Am. Acad. Orthop. Surg.* 2003; 11(6): 413–20.

Kocher, M. S., Zurakowski, D., and Kasser, J. R. Differentiating between septic arthritis and transient synovitis of the hip in children: and evidence-based clinical prediction algorithm. *JBJS* 1999; 81(12): 1662–70.

Pääkkönen, M. and Peltola, H. Bone and joint infections. *Pediatr. Clin. N. Am.* 2013; 60(2): 425–36.

Peltola, H. and Pääkkönen, M. Acute osteomyelitis in children. *NEJM* 2014; 370(4): 352–60.

Pendleton, A. and Kocher, M. S. Methicillin-resistant *Staphylococcus aureus* bone and joint infections in children. *J. Am. Acad. Orthop. Surg.* 2015; 23(1): 29–37.

Plumb, J., Mallin, M., and Bolte, R. G. The role of ultrasound in the emergency department evaluation of the acutely painful pediatric hip. *Pediatr. Emer. Care* 2015; 31(1): 54–61.

Smith, B. G., Cruz, A. I., Milewski, M. D., and Shapiro, E. D. Lyme disease and the orthopaedic implications of lyme arthritis. *J. Am. Acad. Orthop. Surg.* 2011; 19(2): 91–100.

Vander Have, K. L., Karmazyn, B., Verma, M., *et al.* Community-associated Methicillin-resistant Staphylococcus aureus in acute musculoskeletal infection in children: a game-changer. *J. Pediatr. Orthop.* 2009; 29(8): 927–31.

Chapter 54

Pediatric Respiratory Infections

Ghazala Sharieff*

Introduction

Respiratory failure is the most common cause of cardiopulmonary arrest in infants and children. Management varies significantly depending on the etiology, and therefore prompt assessment of pediatric respiratory disease is essential. This chapter will discuss the most common respiratory diseases in children, focusing on epiglottitis, bacterial tracheitis, croup, retropharyngeal abscess, pertussis, bronchiolitis, and pneumonia.

Epiglottitis

Epidemiology and Microbiology

Epiglottitis or supraglottitis is a serious, life-threatening infection of the epiglottis and constitutes an airway emergency. It is more common in the winter, but can occur throughout the year. Peak incidence is in children between 2 and 8 years of age, but epiglottitis also occurs in infants and adults. Since widespread vaccination against *Haemophilus influenzae* type B,

* Thanks to Aleena Shad, research assistant, for her contribution.

Table 54.1 Clinical Features: Epiglottitis

Pathogens	Group A beta-hemolytic *Streptococcus* *Streptococcus pneumoniae* *Klebsiella* *Pseudomonas* *Staphylcoccus aureus*
Signs and symptoms	• Abrupt presentation within 6–24 hours of illness • High fever, irritability, throat pain • "4 Ds" of epiglottitis: drooling, dyspnea, dysphonia, and dysphagia • Symptoms of impending airway obstruction: drooling, stridor, and cyanosis • Tripod positioning
Laboratory and radiographic findings	• Routine laboratory tests are not indicated • Lateral neck radiograph* has classic "thumbprint" sign, but this may be absent in up to 20% of cases. Patients should not be sent out of the ED for radiographic studies • Supraglottic cultures and sensitivities
Treatment	Ceftriaxone 50 mg/kg/dose IV every 12 hours *or* Cefotaxime 50 mg/kg/dose IV every 6 hours *plus* Vancomycin 15 mg/kg/dose IV every 6 hours Steroids are not routinely recommended.

* Radiographs are helpful in ruling out croup, retropharyngeal abscess, and foreign bodies.

previously the most common cause, the incidence has dramatically decreased. The most common identified organisms causing epiglottitis are now group A beta-hemolytic *Streptococcus*, *Streptococcus pneumoniae*, *Klebsiella*, *Pseudomonas*, and *Staphylcoccus aureus*.

Clinical Features

Epiglottitis usually presents abruptly and classically presents with high fever, irritability, and throat pain that may manifest as unwillingness to eat or drink. They may also present with symptoms of impending airway obstruction such as drooling, stridor, cyanosis, marked anxiety, and a toxic appearance. Characteristic voice changes include hoarseness and a muffled voice. These children usually prefer to rest in the tripod position, a sitting position with their jaws thrust forward. As the supraglottic edema worsens, it becomes difficult for the patient to swallow saliva, and drooling is a common complaint. High fevers (e.g. 104 °F or 40.0 °C) and tachycardia may be present. Table 54.1 lists the common features of epiglottitis.

Differential Diagnosis

The differential diagnosis of epiglottitis includes:

- croup
- bacterial tracheitis
- retropharyngeal abscess
- peritonsillar abscess
- vocal cord paralysis

- pharyngitis
- anaphylaxis
- inhaled foreign body

Key features that may help to distinguish epiglottitis are:

- abrupt onset with their appearance
- sore throat with odynophagia and fever
- four D's – drooling, dyspnea, dysphonia, and dysphagia
- these children *do not* cough
- classic "thumbprint sign" on lateral neck radiograph (absent in ~20%)

Laboratory and Radiographic Findings

Routine laboratory tests are not indicated, particularly because agitation of the child prior to definitive airway management is contraindicated. Gentle visualization of the oropharynx may be performed, but without the use of a tongue depressor, because manipulation may result in complete obstruction of the airway. Occasionally, an erythematous epiglottis may be seen protruding at the base of the tongue. Radiographs are helpful in ruling out croup, retropharyngeal abscess, or foreign body. The lateral neck radiograph, especially in hyperextension during inspiration, is the imaging study of choice. The classic finding is the "thumbprint sign," indicative of a round and thick epiglottis (see Figure 54.1). However, this finding may be absent in up to 20% of cases. Once the airway has been secured, cultures and sensitivities should be obtained from the supraglottic region. Blood cultures are typically not helpful, but may be obtained as part of the fever evaluation. Because the airway is so precarious in pediatric epiglottitis, patients should not leave the monitored setting of the ED for radiographs to be taken.

Treatment and Prophylaxis

When a diagnosis of epiglottitis is made by history and physical exam, every effort should be made to avoid any anxiety-provoking procedures, including phlebotomy or extensive intraoral examination. It is imperative to allow the patient to sit in the most comfortable position possible. The confirmatory diagnosis of epiglottitis is made by direct visualization with a laryngoscope, usually during intubation. The mucosa will appear erythematous and pooling of secretions may be present. The supraglottic structures, including the epiglottis, arytenoids, and aryepiglottic folds, may appear cherry red and edematous. Unless there is severe airway compromise requiring immediate emergency department management, laryngoscopy should be performed under sedation, in a controlled setting with the most experienced airway expert and surgical personnel. Broad-spectrum antibiotics such as third-generation cephalosporins should be started as soon as possible after the airway is secured. Steroids are not routinely indicated.

Complications and Admission Criteria

Airway obstruction is the most serious complication of this disease. A surgical airway is necessary if the patient cannot be endotracheally intubated. All children with suspected epiglottitis should be admitted to the intensive care unit (ICU).

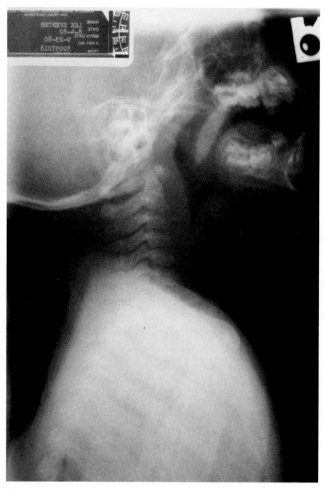

Figure 54.1 Epiglottitis with thumb print sign.
Courtesy of Rady Children's Hospital, San Diego Radiology Department.

Higher pressures may be necessary to adequately ventilate the patient and at minimum an endotracheal tube size smaller than calculated should be used due to airway edema.

Croup

Epidemiology and Microbiology

Croup, or laryngotracheobronchitis, is the most common cause of infectious airway obstruction in children. The most commonly affected age group is 6 months to 4 years. Croup has a peak incidence in early fall and winter, but occasionally may be seen throughout the year. The most common causative organism is parainfluenza virus type I; however, other organisms such as parainfluenza types II and III, *Mycoplasma pneumoniae*, respiratory syncytial virus (RSV), influenza A and B, and adenovirus have been implicated.

Clinical Features

A 1- to 2-day prodrome of nasal congestion, rhinorrhea, and cough is followed by the onset of a harsh, barky cough often described as sounding similar to a seal or a barking dog. The patient may also have stridor, which is typically inspiratory, but may also be biphasic. Biphasic stridor, as well as nasal

Table 54.2 Clinical Features: Croup

Pathogens	Parainfluenza virus type I
	Parainfluenza type II and III
	Mycoplasma pneumoniae
	RSV
	Influenza A and B
	Adenovirus
Signs and symptoms	• Viral prodrome (cough, rhinorrhea, fever)
	• Harsh, barky cough
	• Inspiratory stridor more common than expiratory
	• Tachypnea, hypoxia, and biphasic stridor concerning for respiratory compromise
Laboratory and radiographic findings	• Classic "steeple sign"
	• X-ray can help rule out retropharyngeal abscess, epiglottitis, foreign body, congenital abnormalities
Treatment	Dexamethasone 0.6 mg/kg PO/IM/IV × 1 (maximum 20 mg)
	or
	Budesonide 2 mg via nebulizer × 1
	plus
	Racemic epinephrine: 0.5 mL of a 2.25% solution in 2.5 mL of normal saline via nebulizer × 1

flaring, suprasternal and intercostal retraction, tachypnea, and hypoxia, are indications of severe respiratory compromise. Typical symptom duration is less than 1 week with a peak of 1 to 2 days (see Table 54.2).

Differential Diagnosis

The differential for croup includes:

- foreign body aspiration
- spasmodic croup
- epiglottitis
- bacterial tracheitis
- retropharyngeal abscess
- subglottic stenosis after prolonged endotracheal (ET) tube placement
- laryngeal web
- anaphylaxis with angioedema of the subglottic area
- hemangioma
- neoplasm
- laryngomalacia
- vascular ring
- burn or thermal injuries
- laryngeal papillomatosis

Key features that may help distinguish croup from other respiratory infections are:

- harsh, barky cough
- inspiratory stridor
- classic steeple sign on anteroposterior (AP) neck radiograph (absent in ~50%)

Laboratory and Radiographic Findings

The diagnosis of croup is a clinical one, as complete blood counts (CBCs) tend to be normal. Radiographs may be helpful

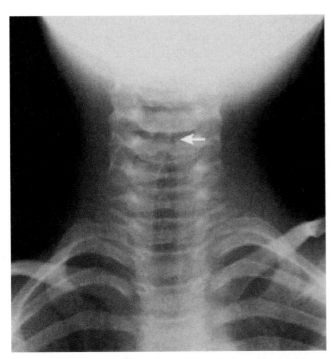

Figure 54.2 Viral croup with steeple sign. (See prior legend for details.)

in differentiation of other disease entities such as epiglottitis, retropharyngeal abscess, congenital abnormalities, foreign body, or hemangioma. Although routine radiographs are not necessary, the classic radiographic finding in a patient with croup is the "steeple sign" (see Figure 54.2) representing subglottic edema. However, the absence of this finding does not rule out croup, as almost half of patients with croup have normal radiographs.

Treatment and Prophylaxis

The management of croup is dependent on the severity of respiratory symptoms. Traditionally, patients with croup have been treated with humidified air, believed to soothe inflamed mucosa and thus decrease coughing. Several studies have shown that mist therapy is not effective in improving clinical symptoms in children presenting to the ED with moderate croup. Because these treatments are harmless, however, many practitioners still use them, particularly in patients who are being held for observation.

Glucocorticoids are used to treat moderate to severe croup because oral or parenteral dexamethasone decreases hospitalization rates. Patients with mild croup also benefit from dexamethasone with faster resolution of symptoms. Although the standard dose of dexamethasone has been 0.6 mg/kg, lower doses of 0.15 mg/kg and 0.3 mg/kg have shown similar efficacy in patients with moderate croup. Because of the long half-life of dexamethasone, there is no need to discharge the patient with additional doses of steroids.

Nebulized budesonide dosed at both 2 mg and 4 mg has also shown efficacy in mild to moderate croup as single-dose therapy. Nebulized racemic epinephrine contains both levo (L) and dextro (D) epinephrine isomers and is the mainstay of treatment for moderate to severe croup. Although racemic

epinephrine does not alter the natural course of croup, it may reduce the need for emergent airway management. The preferred dose is 0.25 to 0.5 mL of the 2.25% solution diluted with normal saline to 3 mLs. Patients who receive nebulized epinephrine should also receive dexamethasone. Patients who receive corticosteroids and demonstrate a sustained response to racemic epinephrine 2 to 3 hours after treatment are generally safe for discharge. If racemic epinephrine is not available, epinephrine can be used in its place. The administration of a mixture of helium and oxygen (heliox) can improve oxygenation in patients with severe croup.

In patients with severe croup that is unresponsive to nebulized epinephrine and corticosteroids, endotracheal intubation and ventilation may be necessary. If intubation is necessary, an endotracheal tube with a diameter smaller than recommended for age and size should be used.

Complications and Admission Criteria

Patients who have persistent tachypnea, hypoxia, or inability to tolerate oral fluids or who require more than two treatments of racemic epinephrine should be admitted. Fortunately, less than 10% of children with croup are hospitalized. Complications include airway compromise and respiratory arrest.

Bacterial Tracheitis

Epidemiology and Microbiology

Bacterial tracheitis, also known as laryngotracheobronchitis, pseudomembranous croup, or bacterial croup, is an uncommon disease, which may be life-threatening. The peak incidence is in the fall and winter in children between 6 months and 8 years of age. Marked subglottic edema and thick mucopurulent (membranous) secretions characterize the illness. The organisms most commonly implicated include *Staphylococcus aureus* and, to a lesser extent, *Streptococcus pneumoniae, Haemophilus influenzae, Moraxella catarrhalis,* and *Pseudomonas.*

Clinical Features

The clinical presentation of bacterial tracheitis has features of both epiglottitis and viral croup. The child may have prodromal viral upper respiratory symptoms such as low-grade fever, cough, and stridor, similar to patients with croup. However, the patient then develops the rapid onset of high fever, respiratory distress, and a toxic appearance. Unlike patients with epiglottitis, these children typically do have a cough, are comfortable lying flat, and do not drool (see Table 54.3).

Differential Diagnosis

Similar to croup, the differential diagnoses to consider include:

- croup
- epiglottis
- foreign body aspiration
- retropharyngeal or peritonsillar abscess

Table 54.3 Clinical Features: Bacterial Tracheitis

Pathogens	*Staphylococcus aureus* (most common) *Streptococcus pneumoniae* *Haemophilus influenzae* *Moraxella catarrhalis* *Pseudomonus*
Signs and symptoms	• Prodromal low-grade fever, cough, and stridor (similar to croup) • Rapid onset of high fevers and respiratory distress; child appears toxic • May or may not have tripod positioning
Laboratory and radiographic findings	• Routine laboratory test are not indicated • CBC may show marked leukocytosis • Blood cultures are typically negative • X-ray is usually normal; AP neck radiograph* may show "steeple sign" or irregularity of the proximal mucosa • Diagnosis is made endoscopically by visualizing normal supraglottic structures with prominent subglottic edema, ulcerations, and copious purulent secretions • Culture secretions
Treatment	Intubation is often required for 3–7 days. Additional endoscopy may be needed to remove the pseudomembrane Vancomycin 15 mg/kg/dose IV every 6 hours *plus* Ceftriaxone 50 mg/kg/dose IV every 12 hours *or* Ampicillin-sulbactam 50 mg/kg/dose IV every 6 hours

* Radiograph in bacterial tracheitis is very similar to that in viral croup, with the marked subglottic narrowing known as the "steeple sign."

Key features that distinguish bacterial tracheitis from epiglottitis and viral croup are:

• comfortable lying flat
• no drooling
• presence of cough

Laboratory and Radiographic Findings

Routine laboratory tests are not indicated; however, a complete blood count may show marked leukocytosis. Blood cultures are typically negative. Radiographically, bacterial tracheitis is similar to croup in that the marked subglottic narrowing known as the "steeple sign" may be present on AP neck films. Occasionally, a slight irregularity of the proximal tracheal mucosa, representing pseudomembranous detachment, may also be seen. If found, these radiographic findings may aid in the diagnosis of bacterial tracheitis; however, their absence does not rule it out. Diagnosis is made endoscopically, by visualizing normal supraglottic structures with prominent subglottic edema, ulcerations, and copious purulent secretions. These secretions should be sent for gram stain and culture.

Treatment and Prophylaxis

When possible, patients in severe respiratory distress should be managed in the operating suite for both the endoscopic

diagnosis and intubation. Copious purulent secretions can be suctioned from the endotracheal tube and should be sent for culture. A tube size smaller than calculated for patient size and age should be utilized due to airway narrowing. If endotracheal intubation is unsuccessful, a tracheostomy may be necessary. In the acute setting, needle cricothyrotomy is the appropriate emergency intervention if endotracheal intubation is unsuccessful. Occasionally, repeat endoscopy may be required to remove pseudomembranous material. Intubation is often required for 3 to 7 days, until the patient is afebrile, there is a decrease in the quantity and viscosity of secretions, and an air leak is present (i.e. there is passage of air around the endotracheal tube, indicating decreased edema). Antibiotics should be initiated early with an initial regimen of vancomycin and a third-generation cephalosporin such as ceftriaxone.

Complications and Admission Criteria

Complications include airway obstruction, pneumothorax, formation of pseudomembranes, and toxic shock syndrome. These patients frequently have concurrent pneumonia. All patients with bacterial tracheitis should be admitted to the ICU for close monitoring.

Retropharyngeal Abscess
Epidemiology and Microbiology

The retropharyngeal space is a potential area located between the anterior border of the cervical vertebrae and the posterior wall of the esophagus; the space contains connective tissues and lymph nodes that receive lymphatic drainage from adjacent structures. A retropharyngeal abscess (RPA) is a life-threatening deep infection of this area. 50% of cases occur in patients between 6 months and 12 months of age. 96% of all cases occur in children less than 6 years of age, as the nodes of Ruvier that drain the retropharyngeal space typically atrophy after this age. There is also a male predominance, in some studies up to 3:1. The most common causative organisms are group A b-hemolytic *Streptococcus*, anaerobic organisms, and *Staphylococcus aureus*.

Clinical Features

The initial clinical picture of retropharyngeal abscess is similar to that of other illnesses such as croup, epiglottitis, tracheitis, and peritonsillar abscess. Patients frequently present with symptoms of an upper respiratory infection, fever, sore throat, neck stiffness, and poor oral intake (see Table 54.4). As purulent material collects, a fluctuant mass may begin to cause airway compromise, and patients may develop drooling, stridor, and respiratory distress. Physical examination may reveal an oropharyngeal mass, though this is only present in half of all children with retropharyngeal abscess. Patients often present with a stiff neck and may be misdiagnosed with meningitis.

Table 54.4 Clinical Features: Retropharyngeal Abscess

Pathogens	Group A b-hemolytic *Streptococcus* Anaerobic organisms *Staphylococcus aureus*
Signs and symptoms	• Initially may have an upper respiratory infection, fever, sore throat • As mass enlarges, drooling, stridor, neck stiffness, and poor intake
Laboratory and radiographic findings	• Routine laboratory tests are not indicated • Radiograph* reveals widening of the retropharyngeal space. Normal prevertebral space parameters are: C2: less than 7 mm C6: less than 14 mm
Treatment	Supportive care, ABCs (airway, breathing, circulation) Clindamycin 10 mg/kg/dose IV every 6–8 hours *or* Ampicillin-sulbactam 50 mg/kg/dose IV every 6 hours

* Radiographs are helpful in ruling out epiglottitis, croup, retropharyngeal abscess, and foreign bodies.

Differential Diagnosis

The differential diagnosis of retropharyngeal abscess includes:

- foreign body ingestion
- tonsillitis
- peritonsillar abscess
- meningitis
- nasopharyngeal mass

Key features that may help distinguish retropharyngeal abscess are:

- neck stiffness
- sore throat
- stridor

Laboratory and Radiographic Findings

Routine laboratory testing is not useful in the diagnosis of a retropharyngeal abscess.

The lateral neck radiograph is very useful in the initial diagnosis of retropharyngeal abscesses. In children, the normal soft tissue should measure no more than 7 mm at the level of the second cervical vertebrae, less than 5 mm anterior to the third and fourth cervical vertebrae (or less than 40% of the AP diameter of the vertebral body), and 14 mm at the sixth cervical vertebrae on a film done with proper neck extension (see Figure 54.3). Retropharyngeal thickening is seen on lateral neck radiograph in 88 to 100% of RPA cases. In clinically stable patients, a computed tomographic (CT) scan of the neck is helpful to delineate whether there is a retropharyngeal cellulitis rather than a true abscess. Ultrasound may also be useful in this differentiation as well.

Treatment and Prophylaxis

Previously, the standard of care for management of RPA was surgical drainage. However, in some cases antibiotic therapy alone is successful. For patients with signs of airway

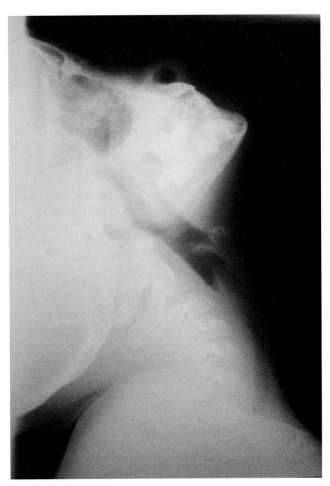

Figure 54.3 Bacterial tracheitis.
Courtesy of Dr. Lee Harvey.

obstruction, endotracheal intubation followed by surgical drainage is still the treatment of choice. When visualizing the airway for endotracheal intubation, care must be taken to avoid abscess rupture. Antibiotic therapy should be initiated in all patients; clindamycin is an appropriate first choice.

Complications and Admission Criteria

Because retropharyngeal abscess is a life-threatening airway illness, all patients should be admitted and closely monitored. Complications include airway compromise, abscess rupture leading to asphyxiation or aspiration pneumonia, or spread of infection to adjacent structures in the neck, including infection of carotid artery sheath, osteomyelitis of the cervical spine, or infection of the structures of the mediastinum.

Pearls and Pitfalls

1. Palpation of the abscess is not recommended as rupture may occur.
2. Peripheral white blood cell count is neither sensitive nor specific in the diagnosis of RPA.
3. Ensure correct positioning of the child for the lateral neck radiograph. Flexion or persistent crying can give the illusion of a large retropharyngeal space.

Table 54.5 Clinical Features: Pertussis

Pathogens	*Bordetella pertussis* *Bordetella parapertussis*, adenovirus, or chlamydia causes a similar clinical syndrome
Signs and symptoms	• Catarrhal phase: cough, coryza, conjunctivitis • Paroxysmal phase: spasmodic cough, infants may have a staccato cough with apnea • Convalescent phase: chronic cough
Laboratory and radiographic findings	• Positive PCR of nasopharyngeal swabs • Chest radiograph may show a shaggy right heart border • Leukocytosis may be present on CBC
Treatment	Azithromycin,* 10 mg/kg/dose PO × 1 on day 1, then 5 mg/kg/dose PO daily × 4 days *or* Clarithromycin,† 15 mg/kg/day PO in divided doses BID × 7 days *or* Erythromycin ethyl succinate,‡ 40 mg/kg/day in divided doses QID × 14 days **Macrolide allergy:** Trimethoprim–sulfamethoxazole,§ 8 mg/kg/day PO in divided doses BID × 14 days

* For infants less than 6 months of age, use 10 mg/kg/dose PO daily for 5 days.

† Not recommended for use in infants less than 6 months of age.

‡ Linked to infantile hypertrophic pyloric stenosis in infants less than 1 month of age.

§ Contraindicated in infants less than 2 months of age.

4. Obtain a CT scan in stable patients to look for retropharyngeal cellulitis.
5. Promptly intubate patients in respiratory distress.

Pertussis

Epidemiology and Microbiology

Pertussis, or whooping cough, is an acute infection of the respiratory tract caused by *Bordetella pertussis*. There are other organisms that may cause a similar clinical syndrome, such as *Bordetella parapertussis*, adenovirus, or chlamydia species. Following the introduction of immunization in the mid-1940s, pertussis incidence declined. However, since then, an increase in disease incidence has been documented.

Clinical Features

Pertussis can be divided into three phases: the first phase (catarrhal) usually is characterized by mild cough, conjunctivitis, and coryza and may last 1 to 2 weeks (see Table 54.5). The second phase, the paroxysmal phase, is characterized by a worsening cough for 2 to 4 weeks. The classic description of the cough in this phase is after a spasmodic cough, the sudden inflow of air produces a "whoop." In infants, the cough is usually a staccato cough with no whoop, and they may present with apneic episodes. Post-tussive emesis is also very common. Fever is rare. Conjunctival hemorrhages and facial petechiae may be caused by harsh coughing. The third phase, the convalescent phase, is characterized by a chronic cough that may last several weeks.

Differential Diagnosis

The differential diagnosis for pertussis is extensive, including:

• asthma
• acute sinusitis with post-nasal drip
• gastroesophageal reflux
• foreign body aspiration
• pneumonia
• bronchiolitis
• tuberculosis
• cystic fibrosis
• other viral illnesses (rhinovirus, adenovirus, RSV, etc.)

Key clinical questions that help to distinguish pertussis include:

• Was the coughing spell prolonged?
• Did the infant have tachypnea?
• Was there a preceding viral illness?
• Is the patient vaccinated?

Laboratory and Radiographic Findings

Bordetella pertussis is a gram-negative, pleomorphic bacterium that can be cultured, though culture is gradually being replaced by polymerase chain reaction (PCR) testing of nasopharyngeal specimens. The chest radiograph in a patient with pertussis is of minimal benefit as it is usually normal, though it may infrequently show a shaggy right heart border. Patients with pertussis may have a lymphocytosis on complete blood count. The leukocytosis may reach 20,000 to 50,000/mm^3; however, this finding is not often seen in children less than 6 months of age. In infants, lymphocytic leukocytosis with pulmonary infiltrates is associated with poor prognosis.

Treatment and Prophylaxis

By the time the paroxysmal phase has begun, treatment has little effect on the clinical course of pertussis. However, treatment should be started in all patients presenting within 3 to 4 weeks of symptom onset to prevent disease spread. Treatment options are erythromycin, azithromycin, or clarithromycin. Trimethoprim-sulfamethoxazole may be used for patients with an allergy to macrolides. Erythromycin use has been associated with a risk of pyloric stenosis when used in infants less than 1 month of age.

Complications and Admission Criteria

Major complications of pertussis infection include pneumonia (20%), encephalopathy and seizures (1%), failure to thrive, and death (0.3%). Pneumonia accounts for 90% of deaths from pertussis. Secondary complications of severe coughing and increased intrathoracic pressure include intracranial hemorrhage, diaphragmatic rupture, pneumothorax, and rectal prolapse. Patients less than 6 months of age with severe symptoms of pertussis generally warrant hospital admission.

Infection Control

Patients with pertussis should be placed in respiratory isolation to prevent transmission. Prophylaxis is recommended for household contacts. Exposed children less than 7 years of age who are unimmunized or have received fewer than four doses of the pertussis vaccine should be evaluated for vaccine initiation or boosting.

Bronchiolitis

Epidemiology

Bronchiolitis is an infection of the upper and lower respiratory tract causing marked inflammation and obstruction of the smaller airways. Although it may occur in all age groups, incidence decreases with age, as the larger airways of older children and adults better accommodate mucosal edema. Severe symptoms are usually seen in children under the age of 2 years. There are approximately 125,000 hospitalizations per year with 80% of admissions occurring in children less than 1 year of age. The most common cause of bronchiolitis is RSV, isolated in 75% of the children less than 2 years of age who are hospitalized for bronchiolitis. Other causes include parainfluenza virus types 1 and 3, influenza B, adenovirus type 1, 2, and 5, *Mycoplasma*, rhinovirus, enterovirus, and herpes simplex virus. In temperate climates, RSV epidemics begin in winter and last until late spring, whereas parainfluenza occurs in the fall.

Clinical Features

Patients with bronchiolitis initially develop mild rhinorrhea, cough, and low-grade fever over the course of 2 to 3 days (see Table 54.6). The illness progresses to an increased cough, which is often paroxysmal, post-tussive emesis, respiratory distress, poor feeding, and increased fussiness. Respiratory distress in these children manifests as tachypnea with respiratory rates as high as 80 to 100 breaths per minute, nasal flaring, intercostal and supraclavicular retractions, apnea, grunting, and cyanosis. Hypoxia may be due to ventilation-perfusion mismatch. Other associated findings are tachycardia and dehydration. The natural course of the illness is about 7 to 10 days, but can last several weeks to a month, and reinfection is possible.

Table 54.6 Clinical Features: Bronchiolitis

Pathogens	Most common cause is RSV Parainfluenza virus types 1 and 3 Influenza B Adenovirus type 1, 2, and 5 *Mycoplasma* Rhinovirus Enterovirus Herpes simplex virus
Signs and symptoms	• Initially, mild rhinorrhea, cough, and low-grade fever • Progresses to increased cough • Develops post-tussive emesis, respiratory distress, poor feeding • Respiratory distress with tachypnea
Laboratory and radiographic findings	• If necessary, may do a rapid ELISA to test for RSV • Chest radiographs may help rule out complications (atelectasis, pneumonia, hyperinflation) • Consider UA and culture for RSV in infants <60 days old
Treatment	• Mostly supportive care with oxygen, hydration, and nasal suctioning • Consider beta-agonists, racemic epinephrine, and steroids in select patients
UA – urinalysis.	

Differential Diagnosis

The differential diagnosis of tachypnea and wheezing with preceding upper respiratory symptoms in a child less than 1 year of age must include:

- pneumonia
- asthma
- congestive heart failure
- foreign body aspiration

Key features that distinguish bronchiolitis from other respiratory problems are:

- upper respiratory tract symptoms with marked nasal congestion
- wheezing

Laboratory and Radiographic Findings

The diagnosis of bronchiolitis in the acute care setting is a clinical one, so routine testing for RSV is not necessary, because it does not change treatment in most cases. In infants or children at high risk for complications, the work-up may include a nasopharyngeal swab for a rapid ELISA to test for RSV. Although a routine chest radiograph is not necessary, it often shows hyperinflation with flattening of the diaphragm and may be helpful in ruling out complications such as atelectasis, hyperinflation, or pneumonia (see Figure 54.4).

Importantly, positive RSV testing in very young febrile infants does not mitigate the need for full evaluation of other causes of fever. It has been shown, for example, that the prevalence of urinary tract infection (UTI) in febrile RSV-positive

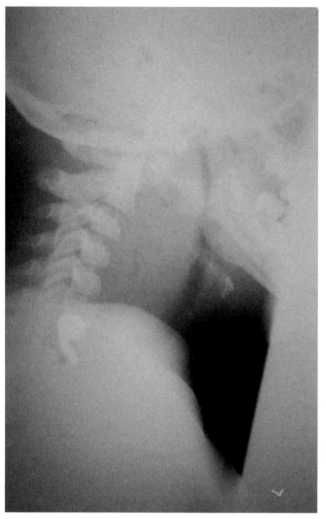

Figure 54.4 Retropharyngeal abscess with widened prevertebral space. Courtesy of Rady Children's Hospital, San Diego Radiology Department.

patients less than 60 days of age is around 2 to 5%, and therefore urinalysis and/or culture may be warranted.

Treatment and Prophylaxis

The mainstay of treatment of bronchiolitis is supportive care, including hydration, oxygenation, and nasal suction, and endotracheal intubation may be necessary in severe respiratory distress. Many therapies have been studied including epinephrine, beta2 agonist bronchodilators, corticosteroids, and ribavirin, but little evidence supports a routine role in management. Nebulized hypertonic saline has recently been demonstrated to reduce the length of hospitalization.

Deep airway suctioning is extremely helpful in infants who present with acute distress. Thick secretions compromise the infant's airway, and this simple therapy can provide immediate relief. Patients with respiratory distress are often quite dehydrated because of insensible losses, and therefore hydration status should be addressed.

Respiratory failure and apnea occur more frequently in children that have underlying conditions such as bronchopulmonary dysplasia, chronic lung disease, congenital heart disease,

or immunodeficiencies. These are a subset of high-risk children that receive palivizumab (Synagis®), a monoclonal antibody that has proven effective in preventing severe bronchiolitis. Palivizumab is given as a monthly IM injection through the RSV season. The American Academy of Pediatrics (AAP) has established guidelines for administration of palivizumab, but in general, it is given to children under the age of 24 months with comorbidities such as prematurity less than 28 weeks, congenital heart disease, severe immune deficiencies, severe neuromuscular disease, or congenital airway abnormalities.

Complications and Admission Criteria

Complications include apnea, respiratory failure, or pneumonia. Patients with persistent hypoxia, respiratory distress, or inability to tolerate fluids, and patients in whom close follow-up cannot be ensured should be admitted. Admission should also be strongly considered in patients less than 2 months of age and premature infants because of the risk of apnea.

Pneumonia

Epidemiology and Microbiology

Community-acquired pneumonia in childhood is a serious infection, leading to significant mortality and morbidity in the United States. The incidence in Europe and North America is about 5 cases per 100 children per year, as defined by fever and acute respiratory symptoms, plus evidence of parenchymal infiltrates on chest radiograph. The most common causative organisms include respiratory viruses and bacteria such as *Mycoplasma*, *Chlamydia trachomatis*, *Streptococcus pneumoniae*, *Staphylococcus aureus*, and *Haemophilus influenzae*, including non-typable strains. The relative frequency of these organisms varies greatly with age and is different for infants, toddlers, and school-age children.

Clinical Features

The clinical features of pneumonia depend on the causative organism, the age of the patient, and the presence of immunosuppression or comorbid disease. Bacterial pneumonia generally has an abrupt onset with fever and chills, productive cough, and chest pain (see Table 54.7). Frequently, respiratory rate and work of breathing are increased, and have been studied as clinical predictors of pneumonia. Upper-lobe pneumonias may evoke suspicion for meningitis as pain may radiate to the neck (see Figure 54.5). The presence of vague abdominal pain and fever should also raise the suspicion for pneumonia. Wheezing is typically associated with viral, *Mycoplasma*, or chlamydial pneumonias.

Differential Diagnosis

Included in the differential are:

- airway foreign body
- aspiration syndromes
- bronchiectasis
- bronchitis

Table 54.7 Clinical Features: Pneumonias

Organisms	Viruses (e.g. influenza, parainfluenza, RSV)
	Mycoplasma
	Chlamydia trachomatis
	Streptococcus pneumoniae
	Staphylococcus aureus
	Haemophilus influenzae
Signs and symptoms	• Fever, chills, productive cough, chest pain (especially bacterial pneumonia)
	• Tachypnea, increased work of breathing
	• Wheezing
	• Abdominal pain and fever
	• Radiating pain to neck (especially upper lobe pneumonias)
Laboratory and radiographic findings	• CBC may show leukocytosis
	• CXR infiltrate
	• Mycoplasma IgM

CXR – chest x-ray.

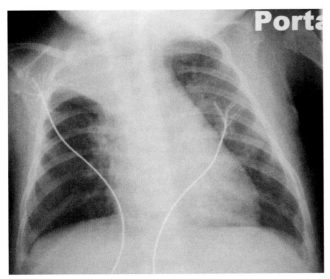

Figure 54.5 Bronchiolitis with right upper lobe atelectasis.
Courtesy of John Amberg, MD.

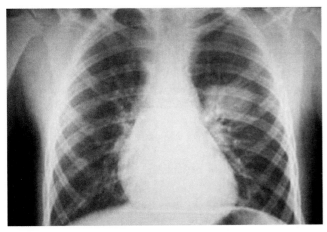

Figure 54.6 Lingular infiltrate.
Courtesy of John Kanegaye, MD.

- reflux
- Goodpasture's syndrome
- hemosiderosis
- congestive heart failure
- pertussis
- pulmonary sequestration
- cystic fibrosis

Key features that may help to distinguish pneumonia are:

- fever
- cough
- infiltrates on radiographs

Laboratory and Radiographic Findings

A peripheral complete blood count may show leukocytosis; however, a normal white blood cell count does not exclude the possibility of bacterial pneumonia. While confirmatory chest X-ray findings are not required to make the diagnosis of pneumonia, particularly in relatively well-appearing children with a consistent clinical presentation, radiographs are generally recommended in the emergency setting, especially in clinically severe disease. Chest X-ray findings include segmental consolidation, diffuse interstitial infiltrate, spherical consolidation, and pleural effusion. Decubitus chest radiographs are helpful in the evaluation of pleural effusions. Children who are dehydrated may not have an infiltrate on initial radiography, and repeat radiography after hydration may be necessary. Serologic tests (e.g. *Mycoplasma* IgM assay) may be helpful.

Treatment and Prophylaxis

Selection of empiric antimicrobial therapy is based on the patient's age and the most likely pathogens in that age group, and whether treatment is on an inpatient or outpatient basis (see Table 54.8). For all pneumonia, supportive care should be initiated with hydration, oxygenation, and continuous cardio-respiratory monitoring for ill-appearing children. Children with large pleural effusions who are ill-appearing or immunocompromised should undergo thoracentesis and chest tube placement. For infants less than 2 months of age, blood, urine, and cerebrospinal fluid cultures should be obtained. Otherwise, blood cultures are rarely positive in pediatric pneumonia. Bronchodilators and steroids should be considered in patients with wheezing or a history of reactive airway disease. An arterial or venous blood gas should be obtained in ill-appearing children and infants in respiratory distress. Endotracheal intubation followed by mechanical ventilation should be initiated in children with respiratory failure.

Complications and Admission Criteria

Infants less than 3 months of age with peumonia should be admitted for intravenous antibiotics because of their high risk for associated sepsis and meningitis. Other criteria for admission include persistent hypoxia, inability to tolerate fluids, outpatient antibiotic failure, or any difficulty ensuring close follow-up. Complications include bacteremia, with associated meningitis, pericarditis, epiglottitis, or septic arthritis.

Table 54.8 Pneumonia Treatment Based on Age and Type

Age	Treatment	Organism
Birth to 1 month	**Inpatient:** Ampicillin* *plus* Gentamicin*	Group B *Streptococcus* Gram-negative enteric bacteria Cytomegalovirus *Listeria monocytogenes*
1 month to 6 months	**Inpatient:** Ceftriaxone 50 mg/kg/dose IV every 24 hours For chlamydia add Azithromycin 10 mg/kg/dose PO/IV daily Dose varies based on severity: Mild – 10 mg/kg on day 1, followed by 5 mg/kg/day on days 2–5 Moderate to severe – 10 mg/kg/day on days 1 and 2, followed by 5 mg/kg/day on days 3–5	*Chlamydia trachomatis* RSV Parainfluenza 3 *Streptococcus pneumoniae* *Bordetella pertussis* *Staphylococcus aureus*
>6 months	**Inpatient:** Ceftriaxone 50 mg/kg/dose IV every 24 hours *plus* Azithromycin 10 mg/kg/dose PO/IV daily **Outpatient:** Amoxicillin 90 mg/kg/day PO in divided doses TID *or* Cefdinir 7 mg/kg/dose PO BID *or* Azithromycin 10 mg/kg/dose PO × 1 on day 1, then 5 mg/kg/dose PO daily × 4 days	RSV Parainfluenza 3 *Streptococcus pneumoniae* *Bordetella pertussis* *Staphylococcus aureus* *Chlamydia trachomatis*

* Neonatal dosing and frequency must be adjusted for weight, postnatal age, and gestational age; consult institutional guidelines for specific dosing recommendations.

Refer to Chapter 46 for oseltamivir, zanamivir, or peramivir selection and dosing for suspected influenza.

Infection Control

Universal precautions should be maintained. A patient should be placed in respiratory isolation in a negative-pressure room if tuberculosis is suspected.

Pearls and Pitfalls

1. Once epiglottis is suspected, minimize patient anxiety.
2. If the patient is in extremis, immediate orotracheal intubation should be performed, preferably with the help of an anesthesiologist or otolaryngologist. If the patient is unable to be intubated, then bag-valve-mask ventilation may still be helpful. Typically high pressures are necessary and therefore a pneumothorax may subsequently occur.
3. If the patient is stable, then the preferred examination and intervention area is the operating room.
4. For patients with suspected epiglottitis, starting an intravenous (IV) line or obtaining blood cultures may exacerbate the patient's condition, and these tests should not be performed in the initial stages of evaluation and treatment.
5. In suspected epiglottitis, treatment should not be delayed for radiographs.
6. Consider anatomical abnormalities or foreign body in patients with recurrent croup.
7. Always administer concurrent steroids to patients ill enough to require nebulized epinephrine.
8. Observe all children receiving nebulized epinephrine for at least 2 to 3 hours.
9. Treat patients with mild croup with dexamethasone to reduce morbidity.
10. Bacterial tracheitis should be considered in an ill-appearing child with high fever and croup-like symptoms that are refractory to conventional treatment with racemic epinephrine and corticosteroids.
11. Intubate patients with bacterial tracheitis promptly.
12. At minimum, an endotracheal tube size smaller than estimated for patient size should be used and suction should be readily available.
13. As in epiglottitis, do not send the patient out of the ED for radiographs.
14. Palpation of a retropharyngeal abscess is not recommended as rupture may occur.
15. Peripheral white blood cell count is neither sensitive nor specific in the diagnosis of RPA.
16. Ensure correct positioning of the child for the lateral neck radiograph. Flexion or persistent crying can give the illusion of a large retropharyngeal space (false positive).
17. Obtain a CT scan in stable patients to look for retropharyngeal cellulitis.
18. Promptly intubate patients in respiratory distress from an RPA.
19. Pertussis should be suspected in infants presenting with apnea or cyanosis after episodes of prolonged coughing.
20. Always treat household contacts who have been exposed to pertussis.

21. Deep suctioning can help in the immediate management of infants with bronchiolitis.
22. Insensible losses contribute significantly to dehydration in infants and small children with respiratory distress.
23. Infants less than 2 months of age are at risk for apnea in the setting of bronchiolitis.
24. Chest radiograph may help rule out other causes of respiratory distress, such as foreign body ingestions, cardiac disease, and pneumothorax.
25. Maintain a high index of suspicion for pneumonia in a child with abdominal or neck pain.
26. Ensure adequate hydration because insensible losses are significant in infants and children with respiratory distress.

References

Chub-Uppakarn, S. and Sangsupawanich, P. A randomized comparison of dexamethasone 0.15 mg/kg versus 0.6 mg/kg for the treatment of moderate to severe croup. *Int. J. Pediatr. Otorhinolaryngol.* 2007; 71(3): 473–7.

Cooper, W. O., Griffin, M. R., Arbogast, P., *et al.* Very early exposure to erythromycin and infantile hypertrophic pyloric stenosis. *Arch. Pediatr. Adolesc. Med.* 2002; 156(7): 647–50.

Craig, F. W. and Schunk, J. E. Retropharyngeal abscess in children: clinical presentation, utility of imaging, and current management. *Pediatrics* 2003; 111(6 Pt. 1): 1394–8.

Dobrovoljac, M. and Geelhoed, G. C. 27 years of croup: an update highlighting the effectiveness of 0.15 mg/kg of dexamethasone. *Emerg. Med. Australas.* 2009; 21(4): 309–14.

Donaldson, D., Poleski, D., Knipple, E., *et al.* Intramuscular versus oral dexamethasone for the treatment of moderate-to-severe croup: a randomized, double blind trial. *Acad. Emerg. Med.* 2003; 10(1): 16–21.

Greenberg, D. P., von Konig, C. H., and Heininger, U. Health burden of pertussis in infants and children. *Pediatr. Infect. Dis. J.* 2005; 24(5 Supp): S39–43.

Gupta, V. K. and Cheifitz, I. M. Heliox administration in the pediatric intensive care unit: an evidence-based review. *Pediatr. Crit. Care Med.* 2005; 6(2): 204–11.

King, V. J., Viswanathan, M., Bordley, W. C., *et al.* Pharmacologic treatment of bronchiolitis in infants and children: a systematic review. *Arch. Pediatr. Adolesc. Med.* 2004; 158(2): 127–37.

Luo, Z., Fu, Z., Liu, E., *et al.* Nebulized hypertonic saline treatment in hospitalized children with moderate to severe viral bronchiolitis. *Clin. Microbiol. Infect.* 2011; 17(12): 1829–33.

Mansbach, J. M., Edmond, J. A., and Camargo, C. A. Bronchiolitis in U.S. emergency departments 1992 to 2000: epidemiology and practice variation. *Pediatr. Emerg. Care* 2005; 21(4): 242–7.

Melendez, E. and Harper, M. B. Utility of sepsis evaluation in infants 90 days of age or younger with fever and clinical bronchiolitis. *Pediatr. Infect. Dis. J.* 2003; 22(12): 1053–6.

Neto, G. M., Kentab, O., Klassen, T. P., and Osmond, M. H. A randomized controlled trial of mist in the acute treatment of moderate croup. *Acad. Emerg. Med.* 2002; 9(9): 873–9.

Plint, A. C., Johnson, D. W., and Wiebe, N. Practice variation among pediatric emergency departments in the treatment of bronchiolitis. *Acad. Emerg. Med.* 2004; 11(4): 353–60.

Scolnik, D. and Coates, A. L. Controlled delivery of high vs. low humidity vs. mist therapy for croup in emergency departments: a randomized controlled trial. *JAMA* 2006; 295(11): 1274–80.

Shah, S. S., Alpern, E. R., Zwerling, L., *et al.* Risk of bacteremia in young children with pneumonia treated as outpatients. *Arch. Pediatr. Adolesc. Med.* 2003; 157(4): 389–92.

Zorc, J. J., Levine, D. A., Platt, S. L., *et al.* Multicenter RSV-SBI Study Group of the Pediatric Emergency Medicine Collaborative Research Committee of the American Academy of Pediatrics. *Pediatrics* 2005; 116(3): 644–8.

Chapter 55

Pediatric Urinary Tract Infections

Jeffrey Bullard-Berent and Steven Bin

Outline

Introduction and Microbiology

Urinary tract infections (UTIs) are a common problem in pediatric patients and an important cause of acute and chronic morbidity. Acute care providers should be well versed in the recognition, basic work-up, and management of this common problem. Although controversy exists in some aspects of the diagnosis, duration of treatment, post-diagnosis imaging, antibiotic prophylaxis, and surgical recommendations, these common infections must be recognized and treated expediently in the acute care setting.

Ascending infections predominate among pediatric UTI, with *Escherichia coli* causing 60 to 80% of cases. In neonates, group B *Streptococcus* should be considered if mothers are colonized. Other pathogens include *Proteus* (more commonly in boys and children with renal stones), *Klebsiella*, *Enterococcus*, and coagulase-negative *Staphylococcus*.

Epidemiology

In the first 8 years of life, 7 to 8% of girls and 2% of boys will have a urinary tract infection. At all ages, girls are more likely to have UTIs than boys, with 3% of girls and 1% of boys being diagnosed with UTI before puberty. The prevalence of urinary tract infection in febrile young children aged 2 months to 2 years without a clinically apparent source is approximately 3 to 7% (see Table 55.1).

Specific risk factors for UTI are dependent on gender. Bathing and wiping patterns have not proven to increase or decrease risk for UTI.

Clinical Features

The American Academy of Pediatrics recommends consideration of urinary tract infection in all febrile children 2 months to 2 years of age, particularly in the toxic-appearing patient. Fever may be the *only* symptom in young children, so consideration of UTI must be part of every work-up of pediatric fever. It is often difficult to differentiate cystitis from pyelonephritis in children, but 60% of children with febrile UTI have signs of pyelonephritis by renal nuclear scans. In females under 2 years of age, the risk likelihood of UTI is increased with the following risk factors: age below 12 months, caucasian, temperature >39°C, fever duration more than 2 days, and absence of another source for fever. In males under 2 years of age, the risk factors include: non-black, temperature >39°C, fever duration more than 24 hours, and uncircumcised. The age of the child greatly affects the clinical presentation (see Table 55.2). In general, older children may articulate symptoms of urinary complaints, whereas infants and small children will present in a myriad of ways.

Differential Diagnosis

Infants and Small Children Younger than 2 Years

Differential diagnosis in febrile infants and toddlers is broad and includes:

- occult bacteremia
- bacterial or viral meningitis
- pneumonia
- acute gastroenteritis
- viral syndromes
- otitis media

It is important to note that the presence of other illnesses that can cause fever (e. g. influenza and bronchiolitis) reduce the probability of UTI, but do not exclude the possibility of a coexistent UTI. Other important diagnoses that should be considered include:

Table 55.1 Prevalence of UTI in Febrile Infants and Children

• 0–3 months	7.2%
• Girls	7.5%
• Circumcised boys	2.4%
• Uncumcised boys	20.1%
• 3–6 months	6.6%
• Girls	5.7%
• Boys	3.3%
• 6–12 months	5.4%
• Girls	8.3%
• Boys	1.7%
• 12–24 months	4.5%
• Girls	2.1%
• Circumcised Boys <1 year	<1%

- vaginitis
- irritant or chemical urethritis
- vaginal foreign body
- sexually transmitted diseases

Older Children

Because older children are better able to differentiate urinary symptoms, the differential includes:

- vaginitis
- vaginal foreign body
- urethritis including sexually transmitted diseases
- ureteral calculi
- dysfunctional elimination
- vulvar ulcerative disease (herpes infections, Behçet's disease)

Children with appendicitis, group A streptococcal disease, and Kawasaki disease can present with fever, pyuria, and abdominal pain. Dysuria may also accompany other more occult sources of fever, including malignancy and autoimmune disease.

Laboratory Diagnosis

The diagnosis of UTI requires a positive urine culture (50,000 CFU/mL) in addition to evidence of pyuria and/or bacteriuria on urinalysis. Urinalysis alone is not sufficient for diagnosing UTI, but can help identify febrile children who should receive empiric antimicrobial treatment while awaiting culture results. The dipstick leukocyte esterase and nitrite test, and microscopy for leukocytes and bacteria can be used to predict culture results (see Table 55.3).

Transurethral bladder catheterization and suprapubic aspiration are the preferred methods of urine specimen collection for children <2 years of age. Suprapubic aspiration is recommended when catheterization is not feasible (e.g. a male infant with phimosis or female with labial adhesions). Bag-collected specimens generally have unacceptable rates of contamination with a false-positive rate of up to 85% and are generally not recommended; however, a negative culture is strong evidence that a UTI is not present.

Table 55.2 Clinical Features: Urinary Tract Infection – Pediatric

Organisms	*Escherichia coli* Group B *Streptococcus* *Klebsiella* *Enterococcus* Coagulase-negative *Staphylococcus*
Clinical presentation	**Young children <2 years old:** • fever • vomiting • diarrhea • irritability • poor feeding • suprapubic tenderness • change in voiding pattern • conjugated hyperbilirubinemia **Children >2 years old:** • fever • dysuria or crying with urination • abdominal pain • urinary frequency • new onset urinary incontinence • hypertension
Laboratory findings (see Table 55.3)	• urine dipstick: positive nitrite, positive • leukocyte esterase • urine microscopy: pyuria and bacteriuria • urine culture: greater than 50,000 CFU/mL Urine obtained via catheter or suprapubic aspiration
Treatment	**Empiric parenteral therapy: infants* <2 months, "toxic" appearing, unable to retain oral intake** Ampicillin 50–200 mg/kg/day divided every 6–8 hours* *plus* Gentamicin 7.5mg/kg/day divided every 8 hours* **Oral therapy: 2–24 months, non-toxic (for 7–14 days)** Cefdinir 7 mg/kg/dose PO BID *or* Cefixime 8 mg/kg/dose PO daily *or* Amoxicillin–clavulanate 20–40 mg/kg/day PO in divided doses TID *or* Trimethoprim–sulfamethoxazole 6–12 mg/kg/day PO in divided doses BID

* Neonatal dosing and frequency must be adjusted for weight, postnatal age, and gestational age; consult institutional guidelines for specific dosing recommendations.

CFU – colony-forming units.

The decision to perform imaging studies to evaluate for vesicoureteral reflux after the first febrile UTI remains controversial, and can usually be deferred to the primary pediatrician. Results will not change clinical management in a febrile child with a primary UTI. The American Academy of Pediatrics recommends a renal and bladder ultrasound (RBUS) for all children aged 2 to 24 months following their first febrile UTI. An update to the AAP guidelines means that they now do not recommend performing voiding cystourethrography (VCUG)

Table 55.3 Diagnostic Value of Urinalysis Tests

Test	Sensitivity (Range) %	Specificity (Range) %
Leukocyte esterase test	83 (67–94)	78 (64–92)
Nitrite test	53 (15–82)	98 (90–100)
Leukocyte esterase or nitrite test	93 (90–100)	72 (58–91)
Microscopy, WBCs (>5/HPF)	73 (32–100)	81 (45–98)
Microscopy, bacteria	81 (16–99)	83 (11–100)
Leukocyte esterase test, nitrite test, or microscopy positive	99.8 (99–100)	70 (60–92)
CFU – colony-forming units.		

routinely after the first febrile UTI unless the RBUS reveals hydronephrosis, scarring, or other findings that would suggest obstructive uropathy or vesicoureteral reflux.

Treatment and Prophylaxis

Empiric treatment pending culture results is recommended for febrile children with suspected UTI and a positive urinalysis. A well-appearing febrile patient with negative urinalysis may follow up with their primary pediatrician for treatment pending urine cultures.

The choice of antibiotics should be based on local antimicrobial susceptibility patterns (if available). Most children older than 2 months who are not vomiting can be treated orally. Cephalosporins, amoxicillin–clavulanic acid, or trimethoprim-sulfamethoxazole are the oral antibiotics most often used (see Table 55.2, Treatment). There is evidence that short-course antimicrobial therapy (1 to 3 days) is inferior to standard duration therapy (7 to 14 days); therefore, the minimal duration selected should be at least 7 to 10 days. Generally, patients with suspected UTI should be started on antibiotic therapy and followed up within 24 to 48 hours for re-evaluation and culture results.

The AAP guidelines do not recommend prophylactic antimicrobials following the first febrile UTI in children aged 2 to 24 months.

Complications and Admission Criteria

Early complications of UTI can include perinephric and retroperitoneal abscesses, pyonephrosis (collection of purulent material in the urinary collecting system), and urinary calculi secondary to stasis or urease-splitting bacteria. Long-term complications include recurrent infection, renal scarring, hypertension, and renal damage. Among children with evidence of pyelonephritis, 10 to 40% will have permanent renal scarring. Retrospective studies suggest a high rate of chronic renal disease, hypertension, and pre-eclampsia. There are few prospective studies of the long-term consequences of UTI, but these suggest a low rate of long-term disease, though they are limited by short study durations. The risk of long-term renal damage is highest in infants and small children (<2 years old) and the diagnosis of UTI in this population can help identify patients with urinary system obstructive anomalies or vesicoureteral reflux (VUR).

Admission is indicated for all toxic-appearing children and in those in whom sepsis is a concern. Other indications for admission include:

- age <2 months
- dehydration requiring intravenous rehydration
- excessive vomiting precluding oral antibiotic therapy
- poor social situation or other barriers to close follow-up
- immunocompromised patient

Pearls and Pitfalls

1. Consider urinary tract infection in all febrile children.
2. Transurethral bladder catheterization and suprapubic aspiration are the preferred methods of urine specimen collection for children <2 years of age.
3. The diagnosis of UTI requires a positive urine culture (50,000 CFU/mL) in addition to evidence of pyuria and/or bacteriuria on urinalysis.
4. Compared to parenteral therapy, oral antimicrobial therapy is as effective in treating UTI.
5. Ensure follow-up within 24 to 48 hours.

References

Finnell, S. M., Carroll, A. E., and Downs, S. M. Subcommittee on Urinary Tract Infection. Technical report – diagnosis and management of an initial UTI in febrile infants and young children *Pediatrics* 2011; 128(3): e749–70.

Montini, G., Tullus, K., and Hewitt, I. Febrile urinary tract infections in children. *N. Engl. J. Med.* 2011; 365(3): 239–50.

Newman, D. H., Shreves, A. E., and Runde, D. P. Pediatric urinary tract infection: does the evidence support aggressively pursuing the diagnosis? *Ann. Emerg. Med.* 2013; 61(5): 559–65.

RIVUR Trial Investigators, Hoberman, A., Greenfield, S. P., Mattoo, T. K., *et al.* Antimicrobial prophylaxis for children with vesicoureteral reflux. *N. Engl. J. Med.* 2014; 370(25): 2367–76.

Roberts, K. B. Urinary tract infection: clinical practice guideline for the diagnosis and management of the initial UTI in febrile infants and children 2 to 24 months. *Pediatrics* 2011; 128(3): 595–610.

Shaikh, N., Borrell, J. L., Evron, J., and Leeflang, M. M. Procalcitonin, C-reactive protein, and erythrocyte sedimentation rate for the diagnosis of acute pyelonephritis in children. *Cochrane Database Syst. Rev.* 2015; 1: CD009185.

Shaikh, N., Craig, J. C., Rovers, M. M., *et al.* Identification of children and adolescents at risk for renal scarring after a first urinary tract infection: a meta-analysis with individual patient data. *JAMA Pediatr.* 2014; 168(10): 893–900.

Shaikh, N., Morone, N. E., Lopez, J., *et al.* Does this child have a urinary tract infection? *JAMA* 2007; 298(24): 2895–904.

Stein, R., Dogan, H. S., Hoebeke, P., *et al.* Urinary tract infections in children: EAU/ESPU guidelines. *Eur. Urol.* 2014; 67(3): 546–58.

Strohmeier, Y., Hodson, E. M., Willis, N. S., *et al.* Antibiotics for acute pyelonephritis in children. *Cochrane Database Syst. Rev.* 2014; 7: CD003772.

Subcommittee on Urinary Tract Infection, Steering Committee on Quality Improvement and Management, and Roberts, K. B. Urinary tract infection: clinical practice guideline for the diagnosis and management of the initial UTI in febrile infants and children 2 to 24 months. *Pediatrics* 2011; 128(3): 595–610.

Chapter

56

Bites (Dogs, Cats, Rodents, Lagomorphs)

Hugh West and Sukhjit S. Takhar

Introduction

Animal and human bites are a common problem in the United States and elsewhere. Acute bite injuries range from minor subcutaneous ecchymoses to life-threatening injuries. Even minor bite wounds are extremely prone to infection. This chapter will focus on treatment of acute bite injuries and preventing infectious complications, as well as treatment of established bite wound infections.

Much has been learned about the microbiology of infected dog, cat, and human bites (see Boxes 56.1 and 56.2). Unlike typical cellulitis in which the organism is usually beta-hemolytic *Streptococcus* or *Staphylococcus aureus*, bite wounds tend to have a more complex microbiology derived from the oral flora of the biting animal. These infections tend to be polymicrobial with various streptococci, *Staphylococcus* spp., gram-negative species, and oral anaerobes. The average infection yields five species of bacteria.

Pasteurella species are the most common pathogens in dog and cat bites. They are found in approximately 75% of cat bites and 50% of dog bites. *Pasteurella* species are found in the oral cavity and gastrointestinal tract of many animals, and may cause a rapid-onset and rapidly progressive infection. The most common infections due to *Pasteurella* involve soft-tissue, but endocarditis, meningitis, septicemia, and pneumonia have all been reported.

Streptococci and staphylococci were found in approximately 40% of bite infections from both dogs and cats. Anaerobic bacteria such as *Bacteroides*, *Fusobacterium*, *Prevotella*, and *Peptostreptococcus* species are often present in mixed infections and foul-smelling wounds. *Capnocytophaga canimorsus* has been associated with severe infections, especially in patients with comorbid conditions such as asplenia, and those on corticosteroids or with liver disease. *Capnocytophaga* species are involved in approximately 5% of dog and cat bite infections.

Infected human bite wounds also tend to be polymicrobial. In the largest case series, an average of four organisms were found in infected human bite wounds. The most common was *Streptococcus anginosus*, which is a *viridans*-like organism with a tendency to form abscesses. *Staphylococcus aureus* was the next most common organism. Anaerobic bacteria are present in about 50% of human bites, and have a tendency to produce beta-lactamase. One major difference in the microbiology of human bite wounds is the presence of *Eikenella corrodens* and the absence of *Pasteurella multocida*. *Eikenella* is a slow-growing gram-negative rod that is often found in combination with other isolates. Much like *Pasteurella*, *Eikenella* is usually sensitive to penicillin and second- or third-generation cephalosporins, while being resistant to first-generation cephalosporins, clindamycin, and oxacillin. Transmission of herpes simplex, hepatitis B and C, and human immunodeficiency virus (HIV) has also been reported from human bites.

Our knowledge of the organisms involved in exotic animal bites is based on case reports and anecdotal data. These reports suggest that exotic animals have oral flora that includes staphylococci, streptococci, and anaerobes, similar to domestic animals. Rodents can transmit a variety of diseases, including rat-bite fever. This rare infection is caused by either *Streptobacillus moniliformis* or *Spirillum minus*. Finally, bites from adult macaque monkeys have been known to transmit the potentially lethal virus Herpesvirus simiae ("monkey B virus").

Epidemiology

Accurate statistics on animal bite injuries are difficult to obtain because of variations in geography, inflicting animals, types of bites, differences in data tracking (e.g. grouping mammalian bites with marine envenomations), and the fact that many bites do not come to medical attention. However, extensive data on dog bites, the most common type of serious bite injury, is collected by the Centers for Disease Control and Prevention

(CDC). The most recent data suggest that approximately 4.5 million bites per year occur in the United States involving nearly 1.5% of the population. Of those, an estimated 885,000 (19%) victims seek medical attention, including over 300,000 emergency department visits.

The incidence of dog bites increases with a dog in the household and increases further yet with multiple dogs. One study quoted a five times higher incidence of dog bites with two or more dogs in the house. Victims are more often male. Dog breeds responsible for the most fatalities include Pit Bulls (59%), Rottweilers (14%), and numerous other breeds with smaller percentages. The most common fatality scenario in the United States is that of an unrestrained dog on the owner's property.

Cat bites are the second most common domestic animal bite. These account for up to 15% of all bite injuries in various studies. In contrast to the dog bite data, cat bite victims tend to be women. Most of these injuries occur in or near the home of the victim.

Human bites are the third relatively frequent form of bite injuries. They can occur in a variety of ways in all age groups. The most common are simple abrasions due to bites among young children, which generally do not become infected. Most serious bite wounds are the result of aggressive behavior. The "fight-bite" or clenched-fist injury (CFI) occurs over the metacarpophalangeal joint when the patient punches another person in the mouth (see Chapter 35, Hand Infections: Fight Bite, Purulent Tenosynovitis, Felon, and Paronychia). Bites may also occur during sexual or sporting activities and they may be self-inflicted in the psychiatric population. Human bite wounds may be somewhat more frequently associated with infection and other complications. This may be due in part to selection bias in that some patients do not seek medical attention until a complication develops.

The remainder of the spectrum of bite injuries includes a wide range of perpetrators from other domestic pets such as ferrets (the third most popular pet in the United States) to domestic herbivores, pigs, rodents, primates, and animals in the wild. Primate bites are the second most common bite in India. In the United States, primate bites may occur in a university setting (research animals). The severity of the injuries varies widely, but all of these types of bites may lead to infection.

Clinical Features

The majority of dog bites (80%) do not seek medical attention. Delayed presentation of bites with established infection or deep structure injuries occurs commonly. Infection of a dog bite arises from a complex interplay between the breed and size of the dog, the type and location of the injury, and patient comorbidities. At the severe end of the injury spectrum are pediatric patients attacked by large or multiple dogs. The most common injury location varies by age. Children younger than 4 years of age commonly sustain bites to the head and neck. In contrast, more than 80% of injuries in patients over the age of 15 occur in the extremities. As might be expected, the lower extremities are more commonly involved than the upper. Infections are

more common and potentially more serious in bite wounds to the hands and feet. Dog bites may injure underlying anatomic structures such as tendon sheaths, tendons, joints, bones, vessels, and nerves. They may penetrate body cavities, puncture the skull, cause open fractures, and result in severe infections such as osteomyelitis.

Cats have slender, sharper canine teeth that can cause deep puncture wounds of a smaller diameter. These make the initial wound management difficult in terms of irrigation and debridement. Most cat bites involve the hand and upper extremity, and they appear to be more likely than dog bites to become infected. Although the true incidence of infection is difficult to determine, studies indicate that up to 67% of cat bites become infected. While it seems reasonable to conclude that cat bites are more likely than dog bites to become infected, there is little reliable data to support this position.

Human bites that become infected most frequently involve the hand or upper extremity (65 to 75%). Human bites elsewhere, usually to well-perfused tissues, are no more likely to become infected than non-bite lacerations. The infection rates for human bites to the hand may range from 25 to 50%. These infections of the hand may be severe, with associated purulent tenosynovitis, septic arthritis, and osteomyelitis. The clenched-fist injury (CFI) or "fight bite" is extemely infection prone. The punching mechanism often involves considerable force, resulting in violation of the tendon sheath, tendon, joint space, and bone of the metatarsal phalangeal region by the victim's teeth, which harbor large numbers of bacteria. To complicate matters, patients with a CFI often present in a delayed fashion, with infections that range from early to well-established, and often are not forthcoming about the mechanism of injury. Bites in children may appear as semicircular erythematous or bruised areas; the issue of non-accidental trauma should always be considered in this age group.

Patients presenting soon after an injury are often concerned about cosmesis. The issue of how or whether to proceed with repair of a contaminated bite wound can be difficult. Rabies prophylaxis may be a concern. When the presentation is delayed and the infection established, there may be signs of the inflammatory response as well as proximal lymphangitis and lymphadenopathy. Infections from animal and human bites may develop rapidly, within 12 to 24 hours of the injury. This may be particularly common with cat bite puncture wounds and *Pasteurella* infections. Fortunately, facial injuries are infected less frequently, probably related to the rich vascular supply.

Pain out of proportion to the exam may indicate serious underlying issues such as necrotizing fasciitis or compartment syndrome. Other serious underlying issues may include septic arthritis or osteomyelitis (see Chapters 33, Adult Septic Arthritis; 37, Osteomyelitis; and 12, Bacterial Skin and Soft-Tissue Infections). Immunocompromised patients may present with fulminant sepsis after a bite wound.

Initial Evaluation

Rare life- and limb-threatening injuries may occur and should be managed accordingly. In the majority of cases, these injuries

Box 56.1 Dog and Cat Bites – Selected Microbiology

Pasteurella species:

- gram-negative coccobacillus
- most common cause of dog and cat bite infections
- can be difficult to culture
- rapid development of an intense inflammatory response
- resistant to many antibiotics that are commonly used to treat cellulitis

Streptococcus species:

- usually of the *viridans* group
- normal oral flora of animal

Capnocytophaga canimorsus

- fastidious gram-negative rod
- can cause fatal infections in immunocompromised hosts (asplenia, chronic steroids, or liver disease) characterized by shock, purpuric lesions, DIC, and gangrene at the bite site
- often found in the normal flora of canines and occasionally in other animals

Anaerobes:

- *Fusobacterium, Bacteroides, Porphyromonas, Prevotella, Propionibacterium,* and *Peptostreptococcus* are commonly isolated from bite wounds
- found in approximately 50% of dog bite wounds and 65% of cat bite wounds
- usually part of mixed infections with aerobic organisms
- variably produce penicillinase
- foul-smelling wounds

DIC – disseminated intravascular coagulation.

Box 56.2 Rare Systemic Infections in Human Bites

hepatitis B and C
syphilis
tetanus
herpes simplex virus
HIV

Box 56.3 Initial Evaluation of Bites

History

- type of animal and behavior and vaccination history of animal
- circumstances leading to the injury
- time elapsed since the bite
- existence of antimicrobial allergies
- tetanus immunization status
- associated medical conditions (liver disease, splenectomy, immunosuppressive medications, HIV, lymphedema, diabetes)

Physical Examination

- temperature
- skin exam for edema, tenderness, erythema, warmth, and lymphangitis
- consider a diagram of the wound, noting depth and location
- perform and document a careful vascular and neurologic exam
- joint range of motion and musculoskeletal exam for tendon, muscle, bone, or intra-articular injury

Studies

- anaerobic and aerobic culture of wound if infected
- radiographs of site if suspected fracture or joint involvement, or to rule out foreign body

---

can be ruled out quickly. A careful history of the circumstances of the bite should be taken (see Box 56.3). This includes the circumstances of the injury (a territorial dog vs. a wandering sick animal) and what led up to the bite. History should also include the patient's comorbid conditions and vaccination status.

A careful physical exam should be performed and documented. Distal neurovascular and tendon examination should be included. After an initial sensory exam, the wound should be well anesthetized and irrigated, and the subsequent motor exam and dry-field exploration should be painless. The wound itself should be well visualized under proper lighting. Dry-field examination refers not only to removal of blood from the field, but also serous oozing and any residual irrigation fluid. The field must be dry if the question of deep structure injury is to be addressed adequately. Proximal tourniquets to the extremity

or the digit may be used, and may be kept in place safely for 15 or 20 minutes. Wound exploration should include a search for foreign bodies, tendon sheath or tendon injuries, joint space violations, and bony injuries (such as chip fractures), as well as injuries to vessels or nerves. It is important to examine tendons throughout the full range of motion as a tendon laceration may not be visible in the exam area, depending on the position of the extremity. In CFIs that occur with the fist clenched, the tendon injury may move proximally when the hand is open.

Plain radiographs are indicated if there is any possibility of fracture and foreign body. Significant bites to the scalp, most often in children, may require CT scan or MRI to further characterize injuries. Vascular injuries may require vascular ultrasound or CT angiography and consultation.

Infected purulent wounds should be cultured (anaerobic and aerobic). Gram stain of infected wounds is rarely useful because of the polymicrobial nature of the infections. Cultures of fresh or non-infected wounds is unnecessary. Blood cultures should be obtained in patients who display systemic manifestations of infection.

Treatment

Initial Management and Prophylaxis of Uninfected Wounds

The location and type of wound, the type of animal, and the medical condition of the patient (comorbidity) may influence

Table 56.1 Antimicrobial Treatment and Prophylaxis for Dog, Cat, or Human Bites

Prophylaxis or treatment of mild infection: adult or child with no PCN allergy	Amoxicillin–clavulanate 875/125 mg PO BID (20 mg/kg/dose PO BID in children)
Prophylaxis or treatment of mild infection: adult with PCN allergy	Ciprofloxacin 500 mg PO BID *plus* Clindamycin 450 mg PO TID
Prophylaxis or treatment of mild infection: child with PCN allergy	Clindamycin 10 mg/kg/dose PO TID *plus* Trimethoprim-sulfamethoxazole 5 mg/kg/dose of TMP compnent PO BID
Treatment: adult or child with no PCN allergy	Ampicillin-sulbactam 3 g IV every 6 hours (50 mg/kg/dose IV every 6 hours in children) *or* Ertapenem 1 g IV every 24 hours (15 mg/kg/dose IV every 12 hours in children, with maximum of 500 mg per dose)
Treatment: adult with a PCN allergy	Clindamycin 600 mg IV every 8 hours *plus* Ciprofloxacin 400 mg IV every 12 hours *Alternative:* Ceftriaxone 1 g IV every 24 hours (if non-life-threatening PCN allergy) *plus* Metronidazole 500 mg PO/IV every 8 hours
Treatment: child with a PCN allergy	Clindamycin 10 mg/kg/dose IV every 8 hours *plus* Trimethoprim-sulfamethoxazole 5 mg/kg/dose of TMP component IV every 12 hours
Treatment: pregnant with PCN allergy	Azithromycin 500 mg IV daily *plus* Clindamycin 600 mg IV every 8 hours

IV – intravenous; PCN – penicillin; PO – by mouth; TMP – trimethoprim.

the likelihood of developing an infection. Infections are more common in the very young, the elderly, and the immunocompromised. None of these factors in isolation, however, can predict a subsequent infection and all bite wounds should be treated as extremely infection-prone. Bite wounds often have been inoculated with multiple bacteria, typically oral flora of the biting animal, in high numbers.

The wound should be irrigated immediately with a large amount of saline at high pressure. This will predictably decrease the bacterial load and eliminate most foreign material. Irrigation can be accomplished by using a large syringe attached to an 18-gauge catheter. All visible foreign material should be removed. Devitalized tissue should be debrided. Whether to proceed with primary wound closure and use of prophylactic antibiotics are two common and controversial issues in bite wound management (see Box 56.4).

Primary closure of bite wounds has been evaluated in multiple studies, which generally support primary closure of selected wounds after careful wound preparation. The fundamental issue involves cosmetic impact versus the risk of infection. Shared decision-making with the patient and family is important. Document the discussion of risks and benefits and the patient's preferences. Facial wounds overall have a low risk of infection; cosmesis is a more significant issue and primary closure is often the correct approach. On the other hand, primary closure is not appropriate for puncture wounds and high-risk hand wounds. Primary closure results in better cosmetic outcome, potentially fewer repeat visits, and better protection

of underlying structures, whereas healing by secondary intention tends to result in more scarring and contraction. Closure in the pretibial area may not be possible without causing tension, compromising perfusion and causing necrosis of tissue and infection. Wounds with exposed tendons, vessels, or bone should not be allowed to heal by secondary intention and generally require consultation.

In delayed primary closure, the wound is cleansed and debrided, left open, and then re-evaluated 3 to 4 days later for suturing. Closure at that time may be appropriate if the wound remains clean and uninfected and may give a better cosmetic result than the long process of closure by secondary intention. Wounds that heal by secondary intention granulate and epithelialize from the edges inward and present a very low risk of infection.

The role of antibiotic prophylaxis remains controversial. In general, prophylactic antibiotics are appropriate for patients with significant comorbidity and those with higher risk wounds such as deep punctures of the hand (see Box 56.5). Cat and human bites, especially those of the hand, generally warrant antibiotic prophylaxis. When antibiotic prophylaxis is used, the regimen should be active against *P. multocida* (dog and cat bites) and *Eikenella* (human bites), staphylococci, streptococci, and anaerobes (see Table 56.1). Oral amoxicillin–clavulanic acid is an excellent single agent choice. First-generation cephalosporins, antistaphylococcal penicillins, and clindamycin show poor activity against *Pasteurella* and *Eikenella* in vitro and are not recommended as single agent prophylaxis.

Box 56.4 Management of Early Non-Infected Bites

Wound Care

- irrigation of wound with large amounts of normal saline
- careful debridement of devitalized tissue
- attention to deeper structures and consultation with a specialist as needed
- wound cultures are not indicated for uninfected wounds

Antibiotic Prophylaxis – Consider for

- hand bites
- immunocompromised patients
- proximity to joint, tendon, or other deep structures
- wounds with devitalized tissue
- wounds closed primarily, or prior to delayed primary closure
- cat bites
- human bites

Wound Closure

- consider risk/benefit analysis for the individual wound
- selected facial wounds and those of cosmetic importance may be primarily closed

Systemic Diseases

- tetanus immunization if necessary
- rabies prophylaxis if necessary
- consider possible hepatitis or HIV exposure for human bites

Discharge Instructions

- stress importance of elevating wound
- return early if any signs of infection
- return in 3 to 4 days for consideration of delayed primary closure

Box 56.5 Conditions Predisposing for a Wound Infection

Host Factors

- age <2 and >50 years
- comorbid medical conditions

Location

- wrist, hand, and foot wounds
- scalp wounds in infants and small children (risk of skull injury)
- injury to tendon, joint, bone, or other deep structures

Wound Type

- crush injuries
- puncture wounds

Biting Animal

- human bite
- cat bite

For penicillin-allergic patients, combination therapy with ciprofloxacin and clindamycin may be used. A short course (3 to 5 days) is common practice, though there are no reliable studies to support this timing.

There is limited data to guide prophylactic antimicrobial treatment for bites by other mammals. While penicillin remains the drug of choice for rat bite fever, rat bites generally have a low rate of infection and routine prophylaxis of rat bites has not been shown to be worthwhile. The best way to manage potential Herpesvirus simiae exposure is by prompt and aggressive local wound lavage. This disease may be contracted from Macaque monkeys and has also been called monkey B virus or herpes virus B. The virus has serologic cross-reactivity with HSV-1 (generally oral) and HSV-2 (genital) in humans. The human case fatality rate is approximately 70%. Macaques may be encountered in academic medical centers where they are used as research animals. Management of a Macaque bite should be undertaken in conjunction with local (university) resources and the CDC. Acyclovir or valacyclovir may be given in high-risk exposures.

Animal bites should be considered tetanus-prone wounds. Patients who have not received a booster within 5 years should be reimmunized. Those who have not completed a primary tetanus series of three doses should be given immune globulin (see Chapter 10, Tetanus) as well. Rabies exposure should also be considered. The epidemiology of animal rabies varies by geographic area. In many areas, animal bites are reported to the local health department and this information may assist with decisions regarding rabies prophylaxis (see Chapter 9, Rabies). For a potential hepatitis B exposure related to a human bite, hepatitis B immunoglobulin and immunization may be appropriate. Post-exposure prophylaxis for HIV may be indicated in human bites if the assailant is HIV positive. A baseline HIV test should be drawn and then repeated in 3 to 6 months.

Treatment of Infected Wounds

Many patients with bite wounds present with an established infection. The normal inflammatory response of wound healing can sometimes be difficult to distinguish from infection. Sutures in infected wounds should be removed. Radiographs should be considered, if they have not already been performed, to evaluate for retained foreign body, missed fractures, or early osteomyelitis. An abscess should be drained if present. Surgical consultation may be warranted for drainage of a particularly large abscess or one in proximity to deeper structures. The infected fluid or tissue should be cultured as this may help direct subsequent antibiotic therapy. Closed fist injury infections require orthopedic consultation for exploration and irrigation of the metacarpophalangeal joint.

Cellulitis associated with bite wounds requires antibiotic treatment. Even when successfully drained, an abscess from a bite wound should also be treated with antibiotics. Antimicrobial agents should be chosen to cover *Pasteurella* species (dog and cat bites) and *Eikenella* (human bites), streptococci, staphylococci, and anaerobic organisms (see Table 56.1). If a patient was previously given prophylactic antibiotics, switching to a broader spectrum agent in another antimicrobial class is recommended. For significant infections, the first dose can be given intravenously. Intravenous (IV) ampicillin-sulbactam is an excellent single agent choice. MRSA coverage is not generally considered necessary in bite wounds. However, in the case of a life- or limb-threatening infection, or patients at high risk for MRSA infection (IDU, prior MRSA infections), adding vancomycin can be considered. A treatment course of 7 to 14 days based on the clinical response is appropriate for most bite-related infections. Osteomyelitis usually requires 4 to 6 weeks of intravenous therapy.

Complications and Admission Criteria

Bite wound infections of the hands and feet and those accompanied by fever should generally be admitted. Complications of bite wounds include septic joint, tenosynovitis, and osteomyelitis. Bacteremia from pathogens such as *Pasteurella* species can result in endocarditis and sepsis.

Pearls and Pitfalls

1. Prophylactic antibiotics may be advisable for high-risk bites or in patients with significant comorbidity.
2. Scrupulous, well-anesthetized dry-field examination of bite wounds provides the single golden opportunity to find foreign bodies, bony injuries, tendon lacerations, or joint space violations.
3. The importance of good wound care, tight follow-up, and shared decision-making cannot be overstated.
4. Good documentation that supports the approach taken is important, since some patients with bite wounds will have adverse outcomes regardless of initial management.

References

Abrahamian, F. M. Dog bites: bacteriology, management, and prevention. *Curr. Infect. Dis. Rep.* 2000; 2(5): 446–52.

Bartholomew, C. F. and Jones, A. M. Human bites: a rare risk factor for HIV transmission. *AIDS* 2006; 20(4): 631–2.

Centers for Disease Control and Prevention (CDC). Dog bite prevention (2011), www.cdc.gov/HomeandRecreationalSafety/Dog-Bites/biteprevention.html.

CDC, Nonfatal dog bite-related injuries treated in hospital emergency departments – United States, 2001. *MMWR Morb. Mortal. Wkly. Rep.* 2003; 52(26): 605–10.

Chen, E., Horing, S., Shepherd, S. M., *et al.* Primary closure of mammalian bites. *Acad. Emerg. Med.* 2000; 7(2): 157–61.

DogsBite.org. Dog bite fatalities (2011), www.dogsbite.org/bite-statistics-fatalities.htm (accessed November 30, 2017).

DogsBite.org. Report: U.S. dog bite fatalities January 2006 to December 2008 (2011), www.dogsbite.org/reports/dogsbite-report-us-dog-bite-fatalities-2006–2008.pdf.

Gilchrist, J., Sacks, J. J., White, D., *et al.* Dog bites: still a problem? *Inj. Prev.* 2008; 14(5): 296–301.

Holmquist, L. and Elixhauser, A. Emergency department visits and inpatient stays involving dog bites 2008 Healthcare Cost and Utilization Project (HCUP) Statistical Briefs (November 2010).

Perron, A. D., Miller, M. D., and Brady, W. J. Orthopedic pitfalls in the ED: fight bite. *Am. J. Emerg. Med.* 2002; 20(2):114–17.

Quinn, J. V., McDermott, D., Rossi, J., *et al.* Randomized controlled trial of prophylactic antibiotics for dog bites with refined cost model. *West J. Emerg. Med.* 2010; 11(5): 435–41.

Schalamon, J., Ainoedhofer, H., Singer, G., *et al.* Analysis of dog bites in children who are younger than 17 years. *Pediatrics* 2006; 117(3): e374–9.

Talan, D. A., Abrahamian, F. M., Moran, G. J., *et al.* Clinical presentations and bacteriological analysis of infected human bites presenting to Emergency Departments. *Clin. Infect. Dis.* 2003; 37: 1481–9.

Talan, D. A., Citron, D. M., Abrahamian, F. M., *et al.* Bacteriologic analysis of infected dog and cat bites. *N. Eng. J. Med.* 1999; 340: 85–92.

Additional Readings

Cohen, J. I., Davenport, D. S., Stewart, J. A., *et al.* Recommendations for prevention of and therapy for exposure to B virus (cercopithecine herpesvirus 1). *Clin. Infect. Dis.* 2002; 35(10): 1191–203.

Cummings, P. Antibiotics to prevent infection in patients with dog bite wounds: a meta-analysis of randomized trials. *Ann. Emerg. Med.* 1994; 23(3): 535–40.

Dwyer, J. P., Douglas, T. S., and van As, A. B. Dog bite injuries in children – a review of data from a South African paediatric trauma unit. *S. Afr. Med. J.* 2007; 97(8): 597–600.

Moscati, R. M., Mayrose, J., Reardon, R. F., *et al.* A multicenter comparison of tap water versus sterile saline for wound irrigation. *Acad. Emerg. Med.* 2007; 14(5): 404–9.

Paschos, N. K., Makris, E. A., Gantsos, A., *et al.* Primary closure versus non-closure of dog bite wounds. A randomized controlled trial. *Injury* 2014; 45(1): 237–40.

Chapter 57

Blood or Body Fluid Exposure Management and Post-Exposure Prophylaxis for Hepatitis B and HIV

Roland C. Merchant

Introduction

Because the effectiveness of prophylactic therapy is considered to be time-dependent, the acute care management of occupational or other blood and body fluid exposures must include rapid determination of the need for prophylaxis, testing, and treatment. Attention to wound care principles and referral for social, medical, or advocacy services remain important in all cases. Clinicians should be mindful that most blood or body fluid exposures will not result in an HIV or hepatitis B or C infection, and therefore post-exposure prophylaxis (PEP) should be prescribed only when indicated.

Exposure Epidemiology and Transmission

Exposure Types

Blood or body fluid exposures can be classified as sexual or non-sexual, or as health-care/public service worker-associated (commonly called "occupational") or non-health-care/public service worker-associated (commonly called "non-occupational"). Sexual exposures include consensual or non-consensual exposures (e.g. sexual assault, sexual abuse, rape). Non-sexual exposures include percutaneous injuries (e.g. needle stick or other sharp injuries) or splashes (e.g. blood or body fluid splashes to mucous membranes). Occupational exposures can occur in medical settings or in the public service, such as exposures sustained by police or correctional officers during their work. Non-occupational exposures are blood or body fluid exposures sustained by lay individuals, such as exposures to blood or body fluids from performing layperson assistance after traumatic injuries.

Hepatitis B

The Centers for Disease Control and Prevention (CDC) estimated in 2014 that 850,000 to 2.2 million people in the United States have a chronic hepatitis B infection. Although 2,953 acute hepatitis B infections were reported in 2014, the CDC estimates that new infections are underreported. After accounting for underreporting, the CDC estimates that there could have been 19,200 acute cases in 2014 in the United States. However, the prevalence and incidence of acute infections have decreased dramatically over the past 25 to 30 years (see Chapter 24, Viral Hepatitis). This reduction is likely due to widespread use of the hepatitis B vaccination, universal precautions in health-care settings, and educational campaigns to increase condom usage and reduce injection-needle sharing. Although it is found in other body fluids (e.g. bile, breast milk, cerebrospinal fluid, saliva, semen, and sweat), hepatitis B is transmitted primarily through contact with blood. Hepatitis B can be transmitted through:

- shared injection-drug use equipment
- unprotected/condomless anal or vaginal sexual intercourse
- perinatal transmission
- percutaneous injuries
- blood or body fluid splashes to mucous membranes or nonintact skin

Table 57.1 Risk of HBV Infection with Antigen Status of Infected Material

Antigen Status	Clinical Hepatitis Risk	Serologic Hepatitis Risk
HBsAg (+) and HBeAg (+)	22–31%	37–62%
HBsAg (–) and HBeAg (–)	1–6%	23–37%

- improper hemodialysis procedures
- transfusions with infected blood products

Among healthy adults acutely infected with hepatitis B, about 95% resolve their infection. The remainder become chronic carriers and about 20% of these develop cirrhosis. The risk of hepatitis B infection from a blood or body fluid exposure is directly related to the infectivity of the source (see Table 57.1). The risk from a percutaneous injury is greatly increased when the source harbors the hepatitis Be (envelope) antigen, which is a marker of active viral replication.

Hepatitis C

According to estimates from the CDC, 2.7 to 3.9 million people in the United States have a chronic hepatitis C infection. In 2014, there were 2,194 new acute hepatitis C infections reported in the United States, but the CDC estimates that due to underreporting of cases, there could have been 30,500 (24,200 to 104,200) new acute infections during 2014. Of evidence to support the efforts to prevent new infections, mortality from hepatitis C infections now exceeds that from the human immunodeficiency virus (HIV) in the United States and many other parts of the world. The mechanisms of hepatitis C transmission are less well understood than those of hepatitis B and HIV, but transmission in the United States is believed primarily to be due to injection-drug use, and less often to needle-stick/sharps injuries and health-care-related exposures from inadequate infection control procedures (e.g. syringe re-use). Hepatitis C likely is transmitted less frequently sexually or perinatally in the United States. Hepatitis C can be transmitted through transfusion of blood products; however, since screening of blood products for hepatitis C began in 1990, this has become a rare form of transmission in the United States. According to the CDC, the average incidence of hepatitis C infection through a percutaneous exposure to a known hepatitis C–infected source is 1.8% (0 to 7%). There are no comparable CDC estimates for other types of exposures to hepatitis C.

HIV

The CDC estimates that approximately 44,073 individuals were infected with HIV in the United States in 2014. The number of estimated new infections has been relatively stable over several years in the United States. Most new infections in the United States are among men who have sexual intercourse with men (MSM).

HIV can be transmitted through:

- unprotected/condomless sexual intercourse
- shared injection-drug use equipment
- perinatal transmission
- percutaneous injuries

Table 57.2 Risk of HIV infection

Exposure Route	Risk per 10,000 Exposures
Screened blood transfusion in the United States	<0.005
Contaminated blood transfusion	9,000
Needle-sharing injection drug use	67
Receptive anal intercourse	50
Percutaneous needle stick	30
Receptive penile-vaginal intercourse	10
Insertive anal intercouse	6.5
Insertive penile-vaginal intercouse	10
Receptive oral intercourse	1
Insertive oral intercourse	0.5

- blood or body fluid splashes to mucous membranes or non-intact skin
- transfusions with HIV-infected blood products

HIV is primarily transmitted through contact with blood, seminal or vaginal fluids, and breast milk. Although HIV can also be recovered from cerebrospinal, synovial, pleural, peritoneal, pericardial, and amniotic fluid, these body fluids are unlikely sources of HIV transmission. Feces, nasal secretions, saliva, sputum, sweat, tears, urine, and vomitus are not considered to be infectious unless they are visibly bloody. Because blood products in the United States have been screened for HIV since the mid-1980s, the risk of HIV-related transfusion transmission is very low. CDC-estimated risks of an HIV infection after selected exposures are shown in Table 57.2. However, these estimates are not meant to be predictive of HIV transmission and instead should be viewed as relative comparatives of transmission risk. Many of these estimates are based on historical data from the early days of the HIV epidemic; much has changed in regards to transmission risk since then. Furthermore, there are many factors that could potentially moderate transmission of these viruses. Some factors that might increase transmission risk are listed in Table 57.3.

Exposure Wound Management

Basic wound care including irrigation with normal saline or clean water should be initiated immediately for patients with percutaneous injuries and for skin and non-genital mucous membrane exposures. Patients with anal or vaginal sexual exposures should not irrigate the sites of their exposure as this may further disrupt mucosa. Hydrogen peroxide and caustic agents (e.g. bleach) should not be used to clean wounds, and there is no evidence that antiseptic solutions reduce transmission. Wounds should not be bled or "milked" or widened, as this may enhance exposures to infectious agents. Since there is no evidence that the timing of closure of open wounds affects infection rates, usual approaches to wound irrigation and closure are appropriate.

Exposure Evaluation

Evaluation begins with a complete history of the exposure and examination of the exposure site to determine whether the

Table 57.3 Factors Moderating Risk of HIV and Hepatitis Transmission

Factor	Non-Sexual Exposures	Sexual Exposures
Volume and type of exposure	For percutaneous exposures: • Large, hollow bore needle • Blood visible on the percutaneous device • Percutaneous device used in artery or vein • Large amount of blood For splash exposures: • Large amount of blood	Exposure involving blood as well as seminal or vaginal fluids Exposure to large amounts of seminal or vaginal fluids
Surface area of exposure site	Deep percutaneous injuries Mucous membrane exposures, particularly eye exposures Non-intact skin	Cervical ectopy Uncircumcised penis Traumatic sexual intercourse (anal and vaginal)
Exposure source and exposure person factors	Higher viral load in source fluid	Higher viral load in source fluid* Sexually transmitted diseases in source and/or exposed person

* Caution: viral load in serum may not be reflective of the viral load in genital secretions; patients may have an undetectable serum viral load, yet have virus in their genital secretions.

exposure could result in transmission of hepatitis or HIV. If transmission is possible, the hepatitis B and C and HIV status of the exposed person and the source should be assessed and prophylaxis considered. Prophylaxis for a given agent is not warranted when the exposed person is known to be already infected with that agent. Because most blood or body fluid exposures will not result in an HIV or hepatitis B or C infection, clinicians should carefully review the indications for PEP and prescribe these medications when they are indicated – not after every exposure.

Assessment of the Hepatitis B, Hepatitis C, and HIV Status of the Source

In most cases, the hepatitis and HIV status of the source will not be known during the patient's ED evaluation. When the source patient is available, he or she should be asked about hepatitis and HIV risk factors and asked to undergo testing unless recent results are already available. There is no accepted rule for deciding when a patient's prior hepatitis B or C or HIV test is current enough for an assessment of their status. As a consequence, all individuals – the source or the exposure and the person exposed – should be offered testing at the time of the exposure. If the source cannot be tested, local prevalence and source population risk factors may provide guidance. Clinicians should be aware of the limitations of applying these estimates to individual cases and rely on actual test results whenever possible. It should be recalled also that a person infected with hepatitis B or C or HIV is usually highly infectious prior to the appearance of serum antibodies and, hence, before antibody-based detection tests become positive. As such, the test results might be negative although the source of the exposure or person exposed is already infected, if they were recently infected. Of reassurance with regard to HIV transmission, per the CDC there is no known instance of a health-care worker exposed on the job becoming HIV-infected after an exposure to a person whose HIV antibody test was negative.

Testing for Hepatitis B and C and HIV

Hepatitis B and C testing involves examining the source's blood for markers of viral infection and for evidence of immunity. Common hepatitis B testing algorithms assess for the presence of the hepatitis B surface antibody (which indicates immunity to hepatitis B), surface(s) antigen (which usually indicates an ongoing infection), and core antibody (which adds further information about the presence of a prior or current infection). There is no US Food and Drug Administration (FDA)-licensed rapid hepatitis B test. Some testing facilities might be able to perform conventional hepatitis B testing in a rapid manner, however, with results available within 1 to 2 hours. Other hepatitis B tests, such as for the envelope (e) antigen (which indicates active viral replication and usually a high viral load), usually require a longer time to receipt of results and hence are not available during the evaluation of individuals with potential exposures to hepatitis B. Consultation with hepatitis B experts on the ordering and interpretation of these additional hepatitis B tests is needed because these tests generally are not recommended in the evaluations of individuals with blood or body fluid exposures.

The interpretation of hepatitis C testing can be complex, thus clinicians should refer to current CDC recommendations for assistance. In general, if the source has a negative antibody test for hepatitis C, then they likely are not infected. A US FDA-approved rapid hepatitis C antibody test is approved for clinical use. Also, some testing facilities might be able to perform conventional hepatitis C antibody testing in a rapid manner, with results available within 1 to 2 hours.

Rapid HIV antibody tests of whole blood, plasma, and oral fluid are now available, and the CDC now recommends these tests as a part of occupational exposure evaluations. The tests provide results within minutes and have test performance characteristics that are similar to conventional tests for HIV. A preliminary positive rapid HIV test result should be confirmed using currently accepted CDC protocols. In addition, rapid

Table 57.4 CDC Hepatitis B Prophylaxis Recommendations

Health-Care Personnel Status	Post-Exposure Testing		Post-Exposure Prophylaxis		Post-Vaccination Serologic Testing†
	Source Patient (HBsAg)	HCP Testing (anti-HBs)	HBIG*	Vaccination	
Documented responder§ after complete series (≥3 doses)	No action needed				
Documented non-responder¶ after six doses	Positive/unknown	–**	HBIG × 2 separated by 1 month	–	No
	Negative	No action needed			
Response unknown after three doses	Positive/unknown	<10mIU/mL**	HBIG × 1	Initiate revaccination	Yes
	Negative	<10mIU/mL	None		
	Any result	≥10mIU/mL	No action needed		
Unvaccinated/incompletely vaccinated or vaccine refusers	Positive/unknown	–**	HBIG × 1	Complete vaccination	Yes
	Negative	–	None	Complete vaccination	Yes

* HBIG should be administered intramuscularly as soon as possible after exposure when indicated. The effectiveness of HBIG when administered >7 days after percutaneous, mucosal, or nonintact skin exposures is unknown. HBIG dosage is 0.06 mL/kg.

† Should be performed 1 to 2 months after the last dose of the HepB vaccine series (and 4 to 6 months after administration of HBIG to avoid detection of passively administered anti-HBs) using a quantitative method that allows detection of the protective concentration of anti-HBs (≥10 mIU/mL).

§ A responder is defined as a person with anti-HBs ≥10 mIU/mL after ≥three doses of HepB vaccine.

¶ A non-responder is defined as a person with anti-HBs <10 mIU/mL after ≥six doses of HepB vaccine.

** HCP who have anti-HBs <10mIU/mL, or who are unvaccinated or incompletely vaccinated, and sustain an exposure to a source patient who is HBsAg-positive or has unknown HBsAg status, should undergo baseline testing for HBV infection as soon as possible after exposure, and follow-up testing approximately 6 months later. Initial baseline tests consist of total anti-HBc; testing at approximately 6 months consists of HBsAg and total anti-HBc.

Anti-HBs – antibody to hepatitis B surface antigen; HBIG – hepatitis B immune globulin; HBsAg – hepatitis B surface antigen; HCP – health-care personnel.

combination antibody/antigen HIV tests are available. Also, in some testing facilities, conventional combination antibody/antigen HIV tests can be performed in a rapid manner, with results available in some cases less than 1 hour. In the absence of these tests, a conventional HIV antibody test can be used to determine the source's HIV status. The use of HIV ribonucleic acid (RNA) instead of HIV antibody testing is not recommended for most exposure evaluations because of their relatively high rates of false-positive test results. However, these tests can be helpful when an acute HIV infection is suspected – that is, when there is evidence of an acute "flu-like" illness with fever, malaise, myalgias, rash, weight loss, and/or adenopathy not explained by another etiology, in the presence of recent high-risk behaviors. Expert consultation is advised when using these tests.

Post-Exposure Prophylaxis for Hepatitis B and HIV

PEP is currently available only for hepatitis B and HIV. There currently is no recommended prophylaxis against hepatitis C. Hepatitis-C-exposed patients should be monitored for seroconversion and referred for treatment if an infection is detected.

Timing of PEP Delivery

If PEP for hepatitis B or HIV is indicated for an exposure, then it should be given as soon as possible after the exposure – ideally, within 1 hour, though this is not possible for many types of exposures. PEP should be initiated in the ED because

the medications are likely more effective when taken soon after exposure. The results of animal and immunologic studies suggest that HIV PEP might not be effective if given more than 72 hours after exposure. The effectiveness of initiating hepatitis B PEP likely wanes over time as well, but PEP may be useful even 1 to 2 weeks post-exposure. All patients who decline PEP when it is recommended should have follow-up scheduled within 24 hours with a clinician experienced in prescribing PEP so that they have a second opportunity to take prophylaxis while it might still be effective.

Hepatitis B PEP Regimens

Hepatitis B prophylaxis (see Table 57.4) consists of post-exposure vaccination alone or vaccination plus hepatitis B immunoglobulin (HBIG). Patients who have been vaccinated adequately and have demonstrated evidence of immunity do not require any prophylaxis. If prophylaxis is required because of lack of immunity, most patients should receive the hepatitis B vaccine. The concept underlying this practice is that the immune system can be adequately stimulated by the vaccine to help contain the virus before it can replicate enough to infect the exposed person. HBIG is reserved for exposures in which the perceived infection risk is high (i.e. when the source has detectable hepatitis B virus DNA, hepatitis B e or s antigen) or when the exposed person will likely not respond to the hepatitis B vaccine (i.e. known prior vaccine non-responders). Clinicians should advise patients who are vaccinated against hepatitis B in the setting of an exposure that they must receive two additional

Table 57.5 CDC Occupational HIV PEP Regimens

Preferred HIV PEP Regimen

Raltegravir (Isentress; RAL) 400 mg PO twice daily

plus

Truvada (Tenofovir DF [Viread; TDF] 300 mg + emtricitbine [Emtriva; FTC] 200 mg) one tab. PO daily

Alternative Regimens

*(May combine one drug or drug pair from the left column with one pair of nucleoside/nucleotide reverse-transcriptase inhibitors from the right column; prescribers unfamiliar with these agents/regimens should consult physicians familiar with the agents and their toxicities)**

Raltegravir (Isentress; RAL) Darunavir (Prezista; DRV) + ritonavir (Norvir; RTV) Etravirine (Intelence; ETR) Rilpivirine (Edurant; RPV) Atazanavir (Reyataz; ATV) + ritonavir (Norvir; RTV) Lopinavir/ritonavir (Kaletra; LPV/RTV)	Tenofovir DF (Viread; TDF) + emtricitabine (Emtriva; FTC); available as Truvada Tenofovir DF (Viread; TDF) + lamivudine (Epivir; 3TC) Zidovudine (Retrovir; ZDV; AZT) + lamivudine (Epivir; 3TC); available as Combivir Zidovudine (Retrovir; ZDV; AZT) + emtricitabine (Emtriva; FTC)

The following alternative is a complete fixed-dose combination regimen, and no additional antiretrovirals are needed: Stribild (elvitegravir, cobicistat, tenofovir DF, emtricitabine).

For consultation or assistance with HIV PEP, contact the National Clinicians' Post-Exposure Prophylaxis Hotline at telephone number 888-448-4911 or visit its website at www.nccc.ucsf.edu/about_nccc/pepline/.

* The alternative regimens are listed in order of prefrence; however, other alternatives may be reasonable based on patient and clinician preference.

DF – disoproxil fumarate; PO – by mouth.

hepatitis B vaccinations at 1 and 6 months to be fully immunized. All health-care workers and others at increased risk of being exposed to blood or body fluids should be vaccinated and have their hepatitis B titers checked 1 to 2 months after the final vaccination to verify immunity. Patients who fail to acquire immunity can receive a second series of hepatitis B vaccination. If they again fail to acquire immunity, they are deemed vaccine "non-responders" and should be given hepatitis B immunoglobulin after any suspected hepatitis B exposure.

HIV PEP Regimens

The optimal regimen for HIV PEP is unknown. Regardless of the regimen, a 28-day course of HIV PEP is recommended, unless severe adverse side effects occur, or the source of the exposure is found to be uninfected. The CDC and other groups offer recommended regimens for "occupational" (health-care/public safety-related) and "non-occupational" (non-health-care/public safety-related) potential exposures to HIV. CDC-recommended regimens for "occupational" exposures are provided in Table 57.5 and additional dosing information for PEP medications is in Table 57.6. Although the CDC-recommended HIV PEP medications for "non-occupational" exposures vary slightly from the "occupational" medications (see Table 57.7), the regimens are all believed to be equally effective. Review current CDC recommendations and local recommendations for any changes to suggested HIV PEP regimens. Local practice guidelines might also suggest different regimens. Because all drugs have adverse side effects, clinicians prescribing HIV PEP should be aware and counsel patients about potential problems that might arise when taking these medications (see Table 57.8).

CDC Non-Occupational HIV PEP Guidelines

CDC non-occupational HIV PEP guidelines specifically address exposures to known HIV-infected persons. Persons who had consensual sex with a known HIV-infected person and a condom failure occurred, or who sustained a needle stick while caring for an HIV-infected person, or an inmate who was sexually assaulted while in prison by another inmate known to be HIV infected are three examples of patients who might present to the ED after an exposure to a known HIV infected person. The management of patients with non-occupational exposures to persons of unknown HIV status is not delineated in these guidelines. Clinicians are advised to consult other non-occupational HIV PEP recommendations from state or other national sources and experts in the provision of HIV PEP for assistance with HIV PEP after exposures to persons of unknown HIV status. The creation of local protocols on non-occupational HIV PEP provision based on available expert resources is recommended.

Discontinuation of HIV PEP

Discontinue HIV PEP:

- if the source of the infection is known or found to be HIV uninfected
- at the completion of 28 days of uninterrupted therapy
- if serious adverse side effects occur

If a source's HIV test at the time of exposure is negative, the CDC recommends that HIV PEP be discontinued. The CDC acknowledges that "although concerns have been expressed regarding HIV-negative sources being in the window period for seroconversion, no case of transmission involving an exposure source during the window period has been reported in the United States." Despite this recommendation, some clinicians and patients may feel uncomfortable deferring or discontinuing HIV PEP when the source is at high risk, even with a negative test at the time of exposure. For these patients, clinicians should attempt to evaluate the source's recent risk factors for HIV (i.e. high-risk sexual and injection-drug behaviors within the prior 3 to 6 months), consider combination HIV antibody and antigen testing (or HIV viral load testing), and be on the alert for any signs or symptoms of an acute HIV infection in

Table 57.6 Dosing on HIV PEP Medications

Drug Name	Dosing (Dosage Form)
Atazanavir (Reyataz; ATV)	• ATV: 300 mg + RTV: 100 mg once daily (preferred dosing for PEP) • ATV: 400 mg once daily without RTV (alternative dosing – may not be used in combination with TDF) • Available as 100-, 150-, 200-, and 300-mg capsules
Darunavir (Prezista)	• DRV: 800 mg once daily + RTV: 100 mg once daily (preferred dosing for PEP) • DRV: 600 mg twice daily + RTV: 100 mg twice daily (alternative dosing) • Avilable as 75-, 150-, 400-, and 600-mg tabs.
Dolutegravir (Tivicay; DTG)	• 50 mg once daily • Avilable as 50-mg tabs.
Emtricitabine (Emtriva; FTC)	• 200 mg once daily; available as 200-mg capsules • Also available as component of fixed-dose combination Atripla, dosed daily (200 mg of FTC + 300 mg of TDF + 600 mg of EFV) • Complera, dosed daily (25 mg of RPV + 300 mg of TDF + 200 mg of FTC) • Stribild, dosed daily (150 mg of EVG + 150 mg of cobicistat + 300 mg of TDF + 200 mg of FTC) • Truvada, dosed daily (200 mg of FTC + 300 mg of TDF)
Etravirine (Intelence; ETR)	• 200 mg twice daily; available as 100- and 200-mg tabs.
Lamivudine (Epivir; 3TC)	• 3TC: 300 mg once daily (preferred dosing for PEP) • 3TC: 150 mg twice daily (alternative dosing) • Available at 150- and 300-mg tabs. • Also available as components of fixed-dose combination generic lamivudine/zidovudine, dosed twice daily (150 mg of 3TC + 300 mg of AZT) • Combivir, dosed twice daily (150 mg of 3TC + 300 mg of AZT) • Epzicom, dosed daily (300 mg of 3TC + 600 mg of ABC) • Trizivir, dosed twice daily (150 mg of 3TC + 300 mg of ABC + 300 mg of AZT)
Lopinavir/ritonavir (Kaletra; LPV/RTV)	• Kaletra: 400/100 mg = two tabs. twice daily (preferred dosing for PEP) • Kaletra: 800/200 mg = four tabs. once daily (alternative dosing) • Available as 200-/50-mg tabs.
Raltegravir (Edurant; RPV)	• 400 mg twice daily; available as 400-mg tab.
Rilpivirine (Edurant; RPV)	• 25 mg once daily; available as 25-mg tab. • Also available as component of fixed-dose combination Complera, dosed daily (25 mg of RPV + 300 mg of TDF +300 mg of FTC)
Ritonavir (Norvir; RTV)	• 100 mg once daily • Also available as component of fixed-dose combinations in Kaletra (lopinavir/ritonavir), see above • Available individually as 100-mg tables, 100-mg soft gelatin capsules, 80-mg/mL oral solution
Tenofovir DF (Viread; TDF)	• 300 mg once daily; available as 300-mg tab. • Also available as component of fixed-dose combination Atripla, dosed daily (200 mg of FTC + 300 mg of TDF + 600 mg of EFV) • Complera, dosed daily (25 mg of RPV + 300 mg of TDF + 200 mg of FTC) • Stribild, dosed daily (150 mg of EVG + 150 mg of cobicistat + 300 mg of TDF + 200 mg FTC) • Truvada, dosed daily (200 mg of FTC + 300 mg of TDF)
Zidovudine (Retrovir; ZDV; AZT)	• AZT: 300 mg twice daily; available as 100-mg capsule or 300-mg tab. • Also available as component of fixed-dose combination generic lamivudine/zidovudine, dosed twice daily (150 mg of 3TC + 300 mg of AZT) • Combivir, dosed twice daily (150 mg of 3TC + 300 mg of AZT) • Trizivir, dosed twice daily (150 mg of 3TC + 300 mg of ABC + 300 mg of AZT)

the source. Consultation with an expert in HIV medicine is advised under these circumstances.

Serious adverse side effects from HIV PEP are uncommon. The most common adverse side effects are gastrointestinal distress (e.g. nausea, diarrhea), fatigue, malaise, and headache. These problems resolve with time for most patients. These problems also might not be due to the medications and could be exacerbated by the stress of the blood or body fluid exposure (e.g. psychological trauma following sexual assault) or the fear of becoming HIV infected. Clinicians should advise patients

who take HIV PEP of stress-induced symptoms and provide encouragement to continue the medications and consider antiemetics, counseling, and referrals for supportive services. As a matter of perspective, it should be recalled that most patients who are HIV infected tolerate their medications quite well and take them for many years without significant problems.

Failure of HIV PEP

Patients being prescribed HIV PEP should be aware that there have been documented prophylaxis failures, though they have

Table 57.7 Primary Side Effects and Toxicities Associated with HIV PEP

Class and Agents	Side Effect and Toxicity
Nucleoside reverse transcriptase inhibitors	
Abacavir	Respiratory symptoms, rash, fever, nausea, vomiting, diarrhea, abdominal pain, malaise
Emtricitabine	Headache, nausea, vomiting, diarrhea, and rash. Skin discoloration (mild hyperpigmentation on palms and soles), primarily among non-whites
Lamivudine	Abdominal pain, nausea, diarrhea, rash, and pancreatitis
Stavudine	Peripheral neuropathy, headache, diarrhea, nausea, insomnia, anorexia, pancreatitis, elevated liver function tests (LFTs), anemia, and neutropenia
Tenofovir DF	Asthenia, headache, diarrhea, nausea, vomiting, nephrotoxicity
Zidovudine	Anemia, neutropenia, nausea, headache, insomnia, muscle pain, and weakness
Transcriptase inhibitors	
Efavirenz	Rash (including cases of Stevens–Johnson syndrome), insomnia, somnolence, dizziness, trouble concentrating, abnormal dreaming, and teratogenicity
Etravirine	Rash (including cases of Stevens–Johnson syndrome), nausea
Rilpivirine	Depression, insomnia, rash, hypersensitivity, headache
Integrase strand transfer inhibitors	
Dolutegravir	Insomnia, headache, fatigue, rash, hepatotoxicity in those with underlying hepatic disease
Elvitegravir	Diarrhea, nausea, headache, nephrotoxicity
Raltegravir	Insomnia, nausea, fatigue, headache, and severe skin, hypersensitivity reactions
Protease inhibitors	
Atazanavir	Hyperbilirubinemia, jaundice, rash, nephrolithiasis
Darunavir	Rash, diarrhea, nausea, headache, hepatotoxicity
Fosamprenavir	Diarrhea, nausea, vomiting, headache, rash
Lopinavir/ritonavir	GI intolerance, nausea, vomiting, diarrhea, PR and QT interval prolongation
Ritonavir	Abdominal pain, asthenia, headache, malaise, anorexia, diarrhea, dyspepsia, nausea, vomiting, circumoral paresthesia, peripheral paresthesia, dizziness, taste perversion
Saquinavir	GI intolerance, nausea, diarrhea, headache, hyperglycemia, and elevated LFTs
Fusion inhibitor	
Enfuvirtide	Local injection site reactions, bacterial pneumonia, insomnia, depression, peripheral neuropathy, and cough
CCR5 coreceptor antagonist	
Maraviroc	Abdominal pain, cough, dizziness, musculoskeletal symptoms, pyrexia, rash, orthostatic hypertension

Table 57.8 CDC Non-Occupational HIV PEP Antiretroviral Regimens

Regimens	Drug Combinations
Preferred	A three-drug regimen consisting of: tenofovir DF 300 mg **and** fixed dose combination emtricitabine 200 mg (Truvada) once daily **with** raltegravir 400 mg twice daily **or** dolutegravir 50 mg once daily
Alternative	A three-drug regimen consisting of: tenofovir DF 300 mg **and** fixed dose combination emtricitabine 200 mg (Truvada) once daily **with** darunavir 800 mg (as two, 400-mg tabs.) once daily **and** ritonavir 100 mg once daily

been reported infrequently. Possible reasons for failure of HIV PEP include:

- exposure to a strain of HIV resistant to the antiretroviral regimen prescribed
- exposure to a large inoculum of virus
- delay to initiation of HIV PEP
- shortened duration of HIV PEP (e.g. non-compliance, early discontinuation)
- factors related to the immune system of the exposed person and the viral strain
- incomplete efficacy of PEP

Expert Consultation

The CDC specifically recommends consulting an expert in HIV PEP under certain circumstances (see Box 57.1). However, consultations should not delay the onset of HIV PEP. If HIV PEP appears warranted, it is better to give the first dose of HIV PEP (unless there are obvious contraindications, such as a medication allergy) and then wait for expert consultation. EDs should establish relationships with local experts in this field, if available, and design protocols that help facilitate rapid consultations. If local experts are not available, ED clinicians are encouraged to seek advice from the 24-hour National

Box 57.1 Situations for Which Expert Consultation for Human Immunodeficiency Virus (HIV) Post-Exposure Prophylaxis (PEP) Is Recommended

Delayed (i.e. later than 72 hours) exposure report

- Interval after which benefits from PEP are undefined

Unknown source (e.g. needle in sharp disposal container or laundry)

- Use of PEP to be decided on a case-by-case basis
- Consider severity of exposure and epidemiologic likelihood of HIV exposure
- Do not test needles or other sharp instruments for HIV

Known or suspected pregnancy in the exposed person

- Provision of PEP should not be delayed while awaiting expert consultation

Breast-feeding in the exposed person

- Provision of PEP should not be delayed while awaiting expert consultation

Known or suspected resistance of the source virus to antiretroviral agents

- If source person's virus is known or suspected to be resistant to one or more of the drugs considered for PEP, selection of drugs to which the source person's virus is unlikely to be resistant is recommended
- Do not delay initiation of PEP while awaiting any results of resistance testing of the source person's virus

Toxicity of the initial PEP regimen

- Symptoms (e.g. gastrointestinal symptoms and others) are often manageable without changing PEP regimen by prescribing antimotility or antiemetic agents
- Counseling and support for management of side effects is very important, as symptoms are often exacerbated by anxiety

Serious medical illness in the exposed person

- Significant underlying illness (e.g. renal disease) or an exposed provider already taking multiple medications may increase the risk of drug toxicity and drug–drug interactions

Expert consultation can be made with local experts or by calling the National Clinicians' Post-Exposure Prophylaxis Hotline (PEPline) at 888-448-4911.

Clinicians' Post-Exposure Prophylaxis Hotline (PEPline) at (888) 448–4911.

Additional Interventions and Prophylaxis

Patients who sustain blood or body fluid exposures are at risk for infections or preventable occurrences besides hepatitis B and HIV. Some additional interventions and prophylaxis that can be provided include:

- emergency contraception: levonorgestrel-only or ethinyl estradiol/norgestrel or ethinyl estradiol/levonorgestrel regimens (first dose should be given in the ED)
- prophylaxis against other sexually transmitted diseases, including gonorrhea, chlamydia, trichomonas, and

Table 57.9 Baseline Post-Exposure Laboratory Testing

Scenario	Labortory Tests
PEP not prescribed	HIV and hepatitis B and C antibodies
Hepatitis B PEP only prescribed	HIV and hepatitis B and C antibodies
HIV PEP prescribed	HIV and hepatitis B and C antibodies
	Complete blood count differential
	Serum chemistry/electrolytes
	Liver enzymes
Conduct pregnancy testing for women of childbearing capacity.	

bacterial vaginosis (see Chapters 30 and 31 on sexually transmitted diseases)

- hepatitis A vaccination at exposure and 6 months post-exposure can be considered for men who have sex with men and others at higher risk

Many of these medications may cause nausea. If HIV PEP is indicated, it should be administered first (if possible), followed by an antiemetic, before emergency contraception and/or other prophylaxes are administered.

ED Laboratory Testing

Table 57.9 provides a list of baseline laboratory tests that should be performed for patients exposed to blood or body fluids. It is not necessary for patients to have an HIV test or a hepatitis panel sample drawn prior to receiving PEP. Most commonly used tests are not affected by recent PEP. Other laboratory tests, such as those for sexually transmitted diseases, may be indicated, depending on the nature of the exposure.

Pearls and Pitfalls

1. Establish and maintain exposure protocols that include:
   - expedited evaluations for PEP – reduce "door-to-drug" time
   - rapid testing or conventional testing with rapid results for hepatitis B and C and HIV
   - regimens available for dispensing in the ED, including starter packs of HIV PEP medications
   - patient information handouts
   - expedited consultation with blood or body fluid and prophylaxis experts
   - facilitated follow-up and referrals to social, mental health, substance abuse counseling, and sexual assault advocacy services, as appropriate
2. Remember that most potential blood or body fluid exposures are not true mucous membrane or non-intact skin exposures and thus do not require PEP.
3. Check the hepatitis B vaccination status on all exposed patients and initiate vaccination in the ED when appropriate.
4. Do not forget to provide prophylaxis against other sexually transmitted diseases and offer emergency contraception to childbearing-age female patients with sexual exposures.
5. Prescribe antiemetics for patients who experience nausea from PEP.

PEP Resources

PEPline: The National Clinicians' Post-Exposure Prophylaxis Hotline. Phone: 1-888-448-4911, available at http://nccc.ucsf .edu/clinician-consultation/post-exposure-prophylaxis-pep/ (accessed November 30, 2017).

National and State PEP Guidelines Websites

CDC

CDC Guidance for Evaluating Health-Care Personnel for Hepatitis B Virus Protection and for Administering Postexposure Management, available at www.cdc.gov/ mmwr/preview/mmwrhtml/rr6210a1.htm (accessed November 30, 2017).

Recommendations for Postexposure Interventions to Prevent Infection with Hepatitis B Virus, Hepatitis C Virus, or Human Immunodeficiency Virus, and Tetanus in Persons Wounded During Bombings and Other Mass-Casualty Events –United States, 2008, available at www.cdc.gov/ mmwr/preview/mmwrhtml/rr5706a1.htm (accessed November 30, 2017).

Sexually Transmitted Diseases Treatment Guidelines, 2015, available at www.cdc.gov/std/tg2015 (accessed November 30, 2017).

Updated Guidelines for Antiretroviral Postexposure Prophylaxis after Sexual, Injection Drug Use, or Other Nonoccupational Exposure to HIV – United States, 2016: from the Centers for Disease Control and Prevention, U.S. Department of Health and Human Services, available at www.cdc.gov/hiv/pdf/ programresources/cdc-hiv-npep-guidelines.pdf (accessed November 30, 2017).

Updated U.S. Public Health Service Guidelines for the management of occupational exposures to HBV, HCV, and HIV and recommendations for postexposure prophylaxis, available at www.cdc.gov/mmwr/preview/mmwrhtml/ rr5011a1.htm (accessed November 30, 2017).

Updated US Public Health Service guidelines for the management of occupational exposures to human immunodeficiency virus and recommendations for postexposure prophylaxis, available at www.jstor.org/ stable/10.1086/672271 (accessed November 30, 2017).

New York

PEP for Non-Occupational Exposure to HIV Guideline, PEP for Occupational Exposure to HIV Guideline, and PEP for Victims of Sexual Assault Guideline, available at www. hivguidelines.org/pep-for-hiv-prevention/.

References

Branson, B. M., Handsfield, H. H., Lampe, M. A., *et al.* for the Centers for Disease Control and Prevention. Revised recommendations for HIV testing of adults, adolescents, and pregnant women in health-care settings. *MMWR Morb. Mortal. Wkly. Rep.* 2006; 55(RR-14): 1–17.

Busch, M. P., Glynn, S. A., Stramer, S. L., *et al.* A new strategy for estimating risks of transfusion-transmitted viral infections based on rates of detection of recently infected donors. *Transfusion* 2005; 45(2): 254–64.

Catalano, S. M. *Criminal Victimization, 2004* (Washington, DC: US Department of Justice, 2005).

Centers for Disease Control and Prevention (CDC). CDC guidance for evaluating health-care personnel for hepatitis B virus protection and for administering postexposure management. *MMWR Morb. Mortal. Wkly. Rep.* 2013; 62(RR-10): 1–24.

CDC. *Epidemiology and Prevention of Vaccine-Preventable Diseases.* W. Atkinson, S. Wolfe, and J. Hamborsky (eds.), 12th edn., 2nd printing (Washington, DC: Public Health Foundation, 2012).

CDC. *HIV Surveillance Report, 2014* (Atlanta, GA, 2015), vol. 26.

CDC. *Laboratory Testing for the Diagnosis of HIV Infection: Updated Recommendations* (Atlanta, GA, 2014).

CDC. Sexually transmitted diseases treatment guidelines, 2015. *MMWR Morb. Mortal. Wkly. Rep.* 2015; 64(RR-3): 1–137.

CDC. *Surveillance for Viral Hepatitis-United States, 2014* (Atlanta, GA, 2015).

CDC. Testing for HCV infection: an update of guidance for clinicians and laboratorians. *MMWR Morb. Mortal. Wkly. Rep.* 2013; 62(18): 362–5.

CDC. Updated U.S. Public Health Service Guidelines for the management of occupational exposures to HBV, HCV, and HIV and recommendations for postexposure prophylaxis. *MMWR Morb. Mortal. Wkly. Rep.* 2001; 50(RR-11): 1–52.

CDC. Updated U.S. Public Health Service Guidelines for the management of occupational exposures to HBV, HCV, and HIV and recommendations for postexposure prophylaxis. *MMWR Morb. Mortal. Wkly. Rep.* 2005; 54(RR-9): 1–17.

CDC, Health Resources and Services Administration, National Institutes of Health, American Academy of HIV Medicine, Association of Nurses in AIDS Care, International Association of Providers of AIDS Care, the National Minority AIDS Council, and Urban Coalition for HIV/AIDS Prevention Services. *Recommendations for HIV Prevention with Adults and Adolescents with HIV in the United States, 2014* (Atlanta, GA, 2014).

Chen, G. X. and Jenkins, E. L. Potential work-related exposures to bloodborne pathogens by industry and occupation in the United States [abstract M2-B1301]. Paper presented at National HIV Prevention Conference (Atlanta, GA, 2005).

Dominguez, K. L., Smith, D. K., Vasavi, T., *et al.* Updated guidelines for antiretroviral postexposure prophylaxis after sexual, injection drug use, or other nonoccupational exposure to HIV – United States, 2016: from the Centers for Disease Control and Prevention, U.S. Department of Health and Human Services, available at https://stacks.cdc.gov/view/cdc/38856 (accessed November 30, 2017).

Ganem, D. and Prince, A. M. Hepatitis B virus infection – natural history and clinical consequences. *N. Engl. J. Med.* 2004; 350(11): 1118–29.

Glynn, M. K. and Rhodes, P. Estimated HIV prevalence in the United States at the end of 2003 [Abstract T1-B1101]. Paper presented at 2005 National HIV Prevention Conference (Atlanta, GA, 2005).

Joyce, M. P., Kuhar, D., and Brooks, J. T. Notes from the field: occupationally acquired HIV infection among health care workers – United States, 1985–2013. *MMWR Morb. Mortal. Wkly. Rep.* 2015; 63(53): 1245–6.

Kruszon-Moran, D. and McQuillan, G. M. Seroprevalence of six infectious diseases among adults in the United States by race/ethnicity: data from the third national health and nutrition examination survey, 1988–94. *Adv. Data* 2005; 352: 1–9.

Kuhar, D. T., Henderson, D. K., Struble, K. A., *et al.* for the US Public Health Service Working Group. Updated US Public Health Service guidelines for the management of occupational exposures to human immunodeficiency virus and recommendations for postexposure prophylaxis. *Infect. Control Hosp. Epidemiol.* 2013; 34(9): 875–92.

Ly, K. N., Xing, J., Klevens, R. M., *et al.* The increasing burden of mortality from viral hepatitis in the United States between 1999 and 2007. *Ann. Intern. Med.* 2012; 156(4): 271–8.

Mast, E. E., Margolis, H. S., Fiore, A. E., *et al.* A comprehensive immunization strategy to eliminate transmission of hepatitis B virus infection in the United States: recommendations of the Advisory Committee on Immunization Practices (ACIP)
part 1: immunization of infants, children, and adolescents. *MMWR Morb. Mortal. Wkly. Rep.* 2005; 54(RR-16): 1–31.

Rich, J. D., Merriman, N. A., Mylonakis, E., *et al.* Misdiagnosis of HIV infection by HIV-1 plasma viral load testing: a case series. *Ann. Intern. Med.* 1999; 130(1): 37–9.

Roland, M. E., Elbeik, T. A., Kahn, J. O., *et al.* HIV RNA testing in the context of nonoccupational postexposure prophylaxis. *J. Infect. Dis.* 2004; 190(3): 598–604.

Roland, M. E., Neilands, T. B., Krone, M. R., *et al.* Seroconversion following nonoccupational postexposure prophylaxis against HIV. *Clin. Infect. Dis.* 2005; 41(10): 1507–13.

Weinbaum, C. M., Williams, I., Mast, E. E., *et al.* for the Centers for Disease Control and Prevention. Recommendations for identification and public health management of persons with chronic hepatitis B virus infection. *MMWR Morb. Mortal. Wkly. Rep.* 2008; 57(RR-8): 1–20.

Outline

Introduction and Unique Considerations in Pregnancy

The work-up and treatment of fever in pregnancy involves several special considerations: the effect of fever itself on the fetus, the impact of the pregnant state on the illness, the impact of the illness on the pregnancy, and the limitations that concerns for fetal well-being may place on diagnostic and therapeutic modalities.

The definition of fever in pregnancy is 100.4 °F or 38.0 °C. The normal fetal heart rate is between 110 and 160 beats per minute and maternal fever can cause a fetal tachycardia up to 180 to 200 beats per minute. It is important to treat maternal fever with antipyretics, especially in the first trimester, to decrease the risk of birth defects. The consequences of an episode of hyperthermia depend on the extent of the temperature elevation, its duration, and the stage of fetal development. Mild maternal febrile illness during the pre-implantation period and more severe episodes during embryonic and fetal development can result in miscarriage. Hyperthermia greater than 2.0 °C above normal can cause a wide range of structural and functional defects in the fetus, ranging from central nervous system defects to growth issues. Although most pregnancies in which there is a maternal infection and fever will result in a normal neonate, all fever in pregnant women should be aggressively controlled. The most commonly used antipyretic is acetaminophen in standard doses. Avoid non-steroidal anti-inflammatory agents, such as ibuprofen, because they have been associated with spontaneous abortions, and at high doses later in pregnancy can affect the fetal kidneys and cause premature closure of the ductus arteriosus.

Besides the important consideration of chorioamnionitis, the differential diagnosis for fever in a pregnant woman is similar to that in a non-pregnant woman. Because of the general suppression of the immune system, however, women are generally more susceptible to infections while pregnant. There are additional considerations depending on the particular etiology and the risk it may pose to the fetus.

Laboratory Considerations

When evaluating fever in pregnancy, alterations in laboratory values that occur must be kept in mind. A mild leukocytosis is normal and will continue approximately 1 week into the postpartum period. There is often a mild anemia and decrease in serum osmolality due to hemodilution. Alkaline phosphatase is produced by the placenta and is usually elevated in pregnancy. Elevation in fibrinogen is also normal in pregnancy, and fibrinogen levels less than 250 mg/dL should raise concern for disseminated intravascular coagulopathy if there is clinical suspicion. Arterial blood gas (ABG) values have different ranges of normal because of changes in maternal physiology: increases in minute ventilation elevate PaO_2 levels and cause a chronic respiratory alkalosis with metabolic compensation. Normal ABG values in pregnancy are as follows: pH 7.4 to 7.45, $PaCO_2$ 27 to 32 mm Hg, serum bicarbonate 18 to

21 mEq/L. Baseline creatinine and blood urea nitrogen (BUN) are typically slightly lower in pregnancy because of an increased glomerular filtration rate.

Changes in physical exam due to pregnancy include a holosystolic murmur at the left upper sternal border due to a 30 to 50% increase in cardiac output and a mild maternal tachycardia. Maternal blood pressure decreases early in pregnancy, with the nadir at 16 to 20 weeks' gestation, and then slowly rises to pre-pregnancy levels near term.

Radiologic Considerations

The need for diagnostic imaging in pregnancy to support a diagnosis must be weighed against concerns about radiation exposure to the fetus (see Table 58.1). Risks to the fetus depend greatly on the amount of radiation exposure and the gestational age at the time of exposure. Small amounts of radiation in utero, typically less than X rads, or fewer than 500 chest X-rays, do not cause an increased risk of birth defects. The risk of childhood leukemias may rise from approximately 1 in 3,000 to 1 in 2,000 after intrauterine exposure to radiation at diagnostic levels. The maximum amount of ionizing radiation that a fetus should be exposed to in utero is a cumulative dose of 5 rad.

In early first trimester (up to 2 weeks, before most women know they are pregnant), the concern for radiation exposure is primarily due to the risk of spontaneous abortion. The risks can be described to the patient as an "all or nothing" risk. During organogenesis, between 2 and approximately 15 weeks, the most important impact is on brain development, malformations, and possible effects on lifetime IQ. However, severe mental retardation has only been seen in very high radiation exposures, such as after the World War II atomic bombs in Hiroshima and Nagasaki. Teratogenic effects on lifetime cancer risk, brain development, adult height, and other malformations still occur during weeks 15 to 26 of gestation, though the amount of radiation needed to cause these effects is much higher than at earlier gestational ages. From 26 weeks' gestation to delivery, the risk of radiation to the fetus is felt to be equivalent to that in the newborn. Increased risk for major anomalies from diagnostic levels of radiation after 26 weeks has not been documented. However, the risk for increased incidence of cancer later in life still exists.

Ultrasound and magnetic resonance imaging (MRI) are felt to be safe in pregnancy with no known teratogenic effects. Gadolinium use in pregnancy has very limited data; gadolinium crosses the placenta, and case reports of its use describe no adverse fetal effects. Gadolinium in pregnancy is usually avoided unless the benefits outweigh the risks.

Treatment Considerations

Medications were historically classified for use in pregnancy as A, B, C, D, or X. In general, medications classified as A and B were considered safe in pregnancy, and class C medications were acceptable to use if the benefit of treatment outweighed the risk. Medications classified as D and X were

Table 58.1 Estimated Fetal Exposure for Various Diagnostic Imaging Methods

Examination Type	Estimated Fetal Dose per Examination (rad)	Number of Examinations Required for a Cumulative 5-rad Dose
Plain films		
Skull	0.004	1,250
Dental	0.0001	50,000
Cervical spine	0.002	2,500
Upper or lower extremity	0.001	5,000
Chest (two views)	0.00007	71,429
Mammogram	0.020	250
Abdominal (multiple views)	0.245	20
Thoracic spine	0.009	555
Lumbosacral spine	0.359	13
Intravenous pyelogram	1.398	3
Pelvis	0.040	125
Hip (single view)	0.213	23
CT scans (slice thickness: 10 mm)		
Head (10 slices)	<0.050	>100
Chest (10 slices)	<0.1	>50
Abdomen (10 slices)	2.6	1
Lumbar (5 slices)	3.5	1
Pelvimetry (1 slice with scout film)	0.250	20
Fluoroscopic studies		
Upper GI series	0.056	89
Barium swallow	0.006	833
Barium enema	3.986	1
Nuclear medicine studies		
Most studies using technetium (^{99m}Tc)	<0.5	>10
Hepatobiliary technetium HIDA scan	0.150	33
Ventilation-perfusion scan (total)	0.215	23
Perfusion portion: Technetium	0.175	28
Ventilation portion: xenon (^{133}Xe)	0.040	125
Iodine (^{131}I) at fetal thyroid tissue	590	Contraindicated in pregnancy
Environmental sources (for comparison)		
Background radiation (cumulative over 9 months)	0.1	N/A

CT – computed tomography; GI – gastrointestinal; HIDA – hepatobiliary iminodiacetic acid.

contraindicated. However, this classification system was not optimal as it resulted in oversimplification of data, and patient and provider confusion. In June 2015, the FDA passed the Pregnancy and Lactation Labeling Rule requiring drug manufacturers to discontinue pregnancy letter categories and provide three sections in a drug's label: 1. detailed information on pregnancy data and exposure registries; 2. drug information for breast feeding mothers; 3. information for patients of reproductive potential.

If surgery is indicated for the treatment of an infection, early intervention is important. This is especially true in the case of appendicitis, because perforation can cause early delivery and maternal, fetal, or neonatal sepsis. General anesthesia is safe during pregnancy, as long as medications and doses are appropriately adjusted.

Pyelonephritis

Epidemiology and Microbiology

Urinary tract infection (UTI) is the most common infection in pregnancy. Hydroureter and mild hydronephrosis is a normal physiological change of pregnancy that persists into the post-partem period. This change is thought to facilitate ascent of bacteria into the bladder, ureters, and kidneys, increasing the incidence of cystitis and pyelonephritis in the setting of bacteriuria.

Cystitis in pregnancy poses a relatively high risk of progressing to pyelonephritis if untreated, and pyelonephritis is the leading cause of septic shock in pregnancy. Therefore, any UTI, even cystitis, is considered complicated in a pregnant

Table 58.2 Urinary Tract Infections in Pregnancy

Organisms	*E. coli* is responsible for 85–90% of infections The remaining 10–15% typically are caused by: • *Klebsiella* • *Enterococcus* • group B *Streptococcus* • *Staphylococcus* • *Proteus*
Cystitis signs and symptoms	Frequency, urgency, dysuria, hematuria Suprapubic tenderness (often abrupt onset) Low back pain Absence of fever or flank tenderness
Pyelonephritis signs and symptoms	May or may not have associated cystitis symptoms Back or flank pain* Fever* and chills Nausea and vomiting Costovertebral angle tenderness

* 85% of women will present with fever and back pain.

patient. The incidence of acute pyelonephritis in pregnancy is 1 to 2.5%. In 10 to 18% of patients, it will recur within the same pregnancy. Risk factors for pyelonephritis include a prior episode of pyelonephritis, asymptomatic bacteriuria (ASB), urinary tract obstructive abnormalities, calculi, pre-gestational diabetes, smoking, nulliparity, and age less than 20 years old.

Asymptomatic bacteriuria (ASB), defined as 10^5 colony-forming units (CFU)/mL *of a single uropathogen* on two successive urine cultures by clean catch or 10^2 CFU *of a single uropathogen* on straight catch, leads to pyelonephritis in 20 to 30% of cases, and widespread prenatal screening to detect and treat ASB has greatly reduced the incidence of acute pyelonephritis in pregnancy.

The etiology of UTI in pregnancy mirrors that in non-pregnant women:

- *Escherichia coli* is the causative organism in 80 to 90% of acute infections.
- Other gram-negative organisms are *Klebsiella, Staphylococcus saprophyticus, Enterobacter, Proteus,* and *Pseudomonas.*
- Group B *Streptococcus* (GBS) is not typically considered pathogenic outside of pregnancy, but untreated GBS UTI is associated with preterm delivery and is treated if diagnosed.

Clinical Features

The following table summarizes the clinical features of UTI in pregnancy.

Differential Diagnosis

Key features that distinguish pyelonephritis from cystitis are:

- fever and back pain
- white blood cell (WBC) casts on urinalysis
- leukocytosis
- nausea and vomiting

Other conditions to consider in pregnant women who present with back pain.

Fever Usually Present	Fever Absent
• appendicitis • cholecystitis • chorioamnionitis • pneumonia	• labor • placental abruption • nephrolithiasis • ovarian torsion • musculoskeletal etiologies

Laboratory Diagnosis

Table 58.3 summarizes the laboratory diagnosis of cystitis versus pyelonephritis.

Treatment and Prophylaxis

Regional antibiotic resistance rates of *E. coli* should be considered when choosing an antibiotic regimen, if possible.

- Cephalosporins and penicillins are considered safe in pregnancy.
- Some sources suggest avoiding sulfonamides near term due to the risk of hyperbilirubinemia in the newborn, though there are no human reports of hyperbilirubinemia in the newborn exposed during the third trimester. Other studies have found associations between sulfonamide use and congenital anomalies, pre-eclampsia, and growth restriction, though the data remains inconclusive. UTIs should generally be treated with other antibiotics that are known safe in pregnancy; however, sulfonamides may be used when no alternative is available.
- Nitrofurantoin is well accepted and commonly used to treat cystitis in pregnancy; however, it is not effective for treating pyelonephritis (though it is used for daily bacteriuria suppression following complete treatment of pyelonephritis). Nitrofurantoin given late in pregnancy may cause hemolytic anemia in a fetus with G6PD deficiency.
- Tetracyclines are contraindicated in pregnancy because of discoloration of fetal teeth and inhibition of bone growth.
- Aminoglycosides are generally avoided in pregnancy because of risk of congenital deafness and nephrotoxicity (data mostly with streptomycin). However, gentamicin has been studied for various infections in pregnant women and may be considered if no alternatives are available.
- Quinolones are rarely used because of potential bone and cartilage abnormalities in the fetus. However, recent safety data show that these risks are low and quinolones may be used in cases of select bacterial resistance.

Initial treatment of pyelonephritis in pregnancy is usually a broad-spectrum cephalosporin administered intravenously until 24 to 48 hours after resolution of fever (see Table 58.4). Continuation of treatment with an oral antibiotic (determined by the urine culture results) for 14 days of therapy is recommended. There is some evidence for safe outpatient therapy for pyelonephritis in pregnancy in select populations. Outpatient regimens include two doses of ceftriaxone, 1 g intramuscularly

Table 58.3 Laboratory Diagnosis of Cystitis versus Pyelonephritis

	Cystitis	Pyelonephritis
Pyuria	+	+
Bacteriuria	+	+
Hematuria	+/−	+/−
Positive urine culture (>100K colonies of a single organism)	+	+
WBC casts on urinalysis	−	+
Leukocytosis	−	+
Positive blood cultures*	−	+/−

* Debatable utility as only 10–15% positive, the same pathogen is almost invariably isolated from the urine, and the duration of treatment is not changed by positive blood cultures. A 2015 Cochrane Collaboration study found no randomized trials of blood cultures in the setting of pylonephritis in pregnancy, and concluded there is not enough data to argue for or against blood cultures in these patients.

Table 58.4 Treatment of UTIs in Pregnancy

Cystitis and asymptomatic bacteriuria	Cephalexin 500 mg PO QID × 7 days or Nitrofurantoin 100 mg PO BID × 7 days or Amoxicillin 500 mg PO TID × 7 days or Fosfomycin 3 g PO × 1 or Trimethoprim-sulfamethoxazole 800/160 mg PO BID × 3 days (avoid in first trimester or use with folate supplementation)
Pyelonephritis	**First-line agents*:** Ceftriaxone 1 g IV or IM every 24 hours or Aztreonam 1 g IV every 8 hours **Second-line agents:** Piperacillin/tazobactam 3.375 g IV every 6 hours or Ertapenem 1 g IV daily (drug of choice for a known ESBL infection) or Ampicillin 2 g IV every 6 hours *plus* Gentamicin 5 mg/kg/day IV daily (*Caution*: due to the theoretical concern of fetal effects, use only if no other alternatives are appropriate) **Prophylaxis until delivery (after 14 days of treatment):** Cephalexin 250–500 mg PO daily or Nitrofurantoin 50–100 mg PO daily

* *Never* start with an oral agent; always use IV or IM antibiotics for initial treatment for 24 to 48 hours, or until afebrile. All intravenous regimens to be followed by an appropriate oral antibiotic for a total treatment of 14 days.

ESBL – extended-spectrum beta-lactamase-producing organism; IV – intravenous; PO – by mouth.

Table 58.5 Prophylaxis for UTIs in Pregnancy

Cystitis	If a pregnant patient has two episodes of cystitis within a single pregnancy, she should be placed on antibiotic suppression for the remainder of the pregnancy.
Pyelonephritis	After completion of a 14-day course of antibiotics determined by the final urine culture, prophylaxis should continue until delivery.

PO – by mouth.

(IM), 24 hours apart, followed by oral antibiotics, chosen based on final urine culture result, to complete a 14-day course.

Complications and Admission Criteria

Recurrence of UTI during the same pregnancy is a significant problem. Therefore, all pregnant patients diagnosed with a UTI should have a repeat "test of cure" urine culture after completing treatment – usually a week after completion of antibiotics. In addition to confirming microbiologic cure, suppressive therapy is used liberally in pregnant patients to prevent recurrence, as outlined in Table 58.5.

In general, pyelonephritis has a more severe course in pregnant than non-pregnant women. Major maternal complications of pyelonephritis in pregnancy include (frequencies among a large pregnancy cohort are given in parentheses):

- respiratory insufficiency or acute respiratory distress syndrome (ARDS) (<1%)
- anemia (26%)
- renal dysfunction (<1%)
- bacteremia (10–15%)

Major fetal complications include:

- preterm labor (14%)
- preterm birth (10%)
- low birth weight (5%)
- fetal demise (<1%)

All pregnant patients with pyelonephritis should be evaluated for admission, and all women more than 24 weeks' gestation require admission. There is some evidence for safe outpatient management of pyelonephritis in pregnancies less than 24 weeks' gestation with strict criteria. The following criteria *exclude* safe outpatient management for patients less than 24 weeks gestation:

- clinical signs of sepsis
- respiratory insufficiency
- initial temperature greater than 39.8 °C
- blood pressure less than 90/50 mm Hg
- sustained pulse greater than 140 bmp
- creatinine greater than 1.4 mg/dL
- WBC greater than 20×10^9/L
- a known allergy to cephalosporins
- inability to tolerate oral intake
- inability to follow instructions
- inability to reliably follow-up
- serious underlying medical illness, including a known renal or urologic problem

Table 58.6 Clinical Features and Treatment: Specific Respiratory Infections

Influenza	Influenza-like illness as defined above
	Sensitivity of rapid antigen flu test is 55–70%
	CBC may show marked leukocytosis
	Blood cultures are negative
	CXR may abnormal in influenza pneumonia or bacterial superinfection
	Treatment:
	Oseltamivir 75 mg PO BID × 5 days
	During influenza season, treatment should be strongly considered when suspision is moderate, even when rapid antigen testing is negative
	Post-exposure prophylaxis:
	Oseltamivir 75 mg PO daily × 7 days for any pregnant woman who has had close contact with an individual infected with influenza
Pneumonia	See Chapter 44, Community-Acquired Pneumonia, for more details
	Chest x-ray with proper shielding has minimal effects on the fetus – do not hesitate to use this modality if needed
	Treatment:
	Antibiotics as indicated. Cephalosporins and macrolides are safe to use in pregnancy. Hospitalize for suspected varicella pneumonia because maternal morbidity is high.

CBC – complete blood count; CXR – chest X-ray; DFA – direct fluorescent antibody.

Respiratory Infections

Epidemiology and Microbiology

Viral upper respiratory infection (URI) is common in pregnant women, and only symptomatic treatment is indicated, including aggressive fever control. The incidence of other respiratory tract infections in women of childbearing age is about 64 per 1,000, ranging from exacerbations of underlying lung disease such as asthma, to bacterial or viral pneumonia. Influenza should be considered in any pregnant women with influenza-like illness during flu season. Pertussis should be considered in pregnant women when prolonged cough is the prominent symptom.

Important respiratory pathogens to consider include the following:

- common respiratory viruses (e.g. rhinovirus and respiratory syncytial virus)
- influenza virus
- *Streptococcus pneumoniae*
- *Mycoplasma pneumoniae*
- *Chlamydia pneumoniae*
- *Bordetella pertussis*
- *Streptococcus pyogenese*

Clinical Features

Viral bronchitis is usually self-limiting (see Table 58.6), though severe or prolonged cough from bronchitis has been associated with placental abruption and premature rupture of membranes and should be treated with beta agonist inhaler. During flu season, influenza infection should be considered in any patient with flu-like illness, defined as fever (>100.0 °F) and sore throat or dry cough. Bacterial pneumonia must also be considered in any pregnant woman with respiratory symptoms and a fever. An oxygen saturation and chest radiograph are indicated when there is suspicion for pneumonia. In a woman with varicella, it is critical to rule out varicella pneumonia, because of significant associated maternal morbidity and mortality. Risk factors for the development of varicella pneumonia in pregnant women include smoking and more than 100 cutaneous lesions.

Differential Diagnosis

Non-infectious causes of respiratory complaints in pregnant women are essential to consider. Pulmonary embolus is the leading cause of maternal death in the United States, and should be on any differential diagnosis for respiratory complaints in pregnancy. Pulmonary edema can also be seen in the third trimester particularly in the setting of pre-eclampsia or peripartum cardiomyopathy. Finally, pyelonephritis in pregnancy is associated with increased risk of respiratory distress syndrome, and can present as fever, cough, chest pain, or dyspnea.

Laboratory Diagnosis

Etiologic testing during flu season is mainly used to confirm the diagnosis since the sensitivity of rapid flu tests is only 55–70% and PCR tests, which perform much better, take more than a day to return. A chest radiograph is generally required for the diagnosis of pneumonia; the radiation exposure is minimal with proper fetal shielding. Other routine laboratory tests are usually not indicated if the chest X-ray is normal. Blood cultures are indicated in pregnant patients requiring admission for pneumonia. In a pregnant patient with a severe respiratory infection and a "normal" adult pCO_2 level, this may indicate ventilatory failure because a respiratory alkalosis is expected in pregnancy.

Treatment

For viral URIs other than influenza, hydration, acetaminophen, and guaifenesin are safe in pregnancy. Pseudoephedrine should not be used during pregnancy as there are reports of increased incidence of limb defects and maternal hypertension. Further, pseudoephedrine may constrict compromised placental blood vessels.

When influenza is suspected, treatment is most effective when started within 48 hours of symptoms. All pregnant woman with influenza-like illness during peak flu season, regardless of immunization status, should be offered immediate treatment since there may be a decreased risk of intensive care unit (ICU) admission with early therapy. Safety data on the use of neuraminidase inhibitors for the treatment of influenza in pregnancy is growing, and there have been no consistently reported adverse events to date. If likelihood of influenza is moderate, the benefits of therapy outweigh the risks. Pregnant women exposed to influenza should be offered post-exposure prophylaxis.

Pregnant women with respiratory symptoms and fever should generally be evaluated for bacterial pneumonia with CXR and treated with antibiotics if there is an infiltrate. As always, consider teratogenicity of antibiotics before choosing a regimen. Cephalosporins and macrolides are safe treatment options for common community-acquired pneumonia in pregnancy.

The approach to possible *Bortadella pertussis* in pregnancy is similar to that outside of pregnancy. However, in pregnancy, the CDC recommends treatment in women up to 8 weeks after the onset of symptoms. Macrolide antibiotics are first-line treatment similar to outside of pregnancy, and sulfonamides are a reasonable alternative.

Pregnant women with varicella pneumonia should generally be admitted to an ICU setting and treated with IV acyclovir because of high associated mortality.

Complications and Admission Criteria

While the rate of complications from respiratory infections is generally similar in pregnant and non-pregnant patients, for a number of reasons the threshold for admission should be lower in pregnant patients. Because of the potential for preterm delivery and low birth weight, clinicians should have a lower threshold for admitting pregnant patients with pneumonia. Preterm premature rupture of the membranes (PPROM) is a complication associated with paroxysmal coughing spasm and significant coughing should be suppressed. Although the placenta usually acts as an excellent filter to prevent infection of the fetus, occasionally transplacental infection will occur, especially in human immunodeficiency virus (HIV)-infected patients.

Importantly, influenza causes significantly higher maternal morbidity and mortality in pregnant women than in non-pregnant women. During the 2009 H1N1 influenza A pandemic, 5% of all deaths from influenza were among pregnant women, though pregnant women represented 1% of the US population. Women in the third trimester are particularly at risk of complications. There is conflicting evidence about the impact of influenza infection on fetal outcomes; some studies suggest an association with increased risk of spontaneous abortion, preterm delivery, and low birth weight.

While a relatively rare infection, mortality from varicella pneumonia in pregnancy has been reported to be 10 to 30%. More recent studies show lower mortality rates, but it remains prudent to admit, closely monitor, and agressively treat varicella pneumonia in pregnancy.

Infection Control

Respiratory precautions in the pregnant population are similar to those in non-pregnant populations. Any patient with suspected varicella pneumonia or influenza should be isolated from other pregnant patients on the hospital floor.

The inactivated flu vaccine is recommended in all trimesters and shows no evidence of harm according to several systematic reviews. Women who are exposed to influenza during pregnancy should be offered post-exposure prophylaxis.

Similarly, prevention of pertussis (and diptheria in developing countries) is very important. According to 2012 recommendations from the CDC Advisory Committee on Immunization Practices (ACIP), all pregnant women should receive a Tdap vaccine (tetanus, diphtheria, pertussis) between 27 and 36 weeks of gestation to maximize the maternal antibody response and passive antibody transfer to the infant. This recommendation is regardless of the timing of the mother's last Tdap immunization. If Tdap is not administered during pregnancy, Tdap should be administered immediately postpartum. If pertussis exposure occurs in unimmunized patients, post-exposure prophylaxis should be offered as in non-pregnant patients.

Appendicitis
Epidemiology and Microbiology

Appendicitis is the most common non-obstetric condition requiring surgery during pregnancy. Because of anatomical changes during pregnancy, diagnosis can be delayed, thereby increasing risk of perforation, preterm labor, preterm delivery, and fetal sepsis and loss. The prevalence of appendicitis in the pregnant population ranges from 0.05 to 0.13%. This is approximately the same rate as in the general population, but the rate of perforation is higher in pregnant women.

Rates of preterm contractions associated with appendicitis are as high as 83% in the third trimester. Preterm labor occurs in up to 13% of pregnant patients with appendicitis in the third trimester. Fetal loss rates in uncomplicated appendicitis are low, ranging from 0 to 1.5%. However, this risk rises significantly in cases of ruptured appendices, ranging from 20 to 35%.

Clinical Features

Appendicitis can present in pregnancy with similar signs and symptoms as in non-pregnant women, including fever, anorexia, nausea, vomiting, periumbilical abdominal pain that migrates to the right lower quadrant, leukocytosis, tachycardia, and abdominal rebound and guarding (see Table 58.7). However, normal pregnancy symptoms such as nausea, vomiting, and anorexia often lower clinicians' suspicion for appendicitis, which can lead to delayed diagnosis. Several anatomic changes in pregnancy alter the classic physical exam findings: displacement of the appendix by the gravid uterus can cause abdominal pain to be localized to any abdominal quadrant, though most often the right upper quadrant, separation of the visceral and parietal peritoneum further decreases the ability to localize abdominal pain, and laxity of the abdominal

Table 58.7 Clinical Features: Appendicitis

Signs and symptoms	**Classic symptoms:**
	Fever, anorexia, nausea, vomiting, periumbilical abdominal pain that migrates to the right lower quadrant, leukocytosis, tachycardia, rebound and guarding on abdominal examination
	Non-classic symptoms:
	Displacement of the appendix by the gravid uterus can cause abdominal pain in any quadrant
	Separation of the visceral and parietal peritoneum in pregnancy further decreases the ability to localize abdominal pain
	Laxity of the abdominal muscles in late pregnancy can reduce rebound tenderness and guarding
Laboratory and radiographic findings	Leukocytosis
	Abdominal ultrasound, CT scan, or MRI with findings consistent with appendicitis
Treatment	**Appendectomy antibiotics:**
	Cefoxitin 2 g IV every 6 hours
	or
	Ampicillin/sulbactam 3 g IV every 6 hours
	or
	Piperacillin/tazobactam 3.375g IV every 6 hours

CT – computed tomography.

muscles in late pregnancy can reduce rebound tenderness and guarding.

Differential Diagnosis

Any intra-abdominal process that causes abdominal pain can occur in pregnancy, so the differential diagnosis is long. Furthermore, some of the symptoms of appendicitis can be considered normal for pregnancy.

Key features that may help distinguish appendicitis from other conditions include:

- **Hyperemesis gravidarum** (refractory anorexia, nausea, and vomiting) is not associated with fever and leukocytosis.
- **Round ligament pain** typically occurs in the second trimester as the uterus continues to grow out of the pelvis. Round ligament pain is classically described by the patient as rapid in onset, sharp, often radiating to the groin and inguinal areas. It is never associated with fever, nausea, vomiting, or any laboratory abnormalities. It will resolve spontaneously, does not require any treatment, and the patient can use acetaminophen as needed for pain control.
- **Labor** may cause intermittent abdominal and uterine pain – it should never cause fever. Severe, continuous, unrelenting uterine pain and tenderness may indicate uterine rupture. Suspicion is higher in the setting of any previous uterine scar.
- **Chorioamnionitis** is accompanied by uterine fundal tenderness and frequently fetal tachycardia. Chorioamnionitis is most frequently diagnosed in the setting of ruptured membranes. Diagnosis may be confirmed with amniocentesis.
- **Pyelonephritis** will almost universally include back pain as a symptom, and the clean catch urinalysis will suggest infection (leukocyte esterase, nitrite, protein, blood).
- **Acute cholecystitis and hepatitis** may present with right upper quadrant pain, fever, and elevated WBC. However, liver function tests can differentiate these diagnoses from appendicitis in pregnancy and right upper quadrant ultrasound will show gallstones in cholecystitis.

- **Ovarian torsion** usually does not occur except in the setting of an enlarged adnexa more than 5 cm in the first or second trimesters. Assisted reproduction technologies increase risk of ovarian torsion, likely due to ovarian hyperstimulation. Pelvic ultrasound can assist in evaluation.
- **Pelvic inflammatory disease** (PID) and tubo-ovarian abscess (TOA) are extremely rare in pregnancy because of the inability of organisms to ascend the genital tract.

Laboratory and Radiologic Diagnosis

Although leukocytosis is usually present in appendicitis and can assist in diagnosis in the non-pregnant population, in pregnancy, mild elevations in WBC can normally be seen, adding to the difficulty of diagnosis. However, an elevated proportion of neutrophils is not normal in pregnancy. Ultrasound is the initial imaging study of choice to evaluate the appendix in pregnancy. However, if diagnosis cannot be confirmed or excluded clinically or with ultrasound, or if obtaining the ultrasound will delay diagnosis in a patient with high suspicion for appendicitis, a CT scan of the abdomen should be strongly considered. At institutions where MRI is readily available and radiologists are experienced in evaluating appendicitis with this modality, MRI can also be used.

Treatment

Ultimately, appendectomy is the treatment of choice for the pregnant woman, as for the general population. In the first half of pregnancy, laparoscopic appendectomy confers the same benefits in pregnancy as in the general population (reduced opioid use, less post-operative pain, early return of bowel function, early ambulation, and less hospitalization time). Data is conflicting on the impact of laproscopic surgery on fetal outcomes. A 2012 meta-analysis found increased risk of fetal loss associated with laparoscopy, but the evidence was low quality and many surgeons still prefer laporoscopy and believe it has benefits. Once a pregnancy is past 26 weeks, however, risk of perforation to the pregnant uterus increases with laparoscopy, and laparotomy may be the preferred approach. Antibiotic coverage for common gastrointestinal organisms can be covered safely in pregnancy.

Complications and Admission Criteria

Complications of appendicitis in pregnancy include perforation, maternal sepsis, preterm labor, preterm delivery, neonatal sepsis, and fetal loss. Any pregnant woman with a confirmed diagnosis or suspicion for appendicitis should be admitted, regardless of gestational age.

Chorioamnionitis

Epidemiology and Microbiology

Chorioamnionitis is an infection of the two membranes of the placenta (the chorion and the amnion) and the amniotic fluid that surrounds the baby. Chorioamnionitis can cause bacteremia and sepsis in the mother and may lead to preterm birth and serious infection in the newborn baby. Other terms for chorioamnionitis include intra-amniotic infection and amnionitis.

Clinical chorioamnionitis occurs in approximately 1 to 2% of term births and in 5 to 10% of preterm births; histologic chorioamnionitis is diagnosed after delivery in nearly 20% of term and 50% of preterm births. Clinical chorioamnionitis has variable definitions, but most frequently is defined as maternal fever greater than 38.0 °C (100.4 °F) that is not attributable to other causes accompanied by purulent amniotic fluid arising from the cervix on speculum exam, sustained fetal tachycardia, or maternal leucocytosis greater than 15,000 in the absence of steroids.

Chorioamnionitis is usually caused by bacteria that reach the uterus through the vagina, and most frequently occurs in the setting of ruptured membranes. Premature rupture of membranes (PROM) happens in 5 to 10% of term pregnancies, and preterm PROM is the initiating event in 30% of preterm births ("premature" refers to prior to the start of labor; "preterm" refers to before 37 weeks' gestation). Risk of neonatal infection increases as the duration of ruptured membranes lengthens. In addition to prolonged rupture of membranes, additional risk factors for chorioamnionitis include prolonged labor, meconium-stained amniotic fluid, and group B Streptococci colonization. Data on correlation between chorioamnionitis and the number of digital exams in the setting of ruptured membranes is conflicting; however, it remains prudent to limit digital exams after artifical or spontaneous amniotomy.

Bacteria causing chorioamnionitis generally reflect the bacteria inhabiting the vaginal environment: group B Streptococci (about 30% of women carry this bacterium in their vaginas), *E. coli*, enterococci, *Gardnerella vaginalis*, and peptostreptococci. The vast majority of chorioamnionitis etiologies are multiorganism infections. Rarely, intra-amniotic infection can occur with intact membranes, likely through transplacental hematogenous transmission of the infectious agent. This is the most common route of infection in the case of *Listeria chorioamnionitis*.

Clinical Features

Any pregnant patient who presents with a fever in the third trimester must be evaluated for uterine tenderness and ruptured membranes (see Table 58.8). A dry, thin layer of vaginal fluid should be evaluated by microscopy for the presence of ferning, which suggests the presence of amniotic fluid and thus rupture of membranes. Sterile indicator paper or swabs can be used to check the pH of the vaginal fluid: resulting blue color indicating a basic pH suggests the presence of amniotic fluid and raises concern for ruptured membranes (though sperm and blood can also increase the pH of vaginal secretions). *Digital exam of the cervix is usually deferred when ruptured membranes are suspected.*

Uterine irritability or frank contractions may be seen. Chorioamnionitis may initiate uteroplacental bleeding or placental abruption. Labor and delivery may be rapid in the presence of chorioamnionitis.

Differential Diagnosis

Key features that may help distinguish chorioamnionitis from other conditions include:

- **Appendicitis:** The abdominal exam may reveal significant rebound and abdominal tenderness distant from the uterus. History reveals persistent nausea and vomiting, and radiological imaging is consistent with appendicitis.
- **Pyelonephritis:** Physical exam often reveals unilateral costovertebral angle tenderness. Urine analysis is suspicious for infection and urine culture confirms the diagnosis of UTI.
- **Musculoskeletal pain:** Should not cause a fever. Pain is not localized to the uterus. Pain may be exacerbated and/or relieved by positional changes.
- **Labor:** Normal labor may cause intermitant abdominal and uterine pain – it should never cause fever. Severe, continuous, unrelenting uterine pain and tenderness may indicate uterine rupture more likely in the setting of a previous uterine scar.
- **Abruption:** May present with bright red vaginal bleeding with associated uterine tenderness. Uterine irritability and/or contractions are common. Fever should not be present, though chorioamnionitis is a risk factor for abruption. There may also be a concealed abruption behind the placenta, which will not present with vaginal bleeding. In abruption there is a signficant risk of maternal consumptive coagulopathy; always send coagulation studies if this is on the differential diagnosis.

Laboratory Diagnosis

Chorioamnionitis is principally a clinical diagnosis. However, several tests may be useful (see Table 58.9).

If not completed in the course of prenatal care, testing for chlamydia, gonorrhea, and GBS should also be done (chlamydia and gonorrhea on cervical or vaginal swabs, and GBS on a swab from the outer third of the vagina and rectum).

Treatment

If ruptured membranes are confirmed (usually all three tests are positive: positive pooling of fluid in the vagina, positive indicator test, and positive microscopic ferning) in the presence of a

Table 58.8 Clinical Features: Chorioamnionitis

Organisms (prevalence %) Often multi-organism	GBS (14.6) *E. coli* (8.2) *Enterococcus* (5.4) *Gardnerella vaginalis* (24.5) *Peptostreptococcus* (9.4) *Bacteroides bivius* (29.4) *Bacteroides fragilis* (3.4) *Fusobacterium* spp. (5.4) *Mycoplasma hominis* (30.4) *Ureaplasma urealyticum* (47.0) *Listeria* is a rare cause of chorioamnionitis, but has serious consequences for the fetus. See section below for more details.
Signs and symptoms	Fever Significant maternal tachycardia (>120 bpm) Sustained fetal tachycardia (>160 bpm for >10 minutes) Tender or painful uterus Malodorous amniotic fluid Maternal leukocytosis (often >15,000) Uterine contractions If ruptured membranes: • leakage of fluid from vagina • pooling of vaginal fluid; fluid is nitrazine positive (blue) on pH paper • ferning of dried amniotic fluid from vagina on microscope slide under magnification
Treatment	**Antibiotic regimen for chorioamnionitis:** Ampicillin 2 g IV every 6 hours *plus* Gentamicin 5 mg/kg IV every 24 hours Consider the addition of clindamycin 900 mg IV every 8 hours especially in the setting of cesarean delivery *or* Ampicillin/sulbactam 3g IV every 6 hours *or* Cefoxitin 2 g IV every 6 hours **Caution:** • Never tocolyze (stop uterine contractions) in the setting of chorioamnionitis, because delivery is always indicated • Limit digital vaginal exams to reduce further ascending infections from the vagina • Delivery • Postpartum antibiotics are generally stopped after vaginal birth and continued after cesarean birth for 24 hours, though data behind dosage and duration of postpartum therapy is limited

Table 58.9 Laboratory Diagnosis of Chorioamnionitis

Study	Anticipated Results in Amnionitis
CBC with differential	Leukocytosis – occurs commonly in normal pregnancy and labor. A significant left shift or neutrophil predominance should raise suspicion for an infection.
Blood cultures	Positive in only 10% of cases. Should only be drawn if there is concern for septic physiology.
Urinalysis and culture	Should be obtained in suspected amnionitis to rule out UTI as an etiology for fever.
Amniocentesis	May be useful in cases of equivocal clinical diagnosis for chorioamnionitis. Should always be performed by an experienced clinician with ultrasound guidance to avoid fetal injury and placental bleeding. Amniotic fluid studies include Gram stain, cell count, culture, glucose, and protein levels. A dye test (injection of dye into the amniotic sac after removal of fluid for analysis) may also assist in diagnosis of ruptured membranes. Leakage of vaginal dye is diagnostic.

CBC – complete blood count.

maternal fever, fetal tachycardia, and uterine tenderness, then the diagnosis is very likely chorioamnionitis and the treatment is delivery regardless of gestational age.

Antibiotics should be started immediately. A second- or third-generation cephalosporin is acceptable. Additional regimens include ampicillin and gentamicin with or without clindamycin. If the pregnancy is viable (generally after 24 weeks), the fetus should be placed on a fetal heart monitor as part of surveillance. Occasionally, a prolapsed umbilical cord can occur with ruptured membranes and will often cause fetal bradycardia. Emergent delivery is indicated in the operating room.

If the pregnancy is less than 34 weeks' gestation and delivery is indicated, maternal betamethasone or dexamethasone should be given to decrease the risk of respiratory distress syndrome and other complications in the newborn. If the pregnancy is less than 32 weeks, maternal intravenous magnesium should be given to reduce the risk of cerebral palsy. Never delay delivery in the setting of chorioamnionitis to wait for the effects of steroids or magnesium.

Complications and Admission Criteria

Complications of chorioamnionitis include PPROM, preterm labor, preterm delivery, maternal sepsis, neonatal sepsis, and fetal loss. Women with chorioamnionitis have increased rates of cesarean delivery, and subsequent postpartum hemorrhage, endometritis, pelvic abscess, and wound infection. The newborns have an increased risk of sepsis, pneumonia, meningitis, cerebral palsy, intraventricular hemorrhage, and periventricular leukomalacia. All pregnant woman with suspected chorioamnionitis should be admitted, at any gestational age.

Infection Control

Follow universal precautions. There is no concern for chorioamnionitis transmission to other individuals.

Special Consideration for Chorioamnionitis: *Listeria*

Listeria infection is a foodborne illness that can present with minimal symptoms or with severe illness in pregnancy. When symptomatic, *Listeria monocytogenes* usually causes gastrointestinal complaints followed by a flu-like illness. It is most commonly diagnosed in the third trimester. If a pregnant patient presents with fever and symptoms of gastroenteritis, it is important to take a careful food history. Foods that have caused *Listeria* outbreaks include unpasteurized dairy products (e.g. soft cheeses, ice cream), deli meats, ready-to-eat foods, and raw fruits and vegetables.

Listeria crosses the placenta to infect the fetus, which may result in miscarriage, fetal death, or neonatal morbidity. Unlike other causative agents of chorioamnionitis, *Listeria* chorioamnionitis often occurs in the setting of intact membranes. Blood culture is the standard method for diagnosing listeriosis in pregnancy; the microbiology lab should be notified of concern for listeriosis. If an amniocentesis is done to rule out chorioamnionitis, the amniotic fluid in *Listeria* infection may be "bright green," and gram-positive rods may be evident on Gram stain. Once the diagnosis is suspected, it is crucial to begin antibiotics immediately to minimize fetal disease. First-line therapy for listeriosis is ampicillin, 2 g IV every 4 hours.

TORCH Infections

The "TORCH" mnemonic describes a group of maternal infections that have teratogenic effects:

- toxoplasmosis
- other infections, such as varicella

- rubella
- cytomegalovirus
- herpes simplex virus

Epidemiology and Microbiology

Toxoplasmosis

Caused by the intracellular parasite *Toxoplasma gondii*, this infection is uncommon in the United States, and congenital infection is rare (0.01 to 0.1% of live births). There is a direct relationship between the likelihood of fetal infection and the gestational age of maternal seroconversion: the probability of congenital infection is 15% with maternal seroconversion at 13 weeks, 44% at 26 weeks, and 71% at 36 weeks, respectively. However, the severity of teratogenic effects is inversely related to gestational age, with more severe effects seen in infections that occur at earlier gestational ages. Infectious sources include raw or undercooked meat, unwashed fruits and vegetables, exposure to soil during gardening or farming, and fresh cat feces. Low socioeconomic status, age over 30, rural residence, and birth outside of the United States are risk factors for acquiring toxoplasmosis.

Varicella (chickenpox)

Varicella is caused by the varicella-zoster virus, a herpes virus. It is a highly contagious virus spread by respiratory droplets and close contact. The incubation period ranges from 10 to 20 days, and individuals are contagious from 2 days *prior* to appearance of the rash until all skin lesions have crusted over. Since the introduction of the varicella vaccination in 1995, the rate of infection has dropped dramatically in the United States. More than 90% of the general population is immune because of previous infection or vaccination, prior to reproductive age. However, maternal varicella infection during pregnancy causes significant risks to the mother (see section on respiratory infections in pregnancy, above), as well as teratogenic risks for the fetus. Because varicella zoster is a reactivation illness in previously exposed persons, there is extremely low risk of infection to the fetus during pregnancy. Cutaneous lesions are infectious regardless of primary or reactivation infection, so skin-to-skin contact with the newborn should be avoided if a woman has lesions postpartum.

Rubella (German Measles)

Since rubella vaccination became available in 1969, the incidence of rubella infections has dropped dramatically. Since 2001, there have been fewer than 25 cases of rubella per year in the United States. Rubella is caused by rubella virus, a member of the Togavirus family, which is spread by respiratory droplets. The risk of a congenital defect is as high as 85% if an intrauterine infection occurs at less than 8 weeks' gestation, and 50% if an intrauterine infection occurs during the ninth to twelfth week of gestation. The risk of congenital rubella syndrome significantly decreases if infection occurs after 20 weeks. Any pregnant woman with a rash and a fever should have serologic testing for rubella, unless she has demonstrated recent antibodies for rubella.

Cytomegalovirus (CMV)

Cytomegalovirus is spread by upper respiratory shedding, close contact, and sexual contact, and most often produces a clinical syndrome of mononucleosis. An estimated 40% of women of reproductive age are susceptible to CMV (not immune), with infection and seroconversion more likely to occur among women of lower socioeconomic status. Most infections are subclinical (90%); thus many infections in pregnancy are missed or often misdiagnosed as mononucleosis. More severe neonatal disease occurs in cases of primary infection as opposed to a recurrent infection during pregnancy. Approximately 0.5 to 2.5% of births in the United States are associated with congenital CMV infection, causing approximately 1,000 neonatal deaths per year, making it the most common intrauterine infection. Surviving infants have a significantly higher disability rate than the unaffected population.

Herpes Simplex Virus (HSV)

Genital HSV outbreaks are most commonly caused by HSV-2; however, about 15% of outbreaks in the genital area can also be caused by HSV-1. Risk of transmission of HSV infection to the neonate is highest during labor, through direct contact. It is very important to ascertain the type of maternal infection during pregnancy, because this has implications for risk to the fetus and neonate. *Primary infection* is an initial infection of either HSV type, without previous exposure producing antibodies. *Non-primary first episode* is an initial outbreak with one HSV type, where the patient has existing antibodies from a prior exposure to the other virus type. *Recurrent infection* is reactivation of latent virus from a previous outbreak and not a new infection. A new primary infection carries the highest risk for the fetus or neonate, with transmission rates as high as 40%. The rate of neonatal infection is less than 1% in the setting of recurrent maternal infection.

Clinical Features

Table 58.10 summarizes the clinical features of TORCH infections.

Differential Diagnosis

Whenever one TORCH infection is suspected, clinicians should be sure to rule out others. Syphilis is an important TORCH infection in the "other" category that does not usually cause fever, but should always be considered. Congenital syphilis is extremely detrimental to the fetus, including intrauterine growth restriction (IUGR), bone abnormalities, ocular abnormalities, non-immune hydrops fetalis, reticuloendothelial abnormalities, significant central nervous system (CNS) anomalies, and stillbirth. Other potentially febrile viral exanthems concerning during pregnancy are coxsackieviruses and parvovirus B19, also known as "fifth disease" or "slapped-cheek" rash (see Chapter 52, Fever and Rash in the Pediatric Population).

Key features that distinguish TORCH infections from coxsackie- and parvoviruses are as follows:

Coxsackieviruses are divided into A and B subtypes – A types rarely have effects on the fetus, whereas B types have both maternal and fetal effects. Maternal coxsackievirus

infection begins as a fever followed by a wide range of possible presentations: myocarditis, meningoencephalitis, pleurodynia, pneumonia, hemolytic uremic syndrome, and hepatitis. Typically, there is not an associated rash. Fetal coxsackievirus type B infections, even in the absence of maternal symptoms, are potentially teratogenic, causing urogenital malformations, cardiac defects and congenital heart disease, digestive tract abnormalities, myocarditis, and neonatal CNS infections. If suspected, the diagnosis can be confirmed with virus isolation from rectal or throat swabs, or from rising maternal antibody titers.

Parvovirus B19 is highly infectious and commonly occurs in outbreaks among day care and school settings. Maternal infection manifests as low-grade prodromal fever and may be followed by the classical erythematous, warm facial "slapped cheek" rash. Rash is less common in adults as opposed to children. Adults are more likely to be asymptomatic (50%) and to develop arthropathy and swollen joints, and they may have a generalized reticular rash on the trunk – thus, if there is any suspicion for a maternal parvovirus B19 infection, even without the textbook "slapped cheek" appearance, a diagnosis should be pursued. Infection in the fetus causes erythroid hypoplasia, shortened red blood cell life span, and hemolysis leading to severe anemia in the fetus, sometimes requiring intrauterine transfusion. Over weeks, the fetus can develop high output cardiac failure leading to hydrops fetalis and intrauterine fetal demise (IUFD). If clinically suspected, parvovirus can be detected by IgM- and IgG-specific enzyme-linked immunosorbent assay (ELISA) antibody tests. Keep in mind that false-positive IgM are relatively common; results should be interpreted with caution and further testing discussed with the laboratory.

Laboratory Findings

Table 58.11 summarizes the laboratory findings of TORCH infections. Fetal ultrasound is often a useful supplement to laboratory evaluation, and sonographic abnormalities may be the first findings that prompt maternal evaluation.

Treatment and Prophylaxis

Table 58.12 summarizes the treatment and prophylaxis of TORCH infections.

Complications and Admission Criteria

Toxoplasmosis

Teratogenic effects include chorioretinitis, intracranial calcifications, intrauterine growth restriction, hydrocephaly, microcephaly, hepatosplenomegaly, and low birth weight in the neonate. Toxoplasmosis has also been associated with spontaneous abortion and prematurity.

Varicella

Congenital varicella can produce spontaneous abortion, stillbirth, limb hypoplasia, cutaneous scars, mental retardation,

Table 58.10 Clinical Features: TORCH Infections

TORCH Infection	Clinical Signs and Symptoms
Toxoplasmosis	• Subclinical infection is common: symptoms are often misdiagnosed as mononucleosis • Fever, fatigue, sore throat • Maculopapular rash • Cervical lymphadenopathy • Hepatosplenomegaly • Ocular (blurriness, photophobia, pain), pulmonary or CNS symptoms in immunocompromised patients
Varicella	• Fever, malaise (precede rash by several days in the adult, are simultaneous in children) • Rash – successive crops progress from macules, to papules, to vesicles, to pustules that eventually form crusts and scabs. Typically starts on face and scalp, spreading to trunk; extremities are minimally involved • Intense pruritis • Respiratory symptoms (second to sixth day after the rash), can rapidly progress to fatal acute respiratory distress syndrome (ARDS) • Chest X-ray: diffuse perihilar nodular or miliary pattern in cases of pneumonia • Symptoms of CNS infection, myocarditis, glomerulonephritis, arthritis
Rubella (defined by the CDC, 1996)	• Temperature >37.2 °C, or 99.0 °F • Acute onset of generalized maculopapular rash (usually starts on face) – about 16–18 days post-exposure • Arthralgias or arthritis • Lymphadenopathy • Conjunctivitis
Cytomegalovirus	• Fever • Leukocytosis (heterophile negative, with lymphocytosis) • Abnormal liver function tests • Malaise, myalgias, chills • Mild pharyngitis • Minimal lymphadenopathy • Absence of hepatosplenomegaly and jaundice
Herpes simplex virus	• Fever, malaise, myalgias, adenopathy, headaches, nausea (systemic symptoms only in primary infections) • Local painful vesicles that progress to ulcerations • Prodromal local symptoms of pain, paresthesias, or pruritis (approximately 2–3 days) • Primary infections average 3 weeks' duration • Recurrent infections average 2–7 days

CNS – central nervous system.

ocular abnormalities, growth retardation, and rudimentary digits. Risk of congenital varicella following maternal infection is low, approximately 1%; however, teratogenic effects can be severe. Neonatal infection has a variable presentation, ranging from mild illness resembling childhood chickenpox to disseminated disease complicated by pneumonia, hepatitis, meningoencephalitis, and death.

Rubella

Although there are very few cases each year in the United States, rubella is a known teratogenic infection, primarily causing cataracts or glaucoma, patent ductus arteriosus, mental retardation, and deafness, all of which comprise congenital rubella syndrome (CRS).

Cytomegalovirus

The teratogenic potential of CMV varies highly. Neonatal disease is more severe when in-utero infection occurs prior to 22 weeks' gestation.

Herpes Simplex Virus

The majority of neonatal herpes infections occur during labor as the infant passes through the birth canal and is exposed

to the virus, resulting in ocular infections, skin lesions, CNS infections, seizures, respiratory difficulties, liver dysfunction, and disseminated intravascular coagulopathy (DIC). Very rarely, in-utero infection can occur, resulting in spontaneous abortion, IUGR, premature birth, skin lesions, and severe CNS malformations such as microcephaly, hydranencephaly, and microphthalmos.

Admission Criteria for TORCH Infections

Serious maternal compromise with a TORCH infection is rare in an immunocompetent host. The most important exception is if there is any concern for varicella pneumonia; in these cases, hospital admission should occur at any gestational age for close maternal monitoring.

Infection Control

Toxoplasmosis

Educate pregnant women to avoid sources of toxoplasmosis such as raw or undercooked meat, unwashed fruits and vegetables, exposure to soil during gardening or farming, and fresh cat feces.

Table 58.11 Laboratory Tests for TORCH Infections

Infection	Laboratory Diagnosis
Toxoplasmosis	• Maternal serum IgM positive (1 week to several months post-infection; however, can persist for years) or IgG positive (1–2 months post-infection for years) • Avidity assay of amniotic fluid through toxoplasmosis reference lab • PCR of amniotic fluid • Complement fixation, Sabin–Feldman dye tests • Toxoplasma antigen detection by immunofluorescence • Histologic diagnosis from lymph node biopsy
Varicella	• IgM or IgG antibodies positive from maternal serum • Isolation of varicella virus from unroofed skin lesion swab or bronchoalveolar lavage • Antigen test from unroofed skin lesion swab or CSF • PCR of CSF sample
Rubella	• Isolation of rubella virus – can be isolated from blood and throat 7–10 days post-infection, shedding continues in throat for approximately 1 week • Significant rise in IgG antibody titers (instruct lab to not report simply "positive" or "negative"; "equivocal" should be considered as susceptible to the virus) • Positive IgM antibody (lasts for 4–5 weeks)
Cytomegalovirus	• Virus isolation by urine or cervical culture (does not distinguish between primary and recurrent infection) • IgM antibody tests (positive if infection occurs in last 4–8 months, may remain positive in up to 10% of women with recurrent CMV) • IgG antibody tests • PCR of amniotic fluid • Avidity assays through a specific CMV reference lab • "Owl's eye" appearance of intranuclear inclusion bodies is pathognomonic for CMV but rare
Herpes simplex virus	• Viral culture • Direct PCR tests • Serum antibodies (serum IgM does not discriminate between acute and chronic infection. Serologies are only useful if conversion is documented from seronegativity to positivity. The presence of IgG indicates that the infection is not primary).

CSF – cerebrospinal fluid; PCR – polymerase chain reaction.

Varicella

Ask all pregnant women if they have had a personal history of varicella. If not, or if prior infection is uncertain, send a varicella antibody test with prenatal labs. If the antibody is negative, vaccinate the mother *postpartum*. If exposure occurred to varicella in the past 96 hours in a woman with a negative antibody titer, offer post-exposure prophylaxis.

Rubella

Send rubella titers with all standard prenatal labs. Vaccinate all non-immune mothers *postpartum*.

Cytomegalovirus

There are no special prophylaxis or prevention strategies for CMV in pregnancy.

Herpes Simplex Virus

Ask all pregnant woman about a personal or partner's history of genital HSV. If a pregnant woman has a history of genital HSV, she should be offered acyclovir 400 mg TID prophylaxis at 36 weeks' gestation until delivery. If the pregnant patient's partner has a history of genital herpes and the patient does not, test for the presence of antibodies in the pregnant patient. If the pregnant patient's antibodies are negative for herpes, counsel the couple to use condoms throughout the pregnancy to avoid a primary infection from asymptomatic shedding. Condoms decrease the risk of transmission, but are not 100% effective; some providers recommend abstinence in the third trimester. The infected partner may be offered suppression in the third trimester; in one study outside of pregnancy, this decreased risk of transmission to the seronegative partner by 48%.

Ask every woman in labor about a history of genital herpes, and if she is taking suppresive medications. Perform a careful peroneal exam on these women, and ask about any current prodromal symptoms. If a lesion is detected directly in the birth canal, discuss with the patient and obstetrical team the option of cesarean delivery. However, if membranes have been ruptured for more than 6 hours, it is unclear if cesarean delivery reduces risk of herpes transmission. If the lesion is near but not in the direct path of the birth canal, cover it with tegaderm and proceed with vaginal delivery if indicated.

Hepatitis

Acute hepatitis is the most frequent cause of jaundice in pregnancy. This section will discuss relevant features of hepatitis A (HAV), hepatitis B (HBV), and hepatitis C (HCV) in pregnancy. For more details on hepatitis, see Chapter 24.

Epidemiology

HAV occurs in approximately 1 in 1,000 pregnancies and is transmitted predominantly through a fecal-oral route.

Table 58.12 Treatment and Prophylaxis of TORCH Infections

Infection	Treatment and Prophylaxis
Toxoplasmosis	• Counsel about risks and clinical features of congenital toxoplasmosis; discuss termination options • Spiramycin for maternal infection (available through the FDA in the United States) or Pyrimethamine and sulfadiazine for fetal treatment (with folic acid); evidence of efficacy with either approach is limited • Avoid cat litter boxes, do not eat undercooked or raw meat, hand wash after touching cats, keep household cats indoors and prevent cats' consumption of mice and raw meat, use gloves with gardening, wash all fruits and vegetables
Varicella	• Provide post-exposure prophylaxis with varicella-zoster immune globulin (VZIG) within 96 hours of exposure. Women previously immunized, who report a history of varicella, or who have positive VZV IgG titers do not require post-exposure prophylaxis. If evidence of maternal rash exists, viremia has already occurred and VZIG is not indicated. • Counsel about risks and clinical features of congenital varicella; discuss termination options • Acyclovir 800 mg PO five times per day for 7 days, or 10–15 mg/kg IV every 8 hours if evidence of systemic severe maternal illness or any respiratory symptoms • Supportive care for severe pulmonary disease • As a live-attenuated vaccine, varicella vaccination should *not* be given in pregnancy, and conception should be avoided for 1 month post-vaccine (though there is currently no evidence of harm if conception occurs sooner). A pregnant woman in the household is *not* a contraindication to varicella vaccination of another individual because the vaccine virus is not transmissible.
Rubella	• Counsel about risks and clinical features of congenital rubella; discuss termination options • Do not culture amniotic fluid as not indicative of fetal infection • The CDC does not recommend routine post-exposure immunoglobulin because it does not prevent viremia. However, the CDC suggests that immune globulin may be useful in exposed non-immune women for whom pregnancy termination is not an option. • As a live-attenuated vaccine, rubella vaccination should *not* be given in pregnancy, and conception should be avoided for 1 month post-vaccine • All rubella non-immune women should receive the MMR vaccine postpartum (safe with breastfeeding)
Cytomegalovirus	• Counsel about risks and clinical features of congenital CMV; discuss termination options • Case reports describe valganciclovir and ganciclovir in pregnancy to treat congenital infection, but data is extremely limited • A trial of CMV hyperimmune globulin before 24 weeks' gestation in women diagnosed with primary CMV to reduce congenital CMV infection is ongoing in 2015
Herpes simplex virus	• Counsel about risks and clinical features of congenital HSV; discuss termination options • Acyclovir has the most data to treat and prevent HSV in pregnancy *For primary infections*: 400 mg PO TID for 7–10 days *For recurrent infections*: 400 mg PO TID for 5 days *For prevention after 36 weeks*: 400 mg PO TID until delivery • Intravenous administration of acyclovir can be used in pregnancy for severe systemic infections • There is currently no available vaccine • Cesarean delivery may be offered to prevent neonatal infection if there is an active lesion directly in the birth canal and membranes have been ruptured for less than 6 hours

CMV – cytomegalovirus; FDA – Food and Drug Administration; MMR – measles, mumps, rubella; PO – by mouth.

The clinical presentation and course are similar to those in non-pregnant women, and there are no reports of transmission to the fetus. There are no known teratogenic effects.

Acute HBV occurs in 1 to 2 in 1,000 pregnancies; approximately 1% of pregnant women in the United States are chronic carriers of HBV. New active infections of HBV in pregnancy have a similar presentation to that in non-pregnant women, and there are no known teratogenic effects. However, acute hepatitis B in pregnancy has been associated with low birth weight and prematurity. Acquisition is by perinatal and sexual routes, with vertical transmission from mother to fetus being the primary concern during pregnancy. Mothers who are co-infected with HIV and/or hepatitis E have higher rates of vertical transmission. Maternal viral load is another important risk factor for transmission. Antiviral therapy has been shown to decrease rates of vertical transmission in women with hepatitis B. Administration of the hepatitis B vaccine and HBIG within 12 hours of delivery further reduce the risk of vertical transmission by 90%. However, cesarean delivery has not been shown to decrease risk of transmission. The American Academy of Pediatrics does not contraindicate breastfeeding in hepatitis B infections. Nevertheless, women should be counseled about the risk of transmission in the setting of cracked or bleeding nipples.

Overall seroprevalence of HCV in pregnant women in the United States is approximately 1%, with higher rates in women co-infected with HIV. Clinical course is usually not affected by pregnancy; however, there is some evidence of postpartum flares. Treatment of hepatitis C in pregnancy is not recommended due to concern for teratogenic effects of therapy. In some studies, chronic HCV was associated with preterm delivery and low birth weight. There are no known teratogenic effects of hepatitis C. The CDC reports rates of perinatal vertical transmission of approximately 5% in HIV-negative

Table 58.13 Clinical Features: Hepatitis

Organisms	Hepatitis A, B, and C
Signs and symptoms	Weakness and malaise
	Nausea, vomiting, anorexia, and right upper quadrant pain, jaundice
	In a small subset of patients, a syndrome similar to serum sickness can occur: fever, an urticarial rash, and migratory polyarticular arthritis

women, and as high as 17% in HIV co-infected women. Only women with detectable Hepatitis C RNA can transmit the virus perinatally. Risk factors for perinatal transmission include co-infection with HIV, viral load, and prolonged rupture of membranes. Cesarean delivery has not been shown to decrease risk of transmission. The American Academy of Pediatrics and the CDC do not recommend against breastfeeding in women with hepatitis C. However, women should be counseled about the risk of transmission in the setting of cracked or bleeding nipples.

Clinical Features

The clinical presentation of acute viral hepatitis in pregnancy is similar for all three viruses and is not affected by pregnancy. Systemic symptoms such as weakness and malaise are common, as well as nausea, vomiting, anorexia, and right upper quadrant pain (see Table 58.13). In a small subset of patients, a syndrome similar to serum sickness can occur, which includes fever, an urticarial rash, and migratory polyarticular arthritis. Immune complex mediated diseases can also occur in the setting of acute viral hepatitis. Icterus occurs in 20 to 50% of acute viral hepatitis infections, usually following onset of systemic symptoms. Mild liver enlargement, right upper quadrant tenderness, rash, warm and tender joints, and spider angiomata can be found on exam. Most concerning is the rare presentation of fulminant viral hepatitis, which can progress to hepatic encephalopathy and coma.

Differential Diagnosis

The differential diagnosis for hepatitis in pregnancy is similar to that in the non-pregnant state. However, there are some special additions and considerations in pregnancy to add to the differential diagnosis.

Key features that help distinguish viral hepatitis from other conditions are as follows:

- **Appendicitis**: Keep in mind that appendicitis in pregnancy can present in atypical locations in pregnancy, such as the right upper quadrant. However, liver function tests are normal in appendicitis.
- **Hyperemesis gravidarum** does not cause fever; however, it can have other symptoms similar to those of acute viral hepatitis, excluding a serum sickness-like presentation.
- At later gestations in pregnancy, diffuse symptoms such as nausea, vomiting, and right upper quadrant pain can be a presentation of **pre-eclampsia**. Pre-eclampsia can reveal abnormal liver function tests, similar to viral hepatitis. However, pre-eclampsia is often (but not always)

accompanied by blood pressures greater than 140/90, and/or proteinuria on urinalysis. Additional symptoms may include headache, visual changes, and dramatic changes in swelling, particularly in the face and hands. Kidney function may or may not be affected. A severe form of pre-eclampsia, **HELLP syndrome** (hemolysis, elevated liver enzymes, and low platelets), is characterized by hemolytic anemia, thrombocytopenia, and elevated liver enzymes, which may or may not be be associated with coagulopathy, hypertension, and proteinuria.

- **Fatty liver of pregnancy** can present in the third trimester with nausea, vomiting, jaundice, abdominal pain, pre-eclampsia, and, in severe cases, mental status changes. Lab values may include elevated liver function tests, elevated ammonia, acute kidney injury, and hypoglycemia.
- Intrahepatic cholestasis of pregnancy (ICP) results in pruritis without a rash and elevated bile acids in the second or third trimesters. Other liver function tests may or may not be elevated. ICP is associated with intrauterine demise.

Laboratory Diagnosis

There are no differences in the laboratory diagnosis of viral hepatitis in the pregnant state. See Chapter 24 on Viral Hepatitis for further details of laboratory diagnosis. Keep in mind that alkaline phosphatase (AP) is produced by the placenta, and is normally elevated in pregnancy; however, aspartate aminotransferase (AST) and alanine aminotransferase (ALT) are unaffected by normal pregnancy. Pregnant women who are HBV or HCV antibody positive should have a hepatic workup similar to any infected, non-pregnant adult, and evaluation should not be delayed because of pregnancy.

Treatment and Prophylaxis

Supportive care is the mainstay of treatment for acute viral hepatitis in pregnancy (see Table 58.14). However, in the case of hepatitis B, treament of lamivudine and tenofovir has been shown to decrease vertical transmission. These drugs are considered safe in pregnancy. In a randomized control trial of women positive for hepatitis B surface antigen and e antigen, tenofovir treatment from 32 weeks until 1 month postpartum reduced infant heptatitis B surface antigen positivity at 6 months from 11% in the placebo arm to 2% in the tenofovir arm. A meta-analysis of similar lamivudine trials showed a risk ratio of 0.31, 95% CI 0.15–0.63 when compared to placebo in infants who also received HBIG.

Furthermore, passive and active immunization of neonates with hepatitis B immune globulin (HBIG) and HBV

Table 58.14 Hepatitis Treatment and Prophylaxis

Hepatitis A	**Treatment:**
	Supportive care
	Prophylaxis:
	HAV if risk of acquisition during pregnancy
Hepatitis B	**Treatment:**
	Supportive care
	Tenofovir 300 mg PO daily
	Lamivudine 100 mg PO daily
	Prophylaxis:
	HBV vaccination if non-immune and at risk during pregnancy
	Vertical transmission prevention:
	Avoid early amniotomy during labor and fetal scalp electrode
	HBIG and HBV vaccine to neonate within 12 hours of birth
	Counsel mother on risk of transmission when breastfeeding in the setting of bleeding or cracked nipples
Hepatitis C	**Treatment:**
	Supportive care
	Vertical transmission prevention:
	Avoid early amniotomy during labor and fetal scalp electrode
	Counsel mother on risk of transmission when breastfeeding in the setting of bleeding or cracked nipples

vaccine given within 12 hours of birth prevents vertical transmission of HBV in 85 to 95% of cases. The World Health Organization (WHO) supports breastfeeding for neonates who have received HBIG and HBV vaccine, because this substantially reduces the risk of HBV perinatal transmission through breast milk.

Vaccines against HAV and HBV are safe to administer during pregnancy. It is essential to inform both the patient and the pediatric team if you have diagnosed hepatitis in pregnancy to take additional measures to prevent neonatal infection, as well as to discuss breastfeeding.

Complications and Admission Criteria

Maternal complications of hepatitis infection are similar in both the pregnant and non-pregnant populations, though there is some evidence of increased risk of hepatitis flares in the postpartum period among chronic carriers of HBV and HCV. Worsening hepatic function and signs of fulminant hepatic failure are criteria for admission in pregnant patients of any gestational age.

Infection Control

Universal precautions should be upheld when taking care of all newborns before their first baths, including babies born to mothers with hepatitis. Hepatitis B vaccinations should be offered to all household contacts of infected mothers. It is also important to identify mothers who are at risk for HCV infection and test for the presence of HCV antibody in order to take

appropriate measures to reduce the risk of vertical transmission in labor and delivery.

HIV

HIV infection in pregnancy and the risk of vertical transmission is a worldwide, important health-care issue. In developed countries like the United States, not only do HIV-infected women frequently test positive for the first time during pregnancy, but increasingly, HIV-infected women are choosing to become pregnant. Women who become infected with HIV during pregnancy are at particularly high risk for perinatal transmission, so it is crucial to identify these patients and aggressively treat to prevent vertical infection. If a pregnant woman is known to be HIV positive and antiretroviral therapy is initiated and viral response is monitored appropriately, the risk of vertical transmission to the infant is less than 1%.

Epidemiology

In the United States, the proportion of HIV-positive individuals who are women has risen to greater than 25%. Women infected with HIV tend to be unemployed and live in socioeconomically disadvantaged communities. The majority (over 80%) of new HIV infections in US women are sexually acquired. While HIV incidence in the United States is declining in most groups, the number of HIV-postitive women giving birth is increasing.

Clinical Features

Manifestations of HIV in pregnant patients, including acute HIV, are similar to those in non-pregnant patients. Acute HIV comonly presents with fever, pharyngitis, rash, myalgias, arthralgias, diarrhea, headache, and lymphadenopathy. Clinicians must have a high index of suspicion to diagnose acute HIV, taking a careful sexual and drug-use history in pregnant patients, and always considering acute HIV in those presenting with the characteristic, but non-specific, symptoms.

Differential Diagnosis

The list of infections that have a similar presentation to acute HIV is broad, including viral illness (most commonly mononucleosis), toxoplasmosis, rubella, syphilis, and viral hepatitis. Diagnosis of another sexually transmitted infection in pregnancy, as well as any unusual (e.g. herpes zoster or tuberculosis) or opportunistic infection, should prompt HIV testing.

Laboratory Diagnosis

Tests used to diagnose HIV, and their accuracy, do not differ in pregnancy. However, pregnancy testing recommendations emphasize the importance of successfully testing all pregnant patients in order to prevent vertical transmission. The CDC recommends "opt out" testing for HIV in all pregnant women in the United States, early in pregnancy. A second test in the third trimester is also recommended for women at high risk of acquisition based on sexual or drug use practices, or based on geographic prevalence. The CDC further recommends that every woman who presents to labor and delivery without a documented prenatal HIV result have a rapid test.

Diagnosis of acute HIV requires special attention. Third-generation HIV antibody tests, currently the most commonly used type of rapid test, have a window period of approximately 18 to 28 days. This is the period when a patient may have acute HIV, but test negative. If a patient has had an exposure within the time period corresponding to the test's window period, a viral load is required to diagnose acute HIV. Fourth-generation tests, which combine an antibody test with a test for HIV p24 antigen, are now recommended and becoming more widespread. These tests detect acute or early infection (previously considered the window period) in about 80% of cases.

Confirmatory testing is also changing, with a move from Western Blot confirmation to use of a HIV-1/HIV-2 antibody differentiation immunoassay. Regardless of the confirmatory test being used, a positive rapid HIV test in a woman during labor should be treated as a true positive until proven otherwise. The national Perinatal HIV Hotline, funded by the Department of Health and Human Services, provides a 24-hour consultation service for providers to call with questions about caring for women with HIV in labor and delivery, as well as throughout pregnancy. See http://nccc.ucsf.edu/clinician-consultation/perinatal-hiv-aids/ or call (888) 448–8765 for details.

Treatment and Prophylaxis

Treatment of HIV in pregnancy is beyond the scope of this chapter, and is rapidly changing. However, guiding principles for treatment of HIV in pregnancy remain the same: treat early and aggressively, because early viral suppression is associated with decreased risk of vertical transmission even in the first trimester. Prophylaxis against opportunistic infections in pregnant patients with AIDS should be approached in the same way as in non-pregant patients. For updated guidelines for the treatment of HIV in pregnancy (including prevention and treatment of opportunistic infections), please refer to the Department of Health and Human Services Guidelines at http://aidsinfo.nih.gov/guidelines/html/3/perinatal-guidelines/0. The national Perinatal HIV Hotline also answers questions about treatment of HIV in pregnancy 24 hours a day, 365 days a year at (888) 448–8765.

For patients in labor, the national perinatal HIV guidelines recommend intravenous zidovudine 2 mg/kg for 1 hour followed by 1 mg/kg until delivery if the viral load is greater than 1,000 to reduce the risk of perinatal transmission. Such women should also be offered cesarean delivery to further reduce risk of transmission if it has been less than 6 hours since onset of labor or rupture of membranes. Infants born to mothers infected with HIV require post-exposure prophylaxis as soon after birth as possible; low-risk exposures may require only zidovudine, but higher-risk exposures require more complex regimens. In the United States, breastfeeding by HIV-infected mothers is not recommended, to minimize risk of perinatal transmission. Obtaining expert opinion is mandatory when caring for HIV-infected women and their newborns in labor, delivery, and the immediate postpartum period. The national HIV perinatal 24/7 hotline number is (888) 448–8765.

All attempts should be made to prevent HIV acquisition during pregnancy. There appears to be an increased risk of HIV acquisition during sex if the woman is pregnant, as well as an eightfold increased risk of vertical transmission to the fetus with acute HIV as compared to chronic HIV. In the acute care setting, any woman with suspected exposure to HIV (sexual exposure, other mucousal exposure such as splash of a bodily fluid to a mucous membrane, or needlestick) must be offered post-exposure prophylaxis. Women with ongoing exposures, such as those in a sexual relationship with an HIV-infected partner, can be offered pre-exposure prophylaxis (PrEP). The areas of post-exposure and pre-exposure prophylaxis to prevent HIV transmission in pregnancy are rapidly evolving; for up-to-date information, contact the national Perinatal HIV Hotline.

Complications and Admission Criteria

HIV in pregnancy does not progress more rapidly than in non-pregnant women, and the risk of acquiring opportunistic infections is the same. However, morbidity and mortality from opportunistic infections may be increased. In pregnant patients with low CD4 counts, prophylaxis is therefore essential. For details on treatment of opportunistic infections in pregnant women with HIV, see the Department of Health and Human Services' Guidelines for the Prevention and Treatment of Opportunistic Infections in HIV-infected Adults and Adolescents.

Women with HIV in pregnancy may also require admission for directly observed therapy to reduce the risk of vertical transmission. If women have persistent viremia in the third trimester despite adherence support in the out-patient setting, many providers use admission for directly observed therapy and frequent viral load monitoring to quickly and aggressively achieve an undetectable viral load, in turn reducing the risk of perinatal HIV transmission.

Infection Control

Women with HIV and their newborns should be cared for using universal precautions.

Malaria in Pregnant Immigrants and Returning Travelers

Malaria

Malaria is an important infectious cause of fever in pregnancy that has a significant effect on both maternal and fetal health (see Chapter 60, Fever in the Returning Traveler). Worldwide, malaria in pregnant women and infants is an enormous problem. In the United States and developing countries, travelers or immigrants from malaria-endemic areas should have malaria ruled out to avoid complications such as preterm birth, low birth weight, spontaneous abortion, stillbirth, IUGR, congenital malaria, and significant maternal anemia.

Table 58.15 Clinical Features: Malaria

Signs and symptoms	• Cyclic fevers every 48–72 hours (late stages) • "Cold stage," followed by "hot stage," followed by "sweating stage" • Tachycardia and tachypnea • Abdominal pain, back pain • Nausea and vomiting • Delirium • Orthostatic hypotension • Jaundice

Epidemiology

In the United States, approximately 1,300 cases of malaria are seen per year. Approximately half of these cases are in US citizens who have recently traveled to malaria-endemic areas, and the other half are seen in non-US citizens. In women from endemic areas, acquired immunity to malaria can be lost or impaired in pregnancy. Because of decreased immune responses in pregnancy, pregnant women are three times more likely to develop severe malarial infections than non-pregnant women with infections from the same region.

Clinical Features

There is a wide spectrum of disease presentation in pregnant women (see Table 58.15). Reactivated latent disease produces a milder illness with less likelihood of fetal infection, whereas new infection in a non-immune woman can be life-threatening with increased risk for stillbirth, spontaneous abortion, and fetal infection. However, fetal infection remains rare.

Differential Diagnosis

In women presenting with recent travel or recent immigrant status, pregnancy, and fever, there is a long differential diagnosis for any infections that are endemic in the region from which the person recently came.

Laboratory Findings

Table 58.16 summarizes the laboratory findings of malaria infections.

Treatment and Prophylaxis

Recommendations for prophylaxis and treatment in pregnant women are similar to those in non-pregnant individuals, with some special considerations regarding teratogenicity and side effects as outlined in Table 58.17. Mefloquine should be used with caution and primaquine and doxycycline are contraindicated. Check for updated prophylaxis regimens based on the destination from the Centers for Disease Control and Prevention website: www.cdc.gov.

Complications and Admission Criteria

All pregnant women with malaria should be admitted. Complications of malarial infections include preterm birth, low birth weight, spontaneous abortion, stillbirth, IUGR, congenital malaria, and maternal anemia.

Table 58.16 Laboratory Test Abnormalities in Malaria

Laboratory Test	Possible Findings
CBC	Anemia – may be severe
Electrolyte panel	Elevated BUN and creatinine Hypoglycemia*
Liver function tests†	Elevated total bilirubin – indicative of hemolysis
Blood smear	Thick – used to identify the presence of parasites Thin – used to make specific diagnosis
ABG	Metabolic acidosis (lactic acidosis)
Chest x-ray	Pulmonary edema
Obstetric ultrasound	Hydrops fetalis in the case of severe fetal anemia due to congenital infection, IUGR

* May be severe with *Plasmodium falciparum*.

† Alkaline phosphatase elevation is normal in pregnancy because of production by the placenta.

CBC – complete blood count.

Table 58.17 Malaria Treatment and Prophylaxis Drugs in Pregnancy

Safe in pregnancy*	Chloroquine, pyrimethamine-sulfadoxine, quinine, quinidine, clindamycin
Use with caution in pregnancy	Mefloquine,† artemisinin derivatives‡
Contraindicated in pregnancy	Primaquine, tetracycline, doxycycline, halofantrine

* Considered safe at therapeutic doses. Some association between chloroquine and retinal or cochleovestibular damage; quinine and ototoxicity; primaquine and hemolysis in glucose-6-phosphate dehydrogenase (G6PD)-deficient patients.

† Single report showing association with increase in stillbirths.

‡ Not well studied in pregnancy.

Infection Control

There are no restrictions or transmission precautions to other pregnant women on the same hospital ward.

Pearls and Pitfalls

1. Acute pyelonephritis is both more common and more severe in pregnant than non-pregnant women.
2. There is an increased risk of respiratory distress syndrome in pregnant women with pyelonephritis.
3. Treat asymptomatic bacteriuria in pregnant women.
4. Fluoroquinolones, commonly used to treat UTI and pneumonia in non-pregnant patients, should be avoided in pregnancy.
5. The risk to the fetus of a chest X-ray is minimal with proper shielding; never withhold a chest X-ray in a pregnant woman if the test is indicated to rule out pneumonia.
6. Influenza in pregnancy is associated with increased risk of ICU admission and death; lower the threshold for treatment and admission; encourage annual influenza vaccination for all pregnant women.
7. Do not delay diagnostic tests and imaging when appendicitis is suspected in a pregnant woman.

8. Appendicitis is the great masquerader in pregnancy because of anatomic changes in the gravid state – it should always be in the differential diagnosis for abdominal pain with or without fever in pregnancy.

9. There are higher rates of perforated appendicitis in pregnancy, likely because of delay to diagnosis in atypical presentations.

10. Every pregnant woman should have a purified protein derivative (PPD) placed during each pregnancy, unless they have a prior history of a positive PPD. Women with a positive PPD and a prior BCG vaccination should be considered as exposed to TB and need a chest radiograph.

11. Every pregnant woman with a positive PPD needs a chest radiograph to rule out evidence of active disease – this can be done in any trimester with the fetus shielded through the postpartum period.

12. Uterine tenderness is never normal and should raise immediate suspicion for chorioamnionitis.

13. Digital vaginal exams should be minimized in the setting of suspected rupture of membranes.

14. Group B *Streptococcus* is an important neonatal pathogen, causing pneumonia, meningitis, enteritis, and sepsis in the newborn – always test for maternal group B *Streptococcus* upon diagnosis of PPROM, preterm labor, or anticipation of early delivery.

15. While maternal sepsis is rare in chorioamnionitis, immediate resuscitation and delivery are crucial and always indicated once the diagnosis is confirmed.

16. Although TORCH infections are relatively rare, never hesitate to send diagnostic tests if there is even a remote suspicion for a TORCH infection, as fetal consequences can be devastating.

17. *Never* give live vaccines in pregnancy (e.g. rubella and varicella). It is safe to give these vaccines to other individuals when there is a pregnant woman in the house, because the vaccine virus is not transmissible. If accidental vaccination occurs during pregnancy, providers should counsel patients on the hypothetical risks of congenital infection.

18. Offer post-exposure prophylaxis to women who are not immune to varicella and who were exposed to varicella in the prior 96 hours.

19. Ask all laboring women about a history of herpes, current lesions, or prodromal symptoms.

20. Send both a thick and thin smear to aid in diagnosis of type of malaria.

21. Take a good travel history and always check for updated information for treatment resistance patterns depending on the area of travel or origin.

22. Pregnant women may have a more severe presentation and course than non-pregnant women because of a mild immunodepressed state.

References

Cantu, J. and Tita, A. T. Management of influenza in pregnancy. *Am. J. Perinatol.* 2013; 30(2): 99–103.

Centers for Disease Control and Prevention (CDC). Measles, mumps, and rubella – vaccine use and strategies for elimination of measles, rubella and congenital rubella syndrome and control of mumps: recommendations of the Advisory Committee on Immunization Practices (ACIP). *MMWR Morb. Mortal. Wkly. Rep.* 1984; 33: 301.

CDC. Guiding principles for development of ACIP recommendations for vaccination during pregnancy and breastfeeding. *MMWR Morb. Mortal. Wkly. Rep.* 2008; 57(21): 580; updates at www.cdc.gov/vaccines/pregnancy/hcp/guidelines.html (accessed April 2, 2018).

CDC. Radiation and pregnancy: a fact sheet for clinicians, https://emergency.cdc.gov/radiation/prenatalphysician.asp (accessed April 2, 2018).

CDC. Treatment of malaria: guidelines for clinicians (United States), www.cdc.gov/malaria/diagnosis_treatment/clinicians3.html (accessed April 2, 2018).

CDC. Recommended antimicrobial agents for the treatment and post-exposure prophylaxis of pertussis: 2005 CDC Guidelines. *MMWR Morb. Mortal. Wkly. Rep.* 2005; 54(RR-14): 1.

CDC. HIV among pregnant women, infants, and children, www.cdc.gov/hiv/pdf/group/gender/pregnantwomen/cdc-hiv-pregnant-women.pdf (accessed April 2, 2018).

Chapman, E., Reveiz, L., Illanes, E., and Bonfill Cosp, X. Antibiotic regimens for management of intra-amniotic infection. *Cochrane Database Syst. Rev.* 2014; 12: Cd010976.

Chen, H. L., Lee, C. N., Chang, C. H., *et al.* Efficacy of maternal tenofovir disoproxil fumarate in interrupting mother-to-infant transmission of hepatitis B virus. *Hepatology* 2015; 62(2): 375–86.

Committee on Obstetric Practice, American College of Obstetricians and Gynecologists, Committee Opinion No. 614: Management of pregnant women with presumptive exposure to Listeria monocytogenes. *Obstet. Gynecol.* 2014; 124(6): 1241–4.

Committee on Obstetric Practice, American College of Obstetricians and Gynecologists, Committee Opinion No. 712: Intrapartum management of intraamniotic infection. *Obstet. Gynecol.* 2017; 130: e95–101.

Dotters-Katz, S. K., Heine, R. P., and Grotegut, C. A. Medical and infectious complications associated with pyelonephritis among pregnant women at delivery. *Infectious Diseases in Obstetrics and Gynecology* 2013; doi 124102.

Farkash, E., Weintraub, A. Y., Sergienko, R., *et al.* Acute antepartum pyelonephritis in pregnancy: a critical analysis of risk factors and outcomes. *Eur. J. Obst. Gynecol. Reprod. Biol.* 2012; 162(1): 24–7.

Fell, D. B., Platt, R. W., Lanes, A., *et al.* Fetal death and preterm birth associated with maternal influenza vaccination: systematic review. *BJOG: Int. J. Obstet. Gynaecol.* 2015; 122(1): 17–26.

Gershan, A. A. Chicken pox, measles and mumps in J. S. Remington and J. O. Klein (eds.), *Infectious Diseases of the Fetus and Newborn* (Philadelphia, PA: WB Saunders, 2001), pp. 683–732.

Gomi, H., Goto, Y., Laopaiboon, M., *et al.* Routine blood cultures in the management of pyelonephritis in pregnancy for improving outcomes. *Cochrane Database Syst. Rev.* 2015; 2: Cd009216.

Guttman, R., Goldman, R., and Koren, G. Appendicitis during pregnancy. *Can. Fam. Physician* 2004; 50: 355–7.

Higgins, R. D., Saade, G., Polin, R. A., et al. Evaluation and management of women and newborns with a maternal diagnosis of chorioamnionitis: summary of a workshop. *Obstet. Gynecol.* 2016; 127(3): 426–36.

Jacquemard, F., Yamamoto, M., Costa, J. M., *et al.* Maternal administration of valaciclovir in symptomatic intrauterine cytomegalovirus infection. *BJOG: Int. J. Obstet. Gynaecol.* 2007; 114(9): 1113–21.

Johns Hopkins. Antibiotic guide, www.hopkins-abxguide.org/ (accessed April 2, 2018).

Kourtis, A. P., Read, J. S., and Jamieson, D. J. Pregnancy and infection. *N. Engl. J. Med.* 2014; 370(23): 2211–18.

McMillan, M., Porritt, K., Kralik, D., *et al.* Influenza vaccination during pregnancy: a systematic review of fetal death, spontaneous abortion, and congenital malformation safety outcomes. *Vaccine* 2015; 33(18): 2108–17.

Panel on Treatment of HIV-Infected Pregnant Women and Prevention of Perinatal Transmission. Recommendations for use of antiretroviral drugs in pregnant HIV-1-infected women for maternal health and interventions to reduce perinatal HIV transmission in the United States, http://aidsinfo.nih.gov/contentfiles/lvguidelines/PerinatalGL.pdf (accessed April 2, 2018).

Puliyanda, D. P., Silverman, N. S., Lehman, D., *et al.* Successful use of oral ganciclovir for the treatment of intrauterine cytomegalovirus infection in a renal allograft recipient. *Transpl. Infect. Dis.* 2005; 7(2): 71–4.

Santos, F., Sheehy, O., Perreault, S., *et al.* Exposure to anti-infective drugs during pregnancy and the risk of small-for-gestational-age newborns: a case-control study. *BJOG: Int. J. Obstet. Gynaecol.* 2011; 118(11): 1374–82.

Smoak, B., Writer, J. V., and Keep, L. W. The effects of inadvertent exposure of mefloquine chemoprophylaxis on pregnancy outcomes and infants of U.S. Army servicewomen. *J. Infect. Dis.* 1997; 176(3): 831–3.

Sperling, R. S., Newton, E., and Gibbs, R. S. Intraamniotic infection in low birth weight infants. *J. Infect. Dis.* 1988; 157: 113.

Sweet, R. and Gibbs, R. Perinatal infections in R. Sweet and R. Gibbs (eds.), *Infectious Diseases of the Female Genital Tract* (Philadelphia, PA: Lippincott Williams & Wilkins, 2002), pp. 449–500.

Sweet, R. and Gibbs, R. Urinary tract infection in R. Sweet and R. Gibbs (eds.), *Infectious Diseases of the Female Genital Tract* (Philadelphia, PA: Lippincott Williams & Wilkins, 2002), pp. 413–48.

Thiebaut, R., Leproust, S., Chene, G., and Gilbert, R. Effectiveness of prenatal treatment for congenital toxoplasmosis: a meta-analysis of individual patients' data. *Lancet* 2007; 369(9556): 115–22.

Toppenberg, K., Hill, A., and Miller, D. Safety of radiographic imaging during pregnancy. *Am. Fam. Physician* 1999; 59(7): 1813–22.

Tracey, M. and Fletcher, H. S. Appendicitis in pregnancy. *Am. Surg.* 2000; 66(6): 555–9.

Ward, K. and Theiler, R. N. Once-daily dosing of gentamicin in obstetrics and gynecology. *Clin. Obstet. Gynecol.* 2008; 51(3): 498–506.

Wilasrusmee, C., Sukrat, B., McEvoy, M., *et al.* Systematic review and meta-analysis of safety of laparoscopic versus open appendicectomy for suspected appendicitis in pregnancy. *Br. J. Surg.* 2012; 99(11): 1470–8.

Wing, D. A., Fassett, M. J., and Getahun, D. Acute pyelonephritis in pregnancy: an 18-year retrospective analysis. *Am. J. Obstet. Gynecol.* 2014; 210(3): 219.e1–6.

Wing, D. A., Hendershott, C. M., Debuque, L., and Millar, L. K. Outpatient treatment of acute pyelonephritis in pregnancy after 24 weeks. *Obstet. Gynecol.* 1999; 94(5 Pt. 1): 683–8.

Additional Readings

Department of Health and Human Services. Guidelines for the prevention and treatment of opportunistic infections in HIV-infected adults and adolescents, http://aidsinfo.nih.gov/guidelines/html/4/adult-and-adolescent-oi-prevention-and-treatment-guidelines/0 (accessed April 2, 2018).

Edwards, M. J. Review: hyperthermia and fever during pregnancy. *Birth Defects Res. A. Clin. Mol. Teratol.* 2006; 76(7): 507–16.

Gabbe, S. G., Niebyl, J. R., and Simpson, J. L. (eds.), *Obstetrics: Normal and Problem Pregnancies*, 4th edn. (New York: Churchill Livingstone, 2002).

Harper, J. T., Ernest, J. M., Thurnau, G. R., *et al.* Risk factors and outcomes of varicella-zoster virus pneumonia in pregnant women. *J. Infect. Dis.* 2002; 185(4): 422–7.

Lim, W. S., Macfarlane, J. T., and Colthorpe, C. L. Treatment of community-acquired lower respiratory tract infections during pregnancy. *Am. J. Respir. Med.* 2003; 2(3): 221.

Chapter 59

Postpartum and Post-Abortion Infections

Lisa Rahangdale and Amy G. Bryant

Introduction

Infections prevalent in the postpartum and post-abortion period include urinary tract and genital tract infections (including endometritis, septic pelvic thrombophlebitis, pelvic inflammatory disease, and tubo-ovarian abscess), as well as mastitis, pneumonia (as a complication of anesthesia), and wound infections. Approximately 6% of women develop infections after vaginal delivery or cesarean section, the majority after hospital discharge. The most common postpartum infections are mastitis and urinary tract infection. This chapter reviews genital tract infections, mastitis, and episiotomy site infections. See Chapters 44, 48, and 63 for a discussion of pneumonia, urinary tract infections, and post-operative infections.

Endometritis

Endometritis is an infection of the uterus that may include the lining of the uterus (endometrium), the muscular layer (myometrium), or the entire organ.

Epidemiology

Postpartum endometritis occur in approximately 5.5% of vaginal deliveries and up to 6.0 to 7.4% of cesarean deliveries. Risk factors for postpartum endometritis include increased duration of labor, cesarean delivery, increased duration of rupture of membranes, increased number of vaginal examinations, increased duration of internal fetal monitoring, manual

removal of the placenta, low socioeconomic status, and diabetes. Delayed-onset endometritis may be associated with prior chlamydia infection.

Postpartum endometritis is thought to occur with exposure of the upper genital tract to vaginal flora at the time of delivery or during operative procedures. It is usually a polymicrobial infection. Pathogens include aerobic and anaerobic gram-positive cocci (group A beta-hemolytic *Streptococcus*, coagulase-positive *Staphylococcus aureus*, group B *Streptococcus*, *Streptococcus pneumoniae*, and *Enterococcus faecalis*), as well as aerobic and anaerobic gram-negative agents (*Escherichia coli*, *Gardnerella vaginalis*, and *Bacteroides fragilis*). In immunocompromised patients, viral pathogens such as herpex simplex virus and cytomegalovirus are also associated with postpartum endometritis.

Approximately 0.1 to 4.7% of surgical abortions worldwide are affected by uterine infection, though it has become an uncommon complication in the United States with widespread use of prophylactic antibiotics. The rate of infection among medical abortions is estimated at 0.006 to 0.9%. Endometritis or pelvic inflammatory disease after surgical abortion may be associated with pre-existing infections such as gonorrhea, chlamydia, or *Mycoplasma*, or be related to retained products of conception or operative trauma such as perforation of the uterus.

A rare, often fatal cause of postpartum as well as post-abortion infection is *Clostridium sordellii*, which causes a toxic shock syndrome.

Table 59.1 Clinical Features and Treatment: Postpartum Endometritis

Incubation period	• Most within first 5 days of delivery • Early onset: with 48 hours of delivery • Late onset: up to 6 weeks after delivery
Signs and symptoms	• Temperature of ≥101 °F *or* • Two separate temperatures of 100.4 °F at least 6 hours apart • Uterine tenderness • Purulent vaginal discharge • Non-specific findings (malaise, abdominal pain, chills, tachycardia)
Laboratory findings	• WBC may be elevated • Possible bacteremia
Treatment	• Gentamicin 1.5 mg/kg/dose IV every 8 hours and clindamycin 900 mg IV every 8 hours Alternative regimens to gentamicin and clindamycin: • Ampicillin–sulbactam 3 g IV every 6 hours • Cefotetan 2 g IV every 12 hours • Cefoxitin 2 g IV every 6 hours • Piperacillin–Tazobactam 3.375 g IV every 6 hours • Levofloxacin 500 mg IV every 24 hours *plus* • Metronidazole* 500 mg IV every 8 hours

* Use of metronidazole is controversial during lactation. Consult current guidelines prior to use.
WBC – white blood (cell) count.

Clinical Features

Postpartum endometritis can develop immediately after delivery in the setting of chorioamnionitis or, more commonly, several days later (see Table 59.1). Clinical signs include temperature of ≥101 °F or two separate temperatures of 100.4 °F at least 6 hours apart, uterine tenderness, and purulent vaginal discharge.

Women who develop infection after abortion or who are having a septic abortion usually present with fever, lower abdominal pain, vaginal bleeding, and possibly passage of products of conception (see Table 59.2). The presentation may be delayed in women who have undergone illegal abortion because of their reluctance to divulge history. These women are at higher risk for infection than those undergoing legal abortion.

In the case of postpartum or post-abortion *Clostridium sordellii* infection and toxic shock, patients are typically afebrile. These infections present with refractory hypotension, edema, pleural effusions, hemoconcentration, and markedly elevated white blood cell counts WBCs.

Differential Diagnosis

In the postpartum or post-abortion patient with a fever, the following sources of infection must be considered:

• genital tract: endometritis, septic pelvic thrombophlebitis, abscess
• urinary tract infection
• mastitis or breast abscess
• anesthesia complications (including aspiration pneumonia)
• wound infection of abdominal incision or episiotomy

Other conditions to consider (if no response within 48 to 72 hours of therapy):

• pelvic abscess
• infected wound or pelvic hematoma
• extensive cellulitis
• retained placenta
• septic pelvic thrombophlebitis
• organism resistant to antibiotic choice

Key features that distinguish endometritis from other conditions are:

• uterine tenderness
• purulent vaginal discharge
• exclusion of other sources of fever

Laboratory and Radiographic Findings

Endometritis is generally a clinical diagnosis based on history, symptoms, and physical examination. Associated laboratory findings may include an elevated WBC and decreased hemoglobin in the setting of vaginal bleeding. However, an elevated WBC count may be normal in postpartum women. Cervical cultures are not routinely performed because of the high likelihood of contamination and the likely polymicrobial nature of the infection. Blood cultures may be obtained in febrile patients.

Ultrasound is useful to evaluate for retained placenta or parametrial abscess or hematoma. Chest X-ray or CT scan of the abdomen and pelvis may detect air in pelvic organs or under the diaphragm in the case of uterine perforation after surgical abortion. CT scan of the pelvis is useful where extensive cellulitis, hematoma, or abscess is suspected.

Table 59.2 Clinical Features: Post-Abortion Endometritis

Incubation period	• Similar to postpartum endometritis
Signs and symptoms	• Lower abdominal pain
	• Vaginal bleeding
	• Fever
	• Tachycardia, tachypnea
	• Bacteremia and blood loss puts patient at more risk for shock
	• Bimanual exam: uterine tenderness, parametrial cellulitis/abscess, crepitus in pelvis consistent with gas gangrene
	• Lacerations to cervix or vaginal wall
Laboratory findings	• WBC count may be elevated
	• Hemoglobin/hematocrit may be low
	• Possible bacteremia

WBC – white blood (cell) count.

Table 59.3 Clinical Features: Septic Pelvic Thrombosis

Incubation period	• Immediately postpartum to 1 month
	• Most common within 1 week postpartum
Signs and symptoms	Ovarian vein thrombosis:
	• Fever up to 103–104 °F
	• Lower abdominal/flank pain localized to one side
	• Rope-like tender abdominal mass possible (more frequently on right)
	• Pelvic exam consistent with uterine tenderness
	• Nausea, ileus, other gastrointestinal symptoms possible
	• No improvement in fever or symptoms despite antibiotics
	Deep septic pelvic vein thrombophlebitis:
	• Fevers despite 48–72 hours of antibiotics
	• Pain improves and appear well in between fever spikes
	• No palpable abdominal masses
Laboratory findings	• WBC count may be elevated

Treatment and Prophylaxis

For postpartum endometritis, the most well-studied treatment regimen is a combination of intravenous gentamicin (1.5 mg/kg/dose IV every 8 hours) and clindamycin (900 mg IV every 8 hours). Peak and trough levels of gentamicin should be obtained to ensure therapeutic dosing. There is research that also supports the use of more convenient once-daily gentamicin and clindamycin, and alternate drugs are listed below (see Table 59.5). Ampicillin can be added when there is inadequate clinical response within 48 to 72 hours, particularly if the mother is known to have clindamycin-resistant group B *Streptococcus* colonization. Additionally, metronidazole can replace clindamycin and be used in combination with ampicillin and gentamicin in these refractory cases.

In cases of treatment failure, the possibility of pelvic abscess or infected hematoma and septic pelvic thrombophlebitis must be considered. Although similar antibiotic regimens will be used, a pelvic abscess may require drainage and septic pelvic thrombophlebitis may require anticoagulation. Endometrial curettage is performed if retained products of conception are suspected.

A first-generation cephalosporin or ampicillin can be given at the time of cesarean section as prophylaxis against postpartum endometritis. The most common choice is cefazolin 1 to 2 g intravenously (IV). Several large studies have consistently shown that giving prophylactic antibiotics 30 to 60 minutes prior to skin incision appears to lower maternal infection risk and presents no adverse effects on the newborn. Prophylaxis against post-abortion infection includes doxycycline 100 mg PO every 12 hours for 1 to 3 days after abortion. In surgical abortion, doxycycline 100 to 200 mg IV is given pre-operatively followed by 200 mg of doxycycline IV/PO 12 hours later. Other regimens, including metronidazole, erythromycin, azithromycin, and ofloxacin, have also been found to be effective.

Septic Pelvic Thrombophlebitis

Septic pelvic thrombophlebitis encompasses two pathologic entities: ovarian vein thrombosis and deep septic pelvic vein thrombophlebitis. Frequently, the two are difficult to distinguish and may occur simultaneously.

Epidemiology and Microbiology

Septic pelvic thrombophlebitis is an unusual condition with an overall prevalence of approximately 1 in 3,000 deliveries. Risk is higher with cesarean section (1 in 800) than with vaginal delivery (1 in 9,000). Predisposing factors for development of septic pelvic thrombophlebitis include cesarean section, pelvic infection, and the hypercoagulable state of pregnancy. Like endometritis, septic pelvic thrombophlebitis is thought to involve seeding from vaginal flora. The microbiology is therefore presumed to be similar to that of endometritis, discussed above.

Clinical Features

Most women with this complication will present with findings consistent with endometritis or pelvic cellulitis. They will usually have lower abdominal pain and fevers within 48 to 96 hours of delivery (see Table 59.3).

Diagnosis is made based on clinical findings, though computed tomographic (CT) scan or magnetic resonance imaging (MRI) can be used to attempt visualization of venous thrombosis. Complications include spread of septic emboli leading to infection of other organ systems, including the lungs.

Differential Diagnosis

Other conditions to consider are:

- appendicitis
- urologic conditions such as kidney stone or pyelonephritis
- gynecologic conditions such as adnexal torsion or degenerating leiomyoma
- broad ligament cellulitis or hematoma
- pelvic cellulitis or abscess

- operative injury to bowel or bladder
- drug fever

Key features that distinguish septic pelvic thrombophlebitis from other conditions are:

- tender rope-like cord in right lower quadrant
- persistent fevers despite broad-spectrum antibiotic therapy
- exclusion of other sources of fever and pain

Laboratory and Radiographic Findings

Diagnosis of septic thrombophlebitis is based in large part on clinical findings such as pain and persistent fever despite antibiotics. Laboratory tests such as WBC may be abnormal, though most are non-specific in the postpartum or post-abortion setting. Blood cultures should be obtained prior to antibiotics if possible. Either CT scan or MRI can be used as the initial diagnostic test; ultrasound does not perform as well as these. CT scan of the pelvis may reveal findings consistent with venous thrombosis, including enlargement of the vein, a low-density mass lumen, or a sharply defined vessel wall enhanced by contrast media. A negative result on imaging does not rule out the diagnosis.

Treatment and Prophylaxis

Treatment of septic pelvic thrombophlebitis involves antibiotic therapy combined with anticoagulation. Similar broad-spectrum antibiotics used for treatment of endometritis are also used for empiric treatment of septic pelvic thrombophlebitis. Persistent fever and pain are criteria for switching regimens. Anticoagulation (unfractionated heparin or enoxaparin) is generally recommended, though there are no placebo-controlled trials. The duration of antibiotic and heparin therapy is usually 1 week, unless signs and symptoms of infection persist. Continuation of anticoagulation beyond antibiotic treatment is unnecessary. Surgical intervention is not routinely required and should be reserved for patients with no response to medical therapy or with other findings requiring surgery.

Lactation Mastitis

Mastitis is acute inflammation of the interlobular connective tissue within the mammary gland. Mastitis is thought to be caused by stagnant milk in the breast that leaks into surrounding breast tissue. The milk itself leads to an inflammatory response and also provides a medium for bacterial growth for maternal skin flora and infant nasal flora. Breast abscess is a complication in 5 to 11% of mastitis cases that presents as a fluctuant or indurated mass and requires drainage.

Epidemiology and Microbiology

It is estimated that between 2 and 33% of breastfeeding women develop lactation mastitis. Although it can occur any time during lactation, most cases occur in the first 12 weeks after delivery. Breast abscess is a complication of mastitis and occurs in 5 to 11% of mastitis cases. Predisposing factors include the following: milk stasis, breast engorgement, history of mastitis, improper nursing technique, maternal stress, and local skin disruption including nipple fissures, sores, and traumatic injuries.

Staphylococcus aureus is the predominant pathogen in both mastitis and breast abscess, with methicillin-resistant *S. aureus* (MRSA) accounting for an increasing proportion of infections. Other pathogens include *Staphylococcus aureus*, coagulase-negative *Staphylococcus*, and less commonly, group A and B beta-hemolytic *Streptococcus*. Infection with gram-negative pathogens has been described, but is unusual.

Clinical Findings

The typical clinical findings in mastitis and breast abscess are listed in Table 59.4.

Differential Diagnosis

Other conditions to consider in the setting of postpartum breast pain include:

- fullness (bilateral, warmth, heavy, hard, no erythema)
- engorgement (bilateral, tender, minimal diffuse erythema, with or without low-grade fever)
- clogged milk duct (painful lump with overlying erythema, no fever, well-appearing, particulate matter in milk)
- galactocele (smooth rounded swelling or cyst)
- inflammatory breast carcinoma (unilateral, diffuse and recurrent, erythema, induration)
- abscess (tender hard breast mass, with or without fluctuance, skin erythema, induration, with or without fever)

Key features that distinguish mastitis from other conditions are:

- tender, hot, swollen wedge-shaped erythema
- fever

Laboratory and Radiographic Diagnosis

Mastitis is generally a clinical diagnosis that does not require laboratory studies. Milk cultures are recommended by some experts, though they can be contaminated with skin or infant nasal flora and often do not change management. The isolation of MRSA can be helpful in determining antibiotic choice. Proper milk cultures are obtained by catching milk in midstream away from the skin. Milk cultures are encouraged in women with hospital-acquired mastitis or recurrent mastitis, or in women who have had not clinical improvement after 2 days of antibiotic treatment.

Suspected breast abscesses that are not clearly fluctuant should undergo ultrasound for confirmation and localization. The pus should be sent for bacterial culture.

Treatment and Prophylaxis

The most important aspects of treatment of mastitis are supportive therapy and continued breast emptying. Continued breastfeeding or expression of breast milk from the affected breast(s) is essential to preventing further milk stasis. Antibiotic therapy is recommended, though high quality evidence of benefit is lacking. Agents listed in Table 59.5 are considered safe during breastfeeding. Needle aspiration is considered the

Table 59.4 Clinical Features: Mastitis and Breast Abscess

Incubation period	Mastitis: • Most common 2–3 weeks postpartum • Can occur any time during lactation Breast abscess: • Most common in first 6 weeks postpartum • Mastitis is predisposing factor
Signs and symptoms	Mastitis: • Systemic illness (fever, chills, malaise) • Fever ≥38.5 °C (102 °F) • Tender, hot, swollen wedge-shaped erythematous area of breast • Usually one breast • Nipple fissure, sharp, shooting pains (fungal infection) Breast abscess: • Fluctuant mass • Fevers despite 48–72 hours of antibiotics
Laboratory findings	• WBC count may be elevated • Skin and milk cultures often contaminated with skin flora

Table 59.5 Treatment of Mastitis and Breast Abscess

	Therapy Recommendation
Mastitis	• Supportive therapy: rest, fluids, pain medication, anti-inflammatory agents • Continue breastfeeding or breast pumping • **Oral antibiotics*** that cover *Staphylococcus aureus* • Dicloxacillin 500 mg PO QID • Cephalexin 500 mg PO QID • Clindamycin 300 mg PO TID • Trimethoprim–sulfamethoxazole† 160/800 mg PO BID **IV therapy:** • Vancomycin 15–20 mg/kg/dose IV every 8–12 hours • Minimum treatment 10–14 days
Breast abscess	• Same as above • Needle aspiration (may be ultrasound-guided) • Incision and drainage less commonly used for treatment

* Safe in lactating women.

† Trimethoprim-sulfamethoxazole should not be used in mothers breastfeeding newborns as it may increase the risk of kernicterus.

PCN – penicillin.

initial drainage method of choice for drainage of most breast abscesses.

Episiotomy Site Infection

Epidemiology and Microbiolgy

Episiotomy infections occur in approximately 0.3% of vaginal deliveries. Infection can occur at the site of a vaginal laceration sustained in the course of delivery or at the site of an incision made by a provider to facilitate delivery. The organisms associated with typical episiotomy site infection include the predominant flora of the vagina or cervix listed above under endometritis. Necrotizing fasciitis is an uncommon but devastating complication. It can rapidly spread along fascial planes to the abdominal wall, buttocks, and thigh. This infection is classically due to group A streptococci, but a combination of aerobic and anaerobic bacteria can cause this condition as well. (See also Chapter 12, Bacterial Skin and Soft-Tissue Infections.)

Clinical Features

Symptoms of episiotomy infection include pain and vaginal discharge. Physical exam findings include localized edema and erythema and drainage. More extensive infection and spread to the deep perineal fascia should be suspected if there is significant surrounding tenderness outside the area of visible skin inflammation. The entire area should be evaluated for signs of necrotizing fasciitis. (See Chapter 12, Bacterial Skin and Soft-Tissue Infections.) Simple episiotomy inflammation is not usually associated with signs of systemic infection such as fever or bacteremia. It is important to obtain aerobic and anaerobic cultures of any exudates, because more aggressive treatment may be considered in the case of group A *Streptococcus* infection.

Differential Diagnosis

Other conditions to consider:
• vulvar hematoma
• generalized edema from delivery, trauma, or pre-eclampsia
• allergic reaction
• necrotizing fasciitis

Key features that distinguish episiotomy site infection from other conditions are:
• erythema, bilateral edema, and exudate localized to superficial layers of the perineum

Laboratory and Radiographic Diagnosis

Diagnosis is made based on physical exam findings, primarily evidence of inflammation local to the site. Aerobic and anaerobic cultures of exudate should be obtained. CT scan should be obtained if there is any suspicion of a necrotizing infection.

Treatment and Prophylaxis

Simple episiotomy site infection should be opened and debrided using local anesthetic. The episiotomy incision should remain open for either healing by secondary intention or repair at a later date once the infection is cleared. Timing of this repair varies, but generally, 1 week is required for healthy tissue to be available for adequate repair. Good hygiene, sitz baths, and stool softeners are useful in promoting healing.

Antibiotics often are not needed. If cellulitis is suspected or extensive infection is noted, the patient should be treated with antibiotics. Surgical exploration is indicated if the wound appearance is suspicious for necrotizing fasciitis, if inflammation extends beyond the labia, if there is significant unilateral edema, if symptoms fail to resolve in 24 to 48 hours, or if the patient shows signs of systemic toxicity.

Infection Control

There are no data to suggest person-to-person transmission of postpartum or post-abortal infections. Therefore, standard precautions are considered adequate for patients with postpartum or post-abortal infections. Patients do not require isolation rooms. Frequent provider hand washing is essential. Mothers and infants do not require separation during treatment for infection.

Pearls and Pitfalls

1. Consider septic pelvic thrombophlebitis in the setting of high fevers and no response to antibiotic treatment for endometritis. However, this disorder is rare among postpartum women and other sources of infection must be ruled out.
2. It is safe and important to continue breastfeeding during treatment for mastitis.
3. Consider coverage of MRSA when treating mastitis or breast abscess without clinical improvement in 48 to 72 hours.
4. Episiotomy site infection is rare, but careful examination is important to assess for serious infections such as necrotizing fasciitis, which requires immediate surgical intervention.

References

Achilles, S. L., Reeves, M. F., and Society of Family Planning. Prevention of infection after induced abortion: release date October 2010: SFP guideline 20102. *Contraception* 2011; 83(4): 295–309.

Aldape, M. J., Bryant, A. E., and Stevens, D. L. Clostridium sordellii infection: epidemiology, clinical findings, and current perspectives on diagnosis and treatment. *Clin. Infect. Diseases.* 2006; 43(11): 1436–46.

American College of Obstetricians and Gynecologists. ACOG Practice Bulletin No. 120: use of prophylactic antibiotics in labor and delivery. *Obstet. Gynecol.* 2011; 117(6): 1472–83.

American College of Obstetricians and Gynecologists. Practice Bulletin No. 143: medical management of first-trimester abortion. *Obstet. Gynecol.* 2014; 123(3): 676–92.

Barbosa-Cesnik, C., Schwartz, K., and Foxman, B. Lactation mastitis. *JAMA* 2003; 289(13): 1609–12.

Brown, C. E., Stettler, R. W., Twickler, D., and Cunningham, F. G. Puerperal septic pelvic thrombophlebitis: incidence and response to heparin therapy. *Am. J. Obstet. Gynecol.* 1999; 181(1): 143–8.

Committee on Health Care for Underserved Women ACoO, Gynecologists. ACOG Committee Opinion No. 361: breastfeeding: maternal and infant aspects. *Obstet. Gynecol.* 2007; 109(2 Pt. 1): 479–80.

Faro, S. Postpartum endometritis. *Clin. Perinatol.* 2005; 32(3): 803–14.

Giraldo-Isaza, M. A., Jaspan, D., and Cohen, A. W. Postpartum endometritis caused by herpes and cytomegaloviruses. *Obstet. Gynecol.* 2011; 117(2 Pt. 2): 466–7.

Ho, C. S., Bhatnagar, J., Cohen, A. L., *et al.* Undiagnosed cases of fatal Clostridium-associated toxic shock in Californian women of childbearing age. *Am. J. Obstet. Gynecol.* 2009; 201(5): 459e1–7.

Jahanfar, S., Ng, C. J., and Teng, C. L. Antibiotics for mastitis in breastfeeding women. *Cochrane Database Syst. Rev.* 2009; 1: CD005458.

Larsen, J. W., Hager, W. D., Livengood, C. H., and Hoyme, U. Guidelines for the diagnosis, treatment and prevention of postoperative infections. *Infect. Dis. Obstet. Gynecol.* 2003; 11(1): 65–70.

Ledger, W. J. Post-partum endomyometritis diagnosis and treatment: a review. *J. Obstet. Gynaecol. Res.* 2003; 29(6): 364–73.

Livingston, J. C., Llata, E., Rinehart, E., *et al.* Gentamicin and clindamycin therapy in postpartum endometritis: the efficacy of daily dosing versus dosing every 8 hours. *Am. J. Obstet. Gynecol.* 2003; 188(1): 149–52.

McGregor, J. A., Soper, D. E., Lovell, G., and Todd, J. K. Maternal deaths associated with Clostridium sordellii infection. *Am. J. Obstet. Gynecol.* 1989; 161(4): 987–95.

Rahangdale, L. Infectious complications of pregnancy termination. *Clin. Obstet. Gynecol.* 2009; 52(2): 198–204.

Sawaya, G. F., Grady, D., Kerlikowske, K., and Grimes, D. A. Antibiotics at the time of induced abortion: the case for universal prophylaxis based on a meta-analysis. *Obstet. Gynecol.* 1996; 87(5 Pt. 2): 884–90.

Smaill, F. M. and Grivell, R. M. Antibiotic prophylaxis versus no prophylaxis for preventing infection after cesarean section. *Cochrane Database Syst. Rev.* 2014; 10: CD007482.

Spencer, J. P. Management of mastitis in breastfeeding women. *Am. Fam. Phys.* 2008; 78(6): 727–31.

Sweet, R. L. and Gibbs, R. S. *Infectious Diseases of the Female Genital Tract*, 5th edn. (Philadelphia, PA: Wolters Kluwer Health/Lippincott Williams & Wilkins; 2009).

Yokoe, D. S., Christiansen, C. L., Johnson, R., *et al.* Epidemiology of and surveillance for postpartum infections. *Emerg. Infect. Dis.* 2001; 7(5): 837–41.

Fever in the Returning Traveler

Bradley W. Frazee and Eric Snoey

Introduction

Each year, hundreds of millions of people travel internationally. US citizens take over 50 million trips outside the country anually, and millions of individuals from outside the United States visit or immigrate. Approximately 8% of travelers from industrialized to developing nations seek medical care during or after travel. In the United States, recent immigrants from developing nations account for up to one-half of visits for travel-related illness. Such travelers and émigrés may have been exposed to numerous exotic pathogens. In the evaluation of the ill traveler, eliciting a detailed travel and exposure history is critical. The first priority in management is early identification of illness that may be rapidly progressive, treatable, or transmissable.

The GeoSentinal Surveillance System monitors the etiology of travel-related infections worldwide, as well as in the United States. Infectious diarrhea is the most common type of infection among travelers, including those who have recently arrived in the United States. This chapter, however, focuses on febrile illnesses. The most common reported cause of fever in returning travelers seeking medical care is malaria. Certain forms of malaria can be rapidly fatal, and a key initial step in evaluation is determining whether the febrile traveler has visited an area where *Plasmodium falciparum* malaria is endemic

and, if so, whether immediate treatment is needed. Other important causes of fever in ill travelers include dengue, enteric fever (also known as typhoid or paratyphoid fever), and rickettsial illnesses. Owing to recent large, sustained outbreaks, Chikungunya virus and Zika virus have also emerged as a common cause of febrile illness in travelers. It is also important to recognize that not all infections in returning travelers are exotic. For example, mononucleosis due to Epstein–Barr virus or cytomegalovirus, which has been acquired abroad, is remarkably common. Upper respiratory tract infections, urinary tract infections, pneumonia, and influenza all remain common causes of fever, even in travelers to developing countries. Finally, sexually transmitted diseases are common among travelers, and acute HIV infection, in particular, should be considered in the differential diagnosis.

This chapter proposes a general approach to the febrile traveler and then discusses in detail malaria, dengue fever, and enteric fever. Rickettsial infection, Chikungunya, mononucleosis and leptospirosis are also covered. Zika virus is discussed in Chapter 73. Ebola virus is discussed in Chapter 72.

Travel History

A thorough travel history should be detailed and include specific questions on all locations visited, dates and duration of visit, potential exposures, their timing, and other factors that may affect the risk of contracting infection:

- precise travel itenerary, including all stops and locations visited
- urban versus rural travel
- type of accomodations
- food and beverage consumed (unfiltered water and ice cubes, uncooked or undercooked foods, and unpeeled fruits and vegetables)
- activities (camping, hiking, fishing, swimming, safari, etc.)
- hygiene practices and availability of soap and toilet facilities
- exposure to animals and insects and use of insect repellant or bed nets
- exposure to fresh water
- exposure to bodily fluids (sexual activity, tattooing, intravenous drug use)
- sexual contact (primarily or secondarily)
- prophylactic medications taken during travel
- vaccination history (including childhood immunizations)
- local medical care received, particularly injectable medication or transfusions

Refining the differential diagnosis also requires knowledge of the patient's precise itinerary, geographic distribution of travel-related illnesses, and information about active outbreaks. A list of major travel-related illnesses that are endemic or epidemic in specific regions of the world is detailed in Table 60.1. The list is not exhaustive and is subject to change. Practitioners can also refer to the Centers for Disease Control and Prevention (CDC) for complete and current information (www.cdc.gov, 1-877-394-8747). Other helpful websites include the World Health Organization (WHO) international travel and health website (www.who.int/ith/en/) and healthmap.org.

Table 60.2 categorizes travel-related diseases by length of time from exposure to onset of symptoms. Table 60.3 relates exposure types and associated illnesses. Several clinical decision-making tools are available to assist physicians with constructing a likely differential diagnosis and ordering appropriate initial tests. A good example is www.fevertravel.ch from the University of Lausanne, Switzerland.

General Approach to the Clinical Evaluation

The first step in evaluation of the febrile traveler is to determine whether there are high-risk findings that require urgent action. These include the following:

1. Hemorrhagic manifestations – signs and symptoms, such as bleeding from gums, bloody stool, urine or hemoptysis, petechial or purpuric rash, should raise suspicion for viral hemorrhagic fevers, meningococcal disease, dengue, rickettsial illnesses, and sepsis. Such patients should be isolated immediately and public health authorities contacted.
2. Neurologic abnormalities – altered mental status should raise suspicion for cerebral malaria, meningococcal disease, or other forms of bacterial meningitis, all of which require emergent treatment. Other considerations include African

trypanosomiasis, leptospirosis, rabies, and certain rickettsial illnesses such as scrub typhus.

3. Acute respiratory distress – severe malaria may present with respiratory distress. Other considerations include influenza, bacterial or fungal pneumonia, tularemia, plague, or Middle East Respiratory Syndrome coronavirus (MERS CoV).

Although febrile illness in the returning traveler is often undifferentiated (lacking localizing signs or symptoms), when present, associated signs and symptoms can help narrow the differential diagnosis and guide management. Additional physical exam pearls include the following:

- *Vital signs*
  - Pulse–temperature dissociation (slow heart rate in spite of high fever) may suggest enteric fever (typhoid or paratyphoid fever), yellow fever, or certain rickettsial illnesses.
  - Paroxysmal fevers may be present with malaria or relapsing fever due to *Borrelia* infections.

- *Dermatologic*
  - Maculopapular rash may be present with dengue, Chikungunya, Zika virus, leptospirosis, scrub typhus, acute HIV infection, acute hepatitis B, infectious mononucleosis, and drug reactions.
  - Rose spots (faint salmon-colored macules typically found on the trunk and abdomen) suggest typhoid fever.
  - An eschar (black necrotic ulcer with erythematous margins) may suggest a rickettsial infection such as rickettsial pox, African tick bite fever, Rocky Mountain spotted fever, or scrub typhus (see Figure 60.1).
  - Jaundice may be present with severe malaria, viral hepatitis, severe dengue, leptospirosis, and viral hemorrhagic fevers.

- *Ocular*
  - Conjunctival suffusion is a classic finding seen in leptospirosis, though also reported with Hantavirus infection.
  - Conjunctival injection may indicate Zika virus or dengue fever.
  - Photophobia and ocular lesions may be seen in roundworm invasion of the eye (onchocerciasis, loaiasis).

- *Abdominal*
  - Abdominal tenderness may be present with enteric fever and hepatitis.
  - Splenomegaly is associated with malaria, infectious mononucleosis, visceral leishmaniasis, or enteric fever.

- *Lymphatic*
  - Cervical lymphadenopathy may be present with infectious mononucleosis or tuberculosis.
  - Generalized lymphadenopathy may be seen with acute HIV infection, enteric fever bartonellosis, and tuberculosis.

Table 60.1 Endemic Infectious Diseases According to Region of Travel

Africa, Central

Diseases – malaria (predominantly chloroquine-resistant *P. falciparum*), yellow fever, traveler's diarrhea (*E. coli* infection, salmonellosis, cholera, parasitic infection), enteric fever, dengue, other viral hemorrhagic fevers (Ebola, Marburg, Crimean-Congo hemorrhagic fever), African trypanosomiasis (sleeping sickness), leishmaniasis, onchocerciasis (river blindness), rickettsioses, Chikungunya, meningococcal disease, echinococcosis (hytadid disease), dracunculiasis, HIV infection, hepatitis A, B, C, or E, tuberculosis, HIV infection, plague, and rabies.

Africa, East

Diseases – malaria (predominantly chloroquine-resistant *P. falciparum*), yellow fever, traveler's diarrhea (*E. coli* infection, salmonellosis, cholera, parasitic infection), dengue, filariasis, leishmaniasis, onchocerciasis (river blindness), schistosomiasis, poliomyelitis (Ethiopia and Somalia), meningococcal disease, rickettsioses, Chikungunya, African trypanosomiasis (sleeping sickness), other viral hemorrahgic fevers (Ebola, Rift Valley fever, Crimean-Congo hemorrhagic fever), dracunculiasis, hepatitis A, B, C, or E, tuberculosis, HIV infection, plague, and rabies.

Africa, North

Diseases – malaria (limited risk), traveler's diarrhea (*E. coli* infection, salmonellosis, cholera, parasitic infection), enteric fever, schistosomiasis, echinococcosis (hytadid disease), hepatitis A, B, C, or E, Middle East Respiratory Syndrome (MERS), tuberculosis, HIV infection, plague, and rabies.

Africa, South

Diseases – malaria (predominantly chloroquine-resistant *P. falciparum*), dengue, traveler's diarrhea (*E. coli* infection, salmonellosis, cholera, parasitic infection), enteric fever, African trypanosomiasis, rickettssioses, Chikungunya, schistosomiasis, echinococcosis (hytadid disease), hepatitis A, B, C, or E, tuberculosis, HIV infection, plague, and rabies.

Africa, West

Diseases – malaria (predominantly chloroquine-resistant *P. falciparum*), yellow fever, traveler's diarrhea (*E. coli* infection, salmonellosis, cholera, parasitic infection), dengue, other viral hemorrhagic fevers (Ebola, Lassa fever, Crimean-Congo hemorrhagic fever), enteric fever, schistomsomiasis, African trypansomiasis, onchocerciasis, leishmaniasis, rickettsioses, Chikungunya, meningococcal disease, poliomyelitis (Nigeria), dracunculiasis, echinococcosis (hytadid disease), paragonomiasis, hepatitis A, B, C, or E, tuberculosis, HIV infection, and rabies.

Asia, East/North

Diseases – malaria (China), traveler's diarrhea (*E. coli* infection, salmonellosis, cholera, parasitic infection), Japanese encephalitis, dengue, ricketsioses, enteric fever, Middle East Respiratory Syndrome (South Korea), leishmaniasis, influenza virus, paragonomiasis, hepatitis A, B, C, or E, tuberculosis, HIV infection, and rabies.

Asia, South

Diseases – malaria (including chloroquine-resistant *P. falciparum*), traveler's diarrhea (*Escherichia coli* infection, salmonellosis, cholera, parasitic infection), enteric fever, dengue, Japanese encephalitis, leptospirosis, Chikungunya, ricketsioses, leishmaniasis, brucellosis, hepatitis A, B, C, or E, HIV infection, tuberculosis, and rabies.

Asia, Southeast

Diseases – malaria (including chloroquine-resistant *P. falciparum*), traveler's diarrhea (*E. coli* infection, salmonellosis, cholera, *Vibrio parahaemolyticus*, parasitic infection), enteric fever, dengue, Japanese encephalitis, Chikungunya, Zika virus, ricketsioses, schistosomiasis, leptospirosis, paragonomiasis, influenza, meliodosis, hepatitis A, B, C, or E, HIV infection, tuberculosis, plague, and rabies.

Australia, New Zealand and Oceania

Diseases – malaria (only in Papua New Guinea, the Solomon Islands, and Vanuatu), traveler's diarrhea (*E. coli* infection, salmonellosis, parasitic infection), enteric fever, dengue, Japanese encephalitis, Ross River virus infection, Murray Valley encephalitis, rickettsioses, Q fever, leptospirosis, brucellosis, meliodosis, Chikungunya, and Zika virus.

Caribbean

Diseases – malaria (Haiti and Dominican Republic only and including *P. falciparum*), traveler's diarrhea (*E. coli* infection, salmonellosis, cholera, parasitic infection), dengue, Chikungunya, yellow fever (Trinidad), leptospirosis, endemic fungal infections (histoplasmosis, coccidioidoycosis, paracoccidioidomycosis, cryptococcosis), hepatitis A, B, C, or E, HIV infection, and rabies.

Mexico and Central America

Diseases – malaria (predominantly *P. vivax*), yellow fever (Panama only), traveler's diarrhea (*E. coli* infection, salmonellosis, cholera, parasitic infection), dengue, Chikungunya, Zika virus, cutaneous leishmaniasis, leptospirosis, Chagas disease, rickettsioses, endemic fungal infections (histoplasmosis, coccidioidoycosis, paracoccidioidomycosis, cryptococcosis, and blastomycosis), hepatitis A, B, C, or E, HIV infection, tuberculsosis, and rabies.

Eastern Europe and Northern Asia

Diseases – malaria (Armenia, Azerbaijan, Georgia, Kyrgyzstan, Tajikistan, Turkmenistan, Uzbekistan), traveler's diarrhea (*E. coli* infection, salmonellosis, cholera, parasitic infection), tick-borne encephalitis, rickettsial infections (particularly *R. prowazekii*), Crimean-Congo hemorrhagic fever, echinococcosis (hydatid disease), diphtheria, influenza, measles, hepatitis A, B, C, or E, HIV infection, tuberculosis, and rabies.

Western Europe

Diseases – measles, mumps, tick-borne encephalitis, *Legionella* infection, traveler's diarrhea (*E. coli* infection, salmonellosis, parasitic infection), Lyme disease, Q Fever.

Middle East

Diseases – malaria (Iran, Oman, Yemen, Saudi Arabia, the Syrian Arab Republic, and Turkey), traveler's diarrhea (*E. coli* infection, salmonellosis, cholera, parasitic infection), Middle East Respiratory Syndrome (MERS), enteric fever, leishmaniasis (cutaneous and visceral), dengue, leptospirosis, poliyomyelitis (the Syrian Arab Republic).

Table 60.1 (cont.)

North America and Hawaii

Diseases – plague, rabies, rickettsioses, including Rocky Mountain spotted fever, tularemia, arthropod-borne encephalitis, influenza, endemic fungi (coccidioidomycosis, histoplasmosis, and blastomycosis), rodent-borne hantavirus pulmonary syndrome, Lyme disease, ehrlichosis, babesisis, anaplasmosis, West Nile fever, enterohemorrhagic *E. coli* infection (*E. coli* O157:H7), salmonellosis, hepatitis A, leptospirosis (Hawaii).

Temperate South America

Diseases – malaria (limited risk, predominantly in Argentina), yellow fever (rural Argentina), traveler's diarrhea (*E. coli* infection, salmonellosis, cholera, parasitic infection), typhoid fever, toxoplasmosis, hepatitis A and B, dengue, American trypanosomiasis (Chagas disease), leishmaniasis, rodent-borne hantavirus pulmonary syndrome, filariasis, onchocerciasis, cryptosporidiosis.

Tropical South America

Diseases – malaria, yellow fever, traveler's diarrhea (*E. coli* infection, salmonellosis, cholera, parasitic infection), dengue, Zika virus, Chikungunya, leishmaniasis (cutaneous and visceral), Chagas disease, rickettsioses including Rocky Mountain spotted fever, leptospirosis, schistosomiasis, bartonellosis (Oroya fever), epidemic typhus (louse-borne), endemic fungi (paracoccidoidomycosis, histoplasmosis).

Table 60.2 Typical Incubation Periods for Travel-related Disease

Incubation Period	Diseases
Short (<2 weeks)	Malaria, dengue, yellow fever, Chikungunya, Japanese encephalitis, West Nile virus, most hemorrhagic fevers (Ebola and Lassa Fever), enteric fever, most gastrointestinal pathogens, many rickettsial illlnesses, leptospirosis, meningococcal disease, bacterial pneumonia, influenza, measles, dysentery, plague, Q fever, relapsing fever
Intermediate (2–3 weeks)	Malaria, tick-borne encephalitis, enteric fever, acute HIV infection, leptospirosis, hepatitis A or E, acute schistosomiasis (Katayama fever), hemorrhagic fevers (Ebola, Lassa Fever, Crimean-Congo), many rickettsia disesaes, leptospirosis, rabies, East African trypansomiasis
Long (>3 weeks)	Amebiasis, brucellosis, filariasis, hepatitis B and C, leishmaniasis, melioidosis, paragonimiasis, rabies, bartonellosis, tuberculosis, Chagas disease, West African trypanosomiasis, some forms of schistosomiasis

Adapted from CDC, Traveler's Health Yellow Book: Health Information for International Travel, 2018, wwwnc.cdc.gov/travel/yellowbook/2018/introduction/planning-for-healthy-travel-cdc-travelers-health-website-and-mobile-applications (accessed December 20, 2017).

Table 60.3 Travel-Related Disease: Exposures and Associated Febrile Illnesses

Exposure	Associated Illnesses
Arthropod bites	
Mosquito	Malaria, yellow fever, dengue, Chikungunya, Zika virus, Japanese encephalitis, West Nile virus, filariasis, Rift Valley fever, Ross River virus, Murray Valley encephalitis
Tse tse fly	African trypanosomiasis
Sand fly	Leishmaniasis
Reduviid bug	Chagas disease
Black fly	Filariasis, onchocerciasis
Tick	Lyme disease, ehrlichiosis, babesiosis, tick-borne encephalitis, Crimean-Congo hemorrhagic fever, many rickettsial illnesses, including Rocky Mountain spotted fever (*R. rickettsii*) and African tick bite fever (*R. africae*)
Louse	Epidemic typhus (*R. prowazekii*)
Mite	Scrub typhus (*O. tsutsugamushi*), Rickettsialpox (*R. akari*), Murine typhus (*R. typhi*)
Animal contact	
Bites and scratches	Rabies (more often from dogs in the developing world; skunks, raccoons, and bats in the United States) Pasteurella species infections (with dog or cat bites), herpes B virus infection (macaque monkey bite)
Rodents	Lassa fever, leptospirosis, plague, hantavirus infections
Livestock	Q fever
Ingestions	
Undercooked or unpasteurized food	Hepatitis A and E, traveler's diarrhea (including that due to salmonella, enterohemorrhagic *E. coli*, cholera *Vibrio parahemolyticus*), enteric fever, brucellosis, listeriosis, toxoplasmosis, paragonamiasis, trichinosis
Untreated water	Cholera, gastrointestinal pathogens as listed above
Infected persons	
Respiratory	Tuberculosis, influenza, Middle East respiratory virus (MERS-CoV), legionellosis, measles, meningococcal disease
Fecal-oral	Poliomyelitis, many gastrointestinal pathogens as listed above
Bodily fluids/sexual contact	HIV infection, hepatis B and C, Ebola virus

(continued)

Initial Laboratory Evaluation

The initial laboratory evaluation should generally include the following:

- thick and thins smear for malaria (if travel to endemic region) or other intracellular parasites
- complete blood count with differential
- chemistry panel (electrolytes, blood urea nitrogen, creatinine)
- liver function tests (alanine aminotransferase, aspartate aminotransferase, total bilirubin, alkaline phosphatase)
- blood cultures
- urinalysis and/or urine cultures
- chest X-ray

Additional tests to consider based on clinical suspicion include:

- stool ova and parasites and culture should be ordered for febrile diarrheal illness and patients at risk for parasites
- serology or PCR testing for suspected pathogens, such as dengue, Zika, Chicungunya, leptospirosis, rickettsial pathogens
- hepatitis serologies
- coagulation studies
- testing for HIV and other sexually transmitted infections
- purified protein derivative (PPD) or interferon-gamma release assay for tuberculosis

Testing for more exotic illnesses should be syndrome and/or exposure specific and may be best made in consultation with a travel medicine or infectious disease specialist. Centers for Disease Control and Prevention provide on-call assistance with the diagnosis and management of parasitic infections at 404-718-4745 for parasitic infections other than malaria or 770-488-7788 (toll-free at 855-856-4713) for malaria, during business hours. After business hours, call the CDC Emergency Operations Center at 770-488-7100.

Malaria

Malaria is an acute, febrile, mosquito-borne illness, present is over 106 countries and territories worldwide. It is estimated that over 3.2 billion people live in areas at risk of transmission, resulting in 214 million clinical episodes and 438,000 deaths in 2015. In the United States, endemic malaria was eradicated in the early 1950s, with only rare, localized outbreaks of mosquito-borne illness occurring when local mosquitos bite individuals carrying malaria from other, endemic areas. Nevertheless, the three species of mosquito responsible for malaria prior to eradication are still prevalent in the United States, underscoring the ongoing risk of a reintroduction of malaria similar to Zika and dengue. Currently, virtually all of the 1,500 to 2,000 annual cases of malaria in the United States involve recent travelers to endemic areas.

Epidemiology and Microbiology

Malaria is caused by one of four species of the protozoan genus *Plasmodium* (*P. falciparum*, *P. ovale*, *P. vivax*, and *P. malariae*) and transmitted by the bite of a female *Anopheles* mosquito. Once inoculated, sporozoites travel to the liver within 1 to 2 hours, after which the individual enters a relatively asymptomatic phase averaging between 7 and 35 days. Symptoms begin in the erythrocytic phase of the life cycle when infected red blood cells rupture and release merozoites prompting fever, malaise, and other manifestations of the disease. Incubation periods will vary based on the plasmodium species, the degree of host defense, and which type of prophylaxis (if any) was used. It would be very unusual for clinical disease to occur less than 7 days post-exposure – a situation that should prompt consideration of an alternative diagnosis. On the other hand, semi-immune individuals or these on inadequate prophylaxis may experience incubation periods of several weeks to months. *P. vivax* and *P. ovale* may have a relapsing course where the disease recurs months or even years after the initial illness due to reactivation of residual hypnozoites in the liver. *P. falciparum* and *P. malariae* have no dormant phase and relapsing symptoms invariably mean re-exposure and infection.

Clinical Features

The initial phase of malaria consists of a non-specific febrile illness in the context of travel to a region where malaria is endemic. In addition to fever, patients may experience malaise, fatigue, muscle aches, headache, vomiting, diarrhea, and abdominal pain. Early in the disease, the pattern of fever is irregular, with daily spikes up to 40 °C, often accompanied by tachycardia and delirium. Later in the disease course, the release of merozoites can synchronize, leading to predictable intervals between fevers. In the case of *P. vivax*, *P. ovale*, and *P. falciparum*, fevers are typically every other day, while febrile episodes with *P. malariae* occur every third day. Physical findings can include evidence of mild anemia, jaundice, and splenomegaly.

Otherwise healthy patients with this general presentation are said to have "uncomplicated malaria." Their parasitic load is <0.1%, or <5,000 parasites/microL of blood. Laboratory abnormalities are limited to mild anemia, thrombocytopenia, elevated transaminase, BUN, and creatinine. Prognosis is excellent with the initiation of appropriate therapy.

Signs of end organ dysfunction herald the development of "severe malaria." Heavier loads of parasitized RBCs (4 to 10%) adhere to vessel walls resulting in obstruction, tissue ischemia, capillary leakage, and multi-organ failure. Patients may experience confusion and seizures, respiratory distress including ARDS, renal and hepatic failure, metabolic acidosis, DIC, hypoglycaemia, and shock. While *P. falciparum* is the species most associated with "severe malaria." *P. vivax* has also been implicated, in particular with ARDS. Groups at greatest risk of complications include non-immune or immunocompromised individuals, those off prophylaxis, pregnant women, and children between 6 and 36 months of age.

Cerebral malaria deserves special consideration because of its potential for rapid deterioration and the critical role of early diagnosis and treatment. The prototypic presentation of cerebral malaria is the child, exposed in an endemic area,

Table 60.4 Clinical Features: Malaria

Organism	*Plasmodium falciparum* *P. vivax* *P. ovale* *P. malariae*
Incubation period	7 days or longer
Signs and symptoms	**Generalized illness:** • fever, chills (a cyclic pattern of febrile episodes may emerge, commonly repeating every 2–3 days) • headache • myalgias, fatigue • vomiting, diarrhea • abdominal pain • hepatosplenomegaly **Severe malaria:** • acute renal and hepatic failure • generalized convulsions • cardiovascular compromise, shock • acute respiratory distress syndrome (ARDS) • metabolic acidosis, DIC, hypoglycemia • altered mental status, coma
Laboratory findings	• thick and thin blood smears: determine presence of malarial parasites, parasitic load, and speciation • rapid diagnostic tests (RDTs): species specific, qualitative tests for presence of parasites, using antigen or antibody assays • mild transaminitis, hyperbilirubinemia • thrombocyctopenia • elevation of BUN/creatinine • mild anemia

with a febrile convulsion, delirium, and impaired consciousness. Cerebral edema and increased intracranial pressure may develop, leading to coma and death. Untreated, cerebral edema is universally fatal; with treatment mortality of 15 to 20%. Many survivors experience profound neurologic sequelae, including hemiplegia, cortical blindness, deafness, and cognitive impairment.

The clinical features of malaria are summarized in Table 60.4.

Differential Diagnosis

The appearance of early, uncomplicated malaria is quite non-specific. Fever, headache, myalgias, and fatigue in the returning traveler can be explained by a variety of infectious etiologies; both exotic and mundane. While laboratory testing will play an important role in confirming the diagnosis (see below), one should seek out distinguishing characteristics to aid in establishing or excluding alternative etiologies.

• Dengue fever: also known as "break-bone fever," severe myalgias are the characteristic feature of this disease, which also demonstrates fatigue, headache, and abdominal pain similar to malaria. A majority of patients will have a rash that would be atypical for malaria. A rare hemorrhagic form of dengue exists. The diagnosis of dengue fever is confirmed with serology.

• Chikungunya (see below): Chikungunya resembles dengue fever with regard to severe myalgias and non-specific maculopapular rash. The clinical course is self-limited with rare clinical deterioration or hemorrhagic complications. The diagnosis is confirmed with serology.

• Typhoid: in addition to fever, patients with typhoid may experience abdominal pain, relative bradycardia, and the characteristic Rose spots rash (faint salmon-colored macules typically found on the trunk and abdomen). The diagnosis of typhoid is confirmed with blood and stool cultures.

• Leptospirosis: a spirochete infection from exposure to the urine of an infected animal. Associated symptoms include fever, rigors, headache, and myalgias that are typically more severe than with malaria. Patients may also experience petechial hemorrhages to the skin and mucosal surfaces. The diagnosis is established by serology.

• Viral hemorrhagic fever: group of several distinct viral illnesses characterized by fever, malaise, petechial rash, and multisystem organ dysfunction. Diagnosis is confirmed via immunoassay or nucleic acid testing.

Laboratory and Radiographic Findings

Any patient with fever and exposure to an area endemic for malaria should undergo confirmatory testing. The principle diagnostic tools are either microscopy for direct visualization of the parasite in stained blood or rapid diagnostic tests (RDTs), which detect malaria-specific antigens or antibodies. Each method has advantages and disadvantages depending on the clinical context.

Microscopy

Direct visualization of parasites with light microscopy allows for diagnostic confirmation, speciation, and determination of parasitic density (correlates with disease intensity and permits monitoring of therapeutic response). Two types of slides are made using a single drop of finger stick whole blood. Thin smear preparations maintain the integrity of the erythrocytes and allow visualization of the parasites species within the RBC. Thick smear preparations use a larger quantity of blood and involve the lysis of the RBCs so that the parasites can be seen independent of the other cellular structures. Because a larger amount of blood is viewed, thick smears are more sensitive for the presence of disease. Light microscopy is labor intensive and requires significant training. Even then, in cases of very low parasite density, the diagnosis may be missed.

RDTs

These antigen/antibody tests are rapidly replacing traditional light microscopy in resource-poor areas due to their accuracy, speed, and ease of use. RDTs are qualitative (yes/no) tests and each is specific for one species of malaria only. They provide no information on parasite density. From a practical standpoint, in endemic areas, the choice of RDT used is determined by the predominant malaria species. Antibody-based RDTs can confirm exposure, but are unable to distinguish acute vs. prior infection. The FDA recently approved an RDT (BinaxNOW Malaria) that is a combination antibody and aldolase (elevated in malaria infections) assay with a sensitivity between 84 and 94%. One study evaluated the ability of patients to self-diagnose using an RDT and found a 97% sensitivity among 153 symptomatic British travelers. Both false-positive and false-negative RDTs have been reported, particularly in cases of very low parasite density.

Treatment and Prophylaxis

Treatment design is dependent on the infecting species, the clinical status of the patient, and likely resistance patterns, based on the geographic regions visited. Identification of the infecting species is critical for several reasons: (1) *P. falciparum* infections require extremely aggressive treatment because of the potential for development of severe clinical malaria; (2) *P. ovale* and *P. vivax* infections generate dormant liver forms (hypnozoites) that may cause recurrent episodes unless treated with primaquine; and (3) geographic drug resistance patterns differ among species.

The treatment information in Table 60.5 is drawn from the CDC guidelines. Clinicians should refer to the CDC recommendations (www.cdc.gov) for the most current and complete information when making patient management decisions. For the management of malaria in pregnant women, refer to the latest CDC guidelines or consult with a specialist via the CDC Malaria Hotline: (770) 488–7788.

See Tables 60.5 and 60.6 for a summary of malaria treatment and prophylaxis.

Complications and Admission Criteria

The majority of malaria patients presenting to non-endemic hospitals are admitted, a practice rooted in part in the relative unfamiliarity with malarial syndromes in these facilities as well as the propensity for *P. falciparum* malaria to deteriorate quickly. In general, patients with non-falciparum malaria can be managed using traditional criteria for admission and discharge decisions. High-risk patient groups (infants 6 to 36 months of age, immunocompromised patients, pregnant women) should be admitted for observation. Similarly, any patients demonstrating features of "severe malaria" need immediate empiric therapy and intensive care observation. Regarding *P. falciparum* malaria without high-risk features, there have been a number of studies looking at various clinical scores. In general, patients with high fever, gastrointestinal symptoms, jaundice, low platelets, and high parasite loads (>2%) required hospital-based care.

Dengue Fever

Dengue is a systemic viral infection with a broad range of clinical severity, from asymptomatic infection to life-threatening dengue hemorrhagic fever. It is among the most common and important mosquito-borne viral infections. Among travelers with a systemic febrile illness, dengue is second only to malaria as an identified etiology. Acute care physicians who may care for travelers should be well versed in the presentation and management of dengue.

Epidemiology and Microbiology

For the most part, dengue viral infection is limited to human and mosquito hosts. The expansion of the current dengue pandemic is linked to several factors, including the expanding distribution of the principle vector, *Aedes aegypti* mosquito, rapid human urbanization crowding, and increasing global travel and trade. It coincides with the emergence of Chicungunga virus and Zika virus infection, also carried by *A. aegypti*.

Dengue is caused by one of four viral serotypes belonging to the flavivirus genus. There is limited cross immunity between serotypes, which means individuals may become ill up to four times when infected with a new serotype. Alterations in microvascular permeability and thromboregulation that are not well understood lead to the severe manifestations of dengue. Severity risk factors include young age, female sex, obesity, and secondary infection or sequential infection with a second serotype.

Clinical Features

The clinical presentation of dengue ranges from asymptomatic to self-limited dengue fever, to life-threatening dengue hemorrhagic fever (DHF) with shock syndrome (see Table 60.7). Asymptomatic infection is less common in adults than children. Symptoms typically develop between 4 and 7 days after exposure, but incubation can extend to 14 days. Thus, it is common for symptoms to begin in travelers after returning home. Classic dengue fever is characterized by abrupt onset of fever often accompanied by headache, retro-orbital pain, extreme fatigue, and marked muscle and joint pains. There may be a maculopapular rash. The severity of musculoskeletal symptoms accounts for its historical name: "breakbone fever." Nausea, vomiting, diarrhea, cough, sore throat, and sinus congestion can be seen. Rare neurological manifestations

Table 60.5 Acute Malaria Treatment

Species	Drug Sensitivity	Adult Treatment*	Pediatric Treatment* (Never to Exceed Adult Dose)
P. falciparum	Chloroquine-sensitive (Central America west of Panama Canal; Haiti; the Dominican Republic; most of the Middle East)	Chloroquine phosphate (Aralen): • 600 mg base PO immediately • 300 mg base PO at 6, 24, 48 hours Second-line alternative: Hydroxychloroquine (Plaquenil): • 620 mg base PO immediately • 310 mg base PO at 6, 24, 48 hours	Chloroquine phosphate (Aralen): • 10 mg base/kg PO immediately • 5 mg base/kg PO at 6, 24, 48 hours Second-line alternative: Hydroxychloroquine (Plaquenil): • 10 mg base/kg PO immediately • 5 mg base/kg PO at 6, 24, 48 hours

	Chloroquine-resistant (all malarious regions except those listed above)	Any of the following three treatment regimens is considered first line:
		1. Artemether-lumefantrine† one tab. BID for 3 days
		  • 5–15 kg: 20/120
		  • 15–25 kg: 40/240
		  • 25–35 kg: 60/360
		  • >35 kg: 80/480
		2. Quinine sulfate plus one of the following: doxycycline, tetracycline, clindamycin:
		  • quinine sulfate: 542 mg base PO TID × 3–7 days
		  • doxycycline: 100 mg PO BID × 7 days
		  • tetracycline: 250 mg PO QID × 7 days
		  • clindamycin: 20 mg base/kg/day PO divided TID × 7 days
		3. Atovaquone-proguanil (Malarone):
		  • four adult tabs PO QD × 3 days
		4. Mefloquine (Lariam):
		  • 684 mg base PO immediately
		  • 456 mg base PO 6–12 hours later
			Any of the following three treatment regimens is considered first line:
			1. Artemether-lumefantrine† one tab. BID for 3 days
			  • 5–15 kg: 20/120
			  • 15–25 kg: 40/240
			  • 25–35 kg: 60/360
			  • >35 kg: 80/480
			2. Quinine sulfate plus one of the following: doxycycline, tetracycline, clindamycin
			  • quinine sulfate: 8.3 mg base/kg PO TID × 3–7 days
			  • doxycycline: 2.2 mg/kg PO BID × 7 days
			  • tetracycline: 25 mg/kg/day PO divided QID × 7 days
			  • clindamycin: 20 mg base/kg/day PO divided TID × 7 days
			3. Atovaquone-proguanil (Malarone):
			  • 5–8 kg: two peds tabs PO QD × 3 days
			  • 9–10 kg: three peds tabs PO QD × 3 days
			  • 11–20 kg: one adult tab PO QD × 3 days
			  • 21–30 kg: two adult tabs PO QD × 3 days
			  • 31–40 kg: three adult tabs PO QD × 3 days
			  • >40 kg: four adult tabs PO QD × 3 days
			4. Mefloquine (Lariam):
			  • 13.7 mg base/kg PO immediately
			  • 9.1mg base/kg PO 6–12 hours later

P. malariae	Chloroquine-sensitive‡	Chloroquine phosphate (as above) Second-line alternative: hydroxychloroquine (as above)	Chloroquine phosphate (as above) Second-line alternative: hydroxychloroquine (as above)
P. vivax, *P. ovale*	Chloroquine-sensitive	Chloroquine phosphate *plus* primaquine phosphate: • chloroquine phosphate (as above) • primaquine phosphate: 30 mg base PO QD × 14 days Second-line alternative: Hydroxychloroquine *plus* primaquine phosphate: • hydroxychloroquine (as above) • primaquine phosphate (as above)	Chloroquine phosphate *plus* primaquine phosphate • chloroquine phosphate (as above) • primaquine phosphate: 0.5 mg base/kg PO QD × 14 days Second-line alternative: Hydroxychloroquine *plus* primaquine phosphate: • hydroxychloroquine (as above) • primaquine phosphate (as above)
P. vivax	Chloroquine-resistant (Papua New Guinea and Indonesia)	Either of the following two treatment regimens are considered first line:	Either of the following two treatment regimens are considered first line:
Severe Infection		**Adult Treatment**	**Pediatric Treatment**
		Quinidine gluconate or Artesunate† plus one of the following: doxycycline, tetracycline, *or* clindamycin • quinidine gluconate: 6.25 mg base/kg loading dose IV over 1–2 hours, 0.0125 mg base/kg/min continuous infusion × at least 24 hours *or* Artesunate† (IV/IM) 2.4 mg/kg, three doses over 24 hours Together with either: • doxycycline (as above) • tetracycline (as above) clindamycin (as above)	Quinidine gluconate or Artesunate† plus one of the following: doxycycline, tetracycline, *or* clindamycin • quinidine gluconate: same as adult *or* Artesunate (IV) 3.0mg/kg Together with either: • doxycycline (as above) • tetracycline (as above) • clindamycin (as above)

(continued)

Table 60.5 (cont.)

* Where applicable, medication dosages have been reported in base form. Conversions to appropriate doses of the corresponding salt can be made using updated CDC treatment guidelines as a reference. Care should taken in making these calculations as they are a common source of error.

† Artemisinin based therapies are now considered first-line by the WHO for treatment of chloroquine resistent *P falciparum*. The CDC recommends oral Artemether–lumefantrine for uncomplicated malaria in the USA and endemic areas. Severe malaria should be treated with parenteral Artesunate. Artesunate is not FDA approved within the USA but can be obtained through the CDC under an investigation protocol (CDC Malaria Hotline: 770-488-7788). The initial 3 doses are followed by oral therapy using standard drugs, as noted above.

‡ There have been no reports to date of chloroquine resistance in any strains of *P. malariae*.

Table 60.6 Prophylactic Antimalarial Regimens

Drug	Use	Adult Dose	Pediatric Dose
Atovaquone–proguanil (Malarone)	Prophylaxis in areas with chloroquine- or mefloquine-resistant *P. falciparum*	One tab. PO, daily. Adult tabs. contain 250 mg atovaquone and 100 mg proguanil hydrochloride.	Pediatric tabs. contain 62.5 mg atovaquone and 25 mg proguanil hydrochloride. Dosing is weight-based: 11–20 kg: one tab. 21–30 kg: two tabs. 31–40 kg: three tabs. 41 kg or more: one adult tab. daily
	Timeline	**Contraindications**	**Notes**
	Begin 1–2 days before travel. Take daily at the same time each day during travel and for 7 days after returning.	Severe renal impairment (creatinine clearance <30 mL/min)	Not recommended for prophylaxis of children <11 kg, pregnant women, or women breastfeeding infants <11 kg. Atovaquone–proguanil should be taken with food or a milky drink
Chloroquine phosphate (Aralen and generic)	Prophylaxis in areas with chloroquine-sensitive *P. falciparum*	5 mg/kg base (8.3 mg/kg salt), up to maximum adult dose of 300 mg base, PO, once per week	
	Timeline	**Contraindications**	**Notes**
	Begin 1–2 weeks before travel. Take weekly on the same day of the week, during travel and for 4 weeks after returning.		May exacerbate psoriasis
Doxycycline	Prophylaxis in areas with chloroquine- or mefloquine-resistant *P. falciparum*	100 mg, PO, daily	For children 8 years old and over, use 2 mg/kg up to adult dose of 100 mg/day
	Timeline	**Contraindications**	**Notes**
	Begin 1–2 days before travel. Take daily at the same time each day while traveling and for 4 weeks after returning.	Contraindicated in pregnant women and children <8 years of age	Patients should be warned about photosensitivity reactions
Hydroxychloroquine sulfate (Plaquenil and generic)	An alternative to chloroquine for prophylaxis in areas with chloroquine-sensitive *P. falciparum*	5 mg/kg base (6.5 mg/kg salt), PO, once per week, up to maximum dose of 310 mg base	
	Timeline	**Contraindications**	**Notes**
	Begin 1–2 weeks before travel. Take weekly on the same day of the week while traveling and for 4 weeks after returning.		
Mefloquine (Lariam and generic)	Prophylaxis in areas with chloroquine-resistant *P. falciparum*	228 mg base (250 mg salt), PO, once per week	Pediatric dosing is weight-based: <10 kg: 4.6 mg/kg base (5 mg/kg salt), once per week 10–19 kg: 1/4 adult tab. once per week 20–30 kg: 1/2 adult tab. Once perweek 31–45 kg: 3/4 adult tab. once per week > 45 kg: one adult tab. once per week

Table 60.6 *(cont.)*

Drug	Use	Adult Dose	Pediatric Dose
	Timeline	**Contraindications**	**Notes**
	Begin 1–2 weeks before travel. Take weekly on the same day of the week while traveling and for 4 weeks after returning.	Contraindicated in persons allergic to mefloquine or related compounds (e.g. quinine and quinidine). Contraindicated in persons with active or recent history of depression, generalized anxiety disorder, psychosis, schizophrenia, other major psychiatric disorders, or seizures.	Not recommended for persons with cardiac conduction abnormalities. May reduce serum levels of common seizure medications
Primaquine	Used for presumptive antirelapse therapy (terminal prophylaxis) to decrease the risk of recurrent illness in *P. vivax* and *P. ovale* infection. Call malaria hotline (770-488-7788) for additional information.	0.6 mg/kg base (1.0 mg/kg salt), up to maximum dose of 30 mg base (52.6 mg salt), PO, daily	
	Timeline	**Contraindications**	**Notes**
	Begin 1–2 days before travel. Take daily at the same time each day while traveling and for 7 days after returning.	May cause hemolytic episode in patients with G6PD deficiency. Contraindicated during pregnancy and lactation, unless the infant being breastfed has a documented normal G6PD level. Use in consultation with malaria experts.	

PO – by mouth.

include encephalopathy, seizures, and acute motor weakness. However, the most common symptoms reported by travelers with dengue are just fever and severe fatigue. Physical exam at this febrile stage may reveal conjunctival injection, pharyngeal erythema, lymphadenopathy, and hepatomegaly. In addition to a brief maculopapular rash, mild petechiae and bruising at venopuncture sites may be evident. The febrile stage typically lasts for 5 to 7 days and most patients recover uneventfully with or without a period of severe fatigue.

As fever wanes, however, a small subset of patients can enter a brief so-called critical phase, characterized primarily by capillary leakage, during which DHF can ensue. A narrowing pulse pressure (with the danger threshold in children and young adults being 20 mmHg) signifies loss of plasma volume and may herald DHF and shock. Other warning signs of the critical phase include worsening abdominal pain, vomiting, development of effusions, marked restlessness or lethargy, and rising hematocrit and falling platelet count.

The five features previously required for the diagnosis of DHF include increased vascular permeability (plasma leakage syndrome, evidenced by 20% or greater rise in hematocrit above baseline value), pleural effusion or ascites, marked thrombocytopenia, fever lasting 2 to 7 days, and hemorrhagic diathesis, including a positive tourniquet test. (This involves inflating a blood pressure cuff around the arm at a pressure midway between systolic and diastolic for 5 minutes. More than 20 petechiae/square inch is positive.) These strict criteria, while helpful for identifying severe disease

manifestations, have recently been abandoned by the WHO. The classification "severe dengue" is now defined by any of the following: plasma leakage resulting in shock, pleural effusion or ascites resulting in respiratory distress, severe bleeding, or severe organ dysfunction. Severe bleeding includes significant skin bleeding, vaginal bleeding, and gastrointestinal bleeding.

Differential Diagnosis

The most important infections to consider in the differential diagnosis of fever and systemic illness in a returning traveler are enumerated above in the malaria section. Because of overlap in their clinical presentation, distinguising between the common arbovirus infections – dengue, Chickungunya, and Zika – can be particularly difficult. However, large case series reveal several differences that may be helpful. Visible arthritis on exam (as opposed to musculoskeletal pain) seems to be fairly specific for chickunguna. Conjunctivitis is specific for Zika virus and maculopapular rash is more common in Zika than the other two infections. Thrombocytopenia and leukopenia are more common in dengue and, most importantly, capillary leak, shock, and hemorrhagic complications are virtually unique to dengue.

Laboratory and Radiographic Features

Laboratory manifestations of dengue which may be uncovered during the standard evaluation of the febrile traveler include

Table 60.7 Clinical Features: Dengue

Organism	Any one of four serotypes of dengue virus (DV1–4)
Incubation period	Typically 4–7, but up to 14 days
Signs and symptoms	**Classic dengue fever (DF):** • fever, abrupt onset • headache, retro-orbital pain • extreme fatigue • marked muscle and joint pain • maculopapular rash • nausea, vomiting, diarrhea • cough, sore throat, sinus congestion • conjunctival injection, pharyngeal erythema • lymphadenopathy • hepatomegaly • encephalopathy, seizures, or acute motor weakness **Dengue hemorrhagic fever (DHF):** • manifestations of increased vascular permeability (hematocrit rise >20%; shock) • pleural effusion or ascites • marked thrombocytopenia (≤100,000 cells/mm³) • spontaneous bleeding (e.g. petechiae, gastrointestinal bleeding) or a hemorrhagic tendency (positive tourniquet test)
Laboratory findings	• thrombocytopenia • moderate elevation (two- to eightfold rise) of serum aspartate transaminase (AST) • leukopenia • viral PCR • MAC-ELISA IgM detetection
Prevention	There is no vaccine currently available, so prevention lies in risk reduction. The *Aedes aegypti* mosquito is most active during the day, so although bed-netting is always a good idea, protective clothing and insect repellent are the most important preventative measures.
Treatment	• There is no specific treatment for dengue virus infection. • The primary goals of therapy are fever reduction, rehydration, volume replacement, and prevention and treatment of hemorrhage and shock. • Because plasma leakage syndrome is the most dangerous complication of DHF, plasma volume replacement is crucial. Shock should be recognized as early as possible.

the following: thrombocytopenia, leukopenia, transaminitis, and hyponatremia. Marked thrombocytopenia and transaminitis, particularly during day 4 to 7 of fever, may signal risk for severe dengue. Patients with suspected dengue should generally undergo daily complete blood count (CBC) and liver function tests (LFT).

Etiologic testing for dengue is somewhat complex, and testing for suspected dengue in returning travelers in the United States should be undertaken in conjuction with public health authorities. The best diagnostic test depends on the duration of illness at the time of testing. During the first 3 days after fever onset, detection of viral nucleic acid by polymerase chain reaction (PCR) is the main test used in the United States, though testing for non-structural protein 1 (NS1) by various methods can also be used at this stage. At or beyond 3 days, an acute-phase serologic test is used. IgM antibiody capture enzyme linked immunosorbant assay (MAC-ELISA) is the most common test used in the United States.

Treatment and Prophylaxis

There is as yet no proven, specific antiviral treatment for dengue, and management remains supportive. Many patients with dengue can be managed as outpatients, though daily

monitoring for signs of severe dengue including CBC and LFT is recommended. Fever should be managed with acetaminophen rather than NSAIDs. In severe dengue, careful intravenous fluid resuscitation and red blood cell and platelet transfusions in cases of hemorrage can be life-saving.

A dengue vaccine is in the late development stage. Although multiple phase three trials have been conducted, more data on long-term efficacy and immunity is required before it can be approved. Vector control is important for prevention in limiting outbreaks. For travelers to endemic areas, prevention of *A. aegypti* bites involves staying indoors or in screened areas during the day, and applying *N,N*-diethyl-*m*-toluamide (DEET) when outdoors.

Complications and Admission Criteria

Most travelers infected with the dengue virus are at low risk for severe dengue because they have no previous infection. Nevertheless, all individuals with suspected dengue should be monitored for signs of severe dengue, which requires hospitalization. Criteria for hospitalization include: hematocrit >50% or rise >20%; platelet <100,000 cells/mm³; marked transaminitis; hemorrhagic signs; abdominal pain, persistent vomiting, or marked lethargy, particularly on days 4 to 7. In addition, hospitalization should be strongly considered in patients with suspected dengue and significant chronic comorbidities, particularly renal disease, or any of the following: infancy, age >65, pregnancy. Complications of dengue include encephalitis, myocarditis, renal failure, and death. Cardiovascular collapse is more common in children and young adults in endemic regions with a prior history of dengue.

Enteric Fever

Enteric fever, or typhoid fever, is a classic cause of prolonged febrile illness in a returning traveler. While less common among US travelers, worldwide enteric fever is the second most common acute and life-threatening infection among travelers, after malaria, and the most common that is vaccine preventable. Enteric fever encompasses a broad range of clinical findings, many of which are subtle, and a range of complications and severity extending to bowel perforation, peritonitis, and death. Acute care physicians caring for febrile travelers need to maintain a high index of suspicion for enteric fever, be familiar with its protean manifestations, and initiate the correct diagnostic and management steps.

Epidemiology and Microbiology

Salmonella, a genus within enterobacteriaciae, has one medically important species, *S. enterica*. *S. enterica* is divided into numerous serotypes. While several non-typhoidal serotypes cause predominantly a food poisoning or diarrheal illness (salmonenolosis) and can infect non-human hosts, only typhi and paratyphi cause enteric fever and are carried exclusively by humans. Although technically classified as serotypes, by convention the pathogens are still referred to as *S. typhi* and *S. paratypi*.

The bacteria are gram-negative rods adapted to survive passage through gastric acid and then penetrate the intestinal epithelium. Lymphatic and hematogenous dissemination throughout the body can occur. Chronic carriage in the biliary and urinary tract, which presents a prolonged risk of transmission, is seen in approximately 5% of cases, and is associated with cholelithiasis and urinary schistosomiasis. Development of drug resistance in *S. typhi* and *S. paratyphi*, and rapid emergence of multidrug-resistant strains where enteric fever is endemic, is an important feature of these pathogens (discussed further in the treatment section, below).

S. typhi and *S. paratyphi* are transmitted by the fecal–oral route via contaminated food or water. Infection occurs predominantly in areas of crowding, poor hygiene, and sanitation. Rare cases acquired within the United States continue to occur, however. Although endemic in developing countries throughout the world, the incidence is highest in the Indian subcontinent (south central Asia). Travelers to India, Nepal, and Pakistan account for the majority of cases. Most travel-associated cases of enteric fever in the United States occur in individuals who have visited friends or relatives. Unvaccinated travelers are at highest risk, though infection in vaccinated travelers can occur, particularly with *S. paratyphi*.

Clinical Features

The incubation period between ingestion and the onset of fever is 5 to 21 days (see Table 60.8). The classic presentation in untreated individuals follows a timed progression. The first week of illness is characterized by increasing fever. Pulse–temperature dissociation is a classic finding. Bacteremia and dissemination occur at this stage. During the second week, mild gastrointestinal symptoms and rose spots develop. Rose spots are described as salmon-colored and appear on the trunk. Abdominal distension, constipation, and diarrhea are all common. The third week of illness is the stage at which severe manifestations appear. These include intestinal bleeding, bowel perforation (related to ileocecal lymphatic hyperplasia), peritonitis, secondary polymicrobial bacteremia, and septic shock.

Neurologic complications are rare, but well described. These include delerium (typhoid encephalopathy), obtundation, myelitis, and rigidity. As a result of bacteremia, focal extraintestinal complications may occur, extending potentially to all organ systems.

Differential Diagnosis

The main differential diagnosis for prolonged fever in a returning traveler is enumerated above in the malaria section.

Laboratory and Radiographic Findings

Initial laboratory findings in enteric fever are non-specific. Complete blood count usually shows a leukocytosis or leukopenia with a left shift. A modest transaminitis (ALT <500) is the norm.

The etiologic diagnosis of enteric fever is made primarily with blood cultures. Therefore, it is essential for acute care providers to obtain two sets of blood cultures before beginning empiric antimicrobial therapy in the febrile traveler. Bone marrow culture is more sensitive than blood culture and may remain positive even after several days of antibiotics. Stool culture may be positive during the early stages of illness. *S. typhi* and *S. paratyphi* isolates should routinely undergo susceptibility testing, particularly for the detection of fluoroquinolone resistance; nalidixic acid resistance can be used as a marker for fluoroquinolone resistance.

Treatment and Prophylaxis

Antimicrobial treatment of confirmed or suspected *S. typhi* and *S. paratyphi* infection is a potentially complex issue because of changing antibiotic resistance pattens in endemic regions. Owing to high levels of resistance to the antimicrobials traditionally used to treat enteric fever (chloramphenicol, ampicillin, and trimethoprim–sulfamethoxazole), flouroquinolones are now the empiric drug of choice for treatment of infection that is acquired in countries outside of Asia. For children with enteric fever, most experts consider the benefits of fluoroquinolones to outweigh the risks. Unfortunately, fluoroquinolone-resistant strains are now common in the Indian subcontinent and are increasing elsewhere in Asia.

Table 60.8 Clinical Features: Enteric Fever

Incubation	5–21 days
Organism	*Salmonella typhi* *S. paratyphi*
Signs and symptoms	• Week 1 – rising "stepwise" fever • Week 2 – abdominal pain, constipation, diarrhea, rose spots • Week 3 – hepatosplenomegaly, intestinal bleeding, bowel perforation • Constipation followed by diarrhea • Relative bradycardia, pulse-temperature dissociation • Uncommon findings include altered level of consciousness, myelitis, rigidity, septic shock
Laboratory findings	• Blood culture isolation of *S. typhi*, *S. paratyphi* is primary means of etiologic diagnosis; antibiotic susceptibility testing is crucial for treatment • Stool cultures may be revealing. If clinical suspicion is high, but blood cultures negative, bone marrow aspiration and culure is recommended. • Leukocytosis, leukopenia • Abnormal liver function tests
Prevention	Two typhoid vaccines (oral and intramuscular) are available. Neither provides protection against paratyphoid infection and neither is completely effective against *S. typhi*.
Treatment	• In all cases, resistance to ampicillin, trimethoprim-sulfamethoxazole, and chloramphenicol should be assumed pending isolate susceptibility. • Fluoroquinolones resistance is common in strains from the Indian subcontinent, and emergeing elsewhere in Asia. • Antibiotic susceptibility testing should be performed and used to guide drug selection from among the list below. • For empiric treatment of severe disease, or when infection has been acquired where fluoroquinolone resistance is common, a parentaral beta-lactam is recommended: Ceftriaxone (2 to 3 g QD parenterally for 7–14 days), cefixime (20–30 mg/kg per day PO, divided into two doses, for 7–14 days) When a fluoroquinolone is appropriate first-line therapy: Ciprofloxacin (500 mg BID), ofloxacin (400 mg BID, either PO or parenterally for 7–10 days) • Azithromycin (1 g PO, single dose, followed by 500 mg QD for 7–14 days) • Chloramphenicol (2–3 g per day PO, divided into four doses, for 14 days) For pediatric patients, the following agents may be used: • Beta-lactam drugs: ceftriaxone (100 mg/kg per day IV, maximum 4 g per day for 10–14 days), cefotaxime (150–200 mg/kg per day IV, maximum 12 g per day for 10–14 days), cefixime (20 mg/kg per day PO, divided into two doses, maximum 400 mg per day for 10–14 days) • Fluoroquinolones: ciprofloxacin (30 mg/kg daily, maximum 1,000 mg per day for 7–10 days), ofloxacin (30 mg/kg daily, maximum 800 mg per day for 7–10 days) For severe typhoid fever (disease with associated mental status changes), corticosteroid therapy is indicated: • Loading dose of 3 mg/kg followed by 1 mg/kg every 6 hours for a total of 48 hours

IV – intravenous; PO – by mouth.

Therefore, for non-severe infections acquired in Asia, oral azithromycin is generally considered the drug of choice. Oral cefixime is another option. Severe illness can be treated with ceftriaxone until susceptibilities return. For isolates that prove susceptible, fluoroquinolones are considered the drug class of choice because of bactericidal activity and tissue and bile penetration. Although data from the post-chloramphenicol era are lacking, for severe disease (delerium, shock) most experts recommend the addition of dexamethasone 3 mg/kg before the first dose of antibiotics, followed by 1 mg/kg every 6 hours for six doses.

Both an oral and parenteral typhoid vaccine are available, which partially protect against *S. typhi*, but not *S. paratyphi*. The CDC recommends that travelers to highly endemic countries (particularly the Indian subcontinent; latest recommendations are available at the CDC website) receive either type of vaccination, though pregnant women and immunocompromised patients should avoid the oral vaccine.

Complications and Admission Criteria

Most cases of enteric fever can be treated on an outpatient basis. Severe disease tends to occur after the second week of illness. The most important complication to consider is ileal perforation. Patients with severe or worsening abdominal pain and distension should undergo CT scanning. Perforation requires immediate laparotomy and broad antibiotic coverage for fecal flora. Altered mental status, other signs of central nervous system involvement, or focal metastatic infection also mandates admission and parenteral antibiotic treatment.

Other Infections

Rickettsial Infections

The rickettsiae (genera Rickettsia and Orientia) are obligate intracellular bacteria, transmitted to humans by bites of ticks, mites, and fleas and distributed worldwide. The expanded use

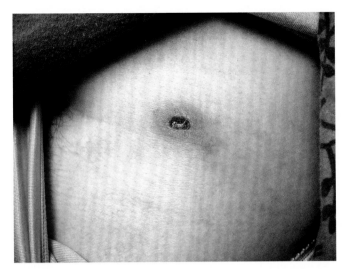

Figure 60.1 Eschar from African tick-bite fever.
Image appears with permission from Jeffrey Callen and VisualDx.

of molecular techniques has improved diagnosis and identification of rickettsiae in both humans and ticks. Rickettsial infections are the fourth most common identified cause of systemic febrile illness in travelers, behind malaraia, dengue, and mononucleosis. The classic presentation of a rickettsial infection consists of acute febrile illness accompanied by a rash of some kind, following a tick bite. Rocky Mountain spotted fever (also known as Brazilian spotted fever), caused by *Rickettsia rickettsii*, is the the prototypical severe rickettsial infection (see Chapter 14). Other important rickettsial infections include African tick-bite fever (*R. africae*), Mediterranean spotted fever (*R. conorii*), scrub typhus (*Orientia tsuhsugamushi*), and murine typus (*R. typhi*).

Risk factors for tick exposure include outdoor activities during spring and summer months, such as big game hunting in southern Africa. The incubation period is typically 1 to 2 weeks, so symptoms may begin after the patient has returned home. The clinical presentation varies greatly by causative pathogen. Typical early symptoms, including fever, headache, and malaise, are non-specific. Hallmark dermatologic signs include maculopapular rash and an eschar surrounded by erythema at the site of the tick bite (see Figure 60.1). Rickettsial infections can be life-threatening. *Rickettsia rickettsii*, for example, invades endothelial cells, causing widespread vasculitis and multi-organ failure.

Laboratory diagnosis is required for definitive identification of Rickettsial pathogens. The CDC rickettsial Zoonoses Branch can be contacted for assistance with diagnosis. Serology and molecular methods are used, but these take days to weeks to return. Initial diagnosis therefore hinges on assessment of travel history and exposure risk, because rickettsial infections are specific to geography and type of vector exposure. Clinical presentation will differ by organism. Relevant information on the rickettsioses and their respective vectors, reservoirs, geographic distributions, and major signs and symptoms are presented in Tables 60.9 and 60.10.

Since rickettsial infections can be life-threatening and definitive diagnosis takes days, immediate empiric therapy is recommended. Tetracyclines, most commonly doxycycline, are the antimicrobials of choice for all forms of rickettsial infection.

Chikungunya Fever

Chikungunya virus is a febrile, mosquito-borne illness endemic to West Africa, with reported outbreaks in Southeast Asia and the Americas. The name comes from the Makonde language in Tanzania meaning "that which bends up, stooped walk" because of the severe myalgias that are a hallmark of the disease. The typical infection presents with an abrupt fever after a mean incubation period of 3 days. Severe arthralgias and myalgias are the dominant feature of this disease, along with a non-specific macular rash over the trunk and abdomen in up to 80% of cases. Complications are uncommon and affect primarily immunocompromised patients, those with underlying heart and lung disease, and those in the extremes of age (very young and very old). Cases of encephalopathy, myocarditis, and multi-organ failure have been described. Hemorrhagic complications are rare and should prompt a search for an alternative diagnosis or concomitant infection with dengue virus.

The diagnosis of Chikungunya is typically clinical; the association of fever, severe myalgias, and an endemic area being highly predictive. Laboratory testing may reveal low lymphocyte count, thrombocytopenia, and mild transaminase elevation. Serologic testing with reverse transcriptase PCR can confirm Chikungunya and is typically done in tandem with IgM antibody testing, and testing for other arboviruses that present similarly, such as Zika and dengue. Treatment of Chikungunya is largely limited to anti-inflammatory drugs for pain control. There is no vaccine, so exposure prevention and vector eradication remain the most important interventions available to travelers and endemic locales.

Infectious Mononucleosis

Infectious mononucleosis (IM) is one of the most common identified causes of systemic febrile illness in returning travelers. In this setting, it is caused primarily (90%) by Epstein–Barr virus (EBV), with a significant subset due to cytomegalovirus (CMV) infection. Initial symptoms of classic IM include malaise, headache, and low-grade fever (see Table 60.11). Tonsillitis, pharyngitis, cervical lymphadenopathy (usually symmetrical, involving the posterior chain), and moderate to high fevers develop subsequently. Severe fatigue is a prominent and characteristic complaint. Tonsillar exudates (white, gray, green, or necrotic in appearance) are common, as are nausea, vomiting, anorexia, and splenomegaly.

Other, less common findings include palatal petechiae, periorbital or palpebral edema, and maculopapular or morbilliform rashes (rashes commonly appear after treatment with ampicillin). Neurologic complications can include Guillain–Barré syndrome, facial nerve palsy, meningoencephalitis, aseptic meningitis, transverse myelitis, peripheral neuritis, and optic neuritis. Potential hematologic abnormalities include hemolytic anemia, thrombocytopenia, aplastic anemia, thrombotic thrombocytopenic purpura, and disseminated intravascular coagulation.

Table 60.9 Clinical Features: Rickettsial Infections

Incubation period	• Generally shorter than 1–4 weeks
Signs and symptoms	• Fever, headache, and malaise • Maculopapular rash • Eschar at the site of bite may be seen in scrub typhus and several of the spotted fevers • Regional adenopathy
Laboratory findings	• Rickettsia do not stain with most conventional methods • Positive DFA, positive ELISA, or a rise in antibody titer are diagnostic Lab abnormalities seen in *R. rickettsii* infection include: • Thrombocytopenia • Mild elevations in hepatic transaminases • Hyponatremia • CSF pleocytosis (with polymorphonuclear or lymphocytic predominance)*
Prevention	Prevention of rickettsial infection is limited to avoidance of the infectious vector. Travelers in endemic regions are advised to use repellents and wear protective clothing. If a tick is detected, rapid and appropriate removal should ensue.
Treatment	Treatment of all rickettsial illness is with a tetracycline (doxycycline 100 mg BID, PO, or IV). In pregnant women, chloramphenicol (50 mg/kg in four divided doses, up to a maximum of 2.0 g) should be used in cases where the clinical course is not expected to be self-limited.

* Laboratory diagnosis of CNS rickettsial infections is difficult and empiric treatment for other causes (e.g. meningococcemia) should be administered until the causative organism is isolated.

CNS – central nervous system; CSF – cerebrospinal fluid; DFA – direct fluorescent antibody; ELISA – enzyme-linked immunosorbent assay; IV – intravenous; PO – by mouth.

Table 60.10 Specific Rickettsial Infections

Disease	Organism	Vector	Reservoir	Geographic Distribution	Signs and Symptoms
Typhus fevers					
Epidemic typhus, sylvatic typhus	*Rickettsia prowazekii*	Human body louse, squirrel flea, squirrel louse	Humans, flying squirrels	Mountainous regions of Africa, Asia, and Central and South America	Headache, chills, fever, prostration, confusion, photophobia, vomiting, rash (generally starting on trunk)
Murine typhus	*Rickettsia typhi*	Rat flea	Rats, mice	Worldwide	Headache, chills, fever, prostration, confusion, photophobia, vomiting, rash (generally appearing first on the trunk), generally less severe than epidemic typhus
Spotted fevers					
Rocky Mountain spotted fever	*Rickettsia rickettsii*	Tick	Rodents	United States (particularly in the southeastern and south central states), Canada, Mexico, Central and South America	Headache, fever, abdominal pain, rash (generally appearing first on the extremities)
Mediterranean spotted fever	*Rickettsia conorii*	Tick	Rodents	Africa, India, Europe, Middle East, Mediterranean	Fever, eschar, regional adenopathy, rash on extremities
African tick-bite fever	*Rickettsia africae*	Tick	Rodents	Sub-Saharan Africa	Fever, eschar, regional adenopathy, rash (subtle or absent)
North Asian tick typhus	*Rickettsia sibirica*	Tick	Rodents	Russia, China, Mongolia	Fever, eschar, regional adenopathy, rash (subtle or absent)
Oriental spotted fever	*Rickettsia japonica*	Tick	Rodents	Japan	Fever, eschar, regional adenopathy, rash subtle or absent
Rickettsial pox	*Rickettsia akari*	Mite	House mice	Russia, South Africa, Korea	Fever, eschar, adenopathy, disseminated vesicular rash
Tick-borne disease	*Rickettsia slovaca*	Tick	Lagomorphs (rabbits, pikas), rodents	Europe	Necrosis, erythema, lymphadenopathy
Aneruptive fever	*Rickettsia helvetica*	Tick	Rodents	Europe, Asia, and Africa	Fever, headache, myalgia

Table 60.10 (*cont.*)

Disease	Organism	Vector	Reservoir	Geographic Distribution	Signs and Symptoms
Cat flea rickettsiosis	*Rickettsia felis*	Cat and dog flea	Domestic cats, opossums	Europe, South America	Headache, chills, fever, prostration, confusion, photophobia, vomiting, rash (generally starting on trunk) generally less severe than epidemic typhus
Queensland tick typhus	*Rickettsia australis*	Tick	Rodents	Australia, Tasmania	Fever, eschar, regional adenopathy, rash on extremities
Flinders Island spotted fever, Thai tick typhus	*Rickettsia honei*	Tick	Not defined	Australia, Thailand	Fever, rash on extremities, eschar and adenopathy are rare
Orientia					
Scrub typhus	*Orientia tsutsugamushi*	Mite	Rodents	Indian subcontinent, Central, Eastern, and Southeast Asia and Australia	Fever, headache, sweating, conjunctival injection, adenopathy, eschar, rash (nascent on trunk), respiratory distress
Coxiella					
Q fever	*Coxiella burnetii*	Most human infections are acquired via inhalation of contaminated aerosols	Goats, sheep, cattle, domestic cats, other	Worldwide	Fever, headache, chills, sweating, pneumonia, hepatitis, endocarditis

Splenic rupture is a rare but potentially fatal complication of IM. Management is similar to other forms of splenic injury. Non-operative treatment with intensive supportive care and splenic preservation has been successfully carried out in select cases, whereas others have required splenectomy. Upper airway obstruction due to massive lymphoid hyperplasia and mucosal edema is another uncommon but serious complication. Corticosteroids may be useful in patients who develop or are at significant risk of obstruction. Principles of emergency airway management should be observed. The vast majority of individuals with IM recover uneventfully. Acute symptoms resolve in 1 to 2 weeks, whereas fatigue often persists for months.

A positive heterophile antibody assay (monospot test) supports the clinical diagnosis of EBV-induced IM (though CMV disease is heterophile negative). Although monospot testing is highly specific, false-negatives are common, especially early in the clinical course. A negative test in the setting of high clinical suspicion warrants either repeat testing or an assay of EBV-specific IgG and IgM (97% sensitivity). A heterophile-negative IM syndrome is seen with CMV, toxoplasmosis, acute HIV infection, hepatitis B, and human herpes virus-6 (HHV-6) infection.

As with EBV, CMV-induced IM can be accompanied by numerous dermatologic manifestations, including maculopapular, rubelliform, morbilliform, and scarlatiniform eruptions (some of these appear with ampicillin use). CMV infection has additionally been associated with neurologic sequelae such as encephalitis, Guillain–Barré syndrome, and various focal deficits (i.e. Horner's syndrome and peripheral neuropathy).

Leptospirosis

Leptospirosis is a zoonosis caused by sprirochetes from the genus Leptospira. It is carried by a variety of wild and domestic mammals, with rats being the most important reservoir. The organism is shed in the animal's urine. Human infection most often occurs from exposure to contaminated water or soil, with the portal of entry being mucosa, conjunctiva, and skin cuts and abrasions. Leptospirosis has a worldwide distribution, but it is more common in tropical regions, and the incidence rises after heavy rainfall and flooding. Infection in travelers usually occurs after recreational water exposure, with several outbreaks reported in triathletes who swam in contaminated fresh water, for example. Southeast Asia is the most high-risk region, though outbreaks have also occured within the United States, in Hawaii and Florida.

The incubation ranges from 2 to 4 weeks, so symptoms often begin after travelers have returned home. Illness ranges from subclinical to fatal. Initial symptoms are non-specific, consisting of fever, headache, myalgias, abdominal pain, and diarrhea. The finding of conjunctival suffusion, a uniform redness with associated chemosis, is considered highly specific for leptospirosis (see Figure 60.2). The disease may progress in up to 10% of patients to a severe phase, with icteris and renal failure, referred to as Weil's disease. Pulmonary hemorrhage is another well-recognized severe manifestation. Hyponatremia and abnormal urinalysis are common; alveolar infiltrates on chest X-ray are a high-risk finding.

Definitive diagnosis is usually made by serology. Real-time PCR tests have been developed, but are not widely available. Like most febrile illnesses in the traveler, early diagnosis requires a careful travel and exposure history combined with a proper index of suspicion and recognition of the clinical syndrome.

The approach to treatment is similar to that of rickettsial infetion: early treatment with doxycycline reduces the severity

427

Table 60.11 Clinical Features: Infectious Mononucleosis

Incubation period	Generally shorter than 4 weeks, but variable
Organism	EBV CMV more rarely HIV (seen in acute infection) *Toxoplasma gondii* Hepatitis B virus HHV-6
Signs and symptoms	**Common:** malaise, headache, fever tonsillitis, pharyngitis (with white, gray, green, or necrotic exudate) symmetrical, posterior chain cervical lymphadenopathy severe fatigue nausea, vomiting, anorexia splenomegaly **Less common:** palatal petechiae periorbital or palpebral edema maculopapular or morbilliform rashes Guillain–Barré syndrome, facial nerve palsy, meningoencephalitis, aseptic meningitis, transverse myelitis, peripheral neuritis, optic neuritis hemolytic anemia, thrombocytopenia, aplastic anemia, thrombotic thrombocytopenic purpura disseminated intravascular coagulation
Laboratory findings	**Virus-specific findings:** EBV – heterophile antibody positive, IgG and IgM serologies CMV – heterophile antibody negative, IgG and IgM serologies, early antigen detection can be accomplished via shell vial cultures **Both:** absolute lymphocytosis with >50% mononuclear cells and >10% atypical lymphocytes reduced haptoglobin levels cold agglutinins elevated rheumatoid factor positive ANA
Prevention	There is no known prophylaxis. Precautions should be taken to avoid contact with body fluids of infected patients.
Treatment	**EBV:** Generally limited to supportive, symptomatic therapy. Use of corticosteroids and acyclovir is controversial, but may be helpful in reducing discomfort from lymphoid and mucosal swelling. Because of the risk of traumatic splenic rupture, patients should be advised not to participate in physical activities that put them at risk for injury. **CMV:** No specific treatment is indicated unless the patient is immunocompromised. In such patients, ganciclovir, valganciclovir, foscarnet, and cidofovir can be used.

ANA – antinuclear antibodies.

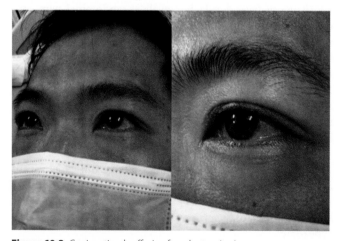

Figure 60.2 Conjunctiveal suffusion from leptospirosis.
Reproduced with permission from *The American Journal of Tropical Medicine and Hygiene*.

of illness and should be initiated immediately once leptospirosis is suspected.

Pearls and Pitfalls

1. Narrowing the differential diagnosis for the cause of fever in a traveler requries taking a precise travel and exposure history and knowing what infectious diseases are prevelent in the countries visited.
2. The immediate priority is prompt diagnosis and treatment of infections that may be rapidly progressive or pose a public health threat.
3. Malaria is the most common identifiable infection in febrile returning travelers; all such patients should have blood smears to rule out malaria.
4. False-negative smears can occur in cases of very low parasite load, partial immunity, or partial prophylaxis.

5. Fever, headache, and altered mental status are cardinal signs of cerebral malaria in an exposed returning traveler, requiring immediate, empiric therapy according to current CDC/WHO guidelines.

6. Patients with *P. falciporum* infection and parasitic loads >2% also require hospitalization and immediate treatment.

7. Onset of malaria-like symptoms less than 7 days post-exposure should prompt a search for alternative, non-malarial etiologies.

8. Dengue, Zika, and Chikungunya have a similar geographic distribution and clinical presentation and, in the United States, are tested for together.

9. Enteric (typhoid and paratyphoid) fever is a particular concern in febrile travelers returning from the Indian subcontinent, where fluoroquinolone resistance is the rule; the diagnosis is made by blood culture.

10. Leptospirosis is associated with adventure sport freshwater exposure in tropical regions.

11. Consider mononucleosis in a returning traveler with fever and lymphadenopathy or history of pharyngitis.

References

Arguin, P. M. and Tan, K. R. Chapter 3 – malaria. CDC health information for international travel, available at wwwnc.cdc.gov/travel/page/yellowbook-home-2014 (accessed December 7, 2017).

Freedman, D. O. Malaria prevention in short term travelers. *N. Engl. J. Med.* 2008; 359(6): 603–12.

Freedman, D. O., Weld, L. H., Kozarsky, P. E., *et al.* Spectrum of disease and relation to place of exposure among ill returned travelers. *N. Engl. J. Med.* 2006; 354(2): 119–30.

Harvey, K., Esposito, D. H., Han, P., *et al.* Surveillance for travel-related disease – Geosentinal Surveillance System, United States, 1997–2011. *MMWR Morb. Mortal. Wkly. Rep.* 2013; 62: 1–23.

Jensenius, M., Han, P. V., Schlagenhauf, P., *et al.* Acute and potentially life-threatening tropical diseases in western travelers – a Geosentinal multicenter study, 1996–2011. *Am. J. Trop. Med. Hyg.* 2013; 88(2): 397–404.

Lin, C. Y., Chiu, N. C., and Lee, C. M. Leptospirosis after typhoon. *Am. J. Trop. Med. Hyg.* 2012; 86(2): 187–8.

McQuiston, J. Chapter 3 - rickettsial (spotted & typhus fevers) & related infections (anasplasmosis & ehrlichiosis). CDC health information for international travel, available at wwwnc.cdc.gov/travel/page/yellowbook-home-2014 (accessed December 7, 2017).

Parry, C. M., Hien, T. T., Dougan, G., *et al.* Typhoid fever. *N. Engl. J. Med.* 2002; 347(22): 1770–82.

Simmons, C. P., Farrar, J. J., Chau, N., *et al.* Dengue. *N. Engl. J. Med.* 2012; 366(15): 1423–31.

Thwaites, G. E. and Dan, N. F. Approach to fever in the returning traveler. *N. Engl. J. Med.* 2017; 376(6): 548–60.

Tomashek, K. M., Sharp, T. M., and Margolis, H. S. Chapter 3 – dengue. CDC health information for international travel, available at wwwnc.cdc.gov/travel/page/yellowbook-home-2014 (accessed December 7, 2017).

Weaver, S. C. and Lecuit, M. Chikungunya virus and the global spread of a mosqito-borne disease. *N. Engl. J. Med.* 2015; 372(13): 1231–9.

WHO. *WHO Guidelines for the Treatment of Malaria*, 3rd edn. (Geneva: WHO, 2013).

Infectious Complications of Injection Drug Use

Bradley W. Frazee and Daniel Schnorr

Outline

Introduction

There are over 700,000 active injection drug users (IDU) in the United States, with heroin being the most common drug used, followed by methamphetamine and cocaine. It is estimated that 3 million Americans have used heroin in their lifetime. Emergency departments (EDs) serve as a regular source of medical care for this patient population. There were approximately 250,000 heroin-related ED visits in the United States in 2011.

The list of infections resulting from IDU spans the entire spectrum of infectious disease – from hepatitis C, HIV and related opportunistic infections, endocarditis caused by a myriad of organisms, skin and soft-tissue infections of every kind, malaria, and diseases caused by Clostridial toxins. This chapter describes the infectious diseases most commonly encountered in the ED in patients who inject drugs. These include infectious endocarditis, cutaneous abscess, necrotizing fasciitis, septic arthritis and osteomyelitis, spinal epidural abscess, wound botulism, and tetanus.

Common to many of the infections discussed in this chapter is the difficulty of making a correct diagnosis and the high risk of morbidity. Soft-tissue infections caused by IDU include not only simple cutaneous abscess and cellulitis, but also necrotizing fasciitis, which may be fatal if not rapidly diagnosed and treated. Wound botulism related to IDU is easily misdiagnosed, and failure to initiate specific therapy can lead to respiratory failure. Similarly, delayed diagnosis of spinal epidural abscess – a notorious complication of IDU that may present simply as back pain – can result in irreversible paralysis.

Roughly 40% of febrile IDUs who present to the ED have no apparent source of fever and seem well enough to be discharged. However, a significant proportion of these patients harbor an occult serious infection, and even a thorough ED work-up cannot exclude the possibility of bacteremia and endocarditis. The issue of appropriate management and disposition of the IDU with fever that has no apparent source is also discussed below.

Injection Drug Use Associated Endocarditis

Epidemiology and Microbiology

Infective endocarditis (IE), defined as a bacterial or fungal infection of the heart valves and perivalvular tissue, is a notorious complication of IDU. Endocarditis due to IDU differs from non-IDU-related disease. In the absence of IDU, community-acquired endocarditis occurs almost exclusively in the setting of underlying valve pathology or intravascular devices, whereas such abnormalities are present in less than 25% of IDU-associated cases (see Chapter 1, Infective Endocarditis). It is speculated that injected material may produce subtle valve damage. The frequent bacteremia caused by IDU, which then leads to IE, results from introduction of skin flora, and less often from contaminated drugs or syringes.

Staphylococcus aureus causes 51 to 82% of cases of IE in IDUs, in contrast to non-IDU cases where viridans Streptococci species are the predominant pathogens. There are numerous reports in the United States and throughout the world of community-associated MRSA IE in IDUs. *Pseudomonas*, a frequent pathogen in some early case series involving IDU, is found in 5 to 10% of cases in recent studies. Other organisms found in IDU-related IE include streptococcal species, *Enterococcus*, enteric gram-negatives, and fungi, particularly *Candida* species. Culture-negative endocarditis, which may be caused by the HACEK organisms or by any organism whose growth is suppressed by prior antibiotic use, accounts for 5 to 10% of cases in IDUs. Finally, IDU is the most important risk factor for polymicrobial endocarditis.

The pattern of valvular involvement in IDU-related endocarditis differs from that in non-IDUs in that vegetations are more commonly located on the tricuspid valve. Right-sided endocarditis has a distinctive pathophysiology and clinical presentation. Left-sided endocarditis usually produces significant mitral or aortic valve regurgitation with an audible murmur and may lead to pump failure. Tricuspid regurgitation is of lesser hemodynamic consequence and may be silent both clinically and on auscultation. Similarly, whereas left-sided IE is associated with prominent vascular and immune phenomena, such as splinter hemorrhages, these findings are absent in isolated right-sided disease. Right-sided endocarditis tends to produce pulmonary signs and symptoms such as chest pain and infiltrates on chest x-ray from septic pulmonary emboli.

Table 61.1 Clinical Features: IDU Endocarditis

Organisms	*Staphylococcus aureus* (MSSA and MRSA)
	Streptococcal species
	Enterococcus species
	Enteric gram-negatives
	Fungi
Signs and symptoms	Fever
	Malaise, weight loss
	Cough (tricuspid)
	Dyspnea
	Chest pain, back pain
	Murmur (30–50% of patients)
	Heart failure (left-sided *S. aureus*)
	Altered mental status (left-sided *S. aureus*)
Laboratory and radiologic findings	Persistent bacteremia
	Echocardiography: oscillating intracardiac mass attached to a valve (definitive), valvular incompetence, reduced ventricular function, perivalvular abscess

Another fairly common form of endocarditis in IDUs is *S. aureus* infection of the aortic or mitral valves, which results in so-called acute bacterial endocarditis. In contrast to isolated tricuspid disease, or subacute bacterial endocarditis with *Streptococcus viridans* species, aortic and mitral valve infection by *S. aureus* is associated with a more aggressive course and high morbidity and mortality (see later discussion). *S. aureus* aortic valve endocarditis results in heart failure, valve destruction requiring surgical replacement, or death in up to 40% of cases. Septic embolization to the brain, coronary arteries, or kidneys can occur. IE presenting with altered mental status or heart failure is considered an ominous sign, indicating likely infection of the aortic valve.

Although a well-recognized complication of IDU, IE is actually fairly uncommon, with an incidence of 1 to 20 per 10,000 users per year. It appears to be on the rise in the United States, however, in parallel with that of prescription opioid abuse, opioid overdoses, and hepatitis C infection. There were over 70,000 cases of IDU-related IE in 2013, accounting for 12% of IE hospitalizations. IDUs who are positive for human immunodeficiency virus (HIV) are at substantial increased risk for IE, and cocaine injection may present a higher risk than heroin.

Clinical Features

Endocarditis typically presents with non-specific symptoms such as arthralgias, malaise, back pain, and weight loss (see Table 61.1). Pulmonary symptoms such as cough, dyspnea, and chest pain are more common in tricuspid disease. Fever is a cardinal sign, found at presentation in more than 90% of patients.

A murmur is heard at the time of presentation in only 30 to 50% of IDU-related cases, and in even fewer of those with isolated right-sided disease. Classic vascular and immune phenomena are often absent in IDU-related disease.

Differential Diagnosis

Rarely is endocarditis obvious at the time of ED presentation. More often, a broad differential for the source of the patient's fever must be considered. Common infections in the IDU population that may present similarly include the following:

- community-acquired pneumonia
- skin and soft-tissue infection
- septic arthritis, osteomyelitis, spinal epidural abscess
- pyelonephritis and pelvic inflammatory disease
- HIV-related opportunistic infections
- transient *S. aureus* bacteremia
- pyrogen reaction to injected material ("cotton fever")

Laboratory and Radiographic Findings

The chest X-ray is an essential diagnostic study in the evaluation of possible endocarditis because the chest radiograph is abnormal in up to 72% of IDUs with IE, likely due to the high proportion of right-sided disease. Septic pulmonary emboli classically appear as multiple round infiltrates that may show evidence of cavitation. Other findings on chest radiograph include non-specific infiltrates, pleural effusions, and pulmonary edema. Laboratory abnormalities that support the diagnosis of IE include hematuria, proteinuria, and anemia. On electrocardiogram (ECG), conduction abnormalities, particularly atrioventricular (AV) block, may be seen because of an associated valve ring abscess that erodes into the conducting system.

Blood cultures are a cornerstone of diagnosis in IE. Endocarditis produces a continuous bacteremia, and blood cultures are positive in 80 to 95% of cases of infectious endocarditis diagnosed by Duke Criteria. The physician must ensure proper blood culture collection prior to administration of antibiotics. At least two separate sets of cultures – and most sources recommend three – should be obtained, each containing 10 mL of blood, though the recommendation that they be separated in time by as much as 1 hour may be difficult to adhere to in the ED.

Echocardiography is used both for definitive diagnosis and to assess complications and prognosis. The finding of an oscillating intracardiac mass attached to a valve is considered definitive evidence of endocarditis. Other possible echocardiographic findings include valvular incompetence, reduced ventricular function, and perivalvular abscess. Diagnostic criteria, such as the Duke Criteria, that incorporate both clinical and echocardiographic findings assist in making the diagnosis of IE.

Treatment and Prophylaxis

Empiric treatment of suspected IE related to IDU should cover *S. aureus* (including MRSA) and streptococcal species. In well-appearing patients, treatment can be delayed until culture results are known; however, empirical treatment should be started for all ill-appearing patients and those with heart failure. Vancomycin is the empiric drug of choice in an IDU with suspected IE. Empiric therapy should be tailored immediately when blood culture results become available. Vancomycin has been shown to be less effective than nafcillin in eradicating methicillin-sensitive *S. aureus*, so patients

Table 61.2 Initial IV Empiric Therapy for IDU Endocarditis

Patient Category	Therapy Recommendation
Adults	Vancomycin 15–20 mg/kg/dose IV every 8–12 hours
Pregnant women	Same as for adults
Immunocompromised	Same as for adults

with methicillin-sensitive strains should receive nafcillin or cefazolin. The addition of gentamicin to nafcillin shortens the time to negative blood cultures and a 2-week course of nafcillin and gentamicin has been shown to effectively treat isolated tricuspid valve IE in IDUs, provided the vegetation is small and there is no evidence of pulmonary emboli (see Table 61.2).

Complications and Admission Criteria

Serious complications of endocarditis are more common with left-sided disease. Intracardiac complications include valvular destruction and resultant heart failure, intracardiac abscess, purulent pericarditis, and septic embolization to the coronary arteries. Septic embolic complications are often seen in left-sided *S. aureus* endocarditis. Septic cerebral emboli may present with delirium or focal neurological findings. Meningitis may occur in association with IE and likely results from microemboli to the meningeal arteries. Spinal epidural abscess is a feared rare complication of IE. Renal sequelae include glomerulonephritis as well as renal infarction. Right-sided IE causes downstream pulmonary complications such as septic pulmonary embolism, pneumonia, empyema, and pyo-pneumothorax. Mortality from endocarditis in IDUs ranges from 2 to 39%. Isolated right-sided disease has a mortality of less than 10%.

Special Considerations – Disposition of the Injection Drug User with a Fever

The proper evaluation and disposition of the IDU with a fever can be difficult. In many cases, there is an underlying infection that requires admission; often, it can be diagnosed after a thorough ED evaluation. Patients should be carefully examined for signs of a soft-tissue infection and a thorough heart and lung exam performed. Any musculoskeletal or neurologic complaint including pain should be viewed as a possible indicator of infection. Findings such as decreased range of motion in a joint, weakness, or numbness may point to an infectious source. The chest radiograph has a high yield in this patient population, because pneumonia and HIV-related diseases such as tuberculosis are common, and because endocarditis frequently produces chest radiograph abnormalities. Occasionally, more advanced diagnostic testing (e.g. magnetic resonance imaging [MRI]) is required to make the correct diagnosis. Despite a thorough work-up, however, in about 40% of IDUs with fever, no apparent source can be found and the patient seems well enough to be discharged. Unfortunately, a significant proportion of these patients harbor an occult serious infection, such as bacteremia or endocarditis.

The problem of proper disposition of febrile but well-appearing IDUs with no apparent source of fever has been examined in four prospective studies involving a total of approximately 500 patients. 6 to 13% of such patients were eventually diagnosed with IE. Unfortunately, these studies show it is difficult to predict which patients actually have endocarditis. Development of a decision rule that can exclude IE in this patient population has so far proved impossible and the potential role of immediated transthoracic echocardiography has yet to be studied. To complicate matters, IDUs may not follow up reliably, for example if blood cultures turn positive after discharge. This forms the basis for the recommendation that all febrile IDUs without an obvious source of fever, even if they appear well, should have two blood cultures drawn and be admitted to the hospital until cultures remain negative for 48 hours. This approach remains the standard of practice at urban teaching hospitals that serve large IDU populations.

Subcutaneous Abscess

Epidemiology and Microbiology

Abscesses are collections of pus or infected material found within the cutaneous or subcutaneous spaces. (See also Chapter 12 on Bacterial Skin and Soft-tissue Infections.) Subcutaneous abscess is by far the most common bacterial complication of IDU. A recent study reported a 32% prevalence of abscess among active IDUs. The practice of subcutaneous injection, or "skin popping," increases the risk of abscess approximately fivefold. Needle licking, another common practice, probably accounts for the high percentage of oral flora found in IDU-related abscesses. Other risk factors for abscess formation include cocaine injection, lack of skin preparation, and use of dirty needles.

Because surgical drainage may be sufficient treatment, antibiotics are not always necessary for cutaneous abscesses. Nonetheless, the bacteriology of IDU abscesses has been well studied. Skin flora and oral flora account for the majority of pathogens. *Staphylococcus aureus* and *Streptococcus* species are the predominant aerobes. MRSA is now a common pathogen in IDU-related abscesses. *Eikenella*, a gram-negative aerobe that is found in "fight bites," is commonly found. *Peptostreptococcus* and *Fusobacterium* are the predominant anaerobes. *Bacteroides fragilis*, an antibiotic-resistant gut anaerobe, is uncommon in abscesses occuring above the diaphragm.

Clinical Features

Most patients complain of a painful mass at a previous injection site (see Table 61.3). Large abscesses that typically occur in the upper arm and gluteal regions may produce a low-grade fever (see Figure 61.1). Erythema, fluctuance, and drainage are confirmatory physical findings, present in a majority of cases. However, early abscesses, or deep subcutaneous or intramuscular collections, may exhibit no fluctuance and are easily misdiagnosed as cellulitis or a septic joint.

Table 61.3 Clinical Features: Subcutaneous Abscesses

Organisms	*Staphylococcus aureus* (MSSA and MRSA) *Streptococcus* species *Eikenella* *Peptostreptococcus* *Fusobacterium*
Signs and symptoms	Pain at a previous injection site Fever (low grade, associated with large abscesses) Erythema Fluctuance Drainage Superficial necrosis
Laboratory and radiologic studies	Blood cultures: positive in approximately 20% of febrile patients Leukocytosis Ultrasound: hypoechoic collection Plain X-ray: foreign body (e.g. needle), gas bubble

MSSA – methicillin-sensitive *Staphylococcus aureus*.

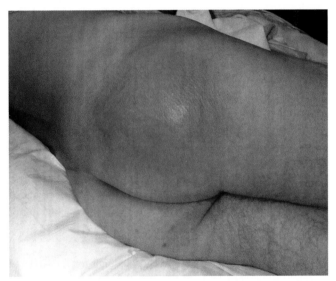

Figure 61.1 Large gluteal abscess due to injection drug use.

Differential Diagnosis

The diagnosis of a subcutaneous abscess is usually straightforward. Complications and coexisting infections can occur, however. These include necrotizing soft-tissue infection, septic arthritis, osteomyelitis, epidural abscess, and endocarditis. Among these, by far the most important is a necrotizing soft-tissue infection, which can appear initially as a simple abscess, yet requires immediate and extensive surgical debridement.

Laboratory and Radiographic Findings

Bedside ultrasound can be indispensable in revealing the correct diagnosis when frank fluctuance or drainage are not apparent. This modality has largely replaced needle aspiration to confirm and localize a pus collection. Abscess cavities are visualized as a hypoechoic mass with posterior acoustic

Table 61.4 Initial Treatment for Abscess Complicated by Cellulitis or Underlying Immunosuppression

Patient Category	Therapy Recommendation
Adults	Incision and drainage required (often sufficient for cure without antibiotics)
	Oral antibiotics (for surrounding cellulitis or underlying diabetes, HIV):
	• TMP-SMX DS one to two tabs. PO BID
	or
	• Clindamycin 300–450 mg PO TID
	IV antibiotics:
	• Vancomycin 15–20 mg/kg/dose IV every 8–12 hours
Pregnant women	Same as for non-pregnant adults
Immunocompromised	Antibiotics are administered in addition to incision and drainage
	Oral antibiotics (for surrounding cellulitis or underlying diabetes, HIV):
	• Same as above

DS – double strength; PO – by mouth.

enhancement. Plain radiographs, though unnecessary in routine management, may reveal a subcutaneous needle or soft-tissue gas. A gas bubble is sometimes seen in an abscess cavity, but gas within the tissues should always raise the possibility of a necrotizing infection.

Abscess cultures from the incision and drainage are generally not indicated, but should be considered if the patient requires hospital admission. Blood cultures are rarely indicated in the management of abscesses. Studies indicate that bacteremia is almost never present, if there is no associated fever. And while bacteremia may be present in up to 20% of patients with large abscesses accompanied by a fever undergoing drainage in the operating room, the results very rarely affect management.

Treatment and Prophylaxis

Incision and drainage is the primary treatment for IDU-related abscess (see Table 61.4). In most cases, this can be performed in the acute care setting. Achieving adequate anesthesia is often challenging for the practitioner. A generous incision should be made and the abscess cavity bluntly dissected and explored. Packing is not needed for small abscesses, and for larger abscesses, loop drainage (see Figure 12.6 in Chapter 12) is an alternative to traditional gauze packing. Patients should be instructed to change the dressing and bathe the affected area in soapy water at least twice daily, and are generally instructed to return at least once, at 24 hours, for a wound check and to review wound care procedures.

The need for prophylactic antibiotics prior to incision and drainage, to suppress bacteremia and prevent endocarditis, is controversial. American Heart Association guidelines list abscess incision and drainage among the procedures for which pre-operative antibiotics should be considered in patients with high-risk cardiac abnormalities. However, there is very little evidence to suggest that abscess incision and drainage actually causes bacteremia in the absence of fever. Pre-incision and drainage antibiotics can be limited to patients at highest risk

for endocarditis: those with a prior history of endocarditis, prosthetic valves, or congenital cardiac abnormalities.

Treatment of uncomplicated abscesses with a course of oral antibiotics, following incision and drainage, is not always indicated. Antibiotics can be reserved for cases with significant surrounding cellulitis and for patients with diabetes or HIV infection, although recent studies do show that routine adjunctive antibiotics provide a small benefit. Adequate staphylococcal (including MRSA) coverage can be achieved with a trimethoprim–sulfamethoxazole (TMP-SMX) or with clindamycin. If TMP-SMX is chosen, it is probably unnecessary to add better streptococcal coverage, even in IDU-related abscesses. Likewise, gram-negative and anaerobic coverage, such as with amoxicillin-clavulanate or a quinolone, is usually not necessary. If the abscess is accompanied by fever or if the patient is ill-appearing, parenteral antibiotics and admission to a surgical service are indicated.

Injection Drug Use Associated Necrotizing Soft-Tissue Infections

(See also Chapter 12 on Bacterial Skin and Soft-Tissue Infections.) Necrotizing soft-tissue infections (NSTIs) include necrotizing fasciitis, myositis, and necrotizing cellulitis. These are rapidly progressive, life-threatening soft-tissue infections involving deep subcutaneous tissue, fascia, and muscle and are associated with systemic toxicity. Immediate surgical exploration is generally required for diagnosis, and if necrotizing fasciitis is found, aggressive debridement is required for cure. A definitive diagnosis is made intraoperatively when there is non-bleeding, friable, necrotic fascia or muscle, or when so-called "dishwater pus" is found.

Epidemiology and Microbiology

Bacteriology studies reveal that 60 to 85% of NSTIs are polymicrobial. Aerobes include *Staphylococcus aureus* and group A *Streptococcus*. The most important anaerobes are *Clostridium sordelli* and gas-forming *Clostridium perfringens*. *Peptostreptococcus* and other oral anaerobes are also common. In cases caused by IDU, staphylococcal species and clostridial species are the dominant pathogens isolated. In community-acquired cases of NSTI (as opposed to hospital-acquired or post-operative cases), the most prevalent risk factor is IDU. Use of black tar heroin, a highly contaminated and adulterated drug produced in Mexico, and the practice of "skin popping" (intradermal or intramuscular injection) are linked to outbreaks of severe NSTI in which clostridial species were isolated in a high proportion of cases (see Figure 61.2).

Clinical Features

The timely diagnosis of NSTI is critical, yet often difficult. Patients typically present with skin and soft tissue symptoms and signs that are non-specific such as pain, warmth, and edema (see Table 61.5). Fever is present at presentation in only about 40%. Findings more specific for NSTI, but often absent, include pain out of proportion to skin findings, skin necrosis, bullae, crepitus from subcutaneous gas, and a cutaneous

Table 61.5 Clinical Features: Necrotizing Soft-Tissue Infections

Organisms	Usually polymicrobial
	Staphylococcus aureus (including MRSA)
	Streptococcus species
	Clostridium species
	Oral anaerobes
Signs and symptoms	Pain (out of proportion to exam)
	Erythema
	Edema (circumferential; "woody")
	Skin necrosis, bullae
	Cutaneous sensory deficit
Laboratory and radiologic findings	WBC >14
	Subcutaneous gas on plain X-ray
	Elevated BUN and sodium <135

BUN – blood urea nitrogen; WBC – white blood (cell) count.

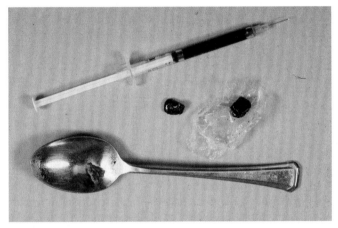

Figure 61.2 Injection drug use paraphernalia and black tar heroin. Courtesy of Dr. Richard Haruff.

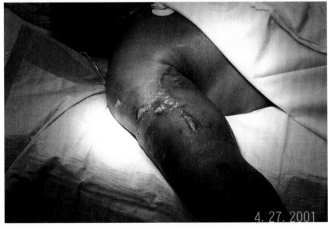

Figure 61.3 Necrotizing fasciitis of the upper extremity from injection drug use. Note skin necrosis and extreme edema extending to the trunk.

sensory deficit. Tense circumferential edema of an extremity, often spreading onto the trunk, is highly characteristic of NSTI due to IDU (see Figure 61.3). Signs of shock or organ dysfunction are found at the time of presentation in up to 40% of cases.

Laboratory and Radiographic Findings

Marked leukocytosis in excess of 20,000/mm³ is highly characteristic of NSTI, particularly IDU-related cases linked to clostridial species. Whereas extreme leukocytosis should raise concern for NSTI, its absence does not exclude the diagnosis. The combination of WBC greater than 15,000/mm³ and serum sodium less than 135 mEq/L is reported to be useful in differentiating necrotizing from non-necrotizing skin infections; however, a reliable clinical decision rule has yet to be validated.

Imaging can help differentiate NSTI from less severe skin infections. Plain film demonstrates subcutaneous gas in a stippled pattern in roughly 25% of cases. Computed tomographic (CT) scan is more sensitive than plain film in demonstrating gas in the tissue and may reveal unsuspected deep fluid collections or phlegmon. The typical CT finding in NSTI is asymmetric thickening of deep fascia associated with gas. MRI has been shown to be useful in differentiating NSTI from non-necrotizing infections, but it is expensive, time-consuming, and inadvisable in potentially unstable patients.

Although a positive result from an imaging study is useful, indicating the need for immediate operation, a negative result cannot be relied on to exclude the diagnosis. Moreover, delays associated with obtaining a CT scan or MRI should not delay surgical exploration, once NSTI is strongly suspected. The proper approach to diagnosis combines the following: a high index of suspicion on the part of the emergency physician, prompt surgical consultation, and a low threshold for operative exploration.

Treatment and Prophylaxis

Initial management of NSTI includes aggressive fluid resuscitation and early broad-spectrum antibiotics (see Table 61.6). Prompt surgical debridement is the cornerstone of therapy. A delay to surgical debridement is the single most important risk for increased morbidity and mortality. Even a 12 to 24 hour delay may increase mortality fourfold.

Complications and Admission Criteria

Death is the major complication of NSTI, with a mortality rate over 20%. Comparison of IDU-related NSTI versus non-IDU NSTI at one institution revealed a lower mortality among IDUs (10% vs. 21%), which may have been explained by the younger age and lack of comorbidities in IDU. Other complications include extremity amputation, which occurs in about 15% of cases, extensive debridement, and prolonged intensive care unit (ICU) stay.

Injection Drug Use Associated Septic Arthritis and Osteomyelitis

Epidemiology and Microbiology

(See Chapters 33 and 37 on Adult Septic Arthritis and Osteomyelitis.) Both septic arthritis (SA) and osteomyelitis (OM) may result from injection drug use, usually arising from hematogenous seeding. Bacteremia may occur transiently after

Table 61.6 Initial IV Therapy for Necrotizing Fasciitis

Patient Category	Therapy Recommendation
Adults	Prompt surgical debridement Aggressive fluid resuscitation Antibiotics: Piperacillin-tazobactam 4.5 g IV every 6 hours *or* Aztreonam 2 g IV every 8 hours *plus* Clindamycin 900 mg IV every 8 hours *plus* Vancomycin 15–20 mg/kg/dose IV every 8–12 hours
Pregnant women	Same as for non-pregnant adults
Immunocompromised	Same as for non-immunocompromised persons and children

Table 61.7 Clinical Features: IDU-Related Osteomyelitis and Septic Arthritis

Organisms	**Septic arthritis:** *Staphylococcus aureus* (including MRSA), *Streptococcus* spp. Gram-negative bacilli **Osteomyelitis:** *Staphylococcus aureus* (including MRSA) Coagulase-negative *Staphylococcus* Gram-negative bacilli
Signs and symptoms	**Septic arthritis:** Joint pain, swelling, tenderness, decreased range of motion, fever **Osteomyelitis:** Back pain, bone pain, fever
Laboratory and radiologic findings	**Septic arthritis:** Elevated WBC Positive arthrocentesis **Osteomyelitis:** Elevated ESR Positive blood cultures Abnormal plain films Abnormal nuclear imaging studies Abnormal MRI

ESR – erythrocyte sedimentation rate.

drug injection or may be due to endocarditis. Bone and joint infections related to IDU typically affect the axial skeleton. In SA, the sacroiliac, costochondral, hip, and sternoclavicular joints are common sites, followed by the knee and shoulder joint. OM occurs more commonly in the lumbar and cervical spines.

The incidence of SA and OM has not been well established, but in one report they together accounted for 4% of IDU-related hospital admissions. SA appears to be more common, occurring five times as often in one case series.

The bacteriology is similar for both infections. *Staphylococcus aureus* predominates, with IDUs being particularly at risk for infection with MRSA. *Streptococcus* spp. are common in SA. Compared to the general population, IDUs are more at risk for infections with gram-negative bacilli, such as *Pseudomonas*, *Escherichia coli*, *Proteus mirabilis*, *Klebsiella*, and *Enterobacter*, as well as, more rarely, fungal organisms.

Clinical Features

Septic arthritis usually presents as an acute infection, with onset of pain, tenderness, and decreased range of motion at a joint, developing over 1 to 2 weeks (see Table 61.7). OM can be more indolent, with patients presenting as late as 3 months after the onset of infection. The shoulder and hip joint are common sites of IDU-related SA. Back pain is the most common chief complaint in spinal OM. Fever is common in both infections, but may be absent at the time of presentation.

Differential Diagnosis

Musculoskeletal complaints in IDUs are often due to infection. SA, OM, and spinal epidural abscess (see below) are primary considerations when an IDU complains of back or joint pain. A high degree of suspicion should be maintained even if the presentation does not include fever or leukocytosis. Gonococcal arthritis remains a consideration in mono- and oligoarticular arthritis in this population. *Mycobacterium tuberculosis* osteomyelitis has been reported in IDU, albeit rarely. Non-infectious entities include gout, pseudogout, and rheumatoid arthritis.

Laboratory and Radiographic Findings

The work-up of both SA and OM includes blood cultures and X-rays of the symptomatic area. Although positive in only 20 to 30% of cases, blood cultures are particularly important in osteomyelitis because they may obviate the need for bone biopsy. A positive blood culture in the setting of SA or OM generally mandates a search for endocarditis.

Serum inflammatory markers are generally elevated, though these findings are non-specific. One retrospective study of patients presenting to the emergency department showed ESR elevation to be 94% sensitive and CRP elevation to be 92% sensitive for SA, using cut-offs of 15 mm/hr and 20 mg/L, respectively. In numerous separate studies, an ESR of greater than 20 mm/hr appears to be greater than 90% sensitive for the diagnosis of OM. Leukocystosis is common in septic arthritis, but less so in OM.

Plain radiographs are insensitive for acute OM, especially early in the disease course, but should be obtained with the goal of ruling out other causes of bone pain. Given its increasing availability, MRI is now considered the modality of choice for the diagnosis of OM, with a reported sensitivity between 78 and 90% and specificity between 60 and 90%. The sensitivity of MRI tends to increase later in the course of the infection. Nuclear imaging modalities, using technetium, gallium, or tagged WBCs to visualize areas of inflammation, are an alternative to MRI, with comparable performance early in the infection.

Arthrocentesis remains the main diagnostic test for suspected SA. Ideally, arthrocentesis is performed before administration of antibiotics. Synovial fluid should be sent for gram stain, culture, leukocyte count with differential, and assessment

Table 61.8 Initial Empirical IV Therapy for Osteomyelitis and Septic Arthritis

Patient Category	Therapy Recommendation
Adults	**Osteomyelitis:** Antibiotics may be sufficient for acute hematogenous osteomyelitis Operative drainage, debridement, and soft-tissue coverage will likely be necessary for chronic osteomyelitis Antibiotics for 6–12 weeks. Initial antibiotics selection should cover methicillin-resistant *Staphylococcus aureus* and gram-negative organisms and be tailored to culture results: Vancomycin (for MRSA) 15–20 mg/kg/dose IV every 8–12 hours *plus* Ceftazidime 2 g IV every 8 hours **Septic arthritis:** Joint drainage with or without irrigation Hold antibiotics until joint aspiration performed and cultures sent Empiric antibiotics after synovial fluid sent for culture and gram stain: Vancomycin 15–20 mg/kg/dose IV every 8–12 hours *plus* Ceftriaxone 1 g IV every 24 hours
Pregnant women	Same as for non-pregnant adults
Immunocompromised	Same as for non-immunocompromised persons and children

for crystals. Likelihood of SA increases with increasing levels of synovial fluid WBC, with most cases of SA exhibiting synovial WBC above 50,000/mm³. A fluid polymorphonuclear cell count of greater than 90% also helps distinguish septic arthritis from other causes of joint inflammation. Gram stain and culture are positive in about roughly one-half and and two-thirds of cases, respectively. Ultrasonography can be invaluable to detect an occult joint effusion and to guide arthrocentesis of the hip and shoulder.

Treatment

Initial treatment for suspected OM is usually empirical (see Table 61.8), though care should be taken to obtain blood cultures and, if possible, bone cultures, before starting antibiotics. In the case of SA, gram stain of synovial fluid can be used to guide initial therapy. If the gram stain is unrevealing, therapy should be directed against *S. aureus*, including MRSA, and gram-negative bacilli, including pseudomonal species. A recent study of vertebral osteomyelitis treatment duration found identical cure rates for a 6-week versus 12-week regimen. Joint drainage is an essential part of therapy for septic arthritis, and options include repeated needle aspiration, arthroscopic drainage, and arthrotomy.

Spinal Epidural Abscess

Epidemiology and Microbiology

Spinal epidural abscess (SEA) is a rare but feared complication of IDU with an incidence that has risen over the last 30 years. SEA is a diagnostic challenge because it may present simply as back pain, because MRI is generally required for diagnosis, and because diagnostic delay can be associated with sudden and irreversible neurologic damage.

SEAs associated with IDU are almost always due to hematogenous seeding of the vertebrae or epidural space. *S. aureus*

(especially MRSA) is the predominant pathogen, implicated in 50 to 70% of cases. *Streptococcus* spp. are the second most common; gram-negative species, while uncommon overall, are more common in IDU-related SEAs. Adjacent bone or soft-tissue infections, such as osteomyelitis, discitis, or psoas abscess, are common.

There are two proposed mechanisms of cord injury in SEA, which may explain the wide variation in the time of onset of neurologic deficits: direct compression and vascular ischemia. Compression of the spinal cord due to mass effect produces a subacute course, whereas thrombosis and vascular injury may result in rapid paralysis.

The incidence of SEA in the general population is estimated at 2.5 to 3 per 10,000 hospital admissions. Depending on the study setting, between 4 and 60% of SEAs are associated with IDU.

Clinical Features

The classic triad of SEA consists of back pain, fever, and neurologic deficit, though presence of all three of these features is rare on initial presentation to the emergency department (see Table 61.9). Neurologic findings on presentation range in severity from radicular pain, urinary incontinence, and leg weakness to para- or quadriplegia. Patients may occasionally present with sepsis or encephalitis, further confounding and delaying the diagnosis.

Differential Diagnosis

The differential diagnosis for spinal epidural abscess includes:

- osteomyelitis and discitis
- psoas abscess
- metastatic cancer
- spinal fracture or disk disease
- meningitis
- herpes zoster

Table 61.9 Clinical Features: Spinal Epidural Abscess

Organisms	*Staphylococcus aureus* (including MRSA) Gram-negative rods Streptococci
Signs and symptoms	Back pain Fever Neurologic findings: radicular pain, weakness, urinary incontinence
Laboratory and radiologic findings	Elevated ESR Positive blood cultures MRI showing phlegmon or frank pus in the epidural space
Treatment	Urgent neurosurgical consultation for possible surgical drainage if cord impingement occurring IV antibiotics

Table 61.10 Initial Therapy for IDU-Related Spinal Epidural Abscess

Patient Category	Therapy Recommendation
Adults	Surgical drainage and decompression Antibiotics: Vancomycin 15–20 mg/kg/dose IV every 8–12 hours *plus* Ceftazidime 2 g IV every 8 hours
Pregnant women	Same as for non-pregnant adults
Immunocompromised	Same as for non-immunocompromised persons and children

Laboratory and Radiographic Findings

With a sensitivity and specificity of over 90%, MRI with gadolinium is the study of choice for diagnosis or SEA. MRI provides images of the abscess and the cord itself, which aids surgical planning, provides prognostic information, and may identify an alternative diagnosis. Plain radiographs cannot be relied on to exclude the diagnosis of SEA, though they may be abnormal if there is associated vertebral osteomyelitis.

ESR is elevated above 20 mm/hr in greater than 90% of patients diagnosed with SEA. In one prospective study examining patients presenting to the emergency department with back pain and at least one risk factor for SEA, such as IDU, an elevated ESR was present in 100% of patients eventually diagnosed with SEA. In the same study, only 33% of patients with a risk factor but no SEA had an elevated ESR. These data suggest that in the case of an IDU with otherwise non-concerning back pain, an ESR less that 20mm/hr can be used to rule out SEA, obviating an MRI. C-reactive protein appears not to perform as well as ESR in this regard.

Blood cultures are positive in greater than 60% of cases of SEA and should be obtained before antibiotic administration in all patients for whom this diagnosis is being considered.

Treatment and Prophylaxis

Surgical decompression is the initial treatment of choice in almost all cases, and a spinal surgeon should be consulted as soon as the diagnosis of SEA is strongly suspected. In one series of IDU-related SEAs, the only modifiable determinant of neurologic outcome was time from presentation to operative decompression. In one study, all patients who had surgery within 36 hours of the development of neurologic deficit showed some degree of recovery, whereas recovery was limited (2 of 11) in those whose surgery was delayed beyond 36 hours. Surgery is followed by 4 to 12 weeks of parenteral antibiotics. Empiric antibiotics should be started only after blood cultures have been drawn, and ideally after surgical specimens have been obtained. The empiric regimen should cover MRSA and gram-negative bacilli.

Wound Botulism

Epidemiology and Microbiology

Botulism is an illness characterized by descending paralysis and autonomic dysfunction due to a neurotoxin produced by *Clostridium botulinum*, a gram-positive rod. (See also Chapter 5, Botulism.) Wound botulism is an increasingly frequent complication of IDU. *Clostridium botulinum* requires anaerobic conditions to germinate and elaborate toxin, and abscess cavities and subcutaneous pockets formed by IDU seem to be an ideal environment. Botulinum toxin binds to the presynaptic terminal, irreversibly blocking acetylcholine release at cranial nerves, autonomic nerves, and neuromuscular junctions.

First reported in an IDU in California in1982, the incidence of wound botulism associated with IDU has risen steadily. IDU now accounts for the vast majority of US cases, and has been linked to several case clusters in Europe. Subcutaneous injection of black tar heroin appears to be the primary risk factor for development of botulism in IDU. Black tar heroin is contaminated by *Clostridium* spores in the process of "cutting" the drug.

Clinical Features

Patients present with three types of neurologic deficits: cranial nerve dysfunction, autonomic dysfunction, and symmetric motor weakness (see Table 61.11). Cranial nerve symptoms include diplopia (88%), dysphagia (82%), and dysarthria/hoarseness (76%). Autonomic dysfunction may manifest as dry mouth, blurry vision, and dilated pupils. 65% of patients complain of shortness of breath. Respiratory muscle weakness, indicated by diminished maximal inspiratory force, is common, and respiratory failure eventually supervenes in up to 70% of patients.

Differential Diagnosis

The diagnosis of botulism remains a clinical one, requiring a very careful history and neurologic exam and an extremely high index of suspicion. There is no rapid confirmatory test currently available. The differential for descending paralysis with prominent bulbar weakness includes myasthenia gravis, Miller–Fisher variant of Guillain–Barré syndrome, brainstem

Table 61.11 Clinical Features: Wound Botulism

Organism	*Clostridium botulinum*
Signs and symptoms	Cranial nerve abnormalities
	Dysphagia
	Dysarthria and hoarseness
	Diplopia
	Autonomic dysfunction
	Dry mouth
	Dilated pupils
	Symmetric motor weakness
Laboratory and radiologic findings	CSF normal
	Wound culture (specify for *Clostridium tetani*)
	Serum mouse bioassay for botulinum toxin

CSF – cerebrospinal fluid.

Table 61.12 Initial IV Therapy for Botulism

Patient Category	Therapy Recommendation
Adults	Botulism antitoxin
	Incision and drainage of cutaneous abscesses
	Penicillin G 24 million units/day IV divided every 6 hours
Pregnant women	Same as for non-pregnant adults
Immunocompromised	Same as for non-immunocompromised persons

stroke, tick paralysis, and hyperkalemic periodic paralysis. In the IDU patient presenting with bulbar symptoms, however, the diagnosis is wound botulism until proven otherwise. Empiric treatment should be initiated while tests to exclude other diagnoses, such as brain imaging and cerebrospinal fluid (CSF) analysis, are undertaken.

Key features that distinguish botulism from other neuromuscular diseases are:

- afebrile illness
- normal mental status
- cranial nerves involved
- descending paralysis
- symmetric bilateral impairment
- absence of paresthesias
- normal CSF studies
- characteristic electromyographic findings

Laboratory and Radiographic Findings

Confirmatory studies include wound cultures for *Clostridium botulinum* and a bioassay for botulinum toxin, performed on patient serum. Anaerobic wound cultures can take weeks to return, and in one report the bioassay was positive in only 68% of clinically diagnosed cases. Results of the edrophonium test for myesthenia gravis can be falsely positive in wound botulism and so should not be used to exclude the diagnosis.

Treatment and Prophylaxis

The management of botulism consists of: (1) minimizing toxin binding, (2) removing the toxin source, and (3) supportive care (see Table 61.12). Heptavalent equine botulism antitoxin (H-BAT) binds toxin subtypes A to G. Since it binds only extraneuronal toxin, it is most effective when given early in the course. Administration in less than 12 hours from the time of diagnosis is associated with a significant reduction in respiratory failure, length of intubation, and overall hospital length of stay. In the United States, antitoxin is obtained from state health departments and the CDC. Unlike older forms of botulinum antitoxin, HBAT resulted in no cases of anaphylaxis among 228 recipients, so pre-treatment skin testing is no longer recommended.

To eliminate ongoing toxin production, all suspicious skin lesions should be drained or excised and IV penicillin given.

Complications and Admission Criteria

The most important complication of botulism is ventilatory failure. Respiratory weakness should be assessed by measuring negative inspiratory force or forced vital capacity. A negative inspiratory force of 20 cm H_2O or less, or a worsening trend, indicates the need for intubation. Ventilatory support is a temporizing measure while synaptic receptors regenerate. Unfortunately, patients may require months of mechanical ventilation before adequate inspiratory strength returns. With the use of mechanical ventilation, mortality due to all forms of botulism has been reduced to approximately 10%. Nonetheless, morbidity remains high because of long-term paralysis and critical care complications.

Injection Drug Use Associated Tetanus
Epidemiology and Microbiology

Tetanus is a rare but dreaded complication of IDU and under-immunization. It is a syndrome of uncontrolled muscle spasm and autonomic dysfunction as a result of *Clostridium tetani* infection and toxin elaboration. (See also Chapter 10, Tetanus.)

Like wound botulism, the pathophysiology of tetanus begins with the introduction of *Clostridium tetani* spores into a wound. Subcutaneous injection of heroin by skin popping is thought to produce favorable conditions for the spore germination and anaerobic bacterial growth. *C. tetani* spores germinate and elaborate the exotoxin tetanospasmin. Tetanospasmin is transported in retrograde fashion to the spinal cord, where the toxin inhibits neurotransmission, ultimately causing muscle spasm and autonomic instability.

Although tetanus is now a rare disease in the United States, IDU remains an important risk factor for developing the disease. Of 176 tetanus cases in the United States between 2001 and 2008 in which drug use history was assessed, 15% were linked to IDU. IDU-related tetanus occurs almost exclusively in un- or under-vaccinated individuals. It is particularly common among foreign-born Hispanic IDUs in California. The United Kingdom also saw 33 IDU-related tetanus cases from 2003 to 2005, with skin popping the dominant form of injection and inadequate antibodies found in 12 of 14 in whom immunity was assessed. Emergency physicians who regularly see IDUs must ensure that this group of patients are immunized.

Table 61.13 Clinical Features: Tetanus

Organism	*Clostridium tetani*
Signs and symptoms	Neck pain
	Back pain
	Trismus
	Opisthotonos
	Risus sardonicus
	Dysphagia and drooling
	Muscle rigidity
	Hyperreflexia
Laboratory and radiologic findings	Initial diagnosis is clinical
	CT negative
	CSF negative
	Tetanus toxoid antibody titers
	Wound culture

Table 61.14 Initial IV Therapy for Tetanus

Patient Category	Therapy Recommendation
Adults	Wound debridement
	Metronidazole 500 mg IV every 8 hours
	Human tetanus immunoglobulin (neutralize unbound toxin)
	Tetanus toxoid (active immunization)
	Treatment of muscle spasm
	Sedatives (diazepam, propofol)
	Neuromuscular blockade (and intubation)
	Treatment of autonomic instability
	Labetalol
	Magnesium
Pregnant women	Same as for non-pregnant adults
Immunocompromised	Same as for non-immunocompromised persons

Clinical Features

Presenting symptoms are due to muscle spasm, which may be localized – so-called cephalic tetanus – or generalized. Trismus and neck or back pain are the initial symptoms in 85% of cases (see Table 61.13). Physical exam reveals palpable muscle rigidity and hyperreflexia. Other findings include opisthotonos (hyperextension and spasm of the neck and back), risus sardonicus (appearance of a sardonic smile from facial muscle spasm), dysphagia, and drooling.

Differential Diagnosis

The diagnosis of tetanus is clinical. Disorders that may present similarly include seizures, meningitis/encephalitis, drug withdrawal, sepsis, and strychnine poisoning. The differential diagnosis of localized tetanus includes peritonsillar abscess, mandibular disorders, and dystonic reactions. The lack of fever, muscle weakness, sensory symptoms, or mental status changes tend to distinguish tetanus from alternate diagnoses. A history and physical consistent with tetanus in an IDU, combined with negative results on CT scan and lumbar puncture, is sufficient to establish the diagnosis.

Laboratory and Radiographic Findings

Wound cultures for *C. tetani* are insensitive. Antibody titers against tetanus toxoid should be ordered, though results will not be available to assist with immediate diagnosis.

Treatment and Prophylaxis

As in wound botulism, the treatment of tetanus primarily involves three strategies (see Table 61.14): (1) Elimination of potential sources of ongoing toxin production is accomplished by draining all skin abscesses and administering antibiotics active against *Clostridium*. Metronidazole is the first-line agent. (2) Clearance of extraneuronal tetanus toxin is achieved by administration of tetanus immunoglobulin (TIG). Intrathecal plus intravenous administration of TIG probably offers an advantage over the intravenous route alone. Active immunization with tetanus toxoid should also be initiated immediately. (3) Aggressive supportive care is critical to prevent morbidity

and mortality. Patients with severe, generalized, or rapidly progressing muscle spasm should be intubated, sedated, and paralyzed if necessary. Long-term ventilatory support and tracheostomy are often required. Muscle spasm is controlled with benzodiazepines or propofol. Labetalol, a combined beta and alpha adrenergic blocker, can be used to manage autonomic instability.

Pearls and Pitfalls

1. IDUs presenting with fever have a serious infection warranting admission about 60% of the time; the majority of these infections can be diagnosed with a thorough ED evaluation.

2. Even if the ED evaluation is negative, these patients generally require hospital admission because occult bacteremia and endocarditis are difficult to exclude.

3. Endocarditis related to IDU often occurs on the tricuspid valve, resulting in pulmonary symptoms and signs and an abnormal chest X-ray.

4. Abscesses may not demonstrate fluctuance; consider the use of bedside ultrasound to identify and localize a pus collection for drainage.

5. Necrotizing soft-tissue infections secondary to IDU are typified by tense edema and extreme leukocytosis.

6. Once the diagnosis of necrotizing fasciitis is entertained, there is no diagnostic test that can reliably exclude the diagnosis, except operative exploration.

7. Mortality in necrotizing soft-tissue infections is directly related to the time between presentation and operative debridement.

8. Musculoskeletal complaints in IDUs are frequently due to an infection; a musculoskeletal complaint plus fever mandates a search for an infection including osteomyelitis or septic arthritis.

9. Back pain plus fever in an IDU mandates evaluation for spinal epidural abscess; the diagnosis should be made prior to the onset of neurologic symptoms; MRI is usually required to exclude the diagnosis.

10. Bulbar neurologic symptoms in an IDU indicate wound botulism until proven otherwise.

11. Prevention of tetanus in IDUs should be possible through careful attention to vaccine status in this population.

References

Binswanger, I. A., Kral, A. H., Bluthenthal, R. N., *et al.* High prevalence of abscesses and cellulitis among community-recruited injection drug users in San Francisco. *Clin. Infect. Dis.* 2000; 30(3): 579–81.

Chandrasekar, P. H. and Narula, A. P. Bone and joint infections in intravenous drug abusers. *Rev. Infect. Dis.* 1986; 8(6): 904–11.

Chen, J. L. Fullerton, K. E., and Flynn, N. M. Necrotizing fasciitis associated with injection drug use. *Clin. Infect. Dis.* 2001; 1(33): 6–15.

Davis, D. P., Salazar, A., Chan, T. C., and Vilke, G. M. Prospective evaluation of a clinical decision guideline to diagnose spinal epidural abscess in patients who present to the emergency department with spinal pain. *J. Neurosurg. Spine* 2011; 14(6): 765–70.

Hecht, S. R. and Berger, M. Right-sided endocarditis in intravenous drug users. *Ann Intern Med* 1992; 117(7): 560–6.

Hariharan, P. and Kabrhel, C. Sensitivity of erythrocyte sedimentation rate and C-reactive protein for exclusion of septic arthritis in emergency department patients. *J. Emerg. Med.* 2011; 40(4): 428–31.

Horowitz, B. Z., Swensen, E., and Marquardt, K. Wound botulism associated with black tar heroin. *JAMA* 1998; 280(17): 1479–80.

Koppel, B. S., Tuchman, A. J., Mangiardi, J. R., *et al.* Epidural spinal infection in intravenous drug abusers. *Arch. Neurol.* 1988; 45(12): 1331–7.

Marantz, P. R., Linzer, M., Feiner, C. J., *et al.* Inability to predict diagnosis in febrile intravenous drug abusers. *Ann. Intern. Med.* 1987; 106(6): 823–8.

Margaretten, M. E., Knohles, J., Moore, D., and Bent, S. Does this patient have septic arthritis? *JAMA* 2007; 297(13): 1478.

Mathew, J., Addai, T., Anand, A., *et al.* Clinical features, site of involvement, bacteriologic findings, and outcome of infective endocarditis in intravenous drug users. *Arch. Intern. Med.* 1995; 155(15): 1641–8.

McGuigan, C. C., Penrice, G. M., Gruer, L., *et al.* Lethal outbreak of infection with *Clostridium novyi* type A and other spore-forming organisms in Scottish injecting drug users. *J. Med. Microbiol.* 2002; 51(11): 971–7.

Samet, J. H., Shevitz, A., Fowle, J., and Singer, D. E. Hospitalization decisions in febrile intravenous drug users. *Am. J. Med.* 1990; 89(1): 53–7.

Sandrock, C. E. and Murin, S. Clinical predictors of respiratory failure and long-term outcome in black tar heroin-associated wound botulism. *Chest* 2001; 120(2): 562–6.

Weisse, A. B., Heller, D. R., Schhimenti, R. J., *et al.* The febrile parenteral drug user: a prospective study in 121 patients. *Am. J. Med.* 1993; 94: 274–80.

Werner, S. B., Passaro, D., McGee, J., *et al.* Wound botulism in California, 1951–1998: recent epidemic in heroin injectors. *Clin. Infect. Dis.* 2000; 31(4): 1018–24.

Wurcel, A. G., Anderson, J. E., and Chiu, K. K. Increasing infectious endocarditis admissions among young people who inject drugs. *Open Forum Infect. Dis.* 2016; 3(3): 1–4.

Additional Readings

Gonzales y Tucker, R. D. and Frazee, B. W. View from the front lines: an emergency medicine perspective on clostridial infections in injection drug users. *Anaerobe* 2014; 30: 108–15.

Mathew, J., Addai, T., Anand, A., *et al.* Clinical features, site of involvement, bacteriologic findings, and outcome of infective endocarditis in intravenous drug users. *Arch. Intern. Med.* 1995; 155(15): 1641–8.

Samet, J. H., Shevitz, A., Fowle, J., and Singer, D. E. Hospitalization decisions in febrile intravenous drug users. *Am. J. Med.* 1990; 89(1): 53–7.

Infections in Oncology Patients

Allison Nazinitsky and Erik R. Dubberke

Introduction

Infection is a leading cause of morbidity and mortality in oncology patients for a number of reasons. Both neoplastic disease and treatment regimens may cause disruption of mucocutaneous barriers, altered immunity, and/or viscus obstruction. The approach to a febrile oncology patient must take into consideration the nature and stage of the underlying disease, past and present treatments, any recent instrumentation or hospitalization, and any recent antibiotic exposures. Acute care providers must be familiar with the unique patterns of infection seen in oncology patients, as well as the careful approach to evaluation and management that is required in these very high-risk patients.

Pathophysiology and Epidemiology

The number of individuals in the United States diagnosed with cancer has risen dramatically from approximately 3 million in the 1970s to over 12 million in 2014. In patients with active disease, susceptibilty to infection results both from direct effects of the cancer itself and from the adverse effects of chemotherapeutic agents. Solid malignancies can directly increase the risk of infection by various means. Obstruction of natural passages leads to inadequate drainage of body fluids, stasis, and increased risk of bacterial colonization and infection. In this setting, infections are typically due to organisms that are a part of the normal flora (e.g. upper respiratory tract flora causing post-obstructive pneumonia, gastrointestinal flora causing

post-obstructive cholangitis). Solid malignancies can invade across tissue planes, leading to conduits between normally sterile areas and the external environment (e.g. rectovesicular fistulas). Central nervous system malignancies can lead to aspiration and subsequent respiratory tract infection by compromising the cough and/or swallow reflex. In addition to these secondary effects, necrotic tissue within a solid tumor itself can act as a nidus for infection.

Although hematologic malignancies (lymphomas, leukemias, and plasma cell dyscrasias) are rarely associated with obstruction or with the invasion of tissue planes, they are often associated with innate, cellular, and/or humoral immune system dysfunction. Lymphomas and T-cell leukemias are associated with T-cell dysfunction that can persist even after complete remission. Diminished T-cell function predisposes to a wide variety of atypical bacteria infections (mycobacterial, *Listeria*, *Nocardia*), viral infections (varicella-zoster virus [VZV], cytomegalovirus [CMV], Epstein–Barr virus [EBV], respiratory syncytial virus [RSV], adenovirus), fungal infections (*Cryptococcus*, *Histoplasma*, *Coccidioides*, *Blastomyces*, *Pneumocystis*), and parasitic infections (*Toxoplasma*, *Giardia*, *Cryptosporidium*, *Strongyloides*). Plasma cell dyscrasias and B-cell leukemias are associated with impaired antibody production, which can lead to sinopulmonary infections due to decreased IgA-mediated mucosal immunity and to increased susceptibility to encapsulated organisms (*Streptococcus pneumoniae*, *Haemophilus influenzae*, *Pseudomonas aeruginosa*, *Cryptococcus*). Anatomic or functional splenectomy, common in hematologic malignancy, increases susceptibility to encapsulated organisms, as well as to the *Capnocytophaga* species, babesiosis, and malaria.

Beyond the direct effects of a neoplastic process, chemotherapeutic agents used in the treatment of both hematologic and solid malignancies may lead to neutropenia. Oncology patients are most likely to develop infections when they are neutropenic. The risk of developing an infection is related to both the severity and the duration of neutropenia. Up to 80% of patients who are neutropenic for at least 1 week develop a fever, and up to 60% of these patients will have a clinically or microbiologically documented infection. Chemotherapy for hematologic malignancies is typically associated with more profound neutropenia and more severe mucositis than chemotherapy for solid malignancies. Approximately 40% of febrile neutropenic patients with solid malignancies will have a documented source of infection and about 30% of these patients will have bacteremia. In contrast, up to 60% of febrile neutropenic patients with hematologic malignancies will have a documented source of infection, of which 50% will be bacteremic.

Whereas gram-negative infections during the neutropenic period predominated two decades ago, gram-positive bacteria, particularly *Staphylococcus aureus*, now account for approximately 60% of microbiologically documented infections. This shift is likely related to increased utilization of central venous catheters and prophylactic antibiotics. Although gram-positive infections predominate, coverage for gram-negative bacteria, and in particular *Pseudomonas aeruginosa*, is still essential in the febrile neutropenic patient. Patients with prolonged neutropenia are also at risk for infections due to environmental molds, such as *Aspergillus*.

Several chemotherapeutic agents can also impair the cellular and humoral immune systems and predispose to opportunistic infections. Corticosteroids inhibit T-cell activation and immunoglobulin production. Purine analogues, such as fludarabine and cladribine, are directly lymphotoxic, particularly to CD4 T-cells. Methotrexate, an inhibitor of dihydrofolate reductase, is highly immunosuppressive to T-cells as well. The immunosuppression due to these medications can last for months after completion of therapy. Alemtuzumab is a monoclonal antibody directed against CD52, a protein expressed on the surface of lymphocytes, natural killer cells, and monocytes. CD4 T-cell counts can remain suppressed for over 12 months after administration of alemtuzumab. Rituximab is another monoclonal antibody, directed against CD20, a protein expressed on B-cells. An ever-expanding list of biological therapies that impair immunity adds to the challenge of evaluating oncology patients with potential infection, and underscores the importance of early communication with the patient's oncologist.

Recent exposure to health-care settings and prophylactic antibiotics increase the risk of developing infections due to antibiotic-resistant organisms. Knowledge of common resistance patterns in the medical facilities and community where the patient has received care are important when selecting empiric antimicrobial therapy for oncology patients.

Clinical Features

Infection should be suspected in any oncology patient presenting with the systemic inflammatory response syndrome or onset of new end-organ dysfunction without an obvious cause. Oncology patients may not present with typical features of infection due to a blunted inflammatory response. On exam, special attention should be given to areas where bacteria are commonly able to evade compromised mucocutaneous defenses: central venous catheter sites, areas of recent invasive procedures, oropharynx and periodontium, lung, and perineum and perianal areas. Whenever possible, clinical specimens should be obtained to microbiologically confirm the diagnosis and direct therapy.

Bacteremia and Fungemia

A sudden onset of fever, often with tachycardia and chills, is associated with a high rate of positive blood cultures (see Table 62.1). Although patients with solid malignancies are likely to have a documented site of infection at the time of bacteremia, 50% of infected patients with hematologic malignancies will have a primary bacteremia. It is thought that the vast majority of early-onset (within 7 days after the onset of neutropenia) febrile episodes in neutropenic patients are due to translocation of intestinal flora across the gut mucosa. The presence of central venous catheters is associated with a higher risk of gram-positive bacteremia. Patients with severe mucositis are at increased risk for bacteremia from oral flora.

Table 62.1 Clinical Features: Bacteremia and Fungemia

Signs and symptoms	May present with sudden onset of fever or evidence of end-organ dysfunction (e.g. mental status changes)
	Tachycardia and chills
	Hypotension frequently seen with gram-negative and *Staphylococcus aureus* bacteremia
	Syndrome of high fevers (≥40°C), refractory hypotension, and ARDS has been associated with *Streptococcus mitis* bacteremia
	Ecthyma gangrenosum is classically associated with *Pseudomonas aeruginosa* bacteremia
	10% of patients with candidal fungemia will develop pinkish subcutaneous nodules
Laboratory findings	10% of bloodstream infections in oncology patients are due to *Candida* species
Treatment	Start empiric treatment for neutropenic fever (see Treatment and Prophylaxis of low- and high-risk patients)
	Local patterns of bloodstream infection isolates are important when choosing empiric therapy

ARDS – acute respiratory distress syndrome.

Table 62.2 Clinical Features: Oropharyngeal Infection

Signs and symptoms	Usually polymicrobial due to loss of oral mucosal integrity
	May present as gingivostomatitis, pharyngitis, Ludwig's angina, or retropharyngeal abscesses
	Oral mucositis predisposes to reactivation of latent HSV and candidal infections
	Thrush is the most common candidal infection of the oropharynx, but invasive disease can occur
Laboratory findings	CT scan of head and neck can be used to identify patients who require surgical intervention
Treatment	If neutropenic, start empiric treatment for neutropenic fever (refer to text)
	If ceftazidime or cefepime is chosen for initial coverage, add metronidazole 500 mg IV every 8 hours for additional anaerobic coverage
	If oral ulcerations are present, add acyclovir 5 mg/kg/dose IV every 8 hours
	If thrush is present, add an echinocandin or an amphotericin product

CT – computed tomography.

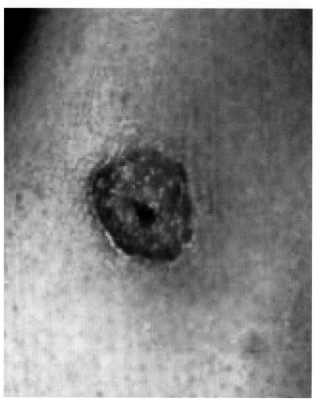

Figure 62.1 Ecthyma gangrenosum in a neutropenic patient with *Pseudomonas aeruginosa* bacteremia.

Image courtesy of Dr. Nigar Kirmani.

Hypotension is most frequently seen with gram-negative and *Staphylococcus aureus* bacteremia. A syndrome of high spiking fevers (≥40 °C), refractory hypotension, and adult respiratory distress syndrome has been associated with *Streptococcus mitis* bacteremia. Ecthyma gangrenosum is classically associated with *Pseudomonas aeruginosa* bacteremia (see Figure 62.1); however, it has also been described with bacteremia due to *Aeromonas* and mold infections of the skin.

Approximately 10% of bloodstream infections in oncology patients are due to *Candida* species. The syndrome is clinically indistinguishable from bacterial bloodstream infections; however, onset is typically later than bacteremia and occurs in patients already receiving broad-spectrum antibiotics. About 10% of patients with candidal fungemia will develop pinkish subcutaneous nodules. Patients with a history of candidal fungemia are at risk for developing hepatosplenic candidiasis, which becomes clinically evident when their neutropenia resolves.

Oropharyngeal Infections

Infections of the oropharynx occur in 15 to 25% of neutropenic oncology patients in whom the source of infection can be identified. Loss of oral mucosal integrity due to chemotherapy provides a portal of entry for oral flora (see Table 62.2 and Box 62.3). Bacterial infections tend to be polymicrobial and can present as gingivostomatitis, pharyngitis, Ludwig's angina, or retropharyngeal abscesses. In addition, oral mucositis predisposes to reactivation of latent herpes simplex virus (HSV) and candidal infections. Reactivated HSV can be severe and can arise in patients without a known history of oral herpes. Thrush is the most common candidal infection of the oropharynx, and invasive disease can occur.

Skin and Soft-Tissue Infections

Infections of the skin and soft tissues account for 10 to 20% of neutropenic oncology patients in whom the source of infection can be identified. Areas of the skin that have been disrupted (e.g. post-venous puncture) and areas that tend to be moist with high bacterial counts (e.g. axilla, perianal area) are predisposed to infection (see Table 62.3 and Box 62.4). Patients initially complain of tenderness with minimal erythema. If left untreated, these infections can rapidly progress and lead to abscess formation, necrosis, and gangrene. The causative organisms are typically local skin flora. *Cryptococcus* can cause a cellulitis in patients on corticosteroids or with impaired T-cell function. As mentioned above, skin lesions may also be the manifestation of a disseminated infection, such as ecthyma gangrenosum in *Pseudomonas* bacteremia or as skin nodules from disseminated candidiasis or fusariosis.

The leading viral cause of skin infections in this population is VZV. Patients typically present with vesicular lesions on an erythematous base limited to one or two dermatomes; patients with impaired T-cell function are at increased risk for disseminated disease and should be placed in negative pressure until dissemination can be ruled out.

Table 62.3 Clinical Features: Skin and Soft-Tissue Infection

Signs and symptoms	Often found in areas of skin disruption (e.g. post-venous puncture) and areas that are moist with high bacterial counts (e.g. axilla, perianal area)
	VZV is the leading viral cause of skin infections in one or two dermatomes (patients with impaired T-cell function are at increased risk for disseminated disease)
Treatment	If neutropenic, start empiric treatment for neutropenic fever (refer to text); add vancomycin 15–20 mg/kg/dose IV every 8–12 hours
	If infection is in an area commonly colonized with anaerobes (e.g. neck, oropharynx, axilla, perianal area) and ceftazidime or cefepime is chosen for initial coverage, add metronidazole 500 mg IV every 8 hours for additional anaerobic coverage
	If concern for VZV, add acyclovir 10 mg/kg/dose IV every 8 hours and place patient in a negative-pressure room

Table 62.4 Clinical Features: Respiratory Tract Infection

Signs and symptoms	Neutropenic patients rarely produce sputum
	Only one-half to two-thirds of oncology patients with radiographic or culture-positive pneumonia will present with typical clinical features (fever, cough, dyspnea, chest pain, sputum production, infiltrates)
	PCP presents more acutely in oncology patients than in patients with AIDS
	Fungal pneumonias typically have an insidious onset with nodular or cavitating disease on CXR or chest CT
	Patients on corticosteroids are at risk for environmental (e.g. *Aspergillus* species) and *Nocardia* infections
Laboratory findings	Diagnostics may include blood and sputum cultures, respiratory viral testing, and serum galactomannan
	Sinusitis with bone erosion may be a sign of fungal sinusitis
	Nodular or cavitating disease on CXR or chest CT are concerning for a mold infection
	Interstitial infiltrates can be seen with atypical bacterial, viral, and PCP
Treatment	If neutropenic, start empiric treatment for neutropenic fever (refer to text)
	If concern for aspiration or post-obstructive pneumonia and ceftazidime or cefepime is chosen for initial coverage, add metronidazole 500 mg IV every 8 hours, for additional anaerobic coverage
	If there is concern for PCP, start trimethoprim-sulfamethoxazole 5 mg/kg/dose of the trimethoprim component IV every 8 hours
	If there are nodules or cavitary lesions, start an antifungal with activity against molds (e.g. amphotericin product, echinocandin, voriconazole, posaconazole)
	If concern for fungal sinusitis, start an amphotericin product

AIDS – acquired immunodeficiency syndrome; PCP – *Pneumocystis* pneumonia.

Respiratory Tract Infections

Respiratory tract infections will be developed by 10 to 15% of neutropenic oncology patients. The list of possible etiologic pathogens is long (see Box 62.5). Because of the impaired inflammatory response, only about one-half to two-thirds of oncology patients with radiographic or culture-positive pneumonia will present with typical clinical features (fever, cough, dyspnea, chest pain, sputum production, discrete infiltrates). Neutropenic patients rarely produce sputum (see Table 62.4). *Pneumocystis jiroveci* pneumonia (formerly *Pneumocystis carinii*) presents more acutely in oncology patients than in patients with AIDS, and signs and symptoms often begin after discontinuation of corticosteroid therapy. Fungal pneumonias typically have an insidious onset with nodular or cavitating disease on chest X-ray (CXR) or chest computed tomography (CT) (see Figure 62.2). Patients at greatest risk for fungal pneumonia due to environmental molds (most commonly *Aspergillus* species) include patients with prolonged neutropenia (≥3 weeks) and corticosteroid therapy.

Patients on corticosteroids are also at risk for *Nocardia* infections. *Nocardia* has a similar pulmonary presentation to mold infections; however, there is an increased likelihood of metastatic infection in the central nervous system. Culture and/or histopathology can differentiate between the two.

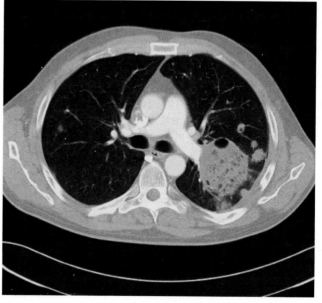

Figure 62.2 Chest CT of a patient with acute lymphoblastic leukemia who had received alemtuzumab 4 months before presentation. The patient presented with 1 week of cough, malaise, and mild left-sided chest pain. The patient's white blood cell count (WBC) was 7.0 with 85% neutrophils. *Aspergillus fumigatus* grew from a bronchial washing.
Image courtesy of Dr. Erik Dubberke.

Table 62.5 Clinical Features: Gastrointestinal Tract Infections

Signs and symptoms	Most common manifestations in the neutropenic patient are esophagitis and enterocolitis
	Odynophagia
	HSV and *Candida* esophagitis can occur in the absence of oral lesions
	Diarrhea, nausea, vomiting, abdominal pain, abdominal distension, and fever commonly occur with colitis
	Neutropenic leukemic patients are at risk for developing neutropenic enterocolitis, also known as typhlitis
Laboratory findings	*C. difficile* testing should be performed if there is concern for colitis
	CT scan of abdomen should be obtained in patients with abdominal pain
Treatment	If patient is neutropenic, start empiric treatment for neutropenic fever (refer to text)
	If ceftazidime or cefepime is chosen for initial coverage, add metronidazole 500 mg IV every 8 hours, for additional anaerobic coverage
	For *C. difficile*, start vancomycin 125 mg PO QID

Table 62.6 Clinical Features: Central Nervous System Infections

Signs and symptoms	Often subtle findings such as headache, confusion, or more remarkable such as seizures, meningismus, changes in behavior, or focal neurological findings
Laboratory findings	Send CSF* for cell count and differential, glucose, protein, bacterial counts, cryptococcal antigen and culture, and HSV PCR
	If neutropenic, neutrophils may not be present in the CSF
Treatment	If neutropenic and there is concern for bacterial meningitis, treat with cefepime 2 g IV every 8 hours, plus vancomycin 15–20 mg/kg/dose IV every 8–12 hours, plus ampicillin 2 g IV every 4 hours.
	If cryptococcal antigen positive, start amphotericin-containing product

* Because of the increased risk for mass lesions, a CT scan of the brain should be obtained before a lumbar puncture is attempted in oncology patients. CSF – cerebrospinal fluid; PCR – polymerase chain reaction.

Although infections of the upper respiratory tract (e.g. otitis, sinusitis) are uncommon, accounting for only 1% of episodes, these infections can be rapidly life-threatening in oncology patients. These infections tend to be caused by *Aspergillus*, *Fusarium* species, and Mucormycosis. Diagnosis of invasive fungal sinusitis requires a high index of suspicion. Boney erosion on sinus CT is highly suggestive. Treatment typically includes early surgical debridement for source control and culture and antifungals.

Gastrointestinal Tract Infections

The gastrointestinal tract is the source of infection in 4 to 8% of oncology patients in whom the source of infection can be identified. The most common manifestations in the neutropenic patient are esophagitis and enterocolitis (see Table 62.5 and Box 62.6). Patients receiving chemotherapy and/or with impaired T-cell function are at increased risk for esophagitis due to HSV or *Candida*. These patients typically present with odynophagia as their primary complaint. The etiological pathogen can be presumed if the patient has oral herpetic lesions or thrush; however, HSV and *Candida* esophagitis can occur in the absence of oral lesions.

Clostridium difficile is the most common infectious cause of colitis. Presenting complaints commonly include diarrhea, nausea, vomiting, abdominal pain, abdominal distension, and fever. Patients with severe colitis may have ileus and thus not have diarrhea. Neutropenic leukemic patients are at risk for developing neutropenic enterocolitis, also known as typhlitis, which can mimic an acute appendicitis. Because of chemotherapy-induced neutropenia and mucosal disruption, intestinal flora are able to invade the gut wall and can cause a life-threatening necrotizing colitis.

Urinary Tract Infections

Urinary tract infections should be considered, but are an uncommon source of infection in oncology patients, accounting for only 1 to 3% of infections. Symptoms are typically minimal, and pyuria is rare because of generalized neutropenia.

Central Nervous System Infections

Although central nervous system infections are an uncommon source of infection in oncology patients, patients with impaired T-cell and splenic function are at increased risk for central nervous system infections due to *S. pneumoniae*, *Listeria*, *Cryptococcus*, *Toxoplasma*, *Nocardia*, and *Aspergillus* (see Box 62.7). Signs and symptoms of central nervous system infections can be subtle in immunocompromised patients, and many agents are associated with indolent infections (see Table 62.6). Patients may present with headache, confusion, seizures, meningismus, changes in behavior, or focal neurological findings. Absence of meningismus, however, cannot be used to exclude CNS infection in this population. Because of the increased risk for mass lesions, a CT scan of the brain should be obtained before a lumbar puncture is attempted in oncology patients.

Differential Diagnosis

Potential Causes of Fever in Oncology Patients

The differential diagnosis of suspected infections in oncology patients is extremely broad. Not only are atypical pathogens

Box 62.1 Differential Diagnosis: Persistent Neutropenic Fever of Unknown Origin in the Oncology Patient*

CMV
EBV
Tuberculosis
Histoplasmosis
Blastomycosis
Coccidioidomycosis

Tumor fever
- Primary or secondary brain tumor
- Primary or secondary liver tumor
- Hypernephroma
- Hematologic malignancies

Acute or delayed transfusion reaction
Drug fever

* The source of fever in patients with persistent neutropenic fever will never be identified in the vast majority of cases, particularly if they are otherwise clinically stable. Evaluation of persistent neutropenic fever of unknown origin should be based on risk factors present and other signs and symptoms.

Box 62.2 Differential Diagnosis: Sepsis Syndrome in the Oncology Patient

Gram-negative infection
S. aureus infection
S. mitis bacteremia
Candidemia
Drug reaction

Thrombotic thrombocytopenic purpura
- mitomycin C

Tumor lysis syndrome
- tamoxifen
- bleomycin
- cytosine arabinoside
- daunomycin

Acute or delayed transfusion reaction
Anaphylaxis
Immune reconstitution after count recovery or steroid weaning

Box 62.3 Differential Diagnosis: Oropharyngeal Infection in the Oncology Patient

Polymicrobial bacterial infection (oral flora)
HSV
Candida
Cryptococcus
Histoplasmosis
Mucositis

Box 62.4 Differential Diagnosis: Skin and Soft-Tissue Infection in the Oncology Patient

Cellulitis
- Bacterial (local flora)
- Deep venous thrombosis
- *Cryptococcus*
- Atypical mycobacteria

Disseminated rash
- Drug reaction
- CMV
- EBV
- Disseminated bacterial infection

Nodular lesion
- Disseminated bacterial infection
- *Cryptococcus*
- *Nocardia*
- Atypical mycobacteria
- Sweet's syndrome

Ulcerative lesion
- HSV
- VZV
- Ecthyma gangrenosum
- Pyoderma gangrenosum
- Environmental mold

possible, but oncology patients are also at high risk for non-infectious complications that mimic infection, including drug and tumor fevers, and transfusion reactions. Most patients with an undocumented source of fever will defervesce within 5 days after initiation of antibiotics. Patients with a documented source of infection typically take longer to respond to antibiotics. Boxes 62.1 through 62.6 list potential causes of fever based on the clinical syndrome.

Laboratory and Radiographic Findings

Two sets of blood cultures should be drawn on all oncology patients with suspected infection. If possible, both sets of blood cultures should be drawn from peripheral veins. Initial diagnostic tests should include a complete blood count with differential, serum electrolytes including creatinine, liver function tests, urinalysis, urine culture, and a chest radiograph (see Table 62.7).

Additional evaluation will depend on the presenting complaint. Patients with diarrhea should have stool tested for *C. difficile* toxin. A CT of the abdomen and pelvis or abdominal ultrasound should be obtained in patients with abdominal tenderness. A CT of the head followed by a lumbar puncture should be obtained in patients with suspected central nervous system infection. CSF should be sent for cell count and differential, glucose, protein, bacterial culture, cryptococcal antigen and culture, and HSV PCR. Unless contraindications exist (e.g. thrombocytopenia), samples should be obtained for Gram stain and culture from areas where infection is suspected. Chronic skin lesions should also be tested for fungi and mycobacteria, and necrotic skin lesions should be tested for fungi. Early bronchoscopy with alveolar lavage and transbronchial biopsy should be considered in patients with suspected or documented pneumonia.

Treatment and Prophylaxis

Choosing the correct empiric antimicrobial therapy in oncology patients, whether for possible bacteremia (febrile neutrapenia)

Box 62.5 Differential Diagnosis: Respiratory Tract Infections in the Oncology Patient

Sinusitis

- Polymicrobial bacterial
- Environmental mold
- Allergy

Focal pulmonary consolidation

- *S. pneumoniae*
- *H. influenzae*
- Gram-negative
- Post-obstructive pneumonia
- *Cryptococcus*
- Pulmonary embolism
- Pulmonary hemorrhage

Interstitial infiltrates

- Respiratory virus
- *Mycoplasma pneumoniae*
- *Chlamydia pneumoniae*
- *Pneumocystis jiroveci*
- Adult respiratory distress syndrome
- Congestive heart failure
- Pericardial effusion
- Drug reaction

    azacitidine

    bleomycin

    busulfan

    chlorambucil

    cyclophosphamide

    cytosine arabinoside

    fludarabine

    melphalan

    methotrexate

    mitomycin

    nitrosoureas

    procarbazine

- Radiation pneumonitis
- Lymphangitic spread of malignancy

Nodules/cavities

- Malignancy
- Environmental mold
- Histoplasmosis
- Blastomycosis
- Coccidioidomycosis
- Tuberculosis
- *Nocardia*

Box 62.6 Differential Diagnosis: Gastrointestinal Infection in the Oncology Patient

Esophagitis

- HSV
- *Candida*
- Radiation esophagitis
- Mucositis
- Bacterial esophagitis
- Malignancy

Enterocolitis

- *Clostridium difficile*
- Typhlitis
- Mucositis
- Radiation poisoning
- Radiation enterocolitis
- Viral gastroenteritis
- *Giardia*
- *Cryptosporidium*

Box 62.7 Differential Diagnosis: Central Nervous System Infection in the Oncology Patient

S. pneumoniae
L. monocytogenes
H. influenzae
Cryptococcus
Nocardia
Carcinomatous meningitis
Brain abscess
HSV
Radiation toxicity
Chemotherapy toxicity

- cytosine arabinoside
- methotrexate
- ifosfamide

Environmental mold
Sedatives/narcotics
Hemorrhage
Diabetes mellitus
Hypercalcemia
Malignancy

or for an identifiable source of infection, can be difficult. Acute care providers are advised to consult both the patient's oncologist and an infectious disease specialist as early as possible in the care of an oncology patient with infection.

Febrile Neutrapenia

The widespread institution of broad gram-negative (in particular, anti-pseudomonal) coverage at the onset of fever in the neutropenic patient has been the single most effective advance in supportive care of oncology patients in the past 30 years. The Infectious Disease Society of America guidelines define febrile neutropenia as a single temperature at or above 38.3 °C or a temperature of 38.0°C to 38.2 °C for 1 hour or longer in patients with a neutrophil count below 500 polymorphonuclear neutrophil leukocytes (PMNs)/mL, or of below 1,000 PMNs/mL with an expected drop to below 500. All neutropenic patients with suspected infection should receive prompt empiric antibiotics.

Patients with febrile neutropenia are often first evaluated in the emergency department. Despite recommendations to administer the first dose of empiric antibiotics within 1 hour, several studies have shown there can be a significant delay in this setting. Many emergency departments and cancer centers have developed protocols to decrease the time to antibiotic

Table 62.7 Baseline Laboratory Assessment of Neutropenic Oncology Patients

Two sets of blood cultures (venipuncture if possible)

Complete blood count with differential

Serum electrolytes

Serum creatinine

Liver function tests

Urinalysis

Urine culture

CXR

Table 62.8 Scoring Index for Identification of Low-Risk Patients Presenting with Neutropenic Fever

Characteristic	Score
Extent of illness (choose one):	
• No symptoms	5
• Mild symptoms	5
• Moderate symptoms	3
No hypotension	5
No chronic obstructive pulmonary disease	4
Solid tumor or no fungal infection	4
No dehydration	3
Outpatient at onset of fever	3
Age 17–60	2

Highest score is 26. Patients with a score between 21 and 26 indicate the patient is at low risk for complications. Adapted from J. Klastersky and M. Paesmans, The Multinational Association for Supportive Care in Cancer (MASCC) risk index score: 10 years of use for identifying low-risk febrile neutropenic cancer patients. Support Care Cancer 2013; 21(5): 1487–95.

treatment and increase the number of blood cultures obtained, which may improve outcomes and reduce length of stay.

Risk Assessment for Oral Therapy

In the past, all febrile neutropenic patients were started on intravenous broad-spectrum antibiotics and admitted to the hospital. More recently, a group of low-risk patients have been identified that may be treated as outpatients with oral antibiotics.

Factors associated with a low risk of adverse outcomes are:
• anticipated duration of neutropenia less than 7 days
• solid malignancy, lymphoma, or myeloma in remission
• no obvious site of infection
• absence of comorbidities

Factors associated with a high risk of complications are:
• anticipated duration of neutropenia greater than 10 days
• acute leukemia
• temperature at or above 39 °C
• rigors
• severe sepsis
• an identified site of infection
• end-organ dysfunction
• presence of comorbidities

Based on these factors, a scoring system was developed and validated prospectively by the Multinational Association for Supportive Care in Cancer (see Table 62.8). A high score from 21 to 26 identified patients with a less than 5% risk of developing severe complications with a positive predictive value of 91%, specificity of 68%, and sensitivity of 71%. Other factors to consider when deciding whether or not to treat a low-risk patient with oral antibiotics include:

• patient adherence
• patient's ability to swallow
• gut motility and absorption
• use of antibiotic prophylaxis

Patients who meet low-risk criteria may be appropriate candidates for oral outpatient therapy (see below). Oncology should be consulted before deciding on oral treatment, and all such patients should have continuous and rapid access to high-level inpatient care.

Treatment of Low-Risk Patients

Oral combination therapy with ciprofloxacin 500 mg PO TID and amoxicillin/clavulanate 500/125 mg PO TID was found to be just as efficacious as intravenous antibiotics in two studies of low-risk patients. This regimen has good coverage of both gram-negative and gram-positive bacteria. Ciprofloxacin and levofloxacin are the only orally available antibiotics that have adequate activity against *Pseudomonas*. Widespread use of oral fluoroquinolones as prophylaxis may limit the efficacy of this regimen. Other factors to consider include the prevalence of antibiotic-resistant organisms in the community (such as community-associated methicillin-resistant *S. aureus* or fluoroquinolone-resistant *E. coli*) and whether the patient has recently been hospitalized.

Treatment of Patients on Prophylaxis

Some oncology patients are treated with a prophylactic regimen of ciprofloxacin or levofloxacin during periods of prolonged neutropenia. This has been shown to reduce the incidence of neutropenic fever and hospitalization. Patients who develop microbiologically proven infections while on fluoroquinolone prophylaxis are more likely to have a fluoroquinolone-resistant organism. Therefore, patients on fluoroquinolone prophylaxis who present with neutropenic fever should not receive a fluoroquinolone as initial treatment and should be admitted and treated with intravenous antibiotics regardless of risk stratification.

Treatment of High-Risk Patients

All high-risk neutropenic patients should be started on broad-spectrum intravenous antibiotics and admitted to the hospital. Choices of empiric intravenous antibiotics include:

• Ceftazidime: 2 g IV every 8 hours plus vancomycin 15–20 mg/kg/dose IV every 8–12 hours
• Cefepime: 2 g IV every 8 hours
• Imipenem-cilastatin: 500 mg IV every 6 hours
• Meropenem: 1 g IV every 8 hours
• Piperacillin-tazobactam: 4.5 g IV every 6 hours

Ceftazidime has poor gram-positive coverage and should be combined with an antibiotic with activity against gram-positive bacteria (e.g. vancomycin). The other agents listed above provide excellent coverage against beta-lactam-sensitive staphylococci and streptococci, though not against MRSA. Choice of agent depends on local sensitivity patterns, formulary availability, and suspected site of infection. Fluoroquinolone monotherapy has not always performed favorably in trials of treatment of neutropenic fever and should be avoided in the absence of severe drug allergies.

Addition of an Aminoglycoside

Although studies of beta-lactam monotherapy versus beta-lactam plus an aminoglycoside have not demonstrated a benefit of combination therapy, combination therapy may be considered in a select group of patients. When possible, aminoglycosides should be avoided in patients at increased risk for adverse events, including the elderly and patients with renal insufficiency, heart failure, or moderate to severe liver disease, as well as patients on other nephrotoxic drugs. Gentamicin or tobramycin 5 mg/kg/dose IV every 24 hours, when indicated, should be considered for patients with:

- severe sepsis
- risk factors for infections due to resistant gram-negative bacteria

Once daily dosing is likely just as efficacious as traditional dosing, but with a lower incidence of nephrotoxicity.

Addition of Vancomycin

Routine empirical use of vancomycin has not been associated with improved patient outcomes. However, there are several settings when empiric vancomycin use should be considered. These include:

- temperature of 40 °C or above
- severe sepsis
- high local rates of penicillin-resistant streptococci
- high local rates of methicillin-resistant *S. aureus*
- catheter exit-site infections
- severe mucositis
- recent fluoroquinolone prophylaxis

Multidrug-Resistant Pathogens

In the past decade, there has been an increased incidence of antimicrobial-resistant infections reported in patients with solid-tumor and hematological malignancies. Organisms associated with nosocomial infections with increased antimicrobial resistance include *Enterococcus faecium*, *Staphylococcus aureus*, *Klebsiella pneumoniae*, *Acinetobacter baumannii*, *Pseudomonas aeruginosa*, and *Enterobacter* spp., and have been called the "ESKAPE" pathogens. *Stenotrophomonas maltophilia* is another often multidrug-resistant pathogen that can be seen in oncologic patients.

Previous infection or colonization with resistant pathogens should be considered when choosing an empiric antibiotic regimen. Hospitals in which multidrug resistant pathogens are endemic should individualize empiric therapy. Inappropriate empiric antibiotics may obviously delay appropriate therapy, which can lead to increased mortality.

It is recommended to use a carbapenem with anti-pseudomonal coverage as first-line antimicrobial if there is concern for extended-spectrum beta-lactamase (ESBL) producing gram-negative bacteria. A polymyxin or tigecycline is recommended if there is concern for a carbapenemase-producing bacteria with *Klebsiella pneumoniae* carbapenemase (KPC) or metallo-beta-lactamase, like the New Delhi metallo-beta-lactamase (NDM-1).

Other Considerations

- Atypical pneumonia pathogen coverage (macrolide or respiratory fluoroquinolone) for patients with interstitial infiltrates.
- *Pneumocystis jiroveci* pneumonia (PCP) coverage for patients with impaired T-cell function or who are on (or have recently discontinued) corticosteroids.
- Antifungal coverage for patients with thrush and esophagitis or nodular/cavitating lesions on CXR.
- Anaerobic coverage for patients with oropharyngeal or intra-abdominal infections.
- Antiviral coverage for patients with oral herpes and esophagitis.
- Ampicillin for patients with meningitis (to cover *Listeria monocytogenes*).
- Oral vancomycin for patients with suspected *C. difficile*-associated disease.
- Patients known to be colonized with resistant pathogens should be placed on isolation to reduce the spread to other patients.

Pearls and Pitfalls

1. Broad-spectrum antibiotics must be started as soon as possible in febrile neutropenic patients.
2. Consulting with the patient's oncologist is imperative to learn about disease status, prophylaxis strategy, recent antimicrobial use, and prior infections.
3. *Pneumocystis jiroveci* is more difficult to diagnose in non-AIDS patients and may require bronchoscopy and transbronchial biopsy to confirm the diagnosis.
4. Neutropenic patients with bacterial pneumonia rarely produce sputum.
5. Patients with a history of invasive fungal infections are at increased risk for reactivation while neutropenic.
6. Invasive fungal sinusitis requires a high index of suspicion and patients may benefit from early surgical debridement.
7. Fungal pneumonia typically has an insidious onset with chest nodules or cavitating lesions on imaging.
8. *Nocardia* infections can involve the brain, lungs, or skin and should be considered in patients on long-term steroids.
9. Skin lesions can be a manifestation of disseminated infection, such as ecthyma gangrenosum due to *Pseudomonas* bacteremia or skin nodules from disseminated candidiasis or fusariosis.

10. Varicella zoster virus is the leading viral cause of skin infections.

11. *Clostridium difficile* is the most common infectious cause of colitis.

12. Because they have a high rate of infection with resistant organisms, patients on fluoroquinolone prophylaxis often require admission and intravenous antibiotics regardless of risk stratification.

13. Early use of carbapenem or a colistin should be considered if history of previous infection or colonization with a multidrug-resistant pathogen.

References

Baden, L. R., Bensinger, W., Angarone, M., *et al.* NCCN clinical practice guidelines in oncology: prevention and treatment of cancer-related infections, Version 2, 2014, available at www.NCCN.org (accessed March 1, 2015).

Behre, G., Link, H., Maschmeyer, G., *et al.* Meropenem monotherapy versus combination therapy with ceftazidime and amikacin for empirical treatment of febrile neutropenic patients. *Ann. Hematol.* 1998; 76(2): 73–80. (Neutropenic fever trial)

Bodey, G. P., Buckley, M., Sathe, Y. S., and Freireich, EJ. Quantitative relationships between circulating leukocytes and infection in patients with acute leukemia. *Ann. Intern. Med.* 1966; 64(2): 328–40. (Study of relationship between severity and length of neutropenia and risk of infection)

Bodro, M., Gudiol, C., Garcia-Vidal, C., *et al.* Epidemiology, antibiotic therapy and outcomes of bacteremia caused by drug-resistant ESKAPE pathogens in cancer patients. *Support Care Cancer* 2014; 22(3): 603–10. (Prospective observational study in oncology patients with bacteremia)

Bow, E. J. There should be no ESKAPE for febrile neutropenic cancer patients: the dearth of effective antibacterial drugs threatens anticancer efficacy. *J. Antimicrob. Chemother.* 2013; 68(3): 492–5. (Review on multidrug-resistant organisms in cancer patients)

Cometta, A., Calandra, T., Gaya, H., *et al.* Monotherapy with meropenem versus combination therapy with ceftazidime plus amikacin as empiric therapy for fever in granulocytopenic patients with cancer. The International Antimicrobial Therapy Cooperative Group of the European Organization for Research and Treatment of Cancer and the Gruppo Italiano Malattie Ematologiche Maligne dell'Adulto Infection Program. *Antimicrob. Agents Chemother.* 1996; 40(5): 1108–15. (Neutropenic fever trial)

Cometta, A., Kern, W. V., de Bock, R., *et al.* Vancomycin versus placebo for treating persistent fever in patients with neutropenic cancer receiving piperacillin-tazobactam monotherapy. *Clin. Infect. Dis.* 2003; 37(3): 382–9. (Neutropenic fever trial)

Cox, A. L., Thompson, S. A., Jones, J. L., *et al.* Lymphocyte homeostasis following therapeutic lymphocyte depletion in multiple sclerosis. *Eur. J. Immunol.* 2005; 35(11): 3332–42. (Study evaluating duration of lymphopenia after alemtuzumab administration)

Dubberke, E. R., Augustine, K., Olsen, M. A., *et al.* Epidemiology of bloodstream infections on a hematopoietic stem cell transplant unit. *Infect. Dis. Soc. Am.* 2004; abstract no. 648. (Study of the epidemiology of bloodstream infections in patients undergoing stem cell transplantation)

Freifeld, A. G., Bow, E. J., Sepkowitz, K. A., *et al.* Clinical practice guideline for the use of antimicrobial agents in neutropenic patients with cancer: 2010 update by the infectious diseases society of america. *Clin. Infect. Dis.* 2011; 52(4): e56–93. (Infectious Diseases Society of America neutropenic fever guidelines)

Freifeld, A., Marchigiani, D., Walsh, T., *et al.* A double-blind comparison of empirical oral and intravenous antibiotic therapy for low-risk febrile patients with neutropenia during cancer chemotherapy. *N. Engl. J. Med.* 1999; 341(5): 305–11. (Study comparing oral antibiotics to IV antibiotics in low-risk febrile neutropenic patients)

Hasbun, R., Abrahams, J., Jekel, J., and Quagliarello, V. J. Computed tomography of the head before lumbar puncture in adults with suspected meningitis. *N. Engl. J. Med.* 2001; 345(24): 1727–33. (Study of which patients should have a CT of the head performed before lumbar puncture)

Kern, W. V., Cometta, A., de Bock, R., *et al.* Oral versus intravenous empirical antimicrobial therapy for fever in patients with granulocytopenia who are receiving cancer chemotherapy. International Antimicrobial Therapy Cooperative Group of the European Organization for Research and Treatment of Cancer. *N. Engl. J. Med.* 1999; 341(5): 312–18. (Study comparing oral antibiotics to IV antibiotics in low-risk febrile neutropenic patients)

Klastersky, J., Paesmans, M., Rubenstein, E. B., *et al.* The Multinational Association for Supportive Care in Cancer risk index: a multinational scoring system for identifying low-risk febrile neutropenic cancer patients. *J. Clin. Oncol.* 2000; 18(16): 3038–51. (Study to identify neutropenic patients at low-risk for complications)

Klastersky, J. and Paesmans, M. The Multinational Association for Supportive Care in Cancer (MASCC) risk index score: 10 years of use for identifying low-risk febrile neutropenic cancer patients. *Support Care Cancer* 2013; 21(5): 1487–95. (Update from previous study on how to identify neutropenic patients at low-risk for complications)

Kyriacou, D. N., Jovanovic, B., and Frankfurt, O. Timing of initial antibiotic treatment for febrile neutropenia in the emergency department: the need for evidence-based guidelines. *J. Natl. Compr. Canc. Netw.* 2014; 12(11): 1569–73.

Montassier, E., Batard, E., Gastinne, T., *et al.* Recent changes in bacteremia in patients with cancer: a systematic review of epidemiology and antibiotic resistance. *Eur. J. Clin. Microbiol. Infect. Dis.* 2013; 32(7): 841–50. (Review of antibiotic resistant bacteremia in cancer patients)

Neuburger, S. and Maschmeyer, G. Update on management of infections in cancer and stem cell transplant patients. *Ann. Hematol.* 2006; 85(6): 345–56. (Review of infections in leukemic patients and patient undergoing stem cell transplantation)

Penack, O., Becker, C., Buchheidt, D., *et al.* Management of sepsis in neutropenic patients: 2014 updated guidelines from the Infectious Diseases Working Party of the German Society of Hematology and Medical Oncology (AGIHO). *Ann. Hematol.* 2014; 93(7): 1083–95. (Review of sepsis in patients with neutropenia and sepsis)

Satlin, M. J., Calfee, D. P., Chen, L., *et al.* Emergence of carbapenem-resistant enterobacteriaceae as causes of bloodstream infections in patients with hematologic malignancies. *Leuk. Lymphoma* 2013; 54(4): 799–806. (Retrospective review of patients with carbapenem-resistant *Enterobacteriaceae* bloodstream infections in patients with hematological malignancies)

Sickles, E. A., Greene, W. H., and Wiernik, P. H. Clinical presentation of infection in granulocytopenic patients. *Arch. Intern. Med.*

1975; 135(5): 715–19. (Study of presentation of neutropenic patients with infections)

Suster, S. and Rosen, L. B. Intradermal bullous dermatitis due to candidiasis in an immunocompromised patient. *JAMA* 1987; 258(15): 2106–7. (Case and review of neutropenic patients who develop subcutaneous nodules after candidemia)

Tamura, K., Matsuoka, H., Tsukada, J., *et al.* Cefepime or carbapenem treatment for febrile neutropenia as a single agent is as effective as a combination of 4th-generation cephalosporin + aminoglycosides: comparative study. *Am. J. Hematol.* 2002; 71(4): 248–55. (Neutropenic fever trial)

Post-Operative Infections

Robert Brown and Siamak Moayedi

Introduction

Each year in the United States, more than 16 million inpatient operations are performed and more than 1 million emergency department (ED) visits are related to surgical complications.[1] Cosmetic procedures conducted at outpatient facilities not subject to government regulations are not well reported, but contribute to the number of complications.[2] Surgical site infections (SSIs), defined as infections that develop near the incision within 30 days after the procedure or within 1 year after a prosthetic implantation, are the most common post-operative infection and the main topic of this chapter.[3] SSIs are classified by the CDC as incisional (superficial or deep) or organ/space infections (see Table 63.1).[4] Other peri-operative infections include catheter-associated urinary tract infections (UTIs), pneumonia, and antibiotic-associated diarrhea.

Epidemiology and Microbiology

SSIs are the most common health-care-associated infection among hospitalized patients. More than 150,000 cases are reported annually in the United States. Mandated reporting demonstrates that SSIs are declining for some operations (cesarean sections, shunts for dialysis) and increasing for others (breast surgery, appendectomy).[5] Among the nearly 1 million total joint replacements per year in the United States, the incidence of SSI ranges from 0.5 to 1% for hips, 0.5 to 2% for knees, and <1% for shoulders.[6] The national incidence of SSI is 1.9% of all surgeries, with an encouraging 19% decrease for ten commonly reported procedures between 2008 and 2013.[7] The wound classification (see Table 63.2) developed by the National Academy of Sciences and the National Research Council predicts that the risk of SSI ranges from 1.3% of clean wounds to 40% of dirty procedures. A variety of factors are associated with SSI, including diabetes, obesity, smoking, and concurrent remote site infections.

According to current guidelines,[8] methicillin-resistant *Staphylococcus aureus* (MRSA) and coagulase-negative *Staphylococcus* are the primary pathogens associated with cardiothoracic, vascular, orthopedic, and neurosurgical site infections,[9] and an increasing number of infections are casused by community-acquired strains of MRSA.[10] Following gastrointestinal surgery, coloform and anaerobes including *Bacteroides* species should be considered.

Clinical Features

The majority of SSIs develop between the third and tenth post-operative days, but some manifest months after the procedure. The risk of delayed presentation is increased with surgeries involving insertion of foreign material such as mesh for hernia repairs.[11] Superficial SSIs are generally evident on direct inspection. Early signs of infection are warmth, tenderness, and erythema that blanches with pressure. It is important to note that even superficial SSIs have the potential to progress to necrotizing infections, leading to high morbidity. Findings that cause concern include early appearance (12 to 48 hours post-operatively) and erythematous streaks proximal to a wound on an extremity. Pain out of proportion to the appearance of the tissue and pain beyond the margins of erythema are the most significant findings and should raise concern for necrotizing soft-tissue infection. Cellulitis can progress to suppuration with superficial abscess formation and skin dehiscence. All incisions with cellulitis should be examined for associated abscesses, which are unlikely to respond to antibiotic therapy alone and require drainage. In the ED, ultrasound is the ideal tool for evaluation of these infections.[12]

Deep incisional SSIs can present at a more advanced stage because patients might not have the visual clues that would typically lead them to seek medical evaluation.[13] As deep

Table 63.1 Post-Operative Infection Types

Surgical Site Infections (SSIs)			Others
Superficial*	**Deep**	**Organ/Space†**	
Involves only the skin or subcutaneous tissue + at least one of the following: • purulent drainage • isolated organism from an aseptically obtained culture • wound is opened by a surgeon for pain, redness, edema, and heat (unless culture is negative)	Extends into the fascial and muscle layers + at least one of the following: • purulent drainage • abscess • spontaneous dehiscence or opening by a surgeon for fever or pain (unless culture is negative)	Involves any anatomy that was opened or manipulated during surgery in addition to the incision + at least one of the following: • purulent drainage from a drain placed through a stab wound‡ • isolated organism aseptically cultured • abscess	Catheter-associated UTIs Pneumonia Antibiotic-associated diarrhea

* Does not include stitch abscesses, episiotomies, circumcision sites, and infected burn wounds (these have additional criteria).

† Does not include infections that drain through the surgical incision, as these are considered deep incisional infections.

‡ Infection around a stab wound is not an SSI, but is considered a skin or soft-tissue infection.

Table 63.2 Classification of Operation Sterility

	Clean	Clean-Contaminated	Contaminated	Dirty
Description	An incision in which no inflammation is encountered during a surgical procedure, without a break in sterile technique, and during which the respiratory, alimentary, and genitourinary tracts are not entered.	An incision through which the respiratory, alimentary, or genitourinary tract is entered under controlled conditions, but with no contamination encountered.	An incision created during an operation in which there is a major break in sterile technique or gross spillage from the gastrointestinal tract, or an incision in which acute, non-purulent inflammation is encountered. Open traumatic wounds that are more than 12–24 hours old also fall into this category.	An incision created during an operation in which the viscera are perforated or when acute inflammation with pus is encountered during the operation (e.g. emergency surgery for fecal peritonitis) Traumatic wounds for which treatment is delayed and that involve fecal contamination or devitalized tissue.
Examples	Inguinal hernia Coronary bypass	Cholecystectomy Lung resection	Colectomy Urinary diversion	Anastomotic leak repair Debridement of necrosis

infection progresses to suppuration, pressure from the collecting pus increases until it dissects through the surgical wound and drains through the skin incision, at which point patients usually present for medical attention. Prolonged deep incisional SSIs can affect the viability of fascial tissues and lead to dehiscence. Among deep SSIs, post-sternotomy wound infections are especially dangerous because of their proximity to the heart and the potential for mediastinitis.

Organ or space SSIs are the most problematic post-operative infections because they cannot drain easily. Spontaneous drainage and decompression occur via fistula formation and/or fascial dehiscence. The two mechanisms accounting for these collections are infection of a hematoma at the operative site and leakage of infectious fluid from an anastomosis or site of viscus closure. Under controlled circumstances, the likelihood of deep organ/space infection depends on the operation, with the highest rates among rectal resection and esophagectomy, as shown in Table 63.3. Following emergency surgery, however, the site makes little difference.

In the abdomen, organ or space SSIs present as secondary peritonitis, with abdominal pain, tenderness, nausea, anorexia, and signs of sepsis. In the chest, SSIs induce pleuritic pain and dyspnea, while mediastinal infections are more likely to cause tachycardia and signs of severe sepsis.

In the setting of infection, output from drainage catheters can either increase (leakage from inflammation) or decrease (catheter occlusion leading to accumulation of infected fluid).

Differential Diagnosis

Normal inflammation during healing may give the appearance of a superficial wound. An incisional hernia that appears to be infected may be misdiagnosed as dehiscence. Whereas dehiscence occurs within the first few weeks after an operation and denotes almost complete failure of the fascia to heal, incisional hernias are isolated defects in healing that occur weeks to months after the operation. Fluid accumulated in a deep space could be a sterile hematoma or serous fluid. In the abdomen, pockets of fluid might be uninfected bilomas and urinomas, while a milky pleural effusion in the chest may represent a chylothorax from thoracic duct injury.

Faced with a febrile post-operative patient, acute care providers should evaluate not only for an SSI, but also consider pneumonia, urinary tract infection, and antibiotic-associated diarrhea. These diagnoses are not always straightforward, however. Shortness of breath, low-grade fever, and tachycardia might represent pulmonary embolism and not pneumonia. Dysuria alone could be nothing more than local,

Table 63.3 Risk of Anastomotic Leak

Gastric bypass	1.7–2.7%
Appendectomy	2–3%
Small bowel resection	3–4%
Bronchoplastic lung resection	3–4%
Gastrectomy	2–5%
Pneumonectomy	4–5%
Colectomy	2.0–5.6%
Urinary diversion	3–8%
Pancreas resection	5–10%
Rectal resection	6.0–13.6%
Esophagectomy	5–16%

sterile inflammation from the catheter. Over-zealous use of post-operative bowel regimens can cause frequent loose stools.

Laboratory and Radiographic Findings

Patients presenting to the ED with possible post-operative infections often will have a complete blood count to evaluate for anemia, leukocytosis, and neutrophilia. It is important to recognize that leukocytosis has poor sensitivity for infection, especially in the elderly and the immunocompromised.

If the patient is febrile, has significant leukocytosis, or is immunosuppressed with constitutional symptoms, then blood cultures should be obtained so that antibiotic therapy can eventually be tailored for the organism(s) present. Cultures from wound swabs are not recommended. Results will be clouded by colonizers, contaminants, and species present in small numbers, which can lead to confusion in treatment. If drainage catheters have been placed recently in otherwise sterile cavities, the fluid can be sent for gram stain and culture.

Fluid from drainage catheters can be sent for other assays that test for the presence of bodily fluids: creatinine for urinary leakage, bilirubin for biliary leakage, amylase and lipase for pancreatic leakage, and triglycerides and lymphocytes for lymph (chyle) leakage.

Imaging is often indicated in SSIs to assess for abscess. Ultrasound can be useful in the evaluation of adults with superficial wounds and in children, but computed tomography is the standard for diagnosing intra-abdominal abscess following surgery. The use of intravenous contrast is ideal, but must be balanced with the risk of renal dysfunction. This risk can be mitigated by pre-treatment with intravenous fluids. Patients who have undergone abdominal operations should also be given enteral contrast. This agent should be water soluble in case of perforation. In complex cases, the choice of imaging modality and use of contrast should be discussed with a radiologist and the surgeon of record.

Chest radiographs should be obtained in all post-thoracic surgery patients and in any post-operative patient with symptoms of dyspnea or cough.

Treatment and Prophylaxis

Superficial surgical site infections are treated primarily with removal of sutures or with incision and drainage. Antibiotics are reserved for wounds with erythema and edema extending beyond the wound and those associated with significant systemic infection. The suggested empiric therapy is a first-generation cephalosporin or antistaphylococcal penicillin. Trimethoprim–sulfamethoxazole, vancomycin, linezolid, daptomycin, telavancin, or ceftaroline may be required for patients at risk for MRSA. Practitioners should consult the local antibiogram to refine the treatment strategy. Cephalosporins or fluoroquinolones with metronidazole are needed to cover gram-negative bacteria and anaerobes for surgical procedures involving the axilla, gastrointestinal tract, perineum, or female genital tract. For patients with health-care-associated intra-abdominal infections, empiric therapy directed against gram-negative aerobes and facultative bacilli may include carbapenems, piperacillin–tazobactam, or a combination of metronidazole with ceftazidime or cefepime.

The cornerstone of managing infected fluid collections is drainage and control of the source. In a superficial wound, this could mean simply probing with a blunt instrument to open the skin and allow pus to escape. Drainage of deep spaces can be accomplished operatively (especially if revision is required) or percutaneously by an interventional radiologist. Until drainage can be established, broad-spectrum antibiotics should be administered. Because drainage is definitive treatment, antibiotics do not need to continue unless the patient has a prosthesis or bacteremia. Guidelines for intra-abdominal wound infections call for operative management if percutaneous drainage is not possible. Surgery may be delayed up to 24 hours if the patient remains hemodynamically stable and appropriate antibiotic therapy has been initiated. In the subset of patients with a well-contained infection, such as a periappendiceal phlegmon, it is possible to treat with antibiotic therapy and close observation.

Prophylactic antibiotics are important for prevention of SSI and recommended for many surgical procedures. Current guidelines call for dosing prophylactic antibiotics within 1 hour before procedure and redosing during long procedures or in the case of significant blood loss. Some evidence indicates timing antibiotics to 15 minutes prior to the procedure might be superior. Post-procedure prophylactic antibiobics are recommended for no more than 24 hours after surgery, even for patients with surgical drains.

Complications and Admission Criteria

The main complications of SSI to consider are abscess formation and necrotizing infection. Recognition and management of skin and soft-tissue infections is covered in Chapter 12.

Many minor SSIs can be managed on an outpatient basis with oral antibiotics. Patients who require an interventional radiology procedure, operative drainage, or removal of implanted material likely need to be managed in the hospial. High-risk patients such as the immunosuppressed and those who have undergone reconstructive operations with soft-tissue flaps also require inpatient management to limit further complications. Transfer to a facility with hyperbaric oxygen therapy capability should be considered early for patients with compromised grafts and flaps.[14]

Other possible indications for admission are sepsis, metabolic acidosis, hypoxia, and the inability to maintain hydration or nutrition. Simple endpoints of therapy are source control and/or drainage, including removal of infected hardware; normalization of leak and pyrexia; and the patient's improved sense of wellness.

Other Post-Operative Infections

Pneumonia

Several aspects of perioperative treatment increase patients' risk of pneumonia. Abdominal and thoracic operations cause pain with chest expansion, so patients splint and hypoventilate. Limited lung inflation leads to atelectasis and poor clearance of airway secretions. Tracheal intubation and prolonged use of nasogastric or orogastric tubes increases the risk of pneumonia by a combination of increased oropharyngeal colonization and microaspiration of oral and gastric bacteria.[15]

Catheter-Associated Urinary Tract Infections

In the United States, UTIs account for millions of ED visits and cost billions of dollars every year when accounting for both treatment and lost work.[16] Indwelling catheters account for up to 80% of complicated UTIs[17] and are the most common cause of secondary bloodstream infections.[18] An increasing proportion of catheter-associated UTIs culture multidrug-resistant organisms. Female sex, old age, and diabetes are the main risk factors for catheter-associated UTIs.[19]

Antibiotic-Associated Diarrhea

Perioperative antibiotics disrupt the protective gut microbiome and permit infection with opportunistic bacteria, which cause antibiotic-associated diarrhea (AAD). Proton pump inhibitors increase this risk, perhaps by allowing easier transit of bacteria through the stomach.[20] Common organisms include *C. difficile*, *C. perfringens*, *S. aureus*, and *K. oxytoca*.[21] The threat of *C. difficile* is especially great because it is now being transmitted in the community[22] among patients formerly thought to be low risk (not elderly, fewer comorbidities).[23] Ironically, treating AAD with antibiotics can cause further dysbiosis and prolong the course of the illness.[24]

Infection Control

Post-operative infections generally do not pose risks for health-care workers. However, health-care workers are vectors for *C. difficile* and multidrug-resistant organisms that pose a threat to other patients. Contact precautions should be exercised strictly and hand hygiene with soap and water should be used when in contact with *C. difficile*. For patients with a history of MRSA or VRE, contact precautions should remain in place until three or more surveillance cultures are negative (1 or 2 weeks for MRSA, 3 weeks for VRE).[25]

Pearls and Pitfalls

1. Infected fluid collections cannot be treated with antibiotics alone. Source control and drainage are paramount.
2. Pain out of proportion to the appearance of the tissue and pain beyond the margins of erythema should raise concern for necrotizing infection.
3. Careful review of a patient's operative report and discharge summary can disclose useful details.
4. Whenever possible, consult the surgical service familiar with the operation because it will need to be involved in follow-up care.

Additional Reading

Infectious Diseases Society of America, Infections by organ system, available at www.idsociety.org/Organ_System/.

Notes

1   Centers for Disease Control and Prevention (CDC), National Center for Health Statistics. National hospital discharge survey, 2010, available at www.cdc.gov/nchs/fastats/inpatient-surgery.htm# (accessed May 9, 2016); CDC, National hospital ambulatory medical care survey: 2011 emergency department summary tables, available at www.cdc.gov/nchs/data/ahcd/nhamcs_emergency/2011_ed_web_tables.pdf (accessed May 9, 2016).

2   A. L. Beaudoin, L. Torso, K. Richards, *et al.*, Invasive group A Streptococcus infections associated with liposuction surgery at outpatient facilities not subject to state or federal regulation. *JAMA Intern. Med.* 2014; 174(7): 1136-42.

3   S. S. Magill, W. Hellinger, J. Cohen, *et al.*, Prevalence of health-care-associated infections in acute care hospitals in Jacksonville, Florida. *Infect. Control Hosp. Epidemiol.* 2012; 33(3): 283-91.

4   A. J. Mangram, T. C. Horan, M. L. Pearson, *et al.*, Guideline for prevention of surgical site infection, 1999. Centers for Disease Control and Prevention (CDC) Hospital Infection Control Practices Advisory Committee. *Am. J. Infect. Control* 1999; 27(2): 97–132.

5   S. S. Magill, J. R. Edwards, W. Bamberg, *et al.*, Multistate point-prevalence survey of health care-associated infections. *N. Engl. J. Med.* 2014; 370(13): 1198-208.

6   CDC, Healthcare-associated infections progress report, last updated March 3, 2016, available at www.cdc.gov/hai/surveillance/progress-report/index.html A(accessed May 9, 2016).

7   A. F. Widmer, New developments in diagnosis and treatment of infection in orthopedic implants. *Clin. Infect. Dis.* 2001; 33(2): S94; J. W. Sperling, T. K. Kozak, A. D. Hanssen, *et al.*, Infection after shoulder arthroplasty. *Clin. Orthop. Relat. Res.* 2001; 382: 206-16.

8   D. Stevens, A. Bisno, J. Wade, *et al.*, Executive summary: practice guidelines for the diagnosis and management of skin and soft tissue infections: 2014 update by the Infectious Diseases Society of America. *Clin. Infect. Dis.* 2014; 59(2): 147-59.

9   A. I. Hidron, J. R. Edwards, J. Patel, *et al.*, NHSN annual update: antimicrobial-resistant pathogens associated with healthcare-associated infections: annual summary of data reported to the National Healthcare Safety Network at the Centers for Disease Control and Prevention, 2006–2007. *Infect. Control Hosp. Epidemiol.* 2008; 29(11): 996-1011.

10 G. J. Moran, A. Krishnadasan, R. J. Gorwitz, *et al.*, Methicillin-resistant S. aureus infections among patients in the emergency department. *N. Engl. J. Med.* 2006; 355(7): 666–74.

11 B. L. Paton, Y. W. Novtsky, M. Zerey, *et al.*, Management of infections of polytetrafluoroethylene-based mesh. *Surg. Infect. (Larchmt.)* 2007; 8(3): 337-42.

12 D. L. Lewis, C. J. Butts, and L. Moreno-Walton. Facing the danger zone: the use of ultrasound to distinguish cellulitis from abscess in facial infections. *Case Rep. Emerg. Med.* 2014; 2014: 935283.

13 J. C. Pham, M. J. Ashton, C. Kimata, *et al.*, Surgical site infection: comparing surgeon versus patient self-report. *J. Surg. Res.* 2016; 202(1): 95-102.

14 R. Baynosa and W. Zamboni, The effect of hyperbaric oxygen on compromised grafts and flaps. *Undersea Hyperb. Med.* 2012; 39(4): 857-65.

15 Z. Shi, H. Xie, P. Wang, *et al.*, Oral hygiene care for critically ill patients to prevent ventilator-associated pneumonia. *Cochrane Database Syst. Rev.* 2013; 8: CD008367; F. Philippart, S. Gaudry, B. Misset, *et al.*, Randomized intubation with polyurethane or conical cuffs to prevent pneumonia in ventilated patients. *Am. J. Resp. Crit. Care Med.* 2015; 191(6): 637-45.

16 B. Foxman, Urinary tract infection syndromes: occurrence, recurrence, bacteriology, risk factors, and disease burden. *Infect. Dis. Clin. North Am.* 2014; 28(1): 1-13.

17 E. Lo, L. E. Nicolle, S. E. Coffin, *et al.*, Strategies to prevent catheter-associated urinary tract infections in acute care hospitals: 2014 update. *Infect. Control Hosp. Epidemiol.* 2014; 35(5): 464-79.

18 A. Flores-Mireles, J. Walker, M. Caparon, *et al.*, Urinary tract infections: epidemiology, mechanisms of infection and treatment options. *Nat. Rev. Microbiol.* 2015; 13(5): 269-84.

19 C. E. Chenoweth, C. V. Gould, and S. Saint, Diagnosis, management, and prevention of catheter-associated urinary tract infections. *Infect. Dis. Clin. North Am.* 2014; 28(1): 105-19.

20 N. Asha, D. Tompkins, and M. Wilcox. Comparative analysis of prevalence, risk factors, and molecular epidemiology of antibiotic-associated diarrhea due to *Clostridium difficile*, *Clostridium perfringens*, and *Staphylococcus aureus*. *J. Clin. Microbiol.* 2006; 44(8): 2785-91.

21 L. V. McFarland, Antibiotic-associated diarrhea: epidemiology, trends and treatment. *Future Microbiol.* 2008; 3(5): 563-78.

22 N. Rouphael, J. O'Donnell, L. McDonald, *et al.* Research: *Clostridium difficile*–associated diarrhea: an emerging threat to pregnant women. *Am. J. Obstet. Gynecol.* 2008; 198(6): 635.e1-6; S. Baker, H. Faden, W. Sayej, *et al.*, Increasing incidence of community-associated atypical Clostridium difficile disease in children. *Clin. Pediatr.* 2010; 49(7): 644-7.

23 D. A. Leffler and J. T. Lamont, *Clostridium difficile* infection. *N. Engl. J. Med.* 2015; 372(16): 1539-48.

24 L. Kyne, *Clostridium difficile* – beyond antibiotics. *N. Engl. J. Med.* 2010; 362(3): 264-5.

25 J. D. Siegel, E. Rhinehart, M. Jackson, *et al.*, Management of multidrug-resistant organisms in health care settings, 2006. *Am. J. Infect. Control* 2007; 35(Suppl. 2): S165-93.

The Febrile Post-Transplant Patient

Justin Bosley and Aparajita Sohoni

Introduction

In the United States, solid organ transplants (SOTs) and hematopoietic stem cell transplants (HSCTs) are increasingly common forms of treatment for a variety of medical conditions. The 1- and 5-year survival rates vary depending on the organ transplanted. In general, kidney, pancreas, and liver transplants have higher survival rates (89 to 99% at 1 year and 77 to 96% at 5 years) than do heart (81% and 69%, respectively), lung (80% and 53%, respectively), or combined heart–lung (63% and 45%, respectively) transplants. Overall, improvements in transplant candidate selection, surgical technique, immunosuppressive regimens, and long-term medical care have resulted in high survival rates from solid organ transplants. As the number of successful transplants increases, so does the number of acute care visits made by these patients. An understanding of the differential diagnosis of fever in a post-transplant patient, and the risk of infection at different times after transplant and at various levels of immunosuppression, can aid in a comprehensive and cost-effective work-up.

Epidemiology

Infectious complications are a serious cause of morbidity and mortality in post-transplant patients, with serious infection occurring in up to two-thirds of organ transplant patients. In one study of renal transplant recipients, the incidence of infection in the first year post-transplant ranged from 25 to 80%. In a separate study of liver transplant patients, up to 67% of recipients had one serious infection, and infection factored in 53% of early post-transplant deaths. Notably, whereas infection must

be ruled out in any febrile transplant patient, not all infected patients will present with a fever, because of therapeutic immunosuppression. And with the increasing use of more potent immunosuppressive agents, susceptibility to opportunistic infections increases. Practitioners should have a high level of suspicion for the presence of serious infectious disease in these patients.

Clinical Features

Infections in transplant patients can best be approached by distinguishing infections associated with SOT and those associated with HSCT.

Infections in Solid Organ Transplant

Solid organ transplant recipients are usually treated with multidrug prophylaxis against rejection for 3 to 12 months after transplant (see Treatment and Prophylaxis section below). Given that the immunosuppressive regimens are similar for all solid organ transplants, there is a general timeline for risk of infection in the post-transplant course. This can be conceptually divided into the early phase (1 month post-transplant), middle phase (1 to 6 months post-transplant), and late phase (more than 6 months post-transplant). Although exceptions are numerous, there is a distinct group of infectious etiologies in each phase (see Figure 64.1).

Early Phase (Less Than 1 Month Post-Transplant)

In the first month post-transplant, the infections are similar to those in a non-immunosuppressed host undergoing a similar

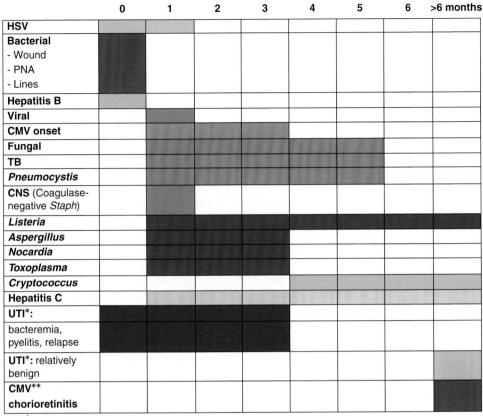

UTI*: Urinary tract infection
CMV**: Cytomegalovirus

Figure 64.1 Infectious etiologies in the Post-Solid Organ Transplant Patient (Month(s) Post-Transplant)

surgical procedure: wound infections, infected hematomas, anastomotic leaks and ischemia, post-surgical pneumonia (either aspiration or due to prolonged intubation), urinary tract infections secondary to indwelling catheters, or bacteremia due to vascular access devices such as central lines. In fact, more than 95% of infections are due to such causes. The risk of infection increases with the duration of intubation or prolonged usage of catheters, vascular access devices, or with the presence of any indwelling catheters or stents. Common pathogens include gram-negative bacilli, *Staphylococcus aureus*, *Staphylococcus epidermidis*, *Enterococcus*, and *Candida* species, including drug-resistant organisms (see Table 64.1). *C. difficile* colitis is increasingly common in this early phase. Opportunistic pathogens are uncommon in the first month after transplantation and, when seen, likely indicate a nosocomial exposure, a severe degree of immunosuppression prior to the transplant, or a pre-existing infection in either the donor or the recipient. Although pre-transplant screening of both the donors and recipients is thorough, transplantation of an infected allograft, contamination of the allograft during transplantation, or unrecognized or inadequately treated pre-transplant infections in the host may occur.

Middle Phase (1 to 6 Months Post-Transplant)

The state of immunosuppression is greatest in the middle phase, as the effects of prolonged T-cell depletion become evident. Most febrile episodes in this period are due to transplant rejection or viral infections. But the top four infectious causes of fever are: cytomegalovirus (CMV), *Listeria monocytogenes*, *Aspergillus* species, and *Pneumocystis jiroveci*. *Nocardia asteroides* and *Salmonella* species are also significant threats to patients in both the middle and late phases post-transplant. New infection with immunomodulatory viruses (such as CMV, Epstein–Barr virus [EBV], hepatitis C virus [HCV], hepatitis B virus [HBV], and human immunodeficiency virus [HIV]), for which these patients are also at risk, may further impair immune responses, resulting in increased susceptibility to opportunistic pathogens such as *Pneumocystis*, *Aspergillus*, and *Listeria*. Each of the most common pathogens is detailed below, with general guidelines for treatment. Specific algorithms should be determined after reviewing individual hospital and community susceptibility patterns, discussion with infectious disease specialists, and examination of all past cultures and biopsy results.

Cytomegalovirus is a member of the *Herpesviridae* and is the most common viral infection in post-transplant patients. Some studies have found CMV infection present in 60 to 90% of all SOT patients. Infection can be asymptomatic or symptomatic. In asymptomatic patients, the disease is usually diagnosed by testing for seroconversion. In symptomatic patients, complaints usually include prolonged fever, anorexia, fatigue, and myalgias. On examination, splenomegaly, elevated transaminases, thrombocytopenia, leukopenia, and atypical lymphocytosis are seen. CMV also can present as pneumonitis,

Table 64.1 Pathogens with Documented Transmission During Transplantation

Class	Pathogen
Bacterial	Enteric gram-negative bacilli
	Pseudomonas aeruginosa
	Staphylococcus aureus
	Bacteroides fragilis
Viral	Cytomegalovirus
	Herpes simplex virus
	Varicella-zoster virus
	Hepatitis B/C viruses
	Human immunodeficiency virus
	Adenovirus
	West Nile virus
	Rabies
	Chagas disease
	Lymphocytic choriomeningitis virus
Fungal	*Candida albicans*
	Histoplasma capsulatum
	Cryptococcus neoformans
	Coccidiodes immitis
	Paracoccidioides brasiliensis
Protozoal	*Toxoplasma gondii*
	Trypanosoma cruzi
	Strongyloides stercoralis
Mycobacterial	*Mycobacterium chelonae*
	Mycobacterium tuberculosis

gastroenteritis, pancreatitis, encephalitis, transverse myelitis, myocarditis, skin ulcerations, or chorioretinitis (more frequently seen in the late phase). The pneumonitis characteristically has bilateral pulmonary infiltrates. Specific allograft injury can occur, such as chronic hepatitis in a liver transplant patient, early atherosclerosis in a heart transplant patient, or bronchiolitis obliterans in a lung transplant patient. Disease is more severe in newly infected patients than in patients who have had CMV infection prior to transplantation. Diagnosis is made via blood culture, bronchoalveolar lavage, or tissue biopsy demonstrating intranuclear inclusions. The approach to prophylaxis and treatment of CMV disease is controversial and should be discussed with available transplant service or infectious disease specialists.

Listeria monocytogenes is a gram-positive bacillus that can cause bacteremia, meningitis, or meningoencephalitis. This organism is one of the most common bacterial causes of central nervous system (CNS) infection in the post-transplant patient. Patients often present with a subacute onset of fever, headache, altered mental status, and sometimes seizures, though frank meningismus is less common. Lumbar puncture often shows an increased opening pressure, and cerebrospinal fluid (CSF) demonstrates a decreased glucose level, neutrophilic pleocytosis, and a negative gram stain. The CSF and blood cultures are key to the diagnosis given that the gram stain is often negative. Recommended treatment is with high-dose intravenous penicillin, ampicillin, or trimethoprim–sulfamethoxazole (in penicillin-allergic patients) for 21 days.

Aspergillus species is a fungus that is a common cause of pneumonia in the severely immunosuppressed patient. Common presentations include fever and non-productive cough and may progress to pleuritic chest pain or pulmonary hemorrhage. Hematogenous dissemination to the CNS can occur, and these patients often present with confusion, altered mental status, and focal neurological findings. A stroke pattern can develop, with computed tomographic (CT) scan findings of low-density lesions. CSF cultures are usually negative and diagnosis is generally made from bronchoscopy with fluid culture, or via biopsy of affected organs, including the lung, liver, or heart. Blood cultures are usually negative, even in patients with hematogenous dissemination. Whereas the mainstay of treatment used to be amphotericin B in life-threatening illnesses, or with itraconazole or voriconazole in less critical disease, recent studies suggest that combination antifungal therapy using caspofungin and voriconazole confers a higher 90-day survival rate in patients with severe infection. This mortality benefit was seen in patients with renal disease as well as with more severe species of *Aspergillus*, such as *A. fumigatus*.

Pneumocystis jiroveci is a protozoa species that causes significant infection in post-transplant patients, especially in heart-lung and lung transplant patients, with up to an 88% rate of infection. Patients characteristically complain of a subacute onset of a non-productive cough, dyspnea, and fever. On examination, exertional hypoxia is seen, with variable pulmonary findings. The chest radiograph classically shows diffuse interstitial infiltrates. Diagnosis is made by examination of induced sputum, bronchoalveolar lavage fluid, or tissue biopsy. First-line prophylaxis and treatment is with trimethoprim–sulfamethoxazole.

Nocardia asteroides is an aerobic, gram-positive, weakly acid-fast staining, branching filamentous bacteria that generally causes pneumonia or brain abscesses in the post-transplant patient. Symptomatic patients generally present with fever (~67% of patients) or cough (>50% of patients). Patients with CNS infection may have fever, headache, or focal neurological signs, though CSF study results are usually non-specific. In patients with pneumonia secondary to this organism, the chest radiograph will often show a focal cavitary or nodular lesion. *Nocardia* has a predilection for vascular sites and can form abscesses within the kidney, liver, bone, joint, eye, skin, or other sites. Blood cultures are rarely positive, and the diagnosis is often made by tissue biopsy of skin lesions, pulmonary cavities, or other affected sites. Treatment is prolonged therapy, up to 1 year, of trimethoprim–sulfamethoxazole.

Salmonella is a gram-negative bacterium that commonly infects the gastrointestinal tract, resulting in gastroenteritis, often causing mucosal ulcerations and hemorrhagic diarrhea. These patients usually present with fever, bacteremia, or sometimes with abscesses secondary to hematogenous spread of the bacillus. Stool, blood, or tissue culture is required to diagnose this infection. Treatment consists of prolonged therapy using amoxicillin, ceftriaxone, trimethoprim–sulfamethoxazole, or ciprofloxacin, depending on the susceptibility of specific isolates.

Late Phase (>6 months Post-Transplant)

To identify a patient's infectious disease risk at this distance from transplantation, it is best to assign patients to one of three categories based on their level of immunosuppression. Patients on minimal immunosuppressive agents (>80% of patients) with good allograft function are susceptible to the same agents as the general community. Opportunistic infections are rarely seen unless there has been either a direct exposure to a contagious host or a probable link to a specific environmental exposure, such as gardening with subsequent development of aspergillosis.

Approximately 10% of patients have chronic or progressive infection with HBV, HCV, CMV, human papilloma virus (HPV), or EBV that can affect the function of the allograft, cause generalized immunosuppression, or predispose to the development of cancer. In these patients, the level of suspicion for any infectious process must remain high and they should be treated aggressively.

Many of the remaining 10% of patients suffer from chronic allograft rejection, are on higher doses of immunosuppressive agents, and are more likely to become infected with opportunistic agents. The source of infection should be aggressively pursued when patients in this group present with fever, given the high likelihood of serious disease.

Infections in Hematopoietic Stem Cell Transplant

In addition to the standard risks of infection from environmental exposures, catheters, tubes, or other vascutionlar access devices, patients who have undergone HSCT also have a unique timetable of infectious risks (see Figure 64.2). This risk of infection is determined by evaluating the degree to which bone marrow and immune reconstitution has occurred, and by assessing the presence or absence of significant graft-versus-host disease (GVHD). The timetable of possible infection in HSCT patients is divided into three phases.

Phase 1: Conditioning Regimen to Engraftment

The conditioning regimen refers to the chemotherapy or irradiation given immediately prior to the HSCT. The purpose of conditioning is to eradicate as much of the patient's disease prior to the transplantation, and also to suppress immune reactions. These regimens usually cause profound granulocytopenia until engraftment occurs. Major risks during this phase are of residual infection from before the transplant (i.e. invasive aspergillosis), or from hematogenous invasion by bacteria or yeast facilitated by breaks in the integrity of mucocutaneous surfaces. Gram-negative bacteria such as *Pseudomonas aeruginosa* and *Enterobacter* and gram-positive cocci such as *Staphylococcus* and *Streptococcus*, along with *Candida* infections, are frequently observed. As the duration of neutropenia lengthens, the risk of invasive fungal infections increases. These patients are at high risk for developing sepsis from these infectious diseases in the setting of almost complete immunosuppression.

Phase 2: Engraftment to Day 100

The major infectious risks during this phase are reactivation of the herpes viruses including CMV, VZV, human herpes virus-6 (HHV-6), and herpes simplex virus (HSV). If engraftment was delayed, then an increased incidence of invasive fungal infections is seen.

Phase 3: More Than 100 Days Post-Engraftment

In this phase, the risk of infection is determined by the presence or absence of GVHD. If GVHD is not occurring, the major infectious threats include varicella-zoster virus (VZV), *Streptococcus pneumoniae*, and respiratory virus infection (including influenza, parainfluenza, and respiratory syncytial virus [RSV]), largely because of the immaturity in function of the reconstituted immune system. Late-onset CMV is also seen, especially in patients who have not received adequate prophylaxis. In patients who have severe GVHD, there is an increased risk of infection with CMV, *Pneumocystis*, invasive fungi, and other organisms.

Differential Diagnosis

The differential diagnosis, aside from infection, for fever in a post-transplant patient (either SOT or HSCT) is:

- allograft rejection or graft-versus-host disease
- drug reaction/hypersensitivity
- thromboembolic disease
- transfusion reaction

Allograft Rejection and GVHD

Fever and isolated organ dysfunction can occur at any time post-transplant. The laboratory abnormalities will be specific to the organ transplanted (i.e. elevated creatinine in renal transplants, elevated bilirubin and alkaline phosphatase in liver recipients, hyperglycemia in pancreatic transplant patients). Pain at the site of the organ graft often occurs in kidney and liver transplant patients. To diagnose rejection, a biopsy of the graft must be obtained. The transplant service should be consulted to perform the graft biopsy.

In GVHD, the immune cells generated by the "graft," or hematopoietic stem cells that were transplanted, attack host tissues. Acute GVHD generally presents 2 to 8 weeks following transplantation. The most commonly involved organs include the skin, intestine, and liver, and patients may present with fever, diarrhea, or skin findings such as bullous lesions and erythematous macules.

In chronic GVHD, attack on host tissues results in inflammation, further complicated by the development of fibrosis or scar tissue. Chronic GVHD necessitates long-term high-dose immunosuppression that predisposes patients to infection with invasive opportunistic pathogens.

Drug Reaction and Hypersensitivity

Post-transplant patients regularly take medications that can cause fever as part of a drug reaction or "drug fever." These include antibiotics and antifungals such as the beta-lactams, sulfonamides, and fluconazole. Other medications that can cause fever include immunosuppressants such as OKT3, azathioprine, cyclosporine, and tacrolimus (FK506). Most febrile

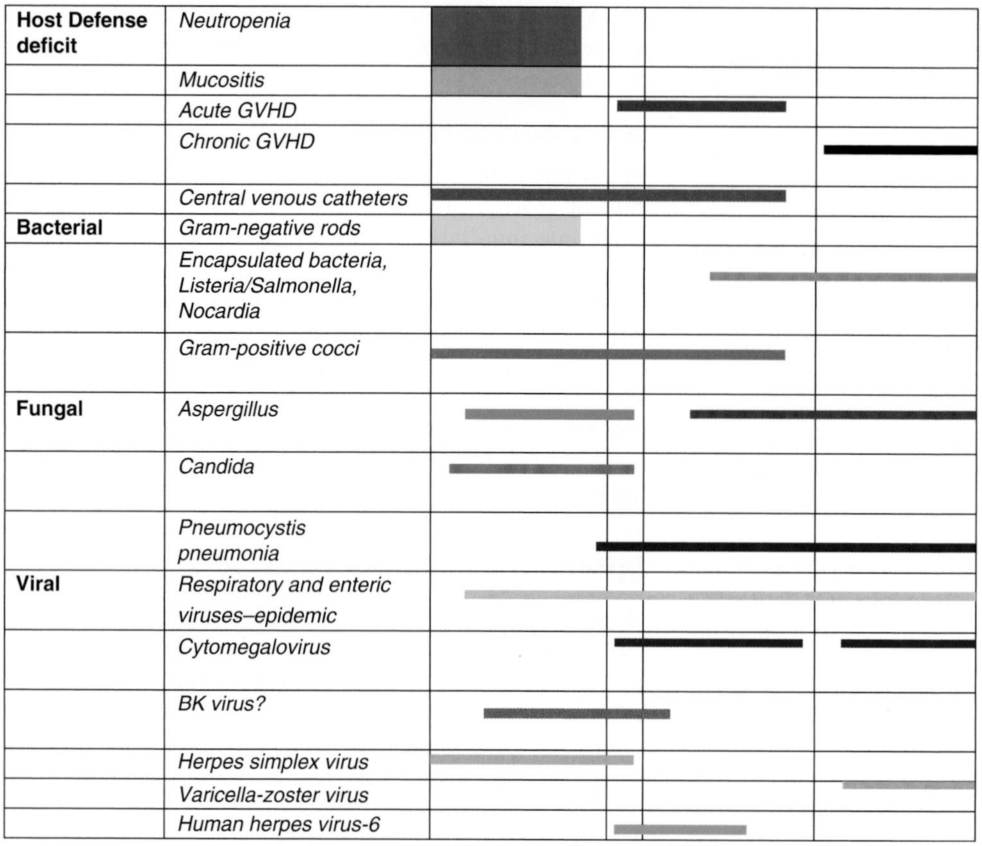

Host Defense deficit	Neutropenia	██████			
	Mucositis	████			
	Acute GVHD		████████		
	Chronic GVHD				████████
	Central venous catheters	████████████			
Bacterial	Gram-negative rods	████			
	Encapsulated bacteria, Listeria/Salmonella, Nocardia			████████	████████
	Gram-positive cocci	████████████			
	Aspergillus	██████		████████	████████
Fungal	Candida	██████			
	Pneumocystis pneumonia		████████████		
Viral	Respiratory and enteric viruses–epidemic		████████████████		
	Cytomegalovirus		████████	████████	
	BK virus?	██████			
	Herpes simplex virus	██████			
	Varicella-zoster virus				████
	Human herpes virus-6		████		

Figure 64.2 Infectious Etiologies in the Post-HSCT Patient

Day #: 0 E* 50 100 365

E* – day of engraftment.

drug reactions will present within 10 days of initial administration. Drug fever generally persists for several days after withdrawal of the offending agent. This diagnosis is difficult to make in the emergency department, especially if past medical records for the patient are unavailable. This diagnosis should be one of exclusion, as infection must be ruled out in any febrile post-transplant patient.

Thromboembolic Disease and Vascular Events

Deep venous thrombosis (DVT) and pulmonary embolisms are important causes of fever in post-operative patients. Other sites of thrombosis are specific to the organ transplantation, such as hepatic artery thrombosis in liver transplant patients. Thrombosis predisposes to bacterial or fungal infection of the allograft or other organ, the development of sepsis, or the seeding of other organs.

Transfusion-Related Fever

Given the high number of blood products generally required in all transplant patients, post-transfusion causes of fever should also be considered. Specifically, hemolytic reactions may be seen in patients with symptoms occurring during a transfusion or with evidence of red blood cell destruction on their peripheral smear. Urticaria may accompany fever in the setting of a transfusion-related hypersensitivity. Transmission of various

organisms via transfusion should also be considered, including CMV, hepatitis B and C, *Treponema pallidum*, *Plasmodium*, *Trypanosoma cruzi*, *Brucella*, *Babesia*, and *Toxoplasma*.

Laboratory and Radiographic Findings

Laboratory Studies

The choice of laboratory studies will be guided by the amount of time since organ transplant and the patient presentation. In patients who are more than 6 months post-transplant, without a significant level of immunocompromise or chronic rejection, and generally well-appearing, the laboratory work-up may be identical to that of a non-transplant patient (i.e. targeted to the chief complaint only).

However, in any post-transplant patient for whom there is concern for level of immunosuppression, function of the graft, significant infection, or who is less than 6 months post-transplant, a thorough laboratory work-up should be performed, regardless of localizing complaints. This work-up should include: complete blood count with differential; chemistries including calcium, magnesium, and phosphate; and liver function tests and urinalysis. These patients should be pan-cultured: send blood samples for bacterial and fungal cultures (at least two sets), urine, sputum, wound cultures, and cultures from any indwelling lines, stents, or tubes that may be accessible. If a lumbar puncture is performed, fluid analysis should include CMV polymerase chain reaction (PCR), culture, gram stain, smear, fungal culture, and acid-fast bacillus (AFB) staining, with other analyses as needed. Serum levels for the following immunosuppressants should be obtained when relevant: cyclosporine, azathioprine, tacrolimus, mycophenolate mofetil, or sirolimus.

Imaging Studies

- Chest radiograph: Pulmonary infection is one of the most common sites of invasive infection in post-transplant patients. Given the immunosuppressed nature of these patients, there may be a significant delay in the development of radiographic findings. CT of the chest should be obtained in the presence of a negative radiograph with a concerning clinical picture, or if the radiograph has early, subtle, or non-specific findings.
- Ultrasound of the transplanted organ (if available): Ultrasound can be used to evaluate for adequate perfusion and drainage of the transplanted organ.
- CT scan: CT scanning may be used to rule out other pathology.

Biopsy

Although a tissue sample is needed to rule out rejection, biopsy should be coordinated by the consulting transplant service.

Treatment and Prophylaxis

Treatment

The use of antibiotics in post-transplant patients is complex mainly due to the interaction of antibiotic agents and immunosuppressive medications. Also, the lengthy courses of antibiotics required for complete treatment necessitate long hospital stays and heighten the risk of renal or hepatic damage, depending on which organ is primarily involved in antibiotic clearance from the circulation.

Treatment for post-transplant patients is summarized in Table 64.2.

The interactions of antibiotics and other medications with the most common immunosuppressive agents are shown in Table 64.3. The emergency department provider should use caution when initiating or altering any drug therapy in an immunosuppressed post-transplant patient.

Prophylaxis

Transplant patients are maintained on complicated antibiotic and immunosuppressive regimens for prophylaxis against infection and rejection. This section covers prophylaxis for infection, while prophylaxis against rejection is addressed next.

For both SOT and HSCT recipients, anti-infection prophylaxis includes influenza immunization and avoidance of environmental hazards including gardening, community cleaning activities, exposure to construction, travel to the developing world, and contact with infected individuals. Additionally, all patients after HSCT must be reimmunized as their immune systems have been reconstituted. Patients who have received a SOT such as liver transplant cannot be exposed to anyone who may be actively shedding a virus, including those who have received live virus vaccines. Any exposures should be reported to the transplant service coordinator.

In SOT patients specifically, prophylaxis against infection by stage includes:

First month:
- perioperative surgical wound prophylaxis
- initiation of trimethoprim-sulfamethoxazole prophylaxis

1–6 months:
- non-contaminated air and water
- low-dose trimethoprim–sulfamethoxazole prophylaxis (prophylaxis against urosepsis, *Pneumocystis*, *Listeria*, *Toxoplasma*)
- CMV prophylaxis or preemptive strategy as determined by transplant service and infectious disease services

After 6 months:
- lowest risk category: no prophylaxis
- in 10% with chronic hepatitis C or B: use of hyperimmune hepatitis B immunoglobulin and antivirals such as lamivudine and adefovir
- in 10% highest risk group: lifelong trimethoprim–sulfamethoxazole and fluconazole prophylaxis

In patients who have received an HSCT, anti-infection prophylaxis includes:

Phase 1:
- mask, gloves, high-efficiency particulate air (HEPA) filters, pneumococcal polysaccharide vaccine (PPV) by healthcare workers
- prophylactic fluoroquinolones, systemic antifungals

Phase 2:
- anti-CMV preventive strategies

Phase 3:
- treatment determined by presentation, no specific prophylaxis

Prophylaxis against rejection consists of three-drug immunosuppressive therapy for 3 to 12 months after transplant; subsequently one of the three drugs is removed, most commonly corticosteroids. Although a full discussion of the immunosuppressive regimens is beyond the scope of this chapter, any alterations or additions to the patient's regimen should only be made after discussion with the transplant center. Table 64.4 lists the most common immunosuppressive agents, their mechanism of action, and common adverse effects.

Complications and Admission Criteria

The major complications facing the febrile transplant patient include severe infection, sepsis, organ failure, and rejection.

Aside from obvious admission criteria, such as hemodynamic instability, sepsis, and so forth, the presence of any of the

Table 64.2 Treatment for Post-Transplant Patients

Patient Category	Therapy Recommendation
Adults	**Bacterial infections:** Broad-spectrum coverage of gram-positive, gram-negative, and anaerobic infections using: • Cefepime 2 g IV every 8 hours *plus* • Vancomycin 15–20 mg/kg/dose IV every 8–12 hours • Consider addition of metronidazole 500 mg IV every 8 hours if intra-abdominal source is suspected **Fungal infections:** • fluconazole 200–400 mg PO/IV daily • Amphotericin B 0.7 mg/kg IV daily • Voriconazole loading dose 6 mg/kg/dose IV every 12 hours × 2 doses, then 4 mg/kg/dose IV every 12 hours maintenance (dose may need to be adjusted based on trough levels) **Viral infections:** • Ganciclovir 5 mg/kg/dose IV every 12 hours • Foscarnet 60 mg/kg/dose IV every 8 hours **Protozoal infections:** • Trimethoprim–sulfamethoxazole 20 mg/kg/day of the trimethoprim component IV divided four times per day (in adults, generally one DS tab. PO BID).
Children*	**Bacterial infections:** Broad-spectrum coverage of gram-positive, gram-negative, and anaerobic infections using: • Ceftazidime 150 mg/kg/day IV divided every 8 hours, maximum 6 g/day • Tobramycin 2.5 mg/kg/dose IV every 8 hours • Vancomycin 15 mg/kg/dose IV every 6 hours, if documented infection with coagulase-negative *Staphylococcus*, *MRSA*, or other aerobic gram-positive cocci is identified, or if patient has had an infected catheter • Meropenem 20/mg/kg/dose IV every 8 hours, can substituted for ceftazidime if high concern for anaerobic infection **Fungal infections:** No history of invasive fungal infections: • Fluconazole 5 mg/kg/dose IV daily, maximum dose 400 mg/day. Adjust dose based on creatinine clearance. Discontinue if LFTs are elevated to two to three times normal, or if itraconazole or liposomal amphotericin B (AmBisome) used. • Amphotericin B 1–1.5 mg/kg/day IV, but if renal insufficiency or toxicity occurs, change to liposomal amphotericin B (if SCr is ≥2 mg/dL, or has doubled in absolute value, or if creatinine clearance is <25 mL/min). In patients with a history of invasive fungal infections, antifungal agent will be determined by past sensitivities. Other agents include: • Voriconazole loading dose 6 mg/kg/dose IV 12 hours × 2 doses, then 4 mg/kg/dose every 12 hours maintenance (dose may need to be adjusted based on age and trough levels) • Itraconazole 3–5 mg/kg/dose IV daily • Caspofungin: < 3 months: 25 mg/m²/dose IV every 24 hours ≥ 3 months: 70 mg/m²/dose IV × 1, then 50 mg/m2/dose IV every 24 hours **Viral infections:** • Ganciclovir 5 mg/kg/dose IV every 12 hours • Foscarnet 60 mg/kg/dose IV every 8 hours **Protozoal infections:** Trimethoprim–sulfamethoxazole prophylaxis: • Pre-transplant: >30 kg: 1 SS tab. PO BID <30 kg: 5 mg/kg/day of TMP component in divided doses BID • Post-transplant: >30 kg: 1 SS tab. PO BID twice weekly on two consecutive days <30kg: 5 mg/kg/day of TMP component PO in two divided doses twice weekly on 2 consecutive days Alternatives: dapsone or IV pentamidine For treatment of active infection with *Pneumocystis jiroveci*, give Trimethoprim-sulfamethoxazole 15–20 mg TMP/kg/day in divided doses IV/PO every 6–8 hours

* High death rates from infection outweigh the relative contraindications of doxycycline and fluoroquinolones in children and pregnant women.

DS – double strength; IV – intravenous; LFT – liver function test; PO – by mouth; SCr – serum creatinine; SS – trimethoprim–sulfamethoxazole single strength tablet 80/160 mg; TMP – trimethoprim.

Table 64.3 Interactions of Common Immunosuppressive Agents and Other Medications

Immunosuppressive Agent	Interacting Drug	Mechanism of Interaction	Possible Adverse Effect/Clinical Implication
Cyclosporine, Tacrolimus, Sirolimus	Diltiazem Verapamil Amiodarone Azoles (keto-, flu-, itra-) Macrolides (erythromycin, azithro-, clarithro-)	Inhibition of hepatic cytochrome P-450, causing an increased level of the immunosuppressive agent	Nephrotoxicity due to elevated cyclosporine or tacrolimus levels; can also enhance adverse effects of each of interacting drugs
Cyclosporine, Tacrolimus, Sirolimus	Phenobarbital Phenytoin Carbamazepine Rifampin Isoniazid	Induction of hepatic cytochrome P-450, causing a decreased level of the immunosuppressive agent	Increased risk of rejection due to a lower level of the immunosuppressive agent
Cyclosporine or Tacrolimus	HMG CoA reductase inhibitors ("statins")	Level of statin increased by immunosuppressive drug	Increased risk of statin-induced rhabdomyolysis
Cyclosporine or Tacrolimus	Aminoglycosides, iodinated radiocontrast, amphotericin B	Synergistic nephrotoxicity of the immunosuppressive agent and the interacting drug	Synergistic nephrotoxicity
Azathioprine	Allopurinol	Xanthine oxidase inhibition by allopurinol causes a decreased metabolism of azathioprine, resulting in increased azathioprine levels	Increased azathioprine levels capable of causing bone marrow suppression

HMG CoA – 3-hydroxy-3-methylglutaryl coenzyme A.

following will likely necessitate admission of the febrile post-transplant patient:

- new-onset graft failure
- patients within 1 year of their transplant
- patients on high levels of immunosuppression
- patients who are non-compliant with medications or poor candidates for independent care

Infection Control

The key measure in the acute care setting is early placement of these patients in reverse isolation if they are found or suspected to be significantly neutropenic or otherwise immunocompromised.

Pearls and Pitfalls

1. Take the risk of infection in these patients seriously. They will often have life-threatening infections and may not present with signs and symptoms typical for an immunocompetent host.
2. Be aggressive with the laboratory and radiographic workups. They are more often positive than negative in this cohort.
3. Start empiric treatments, such as broad-spectrum antibiotics, early in the toxic-appearing patient. However, if the patient is hemodynamically stable, pan-culture the patient prior to administering any antibiotics.
4. Consult the appropriate transplant service early and often.
5. In a generally well-appearing patient, more than 1 year out from transplantation, and on minimal immunosuppressive

therapy, consider outpatient management with close follow-up with the transplant service.

References

Annual Report of the US Organ Procurement and Transplantation Network and the Scientific Registry of Transplant Recipients: transplant data 1998–2007 (Rockville, MD: Health Resources and Services Administration, Healthcare Systems Bureau, Division of Transplantation, 2009).

Fischer, S. A. Infections complicating solid organ transplantation. *Surg. Clin. North Am.* 2006; 86(5): 1127–45, v–vi.

Fischer, S. A., Trenholme, G. M., and Levin, S. Fever in the solid organ transplant patient. *Infect. Dis. Clin. North Am.* 1996; 10(1): 167–84.

Fishman, J. A. Infection in solid-organ transplant recipients. *N. Engl. J. Med.* 2007; 357(25): 2601–14.

Marty, F. M. and Rubin, R. H. The prevention of infection post-transplant: the role of prophylaxis, preemptive and empiric therapy. *Transpl. Int.* 2006; 19(1): 2–11.

Munoz, P., Singh, N., and Bouza, E. Treatment of solid organ transplant patients with invasive fungal infections: should a combination of antifungal drugs be used? *Curr. Opin. Infect. Dis.* 2006; 19(4): 365–70.

Renoult, E., Buteau, C., Lamarre, V., *et al.* Infectious risk in pediatric organ transplant recipients: is it increased with the new immunosuppressive agents? *Pediatr. Transplant* 2005; 9(4): 470–9.

Rubin, R. H., Schaffner, A., and Speich, R. Introduction to the Immunocompromised Host Society consensus conference on epidemiology, prevention, diagnosis, and management of infections in solid-organ transplant patients. *Clin. Infect. Dis.* 2001; 33(Suppl 1): S1–4.

Table 64.4 Immunosuppressive Agent, Mechanism of Action, and Adverse Effects

Agent	Mechanism of Action	Usage	Adverse Effects
Corticosteroids (Prednisone, Methylprednisolone)	Decreases inflammation (suppresses migration of polymorphonuclear leukocytes), reverses increased capillary permeability, suppresses immune system, reduces activity and volume of the lymphatic system. Can cause adrenal suppression, antitumor, or antiemetic effects	Used as part of a triple-drug regimen along with azathioprine and cyclosporine	Weight gain, Cushingoid appearance, cataracts, acne, skin thinning, bruising, osteoporosis, fractures, avascular necrosis of hip or knee, upper gastrointestinal ulceration/bleeding, diabetogenicity, psychologic effects, hyperlipidemia
Cyclosporine (Gengraf, Neoral, Restasis, Sandimmune)	Inhibits production and release of interleukin-2, thereby preventing activation of resting T-cells	Used as part of a triple-drug regimen along with azathioprine and prednisone. Dosage based on trough levels	Acute and chronic nephrotoxicity, hyperkalemia, hypomagnesemia, hyperuricemia/gout, hemolytic-uremic syndrome, hypertension, hyperlipidemia, diabetogenicity, hepatotoxicity, neurotoxicity, hirsutism, gingival hyperplasia
Azathioprine (Azasan, Imuran)	Inhibits B- and T-cell proliferation	Used as part of a triple-drug regimen along with cyclosporine and prednisone	Bone marrow suppression, leukopenia, thrombocytopenia (first weeks after therapy), macrocytosis, with or without anemia, hepatotoxicity (reversible), pancreatitis
Tacrolimus/FK-506, (Prograf, Protopic)	Inhibits T-cell activation	Used either as an induction agent or as rescue therapy for refractory rejection. Dosage based on trough levels	Neurotoxicity more common than with cyclosporine (manifests as tremors, paresthesias, headache, insomnia, and seizures); nephrotoxicity, hyperkalemia, hypomagnesemia, hyperuricemia/gout, hemolytic-uremic syndrome, diabetogenicity, hepatotoxicity, hair loss; less hypertension and hyperlipidemia than with cyclosporine
Mycophenolate mofetil (CellCept, Myfortic)	Inhibits T- and B-cell proliferation	Can be used to replace azathioprine in the triple-drug regimen	Abdominal pain, anorexia, nausea, vomiting, upper gastrointestinal bleeding, diarrhea, anemia, leukopenia, thrombocytopenia
Sirolimus (Rapamune)	Inhibits T-cell activation and proliferation, inhibits antibody production, inhibits acute rejection of allografts, prolongs graft survival	Used in combination with cyclosporine or after withdrawal of cyclosporine	Thrombocytopenia, hyperlipidemia, buccal ulceration, diarrhea, interstitial pneumonitis, less commonly leukopenia/anemia

Savitsky, E. A., Uner, A. B., and Votey, S. R. Evaluation of orthotopic liver transplant recipients presenting to the emergency department. *Ann. Emerg. Med.* 1998; 31(4): 507–17.

Savitsky, E. A., Votey, S. R., Mebust, D. P., *et al.* A descriptive analysis of 290 liver transplant patient visits to an emergency department. *Acad. Emerg. Med.* 2000; 7(8): 898–905.

Slifkin, M., Doron, S., and Snydman, D. R. Viral prophylaxis in organ transplant patients. *Drugs* 2004; 64(24): 2763–92.

Venkat, K. K. and Venkat, A. Care of the renal transplant recipient in the emergency department. *Ann. Emerg. Med.* 2004; 44(4): 330–41.

Chapter

65

Sepsis

David Thompson

Introduction and Microbiology

Sepsis represents a spectrum of pathophysiologic responses to infection. Historically, sepsis has been a feared and poorly understood process. Today, with an enhanced understanding of the complex interplay between microbes and the host immune response, treatment of sepsis has evolved. Advanced antibiotic therapies, respiratory and cardiovascular support, and improved methods for early detection of sepsis are all important interventions. Despite significant progress, mortality associated with severe sepsis has been estimated in some studies as high as 40 to 80%. Because it progresses rapidly, it is imperative that acute care physicians make the diagnosis of sepsis early and manage it aggressively. Additionally, delivering evidence-based care requires that physicians stay abreast of the fast-moving sepsis literature and guidelines.

The identified sites of primary infection leading to sepsis are predominantly lung (47%), followed by unknown/other (28%), peritoneum (15%), and urinary tract (10%). Specific organism identification is challenging, and many cases have non-diagnostic or negative cultures. Most of the existing data on etiologic pathogens come from studies of bloodstream infections. The causative organisms implicated in sepsis have changed over time. Prior to 1987, gram-negative bacteria were the predominant organisms identified. However, in the past 20 years, sepsis caused by gram-positive bacteria has increased markedly, while gram-negative cases have remained steady, such that gram-positive bacteria are now more common. Leading gram-positive pathogens are *Staphylococcus aureus*, coagulase-negative *Staphylococcus*, and beta-hemolytic streptococci. Leading gram-negative pathogens are *E. coli* and *Klebsiella* species. Polymicrobial infections are common and the proportion of isolates that are multidrug resistant is steadily increasing. Additionally, over the past two decades, the incidence of fungal sepsis, in particular from *Candida* species, has increased by over 200%. These changes likely reflect the increased numbers of immunocompromised patients and debilitated surgical patients, the increased use of indwelling catheters and devices, and the emergency of community-associated methicillin-resistant *Staphylococcus aureus* (MRSA).

Epidemiology

The incidence of sepsis appears to be increasing in the United States and worldwide, with rates exceeding 200 cases per 100,000. This is likely due to aging of the population, increasing immunosuppression, and emergence of multidrug-resistant organisms, as well as increased identification of the disorder. The rates of severe sepsis and septic shock are lower. Rates of sepsis increase in the winter months and the disorder is more common in non-white individuals. Patients over the age of 65 account for between 60 and 85% of cases. Meanwhile, sepsis-related mortality has declined in recent years. Whether this is due to improvements in critical care, antimicrobial therapy, or earlier recognition remains uncertain.

Clinical Features

The American College of Chest Physicians and the Society of Critical Care Medicine have developed standardized diagnostic criteria for sepsis, severe sepsis, and septic shock to describe the continuum of evolving physiologic derangement (see Table 65.1). By these criteria, sepsis is defined as systemic

Table 65.1 Sepsis Definitions

SIRS (systemic inflammatory response syndrome)	• Hyperthermia: temperature >38.0 °C *or* • Hypothermia: temperature <36.0 °C • Tachycardia: heart rate >90 • Tachypnea: respiratory rate >20 or PCO_2 <32 • Leukocytosis/leukopenia: WBC >12K or <4K or >10% immature neutrophils
Sepsis	• SIRS *and* • Suspected infectious process
Severe sepsis	• Sepsis *and* • Evidence of organ dysfunction (see Table 65.2)
Septic shock	• Severe sepsis *and* • Persistent hypotension/hypoperfusion despite adequate fluid resuscitation

SIRS – systemic inflammatory response syndrome; WBC – white blood (cell) count.

Table 65.2 Major Organ Dysfunction in Severe Sepsis

Organ	Complications	Clinical Signs and Symptoms
Pulmonary	• ARDS	Tachypnea Hypoxia Respiratory failure
Cardiovascular	• Myocardial depression • Disseminated vasodilation	Tachycardia Hypotension Poor capillary refill Edema
Renal	• Acute renal failure	Oliguria
GI	• Ileus • Hepatic ischemia • Mesenteric ischemia	Abdominal pain or tenderness Decreased bowel sounds Constipation, diarrhea, or vomiting Bleeding
CNS	• Altered mental status	Disorientation Agitation
Hematologic	• DIC • Anemia • Thrombocytopenia • Leukopenia	Bleeding Bruising Petechiae Immunosuppression
Endocrine	• Relative adrenal insufficiency	Hypo/hyperglycemia Persistent hypotension

ARDS – acute respiratory distress syndrome; CNS – central nervous system; DIC – disseminated intravascular coagulation; GI – gastrointestinal.

inflammatory response syndrome (SIRS) plus infection, severe sepsis is defined, in essence, as sepsis plus initial hypotension (systolic blood pressure <90 mm Hg) or lactate greater than 4 mmol/L criteria, and septic shock is defined as sepsis plus persistent hypotension despite fluid resuscitation. Categorization of patients in this system provides vital prognostic information and guides critical disposition and treatment decisions. There is a clear incremental increase in mortality associated with sepsis (16%), severe sepsis (20%), and septic shock (46%). These criteria are well accepted and widely used. In 2015, the US Centers for Medicare and Medicaid (CMS) modified these criteria and expanded the definition of severe sepsis somewhat. In 2016, US and European critical care societies released the Sequential (sepsis-related) Organ Failure Assessment (SOFA), an entirely new system for identifying sepsis and grading its severity. In addition, a quick-SOFA (qSOFA) score was derived and recently validated, which allows rapid identification and risk stratification of sepsis in ED patients with infection. In qSOFA, a point is assigned each for respiratory rate greater than 21 breaths per minute, altered mentation, and systolic blood pressure less than 100 mmHg, with a score greater than 1 associated with poor outcomes and indicating the need for aggressive sepsis management.

Septic patients rarely die in the emergency department (ED). Death tends to occur later from multiple organ failure and its complications. During the initial ED evaluation, however, evidence of organ dysfunction in one or more systems – the result of hyperinflammation, hypercoagulation, and hypoperfusion – is often evident (see Table 65.2). It is the job of the acute care provider to recognize and respond to these signs of organ dysfunction. Prompt recognition and early, aggressive resuscitation can decrease the likelihood of further severe organ dysfunction, such as the adult respiratory distress syndrome (ARDS) and renal failure, and death.

Differential Diagnosis

Many entities can mimic the presentation of severe sepsis (see Table 65.3). Acute coronary syndrome, pancreatitis, medication reactions, and many other conditions can result in systemic inflammatory response and end-organ hypoperfusion that may be difficult to differentiate from severe sepsis.

Laboratory and Radiographic Findings

No single laboratory study confirms or excludes the diagnosis of sepsis. Sepsis can present as a spectrum of laboratory and radiographic study derangements related to primary infection, systemic inflammatory response, or response to end-organ hypo-perfusion (see Table 65.4). Prompt measurement of serum lactate is considered a cornerstone of early severe sepsis recognition.

Treatment and Prophylaxis
Early Goal-Directed Therapy

The landmark study in which a protocol of early goal-directed therapy (EGDT) reduced mortality by 16% established the ED as a focal point for resuscitation of the septic patient. Goals in this treatment strategy refer to hemodynamic and perfusion-related targets (central venous pressure 8 to 12, mean arterial pressure 65 to 90, and central venous oxygenation >70%) to be achieved rapidly and sequentially using fluids, vasopressors,

Table 65.3 SIRS + Hypoperfusion Differential Diagnosis

Diagnosis	Features
• Severe sepsis	Suspected infectious source
• Tumor lysis syndrome	Large tumor burden, chemotherapy
• Jarisch–Herxheimer reaction	Release of endotoxin following microbial cell death in response to antibiotics
• Pulmonary infarction	Dyspnea, pleuritic chest pain, risk factors for pulmonary embolism
• ARDS	Hypoxia, bilateral infiltrates on chest radiograph
• Pancreatitis	Abdominal pain, elevated lipase or amylase
• Myocardial infarction	ECG changes, elevated serum cardiac biomarkers
• Thyrotoxicosis or thyroid storm	Thyromegaly, elevated serum thyroid function tests
• Drug fever	New medication initiation, urticarial rash
• Neuroleptic malignant syndrome or malignant hyperthermia	Muscular rigidity, general anesthesia or dopaminergic medications
• Alcohol withdrawal	Tremulousness, chronic alcohol use
• Acute adrenal insufficiency	Chronic steroid use

ARDS – acute respiratory distress syndrome; ECG – electrocardiogram.

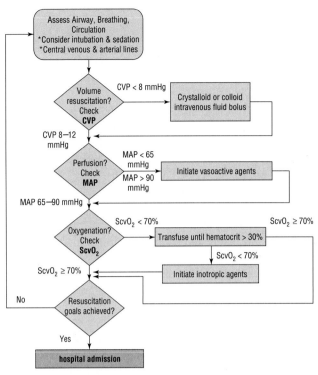

Figure 65.1 Early goal-directed therapy algorithm.

Adapted from E. Rivers, B. Nguyen, S. Havstad, *et al.*, Early goal-directed therapy in the treatment of severe sepsis and septic shock. *N. Engl. J. Med.* 2001; 345(19): 1368–77.

Table 65.4 Common Laboratory and Radiographic Findings in Sepsis

Study	Finding
Complete blood count	• Leukocytosis >12K WBC • Leukopenia <4K WBC • Left shift/bandemia >10% immature neutrophils
Chemistry panel	• Acidosis • Renal failure • Hypo/hyperglycemia
Coagulation	• Elevated INR • Elevated PTT • DIC
Lactate	• Hyperlactemia (>2–4 mmol/L)
Cultures: (blood, urine, cerebrospinal fluid, wound, etc.)	• May identify infection source • Microbial susceptibilities guide antibiotic treatment • Blood cultures frequently negative*
Urine	• Oliguria • Pyuria/urinary tract infection
Chest radiograph	• Diffuse bilateral infiltrates, ARDS • Focal infiltrate, pneumonia

* Negative blood cultures in 31% with septic shock.

ARDS – acute respiratory distress syndrome; DIC – disseminated intravascular coagulation; INR – international normalized ratio; PTT – partial thromboplastin time; WBC – white blood (cell) count.

Table 65.5 Hemodynamic Goals of EGDT

Parameter	Goal	Intervention
1. **CVP**	8–12 mm Hg	Infuse intravenous bolus either crystalloid or colloid for CVP <8 mm Hg
2. **MAP**	65–90 mm Hg	Initiate vasopressors for MAP <65 mm Hg
3. **ScvO$_2$** Central venous oxygen saturation	>70%	Transfuse packed cells to keep HCT above 30 and initiate inotropic agents for ScvO$_2$ <70%

CVP – central venous pressure; HCT – hematocrit; MAP – mean arterial pressure.

blood transfusions, and occasionally ventilatory support with sedation (see Figure 65.1 and Table 65.5).

Three large trials published in 2014 and 2015 comparing EGDT to generally less protocolized and less invasive physician-directed care demonstrated no benefit of EGDT. It is important to recognize that very early sepsis recognition and antibiotic therapy and aggressive fluid resuscitation occurred in all arms of these trials. Emergency departments not enacting a formal EGDT protocol should nonetheless consider two points: (1) primary hemodynamic therapy for septic patients must occur in the ED; (2) prompt fluid resuscitation is the mainstay of therapy and serial reassessments of intravascular volume and perfusion are the mainstays of therapy.

Table 65.6 Ventilation Parameters

	Traditional	Lung Protective
Ventilator mode	Volume assist-control	Volume assist-control
Initial tidal volume	12 cc/kg	6 cc/kg
Plateau pressure	≤50	≤30
Rate settings	6–35	6–35
Inspiratory:expiratory ratio	1:1 to 1:3	1:1 to 1:3
Oxygenation goal	PaO_2 55–88 mm Hg SpO_2 88–95%	PaO_2 55–88 mm Hg SpO_2 88–95%

Table 65.7 Common Vasopressors in Septic Shock

Agent	Action	Dosage range
Norepinephrine	Alpha and beta	1–30 µg/min
Dopamine	Beta Alpha Dopaminergic	5–20 µg/kg/min
Phenylephrine	Alpha	10–200 µg/min
Epinephrine	Beta, alpha	0.05–0.5 µg/kg/min
Vasopressin	V1	0.01–0.04 units/min

Respiratory Support

Attention to the airway and breathing is primary. The hypoxic patient should be given oxygen and the patient who is obtunded and unable to protect his or her airway should be intubated. Many septic patients have a very high work of breathing that can lead to respiratory failure, exhaustive energy expenditure, and lactic acidosis. Many patients with septic shock require respiratory support at some point during hospitalization, and pre-emptive intubation with ventilatory support should be considered.

If mechanical ventilation is initiated, a "lung-protective" strategy should be used (see Table 65.6). Lower tidal volumes (6 mL/kg vs. 10–12 mL/kg) and lower plateau pressure goals (≤30 cm H_2O) may decrease barotrauma and ongoing inflammatory lung damage. This low tidal volume strategy improves survival and decreases ventilator-associated complications of sepsis.

Fluid Resuscitation

Crystalloid fluids are the intravenous fluids of choice for septic patients. They should be delivered in bolus form (500 to 1,000 mL per dose), targeted to a central venous pressure (CVP) greater than 8, and guided by indices of perfusion, such as normalization of serum lactate and urine output. Bicarbonate administration for sepsis-induced lactic acidosis has not been shown to be beneficial and is not recommended.

Vasopressors

Vasopressors should be initiated promptly in patients who have hypoperfusion despite volume resuscitation. All of the vasopressors in Table 65.7 have been shown to be capable of increasing blood pressure in patients with septic shock. Dopamine is used in some centers, though it results in more cardiac dysrhythmias and its putative improved splanchnic blood flow and renal protective effects remain unproven. Norepinephrine has emerged as the most widely accepted first-line agent because of its predominantly vasoconstrictive effects with less tachycardia and fewer dysrhythmias. Initiation of any vasopressor should be viewed as a therapeutic trial. Selection and titration of the agent should be guided by indices of end-organ perfusion.

Antibiotics

The ED physician must initiate prompt and appropriate empiric antibiotic coverage. The Surviving Sepsis Campaign guidelines recommend that empiric antibiotics be given within 1 hour of the diagnosis of severe sepsis and that they should be active against likely pathogens with adequate penetration into presumed sites of infection (see Table 65.8). ED protocols with standardized regimens of pre-mixed antibiotics for common infection sites can facilitate adherence to these guidelines. The specific choice of antibiotic coverage should be guided by suspected source and community-resistance patterns, but in the absence of confirmed infections and microbial sensitivities, broad-spectrum antibiotic coverage of likely pathogens is recommended.

Physiologic Steroid Therapy for Relative Adrenal Insufficiency

Three randomized controlled trials of patients with refractory (vasopressor-requiring) septic shock patients demonstrated marked shock reversal with corticosteroid infusions. One of these studies also showed a decrease in mortality. Thus, for patients in septic shock despite pressors and fluid resuscitation, administration of hydrocortisone 100 mg IV every 8 hours for 7 days is recommended. The practice of formal testing for relative adrenal insufficiency by performing a cosyntropin stimulation test or a random pre-treatment cortisol level remains controversial.

Euglycemia

Glucose levels should be monitored closely, and hyperglycemia should be treated to achieve goal levels <180 µg/dL, with an emphasis on avoiding hypoglycemia.

Complications and Admission Criteria

All patients with severe sepsis should be admitted to an intensive care unit (ICU). In addition to early resuscitation, septic patients require continuous monitoring for the development of end-organ complications.

Acute Respiratory Distress Syndrome

The most common of the organ dysfunctions associated with sepsis is ARDS. Persistent arterial hypoxemia despite treatment with supplemental oxygen is the hallmark (see Box 65.1). The presence of diffuse pulmonary infiltrates and severe hypoxia (defined as $PaO_2/FiO_2 < 200$) in the absence of left atrial hypertension is a currently accepted diagnostic standard for ARDS.

Table 65.8 Common Empiric Antibiotic Regimens for Severe Sepsis

Class	Example
Extended-spectrum penicillin	Piperacillin–tazobactam 4.5 g IV every 6 hours
Carbapenem	Meropenem 1 g IV every 8 hours
Third- or fourth-generation cephalosporin	Cefepime 2 g IV every 8 hours
Beta-lactam plus anti-pseudomonal aminoglycoside	Ceftriaxone 1 g IV every 24 hours *plus* Gentamicin* 5 mg/kg/dose IV every 24 hours
Beta-lactam allergic	Vancomycin 15–20 mg/kg/dose IV every 8–12 hours *plus* Aztreonam 2 g IV every 8 hours
Anti-MRSA agent[†]	Vancomycin 15–20 mg/kg/dose IV every 8–12 hours
Antifungal agent[‡]	Caspofungin 70 mg IV loading dose × 1, then 50 mg IV every 24 hours maintenance dose

* Once daily dosing may not be appropriate in patients with impaired renal function.

[†] Recommended in most US communities where prevalence of MRSA is high.

[‡] Recommended if patient at high risk for invasive candidiasis because of risk factors such as immunocompromise, recent surgery, indwelling catheters or devices, diabetes, parenteral nutrition, or recent broad-spectrum antibiotic use.

IV – intravenous; MRSA – methicillin-resistant *Staphylococcus aureus*.

Box 65.1 Acute Respiratory Distress Syndrome Criteria

- Acute onset
- Bilateral infiltrates on chest radiography
- Pulmonary capillary wedge pressure <18 or absence of clinical evidence for left atrial hypertension
- Acute lung injury is considered if $PaO_2/FiO_2 \leq 300$
- ARDS is considered if $PaO_2/FiO_2 < 200$

Additional features of ARDS include decreased lung compliance and an interstitial, centrally located pattern of opacities.

Although ARDS may be the most evident dysfunction seen in sepsis, it does not predict as grave a prognosis as does failure of other organ systems. Renal failure, central nervous system (CNS) dysfunction, and thrombocytopenia more closely correlate with mortality. This underrecognized point forms part of the basis for current resuscitation protocols in sepsis. Aggressive fluid resuscitation to improve perfusion and prevent renal failure is now favored over cautious fluid support aimed at decreasing pulmonary interstitial fluid.

Myocardial Depression

Severe sepsis may be associated with myocardial depression. Many inflammatory mediators have been implicated and the specific mechanism remains controversial. Unlike acute coronary syndrome, this dysfunction is not believed to be caused by myocardial hypoperfusion and ischemia. Patients who survive severe sepsis with cardiac dysfunction usually regain normal cardiac function in 7 to 10 days. However, patients with underlying coronary artery disease are at risk for acute ischemia from increased cardiac workload, and sepsis may precipitate myocardial infarction.

Renal Failure

Renal failure in sepsis may acutely manifest as oliguria. In severe sepsis, this may reflect decreased renal perfusion due to systemic hypotension. Persistent renal hypoperfusion may result in acute tubular necrosis, renal failure, and may require temporary or ongoing dialysis. As with sepsis-associated cardiac depression, the majority of patients with renal failure who survive do recover baseline renal function. This may suggest the role of inflammatory mediators in temporarily decreasing kidney function without causing irreversible injury.

Infection Control

Communicable agents may cause severe sepsis. Contact precautions should be observed if the primary source of infection is due to soft-tissue infections or skin sources. Cases with suspected high-risk pulmonary sources require respiratory precautions.

Pearls and Pitfalls

1. The first goals in sepsis care are early recognition and aggressive resuscitation.
2. In patients with severe sepsis or septic shock of unclear etiology, broad-spectrum antibiotics should be administered as soon as possible.
3. Early aggressive IV fluid resuscitation is critical. Titrate fluids to perfusion parameters such as, serum lactate, blood pressure, heart rate, and urine output.
4. Septic shock may induce relative adrenal insufficiency. Consider replacement therapy (hydrocortisone 100 mg IV every 8 hours) in cases of hypotension despite fluid resuscitation and vasopressor therapy.
5. Intubate early using lung-protective ventilator settings.
6. Do not withhold fluid resuscitation for possible respiratory compromise.
7. Early drainage or debridement of infected tissue (source control) is crucial in cases of surgically treatable infections.

References

Acute Respiratory Distress Syndrome Network. Ventilation with lower tidal volumes as compared with traditional tidal volumes for acute lung injury and the acute respiratory distress syndrome. *N. Engl. J. Med.* 2000; 342(18): 1301–8.

Angus, D. C. and Wax, R. S. Epidemiology of sepsis: an update. *Crit. Care Med.* 2001; 29: S109–16.

Annane, D., Sebille, V., Charpentier, C., *et al.* Effect of treatment with low doses of hydrocortisone and fludrocortisone of mortality in patients with septic shock. *JAMA* 2002; 288(7): 862–71.

Bochud, P. Y., Bonten, M., Marchetti, O., *et al.* Antimicrobial therapy for patients with severe sepsis and septic shock: an evidence-based review. *Crit. Care Med.* 2004; 32(11 Suppl.): S495–512.

Centers for Disease Control and Prevention (CDC). Increase in national hospital discharge survey rates for septicemia: United States, 1979–1987. *MMWR Morb. Mortal. Wkly. Rep.* 1990; 39(2): 31–4.

Dellinger, R. P. (1), Levy, M. M., Rhodes, A., *et al.* Surviving Sepsis Campaign: international guidelines for management of severe sepsis and septic shock, 2012. *Intensive Care Med.* 2013; 39(2): 165–228.

Forsythe, S. M. and Schmidt, G. A. Sodium bicarbonate for the treatment of lactic acidosis. *Chest* 2000; 117(1): 260–7.

Hotchkiss, R. S. and Karl, I. E. The pathophysiology and treatment of sepsis. *N. Engl. J. Med.* 2003; 348(2): 138–50.

Krishnagopalan, S. Myocardial dysfunction in the patient with sepsis. *Curr. Opin. Crit. Care* 2002; 8(5): 376–88.

Mitchell, M. M., Fink, M. P., Marshall, J. C., *et al.* 2001 SCCM/ESICM/ACCP/ATS/SIS International Sepsis Definitions Conference. *Crit. Care Med.* 2003; 31(4): 1250–6.

Peake, S. L., Delaney, A., Bailey, M., *et al.* Goal-directed resuscitation for patients with early septic shock. *N. Engl. J. Med.* 2014; 371(16): 1496–506.

Rangel-Frausto, M., Pittet, D., Costigan, M., *et al.* The natural history of the systemic inflammatory response syndrome (SIRS): a prospective study. *JAMA* 1995; 273(2): 117–23.

Rivers, E., Nguyen, B., Havstad, S., *et al.* Early goal-directed therapy in the treatment of severe sepsis and septic shock. *N. Engl. J. Med.* 2001; 345(19): 1368–77.

Santacruz, J. F., Zavala, E. D., and Arroliga, A. C.. Update in ARDS management: recent randomized controlled trials that changed our practice. *Cleve. Clin. J. Med.* 2006; 73(3): 217–36.

Van den Berghe, G., Wilmer, A., Milants, I., *et al.* Intensive insulin therapy in mixed medical/surgical intensive care units. *Diabetes* 2006; 55(11): 3151–9.

Ware, L. B. and Matthay, M. A. The acute respiratory distress syndrome. *N. Engl. J. Med.* 2000; 342(18): 1334–49.

Yealy, D. M., Kellum, J. A., Huang, D. T., *et al.* A randomized trial of protocol-based care for early septic shock. *N. Engl. J. Med.* 2014; 370(18): 1683–93.

Additional Readings

Bernard, G. R., Wheeler, A. P., Russell, J. A., *et al.* The effects of ibuprofen on the physiology and survival of patients with sepsis. *N. Engl. J. Med.* 1997; 336(13): 912–18.

Dellinger, R. P. Cardiovascular management of septic shock. *Crit. Care Med.* 2003; 31(3): 946–55.

Vincent, J. L., Fink, M. P., Marini, J. J., *et al.* Intensive care and emergency medicine: progress over the last 25 years. *Chest* 2006; 129(4): 1061–7.

Chapter 66

Infections in Sickle Cell Disease

Suzanne Lippert

Introduction

Sickle cell hemoglobinopathy results from the substitution of a valine for glutamic acid as the sixth amino acid of the beta globin chain. Sickle cell disease (SCD) includes the most severe and most common form, homozygous sickle cell anemia (Hb SS), as well as the heterozygous condition of intermediate severity, S, combined with hemoglobin C (Hb SC). Hemoglobin S is also seen in combination with beta thalassemia producing the more severe form, HbS-β^0 thalassemia, and the less severe HbS-β^+ thalassemia. The heterozygous (carrier) form in which hemoglobin S combines with normal hemoglobin A (Hb AS) is usually asymptomatic.

The sickling of erythrocytes that results from the deoxygenation-induced deformation of the hemoglobin S molecule causes erythrostasis, thrombosis, and ultimately infarction in the spleen of affected patients. SCD patients develop early functional asplenia, usually by 2 to 4 years of age, which leads to susceptibility to encapsulated organisms: *Streptococcus pneumoniae*, *Haemophilus influenzae*, *Mycoplasma pneumoniae*, and *Chlamydia pneumoniae*. Prophylactic penicillin, given as 125 mg orally twice a day until 2 to 3 years of age and 250 mg twice daily until at least 5 years of age, is recommended as prevention against invasive pneumococcal disease.

Sickle cell anemia affects millions throughout the world. According to a 2009 report from the US National Heart, Lung, and Blood Institute, sickle cell anemia affects between 90,000 and 100,000 Americans. The disease occurs in about 1 in every 500 African-American births and 1 in every 36,000 Hispanic-American births. One in 12 African Americans carry the sickle cell allele.

Infection is the primary cause of death in sickle cell patients during childhood, while chronic organ failure from vaso-occlusive disease becomes an equally important cause of mortality in adulthood. However, a 42% reduction in mortality in African-American children with sickle cell disease coincided with the introduction of the 7-valent pneumococcal conjugate vaccine in 2000.

In adult sickle cell patients presenting with fever, it is imperative to consider non-infectious as well as infectious causes of fever. These include vaso-occlusive crisis, bone infarction, pulmonary fat embolism, ischemic cerebrovascular accidents, hepatic or mesenteric infarction, infection with encapsulated organisms, including bacteremia, pneumonia, meningitis, osteomyelitis, and septic arthritis.

The initial diagnostic approach begins with a careful history, review of systems, and physical exam in an attempt to elicit complaints that might localize the source of fever. In particular, the patient should be explicitly questioned about symptoms characteristic of meningitis or stroke, pneumonia, bone or joint infections, urinary tract infections, cholecystitis or cholangitis, viral hepatitis, and mesenteric ischemia.

The initial work-up of all SCD adults with non-localizing fever includes complete blood count with differential, reticulocyte count, lactate dehydrogenase (LDH), urinalysis, blood and urine cultures, respiratory viral panel, and a chest radiograph

(CXR). Further work-up, which may include lumbar puncture (LP), arthrocentesis, and abdominal imaging, is based on signs and symptoms elicited during the history and physical exam as detailed in the subsequent sections on specific infections.

Bacteremia and Sepsis
Epidemiology and Microbiology

Several recent studies have shown bacteremia to be a relatively rare event in SCD adults, on the order of 1.2 episodes per 100 patient-years. Bacteremia in adults is most commonly associated with severe underlying disease and central venous catheters. The most commonly isolated organisms are *Staphylococcus aureus*, including methicillin-resistant *S. aureus* (MRSA) and coagulase-negative staphylococci, followed by gram-negative bacilli, such as *Escherichia coli* and *Klebsiella*.

With widespread use of daily prophylactic penicillin regimens and the pneumococcal vaccine, the incidence of pneumococcal bacteremia in pediatric patients has markedly decreased making pathogens other than pneumococcus responsible for most bacteremic episodes; however, invasive pneumococcal disease continues to pose a serious risk, including a recent surge of non-vaccine serotypes. The incidence of *Haemophilus influenzae* bacteremia, which previously accounted for up to 25% of childhood episodes of SCD bacteremia, has significantly declined since the introduction of the *Haemophilus influenzae* type b (Hib) vaccine. An 18-year retrospective cohort study of pediatric febrile SCD patients completed in 2013 identified a 0.6% risk of bacteremia in contrast to the 3 to 5% risk found in prior studies.

Clinical Features

Bacteremia may present with a myriad of symptoms and signs, most commonly fever or hypothermia, hyperventilation, chills, rigors, diffuse purpuric rash, tachycardia, delirium, decreased urine output, and/or hypotension (see Table 66.1).

Differential Diagnosis

Differential diagnosis includes:

- vaso-occlusive crisis
- acute chest syndrome (ACS)
- aplastic crisis secondary to viral infection (parvovirus B19)
- meningitis
- osteomyelitis
- cholecystitis
- intra-abdominal catastrophe (i.e. mesenteric infarction, perforation)

Laboratory and Radiographic Findings

When bacteremia or sepsis is suspected, blood and urine cultures should be sent and a search for the source of infection initiated. The white blood cell count (WBC) is neither sensitive nor specific for serious infection in this setting. Patients with SCD are also at risk of a hypoplastic or aplastic red blood cell (RBC) crisis in the setting of severe infection, manifesting

in a low reticulocyte count and dropping hemoglobin levels. Severe sepsis commonly results in increasing lactate levels and, secondary to disseminated intravascular coagulation (DIC), low fibrinogen and prolonged prothrombin time (PT) and partial thromboplastin time (PTT). To ensure that an occult source of bacteremia is not overlooked, at a minimum, urinalysis (UA), urine culture, and chest radiography should be obtained. Lumbar puncture and abdominal ultrasound (US) or computed tomographic (CT) scan should be obtained based on clinical suspicion for meningitis or intra-abdominal pathology, respectively.

Treatment

Because bacteremia in adult SCD patients is associated with venous catheters 41 to 80% of the time in various studies, removal of central lines should be considered immediately. Initial antibiotic therapy in children with SCD is a parenteral third-generation cephalosporin to cover *S. pneumoniae*. Initial empiric antibiotics for hospitalized adults or those with venous catheters should cover *S. aureus*, including MRSA, whereas community-acquired bacteremia in SCD adults should initially be treated with antibiotics covering *E. coli*, *S. aureus*, and *S. pneumoniae*. Initial parenteral empiric therapy in adults should begin with vancomycin and ceftriaxone. Levofloxacin may be substituted for ceftriaxone in beta-lactam allergic patients.

Acute Chest Syndrome
Epidemiology and Pathophysiology

ACS is defined by a new alveolar consolidation involving at least one lung segment associated with acute respiratory symptoms, fever, or chest pain. ACS results when a precipitating etiology initiates a proinflammatory cascade causing increasingly severe sickling, thrombosis, and lung injury. The trigger may be a combination of infectious causes (bacterial, viral, or mixed infection) and non-infectious causes (pulmonary fat embolism and pulmonary infarction).

The incidence of ACS is age and genotype dependent, with rates of 25.3 events per 100 patient-years in HbSS children ages 2 to 4 years, decreasing to 8.78 events per 100 patient-years in HbSS adults more than 20 years old. Infection, particularly with viruses, *Chlamydia pneumoniae*, and *Mycoplasma*, are the most frequent cause of ACS in young children. Vascular occlusion and pulmonary fat embolism are thought to be more common causes of ACS in adults because a pneumonia pathogen is less frequently identified and there is a strong association with bone pain.

Clinical Features

Fever above 38.5°C and cough are the most common presenting symptoms in all age groups, though these are more common in children than in adolescents and adults (see Table 66.2). Dyspnea is variably present in all age groups, whereas chest, rib, and extremity pain are more commonly seen in adolescents and adults. On physical exam, children are more likely

Table 66.1 Clinical Features: Bacteremia and Sepsis

	Children	Adults
Organisms	*Streptococcus pneumoniae* *Haemophilus influenzae* *Salmonella* *Escherichia coli,* *Klebsiella*	Community acquired: • *Escherichia coli,* • *Klebsiella* • *Staphylococcus aureus* • *Streptococcus pneumoniae* • *Salmonella* Hospital acquired: • *Staphylococcus aureus,* including MRSA
Risks and associations	• Non-compliance with penicillin prophylaxis • Unvaccinated for *S. pneumoniae* and *H. influenzae*	• Severe immunosuppression • Venous catheter-associated • High frequency of bone and joint infections
Signs and symptoms	• Fever or hypothermia • Chills, rigors • Tachycardia, hypotension • Confusion, delirium • Decreased urine output	
Laboratory and radiographic tests	• CBC: leukocytosis, left shift • Reticulocyte count: aplastic or hypoproliferative crisis • Blood cultures • CXR to rule out ACS • UA with urine culture • Consider LP • Consider abdominal imaging	
Treatment	Ceftriaxone 50 mg/kg/dose IV every 24 hours	Vancomycin 15–20 mg/kg/dose IV every 8–12 hours *plus* Ceftriaxone 1 g IV every 24 hours *or* Levofloxacin 750 mg IV every 24 hours

ACS – acute chest syndrome; CBC – complete blood count; UA – urinalysis.

than adults to exhibit signs of bronchospasm, wheezing, and tachypnea.

Presenting symptoms observed during a patient's first episode of ACS are predictive of symptoms during subsequent events. Nevertheless, clinical assessment alone is unreliable in diagnosing ACS.

Differential Diagnosis

In the Cooperative Study of Sickle Cell Disease (CSSCD) trial, adult patients who were eventually diagnosed with ACS during the same hospitalization most commonly presented with complaints of extremity pain and no evidence of ACS on initial exam. Febrile illness in children and vaso-occlusive pain crises in adults are viewed as precursors to ACS. The differential includes bacterial pneumonia and non-infectious causes of ACS, such as:

• pulmonary fat embolism
• pulmonary infarction
• pulmonary edema
• rib or sternal infarction

Characteristics that may help to distinguish the etiology of ACS are as follows:

• Fat embolism syndrome classically presents with a triad of hypoxemia, neurologic abnormalities, and a petechial rash.

• Pulmonary infarction usually results from in-situ thrombosis secondary to sickling rather than embolic events; therefore, these patients are no more likely to have identifiable deep venous thrombosis (DVT).

• Positive blood cultures in the setting of ACS should be treated as infectious pneumonia until proven otherwise.

Laboratory and Radiographic Findings

Children younger than 10 years old have a higher frequency of upper and middle lobe disease, whereas adults more often have isolated lower lobe infiltrate or multilobar disease. Pleural effusions are seen in more than half of all episodes of ACS, but occur more frequently in adults. In direct comparison with simultaneous high-resolution CT scan, chest radiograph has been shown to underestimate the degree of pulmonary disease in patients presenting with ACS.

At diagnosis, hypoxemia to a mean oxygen saturation of 92% is common. Hemoglobin and white blood cell counts differ markedly from steady-state values. Hemoglobin declines by approximately 0.7 g/dL, while white blood cells increase by an average of 70% in ACS. Platelet counts often decrease throughout the course of the illness, with platelets below 200,000 mm^3 as a strong predictor of morbidity and mortality. The average forced expiratory volume (FEV) is 53% of the predicted value,

Table 66.2 Clinical Features: Bacterial Pneumonia and ACS

	Age <10	Age >10
Organisms	Viral: RSV, rhinovirus *Mycoplasma pneumoniae* *Chlamydia pneumoniae*	*C. pneumoniae* *M. pneumoniae* *S. aureus* *S. pneumoniae*
Signs and symptoms	• Fever >38.5 °C • Cough • Bronchospasm, wheezing • Tachypnea • Dyspnea • Hypoxia	• Fever >38.5 °C • Cough • Chest pain • Dyspnea • Extremity pain • Hypoxia
Laboratory and radiographic tests	• Hb decrease by 0.7 g/dL • WBC increase of 70% • Bacteremia • Secretory phospholipase A$_2$ dramatically increased • CXR: variable with isolated upper and middle lobe disease with or without pleural effusions	• Hb decrease by 0.7 g/dL • WBC increase of 70% • Secretory phospholipase A$_2$ dramatically increased • CXR: variable with lower lobe or multilobar disease with or without pleural effusions
Treatment	Ceftriaxone 1 g IV every 24 hours (50 mg/kg/dose in children) *plus* Azithromycin 500 mg IV every 24 hours (10 mg/kg/dose in children) *or* Levofloxacin 750 mg IV every 24 hours in adults Add vancomycin for large or progressing infiltrates. • Pain control: PCA narcotics, intercostal nerve block • Bronchodilator therapy if reactive airway disease (empiric trial) • Oxygen supplementation • Maintain euvolemia: D5 1/2NS at 1.5–2× maintenance • Incentive spirometry • RBC transfusion if respiratory compromise, significant anemia, clinical deterioration	

PCA – patient-controlled analgesia; RSV – respiratory syncytial virus.

with approximately 25% of patients showing improvement with bronchodilators.

Despite the historically low yield, sputum and blood cultures should be obtained. Bronchoalveolar lavage (BAL) is preferred as it provides higher quality specimens for culture and allows for the examination of fat-laden macrophages characteristic of pulmonary fat embolism. Serologic studies for *Mycoplasma*, chlamydia, and parvovirus and, in children especially, nasopharyngeal samples for viral cultures should be obtained.

Treatment

The treatment of ACS should address the causative agent as well as the host response in order to prevent further pulmonary injury and respiratory compromise. Broad-spectrum antibiotics, proper pain management, alleviation of bronchospasm, oxygen therapy, cautious intravenous fluids (IVF) administration, incentive spirometry, transfusion, and, in severe cases, mechanical ventilation are the fundamentals of therapy in ACS.

Broad-spectrum antibiotics that cover common community-acquired and atypical pathogens, and a macrolide to cover *M. pneumoniae*, are required in all patients. Therapy should begin with a third-generation cephalosporin, cefotaxime or ceftriaxone, in conjunction with a macrolide, or a respiratory fluoroquinolone. In children with SCD, ceftriaxone

should be used with caution as it has been associated with drug-induced immune hemolysis. The CSSD study identified more than 27 unique infectious pathogens as causative agents in ACS; therefore, patients that are rapidly deteriorating should have antibiotic coverage broadened. Local pathogen predominance and sensitivity patterns in community-acquired pneumonia (CAP) should be used to guide initial antibiotic therapy.

Pain management should include patient-controlled analgesia (PCA) and intercostal nerve blocks to minimize narcotic-induced hypoventilation. The use of adrenergic bronchodilators should be attempted in all ACS patients, using caution in adults because of the hypertensive and cardiac effects. Oxygen should be administered in all hypoxic patients and has questionable benefit in other patients presenting with pain. Intravenous fluid administration should be limited to a rate of 1.5 to 2 times maintenance, in order to avoid pulmonary edema from overly aggressive hydration. A hypotonic solution, one-half normal saline (NS) in adults and one-quarter NS in children, should be considered because the osmotic differential supports the primary goal of hydration of erythrocytes. Incentive spirometry, used at least every 2 hours, is recommended in all patients.

Transfusion therapy is recommended if there is clinical deterioration, multilobar infiltrates, or a history of underlying pulmonary or cardiac disease. Exchange transfusion is preferred, whereas simple transfusion should be used for patients

Table 66.3 Clinical Features: Osteomyelitis

Organisms	*Salmonella* *Staphylococcus aureus* Gram-negative enteric bacilli: *Escherichia coli, Enterobacter*
Risks and associations	• Areas of previously infarcted bone
Signs and symptoms*	• Fever • Localized tenderness and swelling • Limitation of movement of joint (septic arthritis) • Commonly involves femur, tibia, humerus
Laboratory and radiographic tests	• ESR elevated • Blood and stool cultures for *Salmonella* • Plain radiographs: non-specific periostitis and osteopenia, lucent areas characteristic of osteomyelitis appear 10–14 days into the course of the illness • CT, MRI, US: locates area of focus for aspiration and identifies possible presence of abscess • Culture of bone aspirate or biopsy remains the gold standard
Treatment	• IVF • Adults: Vancomycin 15–20 mg/kg/dose IV every 8–12 hours *plus* • Ceftriaxone 2 g IV every 24 hours • Children: Oxacillin 100–200 mg/kg/day IV in three to four divided doses *plus* (in areas of high MRSA prevalence) vancomycin 15 mg/kg/dose every 6 hours • Aggressive pain control

* Signs and symptoms are indistinguishable from acute infarction.

ESR – erythrocyte sedimentation rate.

with significant anemia. Leukocyte-poor packed red blood cells matched for Rh, C, E, and Kell antigens should be used to minimize erythrocyte antibody formation. Mechanical ventilation is indicated for respiratory failure.

Osteomyelitis and Septic Arthritis

Epidemiology and Microbiology

Because of their overall increased susceptibility to bacterial infection and bone infarction, patients with SCD have a greater risk of osteomyelitis than the general population. SCD patients with a history of osteonecrosis were shown to have a 2.5- to 3.8-fold greater risk of developing bone and joint infections after bacteremia. The organisms most commonly isolated in SCD-related osteomyelitis are *Salmonella*, *Staphylococcus aureus*, and, less commonly, aerobic gram-negative rods. Despite this increased risk of infection, however, once patients reach adolescence, vaso-occlusive crisis is up to 50 times more likely than osteomyelitis to be the cause of bone pain. Patients with sickle cell disease are also susceptible to septic arthritis, though it occurs less frequently than osteomyelitis. Septic arthritis is generally caused by the same organisms as osteomyelitis, as well as *Streptococcus pneumoniae*, and tends to occur in association with vaso-occlusive crisis.

Clinical Features

Osteomyelitis often presents with fever; persistent and severe bone pain commonly involving the femur, tibia, or humerus; and localized swelling and tenderness over the involved bone (see Table 66.3). Septic arthritis usually presents in the setting of a vaso-occlusive crisis, with fever, swelling, and tenderness of a joint, and a dramatically limited range of motion of the involved joint.

Differential Diagnosis

Bone infarction is extremely difficult to distinguish from osteomyelitis because both present with fever, bone pain, and soft-tissue swelling.

Key features that distinguish bone infarction from osteomyelitis include:

• a history of recurrent bone infarction
• multifocal rather than unifocal bone pain

Pain with joint motion raises suspicion for joint involvement and requires an arthrocentesis to rule out septic arthritis. Plain films, though expected to reveal only non-specific changes, are helpful in excluding pathologic fractures or bone tumors.

Ultrasonography may help diagnose osteomyelitis by demonstrating:

• periosteal elevation
• subperiosteal or intramedullary abscesses
• cortical erosions

Laboratory and Radiographic Findings

In both infarction and osteomyelitis, the complete blood count usually shows leukocytosis, and the ESR is usually elevated. Blood and stool cultures should be obtained as *Salmonella* has been identified as the most prevalent pathogen in osteomyelitis. Plain films may be normal or show the non-specific periostitis and osteopenia consistent with the early stages of both osteomyelitis and bone infarction. The destructive changes of osteomyelitis, appearing as lucent areas on plain radiographs, do not appear until 10 to 14 days after onset. CT, MRI, and bone scintigraphy may help in localizing the area of activity and following the course of the disease; however, no single radiographic modality has shown sufficient specificity to differentiate between infarction and osteomyelitis. There is also significant overlap in the US findings characteristic of infarction and infection; nevertheless, US provides an accessible, non-invasive means of evaluating for obvious elements of infection, such as subperiosteal or intramedullary abscesses. Cultures of the blood, stool, and bone aspirate or biopsy remain the gold standard in the diagnosis of osteomyelitis.

In the case of joint involvement, arthrocentesis with synovial fluid analysis for cell count, Gram stain, and culture should be done to rule out septic arthritis.

Treatment

Empiric parenteral antibiotics covering *Salmonella* and *Staphylococcus aureus* should be initiated in the emergency department for any patient with strongly suspected osteomyelitis. Recommended initial therapy in adult SCD patients is vancomycin plus ceftriaxone, and in children is oxacillin plus (in areas of high MRSA prevalence) vancomycin. In cases of confirmed osteomyelitis, antibiotic treatment tailored to the specific organism and sensitivities should continue for 4 to 6 weeks. Patients not responsive to antibiotics may require surgical debridement and drainage.

Cholecystitis and Cholangitis

Excessive production of bilirubin caused by RBC hemolysis in sickle cell patients often results in pigmented gallstone formation. The incidence of cholelithiasis in sickle cell patients increases with age and corresponds to the rate of hemolysis. One study revealed the prevalence of cholelithiasis to be 58% in HbSS patients aged 10 to 50 years and 17% in HbSC and sickle-thalassemia patients. This increased propensity to form gallstones increases the risk of cholecystitis and, to a lesser degree, cholangitis, in sickle cell patients.

Differential Diagnosis

Abdominal pain is commonly a component of vaso-occlusive crisis and is thought to result from infarcts of the mesentery or abdominal viscera. Although the majority of abdominal pain in sickle cell patients remains idiopathic and resolves spontaneously, acute intra-abdominal infection must be excluded in any sickle cell patient presenting with fever and abdominal pain, or new abdominal symptoms.

Abdominal pain in the sickle cell patient has a broad differential, including acute sickle hepatic crisis, hepatic sequestration and infarction, transfusion-related viral hepatitis and iron overload, and disease resulting from pigmented gallstone formation: cholelithiasis, cholecystitis, and cholangitis. Rarely, acute pancreatitis results from biliary obstruction or ischemic pancreatic injury. Acute splenic sequestration, though primarily a complication in infants, can occur in adults and carries a high mortality. Common causes of abdominal pain, including appendicitis, should not be overlooked.

Laboratory and Radiographic Findings

See Chapter 23, Infectious Biliary Diseases, on biliary pathology for the standard laboratory and radiographic work-up. Additional laboratory tests for SCD patients include reticulocyte count, LDH, UA, and blood and urine cultures.

Complications and Admission Criteria

Adult SCD patients with a history of osteonecrosis were shown to have a 2.5- to 3.8-fold greater risk of developing bone and joint infections 1 to 6 months after suffering an *S. aureus* bacteremia. SCD patients suspected of having bacteremia should be admitted to the hospital for broad-spectrum parenteral antibiotics. Patients exhibiting signs of sepsis should be treated with goal-directed therapy and admitted to the intensive care unit (ICU).

Adults with SCD who were diagnosed with ACS were more likely than children to have complications, such as respiratory failure and neurologic complications, as well as prolonged hospital stays and death. Mortality was four- to ninefold greater in adults older than 20 years. Neurologic complications increased with age and included coma, seizures, anoxic brain injury, and stroke. Febrile illness in children and vaso-occlusive pain crises in adults are viewed as precursors to ACS; therefore, all patients presenting with fever and pain crisis should undergo chest radiography, and patients who exhibit any of the signs or symptoms of ACS should be admitted for serial CXR exams.

Febrile sickle cell patients with severe, persistent musculoskeletal pain should be admitted for diagnostic work-up of osteomyelitis.

Pearls and Pitfalls

1. Adults with SCD are asplenic, raising the risk of fulminant sepsis with encapsulated bacteria.
2. Sepsis is more common in SCD children than adults.
3. Initiate a thorough search for a source of the bacteremia.
4. Rapidly institute broad-spectrum antibiotics for all SCD patients with suspected bacteremia, and initiate goal-directed therapy for septic patients.
5. Febrile illness in children and vaso-occlusive pain crises in adults may be precursors to ACS.
6. Clinical presentation of ACS in adults often includes prominent extremity pain.
7. Platelet count below 200,000 mm^3 is a strong predictor of morbidity and mortality in ACS.
8. Pulmonary infarction usually results from in-situ thrombosis secondary to sickling rather than embolic events; therefore, these patients are no more likely to have identifiable venous thromboembolism.
9. Bone infarction and osteomyelitis are extremely difficult to distinguish from one another; routine laboratory work, plain radiographs, and even CT, MRI, and US will likely not distinguish bone infarction from osteomyelitis.

10. A diagnosis of osteomyelitis is supported by stool and blood cultures positive for *Salmonella*.

11. A diagnosis of bone infarction is supported by a history of recurrent infarction and multifocal bone pain.

12. Perform arthrocentesis and admit all patients with suspected joint involvement.

13. For any patient with strongly suspected osteomyelitis and intractable pain, admission, parental antibiotics, and cultures of bone aspirate are essential.

14. Because of the broad differential for abdominal pain in SCD, febrile patients with abdominal complaints will likely require ultrasound to exclude cholecystitis and abdominal CT scan.

References

Ahmed, S., Shahid, R. K., and Russo, L. A. Unusual causes of abdominal pain: sickle cell anemia. *Best Pract. Res. Clin. Gastroenterol.* 2005; 19(2): 297–310.

Almeida, A. and Roberts, I. Bone involvement in sickle cell disease. *Br. J. Haematol.* 2005; 129(4): 482–90.

Ashley-Koch, A., Yang, Q., and Olney, R. S. Sickle hemoglobin (HbS) allele and sickle cell disease: a HuGE review. *Am. J. Epidemiol.* 2000; 151(9): 839–45.

Bansil, N. H., Kim, T. Y., Tieu, L., and Barcega, B. Incidence of serious bacterial infections in febrile children with sickle cell disease. *Clin. Pediatr.* 2013; 52(7): 661–6.

Baskin, M. N., Goh, X. L., Heeney, M. M., and Harper, M. B. Bacteremia risk and outpatient management of febrile patients with sickle cell disease. *Pediatrics*. 2013; 131(6): 1035–41.

Bond, L. R., Hatty, S. R., Horn, M. E., *et al.* Gall stones in sickle cell disease in the United Kingdom. *Br. Med. J. (Clin. Res. Ed.)* 1987; 295(6592): 234–6.

Burnett, M. W., Bass, J. W., and Cook, B. A. Etiology of osteomyelitis complicating sickle cell disease. *Pediatrics* 1998; 101(2): 296–7.

Castro, O., Brambilla, D. J., Thorington, B., *et al.* The acute chest syndrome in sickle cell disease: incidence and risk factors. The Cooperative Study of Sickle Cell Disease. *Blood* 1994; 84(2): 643–9.

Chulamokha, L., Scholand, S. J., Riggio, J. M., *et al.* Bloodstream infections in hospitalized adults with sickle cell disease: a retrospective analysis. *Am. J. Hematol.* 2006; 81(10): 723–8.

Johnson, C. S. The acute chest syndrome. *Hematol. Oncol. Clin. North Am.* 2005; 19(5): 857–79.

Leikin, S. L., Gallagher, D., Kinney, T. R., *et al.* Mortality in children and adolescents with sickle cell disease. Cooperative Study of Sickle Cell Disease. *Pediatrics* 1989; 84(3): 500–8.

Lottenberg, R. and Hassell, K. L. An evidence-based approach to the treatment of adults with sickle cell disease. *Hematology* 2005; 2005(1): 58–65.

McCavit, T. L., Quinn, C. T., Techasaensiri, C., and Rogers, Z. R. Increase in invasive Streptococcus pneumonia infections in children with sickle cell disease since pneumococcal conjugate vaccine licensure. *J. Pediatr.* 2011; 158(3): 505–7.

Morris, C., Vichinsky, E., and Styles, L. Clinician assessment for acute chest syndrome in febrile patients with sickle cell disease: is it accurate enough? *Ann. Emerg. Med.* 1999; 34(1): 64–9.

Narang, S., Fernandez, I. D., Chin, N., *et al.* Bacteremia in children with sickle hemoglobinopathies. *J. Pediatr. Hematol. Oncol.* 2012; 34(1): 13–16.

National Heart, Lung, and Blood Institute. Disease and conditions index. Sickle cell anemia: who is at risk? (Bethesda, MD: US Department of Health and Human Services, National Institutes of Health, National Heart, Lung, and Blood Institute, 2009), available at www.nhlbi.nih.gov/health/dci/Diseases/Sca/SCA_WhoIsAtRisk.html (accessed December 11, 2017).

Piehl, F. C., Davis, R. J., and Prugh, S. I. Osteomyelitis in sickle cell disease. *J. Pediatr. Orthop.* 1993; 13(2): 225–7.

Vichinsky, E. P., Neumayr, L. D., Earles, A. N., *et al.* Causes and outcomes of the acute chest syndrome in sickle cell disease. National Acute Chest Syndrome Study Group. *N. Engl. J. Med.* 2000; 342(25): 1855–65.

Vichinsky, E. P., Styles, L. A., Colangelo, L. H., *et al.* Acute chest syndrome in sickle cell disease: clinical presentation and course. Cooperative Study of Sickle Cell Disease. *Blood* 1997; 89(5): 1787–92.

William, R. R., Hussein, S. S., Jeans, W. D., *et al.* A prospective study of soft-tissue ultrasonography in sickle cell disease patients with suspected osteomyelitis. *Clin. Radiol.* 2000; 55(4): 307–10.

Wong, A. L., Sakamoto, K. M., and Johnson, E. E. Differentiating osteomyelitis from bone infarction in sickle cell disease. *Pediatr. Emerg. Care* 2001; 17(1): 60–3.

Wong, W. Y., Powars, D. R., Chan, L., *et al.* Polysaccharide encapsulated bacterial infection in sickle cell anemia: a thirty year epidemiologic experience. *Am. J. Hematol.* 1992; 39(3): 176–82.

Yanni, E., Grosse, S. D., Yang, Q., and Olney, R. S. Trends in pediatric sickle cell disease-related mortality in the United States 1983–2002. *J. Pediatr.* 2009; 154(4): 541–5.

Zarrouk, V., Habibi, A., Zahar, J. R., *et al.* Bloodstream infection in adults with sickle cell disease: association with venous catheters, *Staphylococcus aureus*, and bone-joint infections. *Medicine (Baltimore)* 2006; 85(1): 43–8.

Additional Readings

Chang, T. P., Kriengsoontorkij, W., Chan, L. S., *et al.* Clinical factors and incidence of acute chest syndrome or pneumonia among children with sickle cell disease presenting with a fever: a 17-year review. *Pediatr. Emerg. Care.* 2013; 29(7): 781–6.

Inusa, B. P., Oyewo, A., Brokke, F., *et al.* Dilemma in differentiating between acute osteomyelitis and bone infarction in children with sickle cell disease: the role of ultrasound. *PLoS One.* 2013; 8(6): e65001.

Morrissey, B. J., Bycroft, T. P., Almossawi, O., *et al.* Incidence and predictors of bacterial infection in febrile children with sickle cell disease. *Hemoglobin.* 2015; 39(5): 316–19.

Shihabuddin, B. S. and Scarfi, C. A. Fever in children with sickle cell disease: are all fevers equal? *J. Emerg. Med.* 2014; 47(4): 395–400.

Srinivasan, A., Wang, W. C., Gaur, A., *et al.* Prospective evaluation for respiratory pathogens in children with sickle cell disease and acute respiratory illness. *Pediatr. Blood Cancer.* 2014; 61(3): 507–11.

Tordjman, D., Holvoet, L., Benkerrou, M., *et al.* Hematogenous osteo-articular infections of the hand and the wrist in children with sickle cell anemia: preliminary report. *J. Pediatr. Orthop.* 2014; 34(1): 123–8.

Chapter 67

Anthrax

David M. Stier, Mary P. Mercer, and Rachel L. Chin

Introduction

Anthrax is an acute infection caused by *Bacillus anthracis*, a large, gram-positive, spore-forming, aerobic, encapsulated, rod-shaped bacterium. Spores germinate and form bacteria in nutrient-rich environments, whereas bacteria form spores in nutrient-poor environments. The anthrax bacillus produces high levels of two toxins: edema toxin causes massive edema at the site of germination, and lethal toxin leads to sepsis. Severity of anthrax disease depends on the route of infection and the presence of complications. Case fatality ranges from 5 to 95% if untreated.

The Working Group for Civilian Biodefense considers *B. anthracis* to be one of the most serious biological threats. Anthrax has been weaponized and used. It can be fairly easily disseminated to cause illness and death. Of the potential ways that *B. anthracis* could be used as a biological weapon, an aerosol release is expected to have the most severe medical and public health outcomes.

Epidemiology

Naturally Occurring Anthrax

Reservoir

The natural reservoir for *B. anthracis* is soil, and the predominant hosts are herbivores (cattle, sheep, goats, horses, pigs, and others) that acquire infection from consuming contaminated soil or feed. Anthrax spores can persist in soil for years and are resistant to drying, heat, ultraviolet light, gamma radiation, and some disinfectants. Anthrax in animals is endemic in many areas of the world and anthrax outbreaks in animals occur sporadically in the United States.

Mode of Transmission

Anthrax is generally a zoonotic disease. Humans become infected through contact with infected animals and animal products through several mechanisms:

- Contact with infected animal tissues (e.g. veterinarians, animal handlers, meat processors, and other processes that involve animal hides, hair, and bones) or contaminated soil
- Ingestion of contaminated, undercooked meat from infected animals
- Inhalation of infectious aerosols (e.g. those generated during processing of animal products, such as tanning hides, processing wool or bone)

Person-to-person transmission of *B. anthracis* does not occur with gastrointestinal (GI) or inhalational anthrax, but has been reported rarely with cutaneous anthrax.

Worldwide Occurrence

Worldwide, approximately 2,000 cases are reported annually. Anthrax is more common in developing countries with less rigorous animal disease control programs. Cases of human anthrax are most often reported in South and Central America, Southern and Eastern Europe, Asia, Africa, the Caribbean, and the Middle East. The largest reported outbreak of human anthrax occurred in Zimbabwe (1979 to 1985), which involved more than 10,000 individuals and was associated with anthrax disease in cattle.

US Occurrence

Naturally occurring anthrax is rare in the United States, with approximately one to two cases reported each year. The majority of anthrax cases in the United States are cutaneous and acquired occupationally in workers who come into contact with animals or animal products. Only 19 cases of naturally occurring inhalational anthrax have been reported since 1900, and there have been no confirmed gastrointestinal cases. Recent cases of naturally occurring anthrax include the following:

- In 2006, a New York City resident contracted inhalational anthrax while making drums from goat hides imported from Africa. The untanned hides were contaminated with anthrax spores, which may have been aerosolized during removal of hair. The CDC believes that this was an isolated case and considers handling animal skins or making drums to be a low risk for cutaneous anthrax and extremely low risk for inhalational anthrax.
- In 2002, two cases of cutaneous anthrax were reported. A laboratory worker from a Texas lab that processed environmental *B. anthracis* specimens contracted cutaneous anthrax through direct contact with a contaminated surface. The second case occurred in a veterinarian who contracted the infection from a cow during necropsy.
- Two cases of human cutaneous anthrax were reported following epizootics in North Dakota (2000) and southwest Texas (2001). Both cases resulted from exposure during disposal of infected animal carcasses.

Anthrax as a Biological Weapon

Anthrax was successfully used as a biological weapon in the United States in October 2001. Cases resulted from direct or indirect exposure to mail that was deliberately contaminated with anthrax spores. In total, 22 cases were identified: 11 with inhalational (five fatal) and 11 with cutaneous anthrax (seven confirmed, four suspected).

Several countries have had anthrax weaponization programs in the past, including the United States. In 1979, an outbreak of anthrax in the Soviet Union resulted from accidental release of anthrax spores from a facility producing weaponized anthrax. Of 77 reported human cases, all but two were inhalational, and there was an 86% fatality rate.

Experts believe that an aerosol release of weapons-grade spores is the most likely mechanism for use of anthrax as a biological weapon in the future. Anthrax spores could also be used to deliberately contaminate food and water. Spores remain stable in water for several days and are not destroyed by pasteurization.

An intentional release of anthrax may have the following characteristics:

- Multiple similarly presenting cases *clustered in time*:
  ○ Severe acute febrile illness or febrile death
  ○ Severe sepsis not due to predisposing illness
  ○ Respiratory failure with a widened mediastinum on CXR
- Atypical host characteristics: unexpected, unexplained cases of acute illness in previously healthy persons who rapidly develop a progressive respiratory illness
- Multiple similarly presenting cases *clustered geographically*:
  ○ Acute febrile illness in persons who were in close proximity to a deliberate release of anthrax
- Absence of risk factors: patients lack anthrax exposure risk factors (e.g. veterinary or other animal handling work, meat processing, work that involves animal hides, hair, or bones, or agricultural work in areas with endemic anthrax)

Intentionally released anthrax spores may be altered for more efficient aerosolization and lethality (e.g. highly concentrated, treated to reduce clumping and reduce particle size, genetically modified to increase virulence, resist antimicrobials, and reduce vaccine efficacy).

Clinical Features

There are three primary clinical types of anthrax disease, inhalational, cutaneous, and gastrointestinal, which result from the way infection is acquired.

Anthrax infection is a severe clinical illness and can be life-threatening. Case fatality varies by the clinical type of disease. Overall case-fatality rates have declined because of more prompt administration of antibiotics and improved supportive care. Compared to historical rates, mortality has decreased from 86–95% to 45% for inhalational anthrax, 5–20% to less than 1% for cutaneous anthrax, and 25–60% to 12% for gastrointestinal anthrax. Anthrax meningitis case-fatality rates approach 95% even with antibiotic treatment.

In the event of bioterrorism, the method of dissemination would influence the type of clinical disease that would be expected. Following an aerosol release, the majority of cases would be inhalational with some cutaneous cases, whereas use of a small volume of powder could result in both inhalational and cutaneous anthrax cases (as seen in the 2001 attacks). Gastrointestinal cases might occur following contamination of food or water.

Inhalational Anthrax

Inhalational anthrax is caused by inhalation of spores that reach the alveoli, undergo phagocytosis, and travel to regional lymph nodes. The spores then germinate to become bacterial cells, which multiply in the lymphatic system and cause lymphadenitis of the mediastinal and peribronchial lymph nodes. The bacteria release toxins that cause hemorrhage, edema, and necrosis. Bacteria entering the bloodstream can lead to

Table 67.1 Clinical Features: Inhalational Anthrax

Incubation period	1–6 days (range <1 day to 8 weeks)
Transmission	Inhalation of aerosolized spores
Signs and symptoms	• Initial presentation: non-specific symptoms (low-grade fever, chills, non-productive cough, malaise, fatigue, myalgias, profound sweats, chest discomfort) • Intermediate presentation: abrupt onset of high fever, dyspnea, progressive respiratory distress, confusion, nausea or vomiting • Fulminant disease progression, if untreated
Progression and complications	• Severe respiratory distress (dyspnea, stridor, cyanosis), which may be preceded by 1–3 days of improvement • Pleural effusions • Meningitis • Shock
Laboratory and radiographic findings	• Chest CT or radiograph: mediastinal widening (often), pleural effusions that are commonly hemorrhagic (often), infiltrates (rare) • Gram-positive bacilli on unspun peripheral blood smear or CSF • Elevated transaminases • Hypoxemia • Metabolic acidosis • Total WBC count normal or slightly elevated with elevated percentage of neutrophils or band forms

CSF – cerebrospinal fluid; WBC – white blood (cell) count.

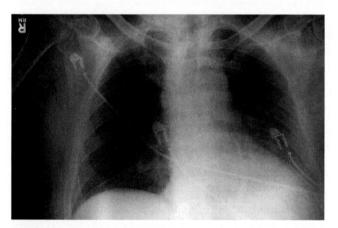

Figure 67.1 Anthrax chest X-ray with mediastinal widening and pleural effusion.

From J. A. Jernigan, D. S. Stephens, D. A. Ashford, *et al.*, Bioterrorism-related inhalational anthrax: the first 10 cases reported in the United States. *Emerg. Infect. Dis.* 2001; 7(6): 933–44.

septicemia, septic shock, and death. Systemic infection following inhalational anthrax is almost always fatal.

One of the key clinical features of inhalational anthrax is evidence of pleural effusion and mediastinal widening on CXR (see Figure 67.1) or chest computed tomographic (CT) scan (see Table 67.1). Based on experience from the 2001 attacks, chest CT (without contrast) was found to be more sensitive than CXR for identification of mediastinal widening typical of inhalational anthrax.

Cutaneous Anthrax

In cutaneous anthrax, spores or bacilli are introduced through cuts or breaks in the skin (see Table 67.2). Spores germinate at the site of contact and release toxins, causing development of a lesion and edema (see Figure 67.2). Organisms may be carried to regional lymph nodes and cause painful lymphadenopathy

and lymphangitis. Septicemic complications of cutaneous anthrax occur in 10 to 20% of untreated cases.

Pediatric Considerations

A case of cutaneous anthrax occurred in a 7-month-old baby during the anthrax attack of 2001. This case was difficult to recognize and rapidly progressed to severe systemic illness despite timely antibiotic treatment. Clinical features included painless draining lesion with edema that developed into an eschar, fever, leukocytosis, severe microangiopathic hemolytic anemia, renal failure, and coagulopathy.

Gastrointestinal Anthrax

Gastrointestinal (GI) anthrax results from ingestion of *B. anthracis* bacteria, such as may be found in poorly cooked meat from infected animals. The incubation period for GI anthrax is 1 to 7 days. Two clinical presentations have been described: intestinal and oropharyngeal.

With *intestinal anthrax*, lesions occur in the ileum or cecum and are followed by regional lymphadenopathy. Symptoms of intestinal anthrax are initially non-specific and include low-grade fever, malaise, nausea, vomiting, anorexia, and fever. As disease progresses, abdominal pain, hematemesis, and bloody diarrhea develop. The patient may present with findings of an acute abdomen. After 2 to 4 days, ascites develop and abdominal pain lessens. Hematogenous spread with resultant septicemia can occur. Mesenteric adenopathy on CT scan is likely, and mediastinal widening on CXR is possible.

In *oropharyngeal anthrax*, a mucosal ulcer occurs initially in the mouth or throat, associated with fever, throat pain, and dysphasia (see Figure 67.3). This is followed by cervical edema and regional lymphadenopathy. Ulcers may become necrotic with development of a white patch covering the ulcer. Swelling can become severe enough to affect breathing. Hematogenous spread, septicemia, and meningitis can occur.

Table 67.2 Clinical Features: Cutaneous Anthrax

Incubation period	3–4 days (range 1–12 days)
Transmission	• Direct skin contact with spores; in nature, contact with infected animals or animal products (usually related to occupational exposure) • Bite of infective arthropod (rare)
Signs and symptoms	• Local skin involvement after direct contact with spores or bacilli (commonly seen on hands, forearms, head, and neck) • Skin lesion with the following progression: (1) development of a papular lesion and localized itching; (2) papule turns into vesicular or bulbous lesion accompanied by painless edema; (3) lesion becomes necrotic and vesicles may surround the ulcer; and (4) lesion develops painless black eschar within 7–14 days of initial lesion • Lymphadenopathy and lymphangitis • Fever and malaise (common)
Progression and complications	• Bacteremia • Meningitis • Extensive edema causing airway compression • Sepsis
Laboratory findings	• Bacilli may be seen on Gram stain of subcutaneous tissue

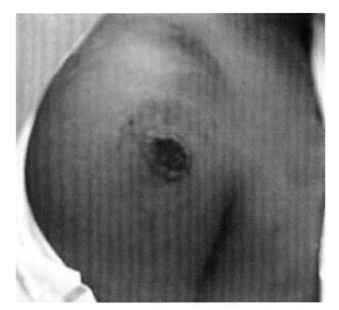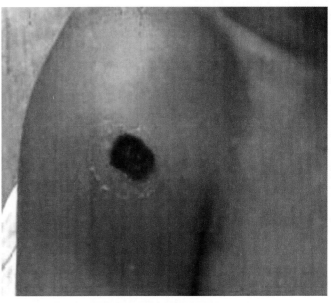

Figure 67.2 Progression of lesion caused by anthrax infection. Note the raised vesicular ring at the perimeter and subsequently the black eschar. From the US Centers for Disease Control and Prevention Emergency preparedness and response. Anthrax: images: cutaneous anthrax.

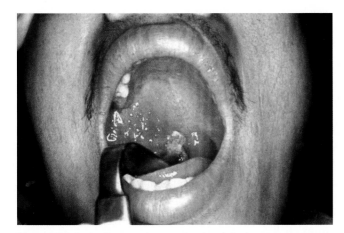

Figure 67.3 Lesion from oropharyngeal anthrax infection. From T. Sirisanthana and A. E. Brown, Anthrax of the gastrointestinal tract. *Emerg. Infect. Dis.* 2002; 8(7): 649–51.

Gram stain of ascitic fluid, oropharyngeal ulcers, or unspun peripheral blood may show gram-positive rods. Leukocytosis with left shift may be present. *B. anthracis* can be cultured from oropharyngeal swabs and stool specimens.

Anthrax Meningitis

Anthrax meningitis can occur as a complication of cutaneous, inhalational, or GI anthrax, but is most commonly seen with inhalational anthrax (up to 50%). Patients may or may not present with symptoms of the primary site of infection. In addition to typical symptoms of bacterial meningitis, anthrax meningitis may involve hemorrhage or meningoencephalitis. Case fatality with anthrax meningitis is greater than 90%. Even one case of anthrax meningitis should alert public health authorities to identify the source of exposure and investigate the possibility of bioterrorism.

Anthrax and Pregnant Women

Maternal and perinatal complications are not completely understood, because anthrax infection is rare, and therefore only a few case reports of infection during pregnancy exist. Preterm delivery may be one of the major complications.

Differential Diagnosis

Because early signs and symptoms are mild and non-specific, a high index of suspicion is necessary to make a timely diagnosis of anthrax. Screening protocols and clinical prediction tools have been proposed and partially evaluated. Prompt administration of antibiotics can be critical to patient survival, hence clinicians should administer appropriate antibiotics as soon as the diagnosis is suspected.

Inhalational Anthrax

Early disease mimics influenza and other respiratory infections. However, nasal symptoms are typically not present and rapid diagnostic tests, such as nasopharyngeal swabs for detection of respiratory virus antigens, would typically be negative.

Key features that distinguish *inhalational* anthrax from other conditions are:

- CXR is abnormal even during early stages of flu-like illness
- CXR or chest CT shows widened mediastinum and pleural effusion, but minimal or no pneumonitis

Characteristics distinguishing inhalational anthrax from influenza are:

- neurological symptoms without headache (e.g. confusion, syncope) and nausea/vomiting are more common in inhalational anthrax
- rhinorrhea and pharyngitis was uncommon in the inhalational anthrax cases from the 2001 US attack

Other conditions to consider are:

- Bacterial pneumonia (*Mycoplasma*, *Staphylococcus*, *Streptococcus*, *Haemophilus*, *Klebsiella*, *Moraxella*, *Legionella*)
- Chlamydia infection
- Influenza
- Other viral pneumonia (respiratory syncytial virus [RSV], cytomegalovirus [CMV], hantavirus)
- Q fever
- Pneumonic plague
- Tularemia
- Primary mediastinitis
- Ruptured aortic aneurysm
- Histoplasmosis
- Coccidioidomycosis
- Silicosis
- Sarcoidosis

Cutaneous Anthrax

Key features that distinguish *cutaneous* anthrax are:

- Painlessness of the lesion itself
- Large extent of local edema

Other conditions to consider include:

- Ecthyma gangrenosum
- Ulceroglandular tularemia
- Bubonic plague
- Cellulitis (staphylococcal or streptococcal)
- Brown recluse spider bite
- Necrotizing soft-tissue infections (e.g. *Streptococcus*, *Clostridium*)
- Coumadin or heparin necrosis
- Rickettsial infection
- Necrotic herpes simplex infection
- Orf virus infection
- Glanders
- Cutaneous leishmaniasis
- Cat scratch fever
- Melioidosis

Gastrointestinal Anthrax

The differential diagnosis for the *intestinal* form of the disease includes:

- Typhoid fever
- Intestinal tularemia
- Acute bacterial gastroenteritis (e.g. *Campylobacter*, *Shigella*, toxicogenic *Escherichia coli*, *Yersinia*)
- Bacterial peritonitis
- Peptic or duodenal ulcer
- Any other causes of acute abdomen

The differential diagnosis for the *oropharyngeal* form of the disease includes:

- Streptococcal pharyngitis
- Infectious mononucleosis
- Diphtheria
- Pharyngeal tularemia
- Other causes of pharyngitis (e.g. enteroviral vesicular, herpetic, anaerobic or Vincent's angina, *Yersinia enterocolitica*)

Anthrax Meningitis

A key feature that distinguishes anthrax meningitis is bloody cerebrospinal fluid (CSF) containing gram-positive bacilli. Other conditions to consider are:

- Subarachnoid hemorrhage
- Bacterial meningitis
- Aseptic meningitis

Laboratory and Radiographic Findings

Diagnosis of anthrax requires a high index and correct use and interpretation of diagnostic tests, ideally in conjunction with public authorities; however, empiric treatment should be started before specific test results return. Routine laboratory and radiographic findings for specific clinical presentations of anthrax are listed in the clinical features tables.

Initial identification and diagnosis of the organism relies on evaluation of infected tissue (blood, sputum, ascites or plural fluid, if present, CSF, fluid collected from an unroofed vesicle, ulcer, eschar, skin lesion scraping, or stool). The gold standard for anthrax diagnosis is direct culture of clinical specimens onto blood agar with demonstration of typical gram stain, motility, and biochemical features. Blood cultures, which are positive nearly 100% of the time in inhalational anthrax, should be obtained prior to antibiotic administration because there is rapid sterilization of blood after a single dose of antibiotics. Because laboratories may view gram-positive bacilli as contaminants and because *B. anthracis* may be a risk to laboratory personnel, clinicians should notify the laboratory when anthrax is suspected.

Although rapid diagnostic tests are not widely available, the public health laboratory system may be able to provide this testing on clinical specimens. Other tests available through the Centers for Disease Control and Prevention (CDC) or the public health laboratory system include polymerase chain reaction (PCR), serologic tests, and immunohistochemistry. Nasal swab cultures have been used to study environmental exposure to aerosolized anthrax; however, they are not recommended for use in the clinical setting. The sensitivity, specificity, and predictive value of nasal swab cultures are not known.

Treatment and Prophylaxis

Treatment of Confirmed or Suspected Anthrax

This section refers to individuals with suspected or confirmed anthrax disease.

The basic components of treatment for anthrax consist of hospitalization with intensive supportive care and IV antibiotics. After obtaining appropriate cultures, antimicrobials should be started *immediately* on suspicion and prior to confirmation of the diagnosis. Patients with inhalational anthrax who received antibiotics within 4.7 days of exposure had a 40% case fatality, compared to a 75% case fatality in those with treatment initiated after 4.7 days.

Because susceptibility data will be delayed, initial antibiotics must be chosen empirically (see Table 67.3). Recommendations for initial empiric therapy of suspected or confirmed anthrax disease are described below. Empiric therapy with at least two agents is recommended because of the potential for infection with strains of *B. anthracis* engineered to be penicillin- and/or tetracycline-resistant. Antibiotic resistance to amoxicillin is of greater concern than resistance to doxycycline or ciprofloxacin; therefore, amoxicillin is not recommended as a first-line agent unless the strain has been proven susceptible. Therapy may be switched to oral antimicrobials when clinically indicated. Therapy should be continued for a total duration of 60 days because spores can persist and then germinate for prolonged periods. There is a possibility that spores could germinate and cause illness up to 100 days after exposure.

Contained Casualty Setting

Parenteral antimicrobial therapy with at least three agents is recommended for *both confirmed anthrax meningitis and for cases in which meningitis cannot be excluded* (see Table 67.3).

Parenteral antimicrobial therapy with at least two agents is recommended for *inhalational and GI anthrax* when individual medical management is available (see Table 67.3). After clinical improvement is noted and a minimum of 2 weeks of parenteral therapy has passed, treatment can be switched to oral therapy for the remainder of the 60 days with ciprofloxacin or doxycycline, based on susceptibilities and clinical considerations (see Table 67.3).

Cutaneous anthrax can be treated with oral antibiotics (see Table 67.3). If in addition to cutaneous lesions there are signs of systemic disease or extensive edema, or if lesions are present on the head or the neck, then the multidrug IV regimen is recommended (see Table 67.3). While a 60-day course is recommended for all cases of bioterrorism-related cutaneous anthrax, only a 7- to 10-day course of treatment is necessary for naturally acquired cutaneous anthrax.

Mass Casualty Setting

Use of oral antibiotics may be necessary if the number of patients exceeds the medical care capacity for individual medical management (see Table 67.3). If pharmaceutical resources permit, therapy with at least two agents is recommended over monotherapy.

Draining of pleural effusions has also been associated with reduced mortality.

Anthrax meningitis can be treated using the inhalational anthrax guidelines; however, IV treatment with a fluoroquinolone plus one to two antimicrobials with good central nervous system (CNS) penetration and activity against *B. anthracis* (e.g. rifampin, vancomycin, penicillin, ampicillin, meropenem) is recommended. The addition of corticosteroids may help manage cerebral edema.

Prophylaxis of Persons Exposed But Without Symptoms

Post-exposure prophylaxis (PEP) is the administration of antibiotics, with or without vaccine, after suspected exposure to anthrax has occurred, but before symptoms are present. (If symptoms are present, see section on treatment, above.) In general, PEP is recommended for persons exposed to an air space or package contaminated with *B. anthracis*. Unvaccinated laboratory workers exposed to *B. anthracis* cultures should also receive PEP. As there is no known person-to-person transmission of inhalational anthrax, prophylaxis should not be offered to contacts of cases, unless also exposed to the original source.

Post-exposure prophylaxis of potential inhalational anthrax consists of oral administration of either ciprofloxacin or doxycycline (see Table 67.3). Therapy should be continued for 60 days. Patients treated for exposure should be informed of the importance of completing the full course of antibiotic prophylaxis regardless of the absence of symptoms. The Food and Drug Administration (FDA) has also approved levofloxacin and penicillin G procaine for PEP of inhalational anthrax. Because of concerns about use of doxycycline or ciprofloxacin in children and about doxycycline use in pregnant women, the CDC has indicated that for prophylaxis, therapy can be

Table 67.3 Anthrax: Treatment and Post-Exposure Prophylaxis Recommendations[1]

	Initial IV Therapy[2, 3] for Systemic Anthrax with Confirmed or Suspected Meningitis	Initial IV Therapy[2, 3] for Systemic Anthrax Without Meningitis Suspected (e.g. Inhalational, GI Anthrax, or Cutaneous Anthrax with Complications[4])	Initial Therapy for Cutaneous Anthrax[2, 4]	Therapy for Anthrax in the Mass Casualty Setting, or Post-Exposure Prophylaxis, or after Clinical Improvement on IV Therapy[5, 6]
Adult	**1st bacteriacidal agent (fluoroquinolone):** Ciprofloxacin, 400 mg IV every 8 hours *or* Levofloxacin 750 mg IV every 24 hours *and* **2nd bactericidal agent (beta-lactam):** Meropenem 2 g IV every 8 hours *or* Imipenem–cilastatin, 1 g IV every 6 hours *and* **3rd agent (protein synthesis inhibitor):** Linezolid 600 mg IV every 12 hours *or* Clindamycin 900 mg IV every 8 hours *or* Chloramphenicol 1 g IV every 6–8 hours	**1st bacteriacidal agent (fluoroquinolone):** Ciprofloxacin 400 mg IV every 8 hours *or* Levofloxacin 750 mg IV every 24 hours *and* **2nd agent (protein synthesis inhibitor):** Linezolid 600 mg IV every 12 hours *or* Clindamycin 900 mg IV every 8 hours *or* Doxycycline 200mg IV × 1, then 100 mg IV every 12 hours *or* Rifampin 600 mg IV every 12 hours	Ciprofloxacin 500 mg PO BID for 60 days *or* Doxycycline 100 mg PO BID for 60 days	Ciprofloxacin[9] 500 mg PO BID for 60 days *or* Doxycycline[10] 100 mg PO BID for 60 days
Children (Age: 1 month and older)	**1st bacteriacidal agent (fluoroquinolone):** Ciprofloxacin[11, 12] 30 mg/kg/dose IV divided every 8 hours (max. 400 mg/dose) *or* Levofloxacin: >50 kg, 500 mg IV every 24 hours <50 kg 10mg/kg/dose IV every 12 hours (max. 250 mg/dose) **2nd bactericidal agent (beta-lactam):** Meropenem 40 mg/kg/dose IV every 8 hours (max 2 g) *or* Imipenem 25 mg/kg/dose IV every 6 hours *and* **3rd agent (protein synthesis inhibitor):** Linezolid: <12 years: 10 mg/kg/dose IV every 8 hours ≥12 years: 15 mg/kg/dose IV every 12 hours (max 600 mg) *or*	**1st bacteriacidal agent (fluoroquinolone):** Ciprofloxacin[11, 12] 30 mg/kg/day IV divided every 8 hours (not to exceed 400 mg/dose) *or* Levofloxacin: <50 kg, 20 mg/kg/day IV divided every 8 hours (not to exceed 250 mg/ dose) >50 kg, 500 mg IV every 24 hours *plus* **2nd agent (protein synthesis inhibitor):** Clindamycin 40 mg/kg/day IV divided every 8 hours (not to exceed 900 mg/dose) *or* Linezolid: <12 years old, 30 mg/kg/day IV divided every 8 hours >12 years old, 30 mg/kg/day IV divided every 12 hours (not to exceed 600 mg/dose) *or* Doxycycline[7, 12, 13]: <45 kg, 4.4 mg/kg/day IV loading dose (not to exceed 200 mg) >45 kg, 200 mg IV loading dose *then* <45 kg, 4.4 mg/kg/day IV divided every 12 hours (not to exceed 100 mg/dose) >45 kg, 100 mg IV given every 12 hours *or* Rifampin 20 mg/kg/day IV divided every 12 hours (not to exceed 300 mg/dose)	Ciprofloxacin 15 mg/kg/dose PO BID (max. 500 mg/dose) for 60 days *or* Doxycycline[7, 12, 13]: ≥45 kg, give 100 mg PO BID for 60 days <45 kg, give 2.2 mg/kg PO BID (max. 200 mg/day) for 60 days	Ciprofloxacin[9] 15 mg/kg PO BID (max. 500 mg/dose) for 60 days *or* Doxycycline[10]: ≥45 kg, give 100 mg PO BID for 60 days <45 kg, give 2.2 mg/kg PO BID (max. 200 mg/day) for 60 days *or* Amoxicillin[14]: 25 mg/kg/dose PO TID for 60 days (not to exceed 1 g/dose)

(continued)

Table 67.3 (cont.)

	Initial IV Therapy[2, 3] for Systemic Anthrax with Confirmed or Suspected Meningitis	Initial IV Therapy[2, 3] for Systemic Anthrax Without Meningitis Suspected (e.g. Inhalational, GI Anthrax, or Cutaneous Anthrax with Complications[4])	Initial Therapy for Cutaneous Anthrax[2, 4]	Therapy for Anthrax in the Mass Casualty Setting, or Post-Exposure Prophylaxis, or after Clinical Improvement on IV Therapy[5, 6]
	Clindamycin 13.3 mg/kg/dose IV every 8 hours *or* Chloramphenicol 25 mg/kg/dose IV every 6 hours			
Pregnant women	Same as for non-pregnant adults[15]	Same as for non-pregnant adults[15]	Same as for non-pregnant adults[15]	Same as for non-pregnant adults *or* Amoxicillin[14] 500 mg PO TID for 60 days
Immuno-compromised persons	Same as for non-immunocompromised persons and children	Same as for non-immunocompromised persons and children	Same as for non-immunocompromised persons and children	Same as for non-immunocompromised persons and children

[1] The treatment recommendations included in this table are adapted from guidance during the 2001 anthrax outbreaks. Therapy recommendations in other situations should be guided by antimicrobial susceptibility.

[2] Ciprofloxacin or doxycycline should be considered an essential part of first-line therapy for inhalational anthrax.

[3] Steroids may be considered an adjunct therapy for patients with severe edema and for meningitis based on experience with bacterial meningitis of other etiologies.

[4] Cutaneous anthrax cases with signs of systemic involvement, extensive edema, or lesions on the head or neck require intravenous therapy, and a multidrug approach is recommended.

[5] Initial therapy may be altered based on clinical course of patient; one or two antimicrobial agents (e.g. ciprofloxacin or doxycycline) may be adequate as patient improves.

[6] If pharmaceutical resources permit in a mass casualty setting, therapy with at least two agents is recommended over monotherapy.

[7] If meningitis is suspected, doxycycline may be less optimal because of poor central nervous system penetration.

[8] Because of concerns of constitutive and inducible beta-lactamases in *Bacillus anthracis* isolates, penicillin and ampicillin should not be used alone. Consultation with an infectious disease specialist is advised.

[9] In vitro studies suggest that ofloxacin (400 mg orally every 12 hours) or levafloxacin (500 mg orally every 24 hours) could be used in place of ciprofloxacin – if supplies were limited in a mass casualty or post-exposure prophylaxis situation.

[10] In vitro studies suggest that 500 mg of tetracycline orally every 6 hours could be used in place of doxycycline – if supplies were limited in a mass casualty or post-exposure prophylaxis situation.

[11] If intravenous ciprofloxacin is not available, oral ciprofloxacin may be acceptable because it is rapidly and well absorbed from the gastrointestinal tract with no substantial loss by first-pass metabolism. Maximum serum concentrations are attained 1 to 2 hours after oral dosing, but may not be achieved if vomiting or ileus is present.

[12] Tetracycline and quinolone antibiotics are generally not recommended during pregnancy or childhood; however, their use may be indicated for life-threatening illness. Ciprofloxacin may be preferred in pregnant women and children up to 8 years of age because of the known adverse event profile of doxycycline (e.g. tooth discoloration). Doxycycline may be preferred in children 8 years and older because of the adverse event profile of ciprofloxacin (e.g. arthropathies).

[13] The American Academy of Pediatrics recommends treatment of young children with tetracyclines for serious infections (e.g. Rocky Mountain spotted fever).

[14] Amoxicillin is not approved by the FDA for post-exposure prophylaxis or treatment of anthrax. However, the CDC has indicated that if the isolate is determined to be susceptible to amoxicillin, it could be used for pregnant women and children for post-exposure prophylaxis or for completion of 60 days' antibiotic therapy after initial treatment with ciprofloxacin or doxycycline. Amoxicillin resistance to anthrax is of greater concern than that of doxycycline or ciprofloxacin, and amoxicillin is not recommended as a first-line agent unless the isolate is proven to be susceptible.

[15] Although tetracyclines are not recommended for pregnant women, their use may be indicated for life-threatening illness. Adverse effects on developing teeth and bones are dose-related; therefore, doxycycline might be used for a short time (7 to 14 days) before 6 months of gestation.

Adapted from: Centers for Disease Control and Prevention, Investigation of bioterrorism-related anthrax and interim guidelines for exposure management and antimicrobial therapy. *MMWR Morb. Mortal. Wkly. Rep.* 2001; 50(42): 909–19; Centers for Disease Control and Prevention, Update: Investigation of anthrax associated with intentional exposure and interim public health guidelines. *MMWR Morb. Mortal. Wkly. Rep.* 2001; 50(41): 889–93; Hendricks, K. A., Wright, M. E., Shadomy, S. V., *et al.* Center for Disease Control and Prevention expert panel meetings on prevention and treatment of anthrax in adults. *Emerg. Infect. Dis.* 2014; 20(2): doi: 10.3201/eid2002.130687; Bradley, J. S., Peacock, G., Krug, S. E., *et al.* Pediatric anthrax clinical management. *Pediatrics* 2014; 133(5): e1411–36.

switched to amoxicillin in these groups if the isolate is determined to be susceptible. Amoxicillin may also be considered for patients allergic to both ciprofloxacin and doxycycline.

The Advisory Committee on Immunization Practices recommends the use of combined antimicrobial prophylaxis and vaccine (Biothrax [formerly Anthrax vaccine absorbed, AVA]). Biothrax is not licensed for this use by the FDA and would need to be given under an Investigational New Drug (IND) application. The recommended regimen is three vaccine doses (given at 0, 2, and 4 weeks after exposure) and at least a 60-day course of antimicrobial therapy. The CDC does not recommend vaccination in pregnant women given lack of data.

Following the 2001 attacks, exposed persons were given the option of: (1) 60 days of antibiotic prophylaxis; (2) 100 days of antibiotic prophylaxis; and (3) 100 days of antibiotic prophylaxis, plus anthrax vaccine (under IND protocol).

Anthrax Vaccine

The anthrax vaccine Biothrax is available, but only in limited supply that is controlled by federal authorities. It is an inactivated cell-free filtrate of an avirulent strain of *B. anthracis*. Local reactions and mild systemic reactions are common. Severe allergic reactions are rare (<1 per 100,000).

The anthrax vaccine is licensed for pre-exposure use to prevent cutaneous anthrax in healthy, non-pregnant adults 18 to 65 years of age who have a high likelihood of coming into contact with anthrax, including certain laboratory workers and animal-processing workers. Biothrax is not currently licensed for post-exposure use and must be given in this context under an FDA investigational drug protocol. The CDC may recommend its use for PEP under some circumstances. Research is underway on new anthrax vaccines.

Other Anthrax Therapeutics

Additional therapeutic candidates for treatment and prophylaxis of anthrax are Anthrax Immune Globulin Intravenous (Human) (Anthrasil), and raxibacumab (ABthrax). Both are FDA approved and use antibodies to neutralize anthrax toxin. The Department of Health and Human Services has purchased the antibody-based therapeutic immune globulin (AIG) and ABthrax for the strategic national stockpile.

Complications and Admission Criteria

Without early antibiotic treatment, inhalational anthrax progresses to pneumonitis marked by severe respiratory distress and cyanosis, and often accompanied by pleural effusion. Patients with anthrax pneumonitis are particularly likely to develop septicemia and septic shock due to hematogenous dissemination of the bacteria. Sepsis may develop as a complication of cutaneous anthrax or gastrointestinal anthrax as well. Anthrax meningitis may occur as a consequence of hematogenous dissemination.

Patients with suspected or confirmed inhalational, gastrointestinal, or meningeal anthrax, as well as those with cutaneous anthrax who exhibit head or neck lesions, extensive edema, or systemic signs of illness, require admission for intravenous antibiotic therapy and supportive care.

Infection Control

Both the HICPAC (Hospital Infection Control Practices Advisory Committee) of the CDC and the Working Group for Civilian Biodefense recommend standard precautions for anthrax patients in a hospital setting without the need for isolation. Person-to-person transmission has only rarely been reported for patients with cutaneous anthrax and standard precautions are considered adequate. Importantly, routine laboratory procedures should be carried out under Biosafety Level 2 (BSL-2) conditions. Clinicians should notify local public health authorities, their institution's infection control professional, and their laboratory of any suspected anthrax cases. Public health authorities may conduct epidemiologic investigations and implement disease control interventions to protect the public.

Decontamination

Contaminated surfaces can be disinfected with commercially available bleach or a 1:10 dilution of household bleach and water. All persons exposed to an aerosol containing *B. anthracis* should be instructed to wash body surfaces and clothing with soap and water.

Pearls and Pitfalls

1. The initial (prodromal) phase of inhalational anthrax resembles an influenza-like syndrome and can be difficult to distinguish from seasonal respiratory illnesses. Nasal congestion and rhinorrhea, however, are common features of seasonal influenza-like syndromes and are unusual with pulmonary anthrax.
2. The classic radiographic findings of inhalational anthrax – CXR showing a widened mediastinum (due to hilar lymphadenopathy) and pulmonary effusion – though not unique to anthrax, should nonetheless prompt a high level of clinical suspicion.
3. The necrotic, edematous, eschar-covered skin lesion of cutaneous anthrax is usually painless, which is an important differentiating feature from a brown recluse spider bite.

References

Bales, M. E., Dannenberg, A. L., Brachman, P. S., *et al.* Epidemiologic response to anthrax outbreaks: field investigations, 1950–2001. *Emerg. Infect. Dis.* 2002; 8(10): 1163–74.

Bell, D. M., Kozarsky, P. E., and Stephens, D. S. Clinical issues in the prophylaxis, diagnosis, and treatment of anthrax. *Emerg. Infect. Dis.* 2002; 8(2): 222–5.

Centers for Disease Control and Prevention (CDC). Anthrax, available at www.cdc.gov/anthrax/ (accessed March 9, 2018).

CDC. Inhalation anthrax associated with dried animal hides – Pennsylvania and New York City, 2006. *MMWR Morb. Mortal. Wkly. Rep.* 2006; 55(10): 280–2.

CDC. Investigation of bioterrorism-related anthrax and interim guidelines for exposure management and antimicrobial therapy, October 2001. *MMWR Morb. Mortal. Wkly. Rep.* 2001; 50(42): 909–19.

CDC. Suspected cutaneous anthrax in a laboratory worker – Texas 2002. *MMWR Morb. Mortal. Wkly. Rep.* 2002; 51(13): 279–81.

CDC. Use of Anthrax vaccine in the United States: Recommendations of the Advisory Committee on Immunization Practices (ACIP), 2009. *MMWR Morb. Mortal. Wkly. Rep.* 2010; 59(RR06): 1–30.

CDC. Considerations for anthrax vaccine absorbed (AVA) postexposure prioritization final (2013), available at www.cdc.gov/anthrax/medical-care/prevention.html (accessed March 19, 2018).

Food and Drug Administration (FDA). Anthrasil [anthrax immune globulin intravenous (human)] www.fda.gov/biologicsbloodvaccines/bloodbloodproducts/approvedproducts/licensedproductsblas/fractionatedplasmaproducts/ucm441234.htm (accessed March 19, 2018).

FDA. Raxibacumab (2012), retrieved March 19, 2018, from www.accessdata.fda.gov/drugsatfda_docs/label/2012/125349s000lbl.pdf.

Freedman, A., Afonja, O., Chang, M. W., *et al.* Cutaneous anthrax associated with microangiopathic hemolytic anemia and coagulopathy in a 7-month-old infant. *JAMA* 2002; 287(7): 869–74.

Hendricks, K. A., Wright, M. E., Shadomy, S. V., *et al.* Centers for Disease Control and Prevention expert panel meetings on prevention and treatment of anthrax in adults. *Emerg. Infect. Dis.* 2014, available at http://dx.doi.org/10.3201/eid2002.130687 (accessed March 20, 2018).

Holty, J. E., Kim, R. Y., and Bravata, D. M. Systematic review: a century of inhalational anthrax cases from 1900 to 2005. *Ann. Intern. Med.* 2006; 144(4): 270–80.

Howell, J. M., Mayer, T. A., Hanfling, D., *et al.* Screening for inhalational anthrax due to bioterrorism: evaluating proposed screening protocols. *Clin. Infect. Dis.* 2004; 39(12): 1842–7.

Huang, E., Pillai, S. K., Bower, W. A., *et. al.* Antitoxin treatment of inhalation anthrax: a systematic review. *Health Security.* 2015; 13(6): 365–77.

Jernigan, J. A., Stephens, D. S., Ashford, D. A., *et al.* Bioterrorism-related inhalational anthrax: the first 10 cases reported in the United States. *Emerg. Infect. Dis.* 2001; 7(6): 933–44.

Kadanali, A., Tasyaran, M. A., and Kadanali, S. Anthrax during pregnancy: case reports and review. *Clin. Infect. Dis.* 2003; 36(10): 1343–6.

Meaney-Delmam, D., Zotti, M. E., Creanga, A. A., *et al.* Centers for Disease Control and Prevention. Special considerations for prophylaxis for and treatment of anthrax in pregnant and postpartum women. *Emerg. Infect. Dis.* 2014, available at wwwnc.cdc.gov/eid/article/20/2/13-0611_article (accessed March 20, 2018).

Meyerhoff, A. and Murphy, D. Guidelines for treatment of anthrax. *JAMA* 2002; 288(15): 1848–9; author reply 1848–9.22.

Sejvar, J. J., Tenover, F. C., and Stephens, D. S. Management of anthrax meningitis. *Lancet Infect. Dis.* 2005; 5(5): 287–95.

Sirisanthana, T. and Brown, A. E. Anthrax of the gastrointestinal tract. *Emerg. Infect. Dis.* 2002; 8(7): 649–51.

Swartz, M. N. Recognition and management of anthrax – an update. *N. Engl. J. Med.* 2001; 345(22): 1621–6.

Additional Readings

Center for Infectious Disease Research and Policy. Anthrax: current, comprehensive information on pathogenesis, microbiology, epidemiology, diagnosis, treatment, and prophylaxis (CIDRAP, 2006), retrieved March 20, 2018 from www.cidrap.umn.edu/infectious-disease-topics/anthrax.

Dixon, T. C., Meselson, M., Guillemin, J., *et al.* Anthrax. *N. Engl. J. Med.* 1999; 341(11): 815–26.

Inglesby, T. V., O'Toole, T., Henderson, D. A., *et al.* Anthrax as a biological weapon, 2002: updated recommendations for management. *JAMA* 2002; 287(17): 2236–52.

Martin, G. J. and Friedlander, A. M. *Bacillus anthracis* (anthrax) in J. E. Bennett, R. Dolin, and M. J. Blaser (eds.), *Mandell, Douglas, and Bennett's Principles and Practice of Infectious Diseases*, 8th edn. (Philadelphia, PA: Elsevier/Saunders, 2015), pp. 2391–409.

Plague

David M. Stier and Mary P. Mercer

Outline

Introduction

Plague is an acute bacterial infection caused by *Yersinia pestis*, a member of the family Enterobacteriaceae. *Y. pestis* is a pleomorphic, non-motile, non-sporulating, intracellular, gram-negative bacillus that has a characteristic bipolar appearance on Wright, Giemsa, and Wayson's stains. There are three virulent biovars – *antiqua*, *mediaevalis*, and *orientalis* – and a fourth avirulent biovar, *microtus*. The *orientalis* biovar is thought to have originated in southern China and caused the most recent pandemic.

The Working Group for Civilian Biodefense considers plague to be a potential biological weapon because of the pathogen's availability "around the world, capacity for its mass production and aerosol dissemination, difficulty in preventing such activities, high fatality rate of pneumonic plague, and potential for secondary spread of cases during an epidemic." Of the potential ways in which *Y. pestis* could be used as a biological weapon, aerosol release would be most likely. This method has been successfully demonstrated to cause disease in rhesus macaques.

Epidemiology

Reservoirs

The natural reservoir for *Y. pestis* is primarily wild rodents. Around the world, the domestic rat has been associated with the most human cases; however, in the western United States,

burrowing rodents (e.g. ground squirrels, rock squirrels, and prairie dogs) are the most important reservoir. Mammals that act as hosts include cats, goats, sheep, camels, and humans. Human plague cases often follow epizootics in local rodent populations.

Mode of Transmission

Humans can become infected in a number of ways:

*   bite of infected rat flea
*   direct contact with infected draining buboes
*   direct contact (including bites or scratches) with infected animals
*   inhalation of respiratory droplets from pneumonic plague-infected humans or animals (within 2 meters)
*   ingestion of bacteria (e.g. eating infected meat)

Human plague cases in nature are most commonly acquired from animal reservoirs via bites of the Oriental rat flea.

Worldwide Occurrence

The first recorded plague pandemic was the Justinian plague (541 to 767 AD), which caused approximately 100 million deaths and is thought to have contributed to the demise of the Roman Empire. The second pandemic, also known as the Black Death, lasted from the fourteenth to the nineteenth centuries and was estimated to have killed between a third and a half of Europe's population. The third and most recent pandemic began in 1894 in China and caused an estimated 12 million deaths. Recent outbreaks in humans have included India (1994), Zambia (1996), Indonesia (1997), Algeria (2003), Uganda (2004), and the Congo (2005). Approximately 1,800 worldwide cases of plague are reported annually to the World Health Organization (WHO), from all continents except Europe and Australia.

Occurrence in the United States

Ships carrying infected rats introduced plague to the Americas via the ports on the Pacific Ocean and Gulf of Mexico in the early 1900s. In San Francisco, urban rats passed the disease to native rodent populations. Eventually, plague spread across the western half of the United States and has been found in the native rodent population, their fleas, and their predators. Naturally occurring plague generally occurs during the summer months in persons exposed to the reservoir. The last urban plague outbreak in the United States occurred in Los Angeles in 1925.

From 1990 to 2005, there has been a median of seven cases of plague reported per year in the United States. In 2006, there were 16 cases based on provisional data.

Plague as a Biological Weapon

In the twentieth century, countries such as the United States, the former Soviet Union, and Japan developed ways for using *Y. pestis* as a weapon. Creating aerosolized plague is technically challenging; however, if an intentional release of aerosolized plague were to take place, an outbreak of pneumonic plague would be likely. This would be of serious concern because of the high case-fatality rate and the potential for person-to-person transmission.

An intentional release of *Y. pestis* would have the following characteristics:

- Clustering in time: multiple similarly presenting cases of severe, progressive multilobar pneumonia, generally 2 to 4 days after release (range of 1 to 6 days)
- Atypical host characteristics: unexpected, unexplained cases of acute illness in previously healthy persons who rapidly develop severe, progressive multilobar pneumonia with hemoptysis and gastrointestinal symptoms
- Unusual geographic clustering: multiple cases in an urban area where naturally occurring plague is not endemic
- Absence of risk factors: patients lack plague exposure risk factors (e.g. recent flea bite; exposure to rodents, especially rabbits, squirrels, wood rats, chipmunks, or prairie dogs; scratches or bites from infected domestic cats)

Intentionally released *Y. pestis* strains may be altered to have enhanced virulence, antimicrobial resistance, or increased ability to evade vaccines and diagnostic tests.

Clinical Features

Human plague occurs in many forms, determined primarily by the route of infection. The most common forms of plague in humans are bubonic plague, septicemic plague, and pneumonic plague. These are presented in detail below.

Table 68.1 Clinical Features: Pneumonic Plague

Incubation period	1–4 days, with a maximum of 6 days
Transmission	• Inhalation of contaminated aerosol • Inhalation of respiratory droplets from pneumonic plague-infected humans or animals (within 2 meters) • Secondary hematogenous spread to the lung
Signs and symptoms	• Acute fever, chills, malaise, myalgia, headache • Productive cough, with sputum becoming increasingly bloody • Chest pain, dyspnea, cyanosis • Tachypnea in children • Gastrointestinal symptoms
Progression and complications	• Refractory pulmonary syndrome • Adult respiratory distress syndrome • Septicemia
Laboratory and radiographic findings	• Leukocytosis with left shift • Gram-negative bipolar bacilli on sputum smear • Elevated creatinine and abnormally high liver enzymes • CXR findings include alveolar infiltrates progressing to lobar consolidation, pleural effusion • Rarely, mediastinal widening on CXR due to adenopathy

CXR – chest X-ray.

Plague infection is a severe clinical illness that can be life-threatening. Case fatality rates vary based on the route of infection. Mortality was historically much higher with nearly 100% mortality for untreated septicemic and pneumonic plague and 50 to 60% mortality for untreated bubonic plague cases. Administration of appropriate antibiotic treatment within the first 18 to 24 hours has decreased mortality rates to 30 to 50% for septicemic plague, 5 to 15% for bubonic plague, and less than 5% for pneumonic plague. Thus, early administration of appropriate antibiotic treatment is critical, because poor outcomes occur with delays in seeking care and/or instituting effective antimicrobial treatment.

Pneumonic Plague

Primary pneumonic plague (see Table 68.1) occurs when the organism is inhaled in respiratory droplets from infected humans or animals or in infectious aerosols accidentally or intentionally produced (e.g. spilled lab specimen or bioterrorism-related release). Secondary pneumonic plague occurs when there is hematogenous spread of the organism to the lung. Primary pneumonic plague causes a more acute and fulminant disease. Pneumonic plague is not highly contagious, but transmission can occur with prolonged close contact (within 2 meters) with a coughing patient in the end stage of illness. In a recent outbreak in Uganda, 1.3 pneumonic plague transmissions per pneumonic plague case were reported. If untreated, pneumonic plague can spread and progress to bubonic or septicemic plague.

Table 68.2 Clinical Features: Bubonic Plague

Incubation period	1–8 days
Transmission	• Bite of infected rat flea • Direct contact with infected draining buboes • Direct contact (including bites or scratches) with infected animals
Signs and symptoms	**Major:** • Sudden onset of chills, high fever, headache, lethargy • Buboes – swollen, red, painful lymph nodes in areas proximal to the inoculation site (e.g. inguinal, axillary, or cervical areas) • Rapid pulse • Hypotension **Other:** • Gastrointestinal discomfort • Restlessness, confusion, lack of coordination • Skin lesion at the site of the flea bite occur in <10% of cases • Buboes may rupture and suppurate in second week
Progression and complications	• Septicemia • Secondary pneumonic plague • Meningitis (rare)
Laboratory findings	• Leukocytosis with left shift • Gram-negative bipolar bacilli on bubo aspirate smear • Elevated creatinine and abnormally high liver enzymes

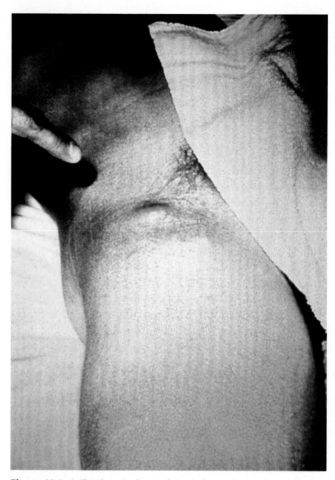

Figure 68.1 Axillary lymphadenopathy, or bubo, and edema caused by plague infection.

From the US Centers for Disease Control and Prevention Public Health Information Library at http://phil.cdc.gov/phil/home.asp. Photograph taken in 1962 by Margaret Parsons and Dr. Karl F. Meyer.

Bubonic Plague

Yersinia pestis can cause bubonic plague in humans via the bite of an infected rodent flea (See Table 68.2). *Y. pestis* survives in the flea midgut after a blood meal from an infected host. The organism is transmitted to a new host when the flea regurgitates during its next feeding. *Y. pestis* migrates to regional lymph nodes where it causes hemorrhagic lymphadenitis, creating the swollen, painful buboes that are characteristic of bubonic plague (see Figures 68.1 and 68.2). The organisms often enter the bloodstream, causing hemorrhagic lesions in distant lymph nodes and organs. If untreated, bubonic plague can spread and progress to pneumonic or septicemic plague. Approximately 80% of cases develop bacteremia, 25% develop clinical septicemia, and 10% develop pneumonia as a complication.

Septicemic Plague

In primary septicemic plague, there is systemic sepsis caused by *Y. pestis*, but without noticeable, preceding lymph node or pulmonary involvement. Up to 25% of naturally occurring plague cases may present with primary septicemic plague (see Figures 68.3 and 68.4). Secondary septicemic plague occurs commonly with either bubonic or pneumonic plague.

Septicemic plague causes a gram-negative sepsis syndrome with multi-organ involvement, disseminated intravascular coagulation (DIC), and shock (see Table 68.3). In the late stages of infection, high-grade bacteremia often occurs, with

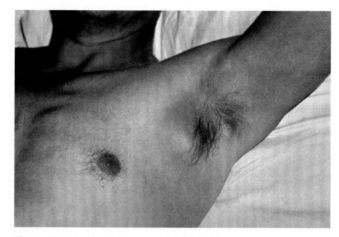

Figure 68.2 Inguinal bubo caused by plague infection.

From the US Centers for Disease Control and Prevention Public Health Information Library at http://phil.cdc.gov/phil/home.asp.

identifiable organisms on peripheral blood smear. Meningitis can occur and is characterized by purulent exudates in cerebrospinal fluid (CSF).

Table 68.3 Clinical Features: Septicemic Plague

Incubation period	1–4 days
Transmission	Site of primary infection may be unknown
Signs and symptoms	• Acute fever, chills, weakness, malaise • Gastrointestinal symptoms • Purpuric skin lesions and gangrene of the distal digits
Progression and complications	• Disseminated intravascular coagulation • Shock • Multi-organ failure
Laboratory findings	• Leukocytosis with left shift and toxic granulation • Gram-negative bipolar bacilli on blood smear • Disseminated intravascular coagulation • Elevated creatinine and abnormally high liver enzymes

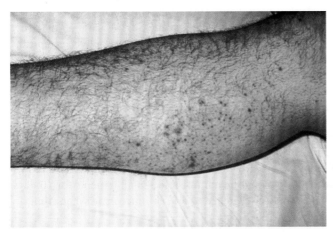

Figure 68.3 Skin hemorrhages due to capillary fragility on the leg of a person with plague.

From the US Centers for Disease Control and Prevention Public Health Information Library at http://phil.cdc.gov/phil/home.asp.

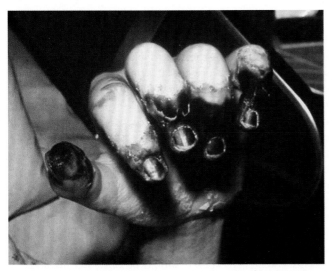

Figure 68.4 Acral necrosis due to abnormal coagulation caused by plague septicemia.

From the US Centers for Disease Control and Prevention Public Health Information Library at http://phil.cdc.gov/phil/home.asp. Photograph taken in 1975 by Dr. Jack Poland.

Other syndromes caused by *Y. pestis* infection include:

- Plague meningitis: Although it is generally a complication of other forms of plague, it can be the presenting clinical syndrome. Plague meningitis results from hematogenous spread of *Y. pestis* organisms. Meningitis is characterized by purulent CSF exudates.
- Plague pharyngitis: Plague pharyngitis generally results from direct inoculation of the pharynx. Eating raw infected meat is a risk factor. Clinically, plague pharyngitis presents as a severe pharyngitis or tonsillitis with cervical adenitis.
- Pestis minor: Pestis minor is a milder form of bubonic plague. Lymph nodes drain and patients convalesce without treatment.

Differential Diagnosis

The diagnosis of plague during the initial stages requires a high index of suspicion because of the non-specific, flu-like picture early in the disease. Early diagnosis is desirable because prompt administration of antibiotics can be critical to survival.

Pneumonic Plague

Consider pneumonic plague in any case of severe gram-negative pneumonia.

Key features that may help to distinguish plague pneumonia are:

Primary pneumonic plague:

- Rapid onset and rapid progression

Secondary pneumonic plague:

- Presence of painful adenitis (buboes)

Primary or secondary pneumonic plague:

- No response to typical antibiotic therapy for community-acquired pneumonia
- Hemoptysis in late stages of disease

Other conditions to consider are:

- Bacterial pneumonia (*Mycoplasma, Legionella, Staphylococcus, Streptococcus, Haemophilus, Klebsiella, Moraxella*)
- Viral pneumonia (influenza, respiratory syncytial virus [RSV], cytomegalovirus [CMV], hantavirus, severe acute respiratory syndrome [SARS])
- Chlamydia infection
- Q fever
- Inhalation anthrax
- Tularemia
- Ricin
- Rickettsial infections
- Aerosolized exposure to staphylococcal enterotoxin B

Bubonic Plague

A key feature that may help to distinguish bubonic plague is:

- Presence of painful adenitis (buboes) progressing to systemic disease

Other conditions to consider are:

- Cat scratch disease (*Bartonella*)
- Ulceroglandular tularemia
- Adenitis due to staphylococcal, streptococcal, or filarial infection
- Tuberculosis
- Non-tuberculosis mycobacterial infection
- Lymphogranuloma venereum
- Capnocytophaga canimorsus infection
- Chancroid
- Primary genital herpes
- Primary or secondary syphilis
- Appendicitis
- Strangulated inguinal or femoral hernia
- Lymphadenopathy (secondary lymphoma, Kikuchi's lymphadenitis, systemic lupus erythematosus, toxoplasmosis, infectious mononucleosis)

Septicemic Plague

Key features that may help to distinguish septicemic plague are as follows:

Primary septicemic plague:

- Absence of painful adenitis (buboes) or pulmonary involvement

Secondary septicemic plague:

- Presence of painful adenitis (buboes)

Other conditions to consider are:

- Gram-negative sepsis
- Gram-positive sepsis (*Staphylococcus*)
- Meningococcemia
- Rickettsial infections
- Malaria
- Louse-borne relapsing fever
- Appendicitis

Laboratory and Radiographic Findings

Routine laboratory and radiographic findings for specific clinical presentations of plague are listed in the clinical features tables.

Initial identification of the organism relies on microscopic evaluation of infected tissue (blood, sputum, cerebrospinal fluid [CSF], or fluid aspirated from a bubo or skin lesion scraping). Staining of the infected tissue may reveal gram-negative bacilli (gram) and bipolar staining (Wright, Giemsa, or Wayson).

Although recommended, culture and isolation may be difficult. Blood and site-specific specimens should be collected prior to antibiotic administration as sterilization can occur rapidly. *Y. pestis* is slow-growing in culture and may not demonstrate growth until 48 hours after inoculation. Also, many commercial bacterial identification systems may misidentify *Y. pestis*. To improve yield and ensure biosafety precautions, clinicians should notify laboratory personnel when plague is suspected.

Although rapid diagnostic tests are not widely available, the public health laboratory system may have rapid diagnostic testing on clinical specimens (e.g. polymerase chain reaction [PCR] or direct fluorescent antibody testing for *Y. pestis* F1 antigen).

Treatment and Prophylaxis

Treatment

Supportive care and timely administration of antibiotics are the keys to successful management of plague (see Table 68.4). Plague pneumonia is often fatal if antibiotics are not begun within 12 to 24 hours of symptoms. Many patients would be expected to require intensive care with respiratory support owing to complications of gram-negative sepsis.

Resistant strains may occur either naturally or intentionally. In 1995, two distinct strains of naturally occurring antibiotic-resistant *Y. pestis* were isolated from human cases of bubonic plague in Madagascar. One strain was resistant to all drugs recommended for plague treatment and prophylaxis, and the other had high-level resistance to streptomycin. Both patients recovered with oral trimethoprim-sulfamethoxazole and intramuscular injections of streptomycin. In addition, in vitro resistance has been seen to imipenem and rifampin.

Contained Casualty Setting

The Working Group recommends parenteral antimicrobial therapy when individual medical management is available. IV antibiotics should be administered to all patients for 10 days. Therapy may be switched to oral antimicrobials when clinically indicated.

Mass Casualty Setting

Replacement with oral antibiotics may be needed if the number of patients exceeds the medical care capacity for individual medical management.

Post-Exposure Prophylaxis

Post-exposure prophylaxis is the administration of antibiotics after suspected exposure to plague has occurred, but before symptoms are present. If symptoms are present, see section above on treatment. Persons thought to have had an infective exposure should receive post-exposure prophylaxis. Infective exposures include household, hospital, or other close contact (less than 2 meters) with a person suspected or confirmed to have pneumonic plague who has received no treatment, less than 48 hours of antimicrobial therapy, or more than 48 hours of antimicrobial therapy without clinical improvement. Post-exposure prophylaxis may be recommended for persons exposed to intentional aerosol releases. In such an event, public health authorities will provide guidance. Regardless of whether post-exposure prophylaxis is recommended or taken, persons potentially exposed should be observed for fever or cough for 7 days after exposure. Any potentially exposed person who develops a fever or cough should seek prompt medical attention and begin treatment. Quarantine is not currently recommended.

Table 68.4 Plague: Treatment and Post-Exposure Prophylaxis Recommendations[1]

		Contained Casualty Setting	Mass Casualty Setting	Post-Exposure Prophylaxis
Duration of Prescription		10 days	10 days	7 days
Adult	Preferred	Streptomycin 1 g IM every 12 hours *or* Gentamicin[2] 5 mg/kg IM/IV every 24 hours	Doxycycline 100 mg PO BID *or* Ciprofloxacin 500 mg PO BID	
	Alternative[8]	Doxycycline[5, 6] 100 mg IV every 12 hours *or* Ciprofloxacin 400 mg IV every 12 hours *or* Chloramphenicol[3] 25 mg/kg IV every 6 hours (max. 4 g/day)	Chloramphenicol[3] 25 mg/kg PO QID (max. 4 g/day)	
Children	Preferred	Streptomycin 15 mg/kg IM every 12 hours (max. 2 g/day) *or* Gentamicin[2] 2.5 mg/kg IM IV every 8 hours	Doxycycline[5, 6]: ≥45 kg, give adult dosage <45 kg, give 2.2 mg/kg PO BID (max. 200 mg/day) *or* Ciprofloxacin,[5, 7] 20 mg/kg/dose PO BID (max. 1 g/day)	
	Alternative[8]	Doxycycline[5, 6]: ≥45 kg, give adult dosage <45 kg, give 2.2 mg/kg IV every 12 hours (max. 200 mg/day) *or* Ciprofloxacin,[5, 7] 10 mg/kg IV every 12 hours (max. 1 g/day) *or* Chloramphenicol[3, 4] 25 mg/kg IV every 6 hours (max. 4 g/day)	Chloramphenicol[3, 4] 25 mg/kg PO QID (max. 4 g/day)	
Pregnant women	Preferred	Gentamicin[2] 5 mg/kg IM/IV every 24 hours	Doxycycline 100 mg PO BID *or* Ciprofloxacin 500 mg PO BID	
	Alternative[8]	Doxycycline[5, 6] 100 mg IV every 12 hours *or* Ciprofloxacin[5] 400 mg IV every 12 hours	Chloramphenicol[3, 4] 25 mg/kg PO QID (max. 4 g/day)	

For plague meningitis, pleuritis, or myocarditis: chloramphenicol should be used for 21 days for conditions when tissue penetration is important. Irreversible marrow aplasia is rare (1 in 40,000 patients).

[1] Treatment recommendations come from the Working Group of Civilian Biodefense and may not necessarily be approved by the US Food and Drug Administration.

[2] Aminoglycoside doses must be further adjusted for newborns, and according to renal function.

[3] Therapeutic concentration is 5–20 µg/mL; concentrations >25 µg/mL can cause reversible bone marrow suppression.

[4] According to the Working Group on Civilian Biodefense, children younger than 2 years of age should not receive chloramphenicol because of risk of "gray baby syndrome"; however, the American Academy of Pediatrics has recommended chloramphenicol as the drug of choice for plague meningitis in children.

[5] Tetracycline and quinolone antibiotics are generally not recommended during pregnancy or childhood; however, their use may be indicated for life-threatening illness.

[6] Ciprofloxacin may be preferred in pregnant women and children up to 8 years of age because of the known adverse event profile of doxycycline (e.g. tooth discoloration).

[7] Doxycylcine may be preferred in children 8 years and older because of the adverse event profile of ciprofloxacin (e.g. arthropathies).

[8] Trimethoprim-sulfamethoxazole has been successfully used to treat plague; however, the Working Group considers this a second-tier choice.

Vaccination

Current killed whole-cell vaccines have been in use for military personnel and have been shown to generate cell-mediated responses lasting at least 15 years; however, they require repeat dosing with adjuvants, have questionable protection against respiratory infections, and are reactogenic. Vaccine production has been discontinued in the United States. Microencapsulated subunit vaccines (of F1 and V proteins) are under development and show the most promise against aerosol exposures and in ease of a single-dose administration.

Complications and Admission Criteria

Whereas primary pneumonic plague results from direct inhalation of plague bacilli, secondary pneumonic plague can manifest as a complication in patients with bubonic plague. Hematogenous dissemination of *Y. pestis* results in plague septicemia, which can be complicated by septic shock, disseminated intravascular coagulation, necrosis of small vessels, and purpuric skin lesions. Plague meningitis due to hematogenous seeding of the meninges occurs infrequently.

Patients with suspected or confirmed pneumonic or bubonic plague require hospitalization for intravenous antibiotics, supportive care, and close monitoring for decompensation and signs of toxemia.

Infection Control

Clinicians should notify local public health authorities, their institution's infection control professional, and their laboratory of any suspected plague cases. Public health authorities may conduct epidemiological investigations and implement disease control interventions to protect the public. Infection control professionals will guide and enforce implementation of infection control precautions within the health-care setting. Laboratory personnel should take appropriate biosafety precautions.

Although not highly contagious, plague can be transmitted person-to-person via respiratory droplets. Both the Healthcare Infection Control Practices Advisory Committee of the CDC and the Working Group on Civilian Biodefense recommend droplet and standard precautions for patients with suspected or confirmed pneumonic plague. These precautions should be maintained until 48 hours of appropriate antibiotics have been administered *and* the patient shows clinical improvement. Close contacts of pneumonic plague patients should be identified, receive prophylaxis, and be monitored for symptoms. For patients with suspected or confirmed bubonic plague or other non-pneumonic plague syndromes, standard precautions are recommended. Aerosol-generating procedures should be avoided if possible. Routine laboratory procedures should be carried out under Biosafety Level-2 conditions; however, manipulation of cultures or other activities that may produce aerosol or droplets (e.g. centrifuging, grinding, vigorous shaking, and animal studies) require Biosafety Level-3 conditions.

Decontamination

In general, environmental decontamination following an aerosol event has not been recommended, because experts have estimated that an aerosol of *Y. pestis* organism would be infectious for only about 1 hour. A recent study demonstrated that *Y. pestis* can survive on selected environmental surfaces for at least several days; however, the potential for re-aerosolization of these organisms was not addressed. Commercially available bleach or 0.5% hypochlorite solution (1:10 dilution of household bleach) is considered adequate for cleaning and decontamination. All persons exposed to an aerosol containing *Y. pestis* should be instructed to wash body surfaces and clothing with soap and water.

Pearls and Pitfalls

1. Bubonic plague is not transmitted directly from one human to another in the absence of lymph node suppuration and drainage. Persons with bubonic plague become more infectious as *Y. pestis* organisms reach the lungs via hematogenous spread. Once pneumonic plague develops, transmission occurs via direct contact with respiratory secretions or inhalation of respiratory droplets.

2. Clinical clues pointing toward a diagnosis of primary pneumonic plague are sudden onset of headache, malaise, and fever, fulminant pneumonitis with rapid progression from dry cough to tachypnea, dyspnea, and productive cough, and in the late stage of disease, hemoptysis with copious amounts of bright red sputum.

References

Begier, E. M., Asiki, G., Anywaine, Z., *et al.* Pneumonic plague cluster, Uganda, 2004. *Emerg. Infect. Dis.* 2006; 12(3): 460–7.

Bin Saeed, A. A., Al-Hamdan, N. A., and Fontaine, R. E. Plague from eating raw camel liver. *Emerg. Infect. Dis.* 2005; 11(9): 1456–7.

Brouillard, J. E., Terriff, C. M., Tofan, A., *et al.* Antibiotic selection and resistance issues with fluoroquinolones and doxycycline against bioterrorism agents. *Pharmacotherapy* 2006; 26(1): 3–14.

Centers for Disease Control and Prevention (CDC). Plague, available at www.cdc.gov/plague/ (accessed March 20, 2018).

CDC. Human plague – United States, 2015. *MMWR Morb. Mortal. Wkly. Rep.* 2015; 64(33): 918–19.

Cono, J., Cragan, J. D., Jamieson, D. J., *et al.* Prophylaxis and treatment of pregnant women for emerging infections and bioterrorism emergencies. *Emerg. Infect. Dis.* 2006; 12(11): 1631–7.

Drancourt, M., Houhamdi, L., and Raoult, D. *Yersinia pestis* as a telluric, human ectoparasite-borne organism. *Lancet Infect. Dis.* 2006; 6(4): 234–41.

Elvin, S. J., Eyles, J. E., Howard, K. A., *et al.* Protection against bubonic and pneumonic plague with a single dose microencapsulated sub-unit vaccine. *Vaccine* 2006; 24(20): 4433–9.

Franz, D. R., Jahrling, P. B., Friedlander, A. M., *et al.* Clinical recognition and management of patients exposed to biological warfare agents. *JAMA* 1997; 278(5): 399–411.

Galimand, M., Carniel, E., and Courvalin, P. Resistance of *Yersinia pestis* to antimicrobial agents. *Antimicrob. Agents Chemother.* 2006; 50(10): 3233–6.

Koirala, J. Plague: disease, management, and recognition of act of terrorism. *Infect. Dis. Clin. North Am.* 2006; 20(2): 273–87, viii.

Kool, J. L. Risk of person-to-person transmission of pneumonic plague. *Clin. Infect. Dis.* 2005; 40(8): 1166–72.

Mwengee, W., Butler, T., Mgema, S., *et al.* Treatment of plague with gentamicin or doxycycline in a randomized clinical trial in Tanzania. *Clin. Infect. Dis.* 2006; 42(5): 614–21.

Rose, L. J., Donlan, R., Banerjee, S. N., *et al.* Survival of *Yersinia pestis* on environmental surfaces. *Appl. Environ. Microbiol.* 2003; 69(4): 2166–71.

Additional Readings

Borio, L. L. , Henderson, A. H., and Hynes, N. A. Bioterrorism: An Overview in J. E. Bennett, R. Dolin, and M. J. Blaser (eds.), *Mandell, Douglas, and Bennett's Principles and Practice of Infectious Diseases*, 8th edn. (Philadelphia, PA: Elsevier/Saunders, 2015), pp. 178–90.

Mead, P. S. *Yersinia* species (including plague) in J. E. Bennett, R. Dolin, and M. J. Blaser (eds.), *Mandell, Douglas, and Bennett's Principles and Practice of Infectious Diseases*, 8th edn. (Philadelphia, PA: Elsevier/Saunders, 2015), pp. 2608–18.

Center for Infectious Disease Research and Policy (CIDRAP). Plague: current, comprehensive information on pathogenesis, microbiology, epidemiology, diagnosis, treatment, and prophylaxis, available at www.cidrap.umn.edu/cidrap/content/bt/plague (accessed March 2, 2018).

Inglesby, T. V., Dennis, D. T., Henderson, D. A., *et al.* Plague as a biological weapon: medical and public health management. Working Group on Civilian Biodefense. *JAMA* 2000; 283(17): 2281–90.

Chapter

69

Smallpox

David M. Stier, Mary P. Mercer, and Rachel L. Chin

Introduction

Smallpox is caused by variola viruses, which are large, enveloped, DNA viruses of the Poxvirus family and the *Orthopoxvirus* genus. Variola major strains cause three forms of disease (ordinary, flat type, and hemorrhagic), whereas variola minor strains cause a less severe form of smallpox. Vaccination with vaccinia virus, another member of the *Orthopoxvirus* genus, protects humans against smallpox because of the high antibody cross-neutralization between orthopoxviruses.

Historically, smallpox was a significant and deadly disease, with a case-fatality rate of 30% or more among unvaccinated persons. However, the virus was declared eradicated worldwide in 1980, following an extensive vaccination campaign led by the World Health Organization (WHO). Nevertheless, because of its lethality and the absence of specific therapy, the Working Group for Civilian Biodefense considers smallpox a dangerous potential biological weapon. Of the potential ways in which smallpox could be used as a biological weapon, an aerosol release is expected to have the most severe medical and public health outcomes because of the virus's stability in aerosol form, low infectious dose, and high rate of secondary transmission. A single case of smallpox would be a public health emergency.

Epidemiology

Reservoirs

The natural reservoir for smallpox was humans with disease; there was no chronic carrier state. When the WHO declared

smallpox eradicated from the world in 1980, it recommended destruction or transfer of all remaining stocks to one of two WHO reference labs, the Centers for Disease Control and Prevention (CDC) in Atlanta, Georgia, and the former Institute of Virus Preparations (later transferred to the Vector Institute) in Russia. Since eradication, there is no natural reservoir for smallpox. Presently, smallpox is officially found only in these designated WHO reference laboratories.

Mode of Transmission

Historically, humans were infected in a number of ways:

- inhalation of droplet nuclei or aerosols originating from the mouths of smallpox-infected humans
- direct contact with skin lesions or infected body fluids of smallpox-infected humans
- direct contact with contaminated clothing or bed linens

Worldwide Occurrence

In 1967, a WHO-led international campaign of mass vaccination, surveillance, and outbreak containment was started in order to eradicate smallpox globally. In 1977, the last community-acquired smallpox case was reported in Somalia, and in 1978, a laboratory accident in England caused the last human case.

Occurrence in the United States

The last case of smallpox in the United States occurred in the Rio Grande Valley of Texas in 1949. The risk of disease was low enough to end routine vaccination of the US population in 1971. Vaccination was previously required for most military personnel, but now is recommended for select military health-care, and emergency workers. Because of the relative frequency and seriousness of vaccine-related complications and the low risk of smallpox outbreak in the United States, routine vaccination is not recommended for the general US population.

In 2002, the CDC recommended pre-event vaccination for local smallpox response teams, consisting of public health, medical, nursing, and public safety personnel, who would conduct investigation and management of initial smallpox cases. Following this recommendation, the Civilian Smallpox Vaccination Program was a vaccination campaign initiated to target this high-risk group of civilian health-care workers (HCWs). Between 2002 and 2004, when the program was reduced, nearly 40,000 HCWs and first responders had been vaccinated, nationally.

Smallpox as a Biological Weapon

Smallpox has been used as a biological weapon in the distant past. More recently, it has been a focus of bioweapons research. In the eighteenth century, British troops in North America gave smallpox-infected blankets to their enemies, who went on to suffer severe outbreaks of smallpox. Defecting Russian scientists describe covert Russian operations during the 1970s and 1980s that focused on bioweapons research and development, including creation of more virulent smallpox strains and development of missiles and bombs that could release smallpox.

Aerosol release of virus (such as into a transportation hub) would likely result in a high number of cases. Other possibilities include use of "human vectors" (i.e. persons who have been deliberately infected with smallpox) and use of fomites (e.g. contamination of letters sent through the mail).

Smallpox is of concern as a biological weapon because:

- Much of the population (80%) is susceptible to infection.
- The virus has a low infectious dose and carries a high rate of morbidity and mortality.
- A vaccine that lacks significant side effects is not yet available for general use; experience has shown that introduction of the virus creates havoc and panic.

An intentional release of smallpox should be suspected in the case of multiple similarly presenting cases clustering in time of fever and rash in mouth and on face, arms, and legs generally 4 days after release. In 2017, the WHO published an "Operational framework for the deployment of the WHO Smallpox Vaccine Emergency Stockpile (SVES) in response to a smallpox event." This document describes the considerations and processes needed for countries to request and distribute the vaccine in the setting of an outbreak.

Clinical Features

Historically, smallpox has been divided into variola major and variola minor based on severity of clinical disease. Variola

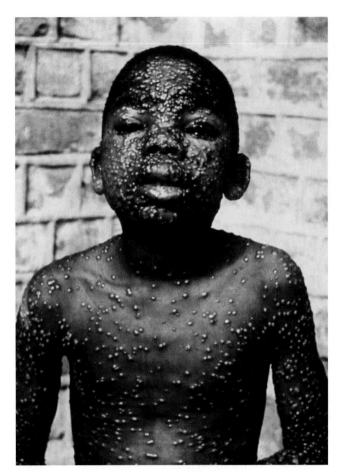

Figure 69.1 Typical distribution of smallpox, with concentration on the face and arms, is seen on this African child.

From the US Centers for Disease Control and Prevention Public Health Information Library.

major was more common and caused more severe disease relative to variola minor. The case mortality was 15 to 45% for variola major and 1% for variola minor.

The infectious dose for smallpox is a few virions. The virus typically enters the body via respiratory or oral mucosa and is carried by macrophages to regional lymph nodes from which a primary asymptomatic viremia develops on the third or fourth day after infection. The reticuloendothelial organs are invaded and overwhelmed leading to a secondary viremia around the eighth to twelfth day after infection. Toxemia and fever onset follow. Seven to 17 days following infection, fever, malaise, and extreme exhaustion begin. A maculopapular rash first presents on the face, mouth, pharynx, and forearms and spreads to the trunks and legs (see Figure 69.1). The rash progresses to a vesicular and pustular stage (round and deeply embedded). Scabs form on the eighth day of the rash. Scars are formed from sebaceous gland destruction and granulation tissue shrinking and fibrosis.

Although most data support communicability with rash onset, some low level of communicability is present prior to rash onset because viral shedding from oral lesions occurs during the 1 to 2 days of fever preceding rash onset. However, secondary transmission peaks 3 to 6 days after fever onset (first

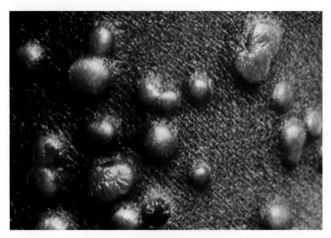

Figure 69.2 Smallpox pustules on day 6 of the rash, located on the thigh of the patient.

From the US Centers for Disease Control and Prevention Public Health Information Library.

week after rash onset), and 91.1% of secondary cases occurred by the ninth day after fever onset (see Figure 69.2). The period of communicability ends when all the scabs have fallen off. Scabs are not very infectious because the tight binding of the fibrin matrix retains the virions; however, secondary cases have been documented through transmission from direct contact with contaminated clothing and bedding.

Secondary bacterial infection and other organ involvement are uncommon. Encephalitis is a possible complication. Mortality is most commonly associated with toxemia of circulating immune complexes and soluble variola antigens and is seen in the second week of illness. Approximately 30 to 80% of unvaccinated close contacts will develop the disease. In addition, 3.5 to 6 transmissions per smallpox case are estimated.

Variola Major

Variola major is associated with the most severe disease and presents as:

- Ordinary (80% or more of cases; mortality is 30% in unvaccinated and 3% in vaccinated patients; see Table 69.1).
- Flat (4 to 6% of cases; mortality is 95% in unvaccinated and 66% in vaccinated patients).
- Hemorrhagic (2 to 3% of cases; mortality is 99% in unvaccinated and 94% in vaccinated patients).
- Modified (13% of cases and low risk of death).
- Variola sine eruptione (30 to 50% of vaccinated contacts of smallpox and low risk of death).

Other forms of smallpox caused by variola major infection include the following:

Flat-type smallpox (also known as *malignant smallpox*) occurred in about 4 to 6% of cases and more frequently in children. It is associated with a late, deficient cellular immune response. It is characterized by a short incubation period, prostrating prodromal illness, severe systemic toxicity, and high mortality (90 to 97%). The lesions do not progress to the pustular stage, instead remaining soft, velvety, and flattened. If the patient survives, the lesions will resolve by desquamation without scabs or scarring.

Hemorrhagic smallpox occurred in about 2 to 3% of cases. Pregnant women are highly susceptible. Similar to flat-type smallpox, it is associated with a defective immune response. It is characterized by a short incubation period, prostrating prodromal illness, severe systemic toxicity, and high mortality (96%). The rash begins as a dusky erythema, followed by extensive petechiae, mucosal hemorrhage, and intense toxemia. Thrombocytopenia and coagulopathy may be present. These patients usually died during week 1 of illness, often before the development of the typical pox lesions.

Modified smallpox occurred in about 13% of cases. It occurred in persons with some immunity. The pre-eruptive illness is typical in duration and severity as ordinary smallpox; however, during the eruption, fever is absent and the skin lesions are superficial, pleomorphic, fewer in number, and evolve rapidly.

Variola sine eruption occurred in about 30 to 50% of vaccinated contacts of smallpox cases. It is characterized by a sudden onset of fever, headache, occasional backache that resolves within 48 hours, influenza-like symptoms, and no rash.

Variola Minor

Variola minor, caused by different strains of variola, is a milder form of smallpox. Compared with variola major, there are milder constitutional symptoms, discrete lesions that evolve a bit more rapidly, lower rates of hemorrhagic disease, and only rare fatal outcomes (less than 1%). The illness may be difficult to distinguish clinically from modified smallpox and variola without eruption. In the 1890s, variola minor spread from South Africa to Florida. In the early 1900s, variola minor became prevalent in the United States, Latin America, and Europe.

Differential Diagnosis

The characteristic features of smallpox need to be differentiated from other illnesses that present with vesicular or pustular rash. One disease that could be confused with smallpox is chickenpox. These may be differentiated clinically as shown in Table 69.2.

Monkeypox is another disease that could be confused with smallpox. In 2003, an outbreak of monkeypox, associated with prairie dog contact, took place in the midwestern United States. Monkeypox in humans presents similarly to ordinary smallpox. However, monkeypox is milder and has prominent lymphadenopathy and a shorter duration of rash.

The CDC has outlined criteria for determining the risk of smallpox when evaluating patients with generalized vesicular or pustular rash (see Table 69.3): www.cdc.gov/smallpox/clinicians/algorithm-protocol.html. Patients deemed to be at high risk present a public health and medical emergency, and in coordination with local public health officials, they should undergo laboratory testing to confirm presence of the disease.

Table 69.1 Clinical Features: Ordinary Variola Major

Incubation period	10–13 days (range 7–19 days)
Transmission	• Inhalation of droplet nuclei or aerosols originating from the mouths of smallpox-infected humans • Direct contact with skin lesions or infected body fluids of smallpox-infected humans • Direct contact with contaminated clothing or bed linens
Signs and symptoms	**Prodromal phase:** • 2–4 days of fever, chills, headache, backache, and often GI symptoms **Rash phase:** • Enanthem (papules, vesicles, then ulcers) of oropharyngeal mucosa beginning 1 day before skin lesions appear • First skin lesions ("herald spots") are often on the face • Lesions spread centrifugally: trunk to proximal extremities to distal extremities • Palms and soles are usually involved, and truncal rash is usually sparse • Lesion progression: maculopapular (days 1–2), vesicular (days 3–5), pustular (days 7–14) • Vesicles and pustules are frequently umbilicated • Pustules can be like small, embedded hard balls or "shotty" • Lesions tend to progress at same rate • Lesions may be discrete, semiconfluent, or confluent • Lesions are typically painful and cause pitted scars as they heal • Lesions gradually scab over during days 13–18
Progression and complications	• Viral bronchitis or pneumonitis • Third spacing of fluid with resulting electrolyte and renal abnormalities • Skin desquamation • Secondary bacterial infection, particularly skin and pulmonary • Spontaneous abortion, stillbirth • Rarely: blindness, keratitis, corneal ulceration, encephalitis, osteomyelitis or arthritis, orchitis • Death may occur during second week of illness, from high-level viremia and circulating immune complexes
Laboratory findings	• Lymphocytopenia and/or granulocytopenia

GI – gastrointestinal.

Table 69.2 Clinical Differentiation of Variola Versus Varicella

Feature	Variola	Varicella
Prodrome	• Duration: 2–4 days • Fever, chills, headache, backache, often GI symptoms	• Commonly does not occur • If present, mild symptoms and duration of 1 day
Rash distribution	• Centrifugal: more dense on face and distal extremities • Frequently involves palms and soles • More involvement of back than abdomen	• Centripetal: more dense on trunk • Spares palms and soles • Back and abdomen equally involved
Lesion evolution	• Usually appear on oropharyngeal mucosa first, then all over within 1–2 days • Progress at same rate; at any point in time, lesions are at same stage of evolution • Lesions progress slowly (7–14 days) from macules to papules to vesicles to pustules to scabs	• Lesions appear in crops • At any point in time, crops of lesions are at different stages of evolution • Lesions progress quickly (1–2 days) from macules to papules to vesicles to scabs
Lesion attributes	• May be semiconfluent or confluent • Deep • May be umbilicated • Often painful; pruritic only as scabs	• Usually discrete • Superficial • Rarely found of palms and soles • Do not umbilicate or dimple • Typically painless; intensely pruritic

The WHO case definition of smallpox includes the same clinical features *and* laboratory confirmation.

Additional considerations in the differential diagnosis of smallpox include:

Macular/papular stage:

- Measles.
- Scarlet fever.
- Rubella.

Vesicular/pustular stage:

- Disseminated herpes zoster.
- Disseminated herpes simplex.
- Molluscum contagiosum.
- Bullous pemphigoid.
- Impetigo (*Streptococcus, Staphylococcus*).
- Human monkey pox.

Table 69.3 Risk of Smallpox in Patients with Generalized Vesicular or Pustular Rash

High	All three major criteria present:
	(a) *Febrile prodrome* 1–4 days before rash onset, with fever >101°F, plus *one or more* of the following: prostration, headache, backache, chills, vomiting, severe abdominal pain
	(b) *Classic smallpox lesions* present (vesicles or pustules that are deep-seated, firm or hard, round, and well-circumscribed; sharply raised and feel like BB pellets under the skin; may become umbilicated or confluent as they evolve)
	(c) Lesions on any one part of the body are in the *same stage of development*
Moderate	Febrile prodrome as in (a) above, plus *either* (b) or (c) above
	or
	Febrile prodrome as in (a) above, plus *at least four* of the following minor criteria:
	• Centrifugal distribution
	• First lesions appeared on the oral mucosa/palate, face, or forearms
	• Patient appears toxic or moribund
	• Slow evolution of lesions from macules to papules to pustules over several days
	• Lesions on the palms and soles
Low	No viral prodrome
	or
	Febrile prodrome as in (a) above, plus fewer than four minor criteria above

Source: CDC, www.cdc.gov/smallpox/clinicians/diagnosis-evaluation.html.

Either stage:

- Erythema multiforme major (Stevens-Johnson syndrome).
- Miscellaneous drug eruptions.
- Secondary syphilis.
- Enteroviral infection (hand, foot, and mouth disease).
- Chickenpox.
- Contact dermatitis.
- Generalized vaccinia (secondary to vaccination or exposure).
- Acne.
- Scabies/insect bites.

Hemorrhagic smallpox may resemble:

- Meningococcemia.
- Rickettsial infections.
- Gram-negative septicemia.

Flat-type smallpox may resemble:

- Hemorrhagic chickenpox.

Laboratory and Radiographic Findings

The diagnosis of smallpox requires a high index of suspicion because the disease has been eradicated and its clinical presentation is similar to other pox viruses. Routine laboratory findings for specific clinical presentations of smallpox are listed in Table 69.1. Radiographic findings do not assist in identification of smallpox.

Diagnosis of smallpox will be clinical initially, but followed by laboratory confirmation. Once smallpox has been confirmed in a geographic area, additional cases can be diagnosed clinically, and specimen testing can be reserved for specific cases in which the clinical presentation is unclear or to assist with law-enforcement activities.

Clinicians should use the CDC-developed tools to assess the likelihood that patients with acute generalized vesicular or pustular rash illnesses have smallpox. The CDC has also developed algorithms for laboratory evaluation of suspect smallpox cases based on the likelihood of disease (www.cdc.gov/smallpox/clinicians/algorithm-protocol.html). If a patient is determined to be at high risk for smallpox, clinicians should call their local public health authorities immediately and obtain photos of the patient. The authorities will provide guidance on specimen collection and packaging and will facilitate transport of specimens to the appropriate public health laboratory.

Multiple tests will be used to evaluate for smallpox. Polymerase chain reaction (PCR) testing will be an important method; however, other methods will also be used, including electron microscopic examination of vesicular or pustular fluid or scabs, direct examination of vesicular or pustular material looking for inclusion bodies (Guarnieri's bodies), culture on egg chorioallantoic membrane, tissue culture, strain analysis with a restriction fragment length polymorphism assay, and serology. Definitive laboratory identification and characterization of the variola virus requires several days.

Treatment and Prophylaxis

Treatment

The management of confirmed or suspected cases of smallpox consists of supportive care, with careful attention to electrolyte and volume status, and ventilatory and hemodynamic support. General supportive measures include ensuring adequate fluid intake (difficult because of the enanthema), alleviation of pain and fever, and keeping skin lesions clean to prevent bacterial superinfection.

Currently, there are no antiviral agents with proven activity against smallpox in humans.

Antiviral agents that have shown some activity in vitro against poxviruses may be available from the CDC under an investigational protocol. Additionally, cidofovir, a nucleoside analogue DNA polymerase inhibitor, might be useful if administered within 1 to 2 days after exposure; however, there is no evidence that it would be more effective than vaccination, and it has to be administered intravenously and causes renal toxicity.

Immunity from Prior Vaccination

Protection from smallpox is estimated to last between 11.7 and 28.4 years after primary vaccination and longer for variola minor than for variola major. Those who were previously vaccinated may retain some protection that could decrease the severity of the disease and allow for greater mobility, thereby complicating public health response.

Post-Exposure Prophylaxis

Post-exposure prophylaxis for smallpox is the administration of vaccinia vaccine after suspected exposure to smallpox has occurred, but before symptoms are present. Immunity generally develops within 8 to 11 days after vaccination with vaccinia virus. Because the incubation period for smallpox averages about 12 days, vaccination within 4 days may confer some immunity to exposed persons and reduce the likelihood of a fatal outcome. Post-exposure vaccination may be particularly important for those vaccinated in the past, provided that revaccination is able to boost the anamnestic immune response. In addition to vaccination, exposed persons should be monitored for symptoms. Temperature should be checked once a day, preferably in evening, for 17 days after exposure for fever (over 38°C).

If a case or cases of smallpox occur, public health authorities will conduct surveillance and implement containment strategies. Ring vaccination will be important and includes identification of contacts of cases and provision of prophylaxis and guidance on monitoring for symptoms. Large-scale voluntary vaccination may be offered to low-risk populations to supplement and address public concerns.

Vaccine Supply, Administration, and Recommendations

The smallpox vaccine previously available in the United States (Dryvax) was withdrawn in 2008 and replaced by ACAM2000, a vaccinia virus vaccine derived from the same strain that was used to manufacture Dryvax. For civilians, ACAM2000 is available only from the US Centers for Disease Control and Prevention (CDC) and should be administered only by trained, vaccinated personnel. Should smallpox vaccination be deemed necessary, it will be coordinated by local, state, and federal health agencies.

ACAM2000 consists of a lyophilized preparation of purified live virus and is reconstituted with a supplied diluent. It is administered in a single dose by the percutaneous route (scarification) using 15 jabs of a stainless steel bifurcated needle that has been dipped into the reconstituted vaccine. Following successful administration of vaccine, ACAM2000 produces vaccination site lesions containing infectious vaccinia virus capable of transmission through autoinoculation and inadvertent inoculation of close contacts of vaccinees. Persons undergoing revaccination may experience modified or greatly reduced vaccination site lesions.

The Advisory Committee for Immunization Practices (ACIP) of the CDC developed guidelines in 2015 for vaccination of health-care and laboratory personnel. Vaccination with ACAM2000 is routinely recommended only for laboratory personnel who directly handle cultures or animals infected with replication-competent orthopoxvirus strains. Health-care personnel whose contact with vaccinia viruses is limited to contaminated dressings and other materials, or who administer ACAM2000 vaccine as part of their duties, do not necessarily require vaccination so long as appropriate infection prevention measures are followed. However, because of a theoretical risk of infection, vaccination with ACAM2000 may be offered to this very limited segment of health-care workers.

Vaccine Contraindications and Complications

Contraindications for non-emergency use of ACAM2000 include:

- History or presence of atopic dermatitis.
- Other active exfoliative skin conditions, such as eczema, burns, severe acne, impetigo, chicken pox, contact dermatitis, severe diaper dermatitis, or Darier disease.
- Conditions associated with immunosuppression due to disease or treatment of disease, including high dose corticosteroids and TNF inhibitors.
- Age <1 year.
- Pregnancy or breastfeeding.
- Known heart disease or at least three known major cardiac risk factors.
- Household contacts with history or presence of atopic dermatitis, other active exfoliative skin conditions, or conditions associated with immunosuppression, or who are age <1 year or pregnant.
- Persons with household contacts.

Smallpox vaccine when administered to millions of individuals in the 1960s was associated with a host of serious and frequent complications related mainly to dissemination of vaccine virus and including generalized vaccinia, eczema vaccinatum, vaccinia keratitis, progressive vaccinia, myopericarditis, fetal vaccinia, and transmission of vaccinia from newly vaccinated persons to susceptible unvaccinated contacts.

Since 2002, data from US military personnel and civilian first responders vaccinated during smallpox vaccination campaigns showed a much lower rate of serious adverse events than was previously reported. ACIP attributed this decrease to stricter exclusion of persons with contraindications, increased use of protective bandages to cover the vaccination site and prevent dissemination, and improved education of vaccinees.

The primary therapy for adverse reactions to smallpox vaccination is vaccinia immunoglobulin (VIG). However VIG is contraindicated in vaccinia keratitis and provides no benefit in post-vaccinial encephalitis. VIG is manufactured from the plasma of persons vaccinated with vaccinia vaccine. An intravenous preparation (VIGIV) was recently licensed by the FDA. Cidofovir and topical ophthalmic antiviral agents are also recommended by some experts. Cidofovir use requires an Investigational New Drug (IND) protocol, and topical ophthalmic agent use is off-label.

Complications and Admission Criteria

Before smallpox was eradicated worldwide, viral bronchitis and pneumonitis were the most frequent complications of ordinary-type smallpox. Cutaneous complications included desquamation, massive subcutaneous fluid accumulation with electrolyte abnormalities and renal failure, or, less commonly, secondary bacterial infection of smallpox lesions. Infrequently, smallpox patients experienced encephalitis, osteomyelitis, corneal ulceration, or ocular keratitis. Ordinary-type smallpox with confluent lesions, rather than discrete lesions, carried a much higher risk of massive exfoliation, tissue destruction, bacterial sepsis, and death. Hemorrhagic-type and flat-type smallpox were nearly always fatal.

Many patients do not require hospitalization. Those with discrete lesions, non-hemorrhagic and non-flat-type, are less likely to become critically ill or require much supportive care and can be more easily managed outside the hospital. These people should be isolated and monitored at home or in a non-hospital facility, and smallpox vaccination should be provided to caregivers and household members. Patients with evidence of severe disease or presentations that suggest progression to severe disease is likely should be considered for admission to a negative-pressure environment with strict maintenance of Airborne Precautions.

Infection Control

Clinicians should notify local public health authorities, their institution's infection control professional, and their laboratory of any suspected smallpox cases. Public health authorities may conduct epidemiological investigations and will implement disease control interventions to protect the public. Infection control professionals will implement infection control precautions within the health-care setting. Laboratory personnel should take appropriate safety precautions.

Smallpox is transmissible from person to person by exposure to respiratory secretions and by direct contact with pox lesions and fomites. Airborne and Contact Precautions in addition to standard precautions should be implemented for patients with suspected smallpox. Health-care workers caring for patients with suspected smallpox should be vaccinated immediately.

Decontamination

Survival of the virus in the environment is inversely proportional to temperature and humidity. All bedding and clothing of smallpox patients should be minimally handled to prevent re-aerosolization and autoclaved or laundered in hot water with bleach. Standard disinfection and sterilization methods are deemed adequate for medical equipment used with smallpox patients and cleaning surfaces and rooms potentially contaminated with the virus. Airspace decontamination (fumigation) is not required.

Pearls and Pitfalls

1. The WHO has developed a number of clinical diagnostic tools to assist with the visual recognition, differential diagnosis, and initial management of suspected smallpox. These resources are available at www.who.int/csr/disease/smallpox/clinical-diagnosis/en/.

2. Hemorrhagic smallpox is rare, but can be confused with invasive meningococcal disease, rickettsial infections, or gram-negative sepsis because of the patient's ill appearance, petechial and purpuric lesions, and hemorrhagic manifestations.

3. Smallpox is most often transmitted through direct contact with respiratory droplets as a result of close (within 2 meters) or face-to-face contact. Viruses can also travel over greater distances as airborne particles, particularly in cases with coughing. Transmission has occasionally been linked to fomites carried on clothing or bedding that has been contaminated by dried respiratory secretions or draining skin lesions.

References

Bhatnagar, V., Stoto, M. A., Morton, S. C., et al. Transmission patterns of smallpox: systematic review of natural outbreaks in Europe and North America since World War II. *BMC Public Health* 2006; 6(126).

Breman, J. G. and Henderson, D. A. Diagnosis and management of smallpox. *N. Engl. J. Med.* 2002; 346(17): 1300–8.

Casey, C. G., Iskander, J. K., Roper, M. H., et al. Adverse events associated with smallpox vaccination in the United States, January–October 2003. *JAMA* 2005; 294(21): 2734–43.

Centers for Disease Control and Prevention (CDC). Acute, generalized vesicular or pustular rash illness testing protocol in the United States, available at www.cdc.gov/smallpox/clinicians/diagnosis-evaluation.html (accessed April 4, 2018).

CDC. Emergency preparedness and response: smallpox, available at www.cdc.gov/smallpox/clinicians/vaccination.html (accessed April 4, 2018).

Cohen, H. W., Gould, R. M., and Sidel, V. W. Smallpox vaccinations and adverse events. *JAMA* 2006; 295(16): 1897–8.

Fenner, F., Henderson, D. A., Arita, I., et al. Smallpox and its eradication (Geneva: World Health Organization, 1988), retrieved February 10, 2007 from http://whqlibdoc.who.int/smallpox/924156.pdf.

Huhn, G. D., Bauer, A. M., Yorita, K., et al. Clinical characteristics of human monkeypox, and risk factors for severe disease. *Clin. Infect. Dis.* 2005; 41(12): 1742–51.

Kim, S.-H., Bang, J.-W., Park, K.-H., et al. Prediction of residual immunity to smallpox by means of an intradermal skin test with inactivated vaccinia virus. *J. Infect. Dis.* 2006; 194(3): 377–84; comments and author reply in 195: 160–2.

Kiang, K. M. and Krathwohl, M. D. Rates and risks of transmission of smallpox and mechanisms of prevention. *J. Lab. Clin. Med.* 2003; 142(4): 229–38.

Military Vaccine Agency – Vaccine Healthcare Centers Network. Office of the Surgeon General. Smallpox vaccination program: questions and answers (July 8, 2014), available at www.usamma.amedd.army.mil/net/assets/doc/pdf/Vaccines/SVP_Q_A_8July2014.pdf (accessed April 4, 2018).

Moore, Z. S., Seward, J. F., and Lane, J. M. Smallpox. *Lancet* 2006; 367(9508): 425–35.

Nishiura, H. Smallpox during pregnancy and maternal outcomes. *Emerg. Infect. Dis.* 2006; 12(7): 1119–21.

Nishiura, H. and Eichner, M. Infectiousness of smallpox relative to disease age: estimates based on transmission network and incubation period. *Epidemiol. Infect.* 2007; 135(7): 1145–50.

Nishiura, H., Schwehm, M., and Eichner, M. Still protected against smallpox? Estimation of the duration of vaccine-induced immunity against smallpox. *Epidemiology* 2006; 17(5): 576–81.

Petersen, B. W., Harms, T. J., Reynolds, M. G., *et al.* Use of vaccinia virus smallpox vaccine in laboratory and health care personnel at risk for occupational exposure to orthopoxviruses – recommendations of the Advisory Committee on Immunization Practices (ACIP). *MMWR Morb. Mortal. Wkly. Rep.* 2016; 65(10): 257–62.

Sejvar, J. J., Labutta, R. J., Chapman, L. E., *et al.* Neurologic adverse events associated with smallpox vaccination in the United States, 2002–2004. *JAMA* 2005; 294(21): 2744–50.

World Health Organization (WHO). Smallpox case definition, available at www.who.int/csr/disease/smallpox/case-definition/en/ (accessed December 22, 2017).

WHO. Operational framework for the deployment of the WHO smallpox vaccine emergency stockpile in response to a smallpox event, available at www.who.int/csr/disease/icg/smallpox-vaccine-emergency-stockpile/en/ (accessed April 4, 2018).

Additional Readings

Borio, L. L., Henderson, D. A., and Hynes, N. A. Bioterrorism, an overview in J. E. Bennett, R. Dolin, and M. J. Blaser (eds.), *Mandell, Douglas, and Bennett's Principles and Practice of Infectious Diseases*, 8th edn. (Philadelphia, PA: Elsevier/Saunders, 2015), pp. 178–90.

Center for Infectious Disease Research and Policy (CIDRAP). Smallpox: current, comprehensive information on pathogenesis, microbiology, epidemiology, diagnosis, treatment, and prophylaxis, retrieved May 18, 2005, from www.cidrap.umn.edu/cidrap/content/bt.

Henderson, D. A., Inglesby, T. V., Bartlett, J. G., *et al.* for the Working Group on Civilian Biodefense. Smallpox as a biological weapon: medical and public health management. *JAMA* 1999; 281(22): 2127–39.

Petersen, B. W. and Damon, I. K. Orthopoxviruses: vaccinia (smallpox vaccine), variola (smallpox), monkeypox, and cowpox in J. E. Bennett, R. Dolin, and M. J. Blaser (eds.), *Mandell, Douglas, and Bennett's Principles and Practice of Infectious Diseases*, 8th edn. (Philadelphia, PA: Elsevier/Saunders, 2015), pp. 1694–702.

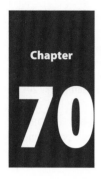

Chapter

70

Tularemia

David M. Stier and Mary P. Mercer

Introduction

Tularemia is a zoonotic disease caused by *Francisella tularensis*, a non-sporulating, non-motile, aerobic, gram-negative coccobacillus. There are several subspecies of *F. tularensis*, with the biovars *tularensis* (type A) and *holarctica* (type B) occurring most commonly in the United States. The clinical syndromes caused by tularemia depend on the route of infection and subspecies of the infecting organism. Tularemia is highly infectious, requiring inhalation or inoculation of as few as ten organisms to cause disease. Although its virulence factors are not well characterized, type A is generally thought to be the more virulent subspecies. However, the virulence of type A subspecies may vary between geographic regions within the United States, with the midwestern and eastern states having more severe infections.

The Working Group for Civilian Biodefense considers tularemia to be a dangerous potential biological weapon because of its "extreme infectivity, ease of dissemination, and its capacity to cause illness and death." Of the potential ways that *F. tularensis* could be used as a biological weapon, an aerosol release is expected to have the most severe medical and public health outcomes.

Epidemiology

Reservoir

The natural reservoirs for *F. tularensis* are small and medium-sized mammals. In the United States, these are primarily lagomorphs (rabbits, hares), but may include beavers, squirrels, muskrats, field voles, and rats. Incidental hosts include some species of mammals (e.g. humans, cats, dogs, cattle), birds, fish, and amphibians. Organisms can survive for weeks in moist environments, including water, mud, and decaying animal tissue.

Mode of Transmission

The primary vectors for infection in the United States are ticks (dog ticks, wood ticks) and flies, such as the deerfly. Humans become infected by a number of mechanisms:

- Bites by infected arthropods (majority of cases).
- Contact with infectious animal tissues or fluids, during, for example, hunting or butchering.
- Ingestion of contaminated food, water, or soil.

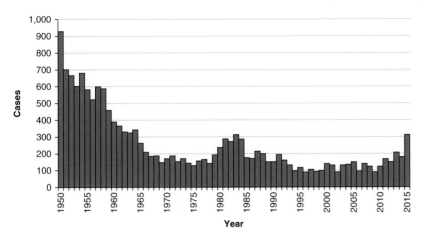

Figure 70.1 Distribution of reported cases of tularemia in the United States, 2001–2015.

From Centers for Disease Control and Prevention (CDC), Statistics, 2015, available at www.cdc.gov/tularemia/statistics/index.html.

- Inhalation of infectious aerosols, including aerosols generated during landscaping activities (e.g. lawn mowing, using a power blower, and brush cutting).
- Exposure in the laboratory (accidental inhalation of aerosol, direct contact with an infectious specimen including accidental parenteral inoculation, or ingestion).

Note: Tularemia is not spread from person to person.

Worldwide Occurrence

Worldwide, human cases of tularemia occur throughout North America, Europe, and Asia. Infections with type A strain are generally only seen in North America. Within Europe and Asia, the greatest numbers of human cases are reported in Scandinavian countries and countries of the former Soviet Union. Recent significant outbreaks of tularemia in humans include Sweden and Finland (2000 to 2011), Kosovo (2005 to 2011), and Turkey (2009 to 2012), the latter with some of the largest volumes of the European outbreaks.

US Occurrence

Nationwide, incidence of tularemia declined from approximately 2,000 annually reported cases during the first half of the twentieth century to an average of 125 cases per year during the 2000s (see Figure 70.1). Most cases occur in rural or semi-rural environments, during the summer months, with the greatest number of cases occurring in Missouri, Oklahoma, South Dakota, Montana, and Martha's Vineyard, Massachusetts. From 1990 to 2000, incidence of tularemia in the United States was highest in children aged 5 to 9 years and adults 75 years and older. Regardless of age, males had a higher incidence of tularemia, potentially because of participation in activities more likely to cause exposures, such as hunting, trapping, butchering, and farming. Recent significant outbreaks include the following:

- In 1978 and 2000, outbreaks of the rare primary pneumonic tularemia occurred on Martha's Vineyard, Massachusetts. These represent the only outbreaks of primary pneumonic tularemia in the United States. Additional cases of tularemia have been reported each year in Martha's Vineyard (2000 to 2006). Exposure is most likely from breathing infectious aerosols generated during landscaping activities. The reservoir in these outbreaks is still unclear, but may involve skunks and raccoons.
- In 2002, tularemia was responsible for a die-off of several hundred prairie dogs caught in the wild in South Dakota and then commercially distributed widely throughout the United States. One human case occurred in an animal handler who cared for the infected animals.
- In September to December 2015 a dramatic increase in cases was reported in Colorado, Wyoming and western South Dakota, and Nebraska, which included a roughly equal number of ulceroglandular, pneumonic, and typhoidal presentations. These approximately 100 cases represented a 200 to 900-fold increase in incidence in those states and was thought to possibly be due to changes in rainfall that might have allowed the bacteria to aerosolize more easily, thereby increasing transmission.

Tularemia as a Biological Weapon

Weaponized *F. tularensis* was developed and stockpiled by the US military, though the supply was destroyed in the 1970s. The Soviet Union is reported to have developed antibiotic- and vaccine-resistant strains of weaponized *F. tularensis*.

Experts believe that an aerosolized release is the most likely intentional use of *F. tularensis* organisms. Exposure to aerosolized *F. tularensis* would cause:

- Via inhalation:
  - primary pneumonic tularemia (majority of patients)
  - typhoidal tularemia (non-specific febrile illness of varying severity)
  - oropharyngeal tularemia
- Via contact with eyes: oculoglandular tularemia
- Via contact with broken skin: glandular or ulceroglandular disease

An intentional release of tularemia would have the following characteristics:

- Multiple similarly presenting cases clustering in time:
  - acute non-specific febrile illness with onset 3 to 5 days after the initial release (range 1 to 14 days)
  - community-acquired atypical pneumonia unresponsive to typical antimicrobials

Table 70.1 Clinical Features: Pneumonic Tularemia

Incubation period	3–5 days (range 1–14 days)
Transmission	• Inhalation of contaminated aerosols • Secondary hematogenous spread to the lung
Signs and symptoms	• Initial presentation as atypical CAP unresponsive to routine antibiotic therapy, which can progress slowly or rapidly to severe disease • Fever (abrupt onset), headache, cough, minimal or no sputum production, dyspnea, pleuritic chest pain, myalgias (often prominent in lower back), bronchiolitis and/or pharyngitis may be present • Generalized maculopapular rash with progression to pustules or erythema-nodosum type rash occurs in 20% • Nausea, vomiting, diarrhea is not uncommon • Hemoptysis (not common)
Progression and complications	• Respiratory failure, ARDS • Severe pneumonia • Lung abscess or cavitary lesions • Sepsis
Laboratory and radiographic findings	• Lobar, segmental, or subsegmental opacities on CXR, pleural effusion, pleural adhesions, Hilar adenopathy • Leukocytosis; differential may be normal • Liver enzymes and/or CK may be abnormal • Sputum Gram stain usually non-specific

ARDS – acute respiratory distress syndrome; CAP – community-acquired pneumonia; CK – creatine kinase; CXR – chest X-ray.

- Atypical host characteristics: unexpected, unexplained cases of acute illness in previously healthy persons who rapidly develop pleuropneumonia and systemic infection, especially if patients develop pleural effusions and hilar lymphadenopathy.
- Unusual geographic clustering: multiple cases in an urban area, where naturally occurring tularemia is not endemic.
- Absence of risk factors: patients lack tularemia exposure risk factors (e.g. outdoor field work or recreational activity, contact with tissues of potentially infected animals).

Intentionally released *F. tularensis* strains may be altered to have enhanced virulence or antimicrobial resistance.

Clinical Features

Human tularemia occurs in six recognized forms, determined primarily by route of infection. Tularemia infection can range from mild to severe clinical illness and can be life-threatening. All forms are accompanied by fever, which can range in severity. Overall case-fatality rates have declined from 5 to 15% in the pre-antibiotic era to approximately 2% currently. Mortality was historically much higher with pneumonic and typhoidal tularemia, with case fatality as high as 30 to 60% if untreated. Administration of appropriate antibiotic treatment typically leads to general symptom improvement within 24 to 48 hours. Recognition of tularemia as a potential etiologic agent is critical, because poor outcomes have been associated with delays in seeking care and/or instituting effective antimicrobial treatment.

Pneumonic Tularemia

Pneumonic tularemia is associated with the most severe disease and intially presents as a non-specific febrile illness that progresses to pleuropneumonitis and systemic infection (see Table 70.1).

Glandular and Ulceroglandular Tularemia

Glandular and ulceroglandular tularemia account for the majority of naturally occurring cases of tularemia (see Table 70.2). In the *ulceroglandular* form, an ulcer is formed at the site of inoculation, with subsequent lymphadenopathy in the proximal draining lymph nodes (see Figures 70.2, 70.3, and 70.4). Occasionally, lymphadenopathy occurs without an ulcer, leading to the designation of *glandular* disease.

Oculoglandular Tularemia

Oculoglandular tularemia results either from ocular inoculation from the hands after contact with contaminated material or from splashes or aerosols generated during handling of infective material (e.g. animal carcasses). This form of tularemia could occur in a bioterrorism setting as a result of an aerosol exposure. Organisms spread from the conjunctiva to regional nodes, where they cause focal necrosis and lesions.

After an incubation period of 3 to 5 (range 1 to 14) days, oculoglandular tularemia presents as a painful "red eye" with purulent exudation, chemosis, vasculitis, and painful regional lymphadenopathy. Additional signs and symptoms may include photophobia, lacrimation, itching, local edema, and changes in visual acuity. There is a potential for lymph node suppuration, hematogenous dissemination, and development of sepsis.

Laboratory values are generally non-specific, and gram stain of conjunctival scrapings may or may not demonstrate organisms.

Oropharyngeal Tularemia

Oropharyngeal or gastrointestinal tularemia occurs via ingestion of contaminated food including undercooked meat, contaminated water or droplets, and oral inoculation from the hands after contact with contaminated material.

Table 70.2 Clinical Features: Glandular and Ulceroglandular Tularemia

Incubation period	3–5 days (range 1–14 days)
Transmission	• Bite of an infective arthropod • Direct contact with infectious material (i.e. contaminated carcass, settled infectious aerosol)
Signs and symptoms	• Ulceroglandular form – local skin involvement at site of exposure that develops into a painful cutaneous papule with subsequent ulceration within several days. Papule becomes necrotic and scars. • Glandular form – no cutaneous lesion occurs • Enlarged and tender regional lymphadenopathy that can persist for months • Fever, chills, malaise, myalgias, arthralgias, headache, anorexia, GI symptoms are common
Progression and complications	• Lymph node suppuration • Secondary pneumonia • Hematogenous spread to other organs • Sepsis
Laboratory findings	• Leukocytosis; differential may be normal • Liver enzymes and/or CK may be abnormal

GI – gastrointestinal.

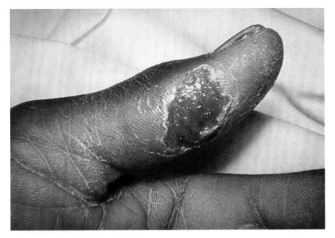

Figure 70.2 Thumb lesion caused by tularemia infection.
From the US Centers for Disease Control and Prevention Public Health Information Library at http://phil.cdc.gov/phil/home.asp. Photograph taken in 1964 by Emory University/Dr. Sellers.

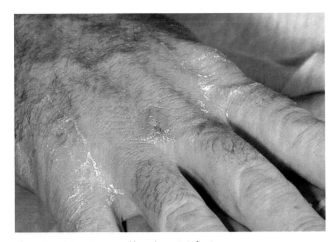

Figure 70.3 Lesion caused by tularemia infection.
From the US Centers for Disease Control and Prevention Public Health Information Library at http://phil.cdc.gov/phil/home.asp. Photograph taken in 1963 by CDC/Dr. Brachman.

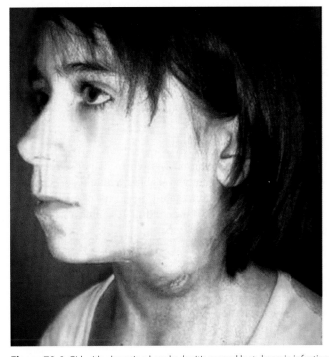

Figure 70.4 Girl with ulcerating lymphadenitis caused by tularemia infection.
From R. Reintjes, I. Dedusha, A. Gjini, *et al.*, Tularemia outbreak investigation in Kosovo: case control and environmental studies. *Emerg. Infect. Dis.* 2002; 8(1): 69–73.

After an incubation period of 3 to 5 (range 1 to 14) days, oropharyngeal tularemia presents either as acute pharyngitis with cervical lymphadenopathy or as ulcerative gastrointestinal lesions with fever, abdominal pain, diarrhea, nausea, vomiting, mesenteric lymphadenopathy, and gastrointestinal bleeding. Severity can range from mild diarrhea to overwhelming ulceration with frank gastrointestinal bleeding and sepsis. A large inoculum (approximately 10^8 organisms) is required to transmit disease orally. There is a potential for lymph node suppuration, hematogenous dissemination, and development of sepsis.

Routine tests are generally non-specific. Leukocytosis may or may not be present.

Table 70.3 Clinical Features: Typhoidal Tularemia

Incubation period	3–5 days (range 1–14 days)
Transmission	• Site of primary infection usually unknown
Signs and symptoms	• Fever, chills, headache, malaise, weakness, myalgias, arthralgias, cough • Prostration, dehydration, hypotension, pharyngitis • Watery diarrhea, anorexia, nausea, vomiting, abdominal pain (children may have more severe GI involvement) • Generalized maculopapular rash with progression to pustules or erythema-nodosum type rash may occur • Splenomegaly and hepatomegaly (not common)
Progression and complications	• Secondary pneumonia • Hematogenous spread to other organs – osteomyelitis, pericarditis, peritonitis, endocarditis, meningitis • Sepsis • Rhabdomyolysis • Cholestasis with jaundice • Renal failure • Debilitating illness lasting several months
Laboratory and radiographic findings	• Pleural effusions • Leukocytosis; differential may be normal • Liver enzymes and/or CK may be abnormal • Sterile pyuria may occur

Typhoidal Tularemia

Typhoidal (septicemic) tularemia is an acute, non-specific febrile illness associated with *F. tularensis* without prominent lymphadenopathy (see Table 70.3).

Differential Diagnosis

A high index of suspicion is required to diagnose tularemia because there are no readily available rapid and specific confirmatory tests. In addition, the various forms of tularemia can have a non-specific appearance and/or resemble a wide range of much more common illnesses.

Pneumonic Tularemia

Many different clinical syndromes can appear similar to the pneumonic form of tularemia, and further history, testing, and empiric treatment for many of these may be indicated early in the evaluative process. The differential diagnosis for pneumonic tularemia includes the following conditions:

- Bacterial pneumonia (*Mycoplasma, Staphylococcus, Streptococcus, Haemophilus, Klebsiella, Moraxella, Legionella*).
- Chlamydia infection.
- Q fever.
- Tuberculosis.
- Inhalational anthrax.
- Pneumonic plague.
- Fungal pulmonary disease (histoplasmosis, coccidioidomycosis).
- Influenza or other viral respiratory illnesses.
- other causes of atypical or chronic pneumonias.

Glandular and Ulceroglandular Tularemia

Many different clinical syndromes can appear similar to glandular and ulceroglandular forms of tularemia, and further history, testing, and empiric treatment for many of these may be indicated early in the evaluative process. The differential diagnosis for glandular and ulceroglandular forms of tularemia includes the following conditions:

- Pyogenic bacterial infections.
- Cat-scratch disease (Bartonella).
- Syphilis.
- Chancroid.
- Lymphogranuloma venereum.
- Tuberculosis.
- Non-tuberculosis mycobacterial infection.
- Toxoplasmosis.
- Sporotrichosis.
- Rat-bite fever.
- Anthrax.
- Plague.
- Herpes simplex virus infection.
- Adenitis or cellulitis (*Staphylococcus* or *Streptococcus*).
- *Pasteurella* infections.
- Rickettsial infections.
- Orf virus infection.

Oculoglandular Tularemia

Many different clinical syndromes can appear similar to the oculoglandular form of tularemia, and further history, testing, and empiric treatment for these may be indicated early in the evaluative process. The differential diagnosis for the oculoglandular form of tularemia includes the following conditions:

- Pyogenic bacterial infections.
- Adenoviral infection.
- Syphilis.
- Cat-scratch disease.
- Herpes simplex virus infection.
- Varicella-zoster virus infection.

- Sporotrichosis.
- Coccidioidomycosis.
- Tuberculosis.

Oropharyngeal Tularemia

Many different clinical syndromes can appear similar to the oropharyngeal form of tularemia. Further history, testing, and empiric treatment for these may be indicated early in the evaluative process. The differential diagnosis for the oropharyngeal form of tularemia includes the following conditions:

- *Streptococcus* pharyngitis.
- Infectious mononucleosis.
- Adenoviral infection.
- Diphtheria.
- Gastrointestinal anthrax.

Typhoidal Tularemia

Many different clinical syndromes can appear similar to typhoidal forms of tularemia. Further history, testing, and empiric treatment for these may be indicated early in the evaluative process. The differential diagnosis for typhoidal forms of tularemia includes the following conditions:

- *Salmonella* spp. infection.
- Brucellosis.
- *Legionella* infection.
- Chlamydia infection.
- Q fever.
- Disseminated mycobacterial or fungal infection.
- Rickettsioses.
- Malaria.
- Endocarditis.
- Leptospirosis.
- Meningococcemia.
- Septicemic plague.
- Septicemia caused by other gram-negative bacteria.
- *Staphylococcus* or *Streptococcus* toxic shock syndrome.
- Other causes of prolonged fever without localizing signs.

Laboratory and Radiographic Findings

The diagnosis of tularemia requires a high index of suspicion because the disease can present with non-specific symptoms and non-specific results of routine lab tests.

Diagnosis is most commonly confirmed by serologic testing. Antibody detection assays include tube agglutination, micro-agglutination, hemagglutination, and enzyme-linked immunosorbent assay (ELISA). IgM and IgG together antibodies appear around the end of the second week of illness, peak at 4 to 5 weeks, and can persist indefinitely. A single titer of 1:160 or greater (by tube agglutination) or 1:128 or greater (by microagglutination) is a presumptive positive; a fourfold rise in titer is required for definitive serologic diagnosis.

Although rapid diagnostic tests are not widely available, the public health laboratory system may be able to provide polymerase chain reaction (PCR) or direct fluorescent antibody (DFA) testing on certain clinical specimens.

Microscopy and culture are difficult and often not fruitful. The organism is rarely seen on stained clinical specimens and is difficult to isolate using routine culture media and conditions. However, isolation is possible from a variety of clinical specimens if culture conditions are optimized. Even still, some strains may require up to a week to develop visible colonies, especially if the patient has been placed on bacteriostatic antibiotic therapy. Because of the need for non-routine laboratory methods and because *F. tularensis* is a risk to laboratory personnel, clinicians should notify the laboratory when tularemia is suspected.

Treatment and Prophylaxis

Treatment

The treatment of choice for all forms of tularemia is streptomycin (see Table 70.4). Gentamicin, which is more widely available, is an acceptable alternative. Other alternatives include tetracycline, chloramphenicol, and ciprofloxacin. Tetracyclines and chloramphenicol are bacteriostatic and their use has produced more relapses than treatment with aminoglycosides. Clinicians should be aware that *F. tularensis* strains released intentionally may be resistant to antimicrobials.

Supportive care, including fluid management and hemodynamic monitoring, should be considered in all patients. Intensive care with respiratory support may be necessary in patients with complications.

Contained Casualty Setting

The Working Group recommends parenteral antimicrobial therapy when individual medical management is available (see Table 70.4). Therapy may be switched to oral antimicrobials when clinically indicated.

Mass Casualty Setting

Use of oral antibiotics may be necessary if the number of patients exceeds the medical care capacity for individual medical management (see Table 70.4).

Post-Exposure Prophylaxis

Antibiotic prophylaxis should begin as soon as possible and preferably within 24 hours after exposure to an infectious aerosol containing *F. tularensis* (see Table 70.4). Post-exposure prophylactic antibiotic treatment of close contacts of tularemia patients is not recommended because human-to-human transmission of *F. tularensis* is not known to occur.

Vaccination

A live, attenuated vaccine was tested in the United States to protect laboratory personnel who work with *F. tularensis*; but failed to receive approval. This vaccine is currently under review by the Food and Drug Administration (FDA) and is unavailable. Attempts to develop a new tularemia vaccine are

Table 70.4 Tularemia: Treatment and Post-Exposure Prophylaxis Recommendations[1]

		Contained Casualty Setting	Mass Casualty Setting or Post-Exposure Prophylaxis
Adult	Preferred	Streptomycin 1 g IM every 12 hours for 10 days *or* Gentamicin[2] 5 mg/kg IM/IV every 24 hours for 10 days	Doxycycline 100 mg PO BID for 14 days *or* Ciprofloxacin 500 mg PO BID for 14 days
	Alternative	Doxycycline 100 mg IV every 12 hours for 14–21 days *or* Chloramphenicol[3] 15 mg/kg/dose IV every 6 hours for 14–21 days *or* Ciprofloxacin 400 mg IV every 12 hours for 10 days	
Children	Preferred	Streptomycin 15 mg/kg/dose IM every 12 hours (max. 2 gm/day) for 10 days *or* Gentamicin[2] 2.5 mg/kg/dose IM/IV every 8 hours for 10 days	Doxycycline[4, 5]: ≥45 kg, give adult dosage twice daily for 14 days <45 kg, give 2.2 mg/kg PO BID (max. 200 mg/day) for 14 days *or* Ciprofloxacin[4, 6] 15 mg/kg PO BID (max. 1 g/day) for 14 days
	Alternative	Doxycycline[4, 5]: ≥45 kg, give adult dosage for 14 days <45 kg, give 2.2 mg/kg IV every 12 hours (max. 200 mg/day) for 14 days *or* Chloramphenicol[3] 15 mg/kg/dose IV every 6 hours for 14–21 days *or* Ciprofloxacin[4, 6] 15 mg/kg/dose IV every 12 hours (max. 1 g/day) for 10 days	
Pregnant women	Preferred	Gentamicin[2] 5 mg/kg IM or IV every 24 hours for 10 days *or* Streptomycin[7] 1 g IM every 12 hours for 10 days	Doxycycline[4, 5] 100 mg PO BID for 14 days *or* Ciprofloxacin[4, 6] 500 mg PO BID for 14 days
	Alternative	Doxycycline[4, 5] 100 mg IV every 12 hours for 14–21 days *or* Ciprofloxacin[4, 6] 400 mg IV every 12 hours for 10 days	

[1] Treatment recommendations come from the Working Group of Civilian Biodefense and may not necessarily be approved by the US Food and Drug Administration.

[2] Aminoglycoside doses must be further adjusted for newborns and according to renal function.

[3] Therapeutic concentration is 5–20 µg/mL; concentrations >25 µg/mL can cause reversible bone marrow suppression.

[4] Tetracycline and quinolone antibiotics are generally not recommended during pregnancy or childhood; however, their use may be indicated for life-threatening illness.

[5] Ciprofloxacin may be preferred in pregnant women and children up to 8 years of age because of the known adverse event profile of doxycycline (e.g. tooth discoloration).

[6] Doxycycline may be preferred in children 8 years and older because of the adverse event profile of ciprofloxacin (e.g. arthropathies).

[7] Streptomycin is not as acceptable as gentamicin for use in pregnant women because of adverse event profile of streptomycin (irreversible deafness in children exposed in utero has been reported).

IM – intramuscular.

underway, but it is not likely that a vaccine will be widely available in the near future.

Complications and Admission Criteria

Disease manifestations and complications are typically related to the portal of entry of *F. tularensis*. Pneumonic tularemia may result in severe pneumonia, lung abscess, or acute respiratory distress syndrome (ARDS). Glandular and ulceroglandular tularemia may progress to lymph node suppuration and secondary pneumonia. Oculoglandular tularemia can cause localized lymph node suppuration, whereas oropharyngeal tularemia has been associated with mesenteric lymphadenitis, gastrointestinal (GI) ulceration, and GI bleeding. Typhoidal tularemia not uncommonly progresses to secondary pneumonia. All forms of human tularemia carry the potential for

hematogenous dissemination of the organism to other organs such as bone, pericardium, and peritoneum, and for progression to sepsis and multi-organ failure.

Admission to the hospital is advisable for patients with any form of tularemia, to administer antibiotics intravenously and to monitor for disease progression.

Infection Control

Clinicians should notify local public health authorities, their institution's infection control professional, and their laboratory of any suspected tularemia cases. Public health authorities may conduct epidemiologic investigations and implement disease control interventions to protect the public. Both HICPAC (Hospital Infection Control Practices Advisory Committee) of the CDC and the Working Group for Civilian Biodefense recommend standard precautions for tularemia patients in a hospital setting without the need for isolation. Routine laboratory procedures should be carried out under Biosafety Level 2 (BSL-2) conditions; however, manipulation of cultures or other activities that may produce aerosol or droplets (e.g. centrifuging, grinding, vigorous shaking) require BSL-3 conditions.

Decontamination

Contaminated surfaces can be disinfected with commercially available bleach or a 1:10 dilution of household bleach and water. All persons exposed to an aerosol containing *F. tularensis* should be instructed to wash body surfaces and clothing with soap and water.

Pearls and Pitfalls

1. The onset of tularemia is usually abrupt, with fever, headache, chills and rigors, generalized body aches, and coryza. A pulse-temperature dissociation has been noted in as many as 42% of patients.

2. Clinicians should familiarize themselves with the local epidemiology of tularemia. The occurrence of human cases may follow a local tularemia epizootic (outbreak of disease in an animal population). Occurrence of pneumonic tularemia in a low-incidence area should prompt consideration of bioterrorism.

3. The diagnosis of tularemia relies heavily on clinical suspicion. Routine laboratory tests are usually non-specific. The organism is usually not apparent on gram-stained smears or tissue biopsies and usually does not grow on standard culture plates. However, *F. tularensis* may be recovered from blood and body fluids using special supportive media. Because of this and its potential hazards to laboratory personnel, the laboratory should be notified if tularemia is suspected.

References

American Public Health Association. Tularemia in J. Chin (ed.), *Control of Communicable Diseases Manual* (Washington, DC: American Public Health Association, 2000), pp. 532–5.

Avashia, S. B., Petersen, J. M., Lindley, C. M., *et al.* First reported prairie dog-to-human tularemia transmission, Texas, 2002. *Emerg. Infect. Dis.* 2004; 10(3): 483–6.

Barry, M. A. Report of pneumonic tularemia in three Boston University researchers. Boston Public Health Commission (2005), available at http://cbc.arizona.edu/sites/default/files/Boston_Univerity_Tularemia_report_2005.pdf.

Berrada, Z. L., Goethert, H. K., and Telford, S. R., 3rd. Raccoons and skunks as sentinels for enzootic tularemia. *Emerg. Infect. Dis.* 2006; 12(6): 1019–21.

Brouillard, J. E., Terriff, C. M., Tofan, A., *et al.* Antibiotic selection and resistance issues with fluoroquinolones and doxycycline against bioterrorism agents. *Pharmacotherapy* 2006; 26(1): 3–14.

Centers for Disease Control and Prevention (CDC). Tularemia, available at www.cdc.gov/tularemia/ (accessed April 4, 2018).

CDC. Tularemia – statistics, available at www.cdc.gov/tularemia/statistics/index.html (accessed April 4, 2018).

CDC. Tularemia – United States, 2001–2010. *MMWR Morb. Mortal. Wkly. Rep.* 2013; 62(47): 963–6.

CDC. Tularemia transmitted by insect bites – Wyoming 2001–2003. *MMWR Morb. Mortal. Wkly. Rep.* 2005; 54(7): 170–3.

Evans, M. E., Gregory, D. W., Schaffner, W., *et al.* Tularemia: a 30-year experience with 88 cases. *Medicine (Baltimore)* 1985; 64(4): 251–69.

Feldman, K. A., Stiles-Enos, D., Julian, K., *et al.* Tularemia on Martha's Vineyard: seroprevalence and occupational risk. *Emerg. Infect. Dis.* 2003; 9(3): 350–4.

Groseclose, S. L., Brathwaite, W. S., Hall, P. A., *et al.* Summary of notifiable diseases – United States, 2002. *MMWR Morb. Mortal. Wkly. Rep.* 2004; 51(53): 1–84.

Gürcan, Ş. Epidemiology of tularemia. *Balkan Med. J.* 2014; 31(1): 3–10.

Hassoun, A., Spera, R., and Dunkel, J. Tularemia and once-daily gentamicin. *Antimicrob. Agents Chemother.* 2006; 50(2): 824.

Johansson, A., Berglund, L., Sjöstedt, A., *et al.* Ciprofloxacin for treatment of tularemia. *Clin. Infect. Dis.* 2001; 33(2): 267–8.

Marohn, M. E. and Barry, E. M. Live attenuated tularemia vaccines: recent developments and future goals. *Vaccine* 2013; 31(35): 3485–91.

Staples, J. E., Kubota, K. A., Chalcraft, L. G., *et al.* Epidemiologic and molecular analysis of human tularemia, United States, 1964–2004. *Emerg. Infect. Dis.* 2006; 12(7): 1113–18.

World Health Organization (WHO). Biological agents in *Health Aspects of Chemical and Biological Weapons*, 2nd edn. (Geneva: WHO, 2004), pp. 250–4.

Additional Readings

Center for Infectious Disease Research and Policy (CIDRAP). Tularemia: current, comprehensive information on pathogenesis, microbiology, epidemiology, diagnosis, treatment, and prophylaxis, retrieved January 8, 2016, from www.cidrap.umn.edu/infectious-disease-topics/tularemia.

Dennis, D. T., Inglesby, T. V., Henderson, D. A., *et al.* Tularemia as a biological weapon: medical and public health management. *JAMA* 2001; 285(21): 2763–73.

Penn, R. L. Francisella tularensis in J. E. Bennett, R. Dolin, and M. J. Blaser (eds.), *Principles and Practice of Infectious Diseases*, 8th edn. (Philadelphia, PA: Elsevier/Saunders, 2015).

World Health Organization (WHO). 2007 guideline on tularaemia, available at www.who.int/csr/resources/publications/WHO_CDS_EPR_2007_7.pdf (accessed April 4, 2018).

Hantavirus

Shruti Kant and Rachel L. Chin

Introduction and Microbiology

Hantaviruses are enveloped, single-stranded RNA viruses belonging to the family *Bunyaviridae*. Hantavirus infection is a zoonosis carried by rodents, and associated with two distinct clinical syndromes: hemorrhagic fever with renal syndrome (HFRS) and hantavirus cardiopulmonary syndrome (HCPS), characterized by often lethal cardiopulmonary collapse.

Named after the Hantaan River in Korea, the virus was first identified in 1976. However, the clinical infection was first identified during the Korean War in the early 1950s, when about 3,000 US and UN soldiers developed a viral illness associated with fever, hypotension, renal failure, thrombocytopenia, and disseminated intravascular coagulation (DIC). The clinical syndrome which befell these soldiers is now recognized as HFRS. Moreover, hantaviruses are believed to have been responsible for outbreaks of hemorrhagic fevers in Russia (1913), Scandinavia (1932 to 1935), and Finland (1945).

Over the past 20 years, hantavirus has become a serious concern in the United States with the recognition of the more virulent HCPS. This syndrome was initially recognized in 1993 in the Four Corners region of the southwestern United States, the intersection formed by the borders of Utah, New Mexico, Arizona, and Colorado. As the cases of HCPS accumulated, a common clinical picture emerged. Patients developed fever, chills, and myalgias, followed by cough and dyspnea, with a rapid progression to cardiovascular collapse, respiratory failure, and death. The initial mortality rate was approximately 80%.

Human infection by hantavirus occurs through inhalation of aerosolized infected rodent urine, droppings, or saliva, resulting in HCPS or HFRS. Both diseases appear to be immunopathologic in nature, and an exuberant inflammatory response contributes to the clinical features. Rodents infected with hantaviruses are chronic carriers without apparent disease. Human-to-human transmission is rarely reported and has only been associated with Andes virus in South America.

Epidemiology

The "Old World" hantaviruses from Asia and eastern Europe cause HFRS. The field mouse (*Apodemus agrarius*) is the primary reservoir of hantaviruses that cause HFRS. These infections are a major public health problem in Asia and eastern Europe, with more than 100,000 cases annually in China and significant numbers in Korea and eastern Russia. HFRS can be caused by any of the Old World hantavirus strains, including Hantaan, Seoul, Dobrava–Belgrade, and Puumala viruses. Fatality associated with these infections can be as high as 10%.

Presently, 13 "New World" hantaviruses have been described. Four of these cause HCPS in North America. Sin Nombre virus (SNV) is the prototypical New World hantavirus and the cause of the vast majority of cases of HCPS in the United States. As of January 2016, a total of 659 cases of HCPS had been identified in 34 states since 1993, with a case fatality rate of 36%. The deer mouse (*Peromyscus maniculatus*) is the primary reservoir of SNV. This small mammal is common and widespread in rural areas throughout much of the United States. Although prevalence varies temporally and geographically, on average about 10% of deer mice tested throughout the range of the species show evidence of infection with SNV. Nearly the entire continental United States falls within the range of one or more of these host species. There are several hantaviruses associated with different rodent populations, but only the deer and white-footed mice are commonly associated with peridomestic environments. Rodent reservoirs of human-pathogenic hantaviruses are not common in cities, making persons with rural residences, occupations, or hobbies the major targets of hantavirus disease because of their increased exposure to rodents or rodent droppings.

Clinical Features

The clinical features of both HFRS and HCPS are directly related to the pathophysiology of the hantaviruses, which preferentially infect the endothelial cells. Endothelial cells in the renal and pulmonary microvasculature are the principle targets in HFRS and HCPS, respectively. Damage to the microvasculature causes capillary leak, fluid extravasation, and eventually organ failure. It has been suggested that immune mechanisms rather than direct viral cytopathic effects are responsible for the capillary leakage seen in both HFRS and HCPS. However, more recent evidence suggests that a virus-cell interaction and an inhibiting interferon type-1 response may also play a role.

Release of an as yet unidentified myocardial depressant also appears central to the pathogenesis of HCPS. This depressant, possibly cytokine mediated, causes cardiogenic shock with an elevated systemic vascular resistance. This cardiogenic depression is exacerbated by hypovolemia secondary to plasma leakage from capillaries, resulting in precipitous cardiopulmonary collapse. The name change from hantavirus pulmonary syndrome to cardiopulmonary syndrome reflects the key contribution to morbidity and mortality made by this myocardial factor.

Hemorrhagic Fever with Renal Syndrome

The clinical features of HFRS consist of a triad of fever, hemorrhagic manifestations, and renal insufficiency. The average incubation period varies from 4 to 45 days. The disease course may range from mild to severe. Severe disease is characterized by hypovolemic shock. Subclinical infections are especially common in children.

Hemorrhagic fever with renal syndrome is characterized by five progressive stages: (a) a febrile stage; (b) a hypotensive stage; (c) an oliguric stage; (d) a polyuric stage; and (e) a convalescent stage (see Table 71.1). Physicians should be aware of the various presentations during each stage. Individual patients may completely skip stages.

The febrile stage is characterized by an abrupt onset of fever with temperatures in the range of 40°C, lasting about 3 to 6 days. Patients may complain of headache, chills, abdominal pain, and malaise. Clinical findings include flushing of the face, neck, and chest due to probable vascular dysregulation, and petechiae in the axilla and on the soft palate. Subconjunctival hemorrhage is noted in one-third of patients. Cardiac manifestations include bradycardia of less than 40 bpm.

The hypotensive stage lasts approximately a few hours to 2 days. It occurs in 11% of patients and coincides with defervescence. Patients may have tachycardia, which may indicate impending shock and an acute abdomen caused by a paralytic ileus. Central nervous system manifestations include convulsions, obtundation, or coma.

The oliguric stage, occurring in 65% of patients, lasts about 3 days to 2 weeks.

This stage is characterized by oliguria, hypertension, bleeding tendency (caused by uremia), and edema. Patients may develop pulmonary edema. Up to 50% of the deaths due to HFRS occur during this phase.

As HFRS progresses, oliguria is followed by diuresis in the range of 3 to 6 L/day. This polyuric stage may lasts up to 2 to 3 weeks. Responsiveness of the collecting duct to vasopressin is reduced. Rapid signs of dehydration and severe shock can occur if fluid replacement is inadequate. The patient's volume status should be closely monitored.

The convalescent stage lasts for 3 to 6 months. Clinical recovery usually begins with gradual resolution of symptoms and azotemia. The concentrating capacity of the renal tubules recovers over many months.

Hantavirus Cardiopulmonary Syndrome

The clinical course of HCPS can be divided into discrete phases: (a) the febrile phase; (b) the cardiopulmonary phase; and (c) the convalescent phase (see Table 71.2).

The Febrile Prodromal Phase

Patients with HCPS typically present with a relatively short febrile prodrome lasting 3 to 5 days. Early symptoms are non-specific and include fever, myalgias, headache, chills, dizziness, non-productive cough, nausea, vomiting, and other gastrointestinal symptoms. The triad of fever, tachypnea (respiratory rate 26 to 30), and tachycardia are often seen on initial presentation. The physical examination is usually otherwise normal. It is not uncommon for patients to be sent home after an initial urgent care or emergency department (ED) visit with these non-specific complaints, only to return hours or a few days later extremely ill. The diagnosis is seldom made at this stage, because cough and tachypnea generally do not develop until approximately day 7.

The Cardiopulmonary Phase

Once the cardiopulmonary phase begins, the disease progresses rapidly, requiring hospitalization. Within 24 hours of initial evaluation, most patients develop hypotension, progressive pulmonary edema, and hypoxia, usually requiring mechanical ventilation. The patients with fatal infections develop severe myocardial depression, which can progress to sinus bradycardia with subsequent electromechanical dissociation, ventricular tachycardia, or fibrillation. Hemodynamic compromise can occur 5 days after symptom onset.

In contrast to HFRS, overt hemorrhage rarely occurs in HCPS, though hemorrhage is occasionally seen in association with DIC. In contrast to septic shock, HCPS patients have a low cardiac output with a raised systemic vascular resistance. Poor prognostic indicators include a plasma lactate of greater than 4.0 mmol/L or a cardiac index of less than 2.2 L/min/m².

Table 71.1 Clinical Features: Hemorrhagic Fever with Renal Syndrome

Incubation period	Up to 45 days after exposure
Organisms	Hantaan Seoul Puumala Dobrava/Belgrade
Transmission	Aerosolized rodent urine, droppings, or saliva
Signs and symptoms	**Febrile stage:** • Sudden onset of fever, chills, malaise, weakness, myalgias • Prostration, dehydration, obtundation • Thirst, nausea, vomiting, abdominal pain • Flushing of the face and V-area of the neck and thorax, subconjunctival hemorrhage • Petechiae, ecchymosis, mucous membrane hemorrhages • Bradycardia **Hypotensive stage:** • Tachycardia • Acute abdomen • Paralytic ileus • Convulsion • Obtundation • Coma **Oliguric stage:** • Oliguria • Bleeding tendencies • Hypertension **Polyuric stage:** • Diuresis: 3–6 L/day • Dehydration • Electrolyte imbalance • Shock **Convalescence:** • Resolution of constitutional symptoms • Resolution of azotemia • Resolution of renal failure
Progression and complications	**Progression:** • Febrile stage lasting 3–6 days • Hypotensive stage lasting from a few hours to 2 days • Oliguric stage lasting few days to 2 weeks • Polyuric stage lasting 2–3 weeks • Convalescent stage of 3–6 months **Complications:** • Hypotension • Shock • Renal failure • Coma
Laboratory and radiographic findings	• Thrombocytopenia • Prolonged bleeding time, PT, aPTT • DIC • Proteinuria, microhematuria • Abnormal urinary sedimentation • Both IgM and IgG hantavirus-specific antibodies are present

aPTT – activated partial thromboplastin time; PT – prothrombin time.

Table 71.2 Clinical Features: Hantavirus Cardiopulmonary Syndrome

Incubation period	Up to 45 days after exposure
Organisms	Sin Nombre virus Black Creek Canal Bayou New York
Transmission	Exposure to aerosolized rodent urine, droppings, or saliva
Signs and symptoms	**Febrile prodromal phase:** • Sudden onset of fever, chills, malaise, weakness, myalgias, headache • Dyspnea, cough, tachypnea, tachycardia • Gastrointestinal complaints such as nausea, vomiting, abdominal pain, diarrhea • Weakness, dehydration
Progression and complications	**Progression to cardiopulmonary phase:** • Pulmonary edema • Large pleural effusions • Respiratory decompensation • Hypotension **Complications:** • Severe cardiopulmonary dysfunction • Myocardial depression • Moderate to severely depressed left ventricular systolic function • Pulmonary edema and hypoxemia • Hypotension and shock • Bradycardia, electromechanical dissociation, arrhythmias
Laboratory and radiographic findings	**Peripheral blood smear triad:** • Thrombocytopenia • Increased immature granulocytes (with elevated white blood cell counts) • Large atypical immunoblastic lymphocytes **Other laboratory findings:** • Hemoconcentration due to intrapulmonary capillary leak *or* • Decreased hematocrit due to fluid administration, *then* • Increased lactate and progressive acidosis • Prolonged partial thromboplastin time and prothrombin time • Both IgM and IgG hantavirus-specific antibodies are present **Radiographic findings:** • Pulmonary edema • Interstitial edema • Severe bilateral airspace disease • Pleural effusions

Pulmonary edema and pleural effusions are common. Fortunately, multi-organ dysfunction is rarely seen, though HCPS patients sometimes have mildly impaired renal function.

The Convalescent Phase

Survivors frequently become polyuric during convalescence and improve almost as rapidly as they decompensated. Of note, symptoms such as fatigue, malaise, and dyspnea can last for months after resolution of the infection.

Differential Diagnosis

HFRS

Differential diagnosis in HFRS includes:

- murine typhus
- hepatitis
- Colorado tick fever
- septicemia
- heat stroke
- DIC
- scrub typhus
- hemolytic uremic syndrome
- other hemorrhagic fevers (e.g. dengue fever, Machupo)

HCPS

HCPS is commonly confused with acute respiratory distress syndrome from other infectious causes, pyelonephritis, intra-abdominal processes, pneumonias, and systemic infections such as rickettsial disease or plague.

Other conditions to consider in HCPS are:

- pneumonias
- influenza
- rickettsial disease
- pneumonic plague
- tularemia
- anthrax
- *Yersinia pestis*
- Colorado tick fever
- lymphocytic choriomeningitis virus infection
- dengue fever
- Rocky Mountain spotted fever
- Q fever
- Lyme disease
- rat-bite fever

Key features that may help to distinguish HCPS are:

- thrombocytopenia
- history of exposure to rodents or rodent droppings
- history of rural exposure

Thrombocytopenia is the single most important finding that should suggest further investigation, but characteristic hematological findings are often absent before onset of respiratory distress. A history of exposure to rodents or rodent droppings is common, but often not elicited. Rural exposure also increases the risk of other acute febrile illnesses associated with animal or arthropod exposure.

Symptoms that make a diagnosis of HCPS *unlikely* include rashes, conjunctival or other hemorrhages, throat or conjunctival erythema, petechiae, and peripheral or periorbital edema.

Laboratory and Radiographic Findings

Providers should contact their local public health authorities promptly if hantavirus-associated illness is suspected. Blood samples should be obtained and forwarded to the state health department for hantavirus antibody testing. In both HFRS and HCPS, a humoral response is detectable during the initial presentation of the patient. Both IgM and IgG hantavirus-specific antibodies are present. Real-time reverse transcriptase-PCR tests have been developed to identify Hantaan, Dobrava, Seoul, and Puumala viruses responsible for HFRS. Definitive diagnosis of HCPS can be made on the basis of one of three serologic assays: an enzyme-linked immunosorbent assay, western blot, and a rapid immunoblot strip assay that detects SNV antibodies in the acute phase of the disease. Local public health agencies will coordinate the diagnostic approach.

HFRS

The hallmark of HFRS is the combination of elevated creatinine (reduced glomerular filtration rate), proteinuria, and microscopic hematuria. Nephrotic range proteinuria can occur. Thrombocytopenia is almost universally seen and laboratory evidence of DIC is common.

HCPS

Numerous laboratory abnormalities may be apparent at initial evaluation. The peripheral blood smear shows a triad of thrombocytopenia, increased immature granulocytes (accompanied with an elevated white blood cell count), and large immunoblastoid lymphocytes. Hemoconcentration may be marked because of intrapulmonary capillary leak, but the hematocrit may be decreased because of pre-existing low red cell mass and fluid administration. Often, there is prolongation of the partial thromboplastin time and the prothrombin time.

On initial chest X-ray, approximately one-third of patients show evidence of pulmonary edema. Although the chest X-ray is usually normal during the prodromal phase, onset of the cardiopulmonary phase causes a characteristic radiologic evolution. Within 48 hours, virtually all patients demonstrate interstitial edema and two-thirds have developed severe bilateral airspace disease. Mild interstitial pulmonary edema, with Kerley B lines and peribronchial cuffing, rapidly progresses to severe bilateral alveolar edema, with a basilar or perihilar pattern. Pleural effusions are commonly observed late in the course of the disease.

Bronchoalveolar lavage fluid is remarkable for its absence of inflammatory cells. The majority of HCPS patients have a PaO_2/FiO_2 of less than 100 (acute respiratory distress syndrome has values of <150). Although gas-exchange abnormalities may become quite severe in many patients, most can be adequately oxygenated.

On electrocardiogram, sinus tachycardia, observed early in the cardiopulmonary phase, may progress to bradycardia, ventricular tachycardia, ventricular fibrillation, and pulseless electrical activity (PEA).

Treatment

Treatment of both HFRS and HCPS is primarily supportive.

HFRS

Successful treatment begins with prompt diagnosis. Shock is usually managed with pressors and judicious fluid

Table 71.3 Treatment of Hantavirus Cardiopulmonary Syndrome

Patient Category	Treatment
Adults/children	Supportive care: early recognition and admission to an ICU
	Respiratory support as indicated, including mechanical ventilation
	Early use of vasopressors to support hypotension
	Cautious use of IV fluids
	ECMO should be considered for cardiopulmonary support, especially for those with poor prognosticators
	No specific antiviral therapy is recommended
	Empiric antibiotic therapy should be started for possible bacterial infection while awaiting confirmation of hantavirus infection

administration; one to two units of human serum albumin may be a useful adjunct. Dialysis reduces the 5 to 15% mortality rate to less than 5% and should be initiated promptly to treat metabolic derangements such as hyperkalemia, volume overload, or uremia. Careful volume control is extremely important because pulmonary edema and intracerebral hemorrhage are two major causes of death in the oliguric stage. Polyuria, in the late phase of the disease, can lead to potentially fatal volume and electrolyte abnormalities.

HCPS

Pre-hospital care of HCPS is supportive. Administer oxygen by nasal cannula, Venturi, or non-rebreather mask, intubate for severe respiratory distress, and support hemodynamics with crystalloids. Rapid transfer to a tertiary care center with intensive care unit (ICU) capabilities is of paramount importance.

Management of HCPS in the acute care setting depends on the stage of the disease. In prodromal HCPS, the provider's main responsibility is to diagnose and admit for close observation. In cases of advanced HCPS, aggressive resuscitation and transfer to an ICU are required. Patients in respiratory failure should be intubated, though hemodynamic status may decline precipitously because of positive pressure ventilation and low intravascular volume status. Fluid resuscitation with crystalloids is indicated for signs of hemodynamic compromise. Inotropic agents such as dobutamine and dopamine should be considered early in the treatment of shock in HCPS patients, together with judicious intravascular volume expansion. Dobutamine is the preferred inotrope, with dopamine added as necessary to maintain blood pressure. Patients with HCPS may require large doses of pressors to maintain a stable blood pressure.

A flow-directed pulmonary artery catheterization (PAC), or Swan–Ganz catheter, is vital to direct fluid resuscitation in severe HCPS. HCPS demonstrates a characteristic hemodynamic profile: in early HCPS, a low pulmonary artery occlusion pressure (consistent with a pulmonary capillary leak) and low cardiac index are apparent. In advanced HCPS, a severe drop in cardiac index is associated with increased systemic vascular resistance. Pulmonary wedge pressures should be maintained in the low-normal range because of the extreme capillary leak.

Extracorporeal membrane oxygenation (ECMO) provides both respiratory and cardiovascular support and has resulted in survival in patients with poor prognostic indicators, such as serum lactate levels exceeding 4 mmol/L and evidence of

cardiogenic shock. Prior to the use of ECMO, a cardiac index of less than 2.5 L/min/m^2 predicted 100% mortality (see Table 71.3).

Studies looking at the use of human immune plasma containing neutralizing antibody (Nab) have shown some promise with a decrease in case fatality rates. However, more studies are needed to confirm its efficacy.

Patients undergoing evaluation for HCPS should be treated with antibiotic regimens designed to treat typical and atypical community-acquired pneumonia and sepsis, including *Yersinia pestis*. Broad-spectrum antibiotics are indicated for all patients presenting with respiratory distress and fever. A third- or fourth-generation cephalosporin plus a respiratory fluoroquinolone or azithromycin are a reasonable start (see Table 71.4).

Currently, no prophylaxis is available against HFRS or HCPS, though studies are underway to develop a vaccine.

Complications and Admission Criteria

Acute complications of HFRS can include hypotension, shock, renal failure, coma, and death. All patients suspected of HFRS should be admitted for stablization and supportive care. HFRS is usually a self-limited disease. Most patients recover without any sequelae; however, in a few patients, neurologic and renal tubular defects may persist. Defective sodium reabsorption has been observed up to 1 year after the illness, causing increased sodium wasting. Long-term monitoring of proteinuria and hypertension is essential. Some patients may develop hypercalciuria and hyperphosphaturia as a result of tubular defects.

Potential acute complications of HCPS include cardiovascular collapse, respiratory and renal failure, anoxic brain injury, PEA, ventricular tachycardia, ventricular fibrillation, and death. All patients suspected of HCPS should be admitted for supportive care as they can deteriorate very rapidly. Those patients who recover from HCPS usually recover without sequelae, though symptoms of fatigue, malaise, and dyspnea can last for months after the illness.

Infection Control and Prophylaxis

Because pneumonic plague is in the differential diagnosis of HCPS, respiratory isolation of patients with suspected cases is recommended even though person-to-person transmission has not been observed.

Human infection by the SNV occurs most commonly through the inhalation of infectious, aerosolized deer mouse

Table 71.4 Empiric Antibiotic Therapy in Hantavirus Cardiopulmonary Syndrome

Patient Category	Therapy Recommendation
Adults: preferred choices	Empiric therapy for possible bacterial infection until diagnosis of HCPS is definitively determined: A beta-lactam *plus* either a respiratory fluoroquinolone or azithromycin: • Ceftriaxone 2 g IV every 24 hours *plus* • Levofloxacin 750 mg IV every 24 hours *or* • Moxifloxacin 400 mg IV every 24 hours Alternatives: • Ceftriaxone 2 g IV every 24 hours *plus* • Azithromycin 500 mg IV every 24 hours For penicillin-allergic patients: • Levofloxacin 750 mg IV every 24 hours *plus* • Aztreonam 2 g IV every 8 hours *and* • Vancomycin 15–20 mg/kg/dose IV every 8–12 hours
Children	Azithromycin 10 mg/kg/dose IV every 24 hours *plus* Ceftriaxone 50 mg/kg/dose IV every 24 hours *or* Meropenem 20 mg/kg/dose IV every 8 hours *or* Piperacillin-tazobactam 100 mg/kg/dose of piperacillin component IV every 8 hours For penicillin-allergic patients: • Vancomycin 15 mg/kg/dose IV every 6 hours *and* • Aztreonam 30 mg/kg/dose IV every 8 hours

saliva or excreta, thus prevention through environmental measures is crucial. Such measures are coordinated by public health authorities. Transmission can occur when dried materials contaminated by rodent excreta are disturbed and inhaled, directly introduced into broken skin or conjunctivae, or, possibly, ingested in contaminated food or water. High risk of exposure has been associated with entering or cleaning rodent-infested structures. Persons have also acquired HFRS or HCPS after being bitten by rodents.

Risk factors for Sin Nombre virus infection include:

- occupying or cleaning actively rodent infested cabins, barns, or outbuildings
- disturbing excreta or rodent nests around the home or workplace
- handling mice without gloves
- keeping captive wild rodents as pets or research subjects
- handling equipment or machinery that has been in storage
- hand plowing or planting
- disturbing excreta in rodent-infested areas while hiking or camping
- sleeping on the ground

Pearls and Pitfalls

1. The early phase of milder hantavirus cases have fewer constitutional symptoms: hypotension is found rather than shock; hemorrhage manifestations may be limited to petechiae; and renal failure can be mild, transient, and readily overlooked. These cases can be easily misdiagnosed.
2. Patients with HCPS can deteriorate quickly. Patients not admitted for observation or treatment should be given careful instructions regarding signs and symptoms that should prompt their immediate return for evaluation.
3. Both HCPS and HFRS show a hemodynamic pattern of low cardiac output and high systemic vascular resistance.
4. Cardiac arrhythmias portend a poor outcome and should be treated aggressively.
5. Most cases of HCPS occur in rural communities, which may lack the facilities for aggressive intensive care.
6. Transport early and quickly: a patient who subsequently "rules out" at a tertiary care center is preferable to a patient who deteriorates suddenly and dies en route.

References

Aitichou, M., Saleh, S. S., McElroy, A. K., *et al.* Identification of DObrava, Hantaan, Seoul and Puumala viruses by one-step real-time RT-PCR. *J. Virol. Methods* 2005; 124(1–2): 21–6.

Centers for Disease Control and Prevention (CDC). Hantavirus pulmonary syndrome – United States: updated recommendations for risk reduction. *MMWR Morb. Mortal. Wkly. Rep.* 2002; 51(RR-9): 1–12.

Dull, S. M., Brillman, J. C., Simpson, S. Q., *et al.* Hantavirus pulmonary syndrome: recognition and emergency department management. *Ann. Emerg. Med.* 1994; 24(3): 530–6.

Dvorscak, L. and Czuchlewski, D. R. Successful triage of suspected hantavirus cardiopulmonary syndrome by peripheral blood smear review. *Am. J. Clin. Pathol.* 2014; 142(2): 196–201.

Hooper, J. W., Moon, J. E., Paolino, K. M., *et al.* A Phase I clinical trial of Hantaan virus and Puumala virus M-segment DNA vaccines for haemorrhagic fever with renal syndrome delivered by electroporation. *Clin. Microbiol. Infect.* 2014; 20(Suppl. 5): 110–17.

Katai, L. H., Williamson, M. R., Telepak, R. J., *et al.* Hantavirus pulmonary syndrome: radiographic findings in 16 patients. *Radiology* 1994; 191(3): 665–8.

Koster, F., Foucar, K., Hjelle, B., *et al.* Rapid presumptive diagnosis of hantavirus cardiopulmonary syndrome by peripheral blood smear review. *Am. J. Clin. Pathol.* 2001; 116(5): 665–72.

Manigold, T. and Vial, P. Human hantavirus infections: epidemiology, clinical features, pathogenesis and immunology. *Swiss Med. Wkly.* 2014; 144: w13937.

Peters, C. J. and Khan, A. S. Hantavirus pulmonary syndrome: the new American hemorrhagic fever. *Clin. Infect. Dis.* 2002; 34(9): 1224–31.

Peters, C. J., Simpson, G. L., and Levy, H. Spectrum of hantavirus infection: hemorrhagic fever with renal syndrome and hantavirus pulmonary syndrome. *Ann. Rev. Med.* 1999; 50: 531–45.

Vial, P. A., Valdivieso, F., Calvo, M., *et al.* A non-randomized multicenter trial of human immune plasma for treatment of hantavirus cardiopulmonary syndrome by ANDV. *Antivir. Ther.* 2014; doi: 10.3851/IMP2875.

Additional Readings

Centers for Disease Control and Prevention (CDC). Hantavirus, available at www.cdc.gov/ncidod/diseases/hanta/hps/index.htm (accessed December 12, 2017).

Mertz, G. J., Miedzinski, L., Goade, D., *et al.* Placebo-controlled, double-blind trial of intravenous ribavirin for the treatment of hantavirus cardiopulmonary syndrome in Northern America. *Clin. Infect. Dis.* 2004; 39(9): 1307–13.

Ramos, M. M., Overturf, G. D., Crowley, M. R., *et al.* Infection with Sin Nombre hantavirus: clinical presentation and outcome in children and adolescents. *Pediatrics* 2001; 108(2): e27, available at www.pediatrics.org/cgi/reprint/108/2/e27.pdf (accessed December 12, 2017).

Chapter

72

Ebola Virus Disease

Edwin Dietrich, Bradley W. Frazee, and Timothy M. Uyeki*

Introduction, Microbiology, and Pathophysiology

Ebola virus disease (EVD) is caused by infection with *Ebolavirus* and has resulted in substantial mortality during sporadic outbreaks primarily in Central and East Africa prior to 2013. The largest EVD outbreak to date is believed to have started in southeastern Guinea in late 2013 and had resulted in greater than 11,300 deaths in West Africa as of April 2016. The West Africa EVD outbreak was a global health crisis, in which the paucity of medical resources and public health infrastructure in West Africa exacerbated the burden of disease. During this outbreak, patients with EVD were diagnosed and managed in the United States for the first time.

Ebola virus disease attracted national attention in August 2014 when two EVD patients were medically evacuated from Liberia to the United States for clinical management at Emory University Hospital, and later when a cluster of three EVD cases were identified at one hospital in Dallas, Texas. The index patient in the cluster, the first patient diagnosed with EVD in the United States, presented initially to an emergency department (ED) with non-specific febrile illness. He had a history of recent contact with a sick person and travel from Liberia was not elicited, but EVD was not suspected, and the patient was discharged home. The patient re-presented to the same ED 2 days later with worsening symptoms, including diarrhea and persistent fever, and *Ebolavirus* infection was confirmed; he later developed multi-organ failure and died. Two nurses who provided care for this patient acquired nosocomial Ebola virus infection. Overall, 11 EVD patients were managed in the United States during 2014 to 2015, including seven medically

evacuated cases, two imported cases, and two secondary cases, with two (18%) deaths.

Acute care providers in the United States and other developed countries must remain aware of *Ebolavirus* infection as a potential cause of fever in patients who have recently travel from an area with an ongoing EVD outbreak. When a patient with suspected EVD is identified, immediate, critical steps include rapid implementation of isolation and recommended infection prevention and control measures, notification of public health authorities, and activation of systems of care that have been established by hospitals and public health agencies.

EVD is caused by infection with viruses belonging to the family *Filoviridae*, genus *Ebolavirus*, which are enveloped, non-segmented, single-stranded negative sense RNA viruses. Four *Ebolavirus* species (*Zaire, Sudan, Bundibugyo, Tai Forest*) are known to cause disease in humans. *Ebolavirus* was discovered in 1976 near the Ebola River in the Democratic Republic of Congo, when an EVD outbreak resulted in 318 confirmed cases and 280 deaths. *Ebolavirus* is similar in structure to Marburg virus, another filovirus that was discovered in 1967 when it caused deaths among primates in research facilities in West Germany.

Pathophysiology

Virulence is mediated through several pathophysiologic effects including direct viral injury, immunosuppression, cytokine dysregulation, increased vascular permeability, and impaired coagulation. Evidence of microscopic hemorrhage is often found, but ranges in severity. Once Ebola virus has entered the patient through mucous membranes, or breaks in the skin, or through percutaneous routes, infection of many cell types occurs,

---

* The findings and conclusions in this report are those of the authors and do not necessarily represent the official position of the Centers for Disease Control and Prevention.

including monocytes, macrophages, dendritic cells, endothelial cells, fibroblasts, hepatocytes, adrenal cortical cells, and epithelial cells. Hepatocellular necrosis is associated with dysregulation of clotting factors and subsequent coagulopathy. Adrenocortical necrosis is associated with hypotension and impaired steroid synthesis. Lymphocytes undergo apoptosis resulting in decreased lymphocyte counts. *Ebolavirus* triggers release of pro-inflammatory cytokines with subsequent vascular leak and impairment of clotting ultimately resulting in multi-organ failure and shock.

Epidemiology

Mortality from Ebola virus disease in sporadic outbreaks primarily in Central and East Africa has ranged from 40 to 88%. The most recent and largest outbreak due to *Zaire* Ebolavirus began in late 2013 in Guinea, with subsequent spread to Liberia and Sierra Leone. By April 2016, ten countries had reported 28,616 suspected, probable, and confirmed cases of EVD and 11,310 deaths, primarily from the three most affected countries in West Africa, though the actual number of cases and deaths is likely higher. Reported mortality in Ebola treatment units during this outbreak ranged from 37 to 74%. Mortality risk factors include very young or older age, and high Ebola viral load at admission to an Ebola treatment unit. The highest mortality was observed in young children. However, among the 27 adult EVD patients who were managed in US or European hospitals during 2014 to 2015, the case fatality proportion was 18.5%.

Ebola virus disease is believed to be a zoonosis, with fruit bats suspected to be the animal reservoir for Ebolaviruses, though Ebolaviruses have not been isolated from bats. *Ebola-virus* infection of mammals such as duikers (forest antelopes) and primates can occur and may also be a source of zoonotic transmission. EVD outbreaks are thought to begin with zoonotic *Ebolavirus* transmission to humans from an infected animal. Subsequent chains of person-to-person *Ebolavirus* transmission can occur through direct contact with blood or other body fluids (including urine, saliva, sweat, feces, vomit, breast milk, or semen) of a symptomatic person with EVD or a corpse that died of EVD (such as during a traditional burial ceremony); nosocomial transmission can also occur through percutaneous exposure to needles and syringes with blood from an EVD patient or through mucous membrane exposure to fomites or contaminated medical equipment. It is believed that EVD patients are not infectious until symptom onset. There is no known airborne transmission of Ebola virus, though cough has been reported in about one-third of EVD cases, and respiratory failure can occur. Ebola viral RNA has been detected in lower respiratory tract specimens from one critically ill patient. Ebola virus RNA is not always detectable in blood at the time of symptom onset, but increases logarithmically during the acute phase of illness to more than 1 million RNA copies/ml serum. Ebola virus RNA levels are highest in blood from critically ill and fatal cases, and the bodies of deceased EVD patients are highly infectious.

Ebola virus is considered to be only moderately transmissible (as compared to respiratory transmitted viruses such as rubeola), with a basic reproductive number (Ro) of approximately 2, even in community settings without access to personal protective equipment. Ebola virus may persist in certain immunologically protected organ tissues (eye, testes, brain) in EVD survivors for unknown duration, and has been isolated from semen, intraocular fluid, and cerebrospinal fluid of survivors. Sexual transmission of Ebola virus from a male survivor to a sexual partner has been reported 179 days after EVD onset in Liberia, and at approximately 470 days after EVD onset in Guinea. Other sporadic cases of suspected *Ebolavirus* transmission from a male EVD survivor to a sexual partner have been reported.

Clinical Features

The mean incubation period is 9 to 11 days, with a range of 2 to 21 days after exposure and infection (typically through mucous membranes). Incubation may be shorter with percutaneous exposure. The early signs and symptoms of EVD are non-specific (fatigue, anorexia, headache, asthenia, myalgia, arthralgia, and fever is often but not always present) (See Table 72.1). Approximately 4 to 7 days after illness onset, gastrointestinal tract symptoms commonly occur (vomiting, diarrhea, abdominal pain). Diarrhea may be profuse, leading to hypovolemia. A maculopapular rash may occur beginning about the fifth illness day. Other less common symptoms may include cough, sore throat, hiccups, and hemorrhagic conjunctivitis. However, frank hemorrhage is less commonly observed. Metabolic abnormalities include hyponatremia, hypokalemia, hypocalcemia, and hypomagnesemia. Hypoalbuminemia and transaminitis with AST elevated two to five times higher than ALT are commonly found. Multi-organ failure (respiratory and renal failure), neurologic abnormalities (coma, encephalitis), and septic shock can occur in critically ill and fatal cases. Mortality risk factors include high Ebola viral load in blood at admission, acute kidney injury, very young or older age, and transaminitis.

Differential Diagnosis

The differential diagnosis for fever in a returning traveler is broad, and includes many diseases far more prevalent than EVD (See Table 72.2). In a traveler returning to the United States from Africa, tropical infectious diseases are a consideration, including malaria, typhoid fever, tickborne rickettsiae, schistosomiasis, and filiariasis (see Chapter 60, Fever in the Returning Traveler). Other community-acquired infections to be considered include enteric and respiratory viral infections, including influenza.

Malaria is by far the most likely cause of febrile illness, and the most common treatable infectious disease in a traveler returning from Africa. EVD signs and symptoms are similar to malaria. Therefore, malaria must be tested for promptly. While *Ebolavirus* and malaria co-infection can occur, testing that confirms malaria can provide the diagnosis in a returned traveler who is febrile without a history of direct contact with the blood or bodily fluids of an EVD patient or corpse.

Laboratory and Radiographic Findings

Patients who are suspected (persons under investigation) to have *Ebolavirus* infection should have blood collected for

Table 72.1 Fever in Returning Traveler from West Africa: Differential Diagnosis

- Community-acquired diseases:
  - Influenza
  - Community-acquired pneumonia
  - Pyelonephritis
  - Acute HIV
  - Hepatitis A, E
  - Viral/bacterial meningitis
- Tropical diseases:
  - Malaria (*P. falciparum, P. vivax*)
  - Tickborne rickettsiae
  - Acute schistosomiasis
  - Filariasis
  - African trypanosomiasis
  - Typhoid fever
  - Dengue

wwwnc.cdc.gov/travel/yellowbook/2016/post-travel-evaluation/fever-in-returned-travelers

Table 72.2 Presenting Signs and Symptoms of Ebola Virus Infection*

Fever	70%
Headache	63%
Weakness	52%
Dizziness	47%
Diarrhea	41%
Abdominal pain	31%
Sore throat	29%
Vomiting	27%
Confusion	15%
Cough	15%
Petechial rash	2%

* Among 44 thoroughly documented cases in 2014 in Sierra Leone, of whom 36 died (J. S. Schieffelin, J. G. Shaffer, A. Goba, *et al.*, Clinical illness and outcomes in patients with Ebola in Sierra Leone. *N. Engl. J. Med.* 2014; 371(22): 2092–100).

Ebolavirus testing while following recommended infection control measures. Blood, serum, and plasma specimens can be tested for Ebola virus RNA by reverse transcription polymerase chain reaction (RT-PCR) at public health laboratories and the CDC. Blood should also be tested for malaria (thick and thin smears, PCR), and other clinical specimens (upper respiratory tract, stool) may be collected and tested by rapid diagnostic test (e.g. for influenza viruses) or by multi-pathogen molecular assays. A complete blood count with differential, metabolic panel liver function tests, and blood cultures should all be obtained. Other tests may be useful depending upon the patient's history and clinical presentation, such as lactic acid, chest X-ray, urinalysis, and urine culture, as well as cerebrospinal fluid studies if there is a concern for meningitis or encephalitis. The local health department, once contacted, will arrange specimen transport for any patient in whom EVD is suspected.

EVD Screening Algorithm

- Triage assessment (CDC Ebola algorithm: www.cdc.gov/vhf/ebola/pdf/ebola-algorithm.pdf):
  - Does the patient have a fever (subjective or >100.4° F) *or* compatible EVD symptoms such as headache, weakness, muscle pain, vomiting, diarrhea, abdominal pain, or hemorrhage?
  - Has the patient traveled to an Ebola virus disease-affected area in the 21 days before illness onset?
- Protocol for patients who screen positive:
  - Isolate in single room with private bathroom
  - Standard, contact, and droplet precautions
  - Notify hospital infection control program
  - Report to the local health department
- Risk assessment for patients who screen positive (CDC evaluation checklist):
  - High-risk exposures:
    - Percutaneous or mucous membrane exposure to blood/body fluids from an EVD patient
    - Direct skin contact with skin, blood, or body fluids from an EVD patient
    - Processing blood or body fluids from an EVD patient without appropriate PPE (personal protective equipment)
    - Direct contact with a dead body in an Ebola virus disease-affected area without appropriate PPE
  - Low-risk exposures:
    - Household members of an EVD patient or others who had brief direct contact with an EVD patient without appropriate PPE
    - Health-care personnel in facilities with EVD patients who have been in care areas of EVD patients without recommended PPE

Treatment and Prophylaxis

In the care of a patient with suspected EVD (person under investigation), medical staff must balance the twin goals of patient care and prevention of disease transmission. Given the high mortality associated with EVD, prevention of nosocomial transmission is a crucial dimension of management. The critical and difficult issue of infection control is discussed further below.

There are no approved medications for treatment of EVD as of early 2018 and clinical management is focused on supportive care: fluid management, correction of electrolyte abnormalities, treatment of co-infections, and advanced organ support for multi-organ failure. This requires critical care nursing and intensive care management. Drugs under investigation include immunotherapy (triple monoclonal antibody – ZMapp, convalescent plasma) and antivirals (favipiravir, GS-5734, TKM Ebola, AVI-7535, BCX-4430), but only one randomized trial of an investigational therapeutic was conducted and clinical benefit was suggested (ZMapp). Post-exposure prophylaxis following suspected percutaneous exposure to *Ebolavirus* has been described using investigational antivirals, immunotherapeutics, and Ebola vaccine, but effectiveness is unknown.

Supportive Care

The early phase of EVD is characterized by intravascular volume depletion from cholera-like gastrointestinal losses. Fluid resuscitation and correction of electrolyte abnormalities is a vital first step, followed by vasopressor support in those with refractory hypotension. Malaria co-infection if present or suspected should be treated as soon as possible because one study reported that malaria co-infection increases the risk of mortality in EVD patients. In patients who progress to septic shock, broad-spectrum antibiotics are recommended to treat potential secondary invasive enteric bacterial infection. As the disease progresses, volume depletion and direct endothelial injury combine to cause end-organ injury, often resulting in respiratory distress syndrome requiring mechanical ventilation or acute renal failure requiring renal replacement therapy.

Frontiers in Care

Although the latest EVD outbreaks in Guinea, Sierra Leone, and Liberia were declared over in late 2015 or early 2016, subsequent emergence of sporadic cases reminded the world of the challenges of controlling EVD epidemics in low-resource settings. In the absence of approved therapeutics, it has been suggested that use of protocolized treatment "packages" consisting of simple and inexpensive interventions, emphasizing early aggressive hydration and control of fluid losses, may help to reduce mortality. Several Ebola candidate vaccines are in Phase II or III clinical trials, and one study of ring vaccination of contacts of EVD patients using an Ebola candidate vaccine reported promising results, suggesting that ring vaccination may be part of a strategy to controlling future EVD outbreaks. In developing countries, regionalizing EVD care could lower costs of preparedness as well as improve effectiveness of the response to the next outbreak. The most recent epidemic in West Africa also prompted a re-evaluation of epidemic response strategies at the WHO and other global health organizations.

Complications and Admission Criteria

All patients with suspected EVD should be admitted to a hospital. Immediate complications of acute Ebola virus infection are enumerated in the Clinical Features section above.

Infection Control

A diagnosis of EVD should be considered in any patient who presents with febrile illness and recent direct exposure to a symptomatic EVD patient or to the blood or bodily fluids of a corpse who died from EVD, and a history of recent travel to a country with widespread Ebola virus transmission (www.cdc .gov/vhf/ebola/healthcare-us/emergency-services/emergency-departments.html; www.cdc.gov/vhf/ebola/healthcare-us/ evaluating-patients/evaluating-travelers.html; www.cdc.gov/

vhf/ebola/healthcare-us/evaluating-patients/discharging.html). An essential first step of evaluation is to immediately place any patient with suspected EVD in isolation (see Side Box). This step precedes and supersedes initial diagnostic evaluation. The CDC has outlined recommended isolation procedures (see EVD Screening Side Box: www.cdc.gov/vhf/ebola/healthcare-us/emergency-services/emergency-departments.html). In addition, the local and state health departments should be immediately contacted for coordination of care and appropriate handling of all patient specimens. If a patient has any high-risk exposure to *Ebolavirus* (see EVD Screening Side Box), the patient is considered a person under investigation and testing for Ebola virus is indicated. Infection prevention and control recommendations should be followed for evaluating persons under investigation (www.cdc.gov/vhf/ebola/healthcare-us/ hospitals/infection-control.html). If a patient has low risk or no exposure, the health department should be consulted to determine if Ebola virus testing and patient isolation is appropriate.

As per the CDC Algorithms (Side Box), proper donning and doffing of recommended personal protective equipment, and implementation of infection control measures is critical to preventing spread of *Ebolavirus* in the health-care setting (www.cdc.gov/vhf/ebola/healthcare-us/ppe/guidance.html).

These measures especially apply to initial emergency medical services (EMS) contact. When EMS personnel encounter a patient with fever and travel to an Ebola-endemic region within 21 days, they must don recommended personal protective equipment (PPE), including gloves, gown, eye protection, and facemask. Invasive procedures and ones likely to involve contact with patient body fluids (such as venipuncture, suctioning of the airway, or endotracheal intubation) should be performed only if absolutely necessary, and under the most controlled circumstances possible (i.e. while vehicle is stopped, but preferably at the destination hospital) (www.cdc.gov/ ebola/healthcare-us/emergency-services/ems-systems.html).

Beyond direct patient contact, additional important infection control measures include safe waste disposal, disinfection of non-disposable supplies, and appropriate handling of a patient's remains in the event of death. These measures have proven essential in controlling the EVD outbreak in West Africa, and are no less vital in a high-resource health-care setting.

Health department authorities must also initiate a thorough investigation of patient contacts. Ebola virus is transmissible as soon as a patient becomes symptomatic. A detailed history of the onset of fever and associated symptoms, and all of a patient's activities and contacts during that period, will provide the basis for identifying other individuals at risk of contracting EVD.

Pearls and Pitfalls

1 As long as *Ebolavirus* transmission among humans in Africa is ongoing, there is a risk that a traveler with undiagnosed EVD could present to an acute care facility outside of Africa.

2. Reducing the risk of EVD in developed countries requires, first and foremost, that sufficient medical resources be deployed in Africa to control future EVD outbreaks.

3. The most important potential pitfall is failure to identify a patient who should be suspected with EVD (person under investigation for EVD) by not obtaining a recent history of exposure to Ebola virus (direct contact with the blood or bodily fluids of an EVD patient or corpse that died of EVD in an area where *Ebolavirus* transmission is occurring). Any patient with signs or symptoms consistent with EVD with potential Ebola virus exposure must be placed in isolation immediately and the local and state health departments should be contacted.

4. Clinical management of EVD is primarily supportive, but investigational therapies may be available in the context of a clinical trial. Potential transport of the patient to a regional care center, supervision of infection control measures, and analysis of contacts should be coordinated by local and state health departments and the CDC.

References

Ansumana, R., Jacobsen, K. H., Sahr, F., et al. *N. Engl. J. Med.* 2015; 372(6): 587–8.

Baize, S., Pannetier, D., Oestereich, L., et al. Emergence of Zaire Ebola virus disease in Guinea. *N. Engl. J. Med.* 2014; 371(15): 1418–25.

Barry, M., Touré, A., Traoré, F. A., et al. Clinical predictors of mortality in patients with Ebola virus disease. *Clin. Infect. Dis.* 2015; 60(12): 1821–4.

Biava, M., Caglioti, C., Bordi, L., et al. Detection of viral RNA in tissues following plasma clearance from an Ebola virus infected patient. *PLoS Pathog.* 2017; 13(1): e1006065.

Chertow, D. S., Kleine, C., Edwards, J. K., et al. Ebola virus disease in West Africa – clinical manifestations and management. *N. Engl. J. Med.* 2014; 371(22): 2054–7.

Diallo, B., Sissoko, D., Loman, N. J., et al. Resurgence of Ebola virus disease in Guinea linked to a survivor with virus persistence in seminal fluid for more than 500 days. *Clin. Infect. Dis.* 2016; 63(10): 1353–6.

Dye, C. and WHO Ebola Response Team. Ebola virus disease in West Africa – the first 9 months. *N. Engl. J. Med.* 2015; 372(2): 189.

Feldmann, H. Ebola – a growing threat? *N. Engl. J. Med.* 2014; 371(15): 1375–8.

Feldmann, H. and Geisbert, T. W. Ebola haemorrhagic fever. *Lancet* 2011; 377(9768): 849–62.

Henao-Restrepo, A. M., Camacho, A., Longini, I. M., et al. Efficacy and effectiveness of an rVSV-vectored vaccine in preventing Ebola virus disease: final results from the Guinea ring vaccination, open-label, cluster-randomised trial (Ebola Ça Suffit!). *Lancet* 2017; 389(10068): 505–18.

Hunt, L., Gupta-Wright, A., Simms, V., et al. Clinical presentation, biochemical, and haematological parameters and their association with out-come in patients with Ebola virus disease: an observational cohort study. *Lancet Infect. Dis.* 2015; 15(11): 1292–9.

Jacobs, M., Aarons, E., Bhagani, S., et al. Post-exposure prophylaxis against Ebola virus disease with experimental antiviral agents: a case-series of health-care workers. *Lancet Infect. Dis.* 2015; 15(11): 1300–4.

Lanini, S., Portella, G., Vairo, F., et al. Blood kinetics of Ebola virus in survivors and nonsurvivors. *J. Clin. Invest.* 2015; 125(12): 4692–8.

Liddell, A. M., Davey, R. T. Jr., Mehta, A. K., et al. Characteristics and clinical management of a cluster of 3 patients with Ebola virus disease, including the first domestically acquired cases in the United States. *Ann. Intern. Med.* 2015; 163(2): 81–90.

Lyon, G. M., Mehta, A. K., Varkey, B., et al. Emory Serious Communicable Diseases Unit. Clinical care of two patients with Ebola virus disease in the United States. *N. Engl. J. Med.* 2014; 371(25): 2402–9.

Mate, S. E., Kugelman, J. R., Nyenswah, T. G., et al. Molecular evidence of sexual transmission of Ebola virus. *N. Engl. J. Med.* 2015; 373(25): 2448–54.

PREVAIL II Writing Group, Multi-National PREVAIL II Study Team, Davey, R. T. Jr., et al. A randomized, controlled trial of ZMapp for Ebola virus infection. *N. Engl. J. Med.* 2016; 375(15): 1448–56.

Rodriguez, L. L., De Roo, A., Guimard, Y., et al. Persistence and genetic stability of Ebola virus during the outbreak in Kikwit, Democratic Republic of the Congo, 1995. *J. Infect. Dis.* 1999; 179(Suppl. 1): S170–6.

Sands, P., Mundaca-Shah, C., and Dzau, V. J. The neglected dimension of global security – a framework for countering infectious-disease crises. *N. Engl. J. Med.* 2016; 374(13): 1281–7.

Schieffelin, J. S., Shaffer, J. G., Goba, A., et al. Clinical illness and outcomes in patients with Ebola in Sierra Leone. *N. Engl. J. Med.* 2014; 371(22): 2092–100.

Tan, K. R., Cullen, K. A., Koumans, E. H., and Arguin, P. M. Inadequate diagnosis and treatment of malaria among travelers returning from Africa during the Ebola epidemic – United States, 2014–2015. *MMWR Morb. Mortal. Wkly. Rep.* 2016; 65(2): 27–9.

Uyeki, T. M., Mehta, A. K., Davey, R. T., Jr., et al., Clinical management of Ebola virus disease in the United States and Europe. *N. Engl. J. Med.* 2016; 374(7): 636–46.

Varkey, J. B., Shantha, J. G., Crozier, I., et al. Persistence of Ebola virus in ocular fluid during convalescence. *N. Engl. J. Med.* 2015; 372(25): 2423–7.

Waxman, M., Aluisio, A. R., Rege, S., and Levine, A. C. Characteristics and survival of patients with Ebola virus infection, malaria, or both in Sierra Leone: a retrospective cohort study. *Lancet Infect. Dis.* 2017; 17(6): 654–60.

WHO Ebola Response Team, Agua-Agum, J., Allegranzi, B., et al. After Ebola in West Africa – unpredictable risks, preventable epidemics. *N. Engl. J. Med.* 2016; 375(6): 587–96.

Wong, K. K., Davey, R. T., Jr., Hewlett, A. L., et al. Use of postexposure prophylaxis after occupational exposure to Zaire Ebolavirus. *Clin. Infect. Dis.* 2016; 63(3): 376–9.

Chapter 73

Zika Virus

Ashley Rider and Bradley W. Frazee*

Introduction and Microbiology

Zika is an arthropod-borne virus carried and transmitted primarily by the *Aedes aegypti* mosquito. It is one of several pathogenic flaviviruses, a genus that includes West Nile virus, yellow fever, tick-borne encephalitis, and dengue virus. Zika virus has recently spread from the location in Africa where it was endemic and emerged explosively to create an international epidemic.

Zika was first isolated from a rhesus monkey in 1947 in Uganda. Human infection received little attention until an outbreak occurred in 2007 on the island of Yap, west of the Philippines. This was followed by an increase in cases of "mild dengue-like syndrome" in French Polynesia and elsewhere in the southern Pacific region. From Easter Island, it spread to Brazil and later to Colombia. Genetic studies of cases in Brazil suggest a single introduction of the virus to the Americas in 2013 coincident with increased air travel to Brazil from the South Pacific. Since then, millions of patients have been infected in South and Central America and the Caribbean. In August 2016, transmission within the continental United States was documented for the first time in South Florida. Three months later, the first case of local mosquito-borne Zika infection was described in Brownsville, Texas. The rapid expansion of Zika is similar to that of dengue and Chickungunya virus, and is likely tied to the spread and success of the *A. aegypti* vector.

Although Zika causes only a mild, self-limiting illness in adults, an alarming association has been established between antenatal infection and microcephaly. The World Health Organization (WHO) has declared Zika "a public health emergency of international concern" due to the nature of infectivity and potentially devastating effects on fetal development. The epidemic is complicated by a broad distribution of mosquitoes that transmit the virus and the need for international coordination to prevent spread.

Acute care providers should be familiar with the typical symptoms of acute Zika to ensure timely diagnosis and management of disease. Early identification of cases in the emergency setting may have a far-reaching public health impact by providing valuable epidemiologic data and preventing disease spread.

Epidemiology

A. aegypti is widely distributed throughout the tropical and subtropical world. It is endemic in Africa, India, Northern Australia, Southeast Asia, Central and South America, southern United States (30 states), Hawaii, the US Virgin Islands, and Puerto Rico. The *A. albopictus* species is also known to carry Zika, and ranges to more temperate climates, including 41 US states.

A. aegypti is the same mosquito species that transmits dengue and Chikungunya viruses. In its original endemic areas in Africa, the Zika virus is believed to circulate between *A. aegypti* mosquitoes and non-human primate hosts, with occasional human infection. In urban areas, however, the transmission cycle is directly from human to mosquito and back to human. *A. aegypti* is adapted to live close to human habitation. It feeds during the day and has an imperceptible bite, making vector control very difficult. Risk of transmission, even to travelers, is relatively low in areas where Zika is endemic and immunity is common (African, Pacific Islands, Asia). Risk of infection is highest when visiting countries where Zika has recently spread, due to low immunity in the population and high levels of transmission.

As of February 15, 2017, 72 countries or territories had documented mosquito-borne transmission. An estimated 25% of Puerto Rican individuals are affected, including 6,000 to

---

*   This work represents the views of the authors.

11,000 pregnant women. In the United States, as of February 15, 2017, there were 220 cases of local mosquito-borne transmission, and 72 cases acquired by other routes (congenital, sexual transmission, laboratory transmission). There were also 4,748 travel-associated infections and 1,455 pregnant women with laboratory evidence of possible Zika infection. While no local transmission has been documented in Canada or Europe, cases have been reported there in returning travelers.

Zika appears to be following a similar history to that of dengue and Chikungunya virus. Chikungunya virus was first described in Africa, then emerged in Asia, and later spread throughout Asia and worldwide. The rapid spread of dengue, Chikungunya, and Zika reflects the successful spread of their common mosquito vector, which is linked to increasing globalization and urbanization. Introduction of virus in previously unexposed populations then leads to epidemic spread.

Although mosquito bites are the principal form of transmission, vertical transmission during early pregnancy is the most feared consequence of Zika, resulting in abnormal fetal development. There is some evidence that peripartum transmission may occur, but effects on the newborn appear to be less severe. Thus far, there is little evidence to suggest that infection can be passed through breast milk.

Zika virus can be sexually transmitted, even when the infected partner is asymptomatic. The viral load can be up to 100,000 times greater in semen than blood or urine and has been detected up to 6 months after symptom onset. Viral RNA has also been detected in female genital tract secretions 14 days after symptom onset. Viral RNA has also been detected in saliva, but it is unknown if Zika can be transmitted through saliva alone. Part of the alarm over Zika stems from the fact that it is the first mosquito-borne virus known to also spread via sexual transmission and cause congenital birth defects.

Finally, there is a risk of transmission via blood products. During the outbreak in French Polynesia, the risk of transmission through blood transfusion was described. More recently, infection by platelet transfusion from an infected donor was reported in Brazil. Similarly, there is evidence of transmission during organ transplantation and laboratory exposure.

Clinical Features

The incubation period of Zika is 3 days to 2 weeks, similar to the Chikungunya and dengue infections. Clinical manifestations occur in only about 20% of infected patients. The high proportion of asymptomatic infections greatly increases the challenge to identifying infected patients and preventing transmission.

According to the WHO and Pan American Health Organization, acute care providers should have a high suspicion for Zika in a patient who presents with the following symptoms: maculopapular rash, fever, non-purulent conjunctivitis, arthralgia/myalgia, malaise, and headache (See Figure 73.1). Symptoms are mild and last 2 to 7 days. Fever is mostly low grade and short-lived. The rash is associated with pruritis; in a study of the Brazilian outbreak, pruritis was the second most common symptom reported. Other less common symptoms of

Table 73.1 Clinical Features: Zika Infection

Organism	Flavivirus
Vector	*Aedes aegypti* or *Aedes albopictus* Sexual transmission Vertical transmission
Incubation period	3–14 days
Symptoms	Pruritic rash Low grade fever Non-purulent conjunctivitis Muscle and joint pain Periarticular edema Malaise Myalgias Headache
Duration of symptoms	2–7 days
Severity	Mild

acute infection are hematospermia, dull hearing, swelling of the distal extremities, and subcutaneous bleeding (see Table 73.1).

Strong observational data suggest a relationship between Zika infection and neurological disease. Most notable is the association with Guillain–Barré syndrome (GBS), but cases of meningitis and meningoencephalitis have also been described. There was a striking increase in GBS cases in both Yap and Brazil that coincided with Zika epidemics. In a case control study from French Polynesia, 98% of patients with GBS had anti-Zika IgM or IgG, and 100% had neutralizing antibodies compared with 56% of controls. The recent Neuroviruses Emerging in the Americas Study (NEAS) documented an increase in the number of GBS cases in Columbia during their recent Zika epidemic, which was not seen during previous outbreaks of Chikungunya and dengue virus. Forty-two patients underwent intensive testing that yielded several important findings: urine was the most likely specimen to test positive for Zika by reverse-transcriptase polymerase-chain-reaction (RT-PCR); GBS was predominantly the classic acute inflammatory polyneuropathy (AIPN) type; bilateral facial palsy was common; and while median time between Zika symptoms and GBS onset was 7 days, 48% of patients had a parainfectious onset, meaning GBS symptoms began immediately following, or slightly overlapped, Zika symptoms.

Maternal infection in the first trimester with Zika seems to be similar to infection with the "TORCH" pathogens, which can cause congenital anomalies due to compromised organogenesis. There is evidence that Zika virus proliferates in the cells of the placenta, and then continues to replicate in the brain of a fetus after birth. Like congenital toxoplasmosis and CMV, Zika is particularly associated with microcephaly (defined as less than third percentile occipitofrontal circumference). The tropism of Zika for neural tissues is supported by the finding of Zika RNA in amniotic fluid and brain tissue of fetuses and infants with microcephaly. A causative link between Zika and microcephaly is now incontrovertible, though the degree of risk remains unclear. In a Brazilian study, 12 of 42 (29%) women with confirmed Zika during pregnancy had abnormal findings on ultrasound, including microcephaly, intracranial calcifications, brain abnormalities, abnormal cerebral artery blood flow, IUGR, and death.

Symptoms in the mother are not predictive of risk to off-spring. In the US Zika in Pregnancy Registry (USZPR), 26 infants from 442 pregnancies had birth defects, including 22 brain abnormalities. The proportion of fetuses with birth defects was the same in symptomatic and asymptomatic mothers. For this reason, all pregnant women living in an area of transmission should be tested for Zika. Acute Zika infection in the first trimester is the most dangerous, but it is possible that fetal transmission can also occur in the second or third trimester.

Ophthalmologic complications have also been described. Abnormalities include vision-threatening pathologies such as focal pigment mottling of the retina, chorioretinal atrophy, optic nerve abnormalities, and coloboma.

Perinatal infection may occur resulting in clinical infection within the first 2 weeks of life. In infants and children who have acquired the virus after birth, infection is similar to that of adults and should be included in the differential diagnosis of a pediatric viral syndrome.

Differential Diagnosis

The diseases that most commonly overlap with Zika are dengue and Chikungunya. Fever, myalgia, and headache are more prominent in dengue, as are thrombocytopenia and neutropenia. Myalgia and arthritis are more commonly described in chikungunya infection. Non-purulent conjunctivitis and arthralgia are more suggestive of Zika infection. Zika should be highly considered if there is conjunctival involvement, as this finding is significantly less common in dengue and Chikungunya. Finally, co-infection with more than one of these viruses can occur.

Other infectious diseases to consider in the differential diagnosis are leptospirosis, malaria, rickettsia, group A *Streptococcus*, rubella, measles, parvovirus, enterovirus, and adenovirus. The provider should inquire about travel history and vaccination status to elucidate the risk for these diseases. The differential diagnosis of fever in the returning traveler is covered in detail in Chapter 60.

Laboratory and Radiographic Findings

Laboratory or imaging studies have a limited role in evaluation of possible Zika infection. Thrombocytopenia, leukopenia, and transaminitis are usually absent or mild; if severe, these lab abnormalities would point toward dengue. Preliminary diagnosis is therefore based on clinical features and travel. Laboratory confirmation should follow.

Zika virus can be detected in whole blood, serum, plasma, urine, cerebrospinal fluid, amniotic fluid, semen, and saliva according to guidelines developed by the WHO (see Figure 73.2). Local public health officials should be notified of all suspected US cases of Zika and can assist with diagnostic testing.

The choice of diagnostic test depends on time from symptom onset. Within 14 days of symptom onset, both urine and serum should be collected for RT-PCR, which detects viral RNA. RT-PCR on serum is most accurate if performed within 1 week of symptom onset, but Zika RNA may be detected in the urine longer, for up to 14 days.

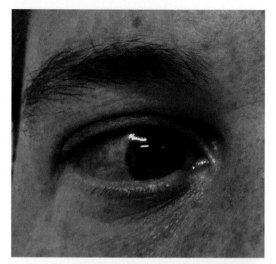

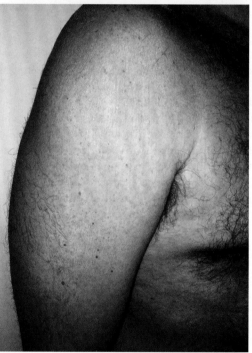

Figure 73.1 Conjunctivitis and maculopapular rash in Zika virus infection
Reproduced with permission from S. M. Derrington, A. P. Cellura, L. E. McDermott, *et al.*, Mucocutaneous findings and course in an adult with Zika virus infection. *JAMA* 2016; 152(6): 691–3. Copyright © (2016) American Medical Association. All rights reserved. Photo credit: Amit Garg MD.

Between 4 days and 12 weeks from symptom onset, serum should also be tested for Zika IgM neutralizing antibodies (MAC-ELISA). IgM antibodies usually emerge after RNA falls to undetectable levels, but serology may be positive as early as 4 days from symptom onset. Simultaneous testing for dengue and chikungunya is also recommended. Serologic Testing for the flaviviruses is imperfect and distinguishing between acute infection with Zika and other flavivirus can be challenging, particularly in patients who may have previously been infected. Although expensive, time-consuming, and susceptible to cross-reactivity, a plaque reduction neutralization test (PRNT) should be forwarded to a CDC laboratory for confirmatory testing.

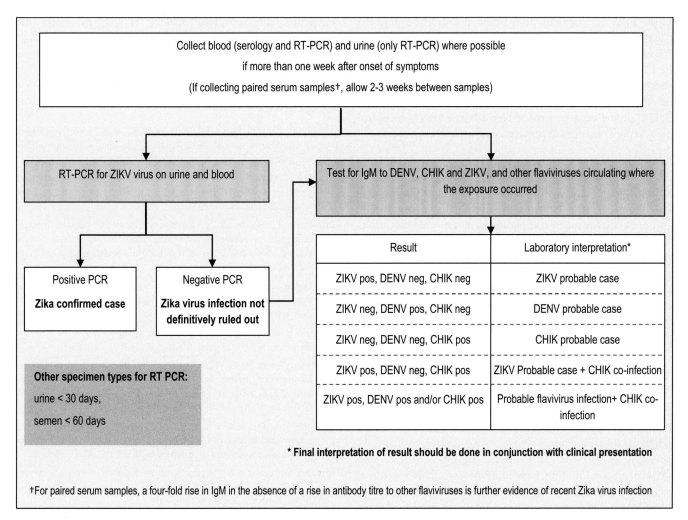

Collect blood (serology and RT-PCR) and urine (only RT-PCR) where possible

if more than one week after onset of symptoms

(If collecting paired serum samples†, allow 2-3 weeks between samples)

RT-PCR for ZIKV virus on urine and blood

Test for IgM to DENV, CHIK and ZIKV, and other flaviviruses circulating where the exposure occurred

Positive PCR
Zika confirmed case

Negative PCR
Zika virus infection not definitively ruled out

Other specimen types for RT PCR:
urine < 30 days,
semen < 60 days

Result	Laboratory interpretation*
ZIKV pos, DENV neg, CHIK neg	ZIKV probable case
ZIKV neg, DENV pos, CHIK neg	DENV probable case
ZIKV neg, DENV neg, CHIK pos	CHIK probable case
ZIKV pos, DENV neg, CHIK pos	ZIKV Probable case + CHIK co-infection
ZIKV pos, DENV pos and/or CHIK pos	Probable flavivirus infection+ CHIK co-infection

* Final interpretation of result should be done in conjunction with clinical presentation

†For paired serum samples, a four-fold rise in IgM in the absence of a rise in antibody titre to other flaviviruses is further evidence of recent Zika virus infection

Figure 73.2 Proposed testing algorithm for suspected cases of arbovirus infection identified within 7 days of onset of symptoms
Proposed testing algorithm for suspected cases of arbovirus infection more than 1 week after onset of symptoms
Reprinted from Laboratory testing for Zika virus infection, interim guidance, WHO Reference number: WHO/ZIKV/LAB/16.1, World Health Organization, http://apps .who.int/iris/bitstream/10665/204671/1/WHO_ZIKV_LAB_16.1_eng.pdf, table located on p. 4. Copyright (23 March 2016).

Diagnosis of Zika infection is obviously of particular importance in pregnant women. All pregnant women should be screened for travel history and symptoms of possible Zika infection at each prenatal visit. Asymptomatic pregnant women living in an area with ongoing Zika transmission should be tested for Zika IgM as a part of routine prenatal care in the first and second trimesters. In those with evidence of infection, amniocentesis may be considered, and serial ultrasounds with a focus on neuroanatomy should be performed every 3 to 4 weeks. Microcephaly and other abnormalities may be detected by 20 weeks.

Treatment and Prophylaxis

There is no specific treatment for Zika. The typically mild symptoms of acute infection can be treated with fluids, analgesics, and antipyretics.

The more pressing concern is how to best limit transmission and adverse pregnancy outcomes. There is a critical need to better understand the clinical consequences of Zika and the pattern of disease spread. The development of better

vector-control strategies, more specific diagnostic tools, and a Zika vaccine are all needed in order to control the current global epidemic. Fortunately, a single vaccine is likely to be protective against all strains of Zika, unlike the case with dengue. Various groups are working on vaccine candidates with different approaches to inducing protective immunity. The World Health Organization also published a Target Product Profile to aid vaccine developers. In February 2017, a group of scientists at University of Pennsylvania reported successful immune responses in mice and monkeys for an mRNA-based vaccine.

It is unclear how long the virus persists and remains infective in urine and semen, but there is evidence that it is significantly longer than in blood and saliva. This uncertainty makes for very conservative recommendations on preventing sexual transmission. Barrier methods or abstinence are recommended for 6 months for males and 8 weeks for females who have traveled to an area with active transmission. If a pregnant woman's partner has lived in or traveled to such an area, the couple should abstain from unprotected sex for the duration of pregnancy.

The FDA recommends that blood donation be deferred at least 120 days after infection. Blood products should be screened or outsourced in regions with active transmission. The FDA now advises that all donated whole blood and blood products in the United States be screened for Zika. The CDC and the Occupational Safety and Health Administration (OSHA) guidelines recommend blood-borne infection control and biosafety practices to prevent occupational exposures.

Complications and Admission Criteria

Zika infection is typically mild and self-limiting. Admission is rarely required and patients can be managed symptomatically as outpatients. The major complications in non-pregnant adults and children are GBS and rare meningoencephalitis. Congenital infection during pregnancy is the most important complication to consider. While the exact risk remains unclear, congenital infection can be neurologically devastating in the unborn fetus. Pregnant women with confirmed infection should be counseled, tested, and treated. Pregnant women living in or traveling to affected areas, or whose partners have done so, should follow recommendations for Zika screening and prevention.

Infection Control

Since there is no specific treatment for Zika, emphasis remains on infection control through prevention of mosquito-borne and sexual transmission, as well as vector control. Measures to prevent *A. aegypti* bites, which occur during the day, include the use of air conditioning, installing window and door screens, wearing long-sleeved pants and shirts, and applying insect repellents on children greater than 2 months of age. Women wishing to get pregnant should postpone travel to countries at altitudes less than 6,500 feet affected by the Zika epidemic. Vector control involves application of larvicides, aerial spraying of insecticides, and elimination of breeding sites such as standing water, but effectiveness of these measures is limited by inconsistent participation of households or cryptic breeding in urban settings. Introduction of genetically modified male *A. aegypti* mosquitos, which produce offspring which die at the larval stage, is a promising though controversial approach.

Pearls and Pitfalls

- Consider Zika in a returning traveler or person living in affected area who presents with fever, rash, pruritus, arthralgias, and conjunctivitis; conjunctivitis in particular may help differentiate Zika from other common arboviruses such as dengue and Chikungunya.
- RT-PCR should be performed if symptoms have been present less than 7 days. Serologic testing should be performed if symptom onset was greater than 4 days but less than 12 weeks prior.
- Pregnant women with suspected Zika should undergo frequent monitoring of fetus, as well as testing at birth.
- Avoidance of travel to affected areas at altitudes less than 6,500 feet, mosquito bite precautions, and protection during intercourse are the best methods to prevent Zika infection.

- Acute care providers working in regions where the *A. aegypti* mosquito is endemic should remain vigilant of Zika-like illness and alert public health authorities early in suspected cases.

References

Abbink, P., Larocca, R. A., de la Barrera, R. A., *et al.* Protective efficacy of multiple vaccine platforms against Zika virus challenge in rhesus monkeys. *Science* 2016; 353(6304): 1129–32.

Brasil, P., Pereira, J. P., Moreira, M. E., *et al.* Zika virus infection in pregnant women in Rio de Janeiro – preliminary report. *N. Engl. J. Med.* 2016; 375(24): 2321–34.

Brooks, J. T., Friedman, A., Kachur, R. E., *et al.* Update: interim guidance for prevention of sexual transmission of Zika virus – United States, July 2016. *MMWR Morb. Mortal. Wkly. Rep.* 2016; 65(29): 745–7.

Cao-Lormeau, V. M., Blake, A., Mons, S., *et al.* Guillain–Barré syndrome outbreak associated with Zika virus infection in French Polynesia: a case-control study. *Lancet* 2016; 387(10027): 1531–9.

Chen, L. H. and Hamer, D. H. Zika virus: rapid spread in the Western Hemisphere. *Ann. Intern. Med.* 2016; 164(9): 613–15.

De Paula Freitas, B., de Oliveira Dias, J. R., Prazeres, J., *et al.* Ocular findings in infants with microcephaly associated with presumed Zika virus congenital infection in Salvador, Brazil. *JAMA Ophthalmol.* 2016; 134(5): 529–35.

Honein, M. A., Dawson, A. L., Petersen, E. E., *et al.* Birth defects among fetuses and infants of US women with evidence of possible Zika virus infection during pregnancy. *JAMA.* 2017; 317(1): 59–68.

Marano, G., Pupella, S., Vaglio, S., *et al.* Zika virus and the never-ending story of emerging pathogens and transfusion medicine. *Blood Transfus.* 2016; 14(2): 95–100.

Motta, I. J. F., Spencer, B. R., Cordeiro da Silva, S. G., *et al.* Evidence for transmission of Zika virus by platelet transfusion. *N. Eng. J. Med.* 2016; 375(11): 1101–3.

Musso, D., Cao-Lormeau, V. M., and Gubler, D. J. Zika virus: following the path of dengue and chikungunya? *Lancet* 2015; 386(9990): 243–4.

Parra, B., Lizarazo, J., Jiménez-Arango, J. A., *et al.* Guillain–Barré syndrome associated with Zika virus infection in Colombia. *N. Eng. J. Med.* 2016; 375(16): 1513–23.

Staples, J. E., Dziuban, E. J., Fischer, M., *et al.* Interim guidelines for the evaluation and testing of infants with possible congenital Zika virus infection – United States, 2016. *MMWR Morb. Mortal. Wkly. Rep.* 2016; 65(3): 63–7.

Villamil-Gómez, W. E., González-Camargo, O., Rodriguez-Ayubi, J., *et al.* Dengue, chikungunya and Zika co-infection in a patient from Colombia. *J. Infect. Public Health* 2016; 9(5): 684–6.

Additional Readings

Long, D., Long, B., and Koyfman, A. Zika virus: what do emergency physicians need to know? *J. Emerg. Med.* 2016; 50(6): 832–8, www.cdc.gov/zika.

Petersen, L. R., Jamieson, D. J., Powers, A. M., and Honein, M. A. Zika virus. *N. Engl. J. Med.* 2016; 374(16): 1552–63.

Shastry, S., Koenig, K. L., and Hirshon, J. M. Zika virus critical information for emergency providers. *Emerg. Med. Clin. N. Am.* 2016; 34(3): e25–37.

Chapter

74

Zoonotic Influenza (Novel Influenza A, including Avian and Swine Influenza A Virus Infections)

Timothy M. Uyeki*

Outline

Introduction and Microbiology

Novel influenza A virus infection refers to human infection with an influenza A virus that is antigenically and genetically distinct from seasonal influenza A viruses circulating among people. Novel influenza A viruses are typically influenza A viruses of animal origin (e.g. circulating among birds or pigs) that have emerged to infect people (zoonotic transmission). Human infections with a novel influenza A virus are of global public health concern because some of these viruses have caused severe and fatal disease from either zoonotic transmission or limited, non-sustained human-to-human transmission, and there is potential for an influenza pandemic if a novel influenza A virus is capable of sustained and efficient transmission, and population immunity to the virus is limited. The range of illness caused by novel influenza A virus infections ranges from mild (e.g. conjunctivitis, upper respiratory tract symptoms) to severe complications (pneumonia, respiratory failure, multi-organ failure). Human illness from infection with swine influenza A viruses has been identified since the 1970s. Since 1997, human illness from infection by different avian influenza A viruses has been increasingly recognized. Influenza pandemics have been caused by direct adaptation of an influenza A virus circulating among birds or pigs (such as the H1N1 virus that caused the 1918 to 1919 "Spanish flu" pandemic resulting in an estimated 20 to 100 million deaths worldwide, or the H1N1pdm09 virus that caused the 2009 pandemic that resulted in an estimated 200,000 respiratory deaths globally) or through genetic reassortment between human and avian influenza A viruses (such as the 1957 H2N2 and 1968 H3N2 pandemic viruses).

Influenza viruses are single-stranded negative sense RNA viruses of the family *Orthomyxoviridae*. Of four known types of influenza viruses, three types (A, B, and C) are known to infect humans, type A and B viruses are associated with epidemics worldwide, but only novel influenza A viruses cause rare influenza pandemics. The genome contains eight gene segments that code for 11 proteins, including the two main surface glycoproteins, hemagglutinin (HA), and neuraminidase (NA). Type A viruses are further classified into subtypes based on the antigenic differences of their HA (referred to as "H") and NA (referred to as "N") proteins. Currently circulating human influenza A subtypes include H1N1pdm09 and H3N2 viruses. Of the 18 HA and 11 NA influenza A virus subtypes that have been identified to date, all have been found in birds except for H17N10 and H18N11 viruses, which were detected in bats. While influenza A viruses have infected a wide range of animals (e.g. birds, pigs, horses, dogs, cats, seals, whales, bats, civet cats, stone martens, tigers, and leopards), the two most important reservoirs are in birds (wild waterfowl) and pigs worldwide.

Avian influenza is caused by infection of the respiratory and gastrointestinal tracts of birds with avian influenza A viruses. Infected birds can excrete avian influenza A viruses in feces that can remain viable for prolonged periods at low temperatures, low humidity, and with abundant fecal matter. The natural reservoir for avian influenza A viruses is wild aquatic birds. Genetic reassortment among avian influenza A viruses occurs frequently. Avian influenza A viruses are dynamic and continue to evolve into new virus strains that are subdivided into clades and subclades on the basis of antigenic diversity.

Avian influenza A viruses are classified as highly pathogenic avian influenza (HPAI) or low pathogenic avian influenza (LPAI) based upon molecular and pathogenicity criteria in experimentally infected chickens. Most avian influenza A

---

* The findings and conclusions in this report are those of the author and do not necessarily represent the official position of the Centers for Disease Control and Prevention.

viruses are LPAI viruses that cause asymptomatic infection of the respiratory and gastrointestinal tracts in wild birds. LPAI virus infection of domestic poultry causes asymptomatic to mild illness (weight loss, reduced egg laying). Some H5 and H7 virus subtypes have been classified as HPAI viruses. HPAI H5 (e.g. H5N1, H5N2, H5N5, H5N6, H5N8) or H7 (e.g. H7N3, H7N7, H7N8, H7N9) virus infections of domestic poultry can result in rapid death within a few days, though some ducks can have asymptomatic infection. HPAI virus infection of wild birds can result in asymptomatic infection to rapid death. Some avian influenza A viruses are considered enzootic (endemic circulation) among poultry in some countries that can lead to epizootics (outbreaks) among poultry in other areas. Both HPAI and LPAI virus infections of domestic poultry are of substantial economic concern to the commercial poultry industry worldwide, and HPAI virus infections of poultry are reportable by countries to the World Organization for Animal Health (OIE).

Pigs are of major importance in the ecology of influenza A viruses because they can be infected with swine influenza A viruses, avian influenza A viruses, and human influenza A viruses, and genetic reassortment between viruses of different species can occur in an infected pig to produce new influenza A viruses. Thus, pigs have been described as "mixing vessels" for influenza A viruses. For example, triple reassortant swine (TRS) influenza A viruses with genes of avian, human, and swine origin, of different subtypes (H1N1, H1N2, and H3N2) have circulated among pigs in North America for many years. Influenza A viruses of swine origin that have infected humans are referred to as "variant" influenza viruses and are designated with a "v" (e.g. H1N1v, H1N2v, and H3N2v). The H1N1pdm09 virus that caused the 2009 influenza pandemic was a reassortant virus that contained genes from swine, human, and avian influenza A viruses.

Since 2003, the epizootic of HPAI A (H5N1) virus among domestic poultry and wild birds has resulted in rare, sporadic, human HPAI H5N1 cases with severe respiratory disease and high mortality in 16 countries of Asia, Europe, the Middle East, and Africa as of March 2017. Six countries (Bangladesh, China, Egypt, Indonesia, India, and Vietnam) were identified as enzootic for HPAI H5N1 virus in poultry by the UN Food and Agriculture Organization in 2011, and epizootic spread to other countries occurs periodically. Most transmission of HPAI H5N1 viruses to humans is believed to be directly from sick or dead birds, but limited non-sustained human-to-human transmission of HPAI H5N1 viruses has been reported.

In contrast, LPAI A (H7N9) virus causes asymptomatic infection of domestic poultry, but can cause severe disease and high mortality in humans. Since 2013, sporadic cases of human infection with LPAI H7N9 virus have been reported in China, with exportation to other countries. Annual epidemic waves of H7N9 cases during the winter and spring months have been reported in China, resulting in mild to critical and fatal illness, primarily attributable to exposures while visiting live poultry markets in urban areas or to backyard poultry in rural areas. Some cases of limited, non-sustained human-to-human transmission of H7N9 viruses have been reported, including nosocomial transmission. In 2017, human infections with HPAI A(H7N9) virus were reported in southern China, including a case identified in Taiwan.

Avian influenza A viruses circulating among wild birds and domestic poultry, as well as swine influenza A viruses circulating among pigs, continue to evolve worldwide, and have the propensity to undergo genetic reassortment to generate new viruses. Geographic and environmental factors may be determinants of seasonality and contribute to distinct genetic and antigenic evolution. Surveillance of influenza A viruses circulating among birds and pigs globally is important for understanding virus evolution, informing agricultural prevention and control measures for poultry and swine production, and to guide public health activities (risk assessment, updating diagnostic tests, antiviral treatment recommendations) and pandemic influenza preparedness (e.g. candidate vaccine development and vaccine stockpiling).

Epidemiology

Sporadic human infections of the respiratory tract with different subtypes of LPAI viruses (H6N1, H7N2, H7N3, H7N7, H7N9, H9N2, H10N7, H10N8) have caused a wide range of reported illness worldwide (see Table 74.1). Most LPAI viruses have caused mild-to-moderate human illness, including conjunctivitis and upper respiratory tract symptoms. However, LPAI H7N9 and H10N8 viruses are unique because they cause asymptomatic or mild illness in infected poultry, but have caused critical and fatal illness in infected humans. Most LPAI virus infections have been linked to direct contact with domestic poultry or indirect exposures while visiting a live poultry market. While some human infections have been linked to exposures during LPAI poultry outbreaks, other cases have occurred after poultry exposure, but without identified outbreaks in birds, and for some human LPAI cases, the source of exposure was unknown. Although most LPAI virus infections have been reported in adults, LPAI H7N9 virus infections have been reported in all ages, and most fatal outcomes have been reported in elderly persons, whereas most reported cases of LPAI H9N2 virus infection have been in children with mild-to-moderate illness in China, Bangladesh, and Egypt. In 2016, one human case of LPAI H7N2 virus infection was identified in a veterinarian who had handled H7N2-virus-infected sick cats in the United States.

More LPAI H7N9 virus infections of humans have been reported than for any other LPAI viruses. Since LPAI H7N9 virus emerged to infect people in eastern China during early 2013, annual seasonal epidemic waves of human infections have occurred primarily in eastern (from the south to the north) and central China during the cooler and lower humidity fall, winter, and spring months, primarily linked to exposures while visiting live poultry markets in urban areas, or to backyard poultry in rural areas. As of March 2017, over 1,300 human cases of H7N9 virus infection with approximately 40% mortality were reported in China since 2013. A large surge in cases occurred during the fifth epidemic wave in 2016 to 2017. Most H7N9 cases have been hospitalized with pneumonia, with a high percentage admitted to an intensive care unit. Other risk

Table 74.1 Infections with Low Pathogenic Avian Influenza A Viruses Reported to Cause Human Illness (as of March 2017)

Subtype	Patient characteristics	Clinical Illness	Illness severity	Countries	Years
H6N1	Young adult	Fever with upper respiratory tract symptoms; mild lower respiratory tract disease	Moderate	Taiwan	2013
H7N2	Adults	Conjunctivitis; fever with upper respiratory tract symptoms; lower respiratory tract disease	Mild to moderate	United States, United Kingdom	2002, 2003, 2007, 2016
H7N3	Adults	Conjunctivitis	Mild	United Kingdom, Canada	2004, 2006
H7N7	Adult	Conjunctivitis	Mild (one case)	United Kingdom	1996
H7N9	All ages	Fever with upper respiratory tract symptoms; lower respiratory tract disease, multi-organ failure	Mild to severe; majority with severe to critical illness with mortality at 40%	China, Hong Kong and Macau Special Administrative Regions of China, cases exported to Taiwan, Malaysia, and Canada	2013–2017
H9N2	Young children and adults	Fever with upper respiratory tract symptoms; lower respiratory tract disease in an immunosuppressed adult	Mild to moderate	China, Hong Kong Special Administrative Region of China, Bangladesh, Egypt	1998, 1999, 2003, 2007, 2008, 2009, 2011, 2013, 2014, 2016
H10N7	Young children and Adults	Conjunctivitis and fever with upper respiratory tract symptoms	Mild	Egypt, Australia	2004, 2010
H10N8	Middle-aged and elderly adults	Severe pneumonia, respiratory failure, multi-organ failure	Critical illness with fatal outcome in two of three cases	China	2013, 2014

factors include having a chronic medical condition (e.g. obesity, chronic obstructive pulmonary disease, immunosuppression), and age over 60 years is associated with fatal outcomes. Clusters of H7N9 cases have been identified in every epidemic wave. Most cluster cases have been attributed to poultry exposures, but limited, non-sustained human-to-human H7N9 virus transmission could not be excluded in some clusters. Furthermore, nosocomial H7N9 virus transmission in unrelated individuals, including patient-to-patient and patient-to-health-care worker, has been reported in multiple clusters. Some cases that acquired H7N9 virus infection in China were exported and identified in Taiwan, Malaysia, and Canada. In 2017, human infections with HPAI H7N9 virus in southern China were identified, including in a fatal case that traveled to Taiwan, indicating that some H7N9 viruses had evolved from a LPAI virus to become pathogenic in poultry.

Sporadic human infections with HPAI viruses of H5 (H5N1, H5N6) and H7 (H7N3, H7N7, H7N9) subtypes have caused a wide spectrum of illness ranging from conjunctivitis, to uncomplicated upper respiratory tract symptoms, to pneumonia and multi-organ failure with fatal outcomes (see Table 74.2). Most human cases of infection with HPAI H5N1 viruses have been among children and young adults and associated with direct contact or indirect poultry exposure (visiting a live poultry market), and a small number of cases were linked to contact with wild birds. As of March 2017, the widespread ongoing epizootic of HPAI H5N1 viruses had resulted in more than 850 human cases and greater than 50% cumulative mortality in 16 countries since 1997. Human cases typically occur during the lower temperature and lower humidity fall and winter months, and are associated with increases in HPAI H5N1

poultry outbreaks. Small clusters of human HPAI H5N1 cases have been reported in several countries among blood-related family members, and some studies have suggested the potential for genetic susceptibility. The majority of these case clusters is thought to represent human infections following common source poultry exposures. However, in several countries, limited, non-sustained human-to-human transmission of HPAI H5N1 viruses has been observed infrequently or could not be excluded in some cases in which very close, prolonged unprotected exposure to a severely ill patient occurred at home or in a hospital. This has occurred primarily, but not exclusively, among blood-related family members. The largest family cluster to date included eight cases with seven deaths and occurred in North Sumatra, Indonesia during May 2006.

Risk factors for human infection with other avian influenza A viruses are similar to those for LPAI H7N9 and HPAI H5N1 viruses, such as direct or close contact with infected poultry. Probable, limited, non-sustained human-to-human transmission of HPAI H7N7 virus was reported in the Netherlands, but as of March 2017, other than LPAI H7N9 and HPAI H5N1 viruses, human-to-human transmission of other avian influenza A viruses has not been reported.

Human cases of variant influenza A virus infection (H1N1v, H1N2v, H3N2v) have been reported sporadically in several countries for several decades (see Table 74.3), with the highest number of cases reported in the United States, likely due to increased surveillance and testing for novel influenza A virus infections over the past 10 years compared with other countries. From 2011 to 2016, more than 380 cases of variant influenza A virus infection were reported in the United States. Variant influenza A virus infections have occurred after direct or close

Table 74.2 Infections with Highly Pathogenic Avian Influenza A Viruses Reported to Cause Human Illness (as of March 2017)

Subtype	Patient Characteristics	Clinical Illness	Illness severity	Countries	Years
H5N1	All ages, primarily children and young adults	Fever with upper respiratory tract symptoms; severe pneumonia, respiratory failure, ARDS, multi-organ failure	Mild to critical illness; majority with severe to critical illness with mortality >50%	Hong Kong Special Administrative Region of China, China, Vietnam, Thailand, Cambodia, Indonesia, China, Turkey, Iraq, Azerbaijan, Egypt, Djibouti, Nigeria, Laos PDR, Pakistan, Myanmar, Bangladesh, Canada (imported from China)	1997, 2003–2017
H5N6	Adults	Severe pneumonia, respiratory failure, multi-organ failure	Mild to critical illness, fatal outcomes	China	2014–2016
H7N3	Adults	Conjunctivitis	Mild	Canada, United Kingdom, Mexico, Italy	2004, 2006, 2012, 2013
H7N7	All ages	Conjunctivitis, fever with upper respiratory tract symptoms, hepatitis, severe pneumonia and respiratory failure, ARDS	Mild to critical illness; majority with conjunctivitis, critical illness with fatal outcome in one adult	United Kingdom, Netherlands	1959, 1996, 2003

Table 74.3 Infections with Variant Influenza A Viruses Reported to Cause Human Illness since 2005 (as of March 2017)

Subtype	Patient Characteristics	Clinical Illness	Illness Severity	Countries	Years
H1N1v	All ages, primarily children and young adults	Upper respiratory tract symptoms – with or without fever, pneumonia, respiratory failure, peritonitis, intestinal necrosis, mesenteric vein thrombosis, hemophagocytosis	Mild to critical and fatal illness	Russia, Switzerland, Netherlands, Hong Kong, Spain, Canada, United States, Italy	1974, 1975, 1976, 1079, 1980, 1982, 1983, 1986, 1988, 1991, 1992, 1993, 1994, 1995, 1998, 1999, 2002, 2005, 2008, 2016
H1N2v	Children and adults	Fever with upper respiratory tract symptoms	Mild to moderate illness	United States	2007, 2012, 2015, 2016
H3N2v	All ages, primarily children and young adults	Upper respiratory tract symptoms – with or without fever	Generally mild to moderate illness; fatal outcomes have been reported rarely	Netherlands, United States, Vietnam	1993, 1999, 2006, 2009, 2010, 2011, 2012, 2013, 2014, 2015, 2016

exposures to infected pigs at farms (while working or living at, or visiting) and other settings, though some cases did not have a history of exposure to pigs. During 2012, more than 300 cases of H3N2v infection were identified in the United States; the main risk factor was exposure to pigs at agricultural fairs during the summer and fall months. Some cases of variant influenza A virus infection have occurred through swine exposures at livestock events or at live animal markets where pigs are sold. Some case clusters have been reported in which limited, non-sustained human-to-human transmission of variant influenza A viruses (H3N2v) was suspected. In 1976, 13 confirmed H1N1v cases with one death occurred in an outbreak in Fort Dix, New Jersey among military recruits without swine exposure, and more than 200 estimated additional cases may have occurred. Most cases of variant virus infection have been reported in children, and most case-patients have experienced mild to moderate disease, not requiring hospitalization. However, a small number of cases of severe illness and deaths associated with variant influenza A virus infection have occurred.

Transmission and Pathogenesis

Avian influenza A viruses that have caused severe pulmonary disease in infected humans (HPAI H5N1, HPAI H5N6, HPAI H7N7, HPAI H7N9, LPAI H7N9, LPAI H10N8) bind primarily to receptors expressed on cells in the lower respiratory tract, though infection of upper respiratory tract tissues can occur. In particular, H7N9 viruses have the ability to also bind to the upper respiratory tract of humans. Some avian influenza A viruses have also been shown to bind to receptors expressed in tissues of the human gastrointestinal tract. In contrast, avian influenza A viruses (most LPAI and some HPAI viruses) that cause mild-to-moderate illness bind primarily to receptors expressed on cells in the upper respiratory tract. Avian influenza A viruses of the H7 subtype can bind to ocular receptors, and conjunctivitis has been reported for cases of H7 virus infection. In addition to specific viral characteristics (receptor binding tropism in the respiratory tract; virulence factors), other potential determinants of disease severity may include age,

Table 74.4 Clinical Features: Novel Influenza A

Incubation period	2–5 days (usually ≤7 days)
Signs and symptoms	Common admission findings: • Fever ≥38 °C, non-productive cough, difficulty breathing, shortness of breath, tachypnea • pulmonary crackles, rhonchi, diminished breath sounds, hypoxia Other findings: • headache, rhinorrhea, sore throat, productive cough, hemoptysis, vomiting, diarrhea, abdominal pain, malaise, myalgias
Laboratory and radiographic findings in severe illness	• Leukopenia, lymphopenia, mild-to-moderate thrombocytopenia, hypoalbuminemia, elevation of hepatic transaminases • Abnormal CXR/CT scan: 　∘ Infiltrates (patchy, interstitial, diffuse), opacities, typically bilateral disease, consolidation (segmental, lobar) 　∘ Pleural effusion
Complications	• Pneumonia with rapid progression to respiratory failure and ARDS • Ventilator-associated pneumonia, pulmonary hemorrhage, pneumothorax • Multi-organ failure, cardiac compromise, renal dysfunction and renal failure • Septic shock • Encephalitis, encephalopathy, obstructive hydrocephalus • Reye syndrome • Hemophagocytosis

underlying medical conditions, genetic susceptibility, route(s) of exposure, exposure dose and frequency of exposures, and immune status. Some sero-surveys have reported low frequencies of antibodies to different avian influenza A viruses in exposed study populations, suggesting that asymptomatic infection or subclinical illness are uncommon. Most variant influenza A viruses bind to receptors in the human upper respiratory tract, and have been generally associated with mild-to-moderate human illness.

Although risk factors for zoonotic transmission of novel influenza A viruses are direct or close contact with well-appearing, diseased, or dead poultry or well-appearing or sick pigs, it is not clear exactly how infection of the respiratory tract is initiated. Inhalation of aerosolized novel influenza A viruses or contact transmission to mucus membranes are thought to be modes of transmission. Limited human-to-human transmission of some novel influenza A viruses can occur through prolonged, unprotected close exposure to a sick, infected person, and has been reported in households and in health-care settings. Data on viral shedding are limited for most novel influenza A viruses, but in uncomplicated illness, viral shedding in the upper respiratory tract is approximately 1 week or less. In patients with viral pneumonia and respiratory failure (HPAI H5N1, HPAI H5N6, HPAI H7N9, and LPAI H7N9 viruses), prolonged viral replication may be detected in lower respiratory tract specimens for more than 2 weeks. Following exposures to birds or pigs, the incubation period for novel influenza A virus infection is similar to or slightly longer than for seasonal influenza, approximately 2 to 5 days up to 7 days, with a mean or median of 3 days, but some studies have suggested longer incubation periods for some avian influenza A viruses. Limited data suggest that the incubation period for human-to-human transmission of some novel influenza A viruses is likely to be approximately 3 to 5 days (HPAI H5N1, LPAI H7N9), but incubation periods of 8 to 9 days or longer have been reported.

The pathogenesis of severe disease caused by novel influenza A virus infection appears to be mediated by high viral replication in the lower respiratory tract that stimulates an over-exuberant host inflammatory response. High viral levels have been correlated with cytokine dysregulation in fatal human cases (HPAI H5N1, LPAI H7N9 viruses). Extrapulmonary dissemination has been reported for fatal cases of HPAI H5N1, with viral RNA detection or virus isolation from serum, plasma, cerebrospinal fluid, and rectal swabs. Neutralizing antibodies to HPAI H5N1 virus in surviving patients can be detected in serum approximately 10 to 14 days after illness onset.

Clinical Features

The signs and symptoms of novel influenza A virus infection cannot be distinguished from those associated with seasonal influenza virus infection. Thus, eliciting a recent history of exposure to poultry or pigs, or to a patient with novel influenza A virus infection, is essential to making a diagnosis of suspected novel influenza A. A wide range of symptoms and clinical complications have been reported for patients with novel influenza A virus infections (see Tables 74.1, 74.2, and 74.4). Diarrhea (non-bloody) has been reported for infection with some avian or variant influenza A viruses.

Patients with lower respiratory tract disease may initially experience fever and upper respiratory symptoms, and present approximately 3 to 6 days after illness onset with continued high fever and hypoxia, non-productive cough, tachypnea, dyspnea, and shortness of breath and rapidly progressive viral pneumonia (HPAI H5N1, HPAI H5N6, HPAI H7N9, LPAI H7N9). Other symptoms that may be present in novel influenza A cases with severe illness include productive cough, hemoptysis, abdominal pain, vomiting, and myalgias. Dehydration may be evident in patients with high fever, tachypnea, and diarrhea. A few HPAI H5N1 cases have presented with diarrhea without obvious respiratory disease, followed later by development of pneumonia. A small number of HPAI H5N1 cases have been diagnosed with encephalitis (seizures, altered mental status) with fatal outcomes. Other complications include respiratory failure, ARDS, septic shock, and renal failure. Bacterial

Table 74.5 Differential Diagnosis: Novel Influenza A

Influenza-like illness with or without lower respiratory tract disease:
- Respiratory viruses (influenza A, influenza B, RSV, rhinovirus, parainfluenzavirus, human metapneumonvirus, adenovirus, non-SARS coronavirus, bocavirus, SARS-CoV, MERS-CoV)
- Dengue virus

Influenza-like illness with diarrhea:
- Respiratory viruses (e.g. influenza A, influenza B, RSV)
- Enteric viruses (e.g. norovirus, rotavirus)
- Bacterial infections (e.g. ETEC, *Salmonella typhi*)

Community-acquired pneumonia:
- Bacterial (*Streptococcus pneumoniae, Hemophilous influenzae, Bordetella pertussis*)
- Respiratory virus co-infection with bacterial pneumonia (*Streptococcus pneumoniae, Hemophilous influenzae*, Group A *Streptococcus pyogenes, Staphylococcus aureus*/MSSA/MRSA)
- Atypical pathogens (*Mycoplasma pneumoniae, Chlamydophila pneumoniae, Legionella pneumophila*; fungi)

Viral pneumonia:
- Influenza A, influenza B, RSV, rhinovirus, parainfluenzavirus, adenovirus (e.g. HAdV-14), human metapneumonvirus, bocavirus, CMV, hantavirus, measles, enterovirus (e.g. EV-D68, EV-71) EBV, VZV, HSV, SARS-CoV, MERS-CoV

co-infection has rarely been reported in novel influenza A patients, though ventilator-associated pneumonia can occur.

Differential Diagnosis

The differential diagnosis is broad and includes infection with respiratory viruses that cause acute febrile upper respiratory tract illness and pathogens that can cause lower respiratory tract disease, including seasonal influenza A and B viruses, and viral and bacterial co-infection (see Table 74.5). It is essential to elicit a recent history of direct (touching) or very close unprotected contact with poultry (well-appearing, diseased, or dead poultry) or wild birds, or pigs, or with a confirmed or highly suspected human case of novel influenza A virus infection. Since some novel influenza A patients have presented with fever and diarrhea with or without subsequent development of lower respiratory disease, the differential diagnosis should also consider infections that cause febrile gastrointestinal illness. In returned travelers, clinicians should also consider common local causes of such diseases in countries where avian influenza A viruses are prevalent among poultry. In patients with pneumonia, viral and bacterial etiologies of community-acquired pneumonia should also be considered.

Laboratory and Radiographic Findings

Hospitalized patients with severe disease due to HPAI H5N1, HPAI H5N6, HPAI H7N9, or LPAI H7N9 virus infection have presented with leukopenia, lymphopenia, and mild-to-moderate thrombocytopenia. Hypoalbuminemia, increased levels of lactate dehydrogenase, and moderate elevation of hepatic transaminases have been described with severe illness due to HPAI H5N1 or LPAI H7N9 virus infections.

Radiographic findings in patients with lower respiratory tract disease due to HPAI H5N1, HPAI H7N9, or LPAI H7N9 virus infection include diffuse, unilateral but more commonly bilateral abnormalities, multifocal or patchy infiltrates, interstitial infiltrates, ground-glass opacities, segmental or lobular consolidation, and pleural effusions.

When novel influenza A virus infection is suspected, the patient should be isolated promptly and recommended infection prevention and control measures should be implemented, including for collection of respiratory specimens. The local and state health department or equivalent public health authorities should be contacted to arrange influenza testing by real-time reverse transcription polymerase chain reaction in a biosafety level 2 (BSL-2) laboratory. In Ill persons with a recent history of exposure to poultry or to a person with avian influenza A virus infection, avian influenza A virus infection may be suspected on the basis of a positive result for detection of influenza A viral RNA, with negative results for detection of seasonal influenza A virus subtypes H3 and H1 (influenza A, not subtypeable). Virus isolation should be attempted only under BSL-3 enhanced laboratory conditions. In the United States, state health departments and some public health laboratories have the ability to perform testing for influenza A virus subtypes H5 and H7. However, the Centers for Disease Control and Prevention (CDC) should be contacted, and respiratory tract specimens and viral RNA extracted from these specimens should be shipped to the CDC for confirmatory testing, sequencing, and virus isolation, identification, and characterization.

In ill persons with a history of exposure to swine or to a person with variant influenza A virus infection, variant influenza A virus infection may be suspected on the basis of: (1) a positive test for detection of influenza A viral RNA and H3, with negative results for H1; or (2) a positive test for detection of influenza A viral RNA, with negative results for H3 and H1 (influenza A, not subtypeable). Respiratory tract specimens and viral RNA extracted from these specimens should be shipped to the CDC for confirmatory testing and sequencing, and virus isolation, identification, and characterization.

Proper respiratory specimen collection is essential. Ideally, respiratory tract specimens should be collected as close to illness as possible. For non-ventilated patients in whom variant influenza A virus infection is suspected, nasopharyngeal and nasal specimens are preferred, or a combined nasal and

Table 74.6 Laboratory Diagnosis: Novel Influenza A

Detection of influenza A viral RNA at public health laboratories; subtyping for seasonal influenza A viruses (H1, H3)	Real-time or conventional reverse-transcription polymerase chain reaction in biosafety level 2 (BSL-2) conditions Best specimens: • Endotracheal aspirate, BAL fluid, chest tube fluid, pleural fluid (from intubated patients) • Nasopharyngeal, nasal, and throat swabs (from non-intubated patients) • Collect specimens from multiple sites on multiple days for testing Note: Some public health laboratories can perform subtyping for influenza A (H5) and (H7) viruses. In the United States, specimens should be shipped to the CDC for confirmatory testing for any influenza A virus identified that is non subtypeable (positive for influenza A, negative for H1 and H3) or from a patient with suspected novel influenza A virus infection.
Isolation of novel influenza A viruses	Embryonated egg or tissue cell culture in biosafety level 3 (BSL-3) enhanced conditions at CDCs or specialized public health laboratories Best specimens: • Endotracheal aspirate, BAL fluid, chest tube fluid, pleural fluid (from intubated patients) • Nasopharyngeal or nasal swabs, and throat swabs (from non-intubated patients)
Serology for detection of antibodies to novel influenza A viruses (retrospective diagnosis)	Multiple assays may be available at specialized public health and research laboratories depending upon the novel influenza A virus strain. Some serological assays may not be standardized. Laboratory requirements may be BSL-2 or BSL-3 enhanced conditions depending upon the serological assay, the virus strain or virus antigen used in the assay, and the severity of human disease associated with the virus strain. Key issues: • Ideally paired acute (within 7 days of illness onset) and convalescent sera (collected 14–21 days later) should be collected and tested together • Serological testing methods may include microneutralization assay using live virus in enhanced BSL-3 conditions (e.g. for HPAI H5N1 virus antibodies), pseudotyped particle-based neutralization assays, ELISA, modified equine RBC HI assay • Standard influenza HI assay is inaccurate (not sensitive and not specific) • In addition to matching the specific virus or virus antigen that the patient was exposed to, serological testing methods must also address the potential for non-specific and specific cross-reactivity that could yield false positive results (e.g. by absorbing potentially cross-reactive antibodies) • To improve accuracy, two serological assays may be utilized (e.g. horse red-blood-cell HI assay for screening sera, followed by microneutralization assay for detection of HPAI H5N1 virus antibodies)
Commercially available influenza tests for seasonal influenza (rapid influenza diagnostic tests, immunofluorescence, commercial molecular assays)	Not recommended for diagnosis of novel influenza A virus infection; not sensitive, not specific. False-negatives are common; a positive influenza A result could indicate human influenza A virus infection, novel influenza A virus infection, or be falsely positive.

BAL – bronchoalveolar lavage; ELISA – enzyme-linked immunosorbent assay; HI – hemagglutinin inhibition; RBC – red blood cell.

throat swab specimen can be collected for testing. For non-ventilated patients in whom avian influenza A virus infection is suspected, a throat swab should be collected in addition to a nasopharyngeal or nasal specimen because throat swabs have higher yield for detection of some avian influenza A viruses (e.g. HPAI H5N1 virus). For intubated patients, endotracheal aspirates should be collected for influenza testing because negative results on influenza testing of upper respiratory tract specimens do not exclude novel influenza A virus infection in patients with severe lower respiratory tract disease. Pleural and bronchioalveolar lavage fluid specimens are also of high diagnostic utility. Collection and testing of multiple respiratory specimens on consecutive days can maximize detection of novel influenza A viruses associated with severe lower respiratory tract disease (e.g. HPAI H5N1, HPAI H5N6, HPAI H7N9, LPAI H7N9).

Influenza testing of respiratory tract specimens for seasonal influenza A viruses by commercially available assays cannot yield a diagnosis of novel influenza A virus infection. Non-molecular influenza assays (e.g. rapid influenza diagnostic tests) have low-to-moderate sensitivity for detection of influenza A viruses. Negative results by commercial assays for seasonal influenza A viruses do not exclude a diagnosis of novel influenza A virus infection.

Serological testing cannot inform clinical management, but novel influenza A virus infection may be diagnosed retrospectively by testing of paired acute and convalescent serum specimens using serological assays with a specific virus antigen (avian or variant influenza A virus strain) performed at CDC and other specialized research laboratories (see Table 74.6).

Antiviral Treatment and Chemoprophylaxis

Any patient with suspected novel influenza A virus infection, especially any hospitalized patient or outpatient who is at high risk for influenza complications, should receive antiviral treatment with a neuraminidase inhibitor (oral oseltamivir, inhaled zanamivir, intravenous peramivir) as soon as possible, without waiting for laboratory testing results. Neuraminidase inhibitor drugs limit the release of influenza viral particles from infected cells. Antiviral treatment with a neuraminidase inhibitor drug is recommended as soon as possible by the CDC for patients infected with novel influenza A viruses that are known to or are related to viruses that have caused severe human disease (e.g. HPAI H5N1, HPAI H5N6, HPAI H7N9, LPAI H7N9) (www.cdc.gov/flu/avianflu/novel-av-treatment-guidance.htm). Oral oseltamivir is the antiviral drug of choice at the same dosage as for seasonal influenza for outpatients and hospitalized patients. Zanamivir is chemically similar to oseltamivir, but is administered as an orally inhaled powder using an inhaler device, and can be given to outpatients. Primary adverse effects associated with inhaled zanamivir are bronchospasm, especially in persons with underlying chronic pulmonary disease.

For patients with severe illness, oseltamivir treatment should be continued beyond the standard 5-day course, and serial testing of respiratory specimens can inform the duration of treatment. Primary side effects associated with oseltamivir include nausea and vomiting. The optimal dosage, duration of therapy, and effectiveness of oseltamivir for treatment of severe disease from HPAI H5N1, HPAI H5N6, HPAI H7N9, or LPAI H7N9 virus infection are unknown. In critically ill patients with novel influenza A virus infection, treatment options include enteric oseltamivir administered via naso or oro gastric tube, or intravenous peramivir or intravenous zanamivir (if available). Inhaled zanamivir should not be administered to hospitalized patients. Observational studies suggest that early initiation of oseltamivir treatment of patients with HPAI H5N1 virus infection can reduce mortality compared to starting treatment later, but late initiation of oseltamivir treatment may still be beneficial compared to no treatment.

Oseltamivir resistance has been documented for some HPAI H5N1, HPAI H7N9, and LPAI H7N9 viruses, and some patients infected with HPAI H7N9 or LPAI H7N9 viruses resistant to the neuraminidase inhibitors oseltamivir and peramivir with reduced susceptibility to zanamivir experienced fatal outcomes. H7N9 virus resistance to oseltamivir and peramivir with reduced susceptibility to zanamivir emerged during treatment with a neuraminidase inhibitor, highlighting the importance of strict adherence to recommended infection prevention and control measures to reduce the risk of nosocomial transmission. Amantadine and rimantadine are not recommended for antiviral treatment of novel influenza A virus infection because of widespread resistance among many avian and variant influenza A viruses. However, when a novel influenza A virus has been determined to be susceptible to amantadine or rimantadine, one of these drugs could be potentially used in combination treatment with a neuraminidase inhibitor. Primary adverse effects associated with amantadine and rimantadine include vomiting, diarrhea, and central nervous system symptoms.

The mainstay of clinical management is supportive care of complications, supplemental oxygen, and mechanical ventilation for respiratory failure, and renal replacement therapy for renal failure. Advanced organ support using extracorporeal membrane oxygenation (ECMO) for LPAI H7N9-associated ARDS and use of vasopressors for refractory shock has been reported for HPAI H5N1, HPAI H7N9, and LPAI H7N9 patients. Corticosteroid therapy is not recommended except for low-dose dexamethasone for septic shock with suspected adrenal insufficiency.

Daily monitoring and post-exposure antiviral chemoprophylaxis of close contacts of patients infected with novel influenza A viruses that are known to be or are related to avian influenza A viruses that have caused severe human disease (e.g. HPAI H5N1, HPAI H5N6, HPAI H7N9, LPAI H7N9) is recommended. Monitoring should be for 10 days, and post-exposure antiviral chemoprophylaxis with a neuraminidase inhibitor should be administered as soon as possible, twice daily (treatment dosing frequency) for 5 days, or 10 days if there is ongoing exposure to close contacts (www.cdc.gov/flu/avianflu/novel-av-chemoprophylaxis-guidance.htm). Similarly, persons exposed to birds (poultry) infected with avian influenza A viruses that are known to be or are related to viruses that have caused severe human disease should be monitored for 10 days after the last known exposure, and post-exposure antiviral chemoprophylaxis with a neuraminidase inhibitor, twice daily (treatment dosing frequency), can be considered depending upon the exposure and whether the exposed person is at high risk for influenza complications. For time-limited exposures that are not ongoing, the duration of twice daily antiviral chemoprophylaxis is 5 days (http://www.cdc.gov/flu/avianflu/guidance-exposed-persons.htm) (see Table 74.7).

Complications and Admission Criteria

Some patients with novel influenza A virus infections have been hospitalized for isolation purposes, but the main reasons for hospital admission in most patients are for supportive care of complications and hypoxemia. Advanced organ support may be needed for respiratory and renal failure, and some patients with LPAI H7N9 in China have been managed with ECMO for refractory hypoxemia. Complications of novel influenza A virus infection include viral pneumonia with progression to respiratory failure and ARDS (e.g. HPAI H5N1, HPAI H5N6, HPAI H7N9, LPAI H7N9). Ventilator-associated pneumonia, pulmonary hemorrhage, and pneumothorax can occur. Septic shock, hypovolemic shock, hemophagocytosis, renal dysfunction, cardiac compromise with arrhythmias, hepatic inflammation, and multi-organ failure (respiratory and renal failure), encephalitis, and obstructive hydrocephalus, have been reported in novel influenza A virus infections. Viremia with extrapulmonary dissemination and isolation of HPAI H5N1 virus from CSF and stool/rectal swab has been reported. Atypical presentations in patients with HPAI H5N1 virus infection include one adult in Thailand who presented with diarrhea before developing pneumonia, one child in Vietnam who presented with diarrhea, seizures, progressed to coma, and was clinically diagnosed with encephalitis, and one child in Hong Kong who developed Reye syndrome after aspirin ingestion.

Infection Control

Infection prevention and control (IPC) measures for symptomatic patients with suspected or confirmed novel influenza A virus infection include addressing three key issues: isolation of the patient, use of recommended personal protective

Table 74.7 Antiviral Treatment for Novel Influenza A

Patient Category	Therapy Recommendation*
Adults	Oseltamivir 75mg PO BID × 5 days is recommended as soon as possible for any outpatient who is at high risk for influenza complications, and any hospitalized patient with suspected novel influenza A; initiate treatment as soon as possible without waiting for influenza testing results. Adverse effects: nausea, vomiting. • Consider higher dosing (especially in patients with diarrhea) and longer duration in patients with severe illness • Can be administered via oro or naso-gastric tube in intubated patients Zanamivir 10mg (two inhalations) BID × 5 days is an option for outpatients without chronic airways disease. Adverse effects: bronchospasm. Intravenous peramivir 600mg IV (single dose) is an option for adult outpatients. Adverse effects: diarrhea. Daily dosing of intravenous peramivir or intravenous zanamivir (if available) can be considered in hospitalized patients, including when enteric oseltamivir administration is contraindicated, using a research protocol.
Children	Oseltamivir‡ (dosing is weight-based by age; dosing frequency and duration is the same as for adults)
Pregnant women	Same as for non-pregnant adults
Immunocompromised	Same as for non-immunocompromised persons

* Primary adverse effects of oseltamivir treatment are nausea and vomiting. Resistance to oseltamivir and peramivir has been reported for some avian influenza A viruses. The primary adverse effect of inhaled zanamivir treatment is bronchospasm; inhaled zanamivir is contraindicated in persons with chronic airways disease, and is not recommended for treatment of influenza in hospitalized patients. The most common adverse effect of intravenous peramivir is diarrhea. Amantadine and rimantadine are not recommended due to a high frequency of resistance among some avian influenza A viruses.

‡ Oseltamivir is approved for treatment of influenza in persons aged ≥14 days in the United States. Dosage is based upon age and weight. An oral suspension is available. Zanamivir is approved for treatment of influenza in persons aged ≥7 years in the United States. The package inserts should be consulted for the appropriate pediatric doses and contraindications. Peramivir is approved for treatment of uncomplicated influenza in persons aged ≥18 years in the United States. Dosage of oseltamivir and peramivir should be adjusted for renal impairment. Inhaled lananimivir and intravenous zanamivir are not approved in the United States, but may be available in other countries.

Source: Centers for Disease Control and Prevention, Interim guidance on the use of antiviral medications for treatment of human infections with novel influenza A viruses associated with severe human disease, available at www.cdc.gov/flu/avianflu/novel-av-treatment-guidance.htm.

equipment (PPE) by all health-care personnel and visiting family members, and strict adherence to infection prevention and control precautions. Nosocomial transmission of H7N9 virus has been reported from patient to patient, and patient to health-care worker in China. Patients with suspected or confirmed infection with novel influenza A viruses that are known to or are related to viruses that have caused severe human disease (e.g. HPAI H5N1, HPAI H5N6, HPAI H7N9, LPAI H7N9) should be placed in an Airborne Infection Isolation Room (AIIR) with negative pressure, or isolated with a facemask in a room with a closed door before transfer to a facility where an AIIR is available (www.cdc.gov/flu/avianflu/novel-flu-infection-control.htm). Contact and airborne precautions should be implemented with recommended personal protective equipment by caregivers (disposable gloves, gowns, eye protection, and fit-tested N95 respirator or equivalent). Environmental infection control should ensure that cleaning and disinfection procedures are implemented. IPC recommendations are available at www.cdc.gov/flu/avianflu/novel-flu-infection-control.htm. IPC recommendations for patients with novel influenza A viruses that have not caused severe human illness are the same as for seasonal influenza, and include implementing contact and droplet precautions: www.cdc.gov/flu/professionals/infectioncontrol/healthcaresettings.htm.

Prevention

No human vaccines for novel influenza A viruses are available outside of a clinical trial. Two H5N1 vaccines are licensed for adults by the Food and Drug Administration in the United States, but are not available for commercial distribution.

Therefore, prevention is focused on avoiding exposure to infected poultry or wild birds, or pigs, and immediately implementing recommended infection prevention and control measures when providing care to a patient with suspected or confirmed novel influenza A virus infection.

Pearls and Pitfalls

- In a patient with acute febrile respiratory illness, including severe illness (fever, cough, shortness of breath, difficulty breathing, tachypnea, pneumonia, diarrhea, leukopenia, lymphopenia, mild-to-moderate thrombocytopenia), elicit a recent history of possible exposures to animals (poultry – well-appearing, sick, or dead poultry, wild birds, pigs, visits to live animal markets, agricultural fairs), sick persons (especially with suspected or confirmed novel influenza A virus infection), or a travel history to an area with avian influenza in poultry or swine influenza in pigs during the week prior to illness onset.

- Cases of human infection with novel influenza A viruses (HPAI H5N1, HPAI H7N9, LPAI H7N9) have been exported from China to other countries where ill patients have presented to health-care facilities, including hospitalization for critical and fatal illness (Malaysia, Taiwan, Canada).

- Seasonal influenza A and B virus infection are the most likely cause of influenza-like illness in any country and among travelers with or without poultry or pig contact. Seasonal influenza A and B viruses circulate year-round in some tropical and subtropical countries, and activity is increased in temperature climates of the Southern

Hemisphere during low influenza periods in the Northern Hemisphere (e.g. summertime). Influenza A and B, and other human respiratory viruses, can cause uncomplicated influenza-like illness, as well as pneumonia and severe respiratory disease.

- Human illness from infection with novel influenza A viruses is uncommon, even among persons with acute febrile respiratory illness who had contact with poultry or pigs.
- Limited, non-sustained human-to-human transmission of novel influenza A viruses is rare, but has been reported in close contacts for HPAI H5N1 and LPAI H7N9 viruses, including health-care personnel, and has been suspected for H3N2v virus.
- Because novel influenza A viruses are dynamic, and new therapies and vaccines are under development, emergency physicians should consult the latest information on surveillance, epidemiology, and clinical characteristics of human infections with avian and variant influenza A viruses, and recommendations on clinical management, diagnostic testing, antiviral treatment, infection prevention and control, and vaccines from websites of the CDC, the Infectious Diseases Society of American (IDSA), and World Health Organization (WHO).

References

Cheng, V. C., Chan, J. F., Wen, X., *et al.* Infection of immunocompromised patients by avian H9N2 influenza A virus. *J. Infect.* 2011; 62(5): 394–9.

Epperson, S., Jhung, M., Richards, S., *et al.* Human infections with influenza A(H3N2) variant virus in the United States, 2011–2012. *Clin. Infect. Dis.* 2013; 57(Suppl. 1): S4–11.

Freidl, G. S., Meijer, A., de Bruin, E, *et al.* Influenza at the animal-human interface: a review of the literature for virological evidence of human infection with swine or avian influenza viruses other than A(H5N1). *Euro. Surveill.* 2014; 19(18): pii: 20793.

Gao, H. N., Lu, H. Z., Cao, B., *et al.* Clinical findings in 111 cases of influenza A (H7N9) virus infection. *N. Engl. J. Med.* 2013; 368(24): 2277–85.

Jhung, M. A., Epperson, S., Biggerstaff, M., *et al.* Outbreak of variant influenza A(H3N2) virus in the United States. *Clin. Infect. Dis.* 2013; 57(12): 1703–12.

Koopmans, M., Wilbrink, B., Conyn, M., *et al.* Transmission of H7N7 avian influenza A virus to human beings during a large outbreak in commercial poultry farms in the Netherlands. *Lancet* 2004; 363(9409): 587–93.

Lai, S., Qin, Y., Cowling, B. J., *et al.* Global epidemiology of avian influenza A H5N1 virus infection in humans, 1997–2015: a systematic review of individual case data. *Lancet Infect. Dis.* 2016; 16(7): e108–18.

Myers, K. P., Olsen, C. W., Gray, G. C. Cases of swine influenza in humans: a review of the literature. *Clin. Infect. Dis.* 2007; 44(8): 1084–8.

Uyeki, T. M. Human infection with highly pathogenic avian influenza A (H5N1) virus: review of clinical issues. *Clin. Infect. Dis.* 2009; 49(2): 279–90.

Writing Committee of the Second World Health Organization Consultation on Clinical Aspects of Human Infection with Avian Influenza A (H5N1) Virus, Abdel-Ghafar, A. N., Chotpitayasunondh, T., *et al.* Update on avian influenza A (H5N1) virus infection in humans. *N. Engl. J. Med.* 2008; 358(3): 261–73.

Wu, P., Peng, Z., Fang, V. J., *et al.* Human infection with influenza A(H7N9) virus during 3 major epidemic waves, China, 2013–2015. *Emerg. Infect. Dis.* 2016; 22(6): 964–72.

Additional Readings

de Jong, M. D., Bach, V. C., Phan, T. Q., *et al.* Fatal avian influenza A (H5N1) in a child presenting with diarrhea followed by coma. *N. Engl. J. Med.* 2005; 352(7): 686–91.

de Jong, M. D., Simmons, C. P., Thanh, T. T., *et al.* Fatal outcome of human influenza A (H5N1) is associated with high viral load and hypercytokinemia. *Nature Medicine* 2006; 12(10): 1203–7.

de Jong, M. D., Thanh, T. T., Khanh, T. H., *et al.* Oseltamivir resistance during treatment of influenza A (H5N1) infection. *N. Engl. J. Med.* 2005; 353(25): 2667–72.

Gaydos, J. C., Top, F. H., Jr., Hodder, R. A., and Russell, P. K. Swine influenza A outbreak, Fort Dix, New Jersey, 1976. *Emerg. Infect. Dis.* 2006; 12(1): 23–8.

Kandun, I. N., Wibisono, H., Sedyaningsih, E. R., *et al.* Three Indonesian clusters of H5N1 virus infection in 2005. *N. Engl. J. Med.* 2006; 355(21): 2186–94.

Ungchusak, K., Auewarakul, P., Dowell, S. F., *et al.* Probable person-to-person transmission of avian influenza A (H5N1). *N. Engl. J. Med.* 2005; 352(4): 333–40.

Yu, H., Cowling, B. J., Feng, L., *et al.* Human infection with avian influenza A H7N9 virus: an assessment of clinical severity. *Lancet* 2013; 382(9887): 138–45.

Methicillin-Resistant *Staphylococcus Aureus* (MRSA)

Tracy Trang and Bradley W. Frazee

Introduction and Microbiology

Staphylococcus is a gram-positive, non-motile, and non-spore-forming bacteria. The *Staphylococcus* genus contains 32 species. Although 16 are capable of causing disease in humans, by far the most prevalent and virulent species is *Staphylococcus aureus*. *Staphylococcus epidermidis* and *Staphylococcus saprophyticus* are other important *Staphylococcus* species that can cause device-related infections and urinary tract infections, respectively.

Two years after the introduction of methicillin in the late 1950s, the first isolate of methicillin-resistant *S. aureus* (MRSA) was discovered. From the 1950s to the 1990s, almost all MRSA infections occurred in hospitals or were associated with health-care settings (now referred to as health-care-associated MRSA or HA-MRSA). Patients typically had recognizable risk factors for HA-MRSA acquisition such as recent hospitalization, hemodialysis, or residence in a nursing home. However, beginning in the mid- to late 1990s, MRSA infections emerged among patients without previous health-care exposure or risk factors. These strains were termed community-associated MRSA (CA-MRSA), and most commonly took the form of skin and soft-tissue infections (SSTIs). However, severe and life-threatening infections due to CA-MRSA, such as pneumonia, osteomyelitis, endocarditis, and bacteremia, were also reported.

The current clinical categorization of *S. aureus* infections, with regard to site of onset and health-care exposure, and the associated acronyms, are presented in Table 75.1.

CA-MRSA can be distinguished from HA-MRSA on the basis of both genotype and antibiotic resistance pattern. The genotype of an MRSA isolate is identified by its clonal family (sequence type) and its methicillin resistance gene. The methicillin resistance gene, which codes for decreased beta-lactam binding affinity, is located on a genetic element referred to as SCCmec. In the United States, HA-MRSA usually belongs to the USA100 and USA200 clonal families and carries SCCmec

types I, II, or III, which confer resistance to not just beta-lactams, but other non-beta-lactam antibiotics. CA-MRSA usually belongs to the USA300 clonal family (less often USA400) and carries SCCmec IV, which confers resistance only to methicillin. Hence, unlike HA-MRSA strains, CA-MRSA strains are usually susceptible to narrow spectrum non-beta-lactam antibiotics such as trimethoprim–sulfamethoxazole and doxycycline.

Although susceptible to narrow spectrum non-beta-lactams, CA-MRSA strains can be highly virulent. Most CA-MRSA strains (USA300) also carry a gene that encodes the Panton–Valentine leukocidin (PVL), a toxin that destroys leukocytes. PVL-positive CA-MRSA has been associated with necrotizing pneumonia and necrotizing fasciitis.

Given the range of infection types potentially caused by *S. aureus*, from abscess to pneumonia to endocarditis, and the prevalence of MRSA now among such infections, the issue of MRSA management arises almost every day in contemporary acute care practice. Providers must have a basic understanding of epidemiology and terminology, be familiar with the types of infections in which MRSA is commonly implicated, and have a solid understanding of the antibiotics to which MRSA is susceptible.

Epidemiology

In the United States, USA300 is the predominant CA-MRSA clone. The explosive emergence of CA-MRSA reflects the remarkable ability of this clone to survive and spread. Before 1997, MRSA infection in patients without risk factors was rarely seen, and USA300 was a rarely isolated genotype. By 2003, USA300 had been identified as the major cause of SSTIs in prison inmates and emergency department (ED) patients across California. A 2004 study carried out in 11 EDs across the United States found that MRSA caused 59% of SSTIs and that 97% of these isolates were USA300.

There are several plausible explanations for the emergence of CA-MRSA, including increased use of fluoroquinolones

Table 75.1 Categorization of MRSA infection

Health-care-associated MRSA (HA-MRSA)	Infection onset more than 48 hours following hospitalization *or* Community onset (or within first 48 hours of hospitalization) with the following health-care exposures in the previous 12 months: surgery, hemodialysis, skilled nursing facility residence
Community-associated MRSA (CA-MRSA)	Community onset (or within first 48 hours of hospital admission) and no health-care exposure
Hospital onset (nosocomial)	Infection begins during hospitalization
Community onset	Infection begins in the community

Box 75.1 Risk Factors Associated with CA-MRSA and Groups at Increased Risk for CA-MRSA

Recent use of antibiotics
Household contacts of a confirmed case
Jail inmates
Military recruits
Children in daycare centers
Athletes (e.g. wrestling, American football, fencing)
Urban underserved communities
Institutionalized adults with developmental disabilities
Men who have sex with men
Intravenous drug users
HIV-infected individuals
Native Americans
Alaska Natives
Pacific Islanders
Veterinarian surgeons, pig farmers, and contact with colonized pets

and the success of pneumococcal vaccination in children and adults. Fluoroquinolones may eliminate methicillin-susceptible *S. aureus* strains from the nasal mucosa, thereby allowing colonization of MRSA strains. Likewise, administration of pneumococcal vaccine may decrease pneumococcal colonization, which leaves a larger niche for CA-MRSA.

CA-MRSA colonizes not only the nares, but the axilla, groin, and gastrointestinal tract, and is also spread directly from draining SSTIs. CA-MRSA tends to survive on fomites and spreads easily within households and other close contact settings, such as prisons and contact sports teams. There have been numerous reports of clustered outbreaks of CA-MRSA SSTIs, with occasional severe infection and bacteremia, among otherwise healthy athletes.

The epidemiology of *S. aureus* infections inside the hospital also has changed in the past three decades, with the proportion of MRSA bacterial isolates steadily increasing. For example, among nosocomial bloodstream infections in the United States, the proportion of isolates that were MRSA increased from 22% in 1995 to 57% in 2001. Very recent surveillance data, however, seem to show a slight decline in the proportion of health-care-associated MRSA infections. This decrease may be attributed to efforts by health-care organizations to curb MRSA transmission through universal precautions and infection control measures.

To complicate matters, CA-MRSA strains are increasingly being isolated from hospital onset infections. Individuals that are colonized with CA-MRSA, and then hospitalized, can develop invasive infections in the hospital, such as catheter-associated bacteremia or ventilator-acquired pneumonia, caused by a community-acquired strain. Patients may also spread the community-acquired strain to staff and other patients. Conversely, a large proportion of community onset infections are actually health-care-associated – whether clinically or genetically (SCCmec I-III) defined.

Several factors have been identified to predict disease caused by CA-MRSA and HA-MRSA. CA-MRSA is prevalent among certain populations, listed in Box 75.1. Physical crowding and hygiene appear to play an important role in determining risk for CA-MRSA infection. Populations at increased risk for HA-MRSA are residents in long-term care facilities, patients undergoing hemodialysis or peritoneal dialysis, and patients with

diabetes, chronic liver, lung, vascular, or renal disease, prolonged hospitalization, intensive care unit (ICU) admission, or indwelling intravascular catheters or medical devices. For the acute care provider, however, attempting to identify patients at increased risk for MRSA is not recommended; since roughly half of *S. aureus* isolates in both community and health-care settings are MRSA, the empiric antimicrobial regimen should always cover MRSA.

MRSA infections are prevalent in other parts of the world as well. Studies have reported a 25 to 50% prevalence of MRSA among *S. aureus* infections in China, Australia, Africa, Portugal, Greece, Italy, and Romania. More recent surveys have found MRSA rates as high as 86% in East Asia (e.g. Sri Lanka, South Korea, Vietnam, Taiwan, and Hong Kong).

Clinical Features

The clinical features of MRSA infections are essentially those of *S. aureus* infections. Although SSTIs and pneumonia caused by the USA300 CA-MRSA clone (that expresses PVL) may differ somewhat from those caused by methicillin-susceptible *S. aureus*, the clinical distinction is not reliable. Nor is assessment of risk factors for MRSA clinically useful in the acute care setting. Given the very high prevalence of MRSA across all geographic regions, health-care settings, and patient types, any infection that could be caused by *S. aureus* should be presumed to be due to MRSA – until a culture with susceptibility proves otherwise.

There are, however, certain infection types that are considered particularly characteristic of CA-MRSA; these are listed in Table 75.2 and discussed briefly below. Most are also discussed in detail elsewhere in this textbook.

Types of community onset SSTIs often caused by MRSA include abscess, furuncle, carbuncle, and purulent cellulitis. Skin abscesses of all sizes, with or without associated purulent cellulitis, are the most common form of CA-MRSA infection. These are discussed in detail in Chapter 12. Furuncles, or boils, are the prototypical CA-MRSA infection. Furuncles are

Table 75.2 Infections with a High Prevalence of CA-MRSA

CA-MRSA common	
Skin and soft-tissue infections	Furuncle
	"Spider bite" lesion (necrotic furuncle)
	Purulent cellulitis
Musculoskeletal infections	Osteomyelitis
	Septic arthritis
	Pyomyositis
Community-acquired pneumonia	Post-influenza
	Necrotizing (hemoptysis, cavitation)
CA-MRSA possible	
Necrotizing skin and soft-tissue infection	
Community-onset staphyloccal bacteremia	
Native valve endocarditis	

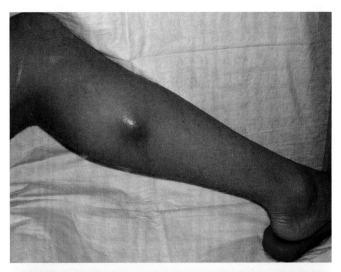

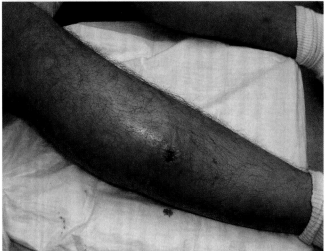

Figure 75.1 (a) Furbuncle; (b) furbuncle after spontaneous drainage (mistaken as a spider bite)

superficial skin abscesses that form in hair follicles and present as inflammatory nodules. After spontaneous drainage, they often form an eschar or necrotic ulcer and patients may present with the chief complaint of spider bite (see Figure 75.1). A cluster of furuncles is known as a carbuncle (see Figure 75.2). Cellulitis refers to a diffuse skin infection that involves the deeper dermis and subcutaneous fat. Cellulitis in the setting of a staphylococcal infection is typically associated with a purulent focus and categorized as purulent cellulitis. MRSA is a possible though uncommon cause of impetigo.

Pyomyositis is an uncommon bacterial infection of muscle, caused by hematogenous spread, which leads to formation of an abscess, typically affecting large muscle groups such as the thigh and pelvic muscles. It is almost exclusively due to *S. aureus*. The incidence of this infection outside of the tropics appears to have increased in recent decades with the emergence of CA-MRSA, which is isolated in approximately 35% of cases.

Staphyococcus aureus is one of the most common pathogens isolated in both hospital onset and community onset bacteremia. MRSA is isolated in over half of community onset, hospital-associated cases. However, the proportion due to MRSA is much lower in patients without recent health-care contact or other risk factors, such as a vascular catheter or injection drug use history. Community-onset MRSA bacteremia is often associated with a metastatic site of infection such as endocarditis, osteomyelitis, or spinal epidural abscess. *S. aureus* is the most common infective endocarditis (IE) pathogen, and approximately 25% of isolates are MRSA.

Septic arthritis and osteomyelitis, particularly childhood and spinal osteomyelitis, are typically caused by hematogenous seeding, and *S. aureus* is the dominant pathogen. CA-MRSA has emerged as a common cause of these infections. There is evidence that PVL-positive MRSA osteoarticular infections tend to be more severe than those caused by MSSA. Post-operative orthopedic infections associated with hardware and prosthetic joint infections are also now commonly caused by MRSA.

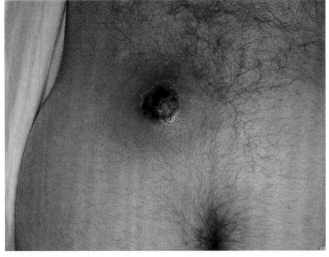

Figure 75.2 Carbuncle with surrounding purulent cellulitis

CA-MRSA community-acquired pneumonia (CAP), usually due to PVL-producing strains, has a prototypical presentation that includes recent or concurrent influenza infection,

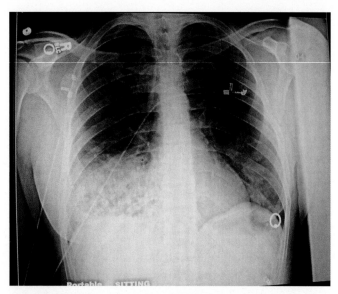

Figure 75.3 Chest X-ray from a case of CA-MRSA pneumonia, showing multilobar involvement and cavitation; the patient presented with hemoptysis

hemoptysis, severe sepsis, leukopenia, and signs of necrosis or cavitation on chest X-ray (see Figure 75.3). Progression to respiratory failure and ARDS is relatively common. However, CA-MRSA pneumonia may also be indistinguishable from that caused by other pathogens like *S. pneumoniae* (see Chapter 44).

Differential Diagnosis

The differential diagnoses for each major infection type that can be caused by MRSA is enumerated in the corresponding chapter in this book: Bacterial Skin and Soft-Tissue Infections (Chapter 12), Infective Endocarditis (Chapter 1), Community-Acquired Pneumonia (Chapter 44), Osteomyelitis (Chapter 37), and Adult Septic Arthritis (Chapter 33).

Laboratory and Radiographic Findings

The clinical and laboratory features of each type of infection commonly caused by MRSA are described in the corresponding chapters in this textbook. The typical findings and specifics of the diagnostic approach are beyond the scope of this chapter. There are, however, several diagnostic issues unique to MRSA, especially regarding etiologic testing, that bear mentioning.

Since the contemporary bacteriology of SSTIs in the United States is well described in the literature, a common question is whether etiologic testing (wound and/or blood cultures) is required. MRSA is known to cause over 50% of purulent SSTIs (i.e. abscesses and purulent cellulitis), whereas its prevalence in non-purulent cellulitis is less than 5%. Empiric oral therapy for uncomplicated outpatient SSTIs is based on this information, and cultures in this setting are not recommended. Cultures are reserved for inpatients who fail to respond to initial outpatient therapy. A culture should generally be obtained in any SSTI severe enough to require admission. If there is purulent material, a wound culture (swab of the material) is usually sufficient. Empiric parenteral MRSA coverage (typically vancomycin) can be stopped if the isolate is methicillin sensitive.

In CAP, the value of sputum culture is debated. However, a sputum gram stain and culture is potentially very useful in cases where MRSA is suspected on clinical grounds. *S. aureus* is not part of normal sputum flora. Isolation of *S. aureus* in sputum, or presence of gram-positive cocci in clusters on gram stain, supports addition or continuation of antibiotics with MRSA activity; absence of *S. aureus* on sputum gram stain or culture can lead to more rapid and confident antibiotic de-escalation, i.e. stopping empiric vancomycin.

The diagnosis of septic arthritis is traditionally based on synovial fluid cell count from an arthrocentesis specimen, with a count greater 50,000 cells/mm³ indicating infection. There is some evidence that CA-MRSA septic arthritis is associated with much lower counts. Sending synovial fluid culture is therefore crucial, and acute care providers should maintain a low threshold for admission and empiric vancomycin therapy if the clinical suspicion for septic arthritis is high despite a cell count less than 50,000 cells/mm³.

Given the tendency for MRSA to cause metastatic infection in the setting of bacteremia, the importance of obtaining blood cultures when invasive MRSA is suspected cannot be overstated. Invasive infections include pneumonia, endocarditis, pyomyositis, osteomyelitis, septic arthritis, and spinal epidural abscess. It is the acute care provider's responsibility to obtain multiple sets of blood cultures before beginning empiric antibiotics when any of these infections are suspected.

The susceptibility pattern of CA-MRSA isolates from SSTIs in the United States is presented in Table 75.3.

There are a number of issues regarding antibiotic susceptibility testing in MRSA isolates that, while important in hospitalized patients, have limited relevance to emergency practice. Isolates initially reported susceptible to clindamycin (but resistant to erythromycin) may develop clindamycin resistance within days of beginning clindamycin treatment. Inducible clindamycin resistance is a fairly uncommon problem, discovered in 2.4 to 10% of CA-MRSA isolates in US studies; however, resultant treatment failures have been reported. Inducible clindamycin resistance is detected in the laboratory by the simple D-zone disk diffusion test, which now is performed routinely in most laboratories.

Rising vancomycin minimum inhibitory concentrations (MICs) among MRSA isolates, and the potential for clinical resistance, has been widely publicized and may occasionally affect inpatient care. In the acute care setting, the main impact of this issue is that it increases the importance of obtaining blood cultures, and other culture specimens whenever possible, before initiating antibiotics.

Treatment and Prophylaxis

Treatment for MRSA in the acute care setting is almost always empiric. Empiric MRSA coverage should be strongly considered for infection types in which it is a known pathogen. However, the threshold for including MRSA coverage in a given infection type is determined not only by the prevalence of MRSA, but also the seriousness of the infection. For example, *S. aureus* is implicated in 10 to 15% of non-purulent cellulitis cases (MRSA in a

Table 75.3 Antimicrobial Susceptibilities of MRSA Strains Isolated from US ED Patients with Purulent Skin and Soft-Tissue Infection in 2008

Antimicrobial	CA- MRSA No. susceptible/total no. tested (%)
Clindamycin	344/366 (94)
Daptomycin	326/326 (100)
Doxycycline	326/326 (100)
Erythromycin	34/350 (10)
Gentamicin	325/326 (99)
Levofloxacin	155/346 (45)
Linezolid	326/326 (100)
Mupirocin	324/326 (99)*
Penicillin	0†
Rifampin	323/326 (99)
Tetracycline	343/350 (98)
Trimethoprim-sulfamethoxazole	366/367 (99)
Vancomycin	326/326 (100)

* Non susceptible strains demonstrated low-level resistance.

† MRSA is resistant to penicillin by definition.

Adapted from Talan, D. A., Krishnadasan, A., Gorwitz, R. J., *et al.* Comparison of Staphylococcus aureus from skin and soft tissue infections in US emergency department patients, 2004 and 2008. *Clin. Infect.* Dis. 2011; 53(2): 144–53.

Table 75.4 Infections Encountered in the Acute Care Setting that Generally Require Empiric CA-MRSA Coverage

Infection Type*	Recommended MRSA Therapy
Skin abscess	Trimethoprim–sulfamethoxazole Clindamycin Doxycycline
Purulent cellulitis	Trimethoprim–sulfamethoxazole Clindamycin
Necrotizing skin and soft-tissue infection	Vancomycin
Severe CAP or HCAP	Vancomycin Clindamycin Linezolid
Septic arthritis	Vancomycin
Osteomyelitis	Vancomycin
Suspected bacteremia (i.e. fever with indwelling intravenous line; community onset, health-care-associated MRSA)	Vancomycin
Suspected infectious endocarditis	Vancomycin

* For some infection types, empiric therapy includes additional agents to cover other likely pathogens besides MRSA. Refer to the corresponding chapters for complete empiric drug selection and dosing.

HCAP – health-care-associated pneumonia.

smaller proportion), but initial empiric treatment for this kind of cellulitis need not cover MRSA, since the infection is not life-threatening. On the other hand, though MRSA is a rare pathogen in necrotizing soft-tissue infections (NSTIs), it is generally recommended that the empiric regimen for these infections include vancomycin, since the consequences of not covering a potential causative pathogen could be dire. Table 75.4 lists the infections for which MRSA coverage is generally recommended. Complete treatment regimens for these infection types can be found in the corresponding chapters elsewhere in this textbook. Table 75.5 provides details on the antibiotics used to treat MRSA in the emergency setting. If available, results of recent, relevant culture results should always be used to select initial antibiotics. Finally, hospital antibiograms, which typically include empiric antibiotic recommendations tailored to local MRSA susceptibilities and pharmacy formulary, should be used to guide empiric treatment whenever possible.

Several points should be borne in mind when choosing an oral agent for skin abscesses and purulent cellulitis. Since *S. aureus* is the predominant pathogen, and over one-half of *S. aureus* isolates are MRSA, antibiotics need only target MRSA. Trimethoprim–sulfamethoxazole is the initial drug of choice in most cases as it is inexpensive, has a narrow spectrum, and has maintained excellent activity against MRSA. Although its β-hemolytic *Streptococcus* activity is considered unreliable, trimethoprim–sulfamethoxazole monotherapy was shown to be as effective as clindamycin in a study of uncomplicated SSTIs of all kinds. Therefore, use of clindamycin or addition of a beta-lactam, "just in case" it is a streptococcal infection, is unnecessary. While a single double-strength tablet twice a day is sufficient in most uncomplicated infections, the largest adult trial of trimethoprim–sulfamethoxazole for simple skin abscesses used two double-strength tablets, and this dosing should be considered in more serious infections (extensive purulent cellulitis) and in obese patients.

With regard to serious and invasive infections requiring parenteral therapy, vancomycin is the drug of choice in the emergency setting in most cases. While there has been a gradual increase in MRSA minimum inhibitory concentrations for vancomycin, related treatment failure is rare and this phenomenon has yet to impact treatment guidelines. Vancomycin underdosing is the most important potential pitfall. Most experts recommend a 20 to 25 mg/kg initial loading dose; the previously common practice of simply giving 1 g is therefore inadequate for most adults. In the case of severe CAP that might be due to MRSA, concerns about achieving adequate vancomycin concentrations in lung tissue and the possible importance of halting toxin synthesis may favor the use of linezolid or clindamycin in this setting, though this is debatable. Vancomycin levels are monitored by measuring trough levels at steady state, usually after three to four doses. For severe infections, a trough of 15 to 20 mg/L is generally recommended, while 10 to 15 mg/L may be appropriate for less serious infections. In the emergency setting, administering an appropriate initial dose expedites the achievement of adequate trough levels.

Decolonization is the main form of prophylaxis for CA-MRSA infections. Although evidence of effectiveness and durability of MRSA eradication is limited, there are situations following treatment for an acute infection where acute care

Table 75.5 Antibiotics Commonly Used to Treat MRSA in the Acute Care Setting

Agent	Usual Dosing	Common Side Effects
Trimethoprim–sulfamethoxazole	Adults: one to two double strength tabs. PO BID Children: 10 mg/kg/day PO divided twice daily	Rash Hyperkalemia
Clindamycin	Adults: 300–450 mg PO TID; 600–900 mg IV every 8 hours Children: 10 mg/kg/dose IV/PO every 8 hours	Nausea, vomiting, diarrhea; strong association with *C. difficile* Poor palatability of oral solution
Doxycycline	Adults: 100 mg PO/IV BID Children: 2 mg/kg/dose PO/IV BID	Photosensitivity Esophagitis
Vancomycin	Adults: 15–20 mg/kg/dose IV every 8–12 hours Children: 15 mg/kg/dose IV every 6 hours	Redman infusion reaction Nephrotoxicity
Linezolid	Adults: 600 mg PO/IV daily Children: 10 mg/kg/dose IV/PO every 12 hours	Headache Diarrhea Blood dyscrasias
Daptomycin	Adults: 4 mg/kg/dose IV daily Children: 6–10 mg/kg/dose IV daily	Increased creatinine phosphokinase

IV – intravenous; PO – by mouth.

providers may wish to attempt to decolonize a patient or to eradicate CA-MRSA from all members of a household. Such situations include:

- Patients who have experienced multiple CA-MRSA SSTIs over a 1-year period
- Households in which multiple members have been infected
- Households with very young, very old, or immunosuppressed members

A common approach to de-colonization is daily dilute bleach baths up to the neck (1/4 cup bleach in a bathtub) plus intranasal mupirocin ointment twice a day for 5 days.

Complications and Admission Criteria

The long list of possible complications from MRSA infection reflects the enormous breadth of infection types caused by *Staphyloccous aureus*. These range from a self-limited infection with no discernable complication, as in the case of a simple furuncle that ruptures on its own, to invasive infection such as pneumonia or endocarditis complicated by rapid development of septic shock and death. Moreover, each type of infection, such as central nervous system abscess or septic arthritis, has its own set of specific complications, which in some cases are more likely when MRSA is the etiology. CA-MRSA CAP, for example, not only causes severe sepsis, with up to 80% of cases requiring ICU admission and a case mortality rate of up to 29%, but it is associated with a high rate of disease-specific complications such as respiratory failure and empyema. Disease-specific complications are discussed in detail in the corresponding chapters in this textbook.

Acute care providers should be aware that *S. aureus* has a unique predilection to cause metastatic infection and suppuration. Therefore, any patient presenting with fever following a recent MRSA bloodstream infection or other invasive infection should be suspected of harboring a new, occult MRSA infection such as osteomyelitis or endocarditis. In such cases, a very low threshold should be maintained for obtaining blood cultures and advanced imaging. Surgical drainage may be required.

Most CA-MRSA SSTIs can be managed on an outpatient basis. Incision and drainage or debridement is required for most of these. Complicated SSTIs, such as those accompanied by fever or a very large area of cellulitis, generally require hospitalization for parenteral antibiotics. Other forms of MRSA infection, including severe or post-influenza CAP, HCAP, suspected indwelling line infection, endocarditis or bacteremia in an injection drug user, septic arthritis, and osteomyelitis – all require blood cultures, hospitalization, and empiric antibiotics with MRSA activity.

Infection Control

In the community setting, MRSA infection control involves enhanced hygiene and disinfection of potential fomites. Specific measures to prevent the spread of CA-MRSA should routinely be included in SSTI discharge instructions; these are listed in Box 75.2. Decolonization is discussed above under prophylaxis. MRSA outbreaks in large cohorts, such as schools or sports teams, should be managed by local health departments.

Developing rational strategies to prevent the spread of CA-MRSA in the ED and hospital setting remains a considerable challenge. The traditional hospital infection control paradigm of nasal swab screening for MRSA, isolation or cohorting of colonized patients, and decolonization therapy, is not well suited for CA-MRSA, nor has it been shown to be effective. Hand hygiene and frequent decolonization of potential fomites are likely the most important measures. Nonetheless, many hospitals require isolation of patients with a history of MRSA infection or a positive nasal swab result, and many require active nasal swab surveillance of patients admitted to the ICU.

Pearls and Pitfalls

1. MRSA now accounts for a significant proportion of *S. aureus* isolates across virtually all types of staphylococcal infections; therefore, empiric *S. aureus* coverage means

Francis, J. S., Doherty, M. C., Lopatin, U., *et al.* Severe community-onset pneumonia in healthy adults caused by methicillin-resistant *Staphylococcus aureus* carrying the Panton–Valentin leukocidin genes. *Clin. Infect. Dis.* 2005; 40(1): 100–7.

Frazee, B. W., Lynn, J., Charlebois, E. D., *et al.* High prevalence of methicillin-resistant *Staphylococcus aureus* in emergency department skin and soft tissue infections. *Ann. Emerg. Med.* 2005; 45(3): 311–20.

Liu, C., Bayer, A., Cosgrove, S. E., *et al.* Clinical practice guidelines by the Infectious Diseases Society of America for the treatment of methicillin-resistant *Staphylococcus aureus* infections in adults and children. *Clin. Infect. Dis.* 2011; 52(3): e18–55.

Miller, L. G., Daum, R. S., Creech, C. B., *et al.* Clindamycin versus trimethoprim–sulfamethoxazole for uncomplicated skin infections. *N. Engl. J. Med.* 2015; 372(12): 1093–103.

Moran, G. J., Krishnadasan, A., Gorwitz, R. J., *et al.* Methicillin-resistant *S. aureus* infections among patients in the emergency department. *N. Engl. J. Med.* 2006; 355(7): 666–74.

Talan, D. A., Krishnadasan, A., Gorwitz, R. J., *et al.* Comparison of *Staphylococcus aureus* from skin and soft-tissue infections in US emergency department patients, 2004 and 2008. *Clin. Infect. Dis.* 2011; 53(2): 144–53.

Talan, D. A., Mower, W. R., Krishnadasan, A., *et al.* Trimethoprim-sulfamethoxazole versus placebo for uncomplicated skin abscess. *N. Engl. J. Med.* 2016; 374(9): 823–32.

Wallin, T. R., Hern, H. G., and Frazee, B. W. Community-associated methicillin-resistant *Staphylococcus aureus*. *Emerg. Med. Clin. N. Am.* 2008; 26(2): 431–55.

Additional Reading

Deresinski, S. Methicillin-resistant *Staphylococcus aureus*: an evolutionary, epidemiologic, and therapeutic odyssey. *Clin. Infect. Dis.* 2005; 40(4): 562–73.

Box 75.2 Patient Instructions to Prevent Spread of CA-MRSA in the Community Setting

Keep draining wounds covered with a clean bandage.

Wash hands frequently with soap and water or alcohol-based hand gel and always wash after touching infected wounds or soiled bandages.

Maintain good general hygiene with regular bathing.

Launder clothing that is contaminated with wound drainage.

Do not share contaminated items like towels, bedding, clothing, and razors.

While there is wound drainage, do not participate in activities involving skin-to-skin contact or in contact sports.

Clean contaminated environmental surfaces and equipment with a detergent or disinfectant that specifies *S. aureus* on the label.

---

empiric MRSA coverage (until cultures return showing the isolate is methicillin susceptible).

2. MRSA risk factor analysis should not be used to limit empiric MRSA therapy.

3. Trimethoprim–sulfamethoxazole is the oral antibiotic of choice for SSTIs.

4. Severe CAP (requiring ICU admission) and influenza-related CAP should be treated with an antibiotic with MRSA activity.

5. Care should be taken not to under-dose vancomycin; the initial loading dose is generally 20mg/kg.

6. Patients presenting with a fever following a recent invasive MRSA infection or bacteremia should be suspected of harboring an occult, metastatic MRSA infection.

References

Dantes, R., Mu, Y., Belflower, R., *et al.* National burden of invasive methicillin-resistant *Staphylococcus aureus* infections, United States, 2011. *JAMA Intern. Med.* 2013; 173(21): 1970–8.

76

Enterococci

Jill Logan and Megan Musselman

Introduction and Microbiology 548
Epidemiology 548
Clinical Features 548
Laboratory Findings 549
Treatment and Prophylaxis 549

Urinary Tract Infections 549
  Bacteremia and Endocarditis 549
  Skin and Soft-Tissue Infections 551
Infection Control 551
Complications and Admission Criteria 551
Pearls and Pitfalls 551
References 551

Introduction and Microbiology

The enterococci are gram-positive cocci, formerly considered group D streptococci, but now recognized to be a unique genus, which commonly colonize the human gastrointestinal and genitourinary tracts. The main pathogenic *Enterococcus* species, *E. faecalis* and *E. faecium*, are well-recognized causes of urinary tract infections, endocarditis, and intra-abdominal infections. Owing to intrinsic resistance to many advanced penicillins, cephalosporins, and clindamycin, the traditional mainstay treatments for enterococcal infections have been ampicillin (or penicillin) and vancomycin. Since many strains exhibit relatively high minimum inhibitory concentrations (MICs) and tolerance to ampicillin, susceptibility to vancomycin is considered crucial in combating enterococcal bloodsteam infections.

Vancomycin-resistant *Enterococcus* (VRE) was first isolated in Europe in the late 1980s, and subsequently spread rapidly through the United States by the late 1990s. Vancomycin impairs gram-positive cell wall synthesis by binding to the terminus of the cell wall precursor. Vancomycin resistance in *Enterococcus* is encoded by a cluster of resistance genes, the most common and well studied of which is termed vanA, which result in production of an altered cell wall precursor that does not bind vancomycin. *E. faeceum* is more often vancomycin resistant than *E. faecalis*.

According to the Infectious Disease Society of America (IDSA), VRE is one of the "ESKAPE" pathogens (the others being *Staphylococcus*, *Klebsiella*, *Acinetobacter*, *Pseudomonas*, and *Enterobacter*), a group of multidrug-resistant organisms (MDROs) that are considered an extremely serious public health problem. While more common in hospitalized patients, VRE infections are also encountered in the emergency setting, particularly in patients with extensive health-care exposure. Acute care providers must be familiar with the risk factors for VRE infections, as well as the approach to management, particularly antibiotic selection, for this emerging pathogen.

Epidemiology

Enterococcus colonizes the gastrointestinal tract of both humans and livestock. The emergence of VRE in Europe was related to use of antibiotics as a cattle feed additive. In humans, VRE colonization of the gastrointestinal tract generally precedes infection. Among risk factors for VRE carriage and infection, use of broad-spectrum antibiotics is by far the most powerful, followed by recent hospitalization. VRE risk factors, categorized as modifiable and non-modifiable, are listed in Table 76.1. Once gastrointestinal colonization is established, the organism is shed in stool and found on skin, urinary catheters, and hospital surfaces. There is no effective means of VRE decolonization, though carriage may wane naturally. Compounding the problem of infection control, *Enteroccocus* survives readily for days on fomites such as hospital surfaces.

Up to 18% of hospital-acquired enterococcal infections are due to VRE. The number of patients with a reported VRE infection at hospital discharge increased from 4.6 to 9.5 per 100,000 hospitalizations in the United States between 2003 and 2006. As of 2010, VRE accounted for 18% of all central line-associated bloodstream infections (CLABSIs), making *Enterococcus* species the second ranking pathogen for all CLABSIs. VRE has been associated with increased mortality when compared to vancomycin-sensitive enterococcal infections (OR 2.32, 95% CI, 1.7–3.2).

Clinical Features

Types of acute VRE infections that might be encountered in the emergency setting include urinary tract infection (UTI), bacteremia, infectious endocarditis (IE), meningitis, and

Table 76.1 Risk Factors for Vancomycin-Resistant Enterococcal Infections

Modifiable Risk Factors	Non-Modifiable Risk Factors

• Indwelling urinary catheters
• Exposure to antibiotics
  ◦ Vancomycin (IV or PO)
  ◦ Cephalosporins
  ◦ Fluoroquinolones
  ◦ Metronidazole
  ◦ Clindamycin
  ◦ Carbapenems
• Exposure to contaminated surfaces
• Proximity to VRE colonized or infected patient
	• Neutropenia/immunosuppression
	• Organ transplant
	• Hemodialysis
	• ICU and hospital length of stay
	• Surgery
	• Severe underlying disease

IV – intravenous; PO – by mouth.

Table 76.2 Clinical and Laboratory Standards Institute Enterococcal MIC Breakpoints to Vancomycin

Classification	MIC
Vancomycin sensitivity	≤4 mcg/L
Vancomycin intermediate	8–16 mcg/L
Vancomycin resistant	≥32 mcg/L

skin and soft-tissue infections, most often in the setting of a chronic wound or ulcer. While there are no distinct clinical features associated with *Enterococcus*, in general *Enterococcus* is less virulent than other uropathogens like *E. coli* and IE pathogens like *S. aureus*. In order to make the diagnosis, acute care providers must be alert to VRE risk factors and previous culture results.

Acute care providers are most likely to encounter VRE UTIs in patients with a recent history of hospitalization, exposure to broad-spectrum antibiotics, and chronic urinary catheters. These patients may arrive from a skilled nursing facility. In many cases, there will be a previous positive urine or stool culture that has grown VRE. The biggest challenge is differentiating acute infection from colonization and asymptomatic bacteriuria, which should not be treated except in pregnant women. Diagnosis of VRE UTI should be made with caution, taking into account presenting signs and symptoms, history of antibiotic use and past culture data, physical exam, and laboratory tests, including a urinalysis and a quantitative urine culture. The threshold for treatment should be lower in patients with compromised immune function (e.g. a history of organ transplant or hematologic malignancy).

Bacteremia and IE due to VRE are often associated with an indwelling intravenous catheter. The issue of IE diagnosis is covered in Chapter 1. A single positive blood culture for VRE in the absence of sepsis need not be treated. Patients with fever or sepsis, however, should begin empiric therapy for endocarditis or catheter-associated bacteremia.

Laboratory Findings

Enterococcus may be isolated from any of several clinical specimens, including blood, urine, cerebrospinal fluid, and wound material. Positive stool cultures merely indicate colonization. Three blood cultures should be obtained to help differentiate skin contamination from bacteremia. In patients with chronic indwelling urinary catheters, urine cultures should be taken from a freshly inserted catheter. The Clinical and Laboratory Standards Institute defines vancomycin resistance using the minimum inhibitory concentration (MIC) as presented in Table 76.2. When evaluating a VRE culture and sensitivity

report, it is important to note susceptibility to ampicillin as this will dictate initial treatment.

Treatment and Prophylaxis

In the acute care setting, it is unlikely that VRE will be suspected as the sole etiology of a UTI, bacteremia, or endocarditis. In most cases, the empiric antibiotic regimen should simply be based on the hospital antibiogram or national guidelines. However, empiric VRE treatment should be considered in patients with a previous positive VRE culture, who are acutely ill with fever or sepsis. In such cases, treatment decisions should be made in conjunction with an infectious disease specialist, if possible. Institutions that restrict the use of specific antimicrobial agents based upon cost or other features should consider placing exceptions in their policy for urgent first-dose administration in the emergency department (see Table 76.3).

Urinary Tract Infections

Treatment options for a VRE UTI depend on whether the infection seems to be cystitis (symptoms but without fever) or pyelonephritis (febrile UTI) and whether or not the isolate is sensitive to ampicillin. In cystitis due to ampicillin-sensitive VRE, oral amoxicillin is the drug of choice. In the case of ampicillin resistance, alternate oral drugs include nitrofurantoin, fosfomycin, doxycycline, or linezolid. In febrile UTIs due to ampicillin-susceptible VRE, ampicillin plus gentamicin (which is used for synergy) is the parenteral regimen of choice. If the isolate is ampicillin resistant, the main choices are daptomycin or linezolid. In all cases, the urinary catheter should be removed or changed.

Bacteremia and Endocarditis

Similar to UTIs, treatment of VRE bacteremia is based on ampicillin susceptibility. For ampicillin-susceptible isolates, ampicillin plus aminoglycoside is often the preferred treatment. The aminoglycoside are added to achieve bactericidal activity in the setting of bloodstream or other life-threatening infection. Although clinical data are limited, daptomycin or linezolid are recommended for ampicillin-resistant VRE strains. The theoretical advantage of daptomycin is its bactericidal activity, while the drawback is its inactivation by lung surfactant, making it less effective if pneumonia is the primary source of bacteremia. Linezolid is bacteriostatic and associated with a host of adverse effects such as peripheral neuropathy and bone marrow toxicity with prolonged administration. In severely ill patients with a suspected catheter-related VRE infection, the catheter should be removed.

Table 76.3 Pharmacologic Treatment of Vancomycin-Resistant Enterococcal Infections*

Drug	Indication and Dosing	Clinical Issues
Ampicillin	1. Ampicillin susceptible UTI: 3–4 g IV every 6 hours or 100–200 mg/kg/day IV divided every 6 hours 2. BSI and endocarditis: 200 mg/kg/day IV divided every 6 hours	• Used for ampicillin-susceptible UTI and BSI and IE, in combination with aminoglycoside • Higher doses may be necessary in life-threatening severe infections • Consider combination with aminoglycoside to improve efficacy: combination therapy recommended for enterococcal endocarditis • Oral amoxicillin may be used if clinically appropriate • Ampicillin/sulbactam useful in cases of penicillinase-producing enterococci • Bacteriostatic as monotherapy; bactericidal when combined with aminoglycosides • Inexpensive
Daptomycin	1. BSI and endocarditis: 6 mg/kg/dose IV daily – doses up to 12 mg/kg/day have been studied 2. SSTI: 4 mg/kg/dose IV daily	• Used for BSI, IE, SSTI • May be used for UTI; however, reserved for highly resistant infections, patients with allergies to alternative therapy, or previous treatment failure • Lower dosing may be used for UTI due to renal clearance of active drug • Suggested weekly or more frequent CPK monitoring with daptomycin • Hold statin therapy while treating with daptomycin • Daptomycin not recommended for treatment of pneumonia • Bactericidal, concentration dependent • Expensive
Fosfomycin	3 g PO × 1	• Used for uncomplicated UTI • Not indicated for complicated or upper UTI therapy; however, dosing every 72 hours × 3 doses has been used • Only available as an oral formulation in the United States • Metoclopramide may decrease efficacy • Bactericidal • Expensive
Linezolid	600 mg IV/PO every 12 hours	• Can be used for UTI, SSTI, BSI, IE, pneumonia • FDA-approved for the treatment of VRE • May be used for UTI; however, reserved for highly resistant infections, patients with allergies to alternative therapy, or previous treatment failure • Risk of serotonin syndrome when given concomitantly with serotonergic medications due to linezolid's inhibition of monoamine oxidase • Hematologic monitoring for myelosuppression with long-term therapy (>2 weeks) • Avoid tyramine containing foods • Bacteriostatic • Expensive
Nitrofurantoin	50–100 mg PO four times per day (immediate release) 100 mg PO BID (Macrobid formulation)	• Only for use in lower tract UTIs • Not effective in end-stage renal disease • Avoid long-term therapy • Use caution in G6PD deficiency • Inexpensive
Quinupristin–dalfopristin	1. UTI: 7.5 mg/kg/dose IV every 8 hours 2. SSTI: 7.5 mg/kg/dose IV every 12 hours	• Can be used for complicated UTI, SSTI • Central line required for administration • Only effective against *E. faecium* (no activity against *E. faecalis*), should not be used empirically • Poor patient tolerability; myalgias and arthralgias common • Previously FDA-approved for the treatment of VRE (*E. faecium*) at the referenced dosing • Expensive
Tigecycline	100 mg IV × 1, followed by 50 mg IV every 12 hours	• Can be used for SSTI and intra-abdominal infections • FDA safety warning for higher all-cause mortality compared to other antimicrobial agents – use when other agents are not feasible • Low serum levels achieved • Bacteriostatic • Expensive

* Dosing for adult patients only. Dosing does not reflect recommended changes for end-organ dysfunction or morbid obesity.

BSI – bloodstream infection; CPK – creatinine phosphokinase; FDA – Food and Drug Administration; G6PD – glucose-6-phosphate dehydrogenase; SSTI – skin and soft-tissue infection.

Antimicrobial dosing data obtained abstracted from H. F. Chambers, G. M. Elipoulos, D. N. Gilbert, and M. S. Saag (eds.), *The Sanford Guide to Antimicrobial Therapy*, 44th edn (Sperryville, VA: Antimicrobial Therapy, 2014).

While other antimicrobial agents have in vitro activity against VRE, they are not usually first-line empiric agents. Quinupristin–dalfopristin lacks activity against *E. faecalis*, the more commonly isolated *Enterococcus* species; however, it may be useful in known *E. faceium* infections. It is associated with numerous adverse effects, including painful arthralgias and myalgias. Tigecycline also has VRE activity; however, poor blood concentrations limit its usefulness in bloodstream infections and endocarditis. Telavancin shows activity only against the vanB gene for enterococcal resistance.

The 2015 American Heart Association (AHA) guidelines recognize the difficulty in treating *Enterococcus* endocarditis. Fortunately, most enterococcal IE is due to *E. faecalis*, which is rarely multidrug resistant. For IE due to a VRE strain that is also aminoglycoside and ampicillin resistant, the AHA recommends linezolid or daptomycin. Antibiotic selection should be managed by an infectious disease specialist in such cases.

Skin and Soft-Tissue Infections

According to the 2014 update to the IDSA skin and soft-tissue infection (SSTI) treatment guidelines, enterococci are the third most prevalent pathogen isolated from diagnostic cultures. VRE SSTIs are typically related to a decubitus ulcer or postoperative wound infection; often a prior wound culture will have grown VRE. In such cases, the recommended treatment is either daptomycin or linezolid.

Infection Control

Standard contact precautions are adequate for the care of patients with VRE infections. These patients should be cared for in a private room or cohorted with other VRE colonized patients. Hospital infection control should be notified.

Complications and Admission Criteria

Standard admission criteria apply to enterococcal infections. Fever and suspected bacteremia or IE generally warrants admission, whereas it is appropriate to treat uncomplicated VRE UTIs with oral antibiotics in the outpatient setting.

Pearls and Pitfalls

1. Recent hospitalization, presence of an indwelling urinary or vascular catheter, and complicated past medical history should alert the acute care provider to possible VRE infection.
2. VRE treatment should be based on susceptibility of a recent VRE isolate when available; review prior culture results carefully.
3. Amoxacillin (PO) or IV ampicillin plus an aminoglycoside are the treatment of choice for ampicillin-susceptible strains.
4. Source control is often important in VRE infections, particularly catheter removal.
5. Empiric treatment with daptomycin or linezolid is reasonable for suspected multidrug-resistant VRE bacteremia.

References

Baddour, L. M., Wilson, W. R., Bayer, A. S., *et al.* Infective endocarditis in adults: diagnosis, antimicrobial therapy, and management of complications: a statement for healthcare professionals from the American Heart Association. *Circulation* 2015; 132(15): 1435–86.

Boucher, H. W., Talbot, G. H., Bradley, J. S., *et al.* Bad bugs, no drugs: no ESKAPE! An update from the Infectious Disease Society of America. *Clin. Infect. Dis.* 2009; 48(1): 1–12.

Chambers, H. F., Eliopoulos, G. M., Gilbert, D. N., and Saag, M. S. (eds.), *The Sanford Guide to Antimicrobial Therapy*, 44th edn (Sperryville, VA: Antimicrobial Therapy, 2014).

Clinical and Laboratory Standards Institute (CLSI). *Performance Standards for Antimicrobial Susceptibility Testing; Twenty-Fifth Informational Supplement*, 3rd edn (Wayne, PA: CLSI, 2015), vol. 35.

DiazGranados, C. A., Zimmer, S. M., Klein, M., and Jernigan, J. A. Comparison of mortality associated with vancomycin-resistant and vancomycin-susceptible enterococcal bloodstream infections: A meta-analysis. *Clin. Infect. Dis.* 2005; 41(3): 327–33.

Heintz, B. H., Halilovic, J., and Christensen, C. L. Vancomycin-resistant enterococcal urinary tract infections. *Pharmacotherapy* 2010; 30(11): 1136–49.

Hooton, T. M., Bradley, S. F., Cardenas, D. D., *et al.* Diagnosis, prevention, and treatment of catheter-associated urinary tract infection in adults: 2009 international clinical practice guidelines from the Infectious Disease Society of America. *Clin. Infect. Dis.* 2010; 50(5): 625–63.

Kullar, R., Davis, S. L., Levine, D. P., *et al.* High-dose daptomycin for treatment of complicated gram-positive infections: a large, multicenter, retrospective study. *Pharmacotherapy* 2011; 31(6): 527–36.

Mermel, L. A., Allon, M., Bouza, E., *et al.* Clinical practice guidelines for the diagnosis and management of intravascular catheter-related infection: 2009 updated by the Infectious Disease Society of America. *Clin. Infect. Dis.* 2009; 49(1): 1–45.

Murray, B. E. Vancomycin-resistant enterococcal infections. *N. Engl. J. Med.* 2000; 342(10): 710–21.

Patel, R. and Gallagher, J. C. Vancomycin-resistant enterococcal bacteremia pharmacotherapy. *Ann. Pharmacother.* 2015; 49(1): 69–85.

Ramsey, A. M. and Zilberberg, M. D. Secular trends of hospitalization with vancomycin-resistant *enterococcus* infection in the united states, 2000–2006. *Infect. Control Hosp. Epidemiol.* 2009; 30(2): 184–6.

Reik, R., Tenover, F. C., Klein, E., and McDonald, L. C. The burden of vancomycin-resistant enterococcal infections in U.S. hospitals, 2003–2004. *Diagn. Microbiol. Infect. Dis.* 2008; 62(1): 81–5.

Sievert, D. M., Ricks, P., Edwards, J. R., *et al.* Antimicrobial-resistant pathogens associated with healthcare-associated infections: Summary of data reported to the national healthcare safety network at the center for disease control and prevention, 2009–2010. *Infect. Control Hosp. Epidemiol.* 2013; 34(1): 1–14.

Extended Spectrum Beta-Lactamase

Colgan Sloan and Christopher J. Edwards

Introduction and Microbiology

Antibiotics belonging to the beta-lactam class all contain a beta-lactam ring in their structure and work by inhibiting bacterial cell wall biosynthesis. This broad class of antibiotics includes the penicillins, cephalosporins, carbapenems, and monobactams. Beta-lactamases are enzymes produced by bacteria that cleave the beta-lactam ring, rendering otherwise effective antibiotics largely powerless. In 1940, even before the widespread clinical use of penicillin, the first beta-lactamase-producing strain of *E. coli* was discovered. Since then, the development of new beta-lactam antibiotics has focused largely on strategies to overcome this important mechanism of bacterial resistance.

The development of third-generation cephalosporins, such as ceftriaxone, in the 1980s was considered a major step forward in the battle against beta-lactamase-producing organisms. Unfortunately, not long after their widespread use, resistance to the third-generation cephalosporins began to develop as a new group of beta-lactamase emerged, termed the extended spectrum beta-lactamases (ESBLs). ESBLs were first reported in *Klebsiella* species in Europe in 1983 and by 1988 had spread throughout the Americas and Asia. These early ESBL infections were particularly alarming because the pathogens were resistant to most antibiotics available at the time to empirically treat serious gram-negative infections.

Over 1,000 unique beta-lactamase enzymes have been subsequently identified that vary in their exact means of genetic transmission and molecular mechanisms of resistance and the types of antibiotics they are capable of inactivating. The common hallmark of ESBL-producing organisms, however, is resistance to third-generation cephalosporins (e.g. ceftriaxone, cefotaxime, ceftazadime). Yet they are susceptible to certain second-generation cephalosporins (e.g. cefoxitin), carbapenams, and in vivo to antibiotics that contain beta-lactamase inhibitors (e.g. pipericillin–tazobactam).

ESBLs are found exclusively in gram-negative bacteria, particularly the *Enterobacteriaceae* species, including the common pathogens *Escherichia coli* and *Klebsiella pneumonia.*

Table 77.1 lists the gram-negative bacterial species in which ESBL production has been found. Although *Pseudomonas* species (which are not *Enterobacteriaceae*) can produce ESBLs, they also exhibit a number of other mechanisms of broad spectrum antibiotic resistance.

ESBL-producing pathogens are theoretically susceptible to other non-beta-lactam antibiotics with gram-negative activity, such as fluoroquinolones and aminoglycosides. However, it is common for ESBL-producing bacteria to acquire mechanisms of resistance to other antibiotic classes (often acquired on the same plasmid that carries the beta-lactamase gene). Thus, ESBL-producing bacteria are usually classified as multidrug-resistant organisms (MDROs).

Compounding the problem of antimicrobial resistance in gram-negative pathogens is the recent emergence of carbapenemase-producing *Enterobacteriaceae*, particularly *Klebsiella* species. Infections with these pathogens leaves clinicians with virtually no available antibiotic treatment. To date, carbapenem resistance remains almost exclusively an inpatient problem.

Since infections with ESBL-producing bacteria can present in the emergency setting, it is important that acute care providers possess a basic familiarity with the biology and epidemiology of these pathogens, as well as know the recommended initial management strategy.

Epidemiology

ESBL-producing bacteria are predominantly carried in the gut and transmitted between patients in the hospital and skilled nursing facility environment. Environmental, animal, and food contamination outside the hospital has also been documented. Fecal ESBL carriage and spread among individuals in a household, with associated urinary tract infections (UTIs), has been reported. Prevalence of ESBL-producing bacteria varies considerably across the globe, with high rates seen in Latin America and parts of Asia, and between regions and hospitals in a given country. ESBL infection rates have risen dramatically

Table 77.1 ESBL-Producing Organisms

Acinetobacter baumanii	*Moraxella (Brahamella)* spp.
Alcaligenes xylosoxidans	*Neisseria gonorrhoeae*
Bacteroides fragilis	*Pasteurella multocida*
Citrobacter freundii	*Proteus mirabilis*
Enterobacter cloacae	*Pseudomonas aeruginosa, putida*
Escherichia coli	*Salmonella typhimurium, enteritidis*
Haemophilus influenza	*Serratia marcescens*
Klebsiella pneumonia	*Klebsiella oxytoca*
Actinobacillus pleuropneumoniae	*Vibrio cholerae*

Adopted from J. E. Bennett, R. Dolin, and M. J. Blaser (eds.), Mandell, Douglas, and Bennett's Principles and Practice of Infectious Diseases, 8th edn. (Philadelphia, PA: Elsevier/Saunders, 2015).

Table 77.2 Risk Factors for ESBL Infection

Prolonged hospitalization	Recent surgery
Recent broad spectrum antibiotic use	Critical illness
Invasive medical devices	Decubitus ulcer
Total parenteral nutrition	Hemodialysis
Diabetes mellitus	Elderly

in the southeastern United States since 2009. Resistance to at least one extended-spectrum cephalosporin (either ceftazidime, cefepime, cefotaxime, or ceftriaxone) is found in over 12% of *Escherichia coli* isolates and over 25% of *Klebsiella* spp. isolates in hospitalized patients with central-line-associated bloodstream infections or catheter-associated UTIs.

Not surprisingly, the risk factors for infection with ESBL-producing pathogens include prolonged hospital stay, critical illness, recent surgery, mechanical ventilation, indwelling catheters and feeding tubes, and recent exposure to broad-spectrum antibiotics, particularly cephalosporins or fluoroquinolones (see Table 77.2). While ESBL-producing organisms are more common in health-care-associated infections, ESBLs are increasing in community-acquired infections as well. Recent US surveillance data from the outpatient setting found that only 1.8% of Klebsiella isolates and 0.4% of E. coli were ceftazidime resistant. However, a 2009 study in a Chicago emergency department found that ESBL-producing bacteria caused 24% of UTIs. Another recent study that characterized E. coli isolates from patients presenting to 10 different US emergency departments with a diagnosis of pyelonephritis (Talan 2016). In this study, rates of ESBL-producing E. coli ranged from 0% to 17.2%. These studies suggest that the incidence of infection with ESBL-producing organisms in the emergency and ambulatory settings is likely to continue to rise.

Although ESBL-producing bacteria are no more virulent than other gram-negative pathogens, their extensive resistance pattern leads to worse outcomes. Multiple studies have documented a delay to inititation of effective antibiotic therapy, longer hospital stays, and higher mortality in patients infected with ESBL-producing isolates.

Clinical Features

The most common type of infection caused by ESBL-producing bacteria is a UTI. Other gram-negative infections that have been associated with ESBL-producing strains include health-care-associated pneumonia, bacteremia, intra-abdominal infections, and wound infections. The clinical features of these infection types can be found in the relevant chapters in this textbook. There are no distinct clinical features associated with ESBL-producing pathogens. In order to make the diagnosis, acute care providers must be alert to ESBL risk factors and previous culture results. For recently hospitalized patients, a thorough review of culture results to look for a previous ESBL isolate is mandatory.

Laboratory Features

The laboratory and radiographic features of the various types of infection caused by ESBL-producing, gram-negative bacteria can be found in the corresponding chapters in this textbook. Urine cultures are by far the most common source of ESBL isolates. For patients with indwelling urinary catheters, it is important to obtain the urine specimen for culture from a newly inserted urinary catheter whenever possible.

Clinical laboratories screen for ESBL production using a variety of phenotypic methods. ESBL screening is typically done on all *E. coli*, certain *Klebsiella* species, and *Proteus mirabilis*. In 2010, new lower minimum inhibitory concentration (MIC) breakpoints for *Enterobacteriaceae* were introduced, which may eliminate the need for specifically identifying and reporting ESBL production. Clinicians may find that laboratories simply report a more complete list of antibiotic susceptibilities, with increased emphasis on calling attention to MDROs. This theoretically reduces the necessity of determining if an organism is capable of producing ESBLs when optimizing an antibiotic regimen.

Genotypic identification of ESBL-producing isolates in research or reference laboratories typically involves PCR amplification of specific genes. PCR-based tests have the potential to identify specific ESBLs prior to culture growth and accurately detect low levels of resistant organisms. Advances in rapid diagnostic tests may soon provide clinicians with relevant information during the patient's initial resuscitation and may guide appropriate antibiotic selection much sooner than traditional methods (Poirel *et al.* 2016). These techniques may also improve the accuracy and efficiency of epidemiologic studies of MDROs and improve infection control measures.

Treatment and Prophylaxis

In the acute care setting, it is unlikely that an ESBL-producing pathogen will be suspected as the sole etiology of a UTI or other gram-negative infection. In most cases, the empiric antibiotic therapy should be selected based on the suspected source of infection, hospital antibiogram or evidence-based guideline recommendations, and clinical judgment. However, immediate empiric ESBL treatment is indicated for patients with a

Table 77.3 Antibiotics Commonly Used to Treat Infections with ESBL-Producing Pathogens

Drug	Dose	Clinical Issues
Imipenem and cilastin	Adults: 500 mg IV every 6 hours Children: 20 mg/kg/dose IV every 6 hours	May lower seizure threshold Broad spectrum of activity Frequent dosing interval
Meropenem	Adults: 1 g IV every 8 hours Children: 20 mg/kg/dose IV every 8 hours	Broad spectrum of activity Frequent dosing interval
Ertapenem	Adults: 1 g IV/IM every 24 hours Children: 15 mg/kg/dose IV/IM every 12 hours	Broad spectrum of activity, but unreliable activity against *Pseudomonas* or *Acinetobacter* The only carbapenem indicated for IM administration Once daily dosing
Fosfomycin	Adults: 3 g PO × 1 Children: not indicated	Only indicated in uncomplicated UTIs Used off-label for outpatient UTIs in men or complicated UTIs (dosed IV formulation not yet available in the United States every 72 hours × 3)
Tigecycline	Adults: 100 mg IV × 1, followed by 50 mg IV every 12 hours Children ≥8 years old: 1.2 mg/kg/dose IV every 12 hours	Similar to tetracyclines, tooth discoloration concern in children Phase III and IV trials raised concern about increased all-cause mortality in patients treated with tigecycline (not ESBL specific)
Ceftazidime-avibactam	Adults: 2.5 g IV every 8 hours Children: not indicated	Newer agent Not often used empirically

previous culture that grew an ESBL-producing isolate, who are now acutely ill with fever or sepsis.

Carbapenems, including imipenem, meropenem, and ertapenem, are the antibiotics of choice for infections with ESBL-producing organisms, with numerous observational studies showing effectiveness. Antibiotics in the new cephalosporin-beta-lactamase inhibitor class show promise, but are not yet widely recommended. Tigecycline has been used effectively in the hospital setting, but is not considered first line. Antibiotics commonly used to treat infections with ESBL-producing pathogens are listed in Table 77.3. Institutions that restrict the use of carbapenems in the emergency setting because of cost should consider placing exceptions in their policy for urgent first-dose administration in certain situations.

Unfortunately, piperacillin–tazobactam, which is a common component of empiric broad-spectrum regimens and is theoretically active against ESBL-producing strains, has been associated with treatment failures. Cefepime in standard doses likewise can lead to treatment failure. Cefoxitin and cefotetan, sometimes used for empiric treatment of intra-abdominal infections, may be effective. ESBL-producing, gram-negative pathogens are often multidrug resistant, with 20 to 70% of isolates also being resistant to fluoroquinolones and aminoglycosides. Agents from these classes may be used if culture results return showing susceptibility.

A frequent problem in the emergency setting is that of non-febrile UTIs in relatively healthy patients – normally treated with oral antibiotics – that are found to be caused by ESBL-producing *Enterobacteriaceae*. An oral fluoroquinolone is a reasonable treatment of such infections if the isolate is known to be susceptible. For isolates that are multidrug resistant, treatment options include oral fosfomycin and intramuscular ertapenem – which requires that patients return daily to the emergency department or clinic (see Table 77.3).

ESBL-producing *E. coli* may be susceptible to nitrofurantoin, though *Klebsiella* is usually resistant.

Infection Control

Standard contact precautions are generally adequate for the care of patients with ESBL infections; however, local infection prevention resources should be engaged in decision making on how best to handle patients identified as having infection or colonization with ESBL-producing organisms.

Complications and Admission Criteria

Standard admission criteria apply to UTIs, suspected bacteremia, and intra-abdominal infections caused by ESBL-producing pathogens.

Pearls and Pitfalls

1. ESBL multidrug-resistant infections are on the rise in the United States and worldwide.

2. The most common ESBL infection emergency providers will encounter are UTIs caused by ESBL-producing *E. coli*.

3. Carbapenems (ertapenem, imipenem-cilastatin, meropenem) are the antibiotics of choice for treatment of complicated ESBL infections. Carbapenems are administered parenterally and require hospitalization or home infusion therapy.

4. One dose of fosfomycin given orally in the emergency department is a treatment for uncomplicated UTIs caused by ESBL-producing *E. coli*.*

References

Abraham, E. P. and Chain, E. An enzyme from bacteria able to destroy penicillin. Nature 1940; 146: 837.

Angelin, M., Forsell, J., Granlund, M., *et al.* Risk factors for colonization with extended-spectrum beta-lactamase producing Enterobacteriaceae in healthcare students on clinical assignment abroad: a prospective study. Travel Med. Infect. Dis. 2015; 13(3): 223–9.

Ben-Ami, R., Rodriguez-Bano, J., Arslan, H., *et al.* A multinational survey of risk factors for infection with extended-spectrum beta-lactamase-producing enterobacteriaceae in nonhospitalized patients. Clin. Infect. Dis. 2009; 49(5): 682–90.

Bush, K. and Fisher, J. F. Epidemiological expansion, structural studies, and clinical challenges of new beta-lactamases from gram-negative bacteria. Ann. Rev. Microbiol. 2011; 65: 455–78.

Curello, J. and MacDougall, C. Beyond susceptible and resistant, part II: treatment of infections due to gram-negative organisms producing extended-spectrum beta-lactamases. J. Pediatr. Pharmacol. Ther. 2014; 19(3): 156–64.

Doi, Y., Park, Y. S., Rivera, J. I., *et al.* Community-associated extended-spectrum β-lactamase-producing Escherichia coli infection in the United States. *Clin. Infect. Dis.* 2013; 56(5): 641–8.

Falagas, M. E. and Karageorgopoulos, D. E. Extended-spectrum beta-lactamase-producing organisms. J. Hosp. Infect. 2009; 73(4): 345–54.

Garrec, H., Drieux-Rouzet, L., Golmard, J. L., *et al.* Comparison of nine phenotypic methods for detection of extended-spectrum beta-lactamase production by Enterobacteriaceae. J. Clin. Microbiol. 2011; 49(3): 1048–57.

Hombach, M., Bloemberg, G. V., and Bottger, E. C. Effects of clinical breakpoint changes in CLSI guidelines 2010/2011 and EUCAST guidelines 2011 on antibiotic susceptibility test reporting of gram-negative bacilli. J. Antimicrob. Chemo. 2012; 67(3): 622–32.

Kantele, A., Laaveri, T., Mero, S., *et al.* Antimicrobials increase travelers' risk of colonization by extended-spectrum betalactamase-producing Enterobacteriaceae. Clin. Infect. Dis. 2015; 60(6): 837–46.

Lin, J. N., Chen, Y. H., Chang, L. L., *et al.* Clinical characteristics and outcomes of patients with extended-spectrum beta-lactamase-producing bacteremias in the emergency department. Int. Emerg. Med. 2011; 6(6): 547–55.

Livermore, D. M. Defining an extended-spectrum beta-lactamase. Clin. Microbiol. Infect. 2008; 14(Suppl. 1): 3–10.

Macdougall, C. Beyond susceptible and resistant, part I: treatment of infections due to gram-negative organisms with inducible beta-lactamases. J. Pediatr. Pharmacol. Ther. 2011; 16(1): 23–30.

National Nosocomial Infections Surveillance. National Nosocomial Infections Surveillance (NNIS) system report, data summary from January 1992 to June 2002, issued August 2002. Am. J. Infect. Cont. 2002; 30(8): 458–75.

Opal, S. M. and Medeiros, A. A. Molecular mechanisms of antibiotic resistance in bacteria in Bennett, J. E., Dolin, R., and Blaser, M.

J. (eds.), *Mandell, Douglas, and Bennett's Principles and Practice of Infectious Diseases*, 8th edn. (Philadelphia, PA: Elsevier/Saunders, 2015), pp. 253–70.

Paterson, D. L. and Bonomo, R. A. Extended-spectrum beta-lactamases: a clinical update. Clin. Microbiol. Rev. 2005; 18(4): 657–86.

Poirel, L. Fernandez, J., and Nordmann, P. Comparison of three biochemical tests for rapid detection of extended-spectrum β-lactamase-producing Enterobacteriaceae. *J. Clin. Microbiol.* 2016; 54(2): 423–7.

Roschanski, N., Fischer, J., Guerra, B., and Roesler, U. Development of a multiplex real-time PCR for the rapid detection of the predominant beta-lactamase genes CTX-M, SHV, TEM and CIT-type AmpCs in Enterobacteriaceae. PloS One. 2014; 9(7): e100956.

Rottier, W. C., Ammerlaan, H. S., and Bonten, M. J. Effects of confounders and intermediates on the association of bacteraemia caused by extended-spectrum beta-lactamase-producing Enterobacteriaceae and patient outcome: a meta-analysis. J. Antimicrob. Chemo. 2012; 67(6): 1311–20.

Schwaber, M. J. and Carmeli, Y. Mortality and delay in effective therapy associated with extended-spectrum beta-lactamase production in Enterobacteriaceae bacteraemia: a systematic review and meta-analysis. J. Antimicrob. Chemo. 2007; 60(5): 913–20.

Sievert, D. M., Ricks, P., Edwards, J. R., *et al.* Antimicrobial-resistant pathogens associated with healthcare-associated infections: summary of data reported to the National Healthcare Safety Network at the Centers for Disease Control and Prevention, 2009–2010. Infect. Cont. Hosp. Epidemiol. 2013; 34(1): 1–14.

Talan, D. A., Takhar, S. S., Krishnadasan, A., *et al.* Fluoroquinolone-resistant and extended-spectrum β-lactamase-producing Escherichia coli infections in patients with pyelonephritis, United States. *Emerg. Infect. Dis.* 2016; 22(9): doi: 10.3201/eid2209.160148.

Tangden, T., Cars, O., Melhus, A., and Lowdin, E. Foreign travel is a major risk factor for colonization with Escherichia coli producing CTX-M-type extended-spectrum beta-lactamases: a prospective study with Swedish volunteers. Antimicrob. Agents Chemother. 2010; 54(9): 3564–8.

Wang, P., Hu, F., Xiong, Z., *et al.* Susceptibility of extended-spectrum-beta-lactamase-producing Enterobacteriaceae according to the new CLSI breakpoints. J. Clin. Microbiol. 2011; 49(9): 3127–31.

Wolfensberger, A., Sax, H., Weber, R., *et al.* Change of antibiotic susceptibility testing guidelines from CLSI to EUCAST: influence on cumulative hospital antibiograms. PloS One. 2013; 8(11): e79130.

Zumla, A., Al-Tawfiq, J. A., Enne, V. I., *et al.* Rapid point of care diagnostic tests for viral and bacterial respiratory tract infections – needs, advances, and future prospects. Lancet 2014; 14(11): 1123–35.

Antimicrobial Overview

Conan MacDougall and Camille Beauduy

Introduction – Principles of Antimicrobial Use

Pharmacokinetics and Pharmacodynamics

Many factors affect the choice of an antimicrobial agent in the acute care setting. Selection of an agent with in vitro activity against the infecting pathogen is necessary but not sufficient for a favorable clinical outcome. Pharmacokinetic (effect of the drug in the body) and pharmacodynamic (effect of the drug on its target) factors must also be taken into account. The most important pharmacokinetic consideration is the concentration of the drug at the site of infection. The physicochemical properties of antimicrobials determine their distribution throughout the body, and these properties may be unfavorable for the penetration of certain tissue compartments.

Sites of particular concern for the adequate penetration of antimicrobials include bone, compartments of the eye, and the central nervous system. Additionally, abscess cavities are poorly penetrated and should be drained regardless of whether systemic antimicrobial therapy is to be used. Even treatment of pulmonary and urinary tract infections (UTIs) depends on site-specific penetration, and recommendations for standard therapies reflect this. Thus, clinicians should rely on standard therapy or use alternative drugs that are documented to achieve effective concentrations at the site of interest. Unfortunately, data as to the relative penetration of different drugs are frequently lacking, though predictions based on physicochemical characteristics (e.g. protein binding) can be made.

An other pharmacodynamic distinction is whether a drug's activity is bactericidal or bacteriostatic. Although the distinction between these is not always absolute (some drugs can be bacteriostatic against certain organisms and bactericidal against others, or bactericidal at some concentrations and bacteriostatic at others), there are a few cases in which bactericidal activity is preferred. Generally, bactericidal activity is necessary in situations where there is minimal contribution from the immune system, either because of restricted access to the tissue compartment or because of the host's immune status. Foremost among these conditions are meningitis and endocarditis, where clinical studies have documented a lower cure rate with bacteriostatic drugs. Other conditions that generally call for bactericidal therapy include osteomyelitis, febrile neutropenia, and septic shock.

Impact of Prior Antimicrobial Use on Choice of Therapy

Prior antimicrobial use increases the risk for infection with drug-resistant organisms and contributes to selection of inappropriate empiric therapy. Thus, obtaining an accurate antimicrobial history is an important consideration for choice of therapy. Although resistance is only one of many possible reasons for therapeutic failure, the most conservative course when a patient has failed therapy with an antimicrobial agent is to assume resistance in the infecting pathogen(s). Subsequent therapy should either move "up the ladder" to a broader-spectrum agent within the same class or move to a different

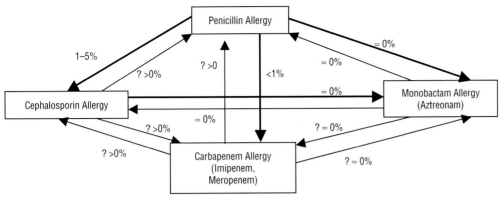

Figure 78.1 Estimated cross-reactivity between beta-lactams. Arrows denote the direction of the exposure (e.g. an arrow from a penicillin to a cephalosporin represents a patient with a penicillin allergy who receives a cephalosporin); the percentage noted indicates the estimated likelihood of a patient experiencing a reaction for that exposure direction.

class that is unlikely to display cross-resistance. If the previously used agent(s) is unknown or if the use of alternative agents is impractical, standard therapy with close monitoring of the patient for signs of therapeutic failure is recommended.

Principles of Antimicrobial Allergy and Toxicity

Antimicrobials, especially beta-lactam drugs, are among the most common agents to which patients report allergies. Specific allergic reactions, however, are often poorly documented in the medical record, are subject to inaccurate recall by patients, vary greatly in their severity and clinical importance, and may change over time. A chart notation of an "allergy to penicillin," for example, is of little practical utility. Documentation of the nature and timing of the initial reaction and whether the patient has been re-exposed to the agent are crucial in determining the clinical significance of an allergy. Patients inaccurately labeled with allergies face a restricted choice of antimicrobials for future infections, possibly leading to suboptimal therapy.

Complicating the matter further is the issue of cross-reactivity between drugs in similar chemical classes, the most important of which are the beta-lactam drugs. Allergies with these drugs may be due to their common pharmacophore, leading to class-wide cross-allergenicity, or to unique elements such as the side chains, which would not generally lead to cross-allergenicity. Estimates of the rates of cross-resistance are indicated in Figure 78.1. Note that estimates of the probability of cross-reactivity are available only for patients with known penicillin allergies who receive cephalosporins or carbapenems, and for immediate hypersenitivity reactions (such as anaphylaxis). For example, the likelihood of cross-reactivity between cephalosporins and carbapenems, or the probability of those with a cephalosporin allergy reacting to a penicillin, is not known. The monobactam class (aztreonam) has a unique pharmacophore and is generally considered to have no cross-reactivity with the other beta-lactams (though ceftazidime, which has an identical side chain to aztreonam, may be an exception). Cross-allergenicity between drugs in other classes (e.g. fluoroquinolones) is even less well defined.

Arrows in Figure 78.1 denote the direction of the exposure (e.g. an arrow from a penicillin to a cephalosporin represents

a patient with a penicillin allergy who receives a cephalosporin); the percentages noted indicate the estimated likelihood of a patient experiencing a reaction for that exposure direction.

Aside from causing allergic reactions, most antimicrobials are relatively well tolerated over the short duration. Other serious toxicities that can occur with antimicrobials include nephrotoxicity (aminoglycosides), hematologic toxicity (penicillins, ganciclovir, linezolid), QT interval prolongation (macrolides, fluoroquinolones, azoles), and hepatotoxicity (macrolides, azoles). Some antimicrobials are prone to drug interactions that may enhance their own toxicity or the toxicity of co-administered drugs. The potential for administration of antimicrobials to lead to "superinfections," such as *Candida* infections or *Clostridium difficile* colitis, should also be considered a potential adverse consequence of their use.

Properties of Antimicrobial Agents

The spectra of activity of commonly used antibacterial and antifungal drugs are reviewed in Table 78.1, with the preferred agents for particular pathogens highlighted. The common uses, pharmacology, and toxicity of the drugs are reviewed in the following text. Emphasis is given to indications and agents likely to be encountered in primary care or emergency settings, and indications are cross-referenced to the corresponding sections in other chapters. Important differences among the agents within a class are highlighted. General dosage ranges for adults are provided, along with recommendations for adjustment in renal or hepatic dysfunction.

Beta-Lactams: Penicillins, Cephalosporins, Carbapenems, and Monobactams

Mechanism of Action

Beta-lactam drugs act by disrupting the bacterial cell wall through inhibition of transpeptidases (penicillin-binding proteins or PBPs), responsible for crosslinking peptidoglycan, the primary structural component of the cell wall. This leads to an imbalance between cell wall autolysis and synthesis. Beta-lactam drugs are generally bactericidal.

Table 78.1 Spectra of Activity of Antibacterial Drugs

Antibacterials	Drug	Gram-Positive								Gram-Negative								Anaerobes		
		Strep. pyogenes	S. pneumoniae (PCN-S or -I)	S. pneumoniae (PCN-R)	S. aureus (MSSA)	S. aureus[1] (MRSA)	Enterococcus faecalis[2]	Enterococcus faecium[2] (VRE)	Listeria	H. influenzae	Neisseria meningitidis	Proteus mirabilis	E. coli[3]	Klebsiella[3]	Pseudomonas aeruginosa	Citrobacter Enterobacter	Serratia	Bacteroides fragilis	Clostridium difficile	Atypicals[4]
Penicillins	**Penicillin G**	++	++	–	–[5]	×	++	–	++	×	++	×	×	×	×	×	×	–	–	×
	Ampicillin/amoxicillin	++	++	+	–[5]	×	++	–	++	+[6]	++	++	–	×	×	×	×	–	–	×
	Nafcillin/dicloxacillin	++	++	–	++	×	–	–	–	×	×	×	×	×	×	×	×	×	–	×
	Amoxicillin/clavulanate	++	++	+	++	×	++	–	++	++	×	++	+	+	×	×	×	++	–	×
	Piperacillin/tazobactam	++	++	–	++	×	+	–	++	++	++	++	++	++	++	++	++	++	–	×
Cephalosporins	**Cefazolin**	++	++	–	++	×	×	×	×	–	–	++	+	+	×	×	×	×	×	×
	Cefuroxime	++	+	–	++	×	×	×	×	++	×	++	+	+	×	×	×	×	×	×
	Cefoxitin	++	+	–	++	×	×	×	×	–	+	++	+	+	×	+	×	+	×	×
	Ceftriaxone	++	++	+	++	×	×	×	×	++	++	++	++	++	×	+	++	×	×	×
	Ceftazidime	++	+	–	–	×	×	×	×	++	×	++	++	++	++	++	++	×	×	×
	Cefepime	++	++	+	++	×	×	×	×	++	×	++	++	++	++	++	++	×	×	×
	Imipenem/meropenem	++	++	+	++	×	+	–	++	++	+	++	++	++	++	++	++	++	×	×
	Aztreonam	×	×	×	×	×	×	×	×	++	×	++	++	++	++	++	++	×	×	×
Fluoroquinolones	**Ciprofloxacin**	++	+	+	+	–	+[7]	–	×	++	++	++	++	++	+	++	++	×	×	+
	Levofloxacin	++	++	++	+	–	+[7]	–	×	++	+	++	++	++	+	++	++	×	–	++
	Moxifloxacin	++	++	++	+	–	–	–	×	++	+	++	++	++	–	++	++	+	–	++
Macrolides	**Erythromycin**	+	+	–	++	–	×	×	–	×	+	×	×	×	×	×	×	×	×	++
	Azithromycin/clarithromycin	+	+	–	++	–	×	×	–	+	×	×	×/+	×/+	×	×	×	×	–	++
	Telithromycin	+	+	+	++	–	×	×	–	+	×	–	–	–	×	×	–	×	–	+
Tetracyclines	**Doxycycline**	++	++	+	++	+	+	+	–	++	–	–	–	–	–	+	–	×	–	++
	Tigecycline	++	++	+	++	+	+	++	–	++	–	+	+	–	–	++	++	++	–	++

(continued)

Table 78.1 (cont.)

Antibacterials		Gram-Positive								Gram-Negative								Anaerobes		
	Drug	Strep. pyogenes	S. pneumoniae (PCN-S or -I)	S. pneumoniae (PCN-R)	S. aureus (MSSA)[1]	S. aureus (MRSA)[1]	Enterococcus faecalis[2]	Enterococcus faecium (VRE)[2]	Listeria	H. influenzae	Neisseria meningitidis.	Proteus mirabilis	E. coli[3]	Klebsiella[3]	Pseudomonas aeruginosa	Citrobacter Enterobacter	Serratia	Bacteroides fragilis	Clostridium difficile	Atypicals[4]
Aminoglycosides	**Gentamicin/ tobramycin**	−[8]	−	−	−[8]	−[8]	−[8]	−[8]	−[8]	+	++	++	++	++	++	++	++	X	X	X
	Amikacin	−	−	−	−	−	−	−	−	+	++	++	++	++	++	++	++	X	X	X
Miscellaneous	**TMP-SMX**	−	+	−	++	++	X	X	++	++	−	++	+	++	X	++	++	X	X	X
	Clindamycin	++	++	−	++	+	X	X	−	X	X	X	X	X	X	X	X	++	−	+
	Metronidazole	X	X	X	X	X	X	X	X	X	X	X	X	X	X	X	X	++	++	X
	Linezolid	++	++	++	++	++	++	++	−	X	X	X	X	X	X	X	X	X	−	++
	Daptomycin	++	++	++	++	++	++	++	−	X	X	X	X	X	X	X	X	X	−	X
	Vancomycin	++	++	++	++	++	++	X	−	X	X	X	X	X	X	X	X	X	++	X

++ = Drug of choice or >90% susceptibility; + = alternative drug or >70% susceptibility; − = minimal clinically useful activity or experience; X = intrinsically resistant.

Bold: Preferred agent under most circumstances, though therapy should be tailored based on the susceptibility of the individual isolate.

[1] Approx. 50% of S. aureus in hospitals are MRSA; 1–50% (and increasing) of community S. aureus are MRSA.

[2] Approx. two-thirds of all enterococci are faecalis, and one-third are faecium (50–75% of which are vancomycin-resistant [VRE]).

[3] Does not include the approx. 1–5% of E. coli and 5–20% of Klebsiella that produce an extended-spectrum beta-lactamase, giving resistance to all beta-lactams (except carbapenems).

[4] Atypical respiratory pathogens: Legionella spp., Mycoplasma pneumoniae, Chlamydophila pneumoniae.

[5] <10% of S. aureus do not produce beta-lactamase and would be susceptible to these drugs.

[6] Non-beta-lactamase-producing H. influenzae (75–90% of isolates) would be susceptible to these drugs.

[7] Fluoroquinolones are only clinically useful in the treatment of enterococcal UTIs where high concentrations can be achieved (moxifloxacin would not be active).

[8] Aminoglycosides are not clinically useful as monotherapy for gram-positive infections; however, they may provide synergistic killing when used in combination with a cell-wall active agent (e.g. nafcillin or vancomycin), especially in endocarditis.

Figure 78.2 illustrates the mechanism of action of antibiotics against the bacterial cell wall. Peptidoglycan is the primary component of the bacterial cell wall, consisting of alternating units of *N*-acetylglucosamine (N-Glu) and *N*-acetylmuramic acid (N-Mur). The N-Mur units are crosslinked by polypeptide chains. Bacterial transpeptidases (also known as PBPs) catalyze this crosslinking (as in pathway 1). Beta-lactam agents irreversibly inhibit the action of PBPs (pathway 2), preventing crosslinking. Glycopeptides (such as vancomycin) bind to the free ends of the polypeptides before crosslinking, sterically inhibiting PBP binding (pathway 3). In pathways 2 and 3, the natural autolytic activity of the bacterial cell leads to the degradation of the cell wall and cell death (beta-lactams may also enhance this autolysis).

Natural Penicillins and Aminopenicillins

The dosages for natural penicillins and aminopenicillins are shown in Table 78.3.

Differences between Agents

The primary differences are in formulation (see Table 78.2): penicillin G is the intravenous form, whereas penicillin V potassium is oral and benzathine penicillin G is an intramuscular (IM), long-acting depot formulation (never to be given intravenously). Likewise, ampicillin and amoxicillin have identical spectra of activity, but ampicillin is available as an intravenous formulation, while amoxicillin is an orally administered drug (though there is an oral form of ampicillin, it is poorly absorbed). In contrast to the natural penicillins, the aminopenicillins have activity against non-beta-lactamase-producing strains of *Haemophilus influenzae* (approximately 60 to 80% of *H. influenzae*).

Table 78.2 Natural Penicillins and Aminopenicillins

Drug	Acute Care Uses	Toxicities
Penicillin G IV Penicillin VK PO Penicillin G benzathine IM	Syphilis Pharyngitis	*Common:* rash, diarrhea *Rare:* anaphylaxis, seizures **Drug interactions**
Ampicillin IV Amoxicillin PO	Meningitis Otitis media	Minimal clinically relevant interactions

IM – intramuscular; IV – intravenous; PO – by mouth.

Cautions

Allergic reactions are the most frequent toxicity encountered with the penicillins. These can range from mild rashes to life-threatening anaphylaxis. Depending on the severity of the reaction, patients can be challenged with a beta-lactam from another class (see Principles of Antimicrobial Allergy and Toxicity, above). A unique entity is the "ampicillin rash," which occurs in patients receiving aminopenicillins and manifests as a self-limited, maculopapular rash. This rash is associated with concurrent infectious mononucleosis or other viral illnesses, or with allopurinol therapy, and does not appear to represent hypersensitivity in the usual sense. Patients considered to have ampicillin rashes (and not true hypersensitivity) may be rechallenged with aminopenicillins in the future.

Pearls and Pitfalls

1. The rise in penicillin resistance has sharply curtailed use of these agents for empiric therapy, except for selected indications (e.g. syphilis, pharyngitis, otitis media). However, if an infecting pathogen is demonstrated to be penicillin- or ampicillin-susceptible, these drugs offer many advantages for definitive therapy: they are narrow-spectrum, are inexpensive, and have rapid bactericidal activity.

2. Whereas penicillin resistance in staphylococci is essentially all or nothing (more than 90% of *S. aureus* are fully penicillin resistant), resistance to penicillins among streptococci tends to occur in a graded fashion. Thus, many penicillin-non-susceptible strains have intermediate or low-level resistance. Because of the very high blood and lung levels attained by penicillins, penicillin or amoxicillin show good cure rates for pneumonia even in the presence of low-level resistance. In meningitis, however, failures have occurred when penicillins are used against pneumococcal strains with intermediate resistance. Thus, penicillin resistance is much more clinically relevant in the treatment of meningitis than in treatment of pneumococcal pneumonia.

Antistaphylococcal Penicillins

Table 78.4 lists acute care uses, toxicities, and drug interactions for antistaphylococcal penicillins. See Table 78.5 for doses.

Table 78.3 Dosages for Natural Penicillins and Aminopenicillins

Drug	Dosage Adjustment for Renal Function (mL/min)			Hepatic Adjust?
	CrCl >50	CrCl 10–50	CrCl <10	
Penicillin G	2–3 million units IV every 4–6 hours	1–2 million units IV every 4–6 hours	1 million units IV every 6 hours	No
Penicillin VK	250–500 mg PO QID	No adjustment	250 mg PO TID	No
Penicillin G benzathine	1.2 million units IM × 1* 2.4 million units IM × 1†	No adjustment	No adjustment	No
Ampicillin	1–2 g IV every 4–6 hours	1–1.5 g IV every 6 hours	1 g IV every 8–12 hours	No
Amoxicillin	500 mg PO TID	250–500 mg PO BID	250–500 mg PO daily	No

* For streptococcal pharyngitis.
† For early syphilis.

Differences between Agents

Nafcillin is an intravenous preparation, whereas dicloxacillin is available for oral administration.

Cautions

Neutropenia is considered to be a potential toxicity of all penicillins and is well documented to occur with nafcillin therapy. Neutropenia usually manifests several days into therapy and is generally considered to be reversible on cessation of the drug. This toxicity may be difficult to differentiate from progression of a severe infection with attendant neutropenia.

Pearls and Pitfalls

1. Nafcillin has superior bacterial killing activity against methicillin-susceptible *Staphylococcus aureus* (MSSA), especially compared to vancomycin. It is generally the preferred therapy for invasive staphylococcal infections, such as endocarditis or osteomyelitis, due to MSSA.

Penicillin–Beta-Lactamase Inhibitor Combinations

Table 78.6 lists acute care uses, toxicities, and drug interactions for penicillin–beta-lactamase inhibitors. See Table 78.7 for doses.

Differences between Agents

Piperacillin–tazobactam has an enhanced gram-negative spectrum compared to the aminopenicillin drugs, with activity against *Pseudomonas* as well as enhanced activity against *Klebsiella* and *Escherichia coli*. Piperacillin–tazobactam is a more appropriate empiric choice than the aminopenicillin-based beta-lactamase inhibitor combinations for patients with severe infections, especially those of suspected nosocomial origin.

Cautions

Piperacillin and other penicillins, especially at high dosages, may have qualitative effects on platelet function. These effects may predispose patients to bleeding, though direct suppression of platelets (thrombocytopenia) is not typically seen. This effect was primarily observed with older, less potent penicillins (ticarcillin, carbenicillin) for which very high doses were required for antipseudomonal activity. The risk with piperacillin is likely to be less, but monitoring for clinically significant bleeding, especially in patients with other risk factors for bleeding, is warranted.

Pearls and Pitfalls

1. The beta-lactamase inhibitors used in these combinations (sulbactam, clavulanate, and tazobactam) serve to expand the activity of their accompanying penicillin by inhibiting bacterial beta-lactamases (enhancing activity against organisms such as *H. influenzae*, *E. coli*, *Klebsiella*, *Moraxella*, and MSSA). They do not add activity where the organism's mechanism of resistance is not beta-lactamase mediated (e.g. MRSA, *Streptococcus pneumoniae*) or where the beta-lactamases are resistant to inhibition by these beta-lacatamase inhibitors (e.g. *Pseudomonas*).

2. The inhibitors are present in fixed ratios to the penicillin for ampicillin–sulbactam (2:1) and piperacillin–tazobactam (8:1), but vary somewhat between the different preparations of amoxicillin–clavulanate (from 4:1 to 16:1). The rationale for the higher amoxicillin:clavulanate ratios

Table 78.4 Antistaphylococcal Penicillins

Drug	Acute Care Uses	Toxicities
Nafcillin IV Dicloxacillin PO	Skin and soft-tissue infections Endocarditis	*Common:* rash *Uncommon:* interstitial nephritis, neutropenia *Rare:* anaphylaxis, seizures
		Drug interactions
		Minimal

Table 78.5 Dosages for Antistaphylococcal Penicillins

Drug	Dosage Adjustment for Renal Function (mL/min)			Hepatic Adjust?
	CrCl >50	CrCl 10–50	CrCl <10	
Nafcillin	1–2 g IV every 4–6 hours	No adjustment	No adjustment	Possibly*
Dicloxacillin	125–250 mg PO QID	No adjustment	No adjustment	No

* Consider reducing dose in hepatic insufficiency if concomitant renal failure.

Table 78.6 Penicillin–Beta-Lactamase Inhibitor Combinations

Drug	Acute Care Uses	Toxicities
Ampicillin–sulbactam IV (Unasyn) Amoxicillin–clavulanate PO (Augmentin) Piperacillin–tazobactam IV (Zosyn)	Intra-abdominal infections Diabetic foot infections Skin and soft-tissue infections Nosocomial infections* Sepsis*	*Common:* GI distress (especially amoxicillin–clavulanate) *Uncommon:* platelet dysfunction, neutropenia **Drug interactions** Minimal

* Use piperacillin–tazobactam.
GI – gastrointestinal.

Table 78.7 Dosages for Penicillin–Beta-Lactamase Inhibitor Combinations

Drug	Dosage Adjustment for Renal Function (mL/min)			Hepatic Adjust?
	CrCl >50	CrCl 10–50	CrCl <10	
Ampicillin–sulbactam (Unasyn)	1.5–3 g* IV every 6 hours	1.5 g IV every 6–8 hours	1.5 g IV every 12 hours	No
Amoxicillin–clavulanate (Augmentin)	500/125 mg† PO TID 875/125 mg PO BID 2000/125 mg PO BID‡	250–500/125 mg PO BID	250–500/125 mg PO daily	No
Piperacillin–tazobactam (Zosyn)§	3.375 g‖ IV every 6 hours or 4.5 g IV every 8 hours	3.375 g IV every 6 hours or 4.5 g IV every 8 hours	2.25 g IV every 8 hours	No

* 1 g ampicillin/500 mg clavulanate or 2 g ampicillin/1 g clavulanate.

† Ratios are amoxicillin to clavulanate (e.g. 500 mg amoxicillin to 125 mg clavulanate).

‡ Extended-release formulation.

§ For documented or suspected *Pseudomonas* infections, use 4.5 g IV every 6 hours for CrCl >20 mL/min.

‖ 3 g piperacillin/0.375 g tazobactam.

Table 78.8 First-Generation Cephalosporins

Drug	Acute Care Uses	Toxicities
Cefazolin IV (Kefzol) Cephalexin PO (Keflex)	Skin and soft-tissue infections UTIs	*Uncommon:* rash *Rare:* anaphylaxis **Drug interactions** Minimal

Table 78.9 Dosages for First-Generation Cephalosporins

Drug	Dosage adjustment for renal function (mL/min)			Hepatic adjust?
	CrCl >50	CrCl 10–50	CrCl <10	
Cefazolin	1–2 g IV every 8 hours	1–2 g IV every 12 hours	0.5–1 g IV every 24 hours	No
Cephalexin	500 mg PO TID–QID	250–500 mg PO TID	250 mg PO BID	No

is that this preparation is often used for respiratory tract infections where *S. pneumoniae* is a concern; increasing the amoxicillin component may overcome low-level penicillin resistance, whereas the beta-lactamase will not add activity.

3. Penicillin–beta-lactamase inhibitor combinations are excellent drugs for mixed infections (e.g. aspiration pneumonia, intra-abdominal infections, diabetic foot infections) by virtue of their coverage of gram-positive, gram-negative, and anaerobic pathogens.

First-Generation Cephalosporins

Table 78.8 lists acute care uses, toxicities, and drug interactions for first-generation cephalosporins. See Table 78.9 for doses.

Differences between Agents

Cephalexin's spectrum of activity is similar to that of cefazolin, making it essentially an oral analogue of cefazolin.

Table 78.10 Second-Generation Cephalosporins

Drug	Acute Care Uses	Toxicities
Cefuroxime IV, PO (Ceftin) Cefprozil PO (Cefzil) Cefoxitin IV (Mefoxin) Cefotetan IV (Cefotan)	Sinusitis* Otitis media* Intra-abdominal infections†	*Uncommon:* rash *Rare:* anaphylaxis **Drug interactions** Minimal clinically relevant interactions

* Use cefuroxime or cefprozil.

† Use cefoxitin or cefotetan.

Cautions

Although these drugs are frequently used for skin and soft-tissue infections, they are not recommended for bite infections because of their lack of activity against *Pasteurella multocida* (dog, cat) and *Eikenella* (human).

Pearls and Pitfalls

1. For serious infections due to MSSA (endocarditis, osteomyelitis), cefazolin is an alternative to nafcillin and may be associated with fewer adverse effects when used for prolonged therapy (e.g. osteomyelitis, endocarditis). However, cefazolin has poor central nervous system (CNS) penetration and should not be used in treatment of MSSA meningitis (nafcillin is preferred).

Second-Generation Cephalosporins

Table 78.10 lists acute care uses, toxicities, and drug interactions for second-generation cephalosporins. See Table 78.11 for doses.

Differences between Agents

Within the second generation of cephalosporins, there are two groups: drugs such as cefuroxime and cefprozil, which are primarily active against respiratory tract organisms (such as *S. pneumoniae* and *H. influenzae*), and cefoxitin and cefotetan, which have activity primarily against gram-negatives and anaerobes.

Table 78.11 Dosages for Second-Generation Cephalosporins

Drug	Dosage Adjustment for Renal Function (mL/min)			Hepatic Adjust?
	CrCl >50	CrCl 10–50	CrCl <10	
Cefuroxime	0.75–1.5 g IV every 8 hours 500 mg PO BID	0.75–1.5 g IV every 12–24 hours 500 mg PO BID	0.5 g IV every 24 hours 250–500 mg PO daily	No
Cefoxitin	1 g IV every 6–8 hours	1 g IV every 8–12 hours	1 g IV every 24 hours	No

Table 78.12 Third- and Fourth-Generation Cephalosporins

Drug	Acute Care Uses	Toxicities
Ceftriaxone IV, IM (Rocephin) Cefotaxime IV, IM (Claforan) Ceftazidime IV (various) Ceftazidime-avibactam IV (Avycaz) Cefepime IV (Maxipime)	Community-acquired pneumonia Acute bacterial meningitis Endocarditis Nosocomial infections Sepsis	*Uncommon:* rash, biliary sludging (ceftriaxone) *Rare:* anaphylaxis **Drug interactions** Minimal

Table 78.13 Dosages for Third- and Fourth-Generation Cephalosporins

Drug	Dosage Adjustment for Renal Function (mL/min)			Hepatic Adjust?
	CrCl >50	CrCl 10–50	CrCl <10	
Ceftriaxone	1 g IV every 24 hours* 2 g IV every 24 hours† 2 g IV every 12 hours‡	No adjustment	No adjustment	No
Cefotaxime	1–2 g IV every 8 hours* 2 g IV every 4 hours‡	1–2 g IV every 8–12 hours	1 g IV every 24 hours	No
Ceftazidime	2 g IV every 8 hours	2 g IV every 12 hours	0.5 g IV every 24 hours	No
Ceftazidime–avibactam (Avycaz)	2.5 g IV every 8 hours±	0.94 g-1.25 g IV every 8–12 hours	0.94 g IV every 24–48 hours	No
Cefepime	2 g IV every 8–12 hours§	1–2 g IV every 12–24 hours	0.5 g IV every 24 hours	No

* Dose for most indications.

† Dose for endocarditis or osteomyelitis.

‡ Dose for meningitis.

± 2 g ceftazidime, 0.5 g avibactam. Each dose infused over 2 hours.

§ Every 8 hours dosing for febrile neutropenia or *Pseudomonas* infections.

Cautions

The second-generation cephalosporins are frequently employed for upper and lower respiratory tract infections. However, their potency against *S. pneumoniae* is less than that of amoxicillin or ceftriaxone. Thus, their use in more severe infections such as community-acquired pneumonia should be restricted to geographic areas where pneumococcal resistance is low.

Pearls and Pitfalls

1. Cefoxitin and cefotetan are used primarily for surgical prophylaxis in gastrointestinal procedures. Although they have activity against gram-negative aerobic and anaerobic organisms, susceptibility rates among *Bacteroides fragilis*, the primary anaerobic pathogen, are unpredictable. Thus, agents such as ampicillin–sulbactam or piperacillin–tazobactam, or combinations such as ceftriaxone and metronidazole, are usually preferred for empiric therapy of intra-abdominal infections.

Third- and Fourth-Generation Cephalosporins

Table 78.12 lists acute care uses, toxicities, and drug interactions for third- and fourth-generation cephalosporins. See Table 78.13 for doses.

Differences between Agents

Third-generation cephalosporins share excellent activity against *Enterobacteriaceae* (e.g. *E. coli*, *Klebsiella*, *Serratia*, *Proteus*), but differ somewhat in their activity against gram-positive cocci and more resistant gram-negative rods (*Pseudomonas*, *Enterobacter*, *Citrobacter*). Ceftriaxone, cefotaxime, and cefepime have potent activity against *S. pneumoniae* and to a lesser extent MSSA, whereas ceftazidime's activity is much less reliable against these organisms. In contrast to ceftriaxone and cefotaxime, ceftazidime and cefepime provide coverage against *Pseudomonas*. Cefepime improves somewhat on ceftazidime's spectrum by virtue of better coverage of *Enterobacter* and *Citrobacter*.

Ceftazidime is now FDA-approved as a co-formulation with a novel beta-lactamase inhibitor, avibactam. The addition of avibactam improves ceftazidime's potency against drug-resistant gram-negative organisms, such as *Enterobacter*, *E. coli*, *Klebsiella*, and *Pseudomonas*; however, it does not substantially improve activity against certain gram-negative aerobic organisms, such as *Burkholderia* and *Acinetobacter* or gram-positive pathogens. It is also unreliable against anaerobic organisms (e.g. *Bacteroides*), so it should be combined with a second agent (preferably metronidazole) when used for empiric treatment of complicated intra-abdominal infections.

Cautions

Exposure to third-generation cephalosporins has been demonstrated to be a risk factor for acquisition of a number of resistant bacteria, including vancomycin-resistant *Enterococcus* (VRE), *Clostridium difficile*, and extended-spectrum beta-lactamase-producing *Klebsiella*. When possible, more narrow-spectrum drugs should be substituted when susceptibility data have been obtained.

Pearls and Pitfalls

1. Dosing of these agents varies by indication, as noted in the dosage table below. Most importantly, for meningitis, higher doses are indicated to compensate for reduced penetration into the CNS. It is unclear whether the new co-formulation ceftazidime–avibactam will effectively treat meningitis, due to limited clinical data; however, animal models suggest potential efficacy.

2. All available cephalosporins (with the exception of cefoxitin and cefotetan) have poor activity against important gram-negative anaerobes such as *B. fragilis*. When used for empiric therapy of intra-abdominal infections, a drug with anaerobic coverage (preferably metronidazole) should be added.

Advanced-Generation Cephalosporins

Two newly approved agents discussed below do not clearly fit into the current cephalosporin generations naming convention (which may need to be revised or discarded). These agents provide activity against some organisms that are typically resistant to other cephalosporins; however, there are substantial differences in spectrum of activity and clinical uses between them. Table 78.14 lists acute care uses, toxicities, and drug interactions. See Table 78.15 for doses of the advanced-generation cephalosporins.

Differences between Agents

The advanced-generation cephalosporins share activity against most *Enterobacteriaceae* (such as *E. coli* and *Klebsiella*), as well as *Haemophilus influenzae*. Ceftaroline has excellent activity against gram-positive organisms such as *Streptococcus pneumoniae* and *Staphylococcus aureus*, including MRSA – a novel characteristic for any beta-lactam. However, it lacks activity against drug-resistant gram-negative pathogens, such as *Pseudomonas* or extended-spectrum beta-lactamase (ESBL)-producing *Enterobacteriaceae*. On the other hand, ceftolozane–tazobactam has shown excellent activity against drug-resistant gram-negative rods, including ESBL-producing *Enterobacteriaceae* and *Pseudomonas*; approximately 70% of multidrug-resistant *Pseudomonas* isolates were found to be susceptible to ceftolozane–tazobactam. It does not have activity against MRSA and is less reliable than earlier generation cephalosporins against *S. pneumoniae*. Unlike piperacillin–tazobactam, ceftolozane–tazobactam is not considered to have adequate activity against gram-negative anaerobic organisms to be used as monotherapy for intra-abdominal infections.

Table 78.14 Advanced-Generation Cephalosporins

Drug	Acute Care Uses	Toxicities
Ceftaroline IV (Teflaro) Ceftolozane–tazobactam IV (Zerbaxa)	Community-acquired pneumonia* Complicated skin and skin structure infections* Complicated intra-abdominal§ infections (in combination with metronidazole) UTIs, pyelonephritis§	*Uncommon:* transaminitis, neutropenia, *C. difficile* disease *Rare:* anaphylaxis **Drug interactions** Minimal

* Uses for ceftaroline.

§ Uses for ceftolozane–tazobactam.

Table 78.15 Dosages for Advanced-Generation Cephalosporins

Drug	Dosage Adjustment for Renal Function (mL/min)			Hepatic Adjust?
	CrCl >50	CrCl 15–50	CrCl <15	
Ceftaroline	600 mg IV every 12 hours	300–400 mg IV every 12 hours	200 mg every 12 hours	No
Ceftolozane–tazobactam	1.5 g IV every 8 hours*	375–750 mg IV every 8 hours	No information	No

* 1 g ceftolozane, 0.5 g tazobactam.

Table 78.16 Carbapenems and Monobactams

Drug	Acute Care Uses	Toxicities
Imipenem IV* (Primaxin) Meropenem IV* (Merrem) Doripenem IV* (Doribax) Ertapenem IV* (Invanz)	Nosocomial infections Sepsis Intra-abdominal infections	*Uncommon:* rash *Rare:* anaphylaxis, seizures **Drug interactions** Minimal
Aztreonam IV† (Azactam)	Nosocomial infections Acute bacterial meningitis	

* Carbapenems.
† Monobactam.

Table 78.17 Dosages of Carbapenems and Monobactams

Drug	Dosage Adjustment for Renal Function (mL/min)			Hepatic Adjust?
	CrCl >50	CrCl 10–50	CrCl <10	
Imipenem	500 mg IV every 6–8 hours	500 mg IV every 8 hours	250–500 mg IV every 12 hours	No
Meropenem	1–2 g IV every 8 hours	0.5–1 g IV every 12 hours	0.5 g IV every 24 hours	No
Doripenem	500 mg IV every 8 hours	250–500 mg IV every 8 hours	250 mg IV every 12 horus	No
Ertapenem	1 g IV every 24 hours	0.5 g IV every 24 hours*	0.5 g IV every 24 hours	No
Aztreonam	2 g IV every 8 hours	2 g IV every 12 hours	1 g IV every 12 hours	No

* For CrCl <30 mL/min.

Cautions

In post-marketing experience, ceftaroline has rarely been associated with profound neutropenia, particularly in patients receiving the drug for a prolonged duration of therapy. It has generally been reversible upon drug discontinuation.

In clinical trials with ceftolozane–tazobactam, patients with baseline impaired renal function had lower cure rates than in the comparator group; however, there were limited numbers included in this sub-group. It remains unclear what significance this will have as clinical experience increases.

Pearls and Pitfalls

1. Being newer agents, both ceftaroline and ceftolozane–tazobactam have few FDA-approved indications. With additional clinical data, these indications may be expanded over time. Certain indications under study utilize higher-than-approved dosages (e.g. ceftaroline 600 mg IV every 8 hours for pneumonia caused by methicillin-resistant *S. aureus* and ceftolozane–tazobactam 3 g IV every 8 hours for ventilator-associated pneumonia).
2. While the ceftolozane–tazobactam combination has promising activity against many drug-resistant gram-negative organisms, it has notable gaps, particularly against organisms producing certain extended spectrum beta-lactamases, such as carbapenemases (e.g. some strains of *Klebsiella pneumoniae*).

Carbapenems and Monobactams

Table 78.16 lists acute care uses, toxicities, and drug interactions of carbapenems and monobactams, and Table 78.17 gives dosing.

Differences between Agents

The most important differences among the carbapenems are between ertapenem and the others (imipenem, meropenem, and doripenem). Ertapenem, unlike the others, lacks clinically significant activity against *Pseudomonas*, *Acinetobacter*, and *Enterococcus*, making it a less attractive choice when these pathogens are a concern. There is little difference in spectrum of activity between imipenem and meropenem. However, meropenem has a lower seizure risk than imipenem (see below) and therefore is the carbapenem of choice for treatment of meningitis or in patients with pre-existing seizure disorders. Doripenem is the newest agent in the carbapenem class; while it has similar activity to imipenem and meropenem, concerns have been raised after a study in nosocomial pneumonias revealed a lower cure rate and increased mortality relative to the comparator group.

Cautions

Carbapenems as a class are associated with a risk of seizures, though it should be noted that other beta-lactam drugs have also caused seizures, especially at high doses. Imipenem appears to be the most epileptogenic of the class, with an incidence of seizure possibly in the range of 1 to 7%. Seizure risk is increased in patients with pre-existing seizure disorders, or with elevated drug levels such as are seen in renal failure without dose adjustment. Meropenem, conversely, has shown to have a low incidence of drug-related seizures and is approved by the Food and Drug Administration (FDA) for the treatment of meningitis. There is less experience with ertapenem; its seizure risk appears to be less than that of imipenem, but it is unclear whether it is as low as that of meropenem.

Table 78.18 Glycopeptides

Drug	Acute Care Uses	Toxicities
Vancomycin IV, PO (various) Telavancin (Vibativ) Dalbavancin* (Dalvance) Oritavancin* (Orbactiv)	Skin and soft-tissue infections Endocarditis Osteomyelitis Meningitis Nosocomial infections *Clostridium difficile* disease§	*Uncommon:* "Red man's syndrome" (histamine release) *Rare:* nephrotoxicity, neutropenia, ototoxicity **Drug interactions** *Aminoglycosides:* possible increase in ototoxicity and nephrotoxicity *Warfarin:* increased INR± *QTc prolonging agents:* additive risk with telavancin

* Skin and soft-tissue infections only.

§ Oral vancomycin only.

± When used with oritavancin.

INR – international normalized ratio.

Table 78.19 Dosages for Glycopeptides

Drug	Dosage Adjustment for Renal Function (mL/min)			Hepatic Adjust?
	CrCl >50	CrCl 10–50	CrCl <10	
Vancomycin	15–20 mg/kg/dose IV every 8–12 hours	10–15 mg/kg IV every 12–24 hours	5–10 mg/kg IV every 24–48 hours	No
Telavancin	10 mg/kg IV every 24 hours	30–50 7.5 mg/kg IV every 24 hours	10–29 10 mg/kg IV every 48 hours	No data	Limited information

Drug	Dosage Adjustment for Renal Function (mL/min)		Hepatic Adjust?
	CrCl >30	CrCl <30	
Dalbavancin	Single dose: 1,500 mg IV once Two dose: 1,000 mg IV once, 500 mg IV 1 week later	Single dose: 1,125 mg IV once Two dose: 750 mg IV once, 375 mg 1 week later	Limited information
Oritavancin	1200 mg IV once	Limited information	Limited information

Pearls and Pitfalls

1. The carbapenems are the most broad-spectrum agents currently in clinical use. To preserve their activity, they should be reserved for use against organisms resistant to other agents. The emergence of carbapenemase-producing *Enterobacteriaceae* (CRE), which are resistant to almost all antimicrobials, is a major threat to public health.

2. Aztreonam's spectrum of activity and pharmacokinetics are similar to those of ceftazidime (though it lacks ceftazidime's weak gram-positive activity). Its primary role in therapy has been in patients with severe beta-lactam allergies, where it is generally safe to administer because of its minimal to absent cross-reactivity. For example, aztreonam would be a reasonable choice for the coverage of *Neisseria meningitidis* in a patient with suspected meningitis and a documented anaphylactic reaction to beta-lactams. Note, however, that cases of cross-allergenicity have been noted if a patient's previous reaction was to ceftazidime, because aztreonam and ceftazidime share an identical side chain (theoretically ceftolozane is a concern as well, since it shares a side chain with ceftazidime).

Glycopeptides

Table 78.18 lists acute care uses, toxicities, and drug interactions of glycopeptides, and Table 78.19 gives dosing.

Mechanism of Action

Inhibition of cell wall synthesis at a different step from beta-lactams (see Figure 78.2), slowly bactericidal, time-dependent killing. Additional mechanisms of action include disruption in membrane potential and cell permeability (telavancin, oritavancin) and inhibition of cell wall crosslinking (oritavancin).

Differences between Agents

Although four agents in the glycopeptide class are currently approved in the United States, vancomycin remains the most widely used, due to extensive clinical experience and lower drug cost. Vancomycin is the only agent which requires monitoring of therapeutic levels. All indications for vancomycin other than treatment of *C. difficile* diseases should use intravenous vancomycin. Oral vancomycin is not appreciably absorbed and is used only for its intracolonic effects in cases of *C. difficile* colitis; note that intravenous vancomycin does not achieve adequate levels in the colon and is insufficient for treatment of *C. difficile* infection.

All these agents have similar in vitro activity against gram-positive pathogens such as streptococci and staphylococci, including MSSA and MRSA. Telavancin, dalbavancin, and oritavancin may retain some activity against vancomycin non-susceptible *S. aureus* isolates (e.g. VISA, VRSA); however, they provide minimal to no advantage over vancomycin in treating

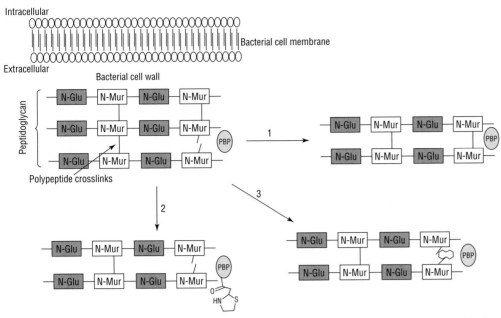

Figure 78.2 Mechanism of action of cell-wall-active antibacterials. Peptidoglycan is the primary component of the bacterial cell wall, consisting of alternating units of N-acetylglucosamine (N-Glu) and N-acetylmuramic acid (N-Mur). The N-Mur units are crosslinked by polypeptide chains. Bacterial transpeptidases (also known as penicillin-binding proteins or PBPs) catalyze this crosslinking (as in pathway 1). Beta-lactam agents irreversibly inhibit the action of PBPs (pathway 2), preventing crosslinking. Glycopeptides (such as vancomycin) bind to the free ends of the polypeptides before crosslinking, sterically inhibiting PBP binding (pathway 3). In pathways 2 and 3, the natural autolytic activity of the bacterial cell leads to the degradation of the cell wall and cell death (beta-lactams may also enhance this autolysis).

VRE. Dalbavancin and oritavancin have only been approved for use in skin and soft-tissue infections, and until further studies are conducted, it is unclear whether they can effectively treat more serious infections (e.g. pneumonia, osteomyelitis, bacteremia). The key distinguishing characteristic of dalbavancin and oritavancin is their extremely long half-life, which enables once-weekly dosing for their approved indication of skin and soft-tissue infection.

Cautions

The most commonly observed adverse effect of vancomycin is "Red man's" (or "Red neck") syndrome, a syndrome of flushing, pruritis, and hypotension (usually mild). The reaction is thought to be the result of histamine release, is reversible on drug discontinuation, and can be reduced or eliminated by slowing the rate of infusion (to >1 hour per gram of drug administered). Pre-medication with a histamine antagonist may be useful in difficult cases. "Red man's syndrome" is not a contraindication to future vancomycin courses, though efforts should be made to differentiate from (much rarer) true hypersensitivity reactions.

Telavancin labeling includes several boxed warnings due to safety concerns, including increased risk of death in patients with baseline moderate to severe renal impairment, new onset nephrotoxicity, and potential teratogenicity. It has also been associated with cardiac conduction abnormalities (prolongation of the QTc interval). Clinical experience with the new long-acting glycopeptides (dalbavancin and oritavancin) is limited, but few serious toxicities were identified at the time of their approval. Oritavancin can inhibit warfarin metabolism, leading to elevated INR; additionally, both oritavancin and telavancin can interfere with certain coagulation tests, leading to falsely elevated levels for about 24 to 48 hours after the antibiotic dose. Caution should be exercised when using these agents concomitantly, as dose titration can be challenging.

Pearls and Pitfalls

1. Vancomycin dosing is based on total body weight. In overweight patients or those with severe infections, dosing should follow a mg/kg approach in order to ensure optimal concentrations, rather than giving a standard 1 g IV every 12 hours dose. Vancomycin levels should be monitored and should be at least 10 mg/L for most indications, with higher levels (in the 15–20 mg/L range) for severe infections (e.g. meningitis, endocarditis, and osteomyelitis).

2. Vancomycin is an important component of empiric therapy because of its activity against MRSA and penicillin-resistant *S. pneumoniae*. However, it has slower bacterial killing compared to the beta-lactam drugs. Thus, beta-lactam agents are preferred for the treatment of infections due to susceptible organisms when intravenous therapy is necessary, despite the dosing convenience offered by vancomycin (BID for vancomycin vs. TID or QID for many beta-lactam drugs).

3. Oritavancin and dalbavancin offer potential benefits for patients who would benefit from intravenous antibiotic therapy, but have no other indication for hospitalization. One dose of oritavancin or one to two doses of dalbavancin are considered therapeutically equivalent to a standard duration of therapy for complicated skin and soft-tissue infections. Their roles for other indications (osteomyelitis, bacteremia) are under study. The cost of these novel

Table 78.20 Fluoroquinolones

Drug	Acute Care Uses	Toxicities
Ciprofloxacin IV, PO (Cipro) Levofloxacin IV, PO (Levaquin) Moxifloxacin IV, PO (Avelox)	UTIs* Community-acquired pneumonia† Bacterial sinusitis† Acute exacerbations of chronic bronchitis† Gonorrhea‡ Nosocomial infections Biliary tree infections Anthrax	*Uncommon:* photosensitivity, headache, dizziness, arthralgias, confusion *Rare:* Achilles tendon rupture, seizures, QT prolongation, dysglycemias **Drug interactions** *Oral cations (Ca, Mg, Fe):* reduced absorption of oral fluoroquinolones

* Use levofloxacin or ciprofloxacin.
† Use levofloxacin or moxifloxacin.
‡ Fluoroquinolones are not recommended for gonorrhea acquired in California, Hawaii, or Asia.

Table 78.21 Dosages for Fluoroquinolones*

Drug	Dosage Adjustment for Renal Function (mL/min)			Hepatic Adjust?
	CrCl >50	CrCl 10–50	CrCl <10	
Ciprofloxacin	400 mg IV every 12 hours *or* 500 mg PO BID 400 mg IV every 8 hours *or* 750 mg PO BID*	200–400 mg IV every 12 hours *or* 250–500 mg PO BID 200–400 mg IV every 8 hours 500–750 mg PO BID*	200 mg IV every 12 hours 250 mg PO BID	No
Levofloxacin	500 mg IV/PO every 24 hours 750 mg IV/PO every 24 hours	250 mg IV/PO every 24 hours 750 mg IV/PO every 48 hours	500 mg IV/PO every 24 hours 500 mg IV/PO every 48 hours†	No
Moxifloxacin	400 mg IV/PO every 24 hours	No adjustment	No adjustment	Possibly

† After 750 mg loading dose.

agents may be a significant factor when using oritavancin or dalbavancin.

Fluoroquinolones

Table 78.20 lists acute care uses, toxicities, and drug interactions of fluoroquinolones, and Table 78.21 gives dosing.

Mechanism of Action

Inhibition of DNA topoisomerases leading to strand breaks and replication failure. Bactericidal, concentration-dependent activity.

Differences between Agents

Ciprofloxacin has less potent gram-positive activity than levofloxacin or moxifloxacin and should not be used for community-acquired pneumonia. Both ciprofloxacin and levofloxacin have antipseudomonal activity (at higher doses), but moxifloxacin does not.

Cautions

Fluoroquinolones are popular drugs for the treatment of respiratory tract infections in the elderly, because they are often at higher risk for resistant respiratory pathogens. However, the elderly may be more predisposed to some of the adverse effects of the fluoroquinolones. Confusion, headache, and dizziness are reported with the fluoroquinolones; the elderly may be at increased risk because of underlying dementias and because of age-related decreases in renal function leading to accumulation of drug to toxic levels. Careful attention should be paid to appropriate dosing. Older patients with heart disease, especially those on anti-arrhythmic drugs (such as amiodarone), may be susceptible to the QT-prolonging effects of the fluoroquinolones. Fluoroquinolones should be used carefully or avoided in these patients. Several studies have reported dysglycemias (hypo- and hyperglycemias) in patients, often elderly, receiving fluoroquinolones. The effect was most pronounced with gatifloxacin, which has subsequently been removed from distribution; however, clinicians should be aware of the possibility with the other fluoroquinolones (especially when the drugs are used in diabetic patients). In 2016, the FDA issued a safety alert warning against prescribing fluoroquinolones for uncomplicated infections (e.g. cystitis, sinusitis, bronchitis) when alternate agents are available due to concerns for toxicities such as tendinopathies or neuropathies, in addition to the above-mentioned CNS and conduction abnormalities.

Pearls and Pitfalls

1. Resistance to fluoroquinolones is rapidly increasing; already these drugs cannot be considered reliable empiric monotherapy for serious *Pseudomonas* infections in many

Table 78.22 Aminoglycosides

Drug	Acute Care Uses	Toxicities
Gentamicin IV (various) Tobramycin IV (various) Amikacin IV (various)	Endocarditis Nosocomial infections UTIs	*Common:* acute renal insufficiency *Uncommon:* ototoxicity (vestibular and cochlear) *Rare:* neuromuscular blockade **Drug interactions** *Other nephrotoxins:* additive nephrotoxicity

Table 78.23 Dosages for Aminoglycosides

Drug	Dosage Adjustment for Renal Function (mL/min)			Hepatic Adjust?
	CrCl >50	CrCl 10–50	CrCl <10	
Gentamicin or tobramycin	*Traditional:* 1.7 mg/kg IV every 8 hours *Extended-interval:* 5–7 mg/kg IV every 24 hours *Gram-positive synergy:* 1 mg/kg IV every 8 hours	*Traditional:* 1.2–1.5 mg/kg IV every 12–24 hours *Extended-interval:* not recommended	1.2–1.5 mg/kg IV every 24–48 hours	No
Amikacin	*Traditional:* 7.5 mg/kg IV every 24 hours *Extended-interval:* 15 mg/kg IV every 24 hours	*Traditional:* 5–7.5 mg/kg IV every 12–24 hours *Extended-interval:* not recommended	5 mg/kg IV every 24–48 hours	No
Aminoglycoside dosing should be based on ideal or adjusted body weight, not total body weight, in obese patients (>120% of their ideal body weight).				

areas. Increasing resistance among *E. coli* threatens their role in UTIs. In patients with urosepsis or pyelonephritis, clinicians might consider third- or fourth-generation cephalosporins as empiric therapy instead, especially if patients have prior exposure to fluoroquinolones or if local resistance to fluoroquinolones is known to be high.

2. Fluoroquinolones have excellent oral bioavailability, making them good drugs for outpatient therapy. However, their absorption is markedly decreased with coadministration of divalent and trivalent cations (calcium, iron, magnesium, etc.). Separate administration of these drugs (as well as multivitamins) by at least 2 hours; or have the patient stop cation-containing drugs for the duration of fluoroquinolone use.

3. Moxifloxacin, by virtue of its non-renal clearance, achieves low urinary concentrations and is thus not indicated for the treatment of UTIs.

4. Fluoroquinolones should generally be reserved for treatment of complicated or drug-resistant infections, or other situations where alternate treatments are not preferred.

Aminoglycosides

Table 78.22 lists acute care uses, toxicities, and drug interactions of aminoglycosides, and Table 78.23 gives dosing.

Mechanism of Action

Ribosomal binding leading to inhibition and mistranslation of bacterial protein synthesis. Bactericidal, concentration-dependent killing.

Differences between Agents

Tobramycin has slightly more potent activity against *Pseudomonas* than gentamicin, whereas gentamicin has somewhat more potent activity against *Serratia*. Amikacin has activity against some gentamicin- and tobramycin-resistant isolates of *E. coli, Klebsiella, Pseudomonas,* and *Acinetobacter* and is a second-line agent for mycobacterial infections. Only gentamicin has been widely studied as synergistic combination therapy with other drugs against gram-positive organisms.

Cautions

Aminoglycosides are among the most predictably toxic antimicrobials in widespread use. Careful dosing and frequent monitoring are necessary to reduce the risk of irreversible nephro- and ototoxicity. The risk-benefit ratio dictates that these drugs should generally not be used for non-severe infections.

Pearls and Pitfalls

1. "Once-daily" or "extended-interval" aminoglycoside dosing leverages the concentration-dependent killing of the drugs to create an equally effective, more convenient, and possibly safer dosing regimen compared to traditional dosing methods. However, there are many populations in which less data exist for once-daily dosing, including the pregnant, the critically ill, those with significant renal dysfunction, and the morbidly obese. Use this dosing method with caution, if at all, in these populations.

2. Aminoglycosides are not clinically useful as single-drug therapy for gram-positive organisms, but may provide synergistic activity against these organisms when used in combination with cell-wall active agents (such as a beta-lactam or glycopeptides). The dosing for gram-positive synergy uses a smaller total daily dose than traditional dosing. The primary established indications are for staphylococcal prosthetic valve endocarditis or severe enterococcal infections.

Table 78.24 Macrolides and Ketolides

Drug	Acute Care Uses	Toxicities
Azithromycin IV, PO (Zithromax) Clarithromycin PO (Biaxin) Erythromycin IV, PO (various) Fidaxomicin PO (Dificid)	Community-acquired pneumonia Bacterial sinusitis Acute exacerbations of chronic bronchitis Otitis media Sexually transmitted diseases (*Chlamydia trachomatis*) *Clostridium difficile* disease*	*Common:* gastrointestinal upset *Rare:* hepatotoxicity, QT prolongation **Drug interactions** *Substrates of CYP P450 enzymes:* increased levels of substrate drugs (erythromycin ~ clarithromycin ~ telithromycin >> azithromycin)

* Fidaxomicin only.

Table 78.25 Dosages for Macrolides and Ketolides

Drug	Dosage Adjustment for Renal Function (mL/min)			Hepatic Adjust?
	CrCl>50	CrCl 10–50	CrCl<10	
Azithromycin	500 mg IV/PO every 24 hours	No adjustment	No adjustment	No
Clarithromycin	500 mg PO BID	No adjustment	250 mg PO BID	No
Erythromycin	500–1,000 mg IV every 6 hours 250–500 mg PO BID	No adjustment	250–500 mg IV every 6 hours	No
Telithromycin	800 mg PO daily	600 mg PO daily	600 mg PO daily	Yes or avoid*
Fidaxomicin	200 mg PO BID	No adjustment	No adjustment	No

* For patients with combined renal and hepatic failure, give 400 mg PO every 24 hours. Consider avoiding in patients with hepatic dysfunction.

Outside of these indications, the toxicity risk of the aminoglycosides should be weighed carefully against the possible benefit of synergistic activity.

3. Aminoglycosides continue to be one of the most active classes of drugs against many gram-negative organisms. For patients with sepsis potentially due to gram-negative organisms (e.g. urosepsis), addition of an aminoglycoside to an empiric regimen will improve the likelihood of covering organisms resistant to other classes. When culture and susceptibility data are available, the aminoglycoside can usually be discontinued and treatment completed with a less toxic drug. Such a strategy balances the excellent coverage of aminoglycosides and their risk of toxicity.

Macrolides and Ketolides

Table 78.24 lists acute care uses, toxicities, and drug interactions of macrolides and ketolides, and Table 78.25 gives dosing.

Mechanism of Action

Binding to 50S ribosome with inhibition of protein synthesis. Bacteriostatic.

Differences between Agents

Erythromycin has fallen out of favor because of its poor tolerance, frequent dosing, drug interactions, and poor coverage of *H. influenzae*. Azithromycin and clarithromycin have similar spectra of activity, though the long half-life of azithromycin allows for once-daily, short-course therapy (e.g. 3 days for sinusitis). Fidaxomicin is a minimally absorbed macrolide that works locally in the gastrointestinal tract and has

been FDA-approved for the treatment of *C. difficile* infection; however, this agent should not be used to treat systemic infections.

Cautions

Other than azithromycin and fidaxomicin, the macrolides and ketolides are potent inhibitors of human drug-metabolizing enzymes (primarily the cytochrome P-450 system), with many possible drug interactions. Patients on multiple medications should be screened for potential interactions when systemic non-azithromycin macrolides are prescribed. Of particular concern is coadministration with drugs that prolong the QT interval, possibly leading to arrhythmias. The macrolides themselves have modest effects on the QT interval; however, when administered with drugs that also prolong the QT interval and are metabolized through enzyme pathways inhibited by the macrolides, the risk of arrhythmias increases substantially.

Pearls and Pitfalls

1. Macrolide resistance in *S. pneumoniae* has become increasingly common, with a number of documented treatment failures, especially in bacteremic disease. Macrolides are generally not recommended as initial monotherapy in patients with severe pneumonia (e.g. those requiring hospitalization).

2. Fidaxomicin was demonstrated to be non-inferior to oral vancomycin in the cure of mild to severe *C. difficile* infections, with fewer recurrent episodes occurring in patients receiving fidaxomicin. It has not been rigorously studied in complicated or multiply recurrent disease.

Table 78.26 Tetracyclines and Glycylcyclines

Drug	Acute Care Uses	Toxicities
Doxycycline IV, PO (various) Tigecycline IV (Tygacil)	Community-acquired pneumonia Anthrax Rickettsial diseases Skin and soft-tissue infections Intra-abdominal infections*	*Uncommon:* photosensitivity, nausea, diarrhea *Rare:* esophagitis **Drug interactions** *Oral cations (Ca, Mg, Fe):* reduced absorption of oral fluoroquinolones

* Tigecycline.

Table 78.27 Dosages for Tetracyclines and Glycylcyclines

Drug	Dosage Adjustment for Renal Function (mL/min)			Hepatic Adjust?
	CrCl >50	CrCl 10–50	CrCl <10	
Doxycycline	100 mg IV/PO every 12 hours	No adjustment	No adjustment	No
Tigecycline	100 mg IV × 1, then 50 mg IV every 12 hours	No adjustment	No adjustment	Yes*

* For severe hepatic disease, loading dose of 100 mg, then 25 mg IV every 12 hours.

Tetracyclines and Glycylcyclines

Table 78.26 lists acute care uses, toxicities, and drug interactions of tetracyclines and glycylcyclines, and Table 78.27 gives dosing.

Mechanism of Action

Binding to 30S ribosome with inhibition of protein synthesis. Bacteriostatic.

Differences between Agents

Doxycycline is generally favored over other tetracycline formulations (tetracycline, minocycline) because of its more convenient dosing and lower incidence of adverse effects. Tigecycline is technically a glycylcycline, a modified version of tetracyclines that evades most tetracycline-resistance mechanisms. Thus, tigecycline has a broader spectrum of activity than the traditional tetracyclines, including activity against many gram-negative aerobic and anaerobic organisms (except for *Pseudomonas* and *Proteus*), as well as staphylococci and enterococci. However, it is only available as an intravenous preparation.

Cautions

Tetracyclines are contraindicated in pregnancy and children under 8 years of age because of their effects on tooth development. However, in the setting of proven or highly probable rickettsial disease, the benefits of a course of tetracyclines are thought to outweigh the risks. Although it has a broad spectrum of activity, clinical use of tigecycline has been limited after FDA labeling was modified to include a boxed-warning after a meta-analysis revealed increased all-cause mortality rates in patients treated with tigecycline.

Pearls and Pitfalls

1. As with the fluoroquinolones, tetracyclines have excellent oral bioavailability, but are chelated by divalent and trivalent cations (Ca, Fe, Mg, etc.). Separate administration of these agents by several hours from oral tetracyclines.

Table 78.28 Lincosamides

Drug	Acute Care Uses	Toxicities
Clindamycin IV, PO (Cleocin)	Skin and soft-tissue infections Aspiration pneumonia	*Uncommon:* diarrhea, *C. difficile* colitis *Rare:* pseudomembranous colitis **Drug Interactions** Minimal

Table 78.29 Dosages for Clindamycin

Drug	Dosage Adjustment for Renal Function (mL/min)			Hepatic Adjust?
	CrCl>50	CrCl 10–50	CrCl<10	
Clindamycin	600–900 mg IV every 8 hours 300–450 mg PO QID	No adjustment	No adjustment	No

2. Tetracyclines have displayed good activity (>90%) against community-acquired MRSA isolates and are an option for oral therapy in skin and soft-tissue infections documented or suspected to be due to MRSA. However, they have variable activity against beta-hemolytic streptococci and are not as reliable as beta-lactams when the likelihood of streptococcal infection is high (e.g. cellulitis).

Lincosamides

Table 78.28 lists acute care uses, toxicities, and drug interactions of lincosamides, and Table 78.29 gives dosing.

Mechanism of Action

Binds to 50S ribosome, with inhibition of protein synthesis. Bacteriostatic.

Table 78.30 Trimethoprim–Sulfamethoxazole

Drug	Acute Care Uses	Toxicities
Trimethoprim–sulfamethoxazole IV, PO (Bactrim, Septra)	UTIs *Pneumocystis* pneumonia *Stenotrophomonas* infections *Nocardia* infections *Listeria* (PCN allergic)	*Uncommon:* rash, hyperkalemia, neutropenia, pseudo-renal failure (asymptomatic increase in SCr) *Rare:* acute renal failure **Drug interactions** *Warfarin:* increased INR

PCN – penicillin; SCr – serum creatinine.

Table 78.31 Dosages of Trimethoprim–Sulfamethoxazole

Drug	Dosage Adjustment for Renal Function (mL/min)			Hepatic Adjust?
	CrCl >50	CrCl 10–50	CrCl <10	
TMP–SMX	10–20 mg TMP/kg/day IV divided every 6–12 hours* 1 DS tab. PO BID†	5–15 mg TMP/kg/day IV divided every 12–24 hours 1 SS PO every 12 hours	2.5–10 mg TMP/kg/day IV every 24 hours 1 SS PO every 24 hours	No

* Higher end of IV dosing range should be used for *Pneumocystis* infections; dosing is based on TMP component.

† Dose for uncomplicated cystitis; oral dose for more severe infections should be based on mg/kg dosing.

DS – double strength; SS – single strength.

Differences between Agents

Not applicable.

Cautions

Diarrhea is one of the most common adverse effects associated with clindamycin. Clindamycin can itself cause a relatively benign, self-limiting diarrhea or can result in more severe diarrhea resulting from superinfection with *Clostridium difficile*. *C. difficile*-associated diarrhea and colitis can occur during or after therapy with any antibacterial agent and can be life-threatening. Clindamycin may be associated with a higher risk of *C. difficile* disease relative to other antibacterials. Patients with diarrhea, especially if it is severe, associated with fever, or persists after the end of clindamycin therapy, need evaluation for *C. difficile* disease.

Pearls and Pitfalls

1. Clindamycin's inhibition of protein synthesis and activity against organisms in stationary-phase growth has been utilized in the treatment of necrotizing fasciitis and other toxin-mediated diseases. Consider the addition of clindamycin to beta-lactam-based therapy when treating these types of serious infections.

2. Clindamycin has good activity against most streptococci and many staphylococci; however, resistance rates have increased, particularly with MRSA. Some strains of staphylococci possess "inducible resistance" – i.e. the organisms appear susceptible to clindamycin in initial in vitro susceptibility testing, but have a high propensity to mutate to a resistant form during therapy. These isolates occur among strains that possess erythromycin resistance; the microbiology lab can perform a screening test (called a "D-test") on erythromycin-resistant, clindamycin-susceptible isolates to determine whether inducible resistance is likely to occur.

Trimethoprim–Sulfamethoxazole

Table 78.30 lists acute care uses, toxicities, and drug interactions of trimethoprim–sulfamethoxazole, and Table 78.31 gives dosing.

Mechanism of Action

Trimethoprim and sulfamethoxazole (TMP–SMX) inhibit sequential steps in the folate biosynthesis pathway. The synergistic combination of the two agents generally results in bactericidal activity.

Differences between Agents

Trimethoprim is available as a single agent and may be used for acute cystitis.

Cautions

TMP–SMX is a frequent cause of rash, most commonly due to the sulfamethoxazole component. Interestingly, the frequency of rash is increased in patients with human immunodeficiency virus (HIV) or acquired immunodeficiency syndrome (AIDS). Life-threatening reactions such as toxic epidermal necrolysis and Stevens–Johnson syndrome have been documented, and patients with a history of rash due to TMP–SMX should generally not be rechallenged because of the risk of severe reactions.

Pearls and Pitfalls

1. For years, TMP–SMX was considered standard first-line therapy for treatment of acute uncomplicated cystitis in women. Recent guidelines suggest, however, that in areas with local resistance rates greater than 15 to 20% in *E. coli*, an alternative drug (e.g. ciprofloxacin or nitrofurantoin) should be used. At a minimum, TMP–SMX should not be used for empiric therapy of more severe UTIs such as pyelonephritis or urosepsis.

Table 78.32 Nitroimidazoles

Drug	Acute Care Uses	Toxicities
Metronidazole IV, PO (Flagyl) Tinidazole PO (Tindamax)	C. difficile disease Trichomoniasis Giardiasis Amebiasis Intra-abdominal infections, in combination with other agents	*Uncommon:* nausea, vomiting, metallic taste *Rare:* peripheral neuropathy **Drug interactions** *Warfarin:* increased INR *Alcohol:* disulfiram-like reaction

Table 78.33 Dosages for Nitroimidazoles

Drug	Dosage Adjustment for Renal Function (mL/min)			Hepatic Adjust?
	CrCl >50	CrCl 10–50	CrCl <10	
Metronidazole	500–750 mg IV/PO every 8 hours 2 g PO × 1*	No adjustment	500 mg IV every 12 hours†	Possibly‡
Tinidazole	2 g PO × 1§ 2 g PO daily × 3–5 days‖	No adjustment	No adjustment	Possibly‡

* For trichomoniasis.

† Dose adjustment required only for patients with CrCl <10 mL/min and not on hemodialysis.

‡ Consider dose reduction in severe hepatic impairment.

§ For trichomoniasis or giardiasis.

‖ For intestinal amebiasis or amebic liver abscess.

2. TMP–SMX comes in a fixed, 5:1 ratio of the two components. The intravenous form is dosed based on the TMP component. The oral form comes in two strengths: single-strength (80:400 mg TMP:SMX) and double-strength (160:800 mg TMP:SMX). TMP–SMX has excellent oral bioavailability, allowing for conversion to oral therapy when patients are tolerating oral medications.

3. Similar to the tetracyclines, TMP–SMX has excellent activity (>95% susceptibility in most series) against community-acquired MRSA, but variable activity against some beta-hemolytic streptococci.

Nitroimidazoles

Table 78.32 lists acute care uses, toxicities, and drug interactions of nitroimidazoles, and Table 78.33 gives dosing.

Mechanism of Action

Nitroreductases (present only in anaerobic bacteria) activate nitroimidazoles to highly reactive, cytotoxic metabolites. Bactericidal.

Differences between Agents

Although the spectrum of activity of the two drugs is similar, clinical efficacy data for tinidazole is available only for its use in parasitic infections. For such infections (including giardiasis, amebiasis, and trichomoniasis), single-dose or short-course therapy appears to be more effective and better tolerated than metronidazole, albeit at a higher cost.

Cautions

Nitroimidazoles have a reputation for causing a disulfiram (Antabuse)-like reaction with the consumption of alcohol, because of their inhibition of aldehyde dehydrogenase. It is recommended to have patients abstain from alcohol while taking nitroimidazoles. Also well described is the interaction with warfarin, in which warfarin's metabolism is inhibited, leading to an increase in anticoagulation. Careful monitoring and warfarin dose reduction may be necessary.

Pearls and Pitfalls

1. Metronidazole is generally considered to be a first-line treatment for initial episodes of C. difficile disease of mild severity. However, clinical studies suggest oral vancomycin is more effective in moderate to severe C. difficile disease. Unlike intravenous vancomycin, intravenous metronidazole does have some role in treatment of patients with C. difficile who cannot take oral medications. In severe or treatment-refractory cases, the combination of intravenous metronidazole and oral vancomycin may be used.

Nitrofurans and Fosfomycin

Table 78.34 lists acute care uses, toxicities, and drug interactions of nitrofurans and fosfomycin, and Table 78.35 gives dosing.

Mechanism of Action

Although not well characterized, nitrofurantoin appears to inhibit bacterial enzyme synthesis. Fosfomycin inhibits bacterial cell wall synthesis via separate mechanism from the action of beta-lactams and glycopeptides. Both are active primarily against uropathogens such as E. coli and Klebsiella.

Differences between Agents

These agents are different chemically, but have similar spectra of activity and clinical uses. There are two preparations of

Table 78.34 Nitrofurans and Fosfomycin

Drug	Acute Care Uses	Toxicities
Nitrofurantoin PO (Macrobid, Macrodantin) Fosfomycin PO (Monurol)	Lower UTI	*Uncommon:* nausea/vomiting *Rare:* pulmonary fibrosis (nitrofurantoin) **Drug interactions** Minimal

Table 78.35 Dosages for Nitrofurans and Fosfomycin

Drug	Dosage Adjustment for Renal Function (mL/min)			Hepatic Adjust?
	CrCl >50	CrCl 10–50	CrCl <10	
Nitrofurantoin macrocrystals	100 mg PO QID	Do not use	Do not use	No
Nitrofurantoin macrocrystal/ monohydrate	100 mg PO BID	Do not use	Do not use	No
Fosfomycin trometerol	3 g PO × 1	Do not use	Do not use	No

Table 78.36 Oxazolidinones and Lipopeptides

Drug	Acute Care Uses	Toxicities
Linezolid IV, PO (Zyvox) Tedizolid IV, PO (Sivextro)*	Skin and soft-tissue infections Pneumonia Nosocomial infections	*Uncommon:* thrombocytopenia *Rare:* optic neuritis, peripheral neuropathy **Drug interactions** *Antidepressants:* risk of serotonin syndrome
Daptomycin IV (Cubicin)	Skin and soft-tissue infections Endocarditis	*Uncommon:* myopathy *Rare:* rhabdomyolysis **Drug interactions** *Statins:* possible increased risk of myopathy

* Tedizolid is approved for use in skin and soft-tissue infections only.

nitrofurantoin: a crystalline form (Macrodantin) and a macrocrystalline/monohydrate form (Macrobid). The former is dosed four times daily for the treatment of cystitis, the latter twice daily. In the United States, fosfomycin is available only as a powder for dissolution in water as a one-time dose for uncomplicated UTI (though some investigators have studied multiple-dosing approaches for complicated UTI).

Cautions

Although generally well tolerated (outside of gastrointestinal upset), there are rare but serious pulmonary adverse effects associated with nitrofurantoin use. These manifest either as an acute pneumonitis or a chronic pulmonary fibrosis. The acute presentation occurs within several days of initiation of the drug and subsides quickly after drug discontinuation. The chronic form is usually associated with long-term nitrofurantoin therapy (as in UTI prophylaxis) and can lead to permanent loss of pulmonary function and death. Patients receiving the drug for prophylaxis should be informed of the need to report any respiratory symptoms immediately.

Pearls and Pitfalls

1. Nitrofurantoin and fosfomycin have good (>90% in most studies) activity against *E. coli*, as well as adequate coverage of other common community-acquired UTI pathogens.

However, their utility is limited to infections of the lower urinary tract, because the drugs require high concentrations for antimicrobial activity, and these are reached only when concentrated in the urine. Thus, nitrofurantoin or fosfomycin should not be used for more severe infections originating in the urinary tract such as pyelonephritis and urosepsis. Also, in patients who have significant renal dysfunction (e.g. a creatinine clearance of <50 mL/min), there may be insufficient accumulation of the drug in the urine for activity.

Oxazolidinones and Lipopeptides

Table 78.36 lists acute care uses, toxicities, and drug interactions of oxazolidinones and lipopeptides, and Table 78.37 gives dosing.

Mechanism of Action

The oxazolidinones linezolid and tedizolid are bacteriostatic inhibitors of protein synthesis, similar to tetracyclines. Daptomycin, a lipopeptide, acts on the bacterial cell membrane to produce a bactericidal effect.

Differences between Agents

Although pharmacologically and mechanistically distinct, these classes are grouped together here because of their

Table 78.37 Dosages for Oxazolidinones and Lipopeptides

Drug	Dosage Adjustment for Renal Function (mL/min)			Hepatic Adjust?
	CrCl >50	CrCl 10–50	CrCl <10	
Linezolid	600 mg IV/PO every 12 hours	No change	No change	No
Tedizolid	200 mg IV/PO every 24 hours	No change	No change	No
Daptomycin	4–6 mg/kg IV every 24 hours*	4–6 mg/kg IV every 48 hours	4–6 mg/kg IV every 48 hours	No

* 4 mg/kg/dose for skin and soft-tissue infections; 6 mg/kg/dose for bacteremia and endocarditis. Some clinical evidence suggests higher, off-label doses (8–10 mg/kg/dose) for serious infections.

Table 78.38 Antifungal Azoles

Drug	Acute Care Uses	Toxicities
Fluconazole IV, PO (Diflucan) Itraconazole IV, PO (Sporanox) Voriconazole IV, PO (Vfend) Posaconazole IV, PO (Noxafil) Isavuconazole IV, PO (Cresemba)	Fungal infections	*Common:* visual disturbances (voriconazole) *Uncommon:* rash, elevated transaminases *Rare:* hepatitis **Drug interactions** *Substrates of CYP P450 enzymes:* increased levels of substrate drugs (voriconazole ~ itraconazole> posaconazole ~ isavuconazole >> fluconazole)

similar spectrum of activity and clinical use. These drugs are active against gram-positive organisms, including those such as MRSA and VRE that are resistant to many other drugs. Linezolid and tedizolid have the advantage of having highly bioavailable oral formulations, whereas daptomycin is rapidly bactericidal in vitro (as opposed to the bacteriostatic oxazolidinones).

Cautions

Linezolid has been associated with more adverse effects when given for extended periods of time (>14 days). Most frequent is a reversible thrombocytopenia, though neutropenia and anemia can be seen. Patients receiving long-term linezolid should have regular complete blood cell counts performed. Recent cases of peripheral and optic neuropathy associated with long-term linezolid have been described; this effect may be due to inhibition of mitochondrial protein synthesis. These toxicities are expected to be less common with tedizolid; however, clinical data are limited, in part because clinical trials used a short duration of therapy (6 days).

Pearls and Pitfalls

1. Linezolid is a moderate inhibitor of monoamine oxidase (MAO) and can cause potentially fatal serotonin syndrome when given concurrently with serotonergic agents such as selective serotonin reuptake inhibitors (SSRIs) – avoid concurrent use if possible. If a patient already on an SSRI requires treatment with linezolid, it may not be feasible to discontinue the SSRI for a short course of linezolid therapy (<10–14 days), because SSRIs generally require tapering rather than abrupt discontinuation. Vigilant monitoring for signs and symptoms of serotonin syndrome should be performed in this case. Tedizolid appears to have less MAO inhibition in vitro, but it may take more experience to know whether this interaction is a concern for this agent.

2. Linezolid has excellent penetration into pulmonary tissue, and may be preferred over vancomycin for some cases of pneumonia due to MRSA. Preliminary pharmacokinetic data suggest that tedizolid lung penetration should be adequate; however, there are limited clinical data to support its use in treatment of pneumonia. In contrast, daptomycin has been shown to be inactivated by lung surfactant and should not be used for pneumonia caused by any pathogen.

Antifungal Azoles

Table 78.38 lists acute care uses, toxicities, and drug interactions of antifungal azoles, and Table 78.39 gives dosing.

Mechanism of Action

Azoles inhibit fungal P-450 enzymes, preventing the synthesis of ergosterol, a crucial component of the fungal cell membrane. These agents are generally fungistatic against yeasts, but voriconazole may be fungicidal against *Aspergillus*.

Differences between Agents

Fluconazole, itraconazole, voriconazole, posaconazole, and isavuconazole all have activity against *Candida* species, with voriconazole, posaconazole, and isavuconazole having the most activity against non-*albicans* species (such as *krusei* and *glabrata*) that may be fluconazole-resistant. Fluconazole has no activity against *Aspergillus* species, while itraconazole has moderate activity, and posaconazole, isavuconazole, and voriconazole have potent activity against *Aspergillus* (with voriconazole currently possessing the most clinical evidence for use in invasive aspergillosis). Fluconazole is cleared renally, whereas the other azoles undergo hepatic metabolism.

Cautions

Similar to many of the agents in the macrolide class, drug interactions are a major concern with the azole antifungals.

Table 78.39 Dosages for Antifungal Azoles

Drug	Dosage Adjustment for Renal Function (mL/min)			Hepatic Adjust?
	CrCl >50	CrCl 10–50	CrCl <10	
Fluconazole	400 mg IV/PO every 24 hours	100–200 mg IV/PO every 24 hours	50–100 mg IV/PO every 24 hours	No
Itraconazole	200 mg IV/PO every 12 hours × 4 doses, then 100–200 mg PO every 12 hours	Avoid intravenous preparation	Avoid intravenous preparation	Possibly
Voriconazole	6 mg/kg/dose IV every 12 hours × 2 doses, then 4 mg/kg IV every 12 hours 400 mg PO BID × 2 doses, then 200 mg PO BID	Caution with intravenous preparation	Caution with intravenous preparation	Yes*
Posaconazole IV or DR tab.	300 mg IV/ PO every 12 hours × 2 doses, then 300mg IV/ PO every 24 hours	Caution with intravenous preparation	Caution with intravenous preparation	No
Posaconazole oral suspension	200 mg PO TID to QID§	No adjustment	No adjustment	No
Isavuconazole	200 mg IV every 8 hours × 3 days, then 200 mg IV/PO every 24 hours	No adjustment	No adjustment	No

* For moderate hepatic dysfunction, reduce maintenance dose by 50%.

§ TID for prophylaxis and QID for treatment.

DR – delayed release.

Table 78.40 Echinocandins

Drug	Acute Care Uses	Toxicities
Caspofungin IV (Cancidas) Micafungin IV (Mycamine) Anidulafungin IV (Eraxis)	Fungal infections	*Uncommon:* phlebitis, elevated transaminases *Rare:* hepatitis **Drug interactions** *Rifampin, phenytoin:* reduced levels of caspofungin

Voriconazole, itraconazole, isavuconazole, and posaconazole are moderate to major inhibitors of drug-metabolizing enzymes, with fluconazole substantially weaker. All these drugs are also substrates of these enzymes to a greater or lesser extent and can have their concentrations affected by other drugs (i.e. there can be two-way interactions). Another similarity to the macrolides is an effect on the QT interval, warranting caution when using these drugs in patients with underlying arrhythmias. Careful screening of these drugs against a patient's current medication list is required to avoid potentially dangerous interactions.

Pearls and Pitfalls

1. Visual disturbances, primarily manifesting as altered color perception, are common with voriconazole administration. The effects generally occur within an hour after dosage administration and subside within an hour or so. They also tend to become less pronounced over longer durations of treatment. Patients should be warned of these effects and should not perform activities such as driving until they become used to the effects of the drug.

2. The intravenous preparations of voriconazole and posaconazole are solubilized with compounds that accumulate in renal failure: voriconazole with a cyclodextran ether and posaconazole with a sulfobutyl ether. Although the deleterious effects of these agents are poorly characterized, the manufacturer recommends avoiding use of the intravenous formulations in patients with CrCl less than 50 mL/min. The oral formulations do not have this issue.

3. Posaconazole is available as an intravenous solution, an oral suspension, and a delayed-release tablet. It is important to distinguish which oral formulation is being prescribed, as dosing and food requirements vary substantially due to differences in absorption.

Echinocandins

Table 78.40 lists acute care uses, toxicities, and drug interactions of echinocandins, and Table 78.41 gives dosing.

Mechanism of Action

Echinocandins inhibit the synthesis of beta-glucan, an important component of the fungal cell wall. They appear to have fungicidal activity against yeasts and fungistatic activity against molds.

Differences between Agents

All three echinocandins have similar spectra of activity and excellent safety profiles. The newer agents (micafungin and anidulafungin) are slightly more potent than caspofungin and have fewer drug interactions, but there is more clinical experience with caspofungin.

Table 78.41 Dosages for Echinocandins

Drug	Dosage Adjustment for Renal Function (mL/min)			Hepatic Adjust?
	CrCl >50	CrCl 10–50	CrCl <10	
Caspofungin	70 mg IV × 1, then 50 mg IV every 24 hours	No adjustment	No adjustment	Yes
Micafungin	100–150 mg IV every 24 hours	No adjustment	No adjustment	No
Anidulafungin	200 mg IV × 1, then 100 mg IV every 24 hours	No adjustment	No adjustment	No

Table 78.42 Polyenes

Drug	Acute Care Uses	Toxicities
Amphotericin B deoxycholate IV (various)	Fungal infections	*Common:* infusion-related toxicities, nephrotoxicity, hypokalemia
Amphotericin B colloidal dispersion IV (Amphotec)		*Uncommon:* hepatitis
Amphotericin B lipid complex IV (Abelcet)		**Drug interactions**
Liposomal amphotericin B IV (AmBisome)		*Aminoglycosides:* enhanced nephrotoxicity

Table 78.43 Dosages for Polyenes

Drug	Dosage Adjustment for Renal Function (mL/min)			Hepatic Adjust?
	CrCl >50	CrCl 10–50	CrCl <10	
Amphotericin B deoxycholate	0.7–1.5 mg/kg IV every 24 hours	No adjustment*	No adjustment*	No
Lipid formulations	3–6 mg/kg IV every 24 hours	No adjustment*	No adjustment*	No

* Although the elimination of amphotericin is unaffected by renal dysfunction, because of the drug's nephrotoxicity consideration should be given to reducing or holding the dose in the setting of renal impairment.

Cautions

Unlike azoles and polyenes, echinocandins lack activity versus *Cryptococcus* species and have no role in the treatment of cryptococcal meningitis.

Pearls and Pitfalls

1. By virtue of their broad spectrum of activity against *Candida* species, echinocandins are a reasonable choice for empiric therapy when these organisms are suspected. If culture results indicate a species of *Candida* that is reliably fluconazole-susceptible (e.g. *C. albicans*), switching to fluconazole may be a cost-effective option because echinocandins have a high acquisition cost.

Polyenes

Table 78.42 lists acute care uses, toxicities, and drug interactions of polyenes, and Table 78.43 gives dosing.

Mechanism of Action

Polyenes disrupt the fungal cell membrane and are generally fungicidal.

Differences between Agents

In addition to "conventional" amphotericin B deoxycholate, three lipid-associated forms of amphotericin are available. Associating amphotericin with a lipid carrier alters the distribution of amphotericin in the body and reduces nephrotoxicity. The lipid complex and liposomal formulations also reduce the incidence of infusion-related reactions, though the colloidal dispersion product does not. The lipid-associated products are all substantially more expensive than conventional amphotericin B.

Cautions

Amphotericin frequently causes dose- and duration-dependent nephrotoxicity. Renal dysfunction is often reversible on discontinuation of amphotericin, but may result in permanent renal failure. Although the lipid-associated forms of amphotericin attenuate this nephrotoxicity somewhat, the risk is not eliminated. Patients receiving any amphotericin product should have frequent monitoring of their renal function, adequate hydration, and, when possible, discontinuation of other potentially nephrotoxic drugs.

Pearls and Pitfalls

1. Although amphotericin has a broad spectrum of antifungal activity and decades of clinical experience, the availability of newer, less toxic antifungals has diminished its role as the "gold standard." Amphotericin continues to be the drug of choice for selected indications such as cryptococcal meningitis and is a reasonable choice for empiric therapy for suspected fungal infections.

Antivirals: Anti-Herpes-Virus Drugs

Table 78.44 lists acute care uses, toxicities, and drug interactions of anti-herpes-virus drugs, and Table 78.45 gives dosing.

Table 78.44 Antivirals: Anti-Herpes-Virus Drugs

Drug	Acute Care Uses	Toxicities
Acyclovir IV, PO (Zovirax) Valacyclovir PO (Valtrex) Famciclovir PO (Famvir) Ganciclovir IV (Cytovene) Valganciclovir PO (Valtrex)	Herpes virus infections	*Uncommon:* headache; neutropenia (ganciclovir, valganciclovir) *Rare:* seizures, nephrotoxicity **Drug interactions** *Additive bone marrow suppression:* other drugs causing marrow suppression (ganciclovir, valganciclovir)

Table 78.45 Dosages for Anti-Herpes-Virus Drugs

Drug	Dosage Adjustment for Renal Function (mL/min)			Hepatic Adjust?
	CrCl >50	CrCl 10–50	CrCl <10	
Acyclovir	5–10 mg/kg IV every 8 hours* 400 mg PO TID†	5–10 mg/kg IV every 12–24 hours No adjustment	2.5–5 mg/kg IV every 24 hours 200 mg PO TID	No
Valacyclovir	500–1,000 mg PO every 12 hours†	500–1,000 mg PO every 12–24 hours	500 mg PO every 24 hours	No
Famciclovir	500 mg PO every 12 hours†	500 mg PO every 12–24 hours	250 mg PO every 24 hours	No
Ganciclovir	5 mg/kg IV every 12 hours‡	1.25–2.5 mg/kg IV every 12–24 hours	1.25 mg/kg IV every 24 hours	No
Valganciclovir	900 mg PO every 12 hours‡	450 mg PO daily (prophylaxis), BID (treatment)	Not recommended	No

* Use higher end of dosing range for herpes encephalitis or varicella-zoster infections.

† Treatment of recurrent genital herpes in HIV-negative adults.

‡ Induction doses for severe CMV disease.

Mechanism of Action

These drugs are nucleoside analogues that inhibit viral DNA synthesis.

Differences between Agents

All these agents have good activity against herpes simplex viruses (HSV) and useful but lower activity against varicella-zoster virus. Only ganciclovir has clinically useful activity against cytomegalovirus (CMV). Because of ganciclovir's greater toxicity, the other agents are preferred for treatment of herpes simplex and varicella-zoster infections. The valine-esterified forms valacyclovir and valganciclovir are oral pro-drugs designed to enhance the absorption of the parent drugs. After absorption, the valine portions are hydrolyzed and acyclovir and ganciclovir are released into the circulation.

Cautions

Ganciclovir (and, by extension, valganciclovir) can cause profound, reversible, dose-related bone marrow suppression. Careful dosing of ganciclovir according to the patient's renal function and avoidance, when possible, of other bone marrow-suppressive drugs is necessary. Nephrotoxicity due to crystallization of acyclovir can be seen when the intravenous formulation is given in doses too high for the patient's renal function, especially if the patient does not receive adequate hydration.

Pearls and Pitfalls

1. Among acyclovir, valacyclovir, and famciclovir, the choice of drug for oral treatment of HSV infections is generally based on cost and frequency of administration (acyclovir is inexpensive, but requires frequent dosing compared to the more expensive valacyclovir and famciclovir).

2. There are a number of different dosing regimens for genital herpes simplex infections, according to whether it is the patient's first or a recurrent episode, whether the drug is being used for suppressive therapy, and whether the patient is HIV-infected. Dosing regimens are also different for herpes zoster infections.

Antivirals: Anti-Influenza Drugs

Table 78.46 lists acute care uses, toxicities, and drug interactions of anti-influenza drugs, and Table 78.47 gives dosing.

Mechanism of Action

Oseltamivir, peramivir, and zanamivir inhibit neuraminidase, which is necessary for the release of virions from infected cells.

Differences between Agents

The neuraminidase inhibitors (oseltamivir, peramivir, and zanamivir) are active against both influenza A and B strains. Oseltamivir is available as an oral agent only, whereas peramivir is only available for IV administration and zanamivir is inhaled.

Cautions

Zanamivir, which is administered via a dry-powder inhaler, has caused bronchospasm in some patients with underlying asthma or chronic obstructive pulmonary disease. For these patients, oseltamivir is preferred.

Table 78.46 Anti-Influenza Drugs

Drug	Acute Care Uses	Toxicities
Oseltamivir PO (Tamiflu) Zanamavir inhalation (Relenza) Peramivir IV (Rapivab)	Influenza	*Uncommon:* bronchospasm (zanamavir), nausea/vomiting *Rare:* confusion **Drug interactions** Minimal

Table 78.47 Dosages for Anti-Influenza Drugs

Drug	Dosage Adjustment for Renal Function (mL/min)			Hepatic Adjust?
	CrCl >50	CrCl 10–50	CrCl <10	
Oseltamivir	75 mg PO BID 75 mg PO daily*	30 mg PO daily BID 30 mg PO every 48–24 hours	No data	No
Zanamavir	2 inhalations BID 2 inhalations daily*	No adjustment	No adjustment	No
Peramivir	600 mg IV once	100–200 mg IV × 1	100 mg IV × 1	No

* Prophylaxis dose.

Pearls and Pitfalls

1. The clinical benefit of neuraminidase inhibitor therapy is time-sensitive; for otherwise healthy patients, efficacy is greatest when given as near to the start of symptoms as possible, becoming minimal after 48 hours have elapsed. Among severely ill patients or those with substantial comorbidities, observational studies suggest a benefit even among patients in whom therapy is delayed more than 48 hours from onset of symptoms.

2. Oseltamivir has been used for the treatment of avian influenza (at doses up to 150 mg every 12 hours) and could be used for mass prophylaxis in the event of an outbreak. However, strains of avian influenza with oseltamivir resistance have been described.

3. Resistance to anti-influenza agents is evolving. Currently, there is minimal resistance to oseltamivir and peramivir among circulating strains of influenza, and zanamivir is active against almost all strains, including most oseltamivir-resistant ones. However, clinicians should keep abreast of the most up-to-date recommendations for treatment and prophylaxis of influenza for every season (available at www.cdc.gov/flu).

References

Bennett, J. E., Dolin, R., and Blaser, M. J. (eds.), *Mandell, Douglas, and Bennett's Principles and Practice of Infectious Diseases*, 8th edn (Philadelphia, PA: Elsevier/Saunders, 2015).

Kucers, A., Crowe, S., Brayson, M. L., and Hoy, J. (eds.), *The Use of Antibiotics* (Boston, MA: Butterworth-Heinemann, 1997).

Yu, V. L., Weber, R., and Raoult, D. (eds.), *Antimicrobial Therapy and Vaccines* (Pittsburgh, PA: ESun Technologies, 2005), vol. II.

Index